ATHLETIC AND SPORT ISSUES IN MUSCULOSKELETAL REHABILITATION

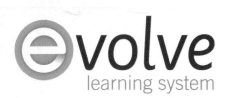 learning system

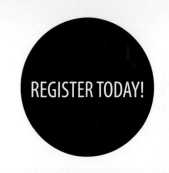 REGISTER TODAY!

To access your free Evolve Resources, visit:

http://evolve.elsevier.com/Magee/athletic

Evolve Student Learning Resources for Magee: Athletic and Sport Issues in Musculoskeletal Rehabilitation offers the following features:

- **References**

  End of chapter References linked to Medline

Evolve Instructor Resources for Magee: Athletic and Sport Issues in Musculoskeletal Rehabilitation offers the following features:

- **Image Collection**

  Search, view and download the large selection of images

  from the textbook

ELSEVIER
SAUNDERS

ATHLETIC AND SPORT ISSUES IN MUSCULOSKELETAL REHABILITATION

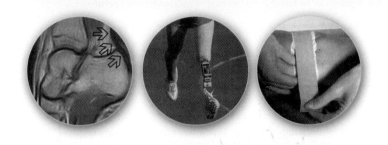

Editors

David J. Magee, PT, PhD
Professor and Associate Dean
Department of Physical Therapy, Faculty of Rehabilitation Medicine
University of Alberta, Edmonton, Alberta, Canada

Robert C. Manske, PT, DPT, SCS, MEd, ATC, CSCS
Associate Professor, Department of Physical Therapy
Wichita State University, Wichita, Kansas

James E. Zachazewski, PT, DPT, SCS, ATC
Clinical Director, Department of Physical and Occupational Therapy
Massachusetts General Hospital, Boston, Massachusetts
Adjunct Assistant Clinical Professor, Program in Physical Therapy
MGH Institute of Health Professions, Boston, Massachusetts

William S. Quillen, PT, PhD, SCS, FACSM
Associate Dean, College of Medicine
Professor and Director, School of Physical Therapy and Rehabilitation Sciences

University of South Florida ,Tampa, Florida

Editorial Consultant

Bev Evjen
Swift Current, Saskatchewan, Canada

ELSEVIER
SAUNDERS

SAUNDERS

3251 Riverport Lane
St. Louis, Missouri 63043

Library of Congress Cataloging-in-Publication Data
Athletic and sport issues in musculoskeletal rehabilitation/editors, David J. Magee . . . [et al.]; editorial
consultant Bev Evjen.
    p. ; cm. -- (Musculoskeletal rehabilitation series)
Includes bibliographical references and index.
ISBN 978-1-4160-2264-0 (pbk. : alk. paper) 1. Sports medicine. 2. Sports injuries--Treatment.
3. Sports--Physiological aspects. 4. Human mechanics. I. Magee, David J. II. Series: Musculoskeletal
rehabilitation series.
[DNLM: 1. Athletic Injuries--rehabilitation. 2. Musculoskeletal Diseases--rehabilitation.
3. Biomechanics. 4. Sports Medicine. QT 261 A8705 2011]
RC1210.A82 2011
617.1'027--dc22

                                                                                              2010024809

Vice President and Publisher: Linda Duncan
Executive Editor: Kathy Falk
Senior Developmental Editor: Christie Hart
Publishing Services Manager: Catherine Jackson
Project Manager: Sara Alsup
Design Direction: Teresa McBryan

Printed in China

Last digit is the print number: 9 8 7 6 5 4 3 2 1

Russell Mark, BS
National Team Performance Support Director
Biomechanics Manager
USA Swimming
Colorado Springs, Colorado

Stephen W. Marshall, PhD
Associate Professor, Department of Epidemiology
Adjunct Associate Professor, Department of Exercise
    and Sport Science
School of Public Health
University of North Carolina at Chapel Hill
Chapel Hill, North Carolina

James W. Matheson, PT, DPT
Board Certified in Sports and Orthopaedic Physical
    Therapy
Minnesota Sport and Spine Rehabilitation
Burnsville, Minnesota

Consultant
EIP Consulting
Savage, Minnesota

Duane G. Messner, MD
Past President
American Orthopaedic Sports Medicine Society
Gunnison, Colorado

Scott T. Miller, PT, MS, SCS, CSCS
Partner/Director of Clinical Operations
Agility Physical Therapy & Sports Performance, LLC
Portage, Michigan

Michael R. Mirabella, MS, ATC, CSCS
Athletic Trainer
Department of Athletics
White Plains High School
White Plains, New York

Athletic Trainer/Physician Extender
Westchester Orthopaedic Associates, PC
White Plains, New York

Elizabeth A. Mooradian, MS
Senior Scientist
Gatorade Sports Science Institute
Barrington, Illinois

Dhiren J. Naidu, MD, FRCP(C), Dip Sport Med
Assistant Professor
Division of Physical Medicine and Rehabilitation
University of Alberta
Edmonton, Alberta, Canada

Education Director, HealthPointe Medical Centre
Sport Medicine Consultant, Glen Sather Sports Medicine
    Clinic
Edmonton, Alberta, Canada

Team Physician, Edmonton Oilers, National Hockey
    League
Team Physician, Edmonton Eskimos, Canadian Football
    League

Juliana Melo Ocarino, BPT, MSc
PhD Candidate in Rehabilitation Sciences
Universidade Federal de Minas Gerais
Belo Horizonte, Minas Gerais, Brazil

Assistant Professor
Centro Universitário de Belo Horizonte (UNI-BH)
Belo Horizonte, Minas Gerais, Brazil

Marilyn M. Pink, PhD, PT
CEO, EDUCATA
Calabasas, California

William S. Quillen, PT, PhD, FACSM
Associate Dean, College of Medicine
Professor and Director, School of Physical Therapy
    and Rehabilitation Sciences
University of South Florida
Tampa, Florida

Mitchell J. Rauh, BSPT, PhD, MPH, FACSM
Associate Professor
Graduate Program in Orthopaedic and Sports Physical
    Therapy
Rocky Mountain University of Health Professions
Provo, Utah

Adjunct Research Faculty
Graduate School of Public Health
School of Exercise and Nutritional Sciences
San Diego State University of Health Professions
San Diego, California

**Michael P. Reiman, PT, DPT, OCS, SCS, ATC,
    FAAOMPT, CSCS**
Assistant Professor
Department of Physical
Wichita State University
Wichita, Kansas

Clinician
Department of Physical Therapy
Via Christi Orthopaedic and Sports Physical Therapy
Wichita, Kansas

Lars C. Richardson, MD
Clinical Instructor in Orthopaedics
Department of Orthopaedics, Harvard Medical School
Boston, Massachusetts

Orthopaedic Surgical Consultant
Department of Orthopaedics, Harvard University Health
    Services
Cambridge, Massachusetts

Clinical Instructor in Orthopaedics
Department of Orthopaedics, Beth Israel Deaconess
    Medical Center
Boston, Massachusetts

Scott A. Riewald, PhD
Senior Sport Technologist
Sport Performance Division
United States Olympic Comittee
Colorado Springs, Colorado

Scott A. Rodeo, MD
Chairman, USA Swimming Sports Medicine Committee
Co-Chief, Sports Medicine and Shoulder Service, Hospital
    for Special Surgery
Professor of Orthopaedic Surgery (Academic Track), Weill
    Medical College of Cornell University
Attending Orthopaedic Surgeon, Hospital for Special
    Surgery
Attending Surgeon (Orthopaedic Surgery),
    The New York-Presbyterian Hospital
Assistant Scientist, Department of Research, Hospital for
    Special Surgery
Associate Team Physician, New York Giants Football
New York, New York

E. Paul Roetert, PhD, FACSM
Managing Director, Coaching Education and Sport
    Science
United States Tennis Association
Boca Raton, Florida

Justin Rohrberg, PT, DPT, ATC
Instructor
Department of Physical Therapy
Wichita State University
Wichita, Kansas

Physical Therapist, Head Athletic Trainer
Player Development Solutions
Wichita, Kansas

Jeffrey A. Russell, MS, ATC
Assistant Professor, Dance Science
Department of Dance
Claire Trevor School of the Arts
University of California, Irvine
Irvine, California

Thales Rezende Souza, BPT, MSc
PhD Student in Rehabilitation Sciences
Universidade Federal de Minas Gerais
Belo Horizonte, Minas Gerais, Brazil

Barry A. Spiering, PhD, CSCS
Department of Kinesiology
California State University, Fullerton
Fullerton, California

William T. Stauber, PT, PhD, FACSM
Division of Physical Therapy
Department of Human Performance and Applied Exercise
    Science
Department of Physiology and Pharmacology
West Virginia University
Morgantown, West Virginia

Alex M. Taylor, PsyD
Neuropsychology Fellow
Department of Sports Medicine
University of Pittsburgh Medical Center
Pittsburgh, Pennsylvania

Benjamin M.J. Thompson, MD
Chief Resident, Orthopaedic Surgery
Department of Orthopaedics and Physical Rehabilitation
University of Massachusetts Medical School
Worcester, Massachusetts

Timothy F. Tyler, MS, PT, ATC
Clinical Research Associate
NISMAT at Lenox Hill Hospital
New York, New York

Anthony A. Vandervoort, PhD
Editor-In-Chief
Journal of Aging and Physical Activity

Professor and Associate Dean (Scholarship)
Faculty of Health Sciences
University of Western Ontario
London, Ontario, Canada

"To Teach is to Learn Twice"

To those who invested in us that we might in turn pass on their knowledge and wisdom to future generations of students.

Contributors

William E. Amonette, MA, CSCS
Fitness and Human Performance Program
School of Human Sciences and Humanities
University of Houston-Clear Lake
Houston, Texas

James R. Andrews, MD
Andrews Sports Medicine and Orthopaedic Center
Birmingham, Alabama

Brant D. Berkstresser, MS, ATC/L
Head Athletic Trainer
Department of Athletics
Harvard University
Boston, Massachusetts

Natália Franco Netto Bittencourt, BPT
MSc Student in Rehabilitation Sciences
Universidade Federal de Minas Gerais
Belo Horizonte, Minas Gerais, Brazil

Physical Therapist
Núcleo de Integração das Ciências do Esporte
Minas Tênis Clube
Belo Horizonte, Minas Gerais, Brazil

Lori A. Bolgla, PT, PhD, ATC
Assistant Professor
Department of Physical Therapy
Medical College of Georgia
Augusta, Georgia

Rich Bomgardner, MS, LAT, ATC, CSCS
Athletic Training Education Coordinator
Department of Human Performance Studies
Wichita State University
Wichita, Kansas

Brian D. Busconi, MD
Associate Professor
Chief of Sports Medicine and Arthroscopy
Department of Orthopedics and Physical Rehabilitation
University of Massachusetts Medical School
Worcester, Massachusetts

W. Lee Childers, MSPO
PhD Candidate
School of Applied Physiology
Georgia Institute of Technology
Atlanta, Georgia

Loren Z.F. Chiu, PhD, CSCS
Assistant Professor
Faculty of Physical Education and Recreation
University of Alberta
Edmonton, Alberta, Canada

Michael W. Collins, PhD
Assistant Professor
Department of Orthopaedic Surgery
Department of Neurological Surgery
University of Pittsburgh Medical Center
Pittsburgh, Pennsylvania

Assistant Director
UPMC Sports Medicine Concussion Program
Pittsburgh, Pennsylvania

Stephen A. Durant, EdD
Instructor
Department of Psychiatry
Harvard Medical School
Boston, Massachusetts

Co-Director
MGH Performance And Character Excellence (PACES)
  Institute of Sports Psychology
Department of Child Psychiatry
Massachusetts General Hospital
Boston, Massachusetts

George T. Edelman, MPT, OCS, MTC
Edelman Spine and Orthopaedic Physical Therapy
Dover, Delaware

Adjunct Professor
Department of Physical Therapy
University of Delaware
Newark, Delaware

Todd S. Ellenbecker, DPT, MS, SCS, OCS, CSCS
Clinic Director, Physiotherapy Associates Scottsdale Sports
  Clinic
National Director of Clinical Research, Physiotherapy
  Associates
Director of Sports Medicine, ATP World Tour
Scottsdale, Arizona

Rafael F. Escamilla, PhD, PT, CSCS, FACSM
Professor
Department of Physical Therapy
California State University, Sacramento
Sacramento, California

Professor
Andrews-Paulos Research and Education Institute
Andrews Institute
Gulf Breeze, Florida

Glenn S. Fleisig, PhD
Research Director
American Sports Medicine Institute
Birmingham, Alabama

Adjunct Professor
Department of Biomedical Engineering
The University of Alabama at Birmingham
Birmingham, Alabama

Sérgio Teixeira Fonseca, BPT, ScD
Associate Professor
Department of Physical Therapy
School of Physical Education, Physical Therapy
 and Occupational Therapy
Universidade Federal de Minas Gerais (UFMG)
Belo Horizonte, Minas Gerais, Brazil

Eileen G. Fowler, PT, PhD
Associate Professor
Peter William Shapiro Chair for the Center for Cerebral
 Palsy
UCLA / Orthopaedic Hospital Department
 of Orthopaedic Surgery
University of California at Los Angeles
Los Angeles, California

Travis L. Francis, MS, LAT, ATC
Via Christi Sports Medicine
Wichita, Kansas

Gary J. Geissler, PT, DPT, SCS, ATC
Clinical Director of Rehabilitation
Athletic Department
Harvard University
Cambridge, Massachusetts

Assistant Professor
Program in Physical Therapy
MGH Institute of Health Professions
Boston, Massachusetts

Physical Therapist
Orthopaedic Physical Therapy Services
Wellesley, Massachusetts

Richard D. Ginsburg, PhD
Instructor
Department of Psychiatry
Harvard Medical School
Boston, Massachusetts

Co-Director
MGH Performance And Character Excellence (PACES)
 Institute of Sports Psychology
Department of Child Psychiatry
Massachusetts General Hospital
Boston, Massachusetts

Gabriela Gomes Pavam Gonçalves, BPT, MSc
Physical Therapist
Núcleo de Integração das Ciências do Esporte
Minas Tênis Clube
Belo Horizonte, Minas Gerais, Brazil

Gary A. Green, MD
Clinical Professor
Division of Sports Medicine
Department of Internal Medicine
David Geffen UCLA School of Medicine
Los Angeles, California

Partner
Pacific Palisades Medical Group
Pacific Palisades, California

Steven A. Greer, MD, CAQ
Program Director, Primary Care Sports Medicine
 Fellowship
Director, Primary Care Sports Medicine
Assistant Professor, Departments of Family Medicine
 and Orthopaedics
Medical College of Georgia
Augusta, Georgia

Robert J. Gregor, PhD, FACSM, FAAKPE
Professor Emeritus
School of Applied Physiology
Georgia Institute of Technology
Atlanta, Georgia

Adjunct Professor
Division of Biokinesiology and Physical Therapy
University of Southern California
Los Angeles, California

Donald W. Groot, MD, FRCP(C), FACP
Clinical Professor of Medicine
Department of Medicine
University of Alberta
Edmonton, Alberta, Canada

Medical Director
Groot DermaSurgery Centre
Edmonton, Alberta, Canada

Michael S. Jellinek, MD
Professor of Psychiatry and of Pediatrics
Harvard Medical School
Boston, Massachusetts

Chief, Child Psychiatry Service
Massachusetts General Hospital
Boston, Massachusetts

President
Newton Wellesley Hospital
Newton, Massachusetts

Patricia A. Johnston, BSc, MClSc, MBA
President, InForum
Edmonton, Alberta, Canada

John P. Kelly, DMD, MD, FACS
Associate Clinical Professor
Department of Surgery
Yale University School of Medicine
New Haven, Connecticut

Chief, Section of Oral and Maxillofacial Surgery
Department of Surgery
Hospital of Saint Raphael
New Haven, Connecticut

W. Ben Kibler, MD, FACSM
Medical Director, Lexington Clinic Sports Medicine
    Center
Medical Director, Shoulder Center of Kentucky
Lexington Clinic
Lexington, Kentucky

Mark S. Kovacs, PhD, CSCS
Senior Manager, Strength and Conditioning/
    Sport Science
United States Tennis Association
Boca Raton, Florida

Richard H. Leu, MD
CAQ Primary Care Sports Medicine
Clinical Associate Professor
Department of Family Medicine
Kansas University School of Medicine
Wichita, Kansas

Faculty Member, Sports Medicine Fellowship, Family
    Medicine Residency Program
Department of Family Medicine
Via Christi Regional Medical Center
Wichita, Kansas

David Lindsay, BHMS, BPhty, MSc
Sport Medicine Centre
University of Calgary
Calgary, Alberta, Canada

Janice Loudon, PT, PhD, ATC, SCS
Associate Professor
Department of Physical Therapy and Rehabilitation
    Science
University of Kansas Medical Center
Kansas City, Kansas

Caroline A. Macera, PhD, FACSM
Professor of Epidemiology
Graduate School of Public Health
San Diego State University
San Diego, California

David J. Magee, BPT, PhD
Professor and Associate Dean
Department of Physical Therapy
Faculty of Rehabilitation Medicine
University of Alberta
Edmonton, Alberta, Canada

Corrie A. Mancinelli, PT, PhD
Associate Professor
Division of Physical Therapy
Department of Human Performance and Applied Exercise
    Science
West Virginia University School of Medicine
Morgantown, West Virginia

**Robert C. Manske, PT, DPT, SCS, MEd, ATC,
    CSCS**
Associate Professor
Department of Physical Therapy
Wichita State University
Wichita, Kansas

Francis Wang, MD
Clinical Instructor
Department of Medicine
Harvard Medical School
Boston, Massachusetts

Physician
Department of Internal Medicine
Harvard University Health Services
Cambridge, Massachusetts

Team Physician
Department of Athletics
Harvard University
Cambridge, Massachusetts

Heidi M. Wells, BS, RD, CSSD, LD
Sports Dietitian/Clinical Dietitian
Via Christi Regional Medical Center
Wichita, Kansas

Kimberly M. White, PhD
Principal Scientist
Gatorade Sports Science Institute
Barrington, Illinois

James E. Zachazewski, PT, DPT, SCS, ATC
Clinical Director
Department of Physical and Occupational Therapy
Massachusetts General Hospital
Boston, Massachusetts

Adjunct Assistant Clinical Professor
Program in Physical Therapy
MGH Institute of Health Professions
Boston, Massachusetts

Jeffrey J. Zachwieja, PhD, FACSM
Gatorade Sports Science Institute
Barrington, Illinois

Contributors to Content Used from
Athletic Injuries and Rehabilitation

Susan Cummings, MS, RD
Mary Jane Rewinski, BS, RD
Scott J. Montain, PhD
Beau J. Freund, PhD
Thomas G. McPoil, PhD, PT, ATC
Mark W. Cornwall, PhD, PT
Frank W. Jobe, MD
James C. Puffer, MD
Ethan Saliba, PhD, ATC, PT, SCS
Susan Foreman, MEd, MPT, ATC
Richard T. Abadie Jr., BA, EMC
Donald Hangen, MD
Andrew W. Nichols, MD
Kathleen A. Curtis, PhD, PT
Robert S. Gailey Jr., MSEd, PT

Preface

Musculoskeletal Rehabilitation Series

Musculoskeletal conditions have an enormous impact on society. Today, musculoskeletal conditions have become the most common cause of disability and severe long-term pain in the industrialized world. As we approach the completion of the Bone and Joint Decade, it is apparent that the knowledge and skill required by the community of health care providers involved in managing the impairments and functional limitations resulting from acute or chronic musculoskeletal injury/illness has grown exponentially as the frequency of visits to practitioners' offices for musculoskeletal system complaints has continued to rise.

The art and science of musculoskeletal rehabilitation began as a consequence of the injuries suffered on the battlefields of Europe during World War I. Since that time, numerous textbooks have been published regarding musculoskeletal rehabilitation. These texts have encompassed the areas of basic science, evaluation, and treatment. However, these books have most often been developed and written in professional "isolation" (ie., from a single discipline's perspective). As a consequence, topics have either been covered in great depth but with a very narrow focus, or with great breadth with very little depth. Our goal in the development and production of this series was to develop a series of textbooks that compliment and build on one another, providing the reader with the needed depth and breadth of information for this critical area of health care.

Volume I of the series is the 5th edition of David Magee's *Orthopedic Physical Assessment.* This now classic text provides the clinician with the most comprehensive text available on this topic. First published in 1987, it has withstood the test of time and is the most widely used text in this area. In 1996, we developed and published the 1000 page textbook *Athletic Injuries and Rehabilitation.* Based upon feedback from both students and clinicians, we have expanded and broadened the scope of *Athletic Injuries and Rehabilitation* into three new volumes comprising approximately 2400 pages of information. *Volume II, Scientific Foundations and Principles of Practice,* provides clinicians with currently available science regarding musculoskeletal issues and principles of practice that should guide clinicians regarding therapeutic intervention. In *Volume III, Pathology and Intervention,* we have attempted to provide readers with a comprehensive text containing information on the most common musculoskeletal pathologies seen and the best evidence behind contemporary interventions directed towards the treatment of impairments and limitations associated with acute, chronic and congenital musculoskeletal conditions which occur across the lifespan. *Volume IV, Athletic and Sport Issues* provides the clinician interested in sport related injuries with specific in-depth information not commonly presented elsewhere. Detailed information is presented regarding non-orthopedic concerns, the biomechanics along with clinical impact of physical activities required for sport and specific patient populations.

International contributors have provided their unique perspectives on current diagnostic methodologies, clinical techniques, and rehabilitative concerns. We hope that our continued use of interdisciplinary author teams has firmly broken down the professional "territorial turf" barriers that have existed in past decades of health care. Health care professionals involved in the contemporary care of musculoskeletal conditions must continue to share and learn from one another to advance the provision of the most time- and cost-efficient care possible in 21st century society.

Each volume in our series is liberally illustrated. Key concepts in each chapter are highlighted in text boxes, which serve to reinforce those concepts for the reader, and numerous tables summarize chapter information for easy reference. Readers will find that references are not contained on printed pages at the end of chapters, but rather contained as part of a comprehensive electronic resource on CD-ROM or EVOLVE site (provided with each volume), which allows the reader to link to MEDLINE abstracts where possible. Because of the comprehensive nature of this multi-volume series, each text, although complete in itself, has been edited to build and integrate with related chapter materials from the other volumes in the series. It is the editors' hope that this series will find its way into use by faculty as a basis for formal coursework as well as a friendly companion and frequently consulted reference by students and those on the front lines of clinical care.

As with our previous collaborations, we look forward to the feedback that only you, our colleagues, can provide, so that we may continue the development and improvement of the *Musculoskeletal Rehabilitation Series.*

David J. Magee
James E. Zachazewski
William S. Quillen
Robert C. Manske

Preface

Athletic and Sport Issues

Athletic and Sport Issues in Musculoskeletal Rehabilitation is the 4th volume in our series *Musculoskeletal Rehabilitation*. For this volume we have added a new editor, Robert Manske. In this volume we have sought to provide the student and practicing clinician with a comprehensive source of information for this topic area not addressed elsewhere in this integrated series. Most texts on sports injuries have a primary focus on musculoskeletal pathology and intervention. Information on these types of problems and conditions are thoroughly addressed in *Volumes 1 – Orthopaedic Physical Assessment, Volume 2 – Scientific Foundations and Principles of Practice and Volume 3 – Pathology and Intervention.* The advantage of *Volume 4 – Athletic and Sport Issues in Musculoskeletal Rehabilitation* being part of an integrated series is that the information the reader will find is summarized and presented in greater depth than most other texts. Because of this, we believe the reader will find this textbook an exceptional resource for their practice.

Volume 4 is divided into four sections:

- **Preparation and Prevention in Sports Medicine** focuses on psychological, nutritional, environmental and pharmacologic factors associated with sport participation and health.
- **Applied Biomechanics of Selected Sport Activities** present in depth reviews of the biomechanics of activities and how they may impact injury development and rehabilitation including clinically relevant points.
- **Management of Sports Injury and Illness** focuses on non-musculoskeletal injury and management factors.
- **Special Populations and Epidemiology** presents information on sport injury concerns based on gender, age or physical ability/disability. Also presented in this section is a comprehensive summary of the epidemiologic injury data by specific sport.

This volume is again liberally illustrated with multiple figures, tables and text boxes to allow the reader to quickly grasp the information being presented. A comprehensive reference list is provided on an Evolve site with links to MEDLINE abstracts where available.

We firmly believe that with the addition of this volume the clinician who practices is the area of "sports medicine" will have a set of resources that provide them with comprehensive information on the management of this patient population.

As we continue to develop this series we welcome the readers' feedback to allow us to continue to enhance the quality and comprehensiveness of the series.

David J. Magee
Robert C. Manske
James E. Zachazewski
William S. Quillen

Acknowledgments

We would like to gratefully acknowledge the ongoing professional assistance of the following individuals who have steadfastly supported this series from its inception.

Kathy Falk – Executive Editor, Health Professions, Elsevier
Christie Hart –Senior Developmental Editor, Elsevier
Megan Fennell – Associate Developmental Editor, Elsevier
Bev Evjen – Editorial Assistant
Ted Huff – Artist

Contents

ROLE OF THE SPORTS MEDICINE TEAM

Richard H. Leu and Robert C. Manske

Introduction

The global term *sports medicine* does not delineate any single career, but describes a vast range of professions and areas of health care that all have a common purpose: to protect the health and well being of athletes. In today's competitive environment, an athlete's care must be provided through a team approach.[1] A *team* is defined as a group or collection of individuals with a common purpose or goal. No one single discipline can care for all of the athlete's varying needs and requirements. "Turf wars" and "profession bashing" waste a significant amount of time and effort that should be spent on the care of athletes. Each team member should have a useful role in ensuring that an athlete can continue to function at his or her peak levels throughout a given sporting season. The primary goal of the sports medicine team is to prevent injury and illness and to arrange for examinations and rehabilitation following injury. Furthermore, the sports medicine team should provide the athlete with the ability to either optimally perform or return to his or her given sport as safely, quickly, and efficiently as possible following injury in such a way that the possibility of reinjury is kept to a minimum. It can clearly be seen that a larger sports medicine team may be of greater benefit to athletes. A larger team can cover an entire group of athletes as a whole with multiple medical disciplines, versus having only a few medical professionals trying to perform all the needed tasks. Multiple disciplines, including but not limited to exercise physiologists, biomechanists, dietitians and nutritionists, sport psychologists, strength and conditioning specialists, nurses, physicians, physician's assistants, dentists, ophthalmologists, athletic trainers, sports physical therapists and chiropractors, may all have a place on the sports medicine team. Building this team approach is as important to the success of an athletic organization as fielding talented athletes.[2] A team approach with direct communication at all levels is best to assist in expediting and facilitating information regarding the athlete's medical status. This chapter discusses the various roles of the "sports medicine team" and provides examples through a case study design describing the "team" approach.

The Sports Medicine Team

- Physician
- Certified athletic trainer
- Sports physical therapist
- Medical specialties
- Chiropractor
- Strength and conditioning specialist
- Sports psychologist
- Dentist
- Physician's assistant
- Biomechanist
- Nutritionist
- Ophthalmologist
- Nurse

Clinical Point

In today's competitive environment, an athlete's care must be provided through a team approach.

Composition of Sports Medicine Team

The sports medicine team consists of five well-defined components which are closely integrated with the athlete as the center of focus (Figure 1-1).[3] The immediate sports

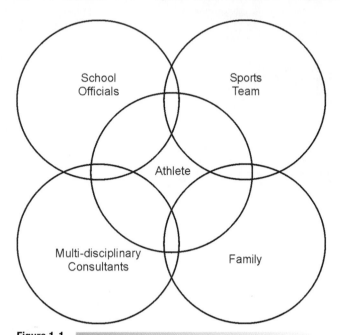

Figure 1-1

The sports team. (Modified from Garfinkel D, Birrer RB: The team physician. In Birrer RB, editor: *Sports medicine for the primary care physician*, ed 2, Boca Raton, FL, 1994, CRC Press.)

medicine team includes the coaching staff, teammates, physician, certified athletic trainer, equipment manager, strength coach, and sports physical therapist.

Certified Athletic Trainer

The certified athletic trainer ("certified athletic therapist" in Canada) is certainly the gate keeper of the day-to-day activities of the athletes. The athletic trainer is the first line of defense for all of the athletes at the high school, college, and professional levels. In other countries, this role may be assumed by a physical therapist, a masseur, or a physician. Because an estimated 20% of all high school athletes develop an injury during their careers, it is imperative that athletic trainers be knowledgeable in all aspects of athletic diagnosis, examination, triage, and treatment.[4] The National Athletic Training Association Board of Certification (NATABOC) has described six practice domains (Box 1-1) that should be

---

Box 1-1 NATABOC Practice Domains

1. Prevention
2. Clinical evaluation and diagnosis
3. Immediate care
4. Treatment, rehabilitation, and reconditioning
5. Organization and administration
6. Professional responsibility

NATABOC, National Athletic Training Association Board of Certification.

---

practiced by all trainers. Almost always, the athletic trainer is the first to see or hear about injuries or potential problems that occur in the athletic environment. It is the athletic trainer who undoubtedly spends the largest amount of time day in and day out with the athletes. Athletic trainers often become very close to these athletes and get to know them on a more personal basis than any other member of the sports medicine team. In addition, athletic trainers commonly have an expertise in bracing, taping, and orthotic and protective equipment used to prevent injury or allow an expedited return to competition that allows an athlete to safely compete even with injuries. Athletic trainers provide sound rehabilitation regimens and are able to apply physical agents to enhance the athletes' healing potential.

An athletic trainer today has to have a 4-year degree from an accredited program and then passes a rigorous three-part examination that has been developed by NATABOC. In addition, athletic trainers are typically licensed or certified through various state boards of health or healing arts.

Sports Physical Therapist

The American Board of Physical Therapist Specialties is the credentialing body of those who possess a Board Certification in sports physical therapy. Only physical therapists are eligible to receive this credential. In Canada, a slightly different process is followed but the outcome and designation are the same. These board-certified specialists have passed an examination that has delineated them as having advanced knowledge that qualifies them to practice in sports medicine settings. Members certified in sports physical therapy typically have experience in performance enhancement; recognition and management of active sports injuries; treatment, rehabilitation, and return to sport; and research of sports injuries. Sports physical therapists have multiple responsibilities. Many physical therapists also hold certifications as athletic trainers. This combination of credentials provides the professional with the opportunity to work with both athletic and general populations. The therapist that holds both credentials is in high demand.[5] The general physical therapist provides rehabilitation of patients and athletes recovering from injuries or medical illnesses resulting from neuromusculoskeletal origin. Physical therapists work in a wide variety of locations, including hospitals, outpatient clinics, private offices, homecare programs and university settings (Figure 1-2). As do athletic trainers, physical therapists work under the direction of a physician. Those therapists with sports specialty certification can also be valuable on the athletic field of play assessing and managing acute injuries. Entry level physical therapist positions require a master's degree as a minimum educational requirement. Most programs are now 2- to 4-year postbaccalaureate degrees ending with either a master's in physical therapy or doctorate of physical therapy.

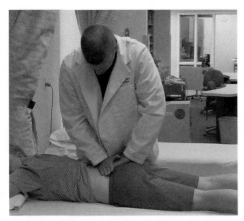

Figure 1-2
Sports physical therapist.

Team Physician by Specialty[1]

- Family Medicine (25.5%)
- Orthopedic Surgery (16.2%)
- Osteopathic Medicine (10.9%)
- Internal Medicine (10.1%)
- General Practice (6.3%)
- Pediatrics (5.4%)
- Emergency Medicine (4.9%)
- General Surgery (4.5%)
- Obstetrics/Gynecology (2.8%)
- Cardiology (2.0%)
- Other (11.5%)

Sports Physical Therapy Competency Areas

- **Rehabilitation and Return to Activity:** Those activities concerned with the rehabilitation of athletes with impairments, functional limitations, or disabilities focusing on the return of athletes to their sport activities.
- **Acute Injury Management:** Those activities concerned with the immediate management of acute injury or illness associated with athletic activity.
- **Sports Science:** Those activities concerned with maximizing the athlete's sports performance, including training considerations and the effect of such factors as nutrition and environment on performance.
- **Medical and Surgical Considerations:** Those activities concerned with the medical and surgical management of athletes.
- **Injury Prevention:** Those activities concerned with injury and disease prevention for athletes.
- **Critical Inquiry:** Those activities concerned with maintaining current knowledge, applying principles of evidence-based practice in sports physical therapy, and contributing to the body of knowledge in sports physical therapy.

Data from American Board of Physical Therapy Specialties Specialty Council on Sports Physical Therapy: *Sports Physical Therapy Description of Clinical Practice*, Alexandria, VA, 2002, American Physical Therapy Association.

Team Physician

The team physician is a licensed physician (medical doctor or doctor of osteopathy) with an interest and additional training in sports medicine. The majority of team physicians are either primary care specialists or orthopedic surgeons; however, a wide variety of specialists devote their expertise and time to caring for athletes at all levels of competition.[2]

It is difficult and impractical to attempt to develop a list of qualifications to become a "team physician." Qualifications depend on the level of competition as well as geographic location. For example, a team physician for a high school in a rural community that participates in eight-man football will most likely be one of the community's primary care physicians who has an interest in sports or has a child as a member of the team.

However, the team physician should have skills in basic life support and a fundamental understanding of the common medical and musculoskeletal conditions that affect athletes. Currently, all family medicine residency training programs in the United States require the equivalent of 1 month of concentrated instruction in sports medicine during the 36-month curriculum. This aspect of a resident's training focuses on performing a complete musculoskeletal examination, use and interpretation of appropriate radiological imaging to assist with diagnoses, recommended therapeutic interventions and "return-to-play guidelines" for common conditions. An established practitioner may have obtained these skills through continuing medical education courses after they complete residency training.

A team physician at the college or professional level has most likely completed a fellowship in either primary care or orthopedic sports medicine, or demonstrated his or her expertise by completion of a Certificate of Added Qualifications in sports medicine. Certification in primary care sports medicine consists of passing a written examination and recertification is on a 10-year cycle. Orthopedic surgeons also have a certification process through the American Board of Orthopedic Surgery. Following the initial few years of its institution, surgeons who want to sit for the examination will have to complete a fellowship in orthopedic sports medicine to be qualified. Recertification is on a 10-year cycle.

It is crucial that these various groups of physicians are not competitors, but work to complement each other and together treat common athletic conditions. There are multiple responsibilities when serving as a team physician. Organized sports are a complex entity that requires multiple interactions by the sports medicine team with a wide range of individuals including the athlete, team, coaching staff, academic institution, and general management depending on the level of competition.

Some Responsibilities of the Team Physician

- Preparticipation physical examination
- Injury assessment and management
- "Return to play" decisions for injured athletes
- Medical coverage of athletic events
- Injury prevention
- Strength training and conditioning
- Substance abuse assessment
- Special population assessment (i.e., youth, elderly, disabled)
- Educating and counseling on sports-related medical issues

The team physician's primary responsibility is to the individual athlete. "Do no harm" is one of the most important Hippocratic oaths medical professionals take upon entering this profession. This must be constantly remembered when athletes are injured during a season. The physician, as do other members of the sports medicine team, has an ethical responsibility to allow the athlete to participate, but must also balance this desire to allow participation with the responsibility of making sure the athlete has been adequately rehabilitated from injury before a return to competition. This does not apply solely to the physical needs of the athlete. The physician must also be an effective communicator and demonstrate empathy and concern toward the athlete; the team physician must be able to recognize the psychological aspects of an injury (e.g., anxiety and depression) and be willing to address these openly with the athlete.

Injuries or illnesses of higher profile athletes at all levels of sports may create discussions in schools, universities, communities, and even at national levels. The team physician must, as must all members of the sports medicine team, maintain confidentiality regarding an athlete's injury without compromising his or her responsibility to the coach, academic institution, general management, or the public.

Clinical Point

The sports medicine team's primary responsibility is to the athlete.

The team physician must always factor in the success and well-being of the entire team when dealing with an individual athlete. It is imperative that the physician demonstrates the same degree of professionalism and understanding to each member of the team regardless of the athlete's abilities.

The coaching staff is ultimately concerned with the success of the team and must be informed and regularly updated regarding an athlete's injury in a timely manner. One of the roles of a team physician is to educate the coaching staff in improvements in medical and preventive care for the team.

The team physician's primary responsibility to an academic institution or general management is protection from liability by screening athletes prior to the start of the competitive season. Furthermore, following injury, the team physician should return an athlete to competition only after the athlete has been adequately rehabilitated. This is accomplished by the team physician fulfilling his or her responsibility to the individual athlete, which will then translate into the success of the team.

The effectiveness of the team physician is built around availability, competence, and the ability to communicate with athletes, coaches, athletic trainers, and other members of the sports medicine team. Obviously, a team physician cannot be physically present at every practice or game event, especially when covering multiple schools or a school with multiple sports.

Clinical Point

To have an effective, efficient sports medicine team, communication is essential.

The team physician or medical associate should always be present for high-risk contact sports such as football, ice hockey, soccer, and wrestling. If a physician cannot be on-site, medical coverage should be provided by a certified athletic trainer or other appropriately trained individual. During these instances in which the team physician is not available on-site, he or she should be readily available by phone in case of suspected emergencies. Team physicians must be flexible and willing to adjust their schedules to evaluate athletes in the training room, the office, or after hours if that is when an injury occurs.

Event coverage and medical supervision of athletes is the most time-consuming aspect of the role as a team physician; however, the most difficult responsibility is the decision on whether and when to return an athlete to play. During event competition the physician must be able to determine quickly if an athlete has full range of motion and demonstrates 90% of normal strength after an injury before returning the athlete back into competition. The athlete returning to competition must also be able to contribute to the success of the team. However, the team physician must also determine whether an athlete is psychologically ready to return to competition. There are times in which an athlete is physically ready, but emotionally not yet ready to compete. This is most often seen following traumatic injuries in which the athlete is still tentative about return even after he or she has been adequately rehabilitated. This may be seen in events such as a triple-jumper wanting to return to his first competition following a distal femur fracture. Although evidence exists of complete fracture healing, and objective data demonstrates full strength and range of motion, this athlete may simply not be sure about landing and jumping off of the leg that was previously fractured because of a fear that the injury may reoccur.

Clinical Point

The most difficult decision the sports medicine team makes is whether and when the athlete should be allowed to return to competition.

Depending on the particular problem, the team physician may use consultation from a multidisciplinary pool of health practitioners. This pool includes medical specialists (e.g., cardiologists, neurosurgeons, general surgeons, dermatologists, orthopedic surgeons, ophthalmologists, and psychiatrists), psychologists, nutritionists, physical therapists, dentists, and podiatrists. The team physician is responsible for coordinating the care provided by these consultants as it pertains to the athlete (Figure 1-3).

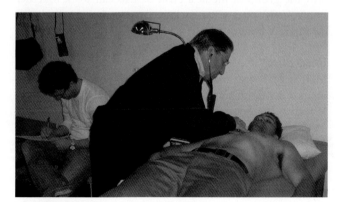

Figure 1-3
Team physician.

Team Approach

Every member of the sports medicine team must demonstrate competence in his or her area of expertise. It is crucial that the selected consultants in the multidisciplinary pool have a special interest and knowledge base relevant to the field of sports medicine as it relates to their particular specialties as well as the sports with which they are involved. Athletes encounter unique problems and have special medical needs that are often different from the general population; consultants must be familiar with these differences. This can commonly be seen during rehabilitation of postsurgical conditions. A general physical therapist who commonly treats all types of orthopedic conditions may only see one or two shoulder labral tears or one or two anterior cruciate ligament (ACL) reconstructions per year, whereas it is not uncommon for a busy sports physical therapist to have six or more of these patients being seen on a daily basis all year round. It is ultimately the responsibility of the team physician to ensure competency in every member of the sports medicine team. For the sports medicine team to work optimally, there must be a mutual respect among all members to function as a "team."

Effective Sports Medicine Team is Built on Three Core Principles

- Competency
- Mutual respect
- Effective communication

Competency is the core ingredient leading to respect for each team member. This respect is sometimes demonstrated through team protocol. A perfect example of teamwork and respect can be seen on the field of play when multiple medical personnel are covering an event and an injury occurs. Typically, protocol requires that initially only the certified athletic trainer go out onto the field to assess an injured athlete. This protocol may differ based on level of competition (high school, college, professional), seriousness of injury, and the personal comfort level of members of the sports medicine team involved. The trainer should signal the physician onto the field if and when needed, at which point the athlete becomes the team physician's patient. It is crucial that the team physician avoid micromanaging every injury to preserve and protect the "team concept." The team physician should understand that he or she is not needed for every incident that occurs during sports participation. Each member of the sports medicine team should recognize his or her own level of expertise and limitations as well as those of other members of the team; the team concept ideally fosters learning among all members of the team. The team physician is always in charge of making medical decisions unless absent, in which case the certified athletic trainer oversees the supervision of the athlete.

Preparticipation Physical Examination

The first step in enabling an athlete to compete safely is the preparticipation physical examination (PPE). The PPE is described in further detail in Chapter 2 of this volume. The purpose of the PPE is to perform a health risk assessment for an individual athlete and start the season-long process of monitoring the health status of the athlete. It is hoped that the PPE will prevent future injury by identifying athletes who may be at risk prior to the season (Figure 1-4[6]).

The PPE takes place in various venues (e.g., training room, mass physicals, private office); it is imperative that an effective means of communication be established between the team physician, athlete, certified athletic trainer, sports physical therapist, coach, and the athlete's parents regarding the need for additional testing for clearance or a decision "not to clear." This may be accomplished with a face-to-face check-out after the examination, a phone call, or clearly delineating the status of the athlete on the PPE form. These lines of communication must remain open as the certified athletic trainer monitors the athlete throughout the season.

Injury Management

A major function of the sports medicine team is to evaluate and manage injuries sustained by an athlete during the season or off-season. The certified athletic trainer and team physician

are typically the members of the team to perform the initial evaluation of the athlete when an injury occurs. The team physician and certified athletic trainer must develop a plan for further evaluation and management of the injury and discuss the plan with the athlete and coach, and family member depending on the age of the athlete. The plan may include additional testing and use of selected consultants. It is imperative that every member of the sports medicine team be "on the same page" regarding the suspected diagnosis and plan of management.

The team physician, with the athlete's permission, informs the coach, certified athletic trainer, and family of pertinent medical information. The coach and certified athletic trainer keep the team physician and family informed of performance problems and other pertinent issues regarding the athlete and his or her injury.

Each encounter with an athlete by the certified athletic trainer, team physician, or consultant must be documented and be incorporated into the athlete's medical file. The technology of electronic health records has greatly facilitated the transfer of medical information. The team's physician can fax or e-mail his or her evaluations to the certified athletic trainer, sports physical therapist, or consultant. The ability to share information among members of the sports medicine team enhances the treatment of the athlete.

The decision to return to play or to end the season must be a "team decision" involving the athlete, team physician, certified athletic trainer, sports physical therapist, coach, and parents. Once again, this requires effective communication among all members of the team and everyone must be "on the same page." Although time consuming, weekly meetings involving the team physician, certified athletic trainer, and sports physical therapist can be most beneficial in staying abreast of the status of injured athletes.

Case Studies

The team approach can be examined and illustrated best by looking at several case studies. These case studies describe how the group of medical professionals can work together as a cohesive "team" to facilitate appropriate medical care for injured athletes.

Case Study 1

M.S. is a 17-year-old male high school soccer goalie who injured his right knee during a game. The athlete was referred to the Sports Medicine Clinic by the high school's certified athletic trainer.

The athlete stated that his right knee was planted and he sustained a blow to the upper torso; he felt his knee "pop" twice. He stated that it felt like the patella was forced to the lateral aspect of his knee and then "popped" back into position. M.S. was unable to continue to participate in the game and noted immediate swelling of his right knee. Initial

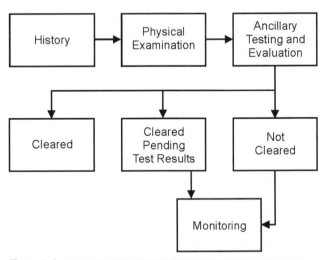

Figure 1-4
Preparticipation physical examination.

treatment by the certified athletic trainer at the high school included rest, ice, elevation, and compression.

M.S. was initially evaluated at the Sports Medicine Clinic 4 days after the initial injury. A moderate effusion was present and there was limited flexion and extension of the knee. The patella apprehension test was negative and the Lachman test had a definite endpoint on the right knee. The working diagnosis was patella subluxation/dislocation of the right knee. M.S. was fitted with a hinged patella-stabilizing brace, instructed in quadriceps strengthening exercises, and referred for formal physical therapy. The physician's evaluation was faxed to the certified athletic trainer and the physical therapist.

The athlete improved with physical therapy but continued to have pain with full-knee flexion and extension. The physical therapist e-mailed the Sports Medicine Clinic with her concern that there was laxity in the ACL of the right knee. M.S. was re-evaluated in the Sports Medicine Clinic 18 days after the initial injury. The Lachman test demonstrated laxity of the right ACL with a soft endpoint. The athlete inquired about being cleared to play goalie in an indoor soccer league scheduled to begin in 3 weeks. A magnetic resonance imaging (MRI) study was ordered to assess the integrity of the ACL ligament.

M.S. returned to the clinic 1 week later to review the MRI results and inquire about clearance to participate. The athlete had been running on the treadmill without pain. He stated that his knee occasionally "popped," but denied locking or a sensation of instability. The MRI showed a bone contusion of the lateral femoral condyle and proximal tibia. There was edema noted in the ACL and the ligament appeared ill-defined but intact. The posterior cruciate ligament and menisci were normal. M.S. was referred to an orthopedic surgeon for a second opinion regarding clearance to play soccer in an indoor soccer league with a possibly deficient ACL ligament. The Sports Medicine Clinic office notes and MRI report were faxed to the consultant's office and the most recent office note was faxed to the certified athletic trainer and physical therapist.

The consultant cleared the athlete to compete in the indoor soccer league. M.S. returned to the consultant's office 4 weeks later with the complaint of a new injury involving the right knee. The athlete stated that he was playing goalie on the day before when he jumped to head a ball. When he landed, his right knee buckled and gave out. The consultant believed that the athlete either sustained a complete tear of the ACL or another patella dislocation with disruption of the vastus medialis oblique. This was discussed with the athlete and his parents and a repeat MRI was ordered.

The MRI confirmed a complete tear of the ACL (Figure 1-5) and a partial tear of the medial collateral ligament; the medial retinaculum appeared intact. M.S. underwent a bone-tendon-bone autograft ACL repair 5 days later. The consultant kept the team updated by

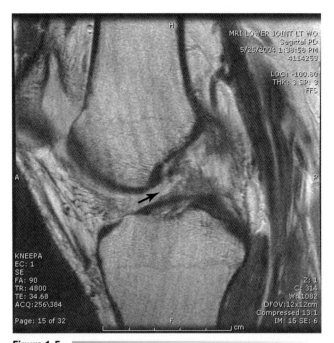

Figure 1-5
Magnetic resonance imaging scan demonstrating torn anterior cruciate ligament.

faxing their office visits as well as the operative report with pictures of the procedure. The most recent visit was 6 months later at which time the consultant cleared M.S. to participate in fall soccer at the high school.

This case illustrates the benefits of effective communication using current technology, which resulted in optimal medical care for this athlete.

Case Study 2

A sports physical therapist working with a freshman high school athlete referred for shoulder rehabilitation because of scapular dyskinesis was seeing terrific gains in scapular strength and stability in the young athlete. After 3 to 4 weeks of consistent rehabilitation, the young athlete was pain-free and back to full sports participation. He missed several recent appointments because of a hand and wrist injury that occurred in football practice a week before. He saw his regular medical doctor regarding his hand injury and had radiographs, which were reported to be negative for any fracture. One week later, the young athlete was brought to therapy for his last physical therapy appointment for his much-improved shoulder. It is noted on that date that he still exhibited hand swelling, increased pain to palpation of the anatomic snuffbox, decreased grip strength, and decreased wrist mobility and strength secondary to pain. These symptoms were duly noted by the sports physical therapists who noticed the clear signs of a potentially disabling scaphoid fracture. An immediate call to the team physician alerted him of the impending problem of this potentially devastating injury. Because of their close relationship and "team" approach the athlete was able to see the team physician first thing the next day. The sports physician reviewed radiographs and had additional images taken and determined that they appeared negative at this point, but, because of the classic symptoms, recommended casting the wrist for 7 to 14 days and scheduled the patient for a follow-up with possible computed tomography (CT) scan in 2 weeks if symptoms were still present. The athlete continued to have hand and wrist pain with active movements and gripping 10 days later. He returned to the sports medicine physician's office where a CT scan was ordered. To his dismay, the athlete actually had a scaphoid fracture that went undetected by early conventional radiographic technique (Figure 1-6). He was placed in a splint and started the arduous process of healing the wrist injury.

These two examples clearly illustrate the team approach and the respect for each of the team members toward one another. Because of this team approach, the athlete was able to see the team physician in an expedited amount of time to get a definitive diagnosis and implement a timely plan of care that was more realistic and appropriate for this form of serious injury.

Conclusion

Members of the sports medicine team clearly have the unique opportunity to establish a relationship with young men and women participating in athletic activities. The team can positively influence these individuals by providing medical, philosophical, and psychological counseling to these athletes regarding academic performance; use of supplements, drugs, and alcohol; and the opposite sex. The implications of the sports medicine team's responsibility and its ability to change these young athlete's lives should not be taken lightly. There is an opportunity for education and demonstration of positive role modeling in every interaction with athletes.

The operative word in the sports medicine team is *team*. In the Navy of old, the acronym TEAM stood for "Treat Everyone as Myself."[7] Another symbolic acronym as it relates to sports is "Together Everyone Achieves More."[8] The effectiveness of the team in enabling an athlete to safely participate in his or her sport is predicated upon competency, mutual respect, and effective communication.

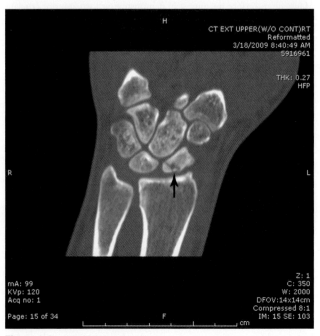

Figure 1-6
Computed tomography scan of scaphoid fracture.

References

1. Mellion MB, Walsh WM, Shelton GL: *The team physician's handbook*, ed 2, Philadelphia, 1997, Hanley & Belfus.
2. Fu FH, Tjoumakaris FP, Buoncristiani A: Building a sports medicine team, *Clin Sports Med* 26:173–179, 2007.
3. Garfinkel D, Birrer RB: The team physician. In Birrer RB, editor: *Sports medicine for the primary care physician*, ed 2, Boca Raton, FL, 1994, CRC Press.
4. Lyznicki JM, Rigg JA, Champion HC: Certified athletic trainers in secondary schools: Report of the Council on Scientific Affairs, American Medical Association, *J Athl Train* 34:272–276, 1999.
5. Prentice WE: *Arnheim's principles of athletic training. A competency-based approach*, ed 12, New York, 2006, McGraw Hill.
6. Matheson G: *Role of preparticipation medical exam: Who can't play*. The Puck Stops Here: Comprehensive Management of Hockey Injuries, Chicago, IL, August 22–24, 2008.
7. Quillen WS: Personal communication, February 8, 2009.
8. Accessed at www.acronymfinder.com/TEAM.html.

PREPARTICIPATION EVALUATION AND PHYSICAL FITNESS PROFILING

PART A: PREPARTICIPATION EVALUATION
David J. Magee and William S. Quillen

PART B: PHYSICAL FITNESS PROFILING
William E. Amonette and Barry A. Spiering

PART A: PREPARTICIPATION EVALUATION

Introduction

The *preparticipation evaluation (PPE),* although generic in some sense, is often designed for a particular activity, sport, or age group.[1-7] Each activity and sport is associated with unique health concerns. For example, football players and runners are at risk for different injuries. In addition, the risks for each activity and sport vary by population, age, and sex.[3,8,9] The sophistication of a PPE can range from a limited physical examination to an extensive evaluation that includes cardiac stress testing, fitness profiling, diagnostic imaging, and other procedures, depending on the practice situation; level of competition; institutional requirements; local, state, or national laws; and insurance policies.[10] Also, more strenuous activities and those involving contact or collision (Box 2-1) commonly require a more extensive evaluation.[11] Ideally, a PPE should occur at least 6 weeks before the intended activity.[12,13] This lead time allows for specialty consultation and an opportunity to treat minor medical problems such as skin disorders, muscle weakness, or acute infections before participation.[10]

PPEs are usually led by a family or team physician who is familiar with the athlete's past medical history and family history as this method is more likely to provide continuity of care. The physician should assess any congenital or developmental problems, immunization status, and recent injuries or illnesses.[12-14] However, many athletes do not have a family physician, or the physician may lack experience or understanding of the proposed activity. Another method for assessing preparticipation health, especially for a specific sport, is to use a team physician who is familiar with the activity requirements and demands. These evaluations are often group efforts, using multiple health care professionals (e.g., athletic trainer, sports physical therapist, nurse) performing selected parts of a multistation evaluation. If properly organized, this method allows for many concurrent screenings; however, some participants may find this method impersonal, confusing, and noisy.[14,15] The PPE is often performed annually, and subsequent PPEs may be less extensive, assessing only body systems affected during the preceding season.[12,13,16-18] For example, strength and functional performance testing may be performed only for those joints affected by injury during the previous season; these evaluations are used primarily to determine if the athlete is ready to resume participation.

McKeag[19] describes five populations that deserve special attention during the PPE. In the prepubescent athlete (i.e., 6 to 10 years old), physicians should examine for previously undetected congenital abnormalities. In pubescent athletes (i.e., 11 to 15 years old), the examination should evaluate physical maturity and good health practices for safe participation. The postpubescent and young adult groups (i.e., 16 to 30 years old) bring the widest variety of skills, levels, and motivation. For this group, discussion of previous injuries and a sport-specific examination are important. For adults (i.e., 30 to 65 years old), the physician should address injury prevention (e.g., overuse), previous injury patterns, and conditioning. Elderly athletes (i.e., 65 years old or older) require an examination based on individual requirements because many elderly athletes increase exercise or physical activity following a medical illness.[5]

Box 2-1 Classification of Sports According to Contact

Contact	Limited Contact	Noncontact
Basketball	Adventure racing[a]	Badminton
Boxing[b]	Baseball	Bodybuilding[c]
Cheerleading	Bicycling	Bowling
Diving	Canoeing or kayaking	Canoeing or
Extreme sports[d]	(white water)	kayaking (flat
Field hockey	Fencing	water)
Football, tackle	Field events	Crew or rowing
Gymnastics	High jump	Curling
Ice hockey[e]	Pole vault	Dance
Lacrosse	Floor hockey	Field events
Martial arts[f]	Football, flag or touch	Discus
Rodeo	Handball	Javelin
Rugby	Horseback riding	Shot-put
Skiing, downhill	Martial arts[f]	Golf
Ski jumping	Racquetball	Orienteering[g]
Snowboarding	Skating	Power lifting[c]
Soccer	Ice	Race walking
Team handball	In-line	Riflery
Ultimate Frisbee	Roller	Rope jumping
Water polo	Skiing	Running
Wrestling	Cross-country	Sailing
	Water	Scuba diving
	Skateboarding	Swimming
	Softball	Table tennis
	Squash	Tennis
	Volleyball	Track
	Weight lifting	
	Windsurfing or surfing	

From Rice SG, Council on Sports Medicine and Fitness: Medical conditions affecting sports participation, *Pediatrics* 121(4):842, 2008. Available at http://aappolicy.aappublications.org/cgi/reprint/pediatrics;121/4/841.pdf.
[a]Adventure racing has been added since the previous statement was published and is defined as a combination of two or more disciplines, including orienteering and navigation, cross-country running, mountain biking, paddling, and climbing and rope skills.
[b]The American Academy of Pediatrics opposes participation in boxing for children, adolescents, and young adults.
[c]The American Academy of Pediatrics recommends limiting bodybuilding and power lifting until the adolescent achieves sexual maturity rating 5 (Tanner stage V).
[d]Extreme sports has been added since the previous statement was published.
[e]The American Academy of Pediatrics recommends limiting the amount of body checking allowed for hockey players 15 years and younger, to reduce injuries.
[f]Martial arts can be subclassified as judo, jujitsu, karate, kung fu, and tae kwon do; some forms are contact sports and others are limited-contact sports.
[g]Orienteering is a race (contest) in which competitors use a map and a compass to find their way through unfamiliar territory.

Five Specific Populations for the Preparticipation Evaluations

- Prepubescent athletes (6 to 10 years of age)
- Pubescent athlete (11 to 15 years of age)
- Young adult athlete (16 to 30 years of age)
- Adult athlete (30 to 65 years of age)
- Masters athlete (> 65 years of age)

Objectives of the Preparticipation Evaluation

- Act as a screening process
- Avoid misinterpretation of findings
- Classify the athlete
- Counsel the athlete
- Determine health status
- Determine if disease is present
- Determine if referral is necessary
- Determine unsuspected correctable conditions
- Develop a musculoskeletal profile
- Develop rapport with the athlete
- Ensure that previous treatments and injury rehabilitation have been completed
- Establish baseline values
- Establish guidelines
- Foster good health practices
- Keep immunizations current
- Meet legal and insurance requirements
- Prevent injuries
- Uncover pre-existing conditions

Objectives of the Evaluation

PPEs have many purposes.[10,12,20,21] The examiner must remember that the purpose is not to disqualify an athlete, but to ensure the health and safety of all athletes.[12] Therefore, an athlete disqualified from specific activities should be counseled to find other activities, exercises, or sports that are more appropriate to the athlete's needs and limitations. Most organizations require PPEs for legal and insurance reasons. PPEs provide some protection in case of litigation, and many insurance companies require them prior to issuing an insurance policy.[10] Often evaluations are performed to uncover pre-existing conditions that could preclude participation for health or safety reasons. These pre-existing conditions range from physical immaturity to organ loss to the presence of specific disease processes.

The PPE helps the sports medicine team develop a current health profile, which is used to determine whether the athlete has the physical attributes necessary for participation. Athletes who have had surgery or an injury must be evaluated physically and psychologically to ensure that they are prepared to endure stresses typically encountered during their return to exercise or sport.[12] In developing a physical fitness profile

(PFP) (Part B of this chapter), the sports medicine team establishes a baseline for the athlete, against which any future injuries may be assessed. The evaluation should not simply include "yes" or "no" answers, but should thoroughly describe the athlete's health and establish appropriate activity levels. This helps decrease the incidence of reinjury and ensures that the athlete can participate at the desired level.

The PPE may be used to determine the athlete's health status before participation or competition. The PPE also helps to identify any abnormalities, physical inadequacies, or poor conditioning that may place the athlete at risk for injury.[22] The examiner may find unanticipated treatable conditions, as well as conditions that prevent safe participation. In addition, the evaluation may uncover pre-existing conditions. Past medical history and records should be reviewed to help establish the presence of pre-existing conditions.

The PPE is important to ensure that previously diagnosed conditions have been properly treated and fully rehabilitated. The PPE also provides an opportunity to diagnose serious or life-threatening medical and surgical conditions so that they may be addressed before participation. For example, those with infectious mononucleosis must avoid contact sports for several weeks because the athlete's enlarged spleen may be easily injured or ruptured. The PPE also ensures that old injuries have properly healed and that recovery and rehabilitation are complete. Athletes may delay or forego treatment for end-season injuries because they believe that the injuries will heal spontaneously with time. The PPE can be used to ensure proper treatment and recovery.

The PPE provides the medical team an opportunity to promote good health practices and fitness. This evaluation allows health care providers to give guidance and to determine the athlete's general state of health. For example, the provider can ensure that weight-class athletes (e.g., wrestlers, weightlifters) maintain healthy weights. At the same time, health team members can discuss with athletes the dangers associated with crash dieting and excessive dehydration.

The PPE enables the health team to bring immunizations up-to-date and to assess athletes for communicable diseases. The reader is referred to the Centers for Disease Control and Prevention for the most up-to-date immunization information (available at http://www.cdc.gov/vaccines/recs/default.htm). Ideally, athletes should have the opportunity to receive age-appropriate vaccinations for diphtheria, tetanus, pertussis, polio, measles, mumps, rubella, varicella, meningococcus, and influenza at their PPE visits.

The evaluation provides an opportunity for the physician and other health care team members to develop rapport with the athlete. The examiners can learn what motivates the athlete while building athlete confidence in the health care team. Every institution or team has a moral and legal obligation to ensure safety and health care if it sponsors particular programs or activities. Meeting this obligation helps to protect the organization from litigation and helps to fulfill insurance requirements.

The evaluation can be used to establish guidelines for athletes, the health care team, coaches, and administrators about health, safety, care, and issues related to performance. It also provides an opportunity to counsel the disabled athlete as to which sports or modified sports would provide suitable activity. The PPE enables a team or organization to restrict from participation anyone whose physical limitations present undue risk. Finally, the PPE may help classify and direct participants by ability.

Structuring the Preparticipation Evaluation

PPEs are structured in a variety of ways. Some participants visit a physician, often their family physician, to obtain "medical clearance" to participate in an activity. Group evaluations are more likely when a large number of athletes need to be seen and in higher level sporting activities in which injury is a bigger risk for unhealthy or unfit persons. These sports are also more likely to provide postseason examinations. Detailed evaluations may include individual stations arranged in a space-available format or a straight-line format (Figure 2-1).[12,23] In the space-available format, athletes register, then proceed from station to station until all evaluations are complete. In the straight-line format, athletes register, then proceed through each station in a predetermined order until all evaluations are complete.

Station Examples for Preparticipation Evaluation

Check-In
- Athlete medical/injury history
- Vital signs
  - Temperature
  - Blood pressure
  - Heart rate
  - Respiratory rate
  - Weight
- Visual examination
- Musculoskeletal examination
- Neurological examination
- Cardiovascular and pulmonary examination
- Additional medical examination
  - Gastrointestinal examination
  - Urogenital examination
  - Dermatological examination
  - Heat illness examination
  - Laboratory examination
- Dental examination
- Physical fitness profile

In group evaluations, each station is designed to evaluate one or more organs or a body system. Not all stations require a physician to conduct the examination. Often administrators or teachers may staff the check-in and check-out stations. The check-in station is where participants complete all legal

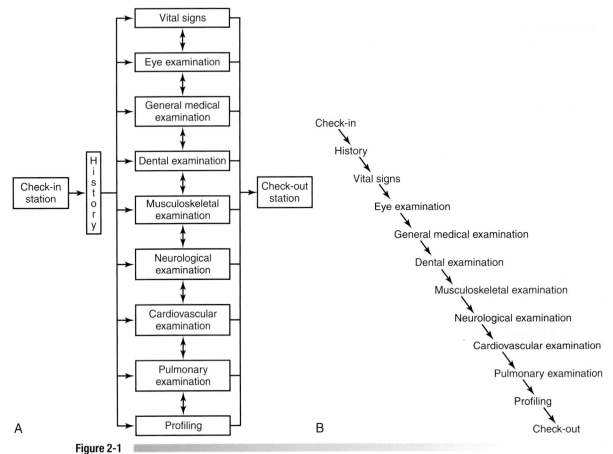

Figure 2-1
Examples of traffic patterns for preparticipation examinations. **A,** Space-available station method.
B, Straight-line station method. (From Magee DJ: *Orthopedic physical assessment,* ed 4, p 964,
Philadelphia, 2002, WB Saunders.)

requirements for the organization and are directed to the other stations. An athletic trainer, sports physical therapist, nurse, or other trained health care provider can obtain vital signs, obtain height and weight data, and perform visual screening. Likewise, a dentist can provide on-site dental screening examinations. The maturity determination and medical examinations should be performed by physicians. At the check-out station, the athlete's file should be reviewed by the team physician to ensure that the athlete has satisfactorily passed all components of the examination, or to determine if further tests or specialty consultation may be required.[12] The athlete should not be told at check-out whether he or she has passed the PPE. This decision should be delayed until the athlete has an opportunity to discuss the evaluation results and final participation decisions with the team physicians.

Preparticipation History

The past medical history plays a central role in the PPE. A complete history can usually identify 60% to 75% of the health issues affecting an athlete.[7,10,24] For young persons,

both the athlete and the parent or guardian should provide past medical history to ensure completeness. The history provides details about health problems and injuries, which enables providers to focus on the most pertinent health issues.[10] Generally, the athlete's history is initiated by asking a series of questions answerable in a "yes/no" format (Figure 2-2). Affirmative responses lead to further questions and investigations. It is important that negative answers also be checked for accuracy. Oral histories are ideal because of increased accuracy, but time may not allow for this approach. The history should include the athlete's past medical history and family history to assess for possible congenital, inherited, or injury problems. It is important that a complete and careful health history be obtained, as athletes may try to conceal past medical or injury information that may prevent participation in the desired activity.[24]

Preparticipation questions cover a wide range of health issues, and specific organ or system evaluations should be performed to corroborate and further explore positive responses. The following evaluation sections are related to specific body systems with positive answers leading to further examinations, tests, or interventions that may need

FHSAA Florida High School Athletic Association

Preparticipation Physical Evaluation (Page 1 of 2)

This completed form must be kept on file by the school. This form is valid for 365 calendar days from the date of the evaluation as written on page 2.

Part 1. Student Information (to be completed by student or parent)

Student's Name: _____ Sex: _____ Age: _____ Date of Birth: ____ / ____ / ____

School: _____ Grade in School: _____ Sport(s): _____

Home Address: _____ Home Phone: (_____) _____

Name of Parent/Guardian: _____ E-mail: _____

Person to Contact in Case of Emergency: _____

Relationship to Student: _____ Home Phone: (___) _____ Work Phone: (___) _____ Cell Phone: (___) _____

Personal/Family Physician: _____ City/State: _____ Office Phone: (___) _____

Part 2. Medical History (to be completed by student or parent). Explain "yes" answers below. Circle questions you don't know answers to.

Yes   No

1. Have you had a medical illness or injury since your last check up or sports physical? ____ ____
2. Do you have an ongoing chronic illness? ____ ____
3. Have you ever been hospitalized overnight? ____ ____
4. Have you ever had surgery? ____ ____
5. Are you currently taking any prescription or non-prescription (over-the-counter) medications or pills or using an inhaler? ____ ____
6. Have you ever taken any supplements or vitamins to help you gain or lose weight or improve your performance? ____ ____
7. Do you have any allergies (for example, to pollen, medicine, food or stinging insects)? ____ ____
8. Have you ever had a rash or hives develop during or after exercise? ____ ____
9. Have you ever passed out during or after exercise? ____ ____
10. Have you ever been dizzy during or after exercise? ____ ____
11. Have you ever had chest pain during or after exercise? ____ ____
12. Do you get tired more quickly than your friends do during exercise? ____ ____
13. Have you ever had racing of your heart or skipped heartbeats? ____ ____
14. Have you had high blood pressure or high cholesterol? ____ ____
15. Have you ever been told you have a heart murmur? ____ ____
16. Has any family member or relative died of heart problems or sudden death before age 50? ____ ____
17. Have you had a severe viral infection (for example, myocarditis or mononucleosis) within the last month? ____ ____
18. Has a physician ever denied or restricted your participation in sports for any heart problems? ____ ____
19. Do you have any current skin problems (for example, itching, rashes, acne, warts, fungus or blisters)? ____ ____
20. Have you ever had a head injury or concussion? ____ ____
21. Have you ever been knocked out, become unconscious or lost your memory? ____ ____
22. Have you ever had a seizure? ____ ____
23. Do you have frequent or severe headaches? ____ ____
24. Have you ever had numbness or tingling in your arms, hands, legs or feet? ____ ____
25. Have you ever had a stinger, burner or pinched nerve? ____ ____

Yes   No

26. Have you ever become ill from exercising in the heat? ____ ____
27. Do you cough, wheeze or have trouble breathing during or after activity? ____ ____
28. Do you have asthma? ____ ____
29. Do you have seasonal allergies that require medical treatment? ____ ____
30. Do you use any special protective or corrective equipment or devices that aren't usually used for your sport or position (for example, knee brace, special neck roll, foot orthotics, retainer on your teeth or hearing aid)? ____ ____
31. Have you had any problems with your eyes or vision? ____ ____
32. Do you wear glasses, contacts or protective eyewear? ____ ____
33. Have you ever had a sprain, strain or swelling after injury? ____ ____
34. Have you broken or fractured any bones or dislocated any joints? ____ ____
35. Have you had any other problems with pain or swelling in muscles, tendons, bones or joints? ____ ____

If yes, check appropriate blank and explain below:

___ Head	___ Elbow	___ Hip
___ Neck	___ Forearm	___ Thigh
___ Back	___ Wrist	___ Knee
___ Chest	___ Hand	___ Shin/Calf
___ Shoulder	___ Finger	___ Ankle
___ Upper Arm	___ Foot	

36. Do you want to weigh more or less than you do now? ____ ____
37. Do you lose weight regularly to meet weight requirements for your sport? ____ ____
38. Do you feel stressed out? ____ ____
39. Record the dates of your most recent immunizations (shots) for:
    Tetanus: _____ Measles: _____
    Hepatitus B: _____ Chickenpox: _____

FEMALES ONLY (optional)

40. When was your first menstrual period? _____
41. When was your most recent menstrual period? _____
42. How much time do you usually have from the start of one period to the start of another? _____
43. How many periods have you had in the last year? _____
44. What was the longest time between periods in the last year? _____

Explain "Yes" answers here: _____
_____
_____
_____

We hereby state, to the best of our knowledge, that our answers to the above questions are complete and correct. In addition to the routine medical evaluation required by s.1006.20, Florida Statutes, and FHSAA Bylaw 9.7, we understand and acknowledge that we are hereby advised that the student should undergo a cardiovascular assessment, which may include such diagnostic tests as electrocardiogram (EKG), echocardiogram (ECG) and/or cardio stress test.

Signature of Student: _____ Date: ___ / ___ / ___ Signature of Parent/Guardian: _____ Date: ___ / ___ / ___

Figure 2-2

Preparticipation physical evaluation form. (Reprinted with permission of the Florida High School Athletic Association.)

Continued

Florida High School Athletic Association

Preparticipation Physical Evaluation (Page 2 of 2)

Revised 06/09

This completed form must be kept on file by the school. This form is valid for 365 calendar days from the date of the evaluation as written on page 2.

Part 3. Physical Examination (to be completed by licensed physician, licensed osteopathic physician, licensed chiropractic physician, licensed physician assistant or certified advanced registered nurse practitioner).

Student's Name: _____   Date of Birth: ____ / ____ / ____

Height: _____   Weight: _____   % Body Fat (optional): _____   Pulse: _____   Blood Pressure: ____ / ____ (____ / ____ , ____ / ____)

Temperature: _____   Hearing: right: P _____ F _____ left: P _____ F _____

Visual Acuity: Right 20/_____   Left 20/_____   Corrected: Yes   No   Pupils: Equal _____   Unequal _____

FINDINGS	NORMAL	ABNORMAL FINDINGS	INITIALS*
MEDICAL			
1. Appearance	_____	_____	_____
2. Eyes/Ears/Nose/Throat	_____	_____	_____
3. Lymph Nodes	_____	_____	_____
4. Heart	_____	_____	_____
5. Pulses	_____	_____	_____
6. Lungs	_____	_____	_____
7. Abdomen	_____	_____	_____
8. Genitalia (males only)	_____	_____	_____
9. Skin	_____	_____	_____
MUSCULOSKELETAL			
10. Neck	_____	_____	_____
11. Back	_____	_____	_____
12. Shoulder/Arm	_____	_____	_____
13. Elbow/Forearm	_____	_____	_____
14. Wrist/Hand	_____	_____	_____
15. Hip/Thigh	_____	_____	_____
16. Knee	_____	_____	_____
17. Leg/Ankle	_____	_____	_____
18. Foot	_____	_____	_____

* – station-based examination only

ASSESSMENT OF EXAMINING PHYSICIAN/PHYSICIAN ASSISTANT/NURSE PRACTITIONER

I hereby certify that each examination listed above was performed by myself or an individual under my direct supervision with the following conclusion(s):

____ Cleared without limitation

____ Not cleared for: _____   Reason: _____

____ Cleared after completing evaluation/rehabilitation for: _____

____ Referred to _____   For: _____

Recommendations: _____

Name of Physician/Physician Assistant/Nurse Practitioner (print): _____   Date: ____ / ____ / ____

Address: _____

Signature of Physician/Physician Assistant/Nurse Practitioner: _____

ASSESSMENT OF PHYSICIAN TO WHOM REFERRED (if applicable)

I hereby certify that the examination(s) for which referred was/were performed by myself or an individual under my direct supervision with the following conclusion(s):

____ Cleared without limitation

____ Not cleared for: _____   Reason: _____

____ Cleared after completing evaluation/rehabilitation for: _____

Recommendations: _____

Name of Physician (print): _____   Date: ____ / ____ / ____

Address: _____

Signature of Physician: _____

Based on recommendations developed by the American Academy of Family Physicians, American Academy of Pediatrics, American Medical Society for Sports Medicine, American Orthopaedic Society for Sports Medicine and American Osteopathic Academy for Sports Medicine.

Figure 2-2, cont'd

to be addressed before the athlete is allowed to participate in a particular physical activity.

Physical Examination

The PPE must be thorough and applicable to the activity, exercise, or sport in which the athlete hopes to participate (see Figure 2-2 for a sample PPE form). Health care professionals should always be alert for concealment, denial, or fabrication of health problems. Depending on the particular activity, certain body sites and structures should be emphasized (e.g., ears in swimmers; upper extremities in racquet sports players; spine, knees, and ankles in football players). The reader is also referred to Chapter 17 of *Orthopedic Physical Assessment*, ed 5, for more information on athlete assessment.

The initial part of the examination establishes the athlete's baseline physiological parameters and vital signs[25] (Table 2-1). This part of the examination can be performed by any health care professional who understands the proper measurement techniques, and includes height and weight, blood pressure, heart rate, respiratory rate, temperature, visual acuity, current medication, allergies, and contact information.

Some General Questions Can be Used to Simultaneously Assess Multiple Areas[10]

- Have you ever been a patient in a hospital, emergency room, or clinic?
- Have you ever seen a physician for an injury or illness?
- Have you ever had an x-ray examination?
- Have you ever had an operation?
- Are you currently taking any medications or pills?
- Do you have any allergies (to medications, insects, food, or other things)?
- What was your last vaccination? What was the vaccination for?
- Have you ever been unable to participate in exercise or sport?
- Have you ever experienced chest pain, dyspnea, or syncope during exercise or sport?
- Have you ever had a seizure?
- Have you ever been told you have high blood pressure?
- Have you ever been told you have high cholesterol?
- Do you have trouble breathing or do you cough during or after exercise?

High blood pressure values should be rechecked at 15- to 30-minute intervals, with the athlete resting between measurements to determine if a high reading is accurate or is caused by anxiety ("white-coat syndrome"). If two consecutive blood pressure measurements are high, the athlete may be hypertensive. If the readings remain high, further investigation is needed.[12,25,26]

Visual Examination

Visual acuity is usually measured by a Snellon or common eye chart. For many sports, peripheral vision and depth perception may also be tested. Any affirmative answers on the health questionnaire or abnormalities detected require further examination. Uncorrected vision worse than 20/40 should be further evaluated.[10,20,27] A visual acuity of 20/40 means that the athlete can read at 20 feet what the average person can read at 40 feet.

Pupil size should also be evaluated before participation. Noting baseline differences in pupil diameter (anisocoria) is important in case of future head injury, which may also affect pupil size.[28]

The health care provider should be aware of eye problems that preclude participation in the chosen activity or sport. Vision in only one eye can impair depth perception, which is detrimental to performance in certain activities. Athletes with monocular vision should only participate in physical activities if they have demonstrated understanding of the dangers and are prepared to accept the risks. Such athletes should only participate in sports that have adequate eye protection. A special consent form outlining the risks and the athlete's acceptance of those risks should be completed prior to participation for such athletes.[10,29]

Lenses that are plastic, polycarbonate, or heat-treated (safety) glass should be used for athletes who wear glasses to prevent shattering during physical activity. Contact lenses should be soft, as hard lenses may shatter.

Myopia (near-sightedness) should be noted because myopic athletes have a greater risk of retinal degeneration and subsequent retinal detachment. A history of retinal detachment may cause the examiner to recommend exclusion from some contact sports. An athlete with a retinal tear should be allowed to compete in strenuous activities only if he or she has a medical letter written by a physician or specialist explaining that the athlete may participate.

Musculoskeletal Examination

The musculoskeletal examination is usually the key element of the PPE for sports. The musculoskeletal examination begins with observation of the athlete's posture to detect any significant asymmetries. Observed asymmetry plus a significant history commonly leads to a detailed evaluation of specific joints. For athletes without obvious asymmetries, the examiner should screen for abnormalities by briefly examining both upper and lower extremities, taking the joints through a full physiological range of motion (ROM). Abnormal movements demonstrating hypomobility, hypermobility, capsular patterns, weakness, abnormal movement patterns, or substitution movements should be noted. Depending on the proposed activity, the examiner may emphasize examination of specific joints.[19]

Table 2-1
Vital Sign Normal Ranges

Age Group	Respiratory Rate	Heart Rate	Diastolic Blood Pressure	Systolic Blood Pressure	Temperature	Weight (kg)	Weight (lb)
Newborn	30-50	120-160	Varies	50-70	97.7°F (36.5°C)	2-3	4.5-7
Infant (1-12 months)	20-30	80-140	Varies	70-100	98.6°F (37.0°C)*	4-10	9-22
Toddler (1-3 years)	20-30	80-130	48-80	80-110	98.6°F (37.0°C)*	10-14	22-31
Preschooler (3-5 years)	20-30	80-120	48-80	80-110	98.6°F (37.0°C)*	14-18	31-40
School Age (6-12 years)	20-30	70-110	50-90	80-120	98.6°F (37.0°C)*	20-42	41-92
Adolescent (13-17 years)	12-20	55-105	60-92	110-120	98.6°F (37.0°C)*	>50	>110
Adults (18+ years)	18-20	60-100	<85	<130	98.6°F (37.0°C)*	Varies	Depends on body size

From Magee DJ: *Orthopedic physical assessment*, ed 5, p 17, St Louis, 2007, Elsevier.
*Ranges from 97.8°F to 99.1°F (36.5°C to 37.3°C).
Remember these points:
The patient's normal range should always be taken into consideration.
Heart rate, blood pressure, and respiratory rate are expected to increase during times of fever or stress.
Respiratory rate for infants should be counted for a full 60 seconds.

Athletes presenting with joint asymmetry, weakness, or other abnormalities, or who have reported previous joint injuries should undergo a more detailed examination of the specific injured area or joint. This evaluation should assess active, passive, and resisted movements, as well as reflexes and sensation if neurological tissue is involved, and available joint play if a joint has been involved. The examiner may also palpate the joint and may consider doing functional or other special tests.

When assessing musculoskeletal health in the PPE, the examiner should consider whether the proposed activity will exacerbate an existing disease or injury, increase an existing deformity, or cause further bone or joint damage. In evaluating orthopedic and musculoskeletal problems, the examiner may, depending on the activity or sport, measure the athlete's flexibility as well as static and dynamic stability, especially if there is the potential for a problem and the problem is easily correctable. For example, spinal instability (especially of the cervical or lumbar spine) or spondylolisthesis may preclude participation in contact, collision, or impact activities. Maturation level, previous injuries, congenital problems, and growth abnormalities should be evaluated for athletes who are still growing.

Neurological Examination and Convulsive Disorders

The neurological examination is very important, especially if the athlete has suffered a concussion or other head injury or neurological injury. Such an examination is especially important prior to contact or collision activities.

When doing the neurological examination, the examiner may assess head injury status, cranial nerve integrity, sensation, and reflexes if problems are suspected. Signs or symptoms suggesting recurrent concussions or nerve palsies should prompt evaluation by a specialist and delay clearance for further activity.

For participants with convulsive disorders, the sports medicine team needs to know the frequency of episodes, whether control of the disorder has been achieved, which medications are used, activating circumstances, and whether the athlete understands the disorder, its hazards, and its predisposing factors. For example, athletes with epilepsy should be discouraged from activities such as skiing, parachuting, and climbing water sports (e.g., swimming alone, scuba diving), auto racing, or any activity in which recurrent head trauma or unexpected falls may cause serious injury (e.g., mountain climbing, working at heights) because of their inherent dangers and the potential of precipitating a convulsive event.[10] Athletes should be restricted from participation if they experience one or more seizures per week, display bizarre forms of psychomotor epilepsy, or experience prolonged postictal (period after seizures) states or states marked by abnormal behavior. It is important to know if athletes can achieve good control of their condition by using medications, not only

in everyday situations, but also in stressful situations. For example, hyperventilation may precipitate epileptic seizures, and seizures tend to occur after exercise, not during the event. It is also important to know if the extent or intensity of the participation poses a significant threat to the athlete's physical condition.

Cardiovascular Examination

Because the athlete needs to remove clothing to permit auscultation, the cardiovascular examination should be performed in a quiet, private area. The examiner should assess for subtle but important cardiac abnormalities to reduce the incidence of sudden death during sports.[13,30-36] More than 90% of sudden deaths in exercise and sports participants younger than the age of 30 involve the cardiovascular system.

If the athlete has experienced dizziness, chest pain, high blood pressure, a heart murmur, raced or skipped beats, or a positive cardiovascular family history, the examiner must consider cardiomegaly, conduction abnormalities, arrhythmias, valvular disease, coronary artery defects, and lung or related problems.[10,37] If cardiovascular problems are suspected, the examiner may order further tests (e.g., electrocardiogram, treadmill stress tests) to detect any cardiac abnormalities.

Abnormal Cardiovascular Findings

- Heart rate faster than 120 beats per minute or inappropriately elevated heart rate for a specific activity
- Arrhythmias or irregular beats
- Midsystolic clicks, indicative of a leaky valve or mitral valve prolapse
- Murmurs that are grade 3 or louder

The health care team should obtain the athlete's history and perform a physical examination for congenital heart abnormalities such as aortic coarctation (aortic stenosis), which can be detected by differences in femoral and brachial pulses. For athletes with aortic coarctation, strenuous activity is contraindicated. Athletes with Marfan syndrome (an autosomal dominant disorder affecting connective tissue) have a 90% prevalence of cardiac abnormalities. The health care team must be aware of atrial-septal defects (abnormal communications between the heart chambers), dextrocardia (heart position is left-to-right reversed within the thoracic cavity), and paroxysmal auricular tachycardia (characterized by short periods of abnormally increased heart rate). Athletes with any of these conditions are disqualified from competitive sports because of the possibility of fainting during physiological stress. The examiner must be aware of heart enlargement resulting from exercise ("athlete's heart"). This condition should not necessarily exclude athletes from participation, but should be investigated further. If any cardiac abnormalities have been surgically corrected, the athlete should be evaluated by a specialist for a decision about the safety of participating in the proposed activity.

Hypertrophic cardiomyopathy is the most common cause of sudden death in athletes, followed by aortic rupture associated with Marfan syndrome, congenital coronary artery anomalies, and atherosclerotic coronary artery disease.[10,38] If any of these conditions are present, strenuous activity should be avoided.

Other cardiovascular problems include thromboembolic disease, heart rate abnormalities, valvular problems such as mitral insufficiency or mitral valve prolapse, and hypertension. A systolic pressure of 140 mm Hg on repeat measurement is considered abnormal.[32] Athletes with labile hypertension (unstable blood pressure characterized by rapid changes) or organic hypertension caused by structural problems should undergo further evaluation. Athletes with hypertension should be assessed for coronary artery disease risk factors. Mild hypertension should not disqualify athletes from exercise or sports participation, but periodic re-evaluation is indicated.[10]

If cardiovascular or cardiopulmonary disease is suspected, an exercise stress test is often recommended.[20] Figure 2-3 provides a flow chart of considerations before conducting such a test. Of those with heart disease, 20% to 35% will have normal stress tests, so it is important to remember that any stress test is only valid to the load at which the heart has been stressed during the test. For runners 40 years and older, 45% have irregular electrocardiogram findings. Furthermore, different types of activity (e.g., static versus dynamic) create different stresses on the heart. Table 2-2 outlines a sports classification based on peak dynamic and static stresses encountered during sports competition.[39]

Pulmonary Examination

The pulmonary examination is often performed concurrently with the cardiovascular examination in a quiet area to determine if the athlete has had long periods of intermittent coughing, shortness of breath, or wheezing during or after activity, exercise, or sport. The examiner should auscultate the lungs to check for clear breath sounds and should observe chest motion for symmetric diaphragmatic excursion.[10] All pulmonary medications should be noted. The ears, nose, and mouth may also be examined at this station. Abnormalities may be further assessed by lung function tests or chest x-ray examination.[40] Respiratory problems such as tuberculosis, uncontrolled asthma, exertional asthma, exercise-induced bronchospasm, pulmonary insufficiency from a collapsed lung, or bronchial asthma deserve special attention and follow-up discussion and evaluation.[20,41,42]

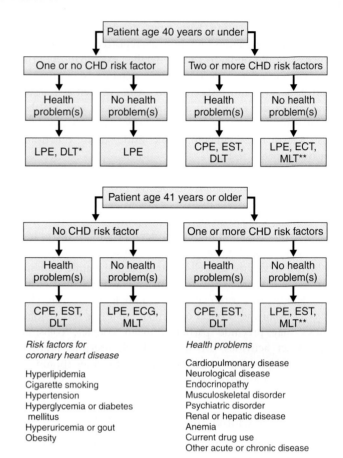

Risk factors for coronary heart disease

Hyperlipidemia
Cigarette smoking
Hypertension
Hyperglycemia or diabetes mellitus
Hyperuricemia or gout
Obesity

Health problems

Cardiopulmonary disease
Neurological disease
Endocrinopathy
Musculoskeletal disorder
Psychiatric disorder
Renal or hepatic disease
Anemia
Current drug use
Other acute or chronic disease

* Exercise stress testing is recommended if patient has cardiopulmonary disease.

** Diagnostic laboratory testing is indicated if CDH risk factors include hyperlipidemia, hyperglycemia, or hyperuricemia.

Figure 2-3

Pre-exercise evaluation flow sheet.
CDH, Coronary heart disease; *CPE,* comprehensive physical examination; *DLT,* diagnostic laboratory testing; *ECG,* resting electrocardiogram; *EST,* exercise stress test; *LPE,* limited physical examination; *MLT,* minimal laboratory testing. (Adapted with permission from Taylor RB, Copyright 1983, Consultants, UBM Medica. All rights reserved.)

Urogenital Examination

The urogenital examination is modified to fit the needs of the male and female athlete. In both males and females, the examiner should determine if the athlete has any problems with his or her kidneys or genitourinary organs, or has been diagnosed as having sugar, albumin, or blood in his or her urine.

The medical team must check for hernias, kidney problems, albuminuria (excessive protein in the urine), and sexually transmitted infections.[43] Athletes with one kidney should be warned of the danger of contact sports, especially if the kidney is abnormally positioned or diseased.[28]

Females may be asked about their menstrual history (e.g., When did it begin? When was the last period?

Table 2-2

Classification of Sports Based on Peak Dynamic and Static Components During Competition

	Low Dynamic	Moderate Dynamic	High Dynamic
Low static	Billiards Bowling Cricket Curling Golf Riflery	Baseball Softball Table tennis Tennis (doubles) Volleyball	Badminton Cross-country skiing (classic technique) Field hockey* Orienteering Race walking Racquetball Running (long-distance) Soccer* Squash Tennis (singles)
Moderate static	Archery Auto racing*† Diving*† Equestrian*† Motorcycling*†	Fencing Field events (jumping) Figure skating* Football (American) Rodeo*† Rugby* Running (sprint) Surfing*† Synchronized swimming†	Basketball* Ice hockey* Cross-country skiing (skating technique) Football (Australian rules)* Lacrosse* Running (middle-distance) Swimming Team handball
High static	Bobsledding*† Field events (throwing) Gymnastics*† Karate/Judo* Luge*† Sailing Rock climbing*† Water skiing*† Weight lifting*† Wind surfing*†	Body building *† Downhill*† Wrestling*	Boxing* Canoeing/kayaking Cycling*† Decathlon Rowing Speed skating

From Mitchell JH, Haskell WL, Raven PB: Classification of sports, *Med Sci Sports Exerc* 26:S242-S245, 1994.
*Danger of bodily collision.
†Increased risk if syncope occurs.

Are there any abnormalities?) or about any gynecological problems. For females, it is important to assess for regular menstruation, because exercise amenorrhea is a significant problem that is associated with low bone density and osteoporosis.[20,44]

For males, the examiner must ask about a history of undescended or atrophied testes or testicular torsion. Males may be given a genital examination to check for abnormalities, hernias, or absence of a testicle.[10]

A urinalysis should be performed if diabetes or kidney disease is suspected. These conditions do not normally preclude activity, exercise, or sport, and may be amenable to treatment. The athlete and sponsoring organization must be made aware of potential dangers caused by these conditions. Dehydration, athletic pseudonephritis (false kidney inflammation), hemoglobinuria (abnormal presence of hemoglobin in the urine), nephroptosis (dropped kidney), and hematuria (abnormal presence of blood in urine) are possible problems of the urogenital system.

Gastrointestinal Examination

The gastrointestinal questions and examination should address digestion, eating habits, and nutrition.[45] Questions are related to eating regularly and having a well-balanced diet; what food groups the athlete does not eat; whether the athlete has been on a diet or views himself or herself as too thin, too fat, or just right; and about weight control, heart burn, and indigestion.

The examiner should palpate the abdomen for masses or organomegaly (enlarged organs).[12] The health care team must ensure that there is no liver or spleen enlargement, especially for contact-sports participants.

For esthetic or weight-conscious sports (e.g., gymnastics, ballet, synchronized swimming, wrestling), the examiner should check the athletes' nutritional status, especially if there is a suspicion of an eating disorder such as anorexia or bulimia.[46] This is best evaluated by asking the athlete to record his or her food intake for at least 3 days and ask a nutritionist to determine if the calculated dietary intake is appropriate for the athlete's activity level (see Chapters 3 and 4 for more information). This also provides an opportunity to find out about any banned or unsafe substances the athletes may be taking.

Dermatological Examination

The PPE is a good opportunity to identify skin conditions that may be amenable to treatment. Questions about acne, rashes, or itching, especially in areas covered by clothes, equipment, or footwear, are appropriate and deal with skin conditions that are usually easily treated. The examiner must ensure that the athlete's skin problems are addressed, because many are contagious. Some common contagious skin problems include bacteria (e.g., boils, impetigo), fungus (e.g., athlete's foot), and viruses (e.g., herpes simplex, herpes gladiatorum, warts).

Examination for Heat Disorders

Examination for prior history of heat disorders should be included if the activity, exercise, or sport will occur in an area with a high temperature, high humidity, or some combination of both. The examiner should determine if the athlete has ever suffered from a heat disorder or muscle cramps; participated in an activity, exercise, or sport in a high-temperature, high-humidity environment; ever passed out or become dizzy in the heat; or is on any medications or drinks large quantities of caffeinated beverages.

Use of antihistamines or excessive caffeine, as well as dehydration (i.e., lack of fluids or electrolytes), can increase the risk of heat disorders. If an athlete has a history of heat-related disorders, the condition should be thoroughly investigated because of the life-threatening potential of these disorders.

General Medical Problems

In addition to the problems previously described, there are general systemic medical problems that deserve evaluation by the health care provider such as systemic diseases, (e.g., diabetes), progressive diseases (e.g., muscular dystrophy, multiple sclerosis, or cancer).

The examiner should be concerned about acute infections, malignancies, and progressive diseases such as multiple sclerosis. Diabetes should not exclude someone from participation, but the examiner must assess the athlete's disease status and control with medications. It must be determined whether the extent or intensity of the activity poses a significant threat to the athlete's physical condition.[47] Acute illnesses tend to be self-limited and usually require that the athlete be temporarily removed from participation, often to protect other participants.[10] Febrile illness often causes dehydration, which can predispose to heat disorders.

Examples of General Medical Problems Requiring Awareness of the Sports Medicine Team

- Athletes with systemic disease (e.g., diabetes)
- Female athlete triad (anorexia or bulimia, amenorrhea, osteoporosis)
- Athletes with progressive disease (e.g., muscular dystrophy, multiple sclerosis)
- Cancer
- Human immunodeficiency virus, acquired immune deficiency syndrome

---

Dental Examination

The dental examination is commonly performed by a dentist. The dentist should determine when the athlete last saw a dentist, whether the athlete has had problems with his or her teeth or gums; whether the athlete has had any teeth knocked out, damaged, or extracted; whether the athlete wears a mouthguard, smokes, or chews tobacco; or whether the athlete has ever had an injury to his or her face or jaw.[27]

When performing the dental examination, the dentist should note the number of teeth the athlete has. This is important because of the potential for liability if teeth are avulsed (knocked out). It also provides an opportunity to fit mouthguards and check dental appliances to ensure good condition.

Examples of Dental Problems Requiring Awareness of the Sports Medicine Team

- Problems with teeth or gums
- History of teeth knocked out, damaged, or extracted
- History of smoking or chewing tobacco
- Previous injury to face or jaw

Laboratory Tests

Laboratory tests are not usually included in the PPE. However, the physician may request diagnostic laboratory tests for suspected problems. For example, if heart disease is suspected or an older athlete is being evaluated, the examiner may order serum cholesterol, triglyceride, or high-density lipoprotein levels.

The incidence of iron deficiency anemia in menstruating female athletes can be as high as 15%. Plasma ferritin may be used to measure iron stores. In males, anemia can occur during growth spurts, with inadequate diet, or with peptic ulcer disease. Hemoglobin is checked if sickle cell anemia is suspected (most commonly in black athletes). Prepubertal hemoglobin should be approximately 11.5 g/dL, and postpubertal values should be at least 14.5 g/dL for males and 12 g/dL for females.

For some sports and some high levels of competition, drug screening may be required; the PPE is an appropriate time for such screening.

Should the Individual be Allowed to Participate?

For any PPE, the athlete's physician should be the final arbitrator. The physician can decide that (1) participation is not allowed; (2) the athlete failed with conditions (i.e., if the conditions are corrected, the decision will be reconsidered); (3) limited participation (in specific sports or activities) is allowed; (4) the decision or recommendation is not possible until additional tests or rehabilitation are completed; or (5) full, unlimited participation is allowed.[13,48] When providing an opinion about participation, health care professionals must realize that almost everyone is suited to some activity, exercise, or sport, and that each person should be matched as nearly as possible to activities appropriate to the athlete's ability, physical fitness, and physical and emotional maturity.

Any recommendations about participation should be based on accurate diagnoses, knowledge of disease processes (Table 2-3), knowledge of the sport, knowledge of the athlete's physical needs, and knowledge about the activity or sport. Sports may be divided in several ways. Level of contact is one way in which sports are divided being divided into contact/collision, limited contact, and noncontact sports (see Box 2-1). A second method is based on level of intensity—high dynamic/high static, high dynamic/low static, low dynamic/high static demands (see Table 2-2). These factors must always be considered when clearing an athlete for competition in a specific sport. Although participation standards are provided, the health care team must make decisions based on an athlete's unique health and safety issues. The physician should document recommendations about the athlete's participation for the athlete's permanent file on the PPE form.

Any athlete with a solitary paired organ, such as an eye, kidney, or testicle, should not participate in contact sports, especially if the organ is abnormal. Children should be encouraged to participate in noncontact sports. High-caliber and older athletes should better understand the risks and will be able to make their own informed decisions after discussions with the health care team.

Criteria for Passing or Failing Preparticipation Evaluation[13,49]

Passed (91%-95% of participants)
- Unconditional
- No reservations
- Cleared for all sports and all levels of exertion or cleared for participation in a specific sport
- No pre-existing or current medical problems
- No contraindications for collision or contact sports

Passed with Conditions
- Has a medical problem needing follow-up
- Can participate in sports at present
- Follow-up must be prior to sports activities
- Athlete may need special treatment on occasion

Passed with Reservations
- No collision sports (hockey, rugby, lacrosse)
- No contact sports (football, basketball, wrestling)

Deferred Clearance
- Further investigation is needed (e.g., dizziness with exercise, asthma history, systolic blood pressure elevation, heart murmur)

Failed with Reservations
- Not cleared for *requested* sport (other sports could be considered)
- Collision not permitted, contact to be limited
- Contact not permitted, noncontact sports allowed

Failed with Conditions
- Can be reconsidered when medical problem is addressed

Failed (< 1% of Participants)
- May prohibit athlete's participation in specific sport
- May be unconditional
- Cannot be cleared for any sport or any level of competition

---

PART B: PHYSICAL FITNESS PROFILING

Introduction

The PPE provides critical information regarding the medical readiness of the athlete; however, it provides little data describing the athlete's ability to successfully perform his or her sport. Therefore, after the sports medicine staff has completed the PPE, they should conduct a PFP of each athlete. A PFP involves developing a battery of physical tests specific to the athlete's sport, administering the test battery to the athlete, and interpreting the resulting data. The interpretation depends on the primary purposes for which the data were collected (discussed in the following text).

To successfully execute the PFP, the sports medicine team should rely on the expertise of the strength and conditioning coordinator. The strength and conditioning coordinator is the member of the sports medicine team who is responsible for overseeing the athlete's physical development with the goal of maximizing the athlete's or team's success during

Table 2-3

Medical Conditions and Sports Participation

Condition	Explanation	Participation
Atlantoaxial instability (instability of the joint between cervical vertebrae 1 and 2)	The athlete needs evaluation to assess the risk of spinal cord injury during sports participation.	Qualified yes
Bleeding disorder	The athlete needs an evaluation.	Qualified yes
Carditis (inflammation of the heart)	Carditis may result in sudden death with exertion.	No
Hypertension (high BP)	Those athletes with significant essential (unexplained) hypertension should avoid weight lifting and power lifting, body building, and strength training. Those with secondary hypertension (hypertension caused by a previously identified disease) or severe essential hypertension need evaluation.*	Qualified yes
Congenital heart disease (structural heart defects present at birth)	Those athletes with mild forms of congenital heart disease may participate fully. Those with moderate or severe forms and those who have undergone surgery need evaluation.†	Qualified yes
Dysrhythmia (irregular heart rhythm)	The athlete needs evaluation because some types of cardiac dysrhythmia require therapy, make certain sports dangerous, or both.	Qualified yes
Mitral valve prolapse (abnormal heart valve)	Those athletes with symptoms (chest pain, symptoms of possible dysrhythmia) or evidence of mitral regurgitation (leaking) on physical examination need evaluation. All others may participate fully.	Qualified yes
Heart murmur	If the murmur is innocent (i.e., it does not indicate heart disease), full participation is permitted. Otherwise, the athlete needs an evaluation (see "Congenital heart disease" and "Mitral valve prolapse").	Qualified yes
Cerebral palsy	The athlete needs an evaluation.	Qualified yes
Diabetes mellitus	If the diabetes is well controlled, the athlete can play in all sports with proper attention to diet, hydration, and insulin therapy. Particular attention is needed for activities that last 30 minutes or more.	Yes
Diarrhea	Unless the disease is mild, no participation is permitted because diarrhea may increase the risk of dehydration and heat illness. (See "Fever.")	Qualified no
Anorexia nervosa, bulimia nervosa	Patients need both medical and psychiatric assessments before sports participation.	Qualified yes
Functionally one-eyed athlete, loss of an eye, detached retina, previous eye surgery, or serious eye injury	A functionally one-eyed athlete has a BCVA of better than 20/40 in the worse eye. These athletes could experience a significant disability if the better eye is seriously injured, as can those athletes who have lost an eye. Athletes who have previously undergone eye surgery or who have had a serious eye injury may be at increased risk of injury because of weakened eye tissue. Use of eye guards approved by ASTM International and other protective equipment may allow the athlete to participate in most sports, but this approach must be judged on an individual basis.	Qualified yes
Fever	Fever can increase cardiopulmonary effort, reduce maximum exercise capacity, make heat illness more likely, and increase orthostatic hypotension during exercise. In rare cases, fever may accompany myocarditis or other infections that may make exercise dangerous.	No
Heat illness, history of	Because of the increased likelihood of the recurrence of heat illness, the athlete needs an individual assessment to determine the presence of predisposing conditions and to arrange a prevention strategy.	Qualified yes

From American Academy of Pediatrics Committee on Sports Medicine and Fitness: Medical conditions affecting sports participation, *Pediatrics* 94:757–760, 1994.

ASTM, American Society for Testing and Materials; *BCVA,* best-corrected visual acuity; *BP,* blood pressure; *HIV,* human immunodeficiency virus.
*National Heart, Lung, Blood Institute: Report of the 2nd task force on blood pressure control in children — 1987, *Pediatrics* 79:1-25, 1987.
†16th Bethesda Conference: Cardiovascular abnormalities in the athlete: recommendations regarding eligibility for competition, *J Am Coll Cardiol* 6:1189-1190, 1985.

Continued

Table 2-3
Medical Conditions and Sports Participation—cont'd

Condition	Explanation	Participation
HIV infection‡	Because of the apparent minimal risk to others, all sports may be played, as allowed by the patient's state of health. In all athletes, skin lesions should be properly covered, and athletic personnel should use universal precautions when handling blood or body fluids with the presence of visible blood.	Yes
Kidney, absence of one	The athlete with one kidney needs individual assessment for contact/collision and limited contact sports.	Qualified yes
Liver, enlarged	If the liver is acutely enlarged, athletic participation should be avoided because of a risk of rupture. If the liver is chronically enlarged, individual assessment is needed before contact/collision or limited contact sports are played.	Qualified yes
Malignancy	The athlete needs an individual assessment.	Qualified yes
Musculoskeletal disorders	The athlete needs an individual assessment.	Qualified yes
History of serious head or spine trauma, severe or repeated concussions, or craniotomy	The athlete needs an individual assessment for participation in contact/collision or limited contact sports and also for noncontact sports if deficits in judgment or cognitions are present. Recent research supports a conservative approach to the management of concussions.	Qualified yes
Convulsive disorder, well controlled	The risk of convulsions during sports participation is minimal.	Yes
Convulsive disorder, poorly controlled	The athlete needs an individual assessment before participation in contact/collision or limited contact sports. Because a convulsion may pose a risk to the athlete or to others, the following noncontact sports should be avoided: archery, riflery, swimming, weight lifting or power lifting, strength training, and sports involving heights.	Qualified yes
Obesity	Because of the risk of heat illness, obese persons need careful acclimatization and hydration.	Qualified yes
Organ transplant recipient	The athlete needs an individual assessment.	Qualified yes
Ovary, absence of one	The risk of severe injury to the remaining ovary is minimal.	Yes
Pulmonary compromise, including cystic fibrosis	The athlete needs an individual assessment, but generally all sports may be played if oxygenation remains satisfactory during a graded exercise test. Patients with cystic fibrosis need acclimatization and good hydration to reduce the risk of heat illness.	Qualified no
Asthma	With proper medication and education, only athletes with the most severe asthma need to modify their participation.	Yes
Acute upper respiratory infection	Upper respiratory obstruction may affect pulmonary function. Athletes, with the exception of those with mild disease, need an individual assessment. (See "Fever.")	Qualified yes
Sickle cell disease	The athlete needs an individual assessment. In general, if the status of the illness permits, the athlete may play all sports except high-exertion, contact/collision sports. Overheating, dehydration, and chilling must be avoided.	Qualified yes

‡American Academy of Pediatrics Committee on Sports Medicine Fitness: Human immunodeficiency virus (acquired immunodeficiency syndrome [AIDS] virus) in the athletic setting, *Pediatrics* 88:640-641, 1991.

Note: This table is designed to be understood by medical and nonmedical personnel. In the Explanation column, a notation that the athlete needs an evaluation means that a physician with appropriate knowledge and experience should determine whether an athlete with the listed medical condition can safely participate in a given sport. Unless otherwise noted, these evaluations are generally recommended because of variations in the severity of disease and in the risk of injury in specific sports.   *Continued*

Table 2-3
Medical Conditions and Sports Participation—cont'd

Condition	Explanation	Participation
Sickle cell trait	Individuals with the sickle cell trait (AS) are unlikely to have an increased risk of sudden death or other medical problems during athletic participation in most conditions. Exceptions include the most extreme conditions of heat; humidity; and, possibly, increased altitude. Like all athletes, those with the sickle cell trait should be carefully conditioned, acclimatized, and hydrated to reduce any possible risk.	Yes
Skin boils, herpes simplex, impetigo, scabies, molluscum contagiosum	During the periods in which the patient is contagious, participation in gymnastics with mats, martial arts, wrestling, or other contact/collision or limited-contact sports is not allowed. Herpes simplex virus is probably not transmitted via mats.	Qualified yes
Spleen, enlarged	Patients with an acutely enlarged spleen should avoid all sports because of the risk of rupture. Those with chronically enlarged spleens need an individual assessment before playing contact/collision or limited-contact sports.	Qualified yes
Testicle, absent or undescended	Athletes in certain sports may require a protective cup.	Yes

competition. His or her specific academic training, professional experience, and certification (e.g., National Strength and Conditioning Association Certified Strength and Conditioning Specialist) makes the strength and conditioning coordinator unique from other members of the sports medicine staff. Therefore, the strength and conditioning coordinator is extremely valuable in designing, administering, and interpreting the PFP test battery.

Clinical Point

A physical fitness profile involves a battery of physical tests that are:
- Specific to an athlete's sport and position
- Designed to determine whether the athlete has the necessary physical and physiological attributes to compete at the desired level
- Designed to establish a baseline and screen for the athlete in case of injury
- Designed to prevent and treat injury or correct poor mechanics
- Designed to predict performance

Needs Analysis

The initial step in designing the PFP is performing a needs analysis. As the name implies, the purpose of the needs analysis is to assess the physical requirements of the sport, and then use this information to design an appropriate PFP test battery. A successful needs analysis requires (1) studying the athlete's games and practices (either live or via video) to identify the physical and physiological needs of the sport, (2) consulting with the team coaching staff to identify the player's or team's strengths and weaknesses, (3) consulting with the sports medicine staff to obtain historical information to identify common sites of injury, and (4) searching the literature for information relevant to the sport. If no direct evidence exists, then the sports medicine staff should consider directly measuring physiological and mechanical demands of the sport and publishing this information. A thorough needs analysis addresses the following questions:

What are the physical and physiological needs of the sport? Each sport requires different physical attributes. The most common characteristics required by a sport are strength, power, speed, acceleration, anaerobic capacity, aerobic capacity, agility, and flexibility. Some sports (e.g., cross-country, shot put) require only one or two physical attributes for success. However, most sports (particularly team sports) require numerous physical attributes. For instance, soccer requires speed to out-run opponents, anaerobic capacity to perform repeated sprints, aerobic endurance to maintain performance throughout the entire match, agility to out-maneuver and successfully defend opponents, strength to hold off opponents and maintain position, and flexibility to kick at various angles and trajectories. To complicate matters, some team sports involve specialized position players whose physical attributes are unique from other team members.[50,51] For instance, soccer goalkeepers depend heavily on explosive power and reaction time for success, yet require relatively little aerobic endurance compared with their teammates. These factors require that the PFP use a battery of tests, as opposed to a single test, to adequately profile the athletes.

Which specific movement patterns are most important for the sport? The PFP battery should consist of tests that are specific to the movement patterns used in the sport. For instance, it has already been stated that a soccer player needs strength and speed to be successful. This does not imply, however, that the test battery developed for soccer players should be the same as the test battery used for football defensive linemen, who also require strength and speed. Defensive linemen require much more upper-body strength and their speed requirements are typically more intermittent and for shorter distances (approximately 5 to 10 yards [4.5-9.1 meters]) compared with soccer players.

What are the common sites of injury for the sport and population? Each sport (e.g., ice hockey, cross-country) and certain populations (e.g., older athletes, women) poses unique injury predispositions. For instance, epidemiological evidence indicates that poor hamstring-to-quadriceps strength ratio may predict noncontact anterior cruciate ligament (ACL) injuries in female athletes.[52] However, this relationship does not necessarily exist in male athletes within similar sports. Therefore, isokinetic testing of knee extension and flexion strength is indicated in female athletes, but might be unnecessary in male athletes participating in similar sports. It is imperative the sports medicine staff consistently read and interpret emerging literature to develop a PFP test battery (and subsequent interventions) that will prevent future injury.

Clinical Point

A physical fitness profile must take into account:
- The physical attributes needed to perform the sport
- The level at which the sport will be played
- The attributes needed to play different positions
- The movement patterns necessary for the sport
- The sport's unique injury patterns
- Muscle actions required for the sport
- The kinetics of the sport

What are the common muscle actions and kinetics of the sport? Each sport requires a unique combination of muscle actions (i.e., concentric, eccentric, and isometric) and kinetics. Downhill or mogul skiing, for example, are sports that require high eccentric and isometric strength.[53,54] Therefore, it is important to incorporate tests that specifically address the eccentric and isometric strength of these athletes to determine their physical readiness for sport.

In contrast, there are few eccentric contractions of the quadriceps in the sport of road cycling. Therefore, tests of eccentric strength in road cyclists would be unnecessary, and would provide irrelevant data.

In addition to the muscle actions, the kinetics of the sport should be considered to provide a sport-specific testing battery. Most sports are played on a field, court, or track that requires an athlete to move his or her body mass or opponent's body mass against gravity. Some sports require an athlete to move a projectile (e.g., discus, shot-put, softball) against gravity. In each of these cases, mass is constant but force varies depending on the acceleration of the mass. The kinetics of these movements are closely simulated using *dynamic constant external resistance* (DCER) testing (i.e., free weights). Swimming is an example of a sport in which the kinetics are not replicated using DCER testing. The resistance encountered in the sport of swimming is predominantly fluid resistance. Therefore, a test more specific to the sport of swimming would incorporate hydraulic resistance testing.

The Importance of a Physical Fitness Profile

The initial profiling session provides critical data that benefits the athlete, sports medicine staff, and strength and conditioning coordinator (Box 2-2). PFP data can be used to establish baseline measures useful in tracking changes in the physical performance of the athlete over time. Comparing these data with results from subsequent tests allows for objective evaluation of the training program. If insufficiencies are identified, then the strength and conditioning coordinator can adjust the training program accordingly.

The PFP also provides baseline data from which initial training loads can be derived. For instance, one-repetition maximum (1-RM) strength tests are commonly used in PFP batteries. Strength and conditioning coaches can use this information to prescribe resistance training loads to induce specific physiological adaptations (e.g., by prescribing squats using loads that are a percentage of 1-RM).

Baseline PFP can also be used for comparative analysis during rehabilitation from injury. An often-used method of assessing an athlete's ability to return to sport after injury is to compare an injured limb with the uninjured limb.[55]

Box 2-2 Select Benefits of Physical Fitness Profiling to the Athlete, Sports Medicine Staff, and Strength and Conditioning Coordinator

Athlete	Sports Medicine Staff	Strength and Conditioning Coordinator
Benchmark with which to set goals	Identify and screen for injuries	Screen for injurious technique during exercise
Data can be compared with team or national norms	Baseline data to describe general physical readiness	Predict success in sport
Gauge of success in training	In case of future injury, data serves as benchmark to determine full recovery	Baseline data for daily exercise prescription
		Monitor effectiveness of training program

Isokinetic knee extension and flexion strength is used by many physicians as a test to determine the physical readiness of an athlete to return to activity after an ACL surgery. Typically, when the strength of the involved limb reaches 75% to 85% of the uninvolved limb, then the athlete is declared ready to return to running activity.[55] However, the inherent flaw in this methodology is that it is possible that the involved limb was significantly stronger or weaker than the uninvolved limb prior to the injury. If baseline data are collected on the athlete prior to injury, the sports medicine staff can quantitatively substantiate "full recovery" in response to rehabilitation.

PFP testing can serve to reveal incompletely rehabilitated injuries that athletes may not have disclosed during the PPE.[56,57] Initial profiling may illuminate muscular asymmetries that increase the risk for injury. As mentioned previously, female athletes often have poor knee flexion strength relative to knee extension strength, which increases the risk for noncontact ACL injuries.[52] As such, in sports with female participants in which there are high numbers of ACL injuries, it is sensible to perform isokinetic knee extension and flexion tests to identify at-risk athletes. Corrective exercise programs can then be implemented to reduce the asymmetries and subsequently reduce the risk of ACL injury. In other sports, asymmetrical flexibility in joints may increase the risk for injury. In baseball pitchers, deficits in internal rotation range of motion of the shoulder (i.e., glenohumeral internal rotational deficit) may indicate capsular changes that predispose the throwing athlete to glenohumeral joint injuries.[58,59] In such cases, specific programs could be implemented to correct range-of-motion imbalances and mitigate these risks.

In addition to screening for asymmetrical muscle strength and flexibility, the initial testing session may be used to screen for injurious technique during key athletic movements. If foundational sport movements (e.g., running, jumping) are performed with poor mechanics, the athlete may be at risk for acute or chronic injuries. Female athletes exhibit different biomechanics compared with males when performing foundational sports skills such as running, jumping, landing, and cutting.[60-67] These unique biomechanics increase valgus stress on the knee joint, contributing to a greater number of noncontact ACL injuries in female athletes. However, if the "at-risk" athletes are identified and specific mechanical training is implemented, the risk of ACL injuries is dramatically reduced.[68]

Finally, the initial testing or profiling session may be used to predict performance. Normative data exist for many standard tests. Therefore, the athlete's scores can be compared against national or international norms for an age group.

Perhaps the most renowned PFP session occurs at the National Football League (NFL) "combine" each April in Indianapolis, Indiana. At the combine, athletes compete in a series of athletic tests specific to the game of football. The data are made available to NFL scouts and they are used to make draft decisions. Sierer and colleagues studied the NFL combine performance scores from 2004 and 2005, comparing the scores of drafted and undrafted players.[69] Furthermore, they divided the players into skill (i.e., wide receivers, running backs, strong safeties, and free safeties), big skill players (i.e., full backs, tight ends, linebackers, and defensive ends), and lineman (i.e., offensive guards, offensive tackles, and defensive tackles). The investigators found that height, body mass, and broad jump did not predict draft status within any of the player categories. Time in the 40-yard sprint, vertical jump, pro-agility drill, and three-cone drill were significantly different in drafted and undrafted skill players. Drafted big skill players had faster 40-yard sprint times and three-cone drills compared with undrafted players. Finally, drafted linemen had faster three-cone drills and 40-yard sprint times, and were able to bench press 225 pounds more times than undrafted linemen. These data indicate that the predictive ability of the combine tests differs across player groups and some of the tests have limited or no predictive ability of draft status. The data also suggest that not all PFP tests are suitable for every athlete. When considering test inclusions and exclusions, data such as these can be used to select appropriate tests for the individual athlete.

The ultimate goal of PFP testing is to actually predict playing ability based on the score of a test. This is complicated given the difficulty of quantifying "playing ability" of sports that are skill-intensive. Some investigators have assessed the predictive ability of a test by comparing starters and nonstarters within a given sport.[70,71] Black and Roundy compiled human performance data from 44 Division I collegiate football strength and conditioning programs.[72] Using biserial correlation coefficients, they compared the scores of starter versus nonstarter football players. Their analysis indicated that body mass, 1-RM back squat and bench press, vertical jump, and 40-yard sprint speed significantly predicted playing status. However, the results differed greatly between positions, suggesting that there are dissimilar qualities needed to play different positions in football. Schmidt also compared the physiological characteristics of starters and nonstarters in football. Using a single Division III collegiate football team (78 players), he demonstrated that the predictive ability of a test differed by playing position.[73] However, his data suggest that seated medicine ball throw and the 1-RM bench press and leg press were the best predictors of playing status. Finally, Fry and Kraemer compared the physical performance of 30 collegiate football programs.[74] They surveyed 10 strength and conditioning programs from Divisions I, II, and III (30 total programs) and compared performance scores between positions. It was determined that 1-RM power clean and bench press, 40-yard sprint, and vertical jump were good predictors of playing level. However, back squat was not a good predictor of playing level.

Sports that are less skill- or strategy-intensive are easier to predict using PFP. Using 20 marathon runners and 23 ultramarathon runners, Noakes and colleagues studied the predictive ability of laboratory maximal aerobic capacity (i.e., maximum oxygen consumption [VO_2 max]) treadmill tests on running distance times in distances from 10 to 90 km (6.2 to 56 miles).[75] They also used shorter distance times to predict long distance times. They found that race time at 10 km (6.2 miles) and 21.1 km (13.1 miles) was the greatest predictor of 42.2 km (26.2 miles) and 90 km (56 miles) run time. However, peak treadmill running velocity, lactate threshold, and percent of VO_2 max at 16 km per hour (9.9 mph) were also highly predictive of marathon and ultramarathon run time ($r > 0.80$). These data suggest the closer the underlying construct is to the actual sport, the better the predictive ability of a test. It also illuminates a potential difficulty of predicting playing ability in more skill-intensive sports (e.g., soccer): few tests actually simulate the skills needed in sport.

> **Clinical Point**
>
> General physical fitness profiles more accurately predict performance in skill- or strategy-intensive sports.

Although PFP has predictive ability for many athletes in various sports, there are always athletes who perform poorly on tests yet are world-class performers in their sport. Therefore, results should be interpreted with caution. PFP testing results should be integrated with other sources of information (e.g., on-field or court performance) to ultimately evaluate the potential success of the athlete.

Administering the Physical Fitness Profile

Unlike many of the screening tools used to assess the medical readiness of the athlete, the PFP has some inherent dangers. Because the sports medicine staff is interested in testing the peak abilities of the athlete, it is possible that injury could occur with such testing. It may be necessary to develop and administer an activity questionnaire to determine the training experience of the athlete. For instance, an athlete who is performing his or her first 1-RM test for an exercise may score low simply because he or she lacks familiarization with the test.[76] In addition, he or she may be at greater risk for injury because of poor technique. Therefore, test familiarization is warranted for athletes who are performing a test for the first time.

> **Testing Safety and Data Quality Considerations for Physical Fitness Profiling**
>
> - Is the environment safe for testing?
> - Is the test safe, or does it place the athlete in any unnecessary danger?
> - Is the athlete familiar with the testing procedures (learning effect)?
> - Is there an adequate number of test operators to ensure the safety of the athlete?
> - Is there sufficient testing time to provide adequate rest between tests?
> - What is the current training status of the athlete (e.g., fatigue)?

Test Classifications

Tests are usually classified as either clinical, laboratory, or field tests. Choosing appropriate tests depends on the qualifications and skills of the rater, the equipment available, and the logistics of testing. Clinical tests (described in the section on PPEs) are often used for medical screening and are outside the realm of the strength and conditioning coordinator, unless he or she also possesses appropriate licensure.

> **Clinical Point**
>
> Physical fitness profiling tests may be classed as:
> - Clinical
> - Laboratory
> - Field tests

Laboratory tests are another category that may be used in the PFP. Generally, these tests are performed in laboratory settings under carefully controlled conditions. The advantages of these tests are that they can precisely quantify the underlying constructs of human performance. For example, aerobic capacity is quantified in the laboratory by measuring oxygen consumption in a maximal exercise condition (VO_2 max test). However, the limitations associated with laboratory tests are that they typically require highly trained professionals, expensive equipment, and substantial time, and in some cases do not necessarily translate to real-world competitive environments. These restrictions often make laboratory tests impractical if attempting to assess large groups of athletes (e.g., a football team). However, when working with a manageable number of athletes, the benefits of laboratory testing might outweigh the costs.

Field tests are normally performed outside of the clinic. The primary advantages of these tests are cost- and time-effectiveness, which makes them practical for testing large groups of athletes. They can also be designed to assess the specific needs of the sport (e.g., agility). However, if field tests are not carefully designed, then the tests will be plagued by poor reliability. The U.S. military provides an excellent example of effective field testing. Because they test more than 1 million soldiers each year, VO$_2$ max testing is not a practical measure of aerobic capacity. Instead, they use 1.5 to 3 mile (2.4 to 4.8 km) run times to extrapolate maximal aerobic capacities of their soldiers and to track fitness over time.[77,78] Even though these tests do not provide precise measures of oxygen consumption, they provide a valid and reliable way to classify aerobic fitness within large groups of individuals.

Profiling Athletic Performance

As stated earlier, the PFP should include tests that are specific to the physical needs of the sport (e.g., energy systems, movement patterns). Generally, the following constructs are tested in athletic profiling: movement screening, muscle strength, muscle endurance, power, speed and acceleration, flexibility and ROM, aerobic capacity, and anaerobic capacity. Many tests are available to evaluate these constructs so it is imperative to remember that the tests chosen should be specific to the demands of the sport.

Clinical Point

Athletic profiling should include:
- Movement screen tests
- Muscle strength tests
- Muscle endurance tests
- Power
- Velocity and acceleration
- Agility and quickness
- Flexibility and range of motion
- Aerobic capacity
- Anaerobic capacity

Movement Screening

Movement screening has little ability to predict human performance but may be a valuable tool in identifying athletes with functional limitations, abnormal biomechanics, or poor ROM during specific sport movements.[79,80] These data could be used to identify athletes at risk for injury. Therefore, movement screening should include the fundamental movements of the sport or those movements that are known to result in injury. Some standardized movement screening tools are available for use.[81] However, most ground-based sports involve some variation of the squat, lunge, jump and land, and running movements; at a

minimum the strength and conditioning coordinator should evaluate mechanics during these movements. Particular emphasis should be placed on the foot, knee, and hip biomechanics. The strength and conditioning coordinator should work together with other members of the sports medicine staff to effectively conduct movement screenings. The team athletic trainer or sport physical therapist can provide helpful insight in the screening process.

Clinical Point

Movement screen tests should include:
- The fundamental movements of the sport
- Movements that could result in injury
- Multiple joints at the same time

Muscular Strength

Most sports require athletes to exert force against an opponent, a projectile, or the ground. Therefore, muscle strength is an important component to sport. Muscle strength can be tested using isometric, isokinetic, or DCER (i.e., free weight) muscle contractions. Further, it can be tested using isolated, single-joint movements that determine the force-generating capabilities of a small group of muscles, or it can be tested using multi-joint movements that determine force capabilities during complex movements. Single-joint muscle strength tests are well controlled, safe, and reliable measures of muscle strength. However, they are dissimilar to most sport movements. Generally, functional sport movement requires the coordination of multiple joints and muscle groups to generate strength and power against the ground or the opponent. Therefore, multi-joint testing is likely more applicable to most sport movements.

The most often used field assessment of strength is 1-RM testing using free weights. Free weights are universally available and can be used to test a variety of functional movements. If performed correctly, 1-RM testing is reliable, safe, and efficient.[82-86] To administer a 1-RM test, the athlete performs a general warm-up, dynamic stretching, and an exercise-specific warm-up. The weight in the exercise is gradually increased until the athlete can no longer perform a single repetition. The highest amount of weight lifted for one repetition through a full ROM using correct technique is recorded as the athlete's 1-RM.

Alternately, 1-RM maximum strength can be estimated using submaximal loads.[87-89] After a general warm-up, dynamic stretching, and exercise-specific warm-up, the athlete performs a single set of the exercise with a submaximal load to failure (multi-RM testing). The number of repetitions performed is used to estimate the 1-RM. The accuracy of multi-RM strength testing differs depending on the number of repetitions performed; it has been suggested that no more than 10 repetitions should be performed to obtain accurate data.[88]

The exercises used in 1-RM or multi-RM testing differ depending on the sport. Generally, the strength and conditioning coordinator should choose multi-joint exercises that are specific to the strength movements required in a sport. It has been suggested that the essential movements in most sports are pushing, pulling, and squatting;[90] therefore, bench press, bench pull, and back squat are appropriate 1-RM test for most sports. For sports that involve high-power movements, it may be appropriate to test 1-RM in the weightlifting exercises (e.g., clean and snatch) as well.

Isokinetic muscle strength testing is a reliable laboratory assessment that determines the force-generating capabilities of a muscle at a fixed angular velocity.[91,92] Because muscle force is indirectly related to velocity of movement,[93] isokinetic testing is able to isolate velocity, eliminating momentum as a factor in completing a movement. Testing typically involves single-joint movements and may involve concentric and eccentric contractions depending on the capabilities of the dynamometer.[94] Data derived from an isokinetic test includes maximum force production, average force production, mechanical work, and other kinetic variables. Each of these kinetic variables (except mechanical work) can also be described at any instantaneous joint angle. Isokinetic testing is useful in describing muscle imbalances between opposing muscle groups[95,96] and may be helpful in screening for certain injuries.[52] It is also correlated with performance in some sports.[97-100]

Isokinetic testing is considered a laboratory test. Therefore, it can be time consuming and is impractical for testing large groups. In addition to the calibration and athlete set-up time, only a single joint is measured with each test. To fully assess the strength of an athlete's lower extremity, it is necessary to test strength at the ankle, knee, and hip. Each of these tests require different machine configurations. In addition, to fully test the capabilities of the muscle, it may be necessary to test at multiple speeds and to perform separate tests of eccentric and concentric strength. Because of these limitations, isokinetic testing is unrealistic for most testing situations and should be used on a limited basis as a tool to screen athletes who are at risk of injury.

Muscle strength can also be assessed by testing the force-generating capabilities against a fixed or immovable object (isometric testing). The advantages of isometric tests are the time requirements (< 5 sec), reliability, and safety of the test.[101] The disadvantage is that it requires force-measuring hardware (i.e., load cell or force plate). Isometric tests can assess single-joint movements or multi-joint movements. The force-generating capabilities of a joint at a given angle are specific to only a 30-degree arc surrounding the joint angle tested.[102] Therefore, to adequately assess the strength of a single joint it is necessary to test at multiple angles, making isometric, single-joint movements impractical.

Whole-body isometric movements are a viable testing option if the sports medicine staff has access to the necessary equipment.[103] The reaction force generated against the ground while pulling against a fixed barbell in the mid-thigh position of the clean exercise (power position for most sports) may be an effective measure of performance in some sport skills.[104-106] This type of isometric testing may be indicated for sports that require ground reaction forces. Furthermore, testing set-up is relatively easy and could be completed on a large number of athletes.

Local Muscle Endurance

Local muscle endurance, or the ability to exert a submaximal force repeatedly, is an important aspect of sports that require continuous activity (e.g., swimming).[107,108] Typically, local muscle endurance is tested using body weight exercises (e.g., push-ups, pull-ups, sit-ups) performed to failure.[77,78,109] It can also be tested by performing a maximal number of repetitions in a certain amount of time or the highest number of repetitions performed using submaximal loads (e.g., maximal number of squat repetitions using a load of 50% of 1-RM).

Power

Newtonian physics defines *power* as the product of force and velocity, or work per unit of time. In practical terms, *power* can be described as the rapid or explosive expression of muscle strength (e.g., maximal jumping, throwing). Because most team sports (e.g., baseball, football, soccer) require fast, explosive movements rather than slow, high-force movements, power is a key indicator of athletic potential.[110-112]

Vertical jump height is the most common field test for muscle power. Vertical jump predicts performance in various sports (e.g., rugby, football)[70,71,74] and is correlated with running speed (Figure 2-4). Vertical jump height is measured as the difference between standing reach height and vertical jump reach height. Because body weight affects vertical jumping performance, methods have been developed to directly (via a force plate) or indirectly (via Sayers's equation for peak power and Harman's equation for average power) measure muscle power during vertical jumps. This allows a strength and conditioning coordinator to compare power output of athletes of different body weights.

Sayers's equation for calculating peak power is:[113]

$$P(W) = (60.7 \times \text{Jump Height [cm]}) + (45.3 \times \text{BM[Kg]}) - 2055.0$$

Harman's equation for calculating average power is:[114]

$$P(W) = (21.2 \times \text{Jump Height [cm]}) + (23.0 \times \text{BM[Kg]}) - 1393.0$$

For sports in which upper-body power is important, an appropriate field test is the medicine ball throw for distance. The throw distance can be measured seated, standing, twisting, or overhead, depending on the mechanics of the sport.[115-118]

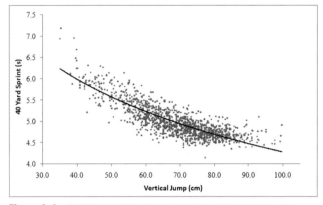

Figure 2-4

Unpublished data from the Human Performance Laboratory at the University of Houston-Clear Lake and Memorial Hermann Sports Medicine Institute displaying the relationship between 40-yard sprint time and vertical jump (r = 0.80). Data were collected on 1250 high school football players.

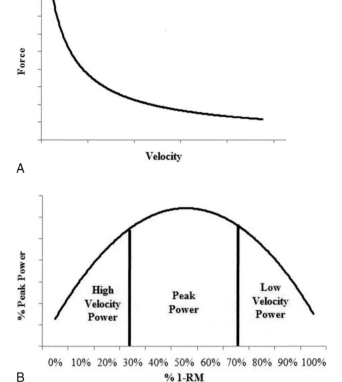

Figure 2-5

Power output that can be achieved when performing maximal-effort resistance exercises at various percentages of one-repetition maximum (1-RM). Because of the inverse relationship of force and velocity (**A**), peak power output is achieved between 30% to 40% of 1-RM for compensatory acceleration lifts and between 40% to 60% of 1-RM for most traditional lifts (**B**).

In the laboratory, peak power can be assessed by having athletes perform maximal, ballistic exercises against a fixed resistance.[119] Because force and velocity are inversely related (Figure 2-5, *A*), power exists on a spectrum with respect to load; the greatest power is generated when force and velocity are optimized (Figure 2-5, *B*). Practically speaking, this means that peak power output occurs when the athletes perform maximal ballistic movements using loads of approximately 30% of 1-RM (depending on the nature of the lift).[120,121] This method, however, requires a force plate, a position transducer, or an accelerometer attached to the barbell.[122,123] The force plate directly measures the kinetics of the lift and provides power and other kinetic variables derived from Newtonian mechanics (e.g., force, work). A position transducer (or linear encoder) measures displacement per unit of time from which velocity and acceleration can be calculated. If a constant mass is used during the lift (i.e., free weights), power can be calculated by multiplying the velocity derived from the position transducer by the known force of the barbell ($m \times g$). Measurement of the kinetics of the lift can provide the coach with an accurate load to train for peak power.[124,125] However, testing power against load may be time-consuming and expensive. In addition, the kinetics of the lift are disrupted if the athlete does not accelerate the barbell through the entire ROM. Magnetic braking systems exist to allow full acceleration through the lift,[126] but these may not be practical in some testing situations.

Velocity and Acceleration

Running velocity (or speed) is a determining factor for success in many team and individual sports. In track events such as the 100-, 200-, and 400-meter sprint, it is the sole determinant of success and in other individual sports, it is an important contributor. For instance, a pole vaulter must sprint at a high speed to develop the kinetic energy to deform the pole on contact with the box. Most team sports also require speed. A running back in American football who breaks into the open field must possess speed to outrun his defensive opponents to the end zone. Therefore, running velocity is included in PFP tests for nearly all sports.

Velocity is the distance covered per unit of time and is typically expressed in meters per second, yards per second, or miles per hour (see the following equation). The distance used to determine running velocity varies by sport. Running velocity of football players is classically tested in timed 40-yard (36.5-m) sprints,[71-74] and basketball players are often tested in a 42-foot (12.8-m) sprint (¾ court; test used at the National Basketball Association combine). A 60-yard (54.8-m) linear sprint is frequently used to test the running velocity of a baseball player;[127] however, a more specific measure of baseball speed is a timed run on the baseball field.[128]

The following equation calculates velocity (V) using distance (d) in meters and time (t) in seconds:

$$\vec{V}\left(M/sec\right) = \frac{d}{t}$$

Some positions in sport rarely require an athlete to achieve top speed. For example, a defensive or offensive lineman infrequently runs at top speed during a game. Therefore, a more important physical profile test may be the measurement of acceleration. Acceleration is the rate of change in velocity over time and is typically expressed as m/sec². The following equation calculates acceleration (a) using the second velocity (V_2) in meters per second, initial velocity (V_1) in meters per second, and time (t) in seconds:

$$a\left(m/sec2\right) = \frac{(V2 - V1)}{t}$$

Velocity and acceleration can be determined using the same test. In the 40-yard (36.5-m) sprint, time can be measured using a stopwatch or timing light system at four different time points (10, 20, 30, and 40 yards [9.1, 18.2, 27.9, and 36.5 m]). Then the average and interval velocity and acceleration can be determined at each time point in the run. These data can be valuable in comparing and evaluating players playing different positions that may rely on interval acceleration more than velocity (Table 2-4).

Agility and Quickness

Agility is the ability to accelerate, decelerate, and change directions in a controlled and rapid manner. Sports such as basketball and soccer require many such movements. Agility is typically measured in a timed drill that requires change of direction. The type of drill used depends on the nature of the sport. Two commonly used tests are the pro-agility test (Figure 2-6, *A*) and T-test (Figure 2-6, *B*) for the sports of football[69] and basketball,[129] respectively. When choosing an agility test, the strength and conditioning coordinator should consider the length of the drill and types of movements needed to perform the drill. For instance, a drill that requires only forward running would appropriately test the agility required for a football defensive lineman; however, a basketball player would be better tested in a drill requiring forward, lateral, and backward movements.

Flexibility and Range of Motion

Flexibility and ROM may be important measurements for predicting injuries and performance limitations in athletes. The type of test and joints measured should be specific to the sport and associated injuries. Furthermore, it should be noted that certain sports require more or less flexibility and ROM for success. Ballet dancers, for instance, may have extreme ROM in the muscles that surround the hip. Their activity necessitates such ROM for performance of many dancing maneuvers. In contrast, distance runners, football players, and baseball players may have far less hip flexibility.

Although there is no conclusive evidence, it is logical to believe that hypomobility could lead to injury.[130-136] Therefore, it is important for strength coaches to determine the baseline flexibility in their athletes. Almost all sports require some hip mobility; therefore, it is vital to document hip flexibility and ROM. The sit-and-reach test is commonly used to measure the flexibility of the hamstrings and lower back musculature,[109] but it does not assess unilateral flexibility. Because athletes may have asymmetries between hips, a more rigorous evaluator of hamstring flexibility may be the lying straight leg raise test. Lying supine with both legs straight, the athlete raises a single leg keeping the knee straight. Using a goniometer, the sports medicine staff measures the peak hip angle just before the opposite leg begins to rise from the floor.[137] Using the straight leg raise test, hip flexibility can be compared between legs.

In addition to testing the flexibility of the hip extensors (i.e., hamstrings), it is important to measure the ROM of the hip flexors. Tight hip flexor muscles (i.e., rectus femoris, iliopsoas) may contribute to injuries and limit sport performance[138] by decreasing the hip extension ROM and

Table 2-4

Theoretical Example of Two Players with Different Velocities and Accelerations During a Timed 40-Yard Sprint

Distance (yd)	Player A			Player B		
	Time (sec)	Average Velocity (m/sec)	Interval Acceleration (m/sec²)	Time (sec)	Average Velocity (m/sec)	Interval Acceleration (m/sec²)
10	1.64	6.10	3.72	1.55	6.45	0.65
20	2.80	7.14	0.10	2.80	7.14	0.07
30	3.70	8.11	0.10	3.90	7.69	0.05
40	4.60	8.70	0.06	5.00	8.00	0.03

Note that the acceleration of Player B is greater than Player A for the first interval, but the acceleration of Player A is greater in the last three intervals. Ultimately, the final velocity of Player A is greater than Player B. Depending on the position, the initial acceleration profile of Player B may be more advantageous than the final velocity of Player A.

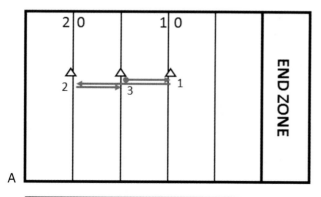

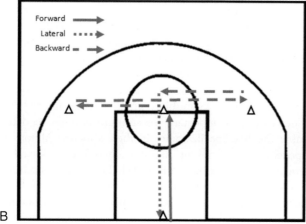

Figure 2-6

A, Pro-agility drill commonly used for testing agility in football.
B, T-test used for testing agility in basketball. The T-test drill can be modified by lengthening the distances for use in soccer agility testing.

subsequently reducing muscle force production (i.e., reducing impulse). The "Thomas test" or "modified Thomas test"[139-141] are commonly used to assess hip flexor flexibility; like the straight leg raise test, the Thomas test can identify limb asymmetries. For overhead athletes (e.g., baseball, softball, swimming, and volleyball), shoulder flexibility, especially internal and external rotation, should be tested to ensure symmetry.[58,59,142]

Metabolic Testing

In addition to testing the physical attributes of an athlete, it is important to test the metabolic capacity of the athlete. During exercise, energy is derived via aerobic or anaerobic metabolic pathways. Depending on the sport, it may be appropriate to test the peak capacity of one or both of the energy systems.

Aerobic Conditioning Tests. Energy derived from the aerobic system is important for sports that require long-duration activity. Long-distance runners and road cyclists derive energy predominantly from the aerobic energy system. In addition to producing energy, the aerobic energy system assists in recovery from anaerobic exercise.[143]

The gold-standard measure of aerobic capacity is to directly measure oxygen consumption during a graded, maximal test.[109] However, several submaximal tests are effective in predicting aerobic capacity (e.g., the 1.5- and 3-mile tests and the Yo-Yo test, discussed in the following text).

Anaerobic Conditioning and Power Endurance Tests. Many sports require sustained long-duration energy production with multiple bouts of high-intensity anaerobic energy production. For example, in a soccer match, athletes may move nonstop for the duration of the competition but have frequent intervals during which they must sprint to a ball or an opponent. Similarly, in basketball, there are many intermittent bouts of high-intensity movement coupled with lower intensity bouts of recovery. For such sports, testing the anaerobic and aerobic energy systems is warranted.

Anaerobic capacity and power endurance can be measured using a single, high-intensity work bout, or repeat high-intensity intervals of work with recovery periods. The Wingate cycle test is an example of a single-bout anaerobic test. After a warm-up, the athlete pedals as fast as possible for 30 seconds while the resistance on the bike is held constant (typically at $0.075 \times$ body mass). Peak power and rate of decline is measured during the 30-second period and used to describe the anaerobic capabilities of the athlete. It is a useful test for describing anaerobic capacity of cyclists, but the mode of exercise is dissimilar to most sports.[109]

For noncyclists, a more appropriate measure of anaerobic power endurance is to repeat vertical jumps for time (20 to 60 sec) or number (10 to 15 repetitions).[144] If available, a force platform or contact mat can be used to measure multiple vertical jump height. Field testing of power endurance is difficult. It may be assessed by measuring the number of times an athlete can touch a submaximal target in 30 to 60 seconds. A target could be set at 85% of the athlete's peak vertical jump height and measure the number of times the athlete contacts the target in 1 minute. Another example of a field test of power endurance is to test the number of times an athlete can jump and contact a fixed target in 30 to 60 seconds. For example, the number of times a basketball player can touch the rim or the backboard of a basketball goal in 1 minute is a sport-specific measure of power endurance.

Power endurance testing allows the coach to describe the peak power exerted during the exercise and can track the decline in power over time. Figure 2-7 describes a theoretical power endurance response of a strength/power athlete and an endurance athlete. Notice the difference in peak power and the rate of decline in power between the two athletes. Because of the metabolic and mechanical properties of type II muscle fibers, which are predominant in strength/power athletes, there is a high peak power generation but an inability to maintain power over time. Relative to the strength/power athlete, the endurance athlete can generate a low peak power but is able to sustain a higher

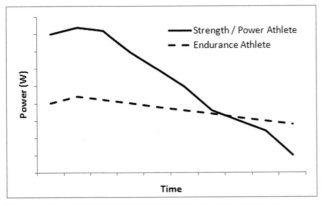

Figure 2-7

Hypothetical comparison of a strength/power and power endurance athlete performing a timed power test.

Table 2-5

Goal Running Times by Position for the 110 Anaerobic Running Test

Position	Goal Time to Run 110 Yards
Wide receivers, safeties, and cornerbacks	15 sec
Quarterbacks, running backs, linebackers	16-17 sec
Offensive and defensive lineman	18 sec

Note: Times were provided by a Division I football program.

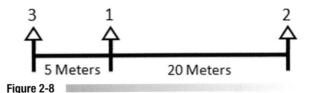

Figure 2-8

Cone dimensions for yo-yo intermittent drill.

power relative to peak over time because of the metabolic properties of his or her skeletal muscle fibers.

An often-used test of anaerobic conditioning in the sport of football is the 110 conditioning test. It is an example of a multiple-bout conditioning test. The 110 test is typically performed on a marked football field. The athlete runs the length of the field from the back of the end zone to the opposite goal line (110 yards). After a 45-second recovery, the athlete repeats the sprint for a total of 16 sprints. The total distance covered in the test is approximately 1 mile. Position-specific times used for football are listed in Table 2-5. Failure to complete a single repetition in the allotted time results in failure of the test.

Sports such as basketball and soccer require both aerobic and anaerobic conditioning. The yo-yo intermittent test is a reliable and effective measure of both energy systems that is similar to discontinuous running sports. To perform the yo-yo test, two cones are spaced 20 meters (21.8 yd) apart; a third cone is spaced 5 meters (5.5 yd) from the second cone (Figure 2-8). An audio recorder is used to play a tape or compact disk (CD) that provides auditory running and recovery commands for the athlete. The tape or CD contains the prerecorded timing intervals for the yo-yo protocol. Beginning at the middle cone, the athlete sprints 20 meters (21.8 yd) forward, touches the cone, and sprints 20 meters (21.8 yd) back (one interval). To successfully complete the interval, the athlete must pass the cone prior to hearing a second "beep." After completing the first interval, the athlete jogs or walks around the third cone until he or she hears the command to begin interval 2. Testing ends when the athlete fails to complete two intervals. The total number of intervals completed is recorded and used to classify the fitness of the athlete.[145-147]

Developing a Testing Battery

A minimal number of tests should be used to describe the physical readiness of the team or athlete (Table 2-6). The strength and conditioning coordinator should ensure that the tests are valid (i.e., that they actually measure the physical constructs they are intended to measure) and reliable (i.e., that they produce repeatable results). To minimize the testing burden on the athlete, the strength and conditioning coordinator should choose single tests that measure multiple underlying constructs. For example, the 40-yard (36.5-m) sprint with timing intervals at 10, 20, 30, and 40 yards (9.1, 18.2, 27.9, and 36.5 m) is a single test that measures two constructs (speed and acceleration). Likewise, the repeat vertical jump test is a single test that measures peak power, power endurance, and anaerobic conditioning. Finally, the strength and conditioning coordinator should choose tests that have good face validity. A test with face validity is one that appears to the athlete to measure a construct important in a sport. For instance, in volleyball, a vertical jump performed on a court, near a volleyball net, has better face validity than a vertical jump performed in a laboratory on a force plate with no reaching target. Ensuring face validity may improve the motivation of the athlete on the test and improve the scoring results.

Conclusion

PFPs provide important benefits to the athlete, sports medicine staff, and strength and conditioning coach. If the sports medicine staff uses due diligence, then injury risks associated with performing PFP can be mitigated. A properly designed PFP should provide baseline data beneficial for identifying talented athletes and for screening for future injury risk.

Table 2-6

Suggested Physical Attributes and Metabolic Testing for Eight Common Sports

	Movement Screening	Muscle Strength	Muscle Endurance	Power	Power Endurance	Speed and Acceleration	Flexibility and ROM	Aerobic Capacity	Anaerobic Capacity	Agility
Football	Running	Iso-pull; 1-RM (squat, bench press and bench pull, power clean)	X	Vertical jump, broad jump, medicine ball throw	X	40-yard sprint (10, 20, 30, 40 yard times)	Sit and reach, Thomas test	X	110 Test	Pro-agility drill
Basketball	Jump and land	Iso-pull; 1-RM (squat, bench press and bench pull, power clean)	Push-up and pull-up to failure	Vertical jump, medicine ball throw	Multi-vertical jump	¾ Court sprint	Sit and reach, Thomas test	1-mile run	Yo-yo intermittent test	Short T-test
Soccer	Jump and land	1-RM (squat, bench press, bench pull)	Push-up and pull-up to failure	Broad jump	Multi-vertical jump	40-Yard sprint (10, 20, 30, 40 yard times)	Sit and reach, Thomas test	3-mile run	Yo-yo intermittent test	Long T-test
Baseball	Running	1-RM (squat, bench press, bench pull)	X	Vertical jump, broad jump, medicine ball throw	X	60-Yard sprint (10, 20, 30, 60 yard times)	Sit and reach, Thomas test, shoulder internal and external rotation	X	X	X
Track and field (distance)	Running	1-RM (squat, bench press, bench pull)	Push-up and pull-up to failure	X	X	X	Sit and reach, Thomas test	Treadmill VO$_2$ max	X	X

Track and field (sprint)	Running	Iso-pull; 1-RM (squat, bench press and bench pull, power clean)	X	Vertical jump, broad jump	X	Distance specific speed and acceleration	Sit and reach, Thomas test	X	X	X
Cycling (track)	X	Iso-pull; 1-RM (squat, bench press and bench pull, power clean)	X	Broad jump	Multi-vertical jump	X	Sit and reach, Thomas test, shoulder internal and external rotation	Cycling VO_2 max	Wingate cycle test	X
Cycling (road)	X	1-RM (squat, bench press, bench pull)	Push-up and pull-up to failure	X	X	X	Sit and reach, Thomas test, shoulder internal and external rotation	Cycling VO_2 max	X	X

1-RM, One-repetition maximum; *iso*, isometric; *ROM*, range of motion; *VO_2 max*, maximum oxygen consumption; *X*, test is not suggested.

Essential to any effective testing battery is a working knowledge of the physical and physiological requirements of sport. Therefore, the strength and conditioning coordinator, the entire sports medicine staff, the sport coaches, and the athletes should all contribute to the development, administration, and interpretation of the PFP.

References

1. Superko HR, Bernauer E, Voss J: Effects of a mandatory health screening and physical maintenance program for law enforcement officers, *Phys Sportsmed* 16:99–109, 1988.
2. Binda C: Precamp physical exams: Their value may be greater than you think, *Phys Sportsmed* 17:167–169, 1989.
3. Gurry M, Pappas A, Michaels J, et al: A comprehensive preseason fitness evaluation for professional baseball players, *Phys Sportsmed* 13:63–74, 1985.
4. Metzel JD: The adolescent preparticipation physical examination—Is it helpful? *Clin Sports Med* 19:577–592, 2000.
5. Kligman EW, Hewitt MJ, Crowell DL: Recommending exercise to healthy older adults—The preparticipation evaluation and exercise prescription, *Phys Sportsmed* 27(11):42–62, 1999.
6. Glover DW, Maron DJ, Matheson GO: The preparticipation physical examination—Steps toward consensus and uniformity, *Phys Sportsmed* 27(8):29–34, 1999.
7. Peltz JE, Haskell WL, Matheson GO: A comprehensive and cost-effective preparticipation exam implemented on the world wide web, *Med Sci Sports Exerc* 31:1727–1740, 1999.
8. Tanji TL: The preparticipation exam: Special concerns for the Special Olympics, *Phys Sportsmed* 19:61–68, 1991.
9. Hudson PB: Preparticipation screening of Special Olympics athletes, *Phys Sportsmed* 16:97–104, 1988.
10. Hunter SC: Preparticipation physical examination. In Griffin LY, editor: *Orthopedic knowledge update: Sports medicine*, Rosemont, IL, 1994, American Academy of Orthopaedic Surgeons.
11. Committee on Sports Medicine: Recommendations for participation in competitive sports, *Pediatrics* 81:737–739, 1988.
12. Sanders B, Nemeth WC: Preparticipation physical examination, *J Orthop Sports Phys Ther* 23:144–163, 1996.
13. American Academy of Orthopaedic Surgeons: *Athletic training and sports medicine*, Rosemont, IL, 1991, American Academy of Orthopaedic Surgeons.
14. Harvey J: The preparticipation examination of the child athlete, *Clin Sports Med* 1:353–369, 1982.
15. DuRaaut RH, Seymore C, Linder CW, et al: The preparticipation examination of athletes: Comparison of single and multiple examiners, *Am J Dis Child* 139:657–666, 1985.
16. Sampler P: Preparticipation exams: Are they worth the time and troubles, *Phys Sportsmed* 14:180–187, 1986.
17. St. Rauss RH, Johnson MD, Kibler WB , et al: Keys to successful preparticipation exams, *Phys Sportsmed* 21:109–123, 1993.
18. Feinstein RA, Soileau EJ, Daniel WA: A national survey of preparticipation physical examination requirements, *Phys Sportsmed* 16:51–59, 1988.
19. McKeag DB: Preparticipation screening of the potential athlete, *Clin Sports Med* 8:373–397, 1989.
20. Stanley K: Preparticipation evaluation of the young athlete. In Stanitski CL, DeLee JC, Drez D, editors: *Pediatric and adolescent sports medicine*, Philadelphia, 1994, WB Saunders Co.
21. Smilkstein G: Health evaluation of high school athletes, *Phys Sportsmed* 9:73–80, 1981.
22. Heidt RS, Sweeterman LM, Carlonas RL, et al: Avoidance of soccer injuries with preseason conditioning, *Am J Sports Med* 28:659–662, 2000.
23. McKeag DB: Preseason physical examination for the prevention of sports injuries, *Sports Med* 2:413–431, 1985.
24. Carek PJ, Futrell M, Hueston WJ: The preparticipation physical examination history: Who has the correct answers? *Clin J Sports Med* 9:124–128, 1999.
25. Kaplan NM, Deveraux RB, Miller HS: Systemic hyperextension, *Med Sci Sports Exerc* 26:S268–S270, 1994.
26. Zabetakis PM: Profiling the hypertensive in sports, *Clin Sports Med* 3:137–152, 1984.
27. Bonci CM, Ryan R: *Preparticipation screening in intercollegiate athletics.* Postgraduate Advances in Sports Medicine, Philadelphia, 1988, University of Pennsylvania Medical School and Forum Medicum, Inc.
28. Halpern B, Blackburn T, Incremona B, et al: Preparticipation sports physicals. In Zachazewski JE, Magee DJ, Quillen WS, editors: *Athletic injuries and rehabilitation*, Philadelphia, 1996, WB Saunders Co.
29. Dorsen PJ: Should athletes with one eye, kidney or testicle play contact sports? *Phys Sportsmed* 14:130–138, 1986.
30. Strong WB, Steed D: Cardiovascular evaluation of the young athlete, *Pediatr Clin North Am* 29:1325–1339, 1982.
31. Huston TP, Puffer JC, Rodney WM: The athletic heart syndrome, *N Engl J Med* 313:24–32, 1985.
32. McGrew CA: Clinical implications of the AHA preparticipation cardiovascular screening guidelines, *Athletic Ther Today* 5:52–56, 2000.
33. Fuller CM: Cost effectiveness analysis of screening of high school athletes for risk of sudden cardiac death, *Med Sci Sports Exerc* 32:887–890, 2000.
34. Maron BJ, Pollac DC, Kaplan JA, et al: Blunt impact to the chest leading to sudden death from cardiac arrest during sports activities, *N Engl J Med* 333:337–342, 1995.
35. Potera C: AHA Panel outlines sudden death screening standards, *Phys Sportsmed* 24(10):27–28, 1996.
36. Fuller CM, McNulty CM, Spring DA, et al: Prospective screening of 5,615 high school athletes for risk of sudden cardiac death, *Med Sci Sports Exerc* 29:1131–1138, 1997.
37. Salem DN, Isner JM: Cardiac screening in athletes, *Orthop Clin North Am* 11:687–695, 1980.
38. Braden DS, Strong WB: Preparticipation screening for sudden cardiac death in high school and college athletes, *Phys Sportsmed* 16:128–144, 1988.
39. Mitchell JH, Hashell WL, Raven PB: Classification of sports, *Med Sci Sports Exerc* 26:S242–S245, 1994.
40. Belman MJ, King RR: Pulmonary profiling in exercise, *Clin Sports Med* 3:119–136, 1984.
41. Ross RG: The prevalence of reversible airway obstruction in professional football players, *Med Sci Sports Exerc* 32:1985–1989, 2000.
42. Rundell KW, Wilber RL, Szmedra L, et al: Exercise-induced asthma screening of elite athletes: Field versus laboratory exercise challenge, *Med Sci Sports Exerc* 32:309–316, 2000.
43. Khosla RK: Detecting sexually transmitted disease—A new role for urinalysis in the preparticipation exam, *Phys Sportsmed* 23(1):77–80, 1995.
44. Lombardo JA: Preparticipation physical evaluation, *Prim Care* 11:3–21, 1984.
45. Johnson MD: Tailoring the preparticipation exam to female athletes, *Phys Sportsmed* 20:61–72, 1992.
46. Slavin JL: Assessing athletes' nutritional status: Making it part of the sports medicine physical, *Phys Sportsmed* 19:79–94, 1991.
47. Nelson MA: The child athlete with chronic disease. In Stanitski CL, DeLee JC, Drez D, editors: *Pediatric and adolescent sports medicine*, Philadelphia, 1994, WB Saunders Co.
48. Magnes SA, Henderson JM, Hunter SC: What conditions limit sports participation: Experience with 10,540 athletes, *Phys Sportsmed* 20:143–160, 1992.

49. American Academy of Pediatrics Committee on Sports Medicine and Fitness: Medical conditions affecting sports participation, *Pediatrics* 94:757–760, 1994.

50. Kraemer WJ, Torine JC, Silvestre R, et al: Body size and composition of National Football League Players, *J Strength Cond Res* 19:485–489, 2005.

51. Kuzmits FE, Adams AJ: The NFL combine: Does it predict performance in the National Football League, *J Strength Cond Res* 22:1721–1727, 2008.

52. Myer GD, Ford KR, Barber Foss KD, et al: The relationship of hamstrings and quadriceps strength to anterior cruciate ligament injury in female athletes, *Clin J Sport Med* 19:3–8, 2009.

53. White AT, Johnson SC: Physiological aspects and injury in elite Alpine skiers, *Sports Med* 15:170–178, 1993.

54. Andersen RE, Montgomery DL: Physiology of Alpine skiing, *Sports Med* 6:210–221, 1988.

55. Paulos L, Noyes FR, Grood E, et al: Knee rehabilitation after anterior cruciate ligament reconstruction and repair, *J Orthop Sports Phys Ther* 13:60–70, 1991.

56. Zazulak BT, Hewett TE, Reeves NP, et al: Deficits in neuromuscular control of the trunk predict knee injury risk, *Am J Sports Med* 35:1123–1130, 2007.

57. Zazulak BT, Hewett TE, Reeves NP, et al: The effects of core proprioception on knee injury: A prospective biomechanical-epidemiological study, *Am J Sports Med* 35:368–373, 2007.

58. Tehranzadeh AD, Fronek J, Resnick D: Posterior capsular fibrosis in professional baseball pitchers: Case series of MR arthrographic findings in six patients with glenohumeral internal rotational deficit, *Clin Imaging* 31:343–348, 2007.

59. Myers JB, Laudner KG, Pasquale MR, et al: Glenohumeral range of motion deficits and posterior shoulder tightness in throwers with pathologic internal impingement, *Am J Sports Med* 34:385–391, 2006.

60. Nagano Y, Ida H, Akai M, et al: Biomechanical characteristics of the knee joint in female athletes during tasks associated with anterior cruciate ligament injury, *Knee* 16:153–158, 2009.

61. Pappas E, Hagins M, Sheikhzadeh A, et al: Biomechanical differences between unilateral and bilateral landings from a jump: Gender differences, *Clin J Sport Med* 17:263–268, 2007.

62. Cowley HR, Ford KR, Myer GD, et al: Differences in neuromuscular strategies between landing and cutting tasks in female basketball and soccer athletes, *J Athl Train* 41:67–73, 2006.

63. Chappell JD, Herman DC, Knight BS, et al: Effect of fatigue on knee kinetics and kinematics in stop-jump tasks, *Am J Sports Med* 33:1022–1029, 2005.

64. Urabe Y, Kobayashi R, Sumida S, et al: Electromyographic analysis of the knee during jump landing in male and female athletes, *Knee* 12:129–134, 2005.

65. Chappell JD, Creighton RA, Giuliani C, et al: Kinematics and electromyography of landing preparation in vertical stop-jump, *Am J Sports Med* 35:235–241, 2007.

66. Joseph M, Tiberio D, Baird JL, et al: Knee valgus during drop jumps in National Collegiate Athletic Association Division I female athletes, *Am J Sports Med* 36:285–289, 2008.

67. Russell KA, Palmieri RM, Zinder SM, et al: Sex differences in valgus knee angle during a single-leg drop jump, *J Athl Train* 41:166–171, 2006.

68. Hewett TE, Lindenfeld TN: The effect of neuromuscular training on the incidence of knee injury in female athletes, *Am J Sports Med* 27:699–706, 1999.

69. Sierer SP, Battaglini CL, Mihalik JP, et al: The National Football League combine: Performance differences between drafted and nondrafted players entering the 2004 and 2005 drafts, *J Strength Cond Res* 22:6–12, 2008.

70. Gabbett T, Kelly J, Ralph S, et al: Physiological and anthropometric characteristics of junior elite and sub-elite rugby league players, with special reference to starters and non-starters, *J Sci Med Sport* 12:215–222, 2009.

71. Young W, Newton R, Doyle T, et al: Physiological and anthropometric characteristics of starters and non-starters and playing positions in elite Australian rules football: A case study, *J Sci Med Sport* 8:333–345, 2005.

72. Black W, Roundy E: Comparisons of size, strength, speed, and power in NCAA Division 1-A football players, *J Strength Cond Res* 8:80–85, 1994.

73. Schmidt WD: Strength and physiological characteristics of NCAA Division III American football players, *J Strength Cond Res* 13:210–213, 1999.

74. Fry AC, Kraemer WJ: Physical performance characteristics of American collegiate football players, *J Appl Sport Sci Res* 5:126–138, 1991.

75. Noakes TD, Myburgh KH, Schall R: Peak treadmill running velocity during the VO_2max test predicts running performance, *J Sports Sci* 8:35–45, 1990.

76. Ploutz-Snyder LL, Giamis EL: Orientation and familiarization in 1RM strength testing in old and young women, *J Strength Cond Res* 15:519–523, 2001.

77. MCO P6100.12: *Marine Corps physical fitness test and body composition program manual*, Washington, DC, 2002, Headquarters Marine Corps.

78. FM 21-20: Physical fitness training, Washington, DC, 1998, Headquarters Department of the Army.

79. Hewett TE, Myer GD, Ford KR, et al: Biomechanical measures of neuromuscular control and valgus loading of the knee predict anterior cruciate ligament injury risk in female athletes a prospective study, *Am J Sports Med* 33:492–501, 2005.

80. Zazulak BT, Hewett TE, Reeves NP, et al: Deficits in neuromuscular control of the trunk predict knee injury risk: a prospective biomechanical-epidemiologic study, *Am J Sports Med* 35:1123–1130, 2007.

81. Murphy C: *Functional movement screening of NCAA Division II male and female athletes*, Eugene, OR, 2001, Microform Publications, University of Oregon.

82. Tagesson SK, Kvist J: Intra- and interrater reliability of the establishment of one repetition maximum on squat and seated knee extension, *J Strength Cond Res* 21:801–807, 2007.

83. Faigenbaum AD, Milliken LA, Westcott WL: Maximal strength testing in healthy children, *J Strength Cond Res* 17:162–166, 2003.

84. Rydwik E, Karlsson C, Frändin K, et al: Muscle strength testing with one repetition maximum in the arm/shoulder for people aged 75+: Test-retest reliability, *Clin Rehabil* 21:258–265, 2007.

85. Phillips WT, Batterham AM, Valenzuela JE, et al: Reliability of maximal strength testing in older adults, *Arch Phys Med Rehabil* 85:329–334, 2004.

86. Levinger I, Goodman C, Hare DL, et al: The reliability of the 1RM strength test for untrained middle-aged individuals, *J Sci Med Sport* 12:310–316, 2009.

87. Kravitz L, Akalan C, Nowicki K, et al: Prediction of 1 repetition maximum in high-school power lifters, *J Strength Cond Res* 17:167–172, 2003.

88. Reynolds JM, Gordon TJ, Robergs RA: Prediction of one repetition maximum strength from multiple repetition maximum testing and anthropometry, *J Strength Cond Res* 20:584–592, 2006.

89. Horvat M, Franklin C, Born D: Predicting strength in high school women athletes, *J Strength Cond Res* 21:1018–1022, 2007.

90. Stone MH, O'Bryant H, Garhammer J: Hypothetical model for strength training, *J Sports Med Phys Fitness* 21:342–351, 1981.

91. Pincivero DM, Lephart SM, Karunakara RA: Reliability and precision of isokinetic strength and muscular endurance for the quadriceps and hamstrings, *Int J Sports Med* 18:113–117, 1997.

92. Moller M, Lind K, Styf J, et al: The reliability of isokinetic testing of the ankle joint and a heel-raise test for endurance, *Knee Surg Sports Traumatol Arthrosc* 13:60–71, 2005.

93. Hill AV: The heat of shortening and the dynamic constants of muscle, *Proc R Soc Lond B Biol Sci* 126:136–195, 1938.

94. Li RCT, Wu Y, Maffulli N, et al: Eccentric and concentric isokinetic knee flexion and extension: A reliability study using the Cybex 6000 dynamometer, *Br J Sports Med* 30:156–160, 1996.

95. Gerodimosa V, Manoua V, Stavropoulos N, et al: Agonist and antagonist strength of ankle musculature in basketball players aged 12 to 17 years, *Isokinet Exerc Sci* 14:81–89, 2006.

96. Hill AM, Pramanik S, McGregor AH: Isokinetic dynamometry in assessment of external and internal axial rotation strength of the shoulder: comparison of two positions, *Isokinet Exerc Sci* 13: 187–195, 2005.

97. Forthomme B, Crielaard JM, Forthomme L, et al: Field performance of javelin throwers: Relationship with isokinetic findings, *Isokinet Exerc Sci* 15:195–202, 2007.

98. Nunes T, Coetzee B: The contribution of isokinetic strength parameters to the performance of cricket batsmen, *Isokinet Exerc Sci* 15:233–244, 2007.

99. Tang WT, Shung HM: Relationship between isokinetic strength and shooting accuracy at different shooting ranges in Taiwanese elite high school basketball players, *Isokinet Exerc Sci* 13: 169–174, 2005.

100. Signorile JF, Sandler DJ, Smith WN, et al: Correlation analyses and regression modeling between isokinetic testing and on-court performance in competitive adolescent tennis players, *J Strength Cond Res* 19:519–526, 2005.

101. Malerba JL, Adam ML, Harris BA, et al: Reliability of dynamic and isometric testing of shoulder external and internal rotators, *J Orthop Sports Phys Ther* 18:543–552, 1993.

102. Kitai TA, Sale DG: Specificity of joint angle in isometric training, *Eur J Appl Physiol Occup Physiol* 58:744–748, 1989.

103. Kawamori N, Rossi SJ, Justice BD, et al: Peak force and rate of force development during isometric and dynamic mid-thigh clean pulls performed at various intensities, *J Strength Cond Res* 20:483–491, 2006.

104. Stone MH, Sands WA, Carlock J, et al: The importance of isometric maximum strength and peak rate-of-force development in sprint cycling, *J Strength Cond Res* 18:878–884, 2004.

105. Stone MH, Stone ME, Sands WA, et al: Maximum strength and strength training: A relationship to endurance? *Strength Cond J* 28:44–53, 2006.

106. Haff GG, Carlock JM, Hartman MJ, et al: Force-time curve characteristics of dynamic and isometric muscle actions of elite women Olympic weightlifters, *J Strength Cond Res* 19:741–748, 2005.

107. Konstantaki M, Swaine IL: Lactate and cardiopulmonary responses to simulated arm-pulling and leg-kicking in collegiate and recreational swimmers, *Int J Sports Med* 20:118–121, 1999.

108. Tesch PA, Wright JE, Vogel AJ, et al: The influence of muscle metabolic characteristics on physical performance, *Eur J Appl Physiol Occup Physiol* 54:237–243, 1985.

109. Whaley MH, Brubaker PH, Otto RM, editors: *ACSM's guidelines for exercise testing and prescription*, ed 7, Baltimore, 2006, Lippincott Williams & Wilkins.

110. Peterson MD, Alvar BA, Rhea MR: The contribution of maximal force production to explosive movement among young collegiate athletes, *J Strength Cond Res* 20:867–873, 2006.

111. Hori N, Newton RU, Andrews WA, et al: Does performance of hang power clean differentiate performance of jumping, sprinting, and changing of direction? *J Strength Cond Res* 22:412–418, 2008.

112. Carlock JM, Smith SL, Hartman MJ, et al: The relationship between vertical jump power estimates and weightlifting ability: A field-test approach, *J Strength Cond Res* 18:534–539, 2004.

113. Sayers SP, Harackiewicz DV, Harman EA, et al: Cross-validation of three jump power equations, *Med Sci Sports Exerc* 31: 572–577, 1999.

114. Harman EA, Posensein MT, Frykman PN, et al: Estimation of human power output from vertical jump, *J Appl Sport Sci Res* 5:116–120, 1991.

115. Mayhew JL, Bird M, Cole ML, et al: Comparison of the backward overhead medicine ball throw to power production in college football players, *J Strength Cond Res* 19:514–518, 2005.

116. Duncan MJ, Al-Nakeeb Y, Nevill AM: Influence of familiarization on a backward, overhead medicine ball explosive power test, *Res Sports Med* 13:345–352, 2005.

117. Ikeda Y, Kijima K, Kawabata K, et al: Relationship between side medicine-ball throw performance and physical ability for male and female athletes, *Eur J Appl Physiol* 99:47–55, 2007.

118. Stockbrugger BA, Haennel RG: Validity and reliability of a medicine ball explosive power test, *J Strength Cond Res* 15: 431–438, 2001.

119. Dugan EL, Doyle TLA, Humphries B, et al: Determining the optimal load for jump squats: A review of methods and calculations, *J Strength Cond Res* 18:668–674, 2004.

120. Siegel JA, Gilders RM, Staron RS, et al: Human muscle power output during upper- and lower-body exercises, *J Strength Cond Res* 16:173–178, 2002.

121. Thomas GA, Kraemer WJ, Spiering BA, et al: Maximal power at different percentages of one repetition maximum: Influence of resistance and gender, *J Strength Cond Res* 21:336–342, 2007.

122. Hori N, Newton RU, Andrews WA, et al: Comparison of four different methods to measure power output during the hang power clean and the weighted squat jump, *J Strength Cond Res* 21:314–320, 2007.

123. Drinkwater EJ, Galna B, McKenna MJ, et al: Validation of an optical encoder during free weight resistance movements and analysis of bench press sticking point during fatigue, *J Strength Cond Res* 21:510–517, 2007.

124. McBride JM, Triplett-McBride T, Davie A, et al: The effect of heavy- vs. light–load jump squats on the development of strength, power, and speed, *J Strength Cond Res* 16:75–82, 2002.

125. Wilson GJ, Newton RU, Murphy AJ, et al: The optimal training load for the development of dynamic athletic performance, *Med Sci Sports Exerc* 25:1279–1286, 1993.

126. Alemany JA, Pandorf CE, Montain SJ, et al: Reliability assessment of ballistic jump squats and bench throws, *J Strength Cond Res* 19:33–38, 2005.

127. Coleman AE, Lasky LM: Assessing running speed and body composition in professional baseball players, *J Appl Sport Sci Res* 6:207–213, 1992.

128. Coleman E, Dupler TL: Changes in running speed in game situations during a season of Major League Baseball, *J Exerc Physiol Online* 7:89–93, 2004.

129. Delextrat A, Cohen D: Physiological testing of basketball players: Toward a standard evaluation of anaerobic fitness, *J Strength Cond Res* 22:1066–1072, 2008.

130. Lawrence H: Effect of stretching on sport injury risk: A review. *Clin J Sport Med* 15:113, 2005.

131. Schwenk TL: Hamstring flexibility decreases overuse injuries, *Phys Sportsmed* 27:26, 1999.

132. Hartig DE, Henderson JM: Increasing hamstring flexibility decreases lower extremity overuse injuries in military basic, *Am J Sports Med* 27:173, 1999.

133. Jones BH, Knapik JJ: Physical training and exercise-related injuries: Surveillance, research and injury prevention in military populations, *Sports Med* 27:111–125, 1999.

134. Gabbe BJ, Finch CF, Bennell KL, et al: Risk factors for hamstring injuries in community level Australian football, *Br J Sports Med* 39:106–110, 2005.
135. Witvrouw E, Mahieu N, Danneels L, et al: Stretching and injury prevention: An obscure relationship, *Sports Med* 34:443–449, 2004.
136. Weerapong P, Hume PA, Kolt GS: Stretching: Mechanisms and benefits for sport performance and injury prevention, *Phys Ther Rev* 9:189–206, 2004.
137. Stutchfield BM, Coleman S: The relationships between hamstring flexibility, lumbar flexion, and low back pain in rowers, *Eur J Sport Sci* 6:255–260, 2006.
138. Young W, Clothier P, Otago L, et al: Relationship between a modified Thomas test and leg range of motion in Australian-rules football kicking, *J Sport Rehabil* 12:343–350, 2003.
139. Harvey D: Assessment of the flexibility of elite athletes using the modified Thomas test, *Br J Sports Med* 32:68–70, 1998.
140. Peeler JD, Anderson JE: Reliability limits of the modified Thomas test for assessing rectus femoris muscle flexibility about the knee joint, *J Athl Train* 43:470–476, 2008.
141. Peeler J, Anderson JE: Reliability of the Thomas test for assessing range of motion about the hip, *Phys Ther Sport* 8:14–21, 2007.
142. Nakamizo H, Nakamura Y, Nobuhara K, et al: Loss of glenohumeral internal rotation in little league pitchers: A biomechanical study, *J Should Elbow Surg* 17:795–801, 2008.
143. Tomlin DL, Wenger HA: The relationship between aerobic fitness and recovery from high intensity intermittent exercise, *Sports Med* 31:1–11, 2001.
144. Sands WA, McNeal JR, Ochi MT, et al: Comparison of the Wingate and Bosco anaerobic tests, *J Strength Cond Res* 18:810–815, 2004.
145. Bangsbo J, Iaia FM, Krustrup P: The yo-yo intermittent recovery test: A useful tool for evaluation of physical performance in intermittent sports, *Sports Med* 38:37–51, 2008.
146. Peter K: The yo-yo intermittent recovery test: Physiological response, reliability, and validity, *Med Sci Sports Exerc* 35:697–705, 2003.
147. Thomas A, Dawson B, Goodman C: The yo-yo test: Reliability and association with a 20-m shuttle run and VO$_2$ max, *Int J Sports Physiol Perform* 1:137–149, 2006.

PSYCHOSOCIAL ASPECTS OF YOUTH SPORTS

Stephen A. Durant, Richard D. Ginsburg, and Michael S. Jellinek

Considerations for Dealing with Today's Young Athletes

Studies assessing the number of American youth playing organized sports between the ages of 6 and 18 vary from 30 million to more than 45 million out of approximately 51 million children.[1,2] The upper estimate comes from a U.S. Department of Health and Human Services report from the Surgeon General in 1996, *Physical Activity and Health,* suggesting 87% of American youth participate in at least one organized sport by the of age 18.[3] Although the true measure of American participation is unclear because many children may be involved in multiple sports across multiple agencies (e.g., Little League baseball, Pop Warner football, Boys and Girls clubs, town or recreational activities, interscholastic teams, club sports), these figures suggest that the great majority of American children are participating in organized sports sometime during their lives. It may be said, then, that youth sports have become the most common ground on which we share a common experience. Sports have become one of the key defining experiences of an American child's physical and emotional development.

As is the case with any powerful and pervasive phenomenon, there is a downside that accompanies the good. Alongside the well-accepted rewards of an organized youth sport program—the fun and friendships; the increased safety; the opportunity for proper instruction and promotion of values such as teamwork, discipline, and fair play—there is also risk. All too often, the pursuit of the spoils of competition (i.e., victories, championships, scholarships, and all the accolades of winning) completely overwhelm the more essential and healthier rewards of youth sport. The dramatic instances revealing the distorted priorities, loss of control, and even violent episodes among adults in youth sport are the observable tip of the iceberg.

The more pervasive, less obvious problems are the physical damage accompanying overuse injuries and the emotional issues that are visited upon children and adolescents in the name of competition and achievement. Physicians, physical therapists, and athletic trainers are often favorably situated at the nexus of youth, high school, and college sports and the physical and emotional problems that can be associated with the intense training and competition that exists at increasingly younger ages. They can, and must be, key agents in the challenging struggle to keep sports appropriately focused on what should be the over-riding mission of youth, high school, and even collegiate sports: promoting healthy physical and emotional development.

Although the numbers clearly demonstrate the pervasive appeal of organized youth sport, statistics also reveal a troubling increase in overuse injuries. Brenner and the American Academy of Pediatrics' Council on Sports Medicine and Fitness[2] state that the incidence of overuse injuries has more than kept pace with the increase in youth sport participation, citing research that 50% of all injuries seen in pediatric sports medicine are from overuse.[4]

Priorities that Physicians, Athletic Trainers, and Sports Physical Therapists Must Set in Caring for Young Athletes

- Ensure the young athlete's overall emotional and cognitive development, in addition to his or her physical development, are crucial factors for the athlete's well-being now and later in life.
- Shield the young athlete from the increased pressures and demands to perform and achieve at an earlier age than athletes of the past. These pressures appear to leave young athletes more vulnerable to injury and emotional burnout.

In addition to physical ailments and injuries associated with overuse and overtraining, the number of young athletes who burn out or drop out of sports has also dramatically increased. Control of children's athletic playtime has effectively become the domain of adults. Informal athletic play has disappeared secondary to the proliferation of organized sports at the earliest of ages and increasing reluctance to leave even older children and young teenagers "unsupervised." The financial, logistical, physical, and psychological strain on the families of young athletes caught in the crucible of increasingly fierce competition in youth sports can be relentless and pervasively consuming. The fight for prep school placement, for college admission, for playing spots on elite travel teams, for finding "just the right coach" on "just the right team" so that "Johnny's" or "Mary's" guaranteed athletic triumph can be secured can be overwhelming for even the most level-headed and emotionally balanced of families. This pressurized, athletic lifestyle appears to be starting earlier and earlier in the lives of young athletes and includes an increasing demand for advanced specialized training as well as demanding expectations for a singular focus in one sport.

These pressures on the young athlete might not always be for the greater good. Several studies suggest there is a growing split in children and adolescents with a small elite moving on to pursue intense athletic coaching and a worrisome majority quitting organized sport, particularly as they enter adolescence. This trend has been reinforced by spending cuts that have limited elementary school, junior high school, and after-school sports programs. As early as 1988, Gould and Petlichkoff reported that the rate for children who dropped out of their organized sport or dropped sport completely ranged up to 35%.[5] According to other studies, the statistics are even more troubling. Up to half of American youth do not engage in regular vigorous exercise according to the Centers for Disease Control.[6] Strikingly, the National Alliance of Youth Sports states that by age 13, 70% of American youth will drop out of sport.[7] Despite the disparity of these findings, there is agreement that one of the chief reasons children give for dropping a sport is simple: it is "no longer any fun."[8] As a result, teens are vulnerable to a sedate life of little or no physical activity that substitutes video games and television for exercise.

The young athletes who completely drop out and quit are reported to be more vulnerable to a slew of physical and emotional problems, including the obvious reduction in physical fitness, increased rates for depression, increased rates for sexual promiscuity for girls, as well as increased vulnerability to drug use and obesity.[9] Those who do not drop out are at risk for premature pressure secondary to becoming mini-sports franchises whose parents act as business managers for their young "free agents." Pediatricians from the Committee on Sports Medicine and Fitness for the American Academy of Pediatrics[10] recognized this pressure when they observed, "unrealistic parental expectations and/or exploitation of young athletes for extrinsic gain can contribute to negative psychological consequences for elite young athletes." Tofler and his colleagues[11] added that parents' behavior in youth sports can become particularly problematic if the parents fail to differentiate between their own needs for success and achievement and their child's emotional needs. The same could certainly be said for coaches and managers of elite teams, whose jobs and livelihoods depend on the performance of a young athlete, as well as on the satisfaction and financial backing of parents.

Injury and emotional overload are certainly not a given, and many young athletes and their parents manage to negotiate these issues to accrue great benefit from their sports participation without serious consequence. However, athletic trainers, sport physical therapists, and physicians are crucial to the health of young athletes and must serve as an early warning system for injury and recognition of emotional stress. A solid appreciation of what is at stake for the sports-oriented family can be critical for understanding the patient, building a good alliance and setting the stage for compliance with proper treatment, and facilitating a reasonable trajectory for the individual child's athletic talents.

The cultural pressures for achievement and the high status of the sports can affect everyone's judgment concerning what is best for the young athlete. They are not mini-adults—they are still developing cognitively and physically, and are actively learning from adult behaviors and values. Parents may push for inappropriate "age-specific" training such as intensive weight training to develop increased muscle mass in a prepubertal child. Parents can also be negative role models for what might be considered unsportsman-like conduct or behavior. More positively, the young athlete still has many developmental tasks such as peer relationships, down time, and, of course, academics (not just so that they are eligible but to learn how to learn for the rest of his or her career).

Clinical Point

All health providers, regardless of their area of expertise or specialty, need to focus on their patient, recognizing that the child and sometimes the parent will lose perspective and consider the next game as "make it or break it" the child's career.

What is the Healthy Focus for Youth Sports?

The answer to this question has very much to do with the age, skills, and the developmental realities of the athlete. As Fraser-Thomas and Cote[12] state in their review of recent findings in youth sport research, "youth sport should lead to physical health, psychosocial development and lifelong recreational or elite sport participation."

Balyi and Hamilton[13] have done interesting and extensive writing (but no substantive research) on a model of long-term athletic development. They have proposed a model that has been promoted as the basis of the national framework for coaching healthy and successful sports participation and achievement in Canada and the United Kingdom.[13] Briefly stated, Balyi and Hamilton stress the importance of recognizing the physical and emotional capabilities and needs of the developing young athlete. Their model (Table 3-1) makes allowances for differences between early specialization sports (e.g., diving, figure skating, gymnastics) and late specialization sports (most team sports as well as cycling, rowing, and racquet sports).[13]

The emphasis early on is for the young athlete to have fun and learn overall motor skills (6 to 10 years of age is the "FUNdamental" stage). As children enter ages 10 to 12 (with some variation for gender differences), the emphasis shifts to building the widest range of fundamental sport skills ("Learning to Train" stage). The "Training to Train" stage, which occurs at roughly 12 to 16 years of age, should aim to build the athlete's aerobic base and improve strength toward the end of the phase while further developing sport-specific skills. In the "Training to Compete" stage (approximately 15 to 18 years of age and beyond), athletes progress toward refining more specialized skills and tactics in their primary sport. This model allows for the gifted athlete who will go on to elite competition while also promoting lifelong fitness and athletic participation for all throughout childhood, adolescence, and adult life.[13] Although the scientific validity of this model as a high-performance template for national development of elite athletes is in dispute, its emphasis on a developmental approach for children and younger adolescent athletes is widely supported. The interested reader is encouraged to review Balyi and Hamilton's work for a more in-depth understanding of the goals of each sport developmental stage from preschool to retirement.[13]

Table 3-1
Bayli's Long-Term Athletic Achievement Model

Early Specialization Model	Late Specialization Model
1. Training to train stage	1. FUNdamental stage
2. Training to compete	2. Learning to train
3. Training to win	3. Training to train
4. Retirement/retainment	4. Training to compete
	5. Training to win
	6. Retirement/retainment

From Balyi I, Hamilton A: *Long-term athlete development: Trainability in childhood and adolescence. Windows of opportunity. Optimal trainability*, Victoria, 2004, National Coaching Institute British Columbia & Advanced Training and Performance Ltd.

Parents may be heavily influenced by recent studies by Ericcson and colleagues,[14] popularized by Malcolm Gladwell's best seller, *Outliers: The Story of Success*.[15] Ericcson found that 10 years or 10,000 hours of practice are required to reach an expert or elite level of performance.[14] These findings were originally based on expert chess players from Herbert Simon's original study in 1973 and virtuoso musicians.[16] Although there may be growing evidence that this "10,000 hour practice rule" holds true in a wide range of athletic endeavors (e.g., Ericcson does cite data supportive of the hypothesis for swimmers and marathon runners), much further study is required before the rule, "Earlier (age) is better and more (practice) is better" can be viewed as a risk-free enterprise for young athletes between the ages of 6 and 18.[14]

Currently, the approach most consistently supported by available research strongly suggests that adults involved in youth sports and parents of athletes from ages 6 to 12 need to encourage fun, friendship, and fitness as the true measures of their children's sporting success. Children in this age range should sample many sport experiences in which the emphasis is on enjoyment and gradually improving fitness and overall athletic skill. As children enter adolescence, they are generally capable of being introduced to more intense competition as well as a more vigorous development of specific sport skill and competencies. Still, it should be reiterated time and again that parents and coaches best serve their teen athletes by promoting, in order of importance, character, camaraderie, and athletic competence. A useful analogy is to think of the young athlete as an automobile: Talent is the engine; the more the talent, the more the horsepower. Good coaching is like the transmission that transforms the power of the engine to make the car move. Good coaching helps the athlete translate his or her talent into real action. But crucially, good character is akin to not only a proper steering mechanism but a well-trained, safe driver. Talent without good coaching will necessarily underperform. Talent and good coaching without proper character may not only underperform, but may also lead the athlete to "recklessly drive into a tree" and self-destruct. The promotion of good character is the ultimate insurance policy that an athlete will have a chance, barring injury, to get the most out of his or her talent. Because the prevalent currents of "win-at-all-costs" and "do everything you can do to play" are swift and powerful, all adults and, most importantly, all health care providers involved in youth and scholastic sports must fully grasp the importance of this mission.

Adults Involved in Youth Sports and Parents Should Stress

- Fun, friendship, and fitness in 6- to 12-year-olds
- Character, camaraderie, and athletic competence in teens

Health care providers can point out to parents that, ironically, the very best sport psychologists seeking to enhance excellent performances in their athletes unanimously emphasize the goal of mastery and the joy of the sport as key components of success. Parents need to be reminded that overspecialization and an overemphasis on outcome may actually decrease the player's confidence and enjoyment and can increase the likelihood that their children will join the ranks of the sporting dropouts, burnouts, and injured.

Key Psychosocial Components to Success in Sport

- Joy of taking part in sport
- Mastery of the sport

What Makes Winning so Special?

There are many factors that make the thrill of "winning" intoxicating and powerful. Biologically, a child or teenager engages the deeply wired "fight or flight" response in many of the competitive sports activities. The experience of the fear, passion, and stress of competition also helps to fuel the sense of pleasure and release that comes with winning. Competition biologically stimulates the physiological state of parents and coaches, as well as young players. All of this biology is embedded in a family that may be under considerable pressure (e.g., time, finances, competing priorities). When the combination of individual parents, who have both high hopes for their children and possibly unfulfilled hopes from their own childhoods, is added to all of the potential cultural rewards of athletic success, there is a powerful effect on the child. Health care providers are frequently at the front lines trying to balance the pressures to win with the realities of what is in the best interests of the child. Winning can be considered so special that it overwhelms other values, priorities, and even sportsmanship. Evidence of undesirable behavior can be seen in steroid use, undue pressure on or by the injured athlete to return prematurely, undue privileges for the gifted star athlete, and the not-so-subtle promotion of a "win-at-all-costs" attitude.

Performance Enhancement

The Essential Questions and Three Steps for Parents of Athletes

One of the key tools of effective sports psychology for performance enhancement is goal setting. Goal setting allows for the mapping and measuring of sports success. But goals must be guided by a broader statement of purpose and ultimate intent, a mission statement. The very first challenge for the parents of young athletes is to answer the following questions to establish their family's sports mission: "When my child is 21 years old, what kind of person do I want him or her to be, and how will sports help us as parents get our child there?"

We advocate that parents focus on three to five virtues that they cherish and make sure that sports always serve to promote and build those virtues. This is effectively done by following the following three steps.

Know Your Child

One would not ask 8-year-olds to baby sit, nor would one expect 12-year-olds to drive a car. Adults easily seem to understand that children need to grow and mature before they are capable of mastering certain skills and responsibilities. However, in sports, parents and coaches often expect consistent, adult-like performances from their young athletes. Adult expectations for young athletes need to be in tune with physical, cognitive, and psychological developmental realities. In addition, children are unique, with different temperaments; idiosyncrasies; rich and varied ethnic, cultural, and family backgrounds; and their own histories. A sports program that *fits the needs of the child* necessarily takes this important knowledge into account.

Key Tools for Parents for Performance Enhancement in Children

- Set goals
- Have a sports mission
- Know your child and his or her stage of physiological and emotional development
- Know yourself and your own personal "baggage"
- Know the child's sport environment
- Know the sport's culture
- Know how to deal with over-involved parents

Know Yourself

Adults, whether acting in the role of parent, coach, or caregiver, each have their own histories of success and failure in the athletic domain. With increasing frequency during the past decades since organized sport participation has blossomed, many adults involved in youth and high school sports carry their own complex narratives about competition with strongly held notions and even scripts of how things should be. Sometimes parents (and even entire communities such as that profiled in the compelling book about Texas high school football by H.G. Bissinger, *Friday Night Lights*[17]) can hope to right the wrongs of their own lives and erase the sting of past or present failures through their children's athletic success. This unresolved psychological baggage makes it extremely difficult for some parents and coaches to truly see what is best for the young athlete. Trainers, physical therapists, and physicians need to be aware of these subtle, unseen issues that cloud what should be a clear history and picture of what the young athlete needs. Sometimes these parental hopes go beyond sports to include college entry, scholarships, and then developing a profile allegedly attractive for a business career.

Know Your Child's Sports Environment and Culture

Our culture places an enormous premium on winning as the ultimate justification and sign of success. Often success in youth and high school sports is seen as the ticket to a good prep school or college placement.

In fact, less than 1% of all high school athletes receive any form of athletic scholarship at the National Collegiate Athletic Association (NCAA) Division 1 level.[18] And only 5.5% of all high school athletes progress to play intercollegiate sports at 4-year institutions.[18] Parents guiding their college-bound athletes need to learn about playing time, the coach's level of training for the sport in question, familiarity with safety procedures and proper injury protocol, as well as background screening for adults in the program. The health care provider associating himself or herself with high school and college programs should be aware of the level of expertise, the common practices, and program philosophy.

By keeping the focus of youth and high school sports on fitness and healthy physical development as well as on the development of specific virtues associated with a good character, such as courage, compassion, perseverance, a sense of justice and fair play, respect for others, dedication, effort, and teamwork, parents ensure that their children will get the most out of their athletic talent over an entire lifespan.

Dealing with the Over-Involved Parent

Parents of young children are often unprepared for an onslaught of unprecedented pressure to enroll their kids in competitive youth sports at a young age. YMCA and community-based programs start at age 4 or 5 and, for the ambitious parent, serve as a path to club soccer, Amateur Athletic Union (AAU) basketball, and elite swimming programs. Summer camps and tournaments throughout the year are "show cases," necessary next steps to ensure talent development and a future college scholarship. The recent financial recession has probably increased these pressures. Some parents fear that failure to start sports participation early and intensely will deprive their children of future happiness and success. As their anxiety mounts, some parents may become zealous about their children's sport activities, which often takes the form of intense over-involvement. As previously mentioned, *Outliers,* by Malcolm Gladwell, has both added and changed the focus of these pressures.[15] Gladwell debunks the myth of unique talent and yet may add to the pressure by pointing out the importance of age and date-of-birth cut off policies in various leagues, the role of opportunity and chance, and the critical effect of culture.[15] All of these influences facilitate the final common pathway to

excellence, which is (allegedly) 10,000 hours of practice at increasingly elite levels.

Much research attention has focused on the role of parents in youth sports. When parents are attentive, positive, and supportive, their children have more fun, have more positive beliefs about their abilities, and are likelier to continue sports participation over time.[19-22] Problems occur when parent involvement becomes distracting or preoccupying to their children. Such involvement can take both overt and subtle forms. In their most recognizable forms, overzealous and over-involved parents may cheer too loudly at athletic contests; be harsh critics of other coaches or referees; offer overly critical feedback to their child before, during, or after practices and games; or burden their children's coaches with comments and suggestions. Their thoughts and behaviors are often well intentioned, but translate into various expressions of pressure to their children. Researchers have found that children experience increased anxiety, greater risk of burnout, and less enjoyment when their parents burden them with pressure and unrealistic expectations.[23,24] The child might feel he or she is not "good enough" to meet the parent's expectations and thus, despite considerable accomplishment, have an underlying sense of low self-esteem. Children and especially teenagers may see quitting a sport as a solution to the pressure.

Parents Should be
• Attentive
• Positive
• Supportive
• Have realistic expectations

More commonly, over-involved parenting evolves subtly over time. An occasional disappointed facial expression or a seemingly benign comment about the child's play contributes to this slowly building pressure. The child is unable to articulate what is bothering him or her and the parent's behavior is too insignificant in an isolated moment for others to take notice. What starts out as mild irritation becomes a deeper burden for the child, gradually undermining the enjoyment of play and the quality of performance. As the child's performance worsens, the parent becomes increasingly concerned and involved, often exacerbating the situation.[25]

Clinicians may detect these subtler forms of pressure by asking key questions of both the child and parent. Observing differences in the child's and parent's responses to these questions can often provide a clearer picture of the child–parent dynamic and reveal how the pressure is being expressed. In the best circumstances, these discussions can lead to greater awareness and prompt healthier adjustments.

Detecting Parental Pressure in Child Athletes: a Clinician's Guide of Questions to Ask Families of a Child Athlete

- Does the child ever feel like skipping practice or even a game?
- Who is the one who most wants the child to play? How much fun is the child actually having when playing?
- Does the intensity of play and competition fit the child's physical and psychological development?
- How would the family feel if the child quit or played a different sport?
- What expectations do family members have about the child's athletic career?
- Is there an expectation that the child will play college sports and what are the chances this will actually happen? (Data from the NCAA indicates that approximately 5% of high school senior athletes continue to play sports at the college level.[18])
- How much time and energy is being consumed by playing sports and how does this fit into the overall schedule for the family?
- Does the child get hurt a lot or sometimes seem to complain more then makes sense for the injury?
- What was your (the parents') experience of sports like when you were growing up?

NCAA, National Collegiate Athletic Association.

Sometimes addressing overzealous and over-involved parenting is a complicated and sensitive endeavor. Parents are frequently so involved and intensely invested in their child's training and competitive play that it is even difficult for them to step back momentarily to reflect on their behavior. Research from Smith and colleagues' seminal study on coaching behaviors[26] reveals that coaches are poor at assessing the effect of their behaviors in the athletic context. Based on this pattern, it is safe to assume that the same is true for parents. They simply cannot see how their behavior may be upsetting those around them in the stands and on the field, and as a result are surprised and even offended when such behavior is brought to their attention.

When clinicians consider confronting the parents of adolescent athletes, they may first try to encourage the athletes to communicate with their parents directly before intervening themselves. As adolescents get older, they need to be encouraged to advocate for themselves and resolve their own problems as they strive for independence, a developmental milestone crucial to their path toward adulthood. For instance, a clinician may suggest that an adolescent boy whose father is pressuring him say, "Dad, when you yell during games, I know you really care, but it makes me nervous. Could you please try to keep it down during the games?" Guiding athletes to recognize and appreciate their parents' involvement initially can help ease the sting of their confrontation. Careful timing may also help such confrontations to succeed. Conversations with parents are most successful long after the game or after the heated moments have passed.

Clinicians working with children or adolescents with particularly difficult parents may have to speak to the parents directly. Frequently, the intensity of the parent involvement is centered on pushing his or her child to perform better or try harder. What makes these parents unconscious or defensive about their over-involvement? For some reason, their child's athletic accomplishment has become so important that it must have roots in the parent's own growing up. The accomplishment, recognition, or fame of their child is seen as belonging to the parents, themselves, rather than as the success and choice of an independent person. Is this because they were harshly driven as a child? Were their parents insensitive to some independent need they had as a child? Did they fail at sports as a child or get an "unfair" break that unjustly ruined their career and they are not going to let that happen to their child? Rigid defensiveness and denial are difficult for us as clinicians and more often reflect a solution parents are using to mask a deeper problem, feeling, or memory that they cannot consciously bear.

Clinicians can be quite effective in alleviating some of these tensions by addressing with the parent the potential physical risks to the young athlete who is being pushed too hard. For example, a clinician may ask, "How hard on a scale of 1 to 10 do you think your daughter is being pushed with the current program? Is this higher or lower than you feel is best? What are the likely rewards and risks? What if I told you that if your daughter or son continues to train and play under this kind of pressure, it increases her or his risk of injury that may not only take her or him out for the season but may also have damaging effects on her or his body as she or he reaches adulthood?"

Clinical Point

Athletic trainers and sports physical therapists typically have tremendous perspective into the inner workings of young athletes and their families. The informal time spent in the training room before and after practice is often when athletes express their feelings or reveal through their behavior and demeanor their level of sport satisfaction. Communication between the therapist or trainer and treating physician can greatly enhance the understanding of young athletes and their family dynamics.

The various perspectives of treating clinicians assist in an overall discussion with the family to help them focus on the present life of their child athlete rather than a somewhat distorted focus on the child's future achievements. Parents may benefit from being grounded in the developmental markers of their growing children to foster more realistic expectations. For example, many young athletes may continue to grow well into their late teen years. Some of these athletes may simply not be ready for the physical and emotional rigors of their present training programs or teams. More rest and fewer demands may be appropriate recommendations.

It is often helpful to ask parents about their short- and long-term goals for their child's athletics: For example, what are their goals for their child's health, discipline, friendships, pleasure, scholarships, professional career, or self-esteem? What are their goals if the child does not hold up under the pressure of regional, state, or national pyramids? Do they appreciate that their child has ultimate control by giving up the sport or even unconsciously over-reacting to an injury, developing disabling psychosomatic illness, or becoming overwhelmed at the next level of competition? A sophisticated discussion about these issues and pathways may help, or nature may have to take its course with a less than optimal outcome. Lastly, it is always helpful to remind families that an enjoyable connection to physical activity is perhaps the most important goal to enhance the long-term health of their children as they progress into adulthood and beyond.

Considerations for Dealing with the Injured Athlete

Insights from research on the psychological responses to physical and emotional trauma as experienced by victims of violence or combat veterans can be useful in assisting the injured athlete. Table 3-2 offers a useful schema for understanding where the injured athlete might be emotionally in the course of injury and recovery.

The Initial Psychological Response to Physical Injury

In the initial shock of an injury, there can be a cluster of overwhelming emotions that flood the injured athlete. This initial cognitive and emotional reaction to the shock of injury and trauma often involves fear, a sense of disconnectedness or sense of things not being real, and a sense of captivity or feelings of being trapped.

Certainly, the injured athlete often experiences a high level of anxiety and fear, which, in the case of serious injuries such as broken bones or torn ligaments, can become gut-wrenching and sickening terror. This is especially true for the young athlete, who may have no history of overcoming real adversity beyond the playing field.

Accompanying the fear can be a sense of captivity, the sense that one is trapped by the injury. Often injury results in a physical inability to move, and in a literal sense the athlete is trapped in a prone or immobilized position. For athletes whose preferred mode of self-expression is the ability to move their body at will with grace and power, this can be psychologically overwhelming. Outbursts of angry frustration, tears, and reckless attempts to over-ride the injury through sheer force of will are not uncommon.

There is often a brief, cognitive disconnectedness from the reality of the trauma, a sense that the injury isn't real—"This can't be happening to me. I never get hurt. I'm bulletproof!" There can also be a powerful urge to engage in protective denial—"It's not that bad. It's only a sprain. I can play." This expectation to "play in pain" is often aided and abetted by coaches, parents, teammates, and fans, who also can be caught up in the heat of competition. We have witnessed an overzealous father who engaged in a heated exchange that threatened to become violent because an athletic trainer refused to clear a high school football player back to the playing field following a concussion. The father only relented when his son plaintively exclaimed, "Dad, it's only a stupid game!" Caregivers in these situations might be the only voice of caution, reason, and firm reassurance that the injured athlete can and will be properly treated.

Psychological Features of the Injured Athlete Following Injury

In the days and weeks directly following a serious injury that results in lost practice and playing time, athletes are likely to experience a characteristic cluster of emotions and behaviors. These include hyperaroused responses, intrusive effects, and emotional withdrawal or avoidance.

Hyperarousal can frequently be understood as an "All hands on deck! Battle Stations!" response, which can be both adaptive yet counterproductive to the healing process. Athletes recovering from the initial shock of their injury might often manifest an intense zeal "to do whatever it takes to get back on the field." This desire can make them amenable to a disciplined approach and a zealous compliance to treatment that the non-athlete might not bring to the doctor's, therapist's, or trainer's office. Such an athlete initially can really be a "super" patient. However, this intense feeling can easily morph into something less than helpful or healthy if frustration arises because the pace of healing isn't what the injured athlete expected. There can be a grandiose self-perception that if the normal healing time is 8 weeks, the athlete will make it in half the time—"I said I'd be back in 4 weeks max! It's been 4 weeks. I'm ready to PLAY NOW!"

Table 3-2

Psychological Response to Injury and Recovery

Event (Initial Response to Injury)	Symptoms (Following Injury)	Recovery (Recovery from Injury)
Terror (Fear in mid- or post-trauma)	Hyperarousal (Forced healing)	Safety (Predictable outcome)
Captivity (No quick fix)	Intrusion (Preoccupied with injury)	Adjustment (Dealing with limits)
Disconnection (Protective denial)	Emotional withdrawal (Depression/despair)	Reconnection (Restoration of health)

Data from Herman, JL: Trauma & Recovery, New York, 1994, Basic Books.

The injured athlete might also be susceptible to intrusive effects that hinder the healing process and undermine his or her overall health. Intrusive effects can manifest as an inability to sleep, a preoccupation with the injury and recovery, an inability to concentrate on school work or other interests, and even an obsessive replaying of the injury with an "if only X had been different, I wouldn't have been hurt" scenario. At its most severe, these intrusive effects can include a startle reflex or a hypersensitivity to any movement involving the injury or even external movement in the vicinity of the injury. For example, a young injured athlete might irritably explode at a sibling or friend who accidentally nudges the crutches or at a parent who doesn't respond quickly enough to a request that is seen as vital in the injured athlete's eyes.

In addition to the intrusive effects of his or her own thoughts, fears, and worries, the injured athlete must also fend off what can feel like an incessant and monotonous litany of inquiries from caring family, friends, and fans. In some professional sports, players are zealously protected from the constant focus and emotionally draining effects of never-ending questions: "How are you feeling? Is your injury getting better? When do you expect to return to play?" Although well intentioned, the constant attention paid to an injury often serves to emotionally exhaust the injured athlete and act as a trigger for negative thoughts about the healing process. Health care professionals serve their athletes well by reviewing this phenomenon with their athletes and strategizing about acceptable ways to diplomatically cocoon them from the intrusive and tiresome questioning they may encounter.

In short, parents, coaches, and health care providers can greatly help the injured athlete by monitoring the fundamentals of good health. Adequate physical and emotional rest; proper hydration and diet; appropriate exercise that does not exacerbate the injury; avoidance of an obsessive focus on the injury; and a balanced approach to home life, academics, and friendships are important factors in the healing process for young athletes.

Finally, it is not unusual for the injured athlete to go through a period of emotional withdrawal or avoidance and possible mini-depression. Just as naval crewmen at battle stations eventually need to stand down lest fatigue and exhaustion overtake them, so too the injured athlete can rarely sustain the gung-ho, hyperaroused "I will force myself to heal sooner" approach to recovery. Eventually, the injured athlete hits the wall of realization that his or her body is well and truly damaged. There will be no magical overnight recovery. Playing time will be lost. This can often hit the young athlete extremely hard.

It is important to remember that young athletes do not have the experience of an adult to fall back on. They have not yet had a life that includes successfully dealing with painful loss, suffering, and adversity and overcoming these trials and tribulations with a fully operational *adult* brain. These patients are in need of clear information on what they can expect, along with ample doses of accurate reassurance and emotional support from knowledgeable health care providers. In addition, trainers, physicians, and sport physical therapists must be able to set firm limits based on sound clinical judgment for the often unrealistic expectations and subtle pressures exerted by parents, coaches, and teammates on their young athletes.

Psychological Features of Recovery for the Injured Athlete

A relative sense of emotional safety is a crucial psychological element in the recovery from trauma. This may take the form of the athlete's recognition that those charged with assisting the healing process are knowledgeable and understand how crucial a return to play is for the injured athlete. The desired outcome of the initial encounter with any health care provider is that sense of recognition of the nature of the injury and course of treatment, but also a sense of reassurance and even relief. "Okay, I am really injured but these guys have helped other athletes with this type of injury so maybe they do know how to help *me*."

This sense of relief and trust in an injured athlete is a function of good "trainer's table" or "bedside" interpersonal skills, as well as effective communication of predictable outcome. The younger the athlete, the more concrete, simple, and repetitive the instructions regarding the course of treatment should be. For example, the health care provider who bluntly orders "Rest!" to the young athletic patient without a more careful step-by-step explanation that outlines the course of recovery, or at least improved functioning, will run the risk of losing the young athlete to a dismissive, noncompliant, and even defiant approach to treatment.

As the injured athlete gradually begins to trust the healing process and builds a sense of trust with his or her doctor, sport physical therapist, and athletic trainer, his or her feelings, comments, and behaviors should begin to reflect a sense that he or she is adapting and adjusting to the process of recovery. This adjustment phase may include some behaviors that are similar to grieving. Comments or behaviors that reflect mourning for the lost playing time or season are not uncommon. For some athletes, there may be a lingering emotional avoidance and withdrawal from all contact with their sport. Other athletes prefer to remain on the sidelines as an observer. The rule of thumb is that people are entitled to grieve in many ways. There is no preferred way to emotionally recover from the losses inflicted by a serious injury. Some behaviors are certainly better than others. Provided the patient is complying with treatment, maintaining healthy relationships, and meeting his or her academic requirements, then the issue of whether an injured young athlete seeks to withdraw from a high level of interaction with the sport should be left to the athlete. For some, an injury can actually provide a surprising window into how life outside the sport can be interesting and fulfilling.

If the recovery process has been successful, then the athlete will enter a phase of reconnection to his or her previous athletic endeavors. This return to the playing field and presumably to the previous level of participation can be as challenging as the earlier stages of injury. This can especially be true for physicians, sport physical therapists, or athletic trainers who must deal with the athlete, parent, and coach who may have a distorted and overly optimistic view of what "recovery" means. The coach who attempts to motivate the recovered athlete by saying, "The doc said you're all better! So you should be good to go!" might not recognize the depth of the athlete's hesitancy and shaky confidence that he or she is fully recovered. The young athlete is also frequently unable to articulate what he or she is feeling and sensing emotionally as well as physically. Therefore, he or she may be unable to express the anxiety being experienced. Furthermore, the athlete may not even be aware that he or she is anxious! For example, the athlete who has recovered from anterior cruciate ligament surgery and the long rehabilitation process still faces a significant hurdle in psychologically trusting his or her repaired knee in the heat of competition. The seasoned coach and caregiver can often detect the hesitancy and tentativeness in the athlete returning from injury.

Clinical Point

Caregivers who can predict, clearly state and normalize some of the difficulties that the returning athlete may experience, can go a long way toward reassuring and calming the jittery, newly healed athlete.

Burnout, Staleness, or Just a Slump?

Burnout has been defined as "state of mental, emotional and physical exhaustion brought on by persistent devotion to a goal whose achievement is dramatically opposed to reality."[28-30] *Burnout* differs from the idea of *staleness*, which has been defined as an early warning sign of possible burnout characterized by diminishing physical and emotional capabilities. The term *slump* usually refers to a diminished performance that may or may not be a function of staleness or burnout. A baseball batter in a slump may in fact be hitting the ball well and not be suffering from staleness or imminent burnout, but in fact may be well-energized and just hitting the ball right at well-positioned fielders. Burnout, staleness, and slump fall under umbrella term of *maladaptive fatigue syndrome.*

Maladaptive Fatigue Syndrome

- Burnout
- Staleness
- A slump

Burnout seems to more frequently occur in quiet, perfectionistic, highly coachable athletes who work too hard and too intensely for too long in unrewarding situations.[31,32] Coakley[24] notes that the external constraints and social limitations placed on athletes hampers the development of a well-balanced, healthy identity and lifestyle and increases the risk of burnout in many collegiate athletic programs. Tofler and colleagues[11] state, "Children should feel that parental love or a relationship with critical adults is not contingent on winning or excelling in any one educational, sporting, career or social goal." Young athletes who are trapped in a situation in which they must live up to the unrealistic expectations of parents, coaches, and the community are at greater risk for burnout and arrested emotional development.

More recent research based on the self-determination theory of Deci and Ryan[33] suggests that burnout occurs when three basic psychological needs—autonomy, competence, and relatedness—have been chronically frustrated. There can be multiple factors that contribute to staleness or burnout. These factors include the length of the season, the monotony of training, lack of positive reinforcement, abusive coaches, overly stringent rules, player boredom, a perception of low achievement and failure, high levels of competitive stress, a sense of being overloaded and helpless to effect constructive change in the sporting environment, and a sense of being trapped in an untenable situation.

Whatever the theoretical underpinning of this phenomenon, health care providers must be well versed in the symptoms of burnout so as to help the struggling athlete and accurately determine when physical complaint is masking a deeper, potentially debilitating emotional and physical exhaustion.

Signs of Burnout in Athletes

- Increased fatigue or prolonged weariness
- Increased irritability or apathy
- Increased somatic complaints or injuries with no apparent pathological cause
- Consistent feelings of intense ambivalence toward practice or competition, including an expressed desire to quit
- Frequent missed practices or skipped games
- Inexplicable pattern of poor athletic performance
- Decreased confidence
- Behaviors that sabotage further athletic participation
- Narrowing of appropriate developmental opportunities in the service of sport commitment (especially for teens)
- Parents who engage in a pattern of risky sacrifice to aid child's athletic career (serious life choices or family decisions seem rashly and overly based on the parents' view of a child's athletic potential)

Treatment for Burnout and Staleness

Review of the literature reveals consistent recommendations for the alleviation of burnout or maladaptive fatigue.[34] These interventions involve appreciating the need for time away from the sport, a mental and physical break or time out. For example, in the professional baseball, hockey, and basketball ranks, "the All Star break" is generally recognized as a time that most players necessarily use to recharge themselves emotionally and physically. In the National Football League and NCAA football, there are often "bye" weeks during which players are given days off completely away from football. The American Academy of Pediatrics[35] outlines specific recommendations that include limiting sporting activity to a maximum of 5 days per week with at least 1 day completely free from organized physical activity. Regularly scheduled breaks from training and competition in any one sport, with time away every 2 to 3 months to cross-train or to focus on other activities are also strongly recommended.[34]

Increased athlete input in decision-making and control can increase motivation and morale and deter burn out. Team captains, in their roles as chief liaison between team and coach, can often assist in informing coaches of the state of individual or team morale. Certainly, athletic trainers, sport physical therapists, and team physicians, who are so often deeply trusted and ever-present confidantes for the athlete, may be in a position to subtly convey to the coaching staff through direct or indirect means the need for an emotional break or change in routine to re-energize the athlete.

Improved management of postcompetition tension is also cited as an important area for reducing burnout, staleness, and team friction. This includes protecting athletes from overly emotional responses to victory or defeat and reducing overall postgame stimuli as well as overly critical individual, player-to-player, and coach-to-player responses. Again, athletic trainers, sport physical therapists, and physicians may be in a position to quietly recommend practices that protectively cocoon the athlete and help diffuse postgame emotional overload. As we have previously highlighted, the preservation of enjoyment (Henschen calls it the "fun factor")[34] is an indispensable tool in preventing burnout and staleness. Athletes who are having fun do not burn out. Increased input from players; adequate physical and emotional time away from the grind to relax and recharge the body, mind, and spirit; as well as keeping practices up-tempo, interesting, and fun all serve to prevent and address sports staleness and burnout.

Burnout and Depression

In addition to identifying potential cases of burnout, the health care provider must be prepared for the possibility that an athlete may be dealing with a more serious emotional issue beyond burnout or staleness such as major depression. Because the burned-out athlete might be reacting to stressors from a home environment and areas of life outside of the sports domain, discerning where burnout ends and major depression begins can be difficult. For example, it is not unusual for young athletes to be painfully caught between competing emotional pulls from separating or divorcing parents. This tension can frequently be played out at the sports venue as athletes nervously try to gauge who is there and what will be required to appease each parent and keep the peace. "Who do I acknowledge first? What will each parent want from me? How will I juggle their irreconcilable requests?" Athletes in these situations often get worn down by being forced to sacrifice their sporting life to their parents' needs. This social dilemma meets the criteria for potential burnout with an untenable, unwinnable, trapped situation in which the athlete in question cannot live up to others' expectations. Burnout certainly could result from such a scenario, but so too could a reactive depression emerge if the untenable situation exists in other areas of life and is not addressed. If burnout continues unabated for the athlete, then major depression can result.

As Coakley points out,[24] the social landscape of competitive sports often lends itself to a limited and fragile, one-dimensional identity: "I am first and foremost, a basketball player. If I am failing at that, I am a failure". In this type of culture, just as unchecked staleness can lead to burnout, unaddressed burnout can lead to a deeper depression. In general, however, depression most often differs from burnout or staleness in that the negative emotional state exists in virtually all areas of the athlete's life and is not alleviated by addressing the conditions on the team or in the environment that have caused the sports malaise.

The eight symptoms for a major depression cued by the mnemonic "SIGECAPS" are listed in Box 3-1. If the conditions of burnout have been addressed and five of the eight symptoms listed in Box 3-1 have been present for 2 weeks, then the athlete in question should be referred to his or her physician and then on to a mental health professional.

Box 3-1 Signs of Depression (SIGECAPS)[36]

1. **Sleep** (increase or decrease)
2. **Interest/pleasure** (socially less active, reduced libido)
3. **Guilt** or ruminations (self-blame): possibly manifested as irritability
4. **Energy** (decreased/not motivated): indifference
5. **Concentration** (cannot focus or make decisions)
6. **Appetite** (increase or decrease)
7. **Psychomotor** (agitation [adolescents] or lethargy)
8. **Suicide** (thoughts and/or plans about death and dying)

Note: Five symptoms over a 2-week period constitute a major depressive episode.

Dealing with Athletes with Attention Deficit Disorder

Attention deficit disorder and *attention deficit hyperactivity disorder* (ADD/ADHD) are psychological conditions that exist in approximately 3% to 5% of the population,[36] but some experts cite higher incidence rates.[37] The prevalence is higher for boys than girls. ADD/ADHD can be diagnosed by the presence of a cluster of symptoms that include significantly elevated levels of distractibility, inattentiveness, and cognitive or behavioral impulsivity.[36] These weaknesses often undermine academic performance and can affect athletic performance as well as compliance to medical treatment.

Often, there are secondary psychological features of ADD or ADHD, including difficulty with organizational and executive tasks such as fluidly handling transitions or following through on multistep tasks.[36] It is important to note that often individuals with ADD/ADHD may be more prone to engage in high-risk or thrill-seeking behaviors. This may be especially true for boys. Untreated ADD/ADHD may place the individual at risk for addictive, self-medicating behaviors such as substance abuse, sexual acting out, fighting, and gambling. Anecdotally, there is some evidence to suggest that athletes as a group may manifest a much higher incidence rate of ADD/ADHD and the behaviors that have come to be associated with the condition.

It is easy to understand how the constellation of these symptoms in an athlete might pose both a threat to the maintenance of consistent good health and training practices as well as an impediment to the successful implementation of therapeutic treatment and preventative or rehabilitative work. The ADD/ADHD pattern of inattentiveness, impulsivity, risk-taking, and stubbornly rigid thinking or hyperfocus leaves these athletes more vulnerable to accident and injury. They may miss important information from coaches and health care providers, which in turn may decrease consistent compliance with preventative conditioning practices as well as proper playing technique. Ironically, the athlete with ADD/ADHD might be more likely to both over-do it and under-do it because they may manifest both a stubborn, single-mindedness and a reckless, haphazard style as they follow the beat of their own drummer.

In general, the pressures that exist for the injured athlete as outlined earlier in the chapter can be presumed to exist to a greater degree in the athlete with ADD or ADHD. The impatience, impulsivity, inattention, and possible poor judgment that so often exists with ADD/ADHD increases the likelihood of ignoring treatment protocols, recklessly forcing "a rush to health," and seeking alternative and possibly contraindicated therapies.

Untreated ADD/ADHD can result in underperformance and behavioral problems in school, home, and in the community in general. These individuals may be more likely to get depressed in response to a persistent pattern of relative failure and subsequent interpersonal difficulties with teachers, parents, coaches, and even peers.

It is recommended that caregivers take careful histories when dealing with their athletes to determine whether their patients are currently being treated for ADD/ADHD. Often athletes avoid taking prescribed medication when training or competing as they may identify their problems as being solely a school-based phenomenon. Parents concerned about unnecessarily medicating children may at times put pressure on their child athlete to forego the use of their prescribed medicine. This practice of not medicating during athletics or recreational activities may or may not be appropriate. The student-athlete with ADD/ADHD may need and benefit from medication for endeavors outside of the academic domain. The issues regarding athletes' use of medication for treatment of ADD/ADHD need to be addressed on a case-by-case basis in consultation with the athlete's primary care physician or treatment specialist.

Athletes with undiagnosed ADD/ADHD can pose a coaching, parenting, and treatment problem that may present in several ways. These patients may appear as the athlete whose inattentiveness or impulsivity leads to dangerous, high-risk play in practice and competition and therefore frequent injury or physical complaint. In noncontact sports, this risky behavior may present as overtraining to the point of physical burnout or overuse injury.

Sometimes the inattentiveness and problems with following multitask instruction might give the athlete a reputation for being "spacey" or unintelligent. Female athletes with undiagnosed ADD/ADHD can be mislabeled in such a manner because, perhaps for cultural reasons, they may not display the higher risk behaviors or impulsive outbursts of anger that can typify the ADHD presentation in the male athlete. Finally, the stubborn, noncompliant athlete who routinely presents as being unable to contain his or her irritability at the treatment regimen and fails to follow medical advice may also be exhibiting signs of ADD/ADHD. For example, although many injured athletes wearing a cast for a fractured limb express deep dissatisfaction and threaten to forcibly remove the cast, it stands to reason that the ADD/ADHD athlete is more likely to act on that irritability and impulsively remove the protective cast against all medical advice. There are multiple anecdotes of athletes who cut off their casts so they could play. These stories unfortunately can serve to glorify the physical and mental toughness of the athlete and can be passively condoned by coaches, teammates, parents, and supporters. These athletes, as well as their extended network of relationships, need vigilant follow-up supervision with ongoing reassurance regarding the efficacy of the treatment plan. Frequent reminders that such impulsive acts expose the athlete to chronic injury or possible career-ending debilitation may be necessary.

In conclusion, athletes with a history of inexplicable academic difficulty, as well as problems associated with inattentiveness, distractibility, impulsive behaviors, and a pattern of reckless or thrill-seeking acts should be referred to their primary care physician or a mental health specialist for appropriate evaluation and possible treatment.

Possible Risks Associated with ADD/ADHD in Athletes Recovering from Injury

- Pattern of thrill-seeking or risk-taking behaviors
- Noncompliance or impatience with recovery (may seek alternative therapies)
- Increased substance use
- Increased irritability, oppositional defiance, or fighting
- Increased addictive behaviors (e.g., sex, gambling, video games)
- Increased depressive symptoms
- Decreased academic performance
- Recurring injury, accident, or other trauma

ADD, Attention deficit disorder; *ADHD*, attention deficit hyperactivity disorder.

Dealing with the Concussion: Psychological Considerations

Sports-related concussions that include a loss of consciousness are estimated to occur in 300,000 athletes in the United States each year.[38] Because, by definition, concussions can occur without a loss of consciousness, many researchers view these numbers as a gross underestimate of the problem by as much as 50%.[39] All sports-related concussions should be viewed as serious because they pose a threat to the young athlete that only in recent years is being fully realized. Young athletes appear more susceptible to *second-impact syndrome,* a condition that results from a second head injury before full recovery from an initial concussion. This phenomenon can lead to acute and long-term neurological and neuropsychological problems that in rare cases have been fatal in athletes, especially athletes 18 and younger. Because of the hidden nature of head injury, many concussions are unseen, unrecognized, unreported, and therefore undiagnosed and untreated. Because a blow to the head might result in a dazed or confused state, many athletes might not remember or understand the importance of their symptoms. Athletes are trained and conditioned to ignore pain and physical adversity. Even the language of athletes serves to downplay potentially serious head injury: "I'm okay, I just got a ding." At times, the nature of competitive sports is such that the athlete may intentionally hide the injury from the training and medical staff for fear of loss of playing time or loss of status with his or her peers or coach.

The competitive pressure to continue to compete even in the presence of a concussion that includes a loss of consciousness is a very powerful phenomenon. Recently, in an international rugby match between Scotland and Wales in 2009, a player was seriously concussed while making a tackle. It was clear on video, replayed on the stadium screen, that the player in question had knocked himself unconscious as his head hit an opposing player in a violent tackle. The player's body went limp upon impact but, fortunately, he was cushioned from an unprotected, face-first fall by the body of his opponent. Six to seven medical staff attended the injured rugby player for several minutes, during which time it was obvious to the television commentators and spectators that the player had been rocked in the tackle and that, at least initially, the player was dazed and unsteady on his feet. Despite his symptoms, including a brief loss of consciousness, the player was allowed to continue play for another 10 minutes. During this time, he was involved in further physical contact on at least five occasions while both tackling and running with the ball. It was left to the match referee to order the player off the pitch after he witnessed the player on his knees vomiting. The referee was distinctly heard to say, "He still hasn't recovered from the tackle. I'm not happy with that at all. I want him off!" Hence, it was left to a neutral, nonmedical official to accurately recognize the danger the injured player was in and act in his best interest. This unfortunate but perhaps not uncommon example of trained medical personnel allowing a concussed athlete back in a highly competitive, passionately contested contact sport sends a bad message to athletes at all age levels, coaches, parents, and fans. **"Do no harm"** is the mission, and concussed athletes placed back in the fray will necessarily be in harm's way; the younger the athlete, the greater the short- and long-term risk, a risk that can be fatal.

Clinical Caution

Young athletes are more susceptible to second-impact syndrome following concussions.

Significant damage and risk can be present for the young athlete who has sustained a concussion even without a loss of consciousness. Headache and dizziness are the most commonly reported symptoms of concussion. Because there may be other reasons that young athletes might experience headache or dizziness such as dehydration, fatigue, or inadequate nutrition, the accurate diagnosis of a sports-related concussion requires keen and ongoing observation.

Signs and Symptoms of Sports-Related Concussion[39]

- Headache
- Dizziness
- Amnesia (retrograde or antegrade)
- Inability to recall plays, rules, assignments, date, venue, score, or opponent
- Disorientation or confusion
- Drowsiness
- Irritability, sadness, or emotionality that does not seem to fit the situation
- Lack of balance or diminished physical coordination
- Slow verbal response or hyperaroused, pressured, or rambling verbal output
- Tinnitus (ringing in the ears)
- Difficulty with vision
- Nausea or vomiting
- Sensitivity to light or sound
- Trouble with concentration

It should be noted that previously used grading scales for assessing the concussed athlete have been abandoned for a diagnostic classification of either simple or complex concussion. Complex concussions may involve a loss of consciousness for longer than 1 minute; convulsions; and prolonged symptoms that include impaired cognitive function, multiple concussions, or persistent, unresolved symptoms as detailed in the box "Signs and Symptoms of Sports-Related Concussion."[39] A simple concussion is one in which symptoms are resolved in 1 week to 10 days.

The procedure for proper assessment and treatment of sports-related concussion is currently a hot topic of medical debate and has been well-reviewed in a recent article by Meehan and Bachur[39] from which we have drawn much of the information for this section. Because the focus of this chapter is addressing the psychological considerations for dealing with young athletes, we leave medical protocol in these matters to those far more qualified. The American Academy of Pediatrics unequivocally recommends that no player should be cleared to play until all symptoms have resolved completely.[39] Return-to-play protocols as outlined by the Second International Conference in Sport[40] offer clear, gradual steps that can be closely monitored for the protection and health of the young athlete. From a psychological standpoint, these are crucial protocols because they clarify and reduce conflict or confusion about decision-making as well as reducing pressure on the young, impressionable injured athlete to prematurely return to play.

The clinician can presume that in recovery, the concussed athlete may manifest all of the secondary psychological and emotional responses to injury that have been previously outlined in this chapter. The hidden, unseen, and confounding overlap with other psychological issues can make treatment and management an even more complex matter. The advent of neuropsychological testing, aided by more easily administered computer applications, provides useful, standardized measures of baseline neurological and neuropsychological functioning. This use of new technology has alleviated some of the difficulties inherent in treating the concussed athlete, but these measures are not yet in widespread use and more research is required to more fully understand their strength and limitations. Regardless of technology, it falls on the clinician to guide, support, counsel and educate the concussed young athlete as well as the athlete's extended competitive and social network toward a safe recovery.

Health care providers can play a significant role in counseling concussed athletes and their parents, coaches, and teachers about the healthy management of this condition. Aside from the obvious cautioning about the avoidance of activities that could exacerbate the head injury such as elevation of the heart rate or the use of aspirin or nonsteroidal anti-inflammatory drugs, there are also aspects of this condition that may further affect the athlete's emotional well-being. Strenuous cognitive activity like the academic demands required of high school or college may need to be avoided or curtailed. This further loss or reduction in normal function may be another emotional slap to the self-esteem of the athlete. For anxious students and parents who are overly-concerned about meeting what they perceive to be the unyielding high performance necessary for acceptance into top-tier universities or colleges, this forced academic cutback might be initially hard to accept and implement. However, cognitive rest has been documented to be a crucial need in young athletes that are still symptomatic with a sports-related concussion.

Clinical Point

Failure by the clinician and family to provide the necessary information and structure to implement a slow-down in physical, cognitive, and academic demand on the injured youngster can delay the healing process and prolong the athlete's suffering.

Concussions are invisible. There is no cast or brace that communicates the "real" nature of the injury. Concussed athletes may need to be protected emotionally, cocooned from what can be a virtual bombardment of well-intentioned inquiries that serve to exhaust and negatively overstimulate the athlete with unending reminders that he or she is hurt. Anecdotally, we have routinely noticed that athletes from all levels, ranging from high school to professional sports, recovering from serious injury frequently complain about how often they have to "tell their injury story" and provide ongoing updates to coaches, teammates, friends, peers, the press, family, significant others, and even the treating physician and health care team. As one injured professional athlete stated, "It tires me out as much as anything during the day, repeating the same damn thing over and over and trying not to be rude to people who care about me. I just wanted to get away by myself."

Screening for Substances Abuse

Alcohol is the most widely used drug and poses a health risk for young athletes. It is widely acknowledged to increase thrill-seeking and risk-taking behavior that can result in a number of life-threatening situations such as drunk driving, violence, and risky sexual practice. In a 2007 Centers for Disease Control report,[41] it was estimated that there were approximately 11 million underage drinkers in the United States. In addition, prevalence of illicit drug use in children older than the age of 12 was estimated at 8% of the population.[41] Research from Pate and colleagues[9] demonstrated that although sports participation in teens was associated with numerous positive health benefits, including a decreased likelihood to engage in some risky behaviors such as drug use, these findings were not substantiated for binge drinking in teen athletes. According to their findings, participation in sports therefore showed no effect on reducing the incidence of binge drinking in the adolescent athlete.[9] Therefore, the odds are high that health care providers associated with youth, high school, and collegiate sports will encounter young athletes who are engaged in substance abuse and are at risk for serious medical and psychological problems as a result of their use.

Athletes need to be educated about the damaging effects of alcohol or similar illegal substances on peak athletic performance as well as the detrimental effect substance abuse may have in the healing process. Certainly substance abuse can have grave consequences for athletes who have been diagnosed with sports-related concussion. In addition, the disinhibiting effects of alcohol or drugs can dangerously increase the potential for poor judgment; impulsivity; and risky, thrill-seeking behaviors in athletes who have been diagnosed with ADD or ADHD. The "CRAFFT" screening tool presented in Box 3-2 has been developed for use with adolescents and young adults for assessing risk for serious problems with substance use.[42] A score of 2 or more on this tool indicates that referral for further assessment and treatment of substance use is strongly indicated.

Eating Disorders

Unfortunately, the pressures and demands in youth sports can overwhelm the ability of some young athletes to cope. Their "solution" to adapting to their inner stress, anxiety, and ambivalence can have dangerous health consequences. Vulnerable adolescents may damage their bodies through food restriction in a mistaken attempt to improve appearance or, for a few, as the only "acceptable" way out of what

---

Box 3-2 CRAFFT Screening Tool for Substance Abuse

C Have you ever ridden in a <u>Car</u> driven by someone (including yourself) who was high or had been using alcohol or drugs?

R Do you ever use alcohol or drugs to <u>Relax</u>, feel better about yourself, or fit in?

A Do you ever use alcohol or drugs while you are <u>Alone</u>?

F Do you ever <u>Forget</u> things you did while using alcohol or drugs?

F Do your <u>Family or Friends</u> ever tell you that you should cut down on your drinking or drug use?

T Have you ever gotten into <u>Trouble</u> while you were using alcohol or drugs?

From Knight JR, Sherritt L, Shrier LA et al: Validity of the CRAFFT substance abuse screening test among adolescent clinic patients, Arch Pediatr Adolesc Med 156(6):609, 2002.

---

is experienced as a "no-win" situation (e.g., conflict with parents, a coach, or wanting to quit the sport). Eating disorders involving food restriction and binge eating are more commonly expressed in girls who are experiencing a combination of stresses stemming from home life as well as school, athletic, and social pressures. Ironically, such efforts among these young athletes to control their appearance and performance can have an opposite effect, making them sick, weak, and vulnerable to life-threatening consequences.

Detection and treatment of eating disorders are often difficult, raising significant challenges for health care providers. Secrecy is common for eating disorders as part of the syndrome. The most common ways orthopedic or primary care physicians may detect an eating disorder in young girls is when they observe repeated stress fractures, for example, in track or cross country athletes. A 17-year-old track athlete may return several times to a clinician's office for unresolved shin splints, which should raise a red flag that there is a possible underlying eating disorder that is accompanying the physical injury. The possibility of an eating disorder then requires a series of steps and considerations including interviews during which indignant denial is more likely than full disclosure.

The level and direction of inquiry for physicians suspicious of eating disorders in female athletes are guided by what is called the *female athlete triad,* a term used in sports medicine to describe a set of physical and behavioral symptoms that include disordered eating, amenorrhea (absence of menstruation), and osteoporosis (weakening and thinning of bones).[43] Therefore, as part of their clinical interview assessing a possible eating disorder, physicians also need to ask about the frequency and regularity of menstruation and eating patterns. Although adolescent girls may be able to get past their embarrassment to talk about their menstrual cycles, they are much less likely to discuss their eating patterns, particularly if they have an eating disorder.

Medical Complications of Eating Disorders

- For women—irregular periods, cessation of periods (amenorrhea), reproductive complications
- Lowered metabolism
- Fatigue
- Weakness
- Cold intolerance
- Muscle wasting (including heart tissue)
- Anemia
- Dehydration
- Electrolyte abnormalities: dizziness, lightheadedness, weakness
- Fluid retention
- Delayed gastric emptying (i.e., bloating, early fullness, indigestion)
- Constipation
- Diarrhea
- Hypoglycemia
- Stomach pain
- Esophageal tears
- Sore throat
- Dental erosion
- Parotid gland enlargement
- Rectal bleeding
- Frequent bruising
- Slow bone or wound healing
- Night blindness
- Dry skin and lips
- Dry, dull hair or significant hair loss

Clinical Point

All health care providers who work with athletes must be sensitive to the great amount of secrecy and shame that accompanies eating disorders and the potential denial that exists in the family.

The Diagnostic and Statistical Manual–IV,[36] which describes symptoms of all recognized psychiatric disorders and conditions, also identifies several forms of eating disorders. The two most common eating disorders are anorexia nervosa (restricted eating) and bulimia nervosa (binge eating followed by either purging, extreme exercise, or medicines used to prevent weight gain).[36] Severely anorexic athletes are easier to detect because of their extreme weight loss. If the young 17-year-old track athlete with repeated stress fractures has a normal weight of 130 lb (59 kg) but now weighs less than 85% of her weight (110 lb/[50 kg]), the treating clinician would almost definitely diagnose anorexia nervosa. Additional symptoms to support this diagnosis include a tremendous fear of becoming fat and a highly self-critical view of appearance. This young track athlete may be in incredible cardiovascular shape but she is still quite dissatisfied with her body and sees a fat person when she looks in the mirror. In the most serious cases, her view of her body is so distorted that she is completely detached from a reality regarding food, body image, and weight, making her so vulnerable to continued starvation that she may require emergent care and hospitalization.

Abnormal Eating Patterns in Anorexia Nervosa[44-46]

- Food intake is restricted and constant in content from day-to-day.
- Hunger is controlled by high-bulk, low-calorie, calorie-free, or strongly flavored food (e.g., lemon juice, vinegar, pepper, mustard).
- Large amounts of caffeine or carbonated beverages, chewing gum, or hard candy may be consumed to control hunger.
- Fat-containing food is stringently avoided.
- Food may be prepared and eaten in a ritualistic manner that may appear bizarre.
- Claims to be vegetarian may be a guise to avoid fat-containing animal protein.
- There is often a complex interplay between calories consumed, amount of hunger-suppressing foods eaten, amount of exercise performed, and the amount of strongly flavored foods eaten.

Bulimic athletes are harder to detect because they generally look quite normal, as they may remain at normal weight and typically hide their purging behaviors. In these circumstances, clinicians may notice other revealing symptoms in a young woman such as broken blood vessels under her eyes and scratches from her teeth on the back of her fingers and knuckles from vomiting. The stomach acid from vomiting may also cause decay in the enamel of her teeth. She may experience chronic chest pains and sore throats from vomiting and at times look tired and even depressed. Clinicians may also notice that her skin is turning a pale yellowish color from malnutrition. In some instances, she may report that her performance has declined and that she is more isolated from friends. At the extremes, the diagnosis may be obvious. However, many women athletes are very thin secondary to their body type and training. Therefore, clinicians must be sensitive to eating disorders and be ready to consult others if they have a serious suspicion.

Frequently, the treatment for eating disorders requires a multidisciplinary team. Because of the severe health risk from malnutrition, electrolyte levels and weight need to be monitored by a physician's office. A nutritionist, athletic trainer, and mental health counselor are also needed to work with the individual and the family to begin the treatment process. Athletic trainers may also play a key role in solidifying the diagnosis, because it is frequently the case that other members of her team may be discussing their concerns informally. The athletic trainer may be the first clinician to detect a problem. As the treatment progresses, physicians can play a crucial role in setting limitations on exercise and training while setting parameters for health and weight before full return to play.

Abnormal Eating Patterns in Bulimia Nervosa[44-46]

- May have regular pattern, albeit restricted, of food intake and regular binging and purging patterns.
- Food intake, binging, and purging patterns may be chaotic.
- Often relies on similar hunger-suppressing foods and substances as in anorexia nervosa.
- Late afternoon and evening are common time frames for extreme hunger to override control and result in binging and purging.
- Binging can last for minutes to hours before purging, or there can be several binges and purges in succession.
- Binges are highly variable in caloric content; 1200 to 11,500 kcal per episode have been reported.
- Fat-containing food is stringently avoided, and as in anorexia nervosa, the individual may claim to be vegetarian to avoid fat-containing animal protein.

The treatment team can also be quite useful in communicating with a family in which there is a suspected eating disorder. Confronting an eating-disordered patient requires great sensitivity and experience. Frequently, helping young women envision how they can strengthen their bodies and begin to feel better physically and emotionally is a much more effective approach than pathologizing the eating behavior. Changing disordered patterns of eating behavior is very difficult for the young person, and the desire to be strong and healthy for sports participation may be one of the few incentives that may motivate change. One must understand the underlying psychological dynamics before deciding whether to use participation as an incentive. If the deeper motive is to escape the sport, that leads to a very different approach than if performance or participation, maybe with less stress, is the young athlete's true wish. At times, eating disorders among young women mask broader family problems that may need additional attention. Consequently, steps to treat the whole family (including family and parent counseling) may also be necessary to appropriately address the disordered eating.

In some circumstances, when the team has fewer support systems in place, including the absence of a regular athletic trainer, detection and treatment of eating disorders may be even more challenging. For those clinicians who may work with these types of teams, it is crucial that they periodically check with the coaching staff and sometimes even team captains about potential problematic eating and poor body-image issues as well as being particularly sensitive to evidence of chronic injuries that may be caused by malnutrition. When the presence of an eating disorder is unclear, it is wise to consult with an eating disorder specialist to assess whether further steps are needed. Because eating disorders are common among female athletes, particularly in endurance sports, developing a relationship with a local eating disorder specialist

may help facilitate the speed and sensitivity of more effective detection and treatment.

Steroid Abuse

The recent tabloids on steroid use in top professional baseball players, as well as numerous top professional athletes in a variety of sports, illustrate the level at which steroid use is permeating our sport culture and unfortunately setting a dangerous precedent for our youth. Driven by the desire to increase strength and improve performance in dramatically short periods to gain a competitive edge much like the professional athletes, young boys and girls are dangerously experimenting with steroids despite significant risks to their minds and bodies. Although steroid use is more commonly associated with boys and men, there are reports that girls and young women are also using steroids. Data from the National Institute on Drug Use between the years 1999 and 2003[47] reveals that steroid use among boys and girls in grades 8 through 12 ranged from 1.8% to 2.5%, with boys using steroids at a higher rate. Although these numbers appear relatively small, many believe that adolescents and adults are using steroids at a much higher rate than is reported.

Drug use is frequently secretive and individuals, even when asked anonymously, are less likely to reveal their drug use and potentially illegal practices. These patterns of lying and secrecy are evident in the numerous occasions in which professional athletes have lied privately as well as in court and television appearances to confine and protect their behavior.

Although it is difficult to estimate the actual prevalence of steroid use in young athletes, the effects of using these drugs are dramatic. It is widely known that anabolic steroids cause an increase in appetite and trigger the bulking of muscle mass and noticeable weight gain. The risks of steroid use are less commonly recognized. Anabolic steroids can cause damage to the liver, heart, and brain. Steroid use can interfere with normal growth (i.e., early closure of the epiphysis), including sexual development and functioning, as well as trigger severe acne and male baldness. Approximately 10% of steroid users experience what is called "roid rage," terrifying violent outbursts that may surface unpredictably.[47] Steroid users are susceptible to lower levels of self-esteem as well as elevated rates of depression and suicide attempts.[47]

Although steroid users can be of any age or gender, adolescent boys who are trying to work their way up the competitive athletic hierarchy constitute a population particularly vulnerable to potential steroid abuse. As the size and speed of athletes at high school, collegiate, and professional levels continues to rise, young male athletes are under increasing pressure to "bulk up" and strengthen rapidly. For example, a 15-year-old boy who is told that he needs to gain 20 pounds (9 kg) over the summer if he is to have a chance to make the high school football team in the fall may take cycles of steroids to accomplish this unreasonable physical goal. If this boy is also socially isolated and has low self-esteem, then he may place even greater value on making the school team, as it represents a form of identity and validation. Driven to feel better about himself, he may be willing to experiment with steroids despite the risks to his physical and psychological well-being. In particular, the mindset of an adolescent male—namely, the belief that "I am bulletproof"—makes health risks feel remote and the potential benefits of getting stronger and faster much more compelling. The fact that some athletes use steroids, lie about it, and then face minimum consequences while maintaining multi-million dollar contracts only makes steroid use among our youth more compelling and worth the risk. Further feeling of being "bullet-proof" might encourage risk taking in other areas of life beyond sports such as driving or drinking.

Unfortunately, desperation to get immediate results may lead to dangerous and unregulated experimentation with steroid use, including ordering steroids through the Internet or acquiring the drugs through other steroid users at local gyms. Intravenous steroid users have obvious risks of infection, including human immunodeficiency virus (HIV) and hepatitis.[48] Because the drugs are obtained and used in secrecy, adequate education is not provided, much like the case of many professional athletes, leaving the adolescent similarly isolated in his dangerous experimentation.

Detection of steroid use may occur through joint observations by parents, coaches, sport physical therapists, athletic trainers, and physicians. Parents may notice changes in mood, increased secrecy about weight training and in particular time spent at the gym. However, much like the difficulty parents with eating-disordered daughters may have in noticing significant weight loss, parents of steroid-using boys may not be able to detect the rapid weight gain and muscle mass while living with their son every day. A sport physical therapist, athletic trainer, or coach who may see the athlete less frequently over the course of the summer may be better able to recognize unexpected and troubling changes. A physician may also track significant changes in weight as well as increased acne.

Much like addressing concerns around eating and body image, a collaborative approach between parents and clinicians is likely to be most effective in treating steroid abuse. Adolescents using steroids may experience a tremendous amount of shame and fear. Therefore, clinicians will be most effective when being tactful about how they raise their concerns. In particular, it is crucial that they recognize the importance of sports in these young athletes' lives and the intoxicating power of the immense improvements in strength and speed caused by steroid use, even while expressing strong concern about their health. Making specific references to immediate health risks may be a potentially effective deterrent. For young males, mentioning the fact that their testicles may shrink to the size of raisins or that they may develop feminine-appearing breasts, perhaps through shock value, can trigger some change in their behavior.

Young steroid users need to understand that there are healthy ways to build strength. Sport nutritionists can advise youth and their families about healthy eating and nutrition. Connecting young athletes with well-educated sport physical therapists and athletic trainers can help expose them to proper weight training regimens, supervised by caring adults. Redirecting youth away from gyms where there is unsupervised interaction with unqualified adults (who are possibly using steroids) is also advisable. And in certain cases, when the self-esteem of the adolescent is considerably low or his or her investment in athletics is imbalanced, a referral to a sports or clinical counselor may be appropriate.

Of course, steroid use, much like eating disorders, can take place in the context of a culture and team. Assessing the team's values, including pressure relating to performance, appearance, interpersonal dynamics, and quality of coaching, are all relevant to assessing the individual athlete and are critical if the clinician has an ongoing role with the team.

Conclusion

The benefits of athletics—physical, emotional, psychological, and developmental—are clear. Parents and health professionals want the health benefits, the self-esteem, friendships, mentoring, and opportunities that come with every level of participation. As we strive for these worthy goals, we must always keep in sight the individuality, abilities, aspirations, and needs of the child and adolescent. Lastly, we must be aware of the risks that are intrinsically linked with the benefits and recognize psychological and medical issues that may interfere with the very worthy goals of athletic competition.

References

1. Smoll F, Smith J: *Children and youth in sport*, ed 2, Dubuque, 2002, Kendall Hunt Publishing.
2. Brenner J, Council on Sports Medicine and Fitness: Overuse injuries, overtraining, and burnout in child and adolescent athletes, *Pediatrics* 119:1242–1245, 2007.
3. U.S. Department of Health and Human Services: *Physical activity and health: A report of the surgeon general* (S/N 0-7-023-00196-5), Atlanta, 1996, Superintendent of Documents.
4. Dalton SE: Overuse injuries in adolescent athletes, *Sports Med* 13:58–70, 1992.
5. Gould D, Petlichkoff L: Participation motivation and attrition in young athletes. In Smoll FL, Magill RA, Ash MJ, editors: *Children in sport*, ed 3, Champaign, IL, 1988, Human Kinetics.
6. Centers for Disease Control and Prevention: *Adolescents and young adults*. Retrieved on October 10, 2004, from http://www.cdc.gov/nccdphp/sgr/adoles.htm.
7. National Alliance for Youth Sports: http://www.nays.org, 2009.
8. Seefeldt V, Ewing M, Walk S: *Overview of youth sports programs in the United States*, Washington, DC, 1992, Carnegie Council on Adolescent Development.

9. Pate RR, Trost SG, Levin S, Dowda M: Sports participation and health-related behaviors among US youth, *Arch Pediatr Med* 154(9):904–911, 2000.

10. Committee on Sports Medicine and Fitness: Intensive training and sports specialization in young athletes, *Pediatrics* 106(1):154–157, 2000.

11. Toffler IR, Knapp R, Penelop K, Dell MJ: The achievement by proxy spectrum in sports: Historical perspective and clinical approach to pressured and high-achieving children and adolescents, *Child Adolesc Psychiatr Clin North Am* 7(4):725–744, 1998.

12. Fraser-Thomas J, Cote J: Youth sports: Implementing findings and moving forward with research, *Athletic Insight* 8(3):12–27, 2006.

13. Balyi I, Hamilton A: *Long-term athlete development: Trainability in childhood and adolescence. Windows of opportunity.* Optimal trainability, Victoria, 2004, National Coaching Institute British Columbia & Advanced Training and Performance Ltd.

14. Ericcson KA, Krampe RT, Tesch-Rommer C: The role of deliberate practice in the acquisition of expert performance, *Psychol Rev* 100(3):363–406, 1993.

15. Gladwell M: *Outliers: The story of success.* New York, 2008, Little & Brown.

16. Simon HA, Chase WG: Skill in chess, *Am Sci* 61:394–403, 1973.

17. Bissinger HK: *Friday Night Lights: A town, a team and a dream*, Cambridge, 1990, DaCapo Press.

18. NCAA Data: *Estimated Probability of competing in athletics beyond the high school interscholastic level*, 2007. Retrieved November 1, 2008, *from* http://www.ncaa.org/wps/ncaa?ContentID=279.

19. Anderson J: *Parental support and pressure: Relationships with children's experience of extracurricular activities*, Dissertation Abstracts International, Section B, The Sciences and Engineering 65:3696, 2005.

20. Babkes ML, Weiss MR: Parental influence on cognitive and affective responses in children's competitive soccer participation, *Pediatr Exerc Sci* 11:44–62, 1999.

21. Hayashi SW: *Understanding youth sport participation through perceived coaching behaviors, social support, anxiety and coping*, Dissertation Abstracts International 59(7-A):2418, 1999.

22. Hoyle RH, Leff SS: The role of parental involvement in youth sport participation and performance, *Adolescence* 32(125):233–243, 1997.

23. Stein GL, Raedeke TD, Glenn SD: Children's perceptions of parental sport involvement: It's not how much but to what degree that's important, *J Sport Behav* 22:591–601, 1999.

24. Coakley J: Burnout among adolescent athletes: A personal failure or social problem? *Sociol Sport J* 9:271–285, 1992.

25. Ginsburg RD, Durant S, Baltzell A: *Whose game is it, anyway? A guide to helping your child get the most from sports, organized by age and stage*, Boston, 2006, Houghton Mifflin Company.

26. Smith RE, Smoll FL, Curtis B: Coaching behaviors in Little League baseball. In Smoll FL, Smith RW, editors: *Psychological perspectives in youth sports*, Washington, DC, 1978, Hemisphere Publishing.

27. Herman JL: *Trauma & recovery*, New York, 1994, Basic Books.

28. Freudenberger HJ, Richelson G: Burnout: *how to beat the high cost of success*, New York, 1981, Bantam Books.

29. Maslach C: Understanding burnout: definitional issues in analyzing a complex phenomenon. In Paine WS, editor: *Job stress and burnout: Research, theory and intervention perspectives*, Beverly Hills, 1982, Sage.

30. Pines A, Aronson E: *Career burnout*, New York, 1988, Free Press.

31. Fender LK: Athlete burnout: Potential for research and intervention strategies, *Sport Psychol* 3:63–71, 1989.

32. Maslach C, Pines A: The burnout syndrome, *Child Care Q* 6:100–114, 1977.

33. Deci EL, Ryan RM: Self-determination theory: A macrotheory of human motivation, development and health, *Can Psychol* 49(3):182–185, 2008.

34. Henschen K: Maladaptive fatigue syndrome and emotions in sport. In Harris YL, editor: *Emotions in sport*, Champaign, IL, 1999, Human Kinetics.

35. Committee on Sports Medicine and Fitness, Committee on School Health: Intensive training and sport specialization in young athletes, *Pediatrics* 106(1):154–157, 2000.

36. American Psychiatric Association: *Diagnostic and statistical manual of mental disorders-IV*, Washington, DC, 1994, American Psychiatric Association.

37. Hallowell E, Ratey J: *Driven to distraction*, New York, 1994, Pantheon Books.

38. Martineau C, Kingma JJ, Bank L, McLeod TCV: Guidelines for treatment of sport-related concussions, *J Am Acad Physician Assist* 20(5):123–132, 2007.

39. Meehan WP, Bachur RG: Sport-related concussion, *Pediatrics* 123:114–123, 2009.

40. McCory P, Johnson K, Meeuwise W: Summary and agreement statement of the 2nd International Conference on Concussion in Sport, Prague, 2004, *Br J Sport Med* 39(4):196–204, 2005.

41. Centers for Disease Control: *National Center for Health Statistics Health*, United States, 2007: With Chartbook on Trends in the Health of Americans, Hyattsville, 2007, CDC.

42. Knight JR, Sherritt L, Shrier LA et al: Validity of the CRAFFT substance abuse screening test among adolescent clinic patients, *Arch Pediatr Adolesc Med* 156(6):607–614, 2002.

43. Hobart JA, Smucker DR: The female athlete triad, *Am Fam Physician* 61:3357–3367, 2000.

44. Luder E, Schebendach J: Nutrition management of eating disorders, *Top Clin Nutr* 8:48–63, 1993.

45. Rock CL, Yager J: Nutrition and eating disorders: A primer for clinicians, *Int J Eat Disord* 6:267–280, 1987.

46. Reiff DW, Reiff KKL: *Eating disorders: Nutrition therapy in the recovery process*, Gaithersberg, MD, 1992, Aspen.

47. National Institute on Drug Abuse: *Monitoring the future study, 2003*. Retrieved June 1, 2007 from http://www.nida.nih.gov/Infofax/HSYouthtrends.html.

48. Volkow N, The National Institute on Drug Abuse: *Consequences of the abuse of anabolic steroids*, 2005. Retrieved November 15, 2008, from http://www.drugabuse.gov/about/welcome/MessageSteroids305.html.

NUTRITION COUNSELING AND ATHLETES

Heidi M. Wells

Introduction

Optimal athletic performance is a common goal among all athletes. Each athlete strives to be the biggest, strongest, and fastest within his or her sport. For this reason, the athlete is particularly vulnerable to health claims that may or may not supply accurate information. Misleading nutritional information may affect the athlete's ability to make appropriate decisions regarding nutritional intake. Unfortunately, it seems that new claims are made just as fast as old claims are disproved. The objective of this chapter is to provide nutritional information based on current scientific findings, as well as to provide a guide for assessing an athlete's intake for the development of an individualized nutrition plan aimed toward helping the athlete achieve his or her optimal athletic performance.

Components of Nutritional Assessment

A nutritional assessment of an athlete is made up of multiple components. Health screens by a primary care physician are recommended to determine an athlete's current health status (see Chapter 2). Health screens can help determine medical risks and any nutritional complications that may be associated with these health risks, which can serve as a starting point for the development of a dietary regimen.[1] Information obtained during a health screen should include laboratory data providing objective information that may substantiate physical findings and dietary deficiencies or excesses noted in the dietary intake analysis. Anthropometric data such as height, weight, body mass index (BMI), and body composition should also be determined at baseline.

Note: This chapter includes content from previous contributions by Susan Cummings, MS, RD, and Mary Jane Rewinski, BS, RD, as it appeared in the predecessor of this book—Zachazewski JE, Magee DJ, Quillen WS, editors: *Athletic Injuries and Rehabilitation*, Philadelphia, 1996, WB Saunders.

These values can then be used as a standard to measure body composition changes and as guidance for individual training strategies for the athlete. A comprehensive medical history, including both current and past medical events, should also be a vital part of nutritional assessment.

Energy Needs

The longer and more effectively an athlete trains, the more efficient the body becomes at burning calories and using oxygen. *Efficiency of energy burned* refers to the quantity of energy required to perform a particular task in relation to the actual work that is accomplished.[2]

To obtain optimum efficiency of energy, or athletic performance, energy intake must be adequate. In other words, there should be a balance between energy brought into the body and energy being expended by the body.[3] If inadequate energy is brought into the body and energy expenditure exceeds energy intake, performance and benefits of training will be compromised, forcing the body to tap into fat and lean muscle mass stores for energy.[3]

Highly trained endurance athletes burn energy more efficiently than less-well-trained athletes. They also burn a large number of calories simply because of the extended time spent in training. Table 4-1 lists caloric expenditure for various physical activities.

Determining Nutrient Intake

Once a good physical assessment of the athlete has been established, attention must be turned to focus on his or her dietary habits. Achieving the most accurate depiction of a typical nutrient and food intake of an individual is the primary goal of conducting a dietary assessment. However, this can also be the most difficult goal to accomplish because of multiple outside co-factors that often decrease the accuracy of the information obtained. Therefore, one should choose the dietary assessment method appropriate for the particular individual or population for which the assessment is being conducted. Valid, reliable dietary assessment tools appropriate for the individual or population for which the assessment is being conducted will help achieve the most accurate results possible. Other factors to consider when choosing the appropriate dietary assessment tool include objectives of the assessment, dietary information of interest (i.e., energy, specific nutrients, food groups, and dietary patterns), the timeframe involved, cost, and the interviewer's qualifications and experience.[1]

Clinical Point

The primary goal of a dietary assessment is to determine the most accurate and typical nutrient and foot intake of an individual.

The 24-Hour Recall

The 24-hour recall method is best conducted as a face-to-face interview with the athlete to recall and report all foods and beverages the athlete has consumed in a 24-hour period, beginning with the first bite or sip in the morning and continuing throughout the day. If available, food models and other measuring tools (e.g., cups, spoons, visuals) can help obtain a better estimate of portion sizes reported. Time, food, portion, and activities should all be accounted for. Because the 24-hour recall assessment relies on memory and may not be representative of a typical or even average day, combining it with questions regarding food frequency may provide a more complete overview of the athlete's usual intake. For example, how many times in a week do you eat cereal for breakfast? If you didn't have cereal, what would you have instead? How many times in a week do you skip breakfast?

Methods of Nutritional Assessment

- 24-hour recall
- Food frequency questionnaire
- Food record

The Food Frequency Questionnaire

A food frequency questionnaire is designed to obtain both qualitative and semi-quantitative descriptive information about usual food intake.[1,4] This is accomplished by assessing the frequency with which foods are eaten during a specified time (e.g., daily, weekly, monthly, or yearly). The advantages of a food frequency questionnaire are that it is relatively inexpensive, and can be administered by nonprofessionals or can be self-administered. One disadvantage to its

use is that it is fairly time-consuming. Another disadvantage is that the accuracy depends on either a trained person sitting with the individual to define portion sizes and quantities, or the individual's understanding of the questionnaire and how accurately he or she self-assesses portions and frequency.

One may also use an abbreviated version of the food frequency questionnaire by going through the food groups in the food guide pyramid (i.e., grains, fruits, vegetables, dairy, meat and beans, and fats) (Figure 4-1) and question how often and in what quantity the athlete eats these foods, including what foods and beverages the athlete consumed prior to and just after exercise, training, and an event; what typical snack foods are eaten; and what, if any nutritional supplements the athlete takes.

The Food Record

A food record is best explained as a diary of food and beverage intake maintained by an individual. Food records consist of the exact quantity of food eaten within a specified period, usually at least 3 to 7 days, including at least 2 usual weekdays and 1 weekend day. Accuracy depends on the individual's diligence and integrity. During a specified time, this method provides a fairly accurate estimate of food consumption.

By keeping a food record for 7 days, total caloric intake can be found and compared with weight changes to determine the level of exercise and caloric intake that produces weight maintenance, weight loss, or weight gain.

Evaluation of Nutrient Intake
Computer Programs

Nutrient analysis programs have come a long way in the past 5 to 10 years. Currently, there are numerous computerized diet analysis programs out on the market for purchase, as well as online programs and databases—both free or for a fee. For example, the Healthy Eating Index, developed and maintained by the U.S. Department of Agriculture, is an example of a high-quality internet resource.[4] This program incorporates the food guide pyramid recommendations and guidelines to evaluate the dietary intake of an individual.

When considering which program best suits the athlete's needs, an accurate database is essential. The source of the database, its completeness in terms of the range of foods listed, and the availability of nutrient values for individual foods must be determined. The validity of the computer program for calculating nutrient intakes must also be assessed. Diet analysis software packages should provide total nutrients per meal, total nutrients for each day, average daily nutrient intake per major food group and subgroups, and average frequency of consumption of major food groups and subgroups.

text cont'd on page 66

Table 4-1
Caloric Expenditure for Various Physical Activities

Body Weight (kcal · min⁻¹ · kg⁻¹)

Kg	45	48	50	52	55	57	59	61	64	66
Pounds	100	105	110	115	120	125	130	135	140	145
Sedentary Activities										
Lying quietly	.99	1.0	1.1	1.1	1.2	1.3	1.3	1.4	1.4	1.5
Sitting and writing, card playing, etc.	1.2	1.3	1.4	1.5	1.5	1.6	1.7	1.7	1.8	1.8
Standing with light work, cleaning, etc.	2.7	2.9	3.0	3.1	3.3	3.4	3.5	3.7	3.8	3.9
Physical Activities										
Archery	3.1	3.3	3.5	3.6	3.8	4.0	4.1	4.3	4.5	4.6
Badminton										
Recreational singles	3.6	3.8	4.0	4.2	4.4	4.6	4.7	4.9	5.1	5.3
Social doubles	2.7	2.9	3.0	3.1	3.3	3.4	3.5	3.7	3.8	3.9
Competitive	5.9	6.1	6.4	6.7	7.0	7.3	7.6	7.9	8.2	8.5
Baseball										
Player	3.1	3.3	3.4	3.6	3.8	4.0	4.1	4.3	4.4	4.5
Pitcher	3.9	4.1	4.3	4.5	4.7	4.9	5.1	5.3	5.5	5.7
Basketball										
Half court	3.0	3.1	3.3	3.5	3.6	3.8	3.9	4.1	4.2	4.4
Recreational	4.9	5.2	5.5	5.7	6.0	6.2	6.5	6.7	7.0	7.2
Vigorous competition	6.5	6.8	7.2	7.5	7.8	8.2	8.5	8.8	9.2	9.5
Bicycling, level										
(mph) (min/mile)										
5 12:00	1.9	2.0	2.1	2.2	2.3	2.4	2.5	2.6	2.7	2.8
6 10:00	2.7	2.8	3.0	3.1	3.2	3.4	3.5	3.6	3.8	3.9
8 7:30	3.4	3.6	3.8	4.0	4.1	4.3	4.5	4.7	4.8	5.0
10 6:00	4.2	4.4	4.6	4.8	5.1	5.3	5.5	5.7	5.9	6.1
11 5:28	5.0	5.2	5.5	5.7	6.0	6.2	6.5	6.7	7.0	7.2
12 5:00	5.7	6.0	6.3	6.6	6.9	7.2	7.5	7.8	8.1	8.4
13 4:37	6.8	7.1	7.5	7.8	8.2	8.5	8.8	9.2	9.5	9.9
Bowling	2.7	2.8	3.0	3.1	3.3	3.4	3.5	3.7	3.8	3.9
Calisthenics										
Light type	3.4	3.6	3.8	4.0	4.1	4.3	4.5	4.7	4.8	5.0
Timed vigorous	9.7	10.1	10.6	11.1	11.6	12.1	12.6	13.1	13.6	14.1
Canoeing										
(mph) (min/mile)										
2.5 24	1.9	2.0	2.1	2.2	2.3	2.4	2.5	2.6	2.7	2.8
4.0 15	4.4	4.6	4.9	5.1	5.3	5.5	5.8	6.0	6.2	6.4
5.0 12	5.7	6.0	6.3	6.6	6.9	7.2	7.5	7.8	8.1	8.4
Dancing										
Moderate (waltz)	3.1	3.3	3.5	3.6	3.8	4.0	4.1	4.3	4.5	4.6
Active (square, disco)	4.5	4.7	5.0	5.2	5.4	5.6	5.9	6.1	6.3	6.6
Aerobic (vigorous)	6.0	6.3	6.7	7.0	7.3	7.6	7.9	8.2	8.5	8.8
Fencing										
Moderate	3.3	3.5	3.6	3.8	4.0	4.1	4.3	4.5	4.6	4.8
Vigorous	6.6	7.0	7.3	7.7	8.0	8.3	8.7	9.0	9.4	9.7
Field hockey	5.0	6.3	6.7	7.0	7.3	7.6	7.9	8.2	8.5	8.8
Football										
Moderate	3.3	3.5	3.6	3.8	4.0	4.1	4.3	4.5	4.6	4.8
Touch, vigorous	5.5	5.8	6.1	6.4	6.6	6.9	7.2	7.5	7.8	8.0
Golf										
Twosome (carry clubs)	3.6	3.8	4.0	4.2	4.4	4.6	4.7	4.9	5.1	5.3
Foursome (carry clubs)	2.7	2.9	3.0	3.1	3.3	3.4	3.5	3.7	3.8	3.9
Power cart	1.9	2.0	2.1	2.2	2.3	2.4	2.5	2.6	2.7	2.8

68 150	70 155	73 160	75 165	77 170	80 175	82 180	84 185	86 190	89 195	91 200	93 205	95 210	98 215	100 220
1.5	1.5	1.6	1.6	1.7	1.7	1.8	1.8	1.9	1.9	2.0	2.0	2.1	2.1	2.2
1.9	2.0	2.0	2.1	2.2	2.2	2.3	2.4	2.4	2.5	2.5	2.6	2.7	2.7	2.8
4.1	4.2	4.4	4.5	4.6	4.8	4.9	5.0	5.2	5.3	5.4	5.6	5.7	5.9	6.0
4.8	4.9	5.1	5.3	5.4	5.6	5.7	5.9	6.0	6.2	6.4	6.5	6.7	6.9	7.0
5.4	5.6	5.8	6.0	6.2	6.4	6.6	6.7	6.9	7.1	7.3	7.4	7.6	7.8	8.0
4.1	4.2	4.4	4.5	4.6	4.8	4.9	5.0	5.2	5.3	5.4	5.6	5.7	5.9	6.0
8.8	9.1	9.4	9.7	10.0	10.3	10.6	10.9	11.2	11.5	11.8	12.1	12.4	12.7	13.0
4.7	4.8	5.0	5.2	5.3	5.5	5.6	5.8	5.9	6.1	6.3	6.4	6.6	6.8	6.9
5.9	6.0	6.3	6.5	6.7	6.9	7.1	7.3	7.4	7.7	7.9	8.0	8.2	8.5	8.6
4.5	4.7	4.8	5.0	5.1	5.3	5.4	5.6	5.7	5.9	6.0	6.2	6.4	6.5	6.7
7.5	7.7	8.0	8.2	8.5	8.7	9.0	9.2	9.5	9.7	10.0	10.2	10.5	10.7	11.0
9.9	10.2	10.5	10.9	11.2	11.5	11.9	12.2	12.5	12.9	13.2	13.5	13.8	14.2	14.5
2.9	3.0	3.1	3.2	3.3	3.4	3.5	3.6	3.7	3.8	3.9	4.0	4.1	4.2	4.3
4.0	4.2	4.3	4.4	4.6	4.7	4.9	5.0	5.1	5.3	5.4	5.5	5.7	5.8	6.0
5.2	5.4	5.5	5.7	5.9	6.1	6.3	6.4	6.6	6.8	6.9	7.1	7.3	7.5	7.7
6.4	6.6	6.8	7.0	7.2	7.4	7.6	7.9	8.1	8.3	8.5	8.7	8.9	9.1	9.4
7.5	7.8	8.0	8.3	8.5	8.8	9.0	9.3	9.5	9.8	10.0	10.3	10.6	10.8	11.1
8.7	9.0	9.3	9.5	9.8	10.1	10.4	10.7	11.0	11.3	11.6	11.9	12.2	12.5	12.8
10.2	10.6	10.9	11.3	11.6	12.0	12.3	12.6	13.0	13.3	13.7	14.0	14.4	14.7	15.0
4.1	4.2	4.4	4.5	4.6	4.8	4.9	5.0	5.2	5.3	5.5	5.6	5.7	5.9	6.0
5.2	5.4	5.5	5.7	5.9	6.1	6.3	6.4	6.6	6.8	7.0	7.1	7.3	7.5	7.7
14.6	15.1	15.6	16.1	16.6	17.1	17.6	18.1	18.6	19.1	19.6	20.0	20.5	21.0	21.5
2.9	3.0	3.1	3.2	3.3	3.4	3.5	3.6	3.7	3.8	3.9	4.0	4.1	4.2	4.3
6.7	6.9	7.1	7.4	7.6	7.8	8.0	8.2	8.5	8.7	8.9	9.1	9.4	9.6	9.8
8.7	9.0	9.3	9.5	9.8	10.1	10.4	10.7	11.0	11.3	11.6	11.9	12.2	12.5	12.8
4.8	4.9	5.1	5.3	5.4	5.6	5.7	5.9	6.0	6.2	6.4	6.5	6.7	6.9	7.0
6.8	7.0	7.3	7.5	7.7	7.9	8.2	8.4	8.6	8.9	9.1	9.3	9.5	9.8	10.0
9.1	9.4	9.7	10.0	10.3	10.6	10.9	11.2	11.5	11.8	12.1	12.4	12.7	13.0	13.3
5.0	5.2	5.3	5.5	5.7	5.8	6.0	6.2	6.3	6.5	6.7	6.8	7.0	7.1	7.3
10.0	10.4	10.7	11.0	11.4	11.7	12.1	12.4	12.7	13.1	13.4	13.8	14.1	14.4	14.8
9.1	9.4	9.7	10.0	10.3	10.6	10.9	11.2	11.5	11.8	12.1	12.4	12.7	13.0	13.3
5.0	5.2	5.3	5.5	5.7	5.8	6.0	6.2	6.3	6.5	6.7	6.8	7.0	7.1	7.3
8.3	8.6	8.9	9.2	9.4	9.7	10.0	10.3	10.6	10.8	11.1	11.4	11.7	12.0	12.2
5.4	5.6	5.8	6.0	6.2	6.4	6.6	6.7	6.9	7.1	7.3	7.4	7.6	7.8	8.0
4.1	4.2	4.4	4.5	4.6	4.8	4.9	5.0	5.2	5.3	5.4	5.6	5.7	5.9	6.0
2.9	3.0	3.1	3.2	3.3	3.4	3.5	3.6	3.7	3.8	3.9	4.0	4.1	4.2	4.3

Continued

Table 4-1

Caloric Expenditure for Various Physical Activities—cont'd

Body Weight (kcal · min^{-1} · kg^{-1})

Kg		45	48	50	52	55	57	59	61	64	66
Pounds		100	105	110	115	120	125	130	135	140	145
Handball											
Moderate		6.5	6.8	7.2	7.5	7.8	8.2	8.5	8.8	9.2	9.5
Competitive		7.7	8.0	8.4	8.8	9.2	9.6	10.1	10.4	10.8	11.1
Hiking, pack (3 mph)		4.5	4.7	5.0	5.2	5.4	5.6	5.9	6.1	6.3	6.6
Hockey, ice		6.6	7.0	7.3	7.7	8.0	8.3	8.7	9.0	9.4	9.7
Horseback riding											
Walk		1.9	2.0	2.1	2.2	2.3	2.4	2.5	2.6	2.7	2.8
Sitting to trot		2.7	2.9	3.0	3.1	3.3	3.4	3.5	3.7	3.8	3.9
Posting to trot		4.2	4.4	4.6	4.8	5.1	5.3	5.5	5.7	5.9	6.1
Gallop		5.7	6.0	6.3	6.6	6.9	7.2	7.5	7.8	8.1	8.4
Horseshoes		2.5	2.6	2.8	2.9	3.0	3.1	3.3	3.4	3.5	3.7
Jogging (see running)											
Judo		8.5	8.9	9.3	9.8	10.2	10.6	11.0	11.5	11.9	12.3
Karate		8.5	8.9	9.3	9.8	10.2	10.6	11.0	11.5	11.9	12.3
Mountain climbing		6.5	6.8	7.2	7.5	7.8	8.2	8.5	8.8	9.2	9.5
Paddle ball		5.7	6.0	6.3	6.6	6.9	7.2	7.5	7.8	8.1	8.4
Pool (billiards)		1.5	1.6	1.6	1.7	1.8	1.9	1.9	2.0	2.1	2.2
Racquetball		6.5	6.8	7.1	7.5	7.8	8.1	8.4	8.8	9.1	9.4
Roller skating (9 mph)		4.2	4.4	4.6	4.8	5.1	5.3	5.5	5.7	5.9	6.1
Running (steady state)											
(mph)	(min/mile)										
5.0	12:00	6.0	6.3	6.6	7.0	7.3	7.6	7.9	8.2	8.5	8.8
5.5	10:55	6.7	7.0	7.3	7.7	8.0	8.4	8.7	9.0	9.4	9.7
6.0	10:00	7.2	7.6	8.0	8.4	8.7	9.1	9.5	9.8	10.2	10.6
7.0	8:35	8.5	8.9	9.3	9.0	10.2	10.6	11.0	11.5	11.9	12.3
8.0	7:30	9.7	10.2	10.7	11.2	11.6	12.1	12.6	13.1	13.6	14.1
9.0	6:40	10.8	11.3	11.9	12.4	12.9	13.5	14.0	14.6	15.1	15.7
10.0	6:00	12.1	12.7	13.3	13.9	14.5	15.1	15.7	16.4	17.0	17.6
11.0	5:28	13.3	14.0	14.6	15.3	16.0	16.7	17.3	18.0	18.7	19.4
12.0	5:00	14.5	15.2	16.0	16.7	17.4	18.2	18.9	19.7	20.4	21.1
Sailing, small boat		2.7	2.9	3.0	3.1	3.3	3.4	3.5	3.7	3.8	3.9
Skating, ice (9 mph)		4.2	4.4	4.6	4.8	5.1	5.2	5.5	5.7	5.9	6.1
Skiing, cross-country											
(mph)	(min/mile)										
2.5	24:00	5.0	5.2	5.5	5.7	6.0	6.2	6.5	6.7	7.0	7.2
4.0	15:00	6.5	6.8	7.2	7.5	7.8	8.2	8.5	8.8	9.2	9.5
5.0	12:00	7.7	8.0	8.4	8.8	9.2	9.6	10.0	10.4	10.8	11.1
Skiing, downhill		6.5	6.8	7.2	7.5	7.8	8.2	8.5	8.8	9.2	9.5
Soccer		5.9	6.2	6.6	6.9	7.2	7.5	7.8	8.1	8.4	8.7
Squash											
Normal		6.7	7.0	7.3	7.7	8.0	8.4	8.7	9.1	9.5	9.8
Competition		7.7	8.0	8.4	8.8	9.2	9.6	10.0	10.4	10.8	11.1
Swimming (yards/min)											
Backstroke											
25		2.5	2.6	2.8	2.9	3.0	3.1	3.3	3.4	3.5	3.7
30		3.5	3.7	3.9	4.1	4.2	4.4	4.6	4.8	4.9	5.1
35		4.5	4.7	5.0	5.2	5.4	5.6	5.9	6.1	6.3	6.6
40		5.5	5.8	6.1	6.4	6.6	6.9	7.2	7.5	7.8	8.0
Breaststroke											
20		3.1	3.3	3.5	3.6	3.8	4.0	4.1	4.3	4.5	4.6
30		4.7	5.0	5.2	5.4	5.7	5.9	6.2	6.4	6.7	6.9
40		6.3	6.7	7.0	7.3	7.6	8.0	8.3	8.6	8.9	9.3

68 150	70 155	73 160	75 165	77 170	80 175	82 180	84 185	86 190	89 195	91 200	93 205	95 210	98 215	100 220
9.9	10.2	10.5	10.9	11.2	11.5	11.9	12.2	12.5	12.9	13.2	13.5	13.8	14.2	14.5
11.5	11.9	12.3	12.7	13.1	13.5	13.9	14.3	14.7	15.0	15.4	15.8	16.2	16.6	17.0
6.8	7.0	7.3	7.5	7.7	7.9	8.2	8.4	8.6	8.9	9.1	9.3	9.5	9.8	10.0
10.0	10.4	10.7	11.0	11.4	11.7	12.1	12.4	12.7	13.1	13.4	13.8	14.1	14.4	14.8
2.9	3.0	3.1	3.2	3.3	3.4	3.5	3.6	3.7	3.8	3.9	4.0	4.1	4.2	4.3
4.1	4.2	4.4	4.5	4.6	4.8	4.9	5.0	5.2	5.3	5.4	5.6	5.7	5.9	6.0
6.4	6.6	6.8	7.0	7.2	7.4	7.6	7.9	8.1	8.3	8.5	8.7	8.9	9.1	9.4
8.7	9.0	9.3	9.5	9.8	10.1	10.4	10.7	11.0	11.3	11.6	11.9	12.2	12.5	12.8
3.8	3.9	4.0	4.2	4.3	4.4	4.5	4.7	4.8	4.9	5.2	5.2	5.3	5.4	5.6
12.8	13.2	13.6	14.1	14.5	14.9	15.4	15.8	16.2	16.6	17.1	17.5	17.9	18.4	18.8
12.8	13.2	13.6	14.1	14.5	14.9	15.4	15.8	16.2	16.6	17.1	17.5	17.9	18.4	18.8
9.8	10.2	10.5	10.8	11.2	11.5	11.8	12.1	12.5	12.8	13.1	13.5	13.8	14.1	14.5
8.7	9.0	9.3	9.5	9.8	10.1	10.4	10.7	11.0	11.2	11.6	11.9	12.2	12.5	12.8
2.2	2.3	2.4	2.5	2.6	2.6	2.7	2.8	2.9	2.9	3.0	3.1	3.2	3.2	3.3
9.8	10.1	10.4	10.7	11.1	11.4	11.7	12.0	12.4	12.7	13.0	13.4	13.7	14.0	14.4
6.4	6.6	6.8	7.0	7.2	7.4	7.6	7.9	8.1	8.3	8.5	8.7	8.9	9.1	9.4
9.1	9.4	9.7	10.0	10.3	10.6	10.9	11.2	11.6	11.9	12.2	12.5	12.8	13.1	13.4
10.0	10.4	10.7	11.1	11.4	11.7	12.1	12.4	12.8	13.1	13.4	13.8	14.1	14.5	14.8
10.9	11.3	11.7	12.0	12.4	12.8	13.1	13.5	13.8	14.3	14.6	15.0	15.4	15.7	16.1
12.8	13.2	13.6	14.1	14.5	14.9	15.4	15.8	16.2	16.6	17.1	17.5	17.9	18.4	18.8
14.6	15.1	15.6	16.1	16.6	17.1	17.6	18.1	18.5	19.0	18.5	20.0	20.5	21.0	21.5
16.2	16.8	17.3	17.9	18.4	19.0	19.5	20.1	20.6	21.2	21.7	22.2	22.8	23.3	23.9
18.2	18.8	19.4	20.0	20.7	21.3	21.9	22.5	23.1	23.7	24.2	24.8	25.4	26.0	26.7
20.0	20.7	21.4	22.1	22.7	23.4	24.1	24.8	25.4	26.1	26.8	27.5	28.1	28.8	29.5
21.9	22.6	23.3	24.1	24.8	25.6	26.3	27.0	27.8	28.5	29.2	30.0	30.7	31.5	32.2
4.1	4.2	4.4	4.5	4.6	4.8	4.9	5.0	5.2	5.3	5.4	5.6	5.7	5.9	6.0
6.4	6.6	6.8	7.0	7.2	7.4	7.6	7.9	8.1	8.3	8.5	8.7	8.9	9.1	9.4
7.5	7.8	8.0	8.3	8.5	8.8	9.0	9.3	9.5	9.8	10.0	10.3	10.6	10.8	11.1
9.9	10.2	10.5	10.9	11.2	11.5	11.9	12.2	12.5	12.9	13.2	13.5	13.8	14.2	14.5
11.5	11.9	12.3	12.7	13.1	13.5	13.9	14.3	13.7	15.0	15.4	15.8	16.2	16.6	17.0
9.9	10.2	10.5	10.9	11.2	11.5	11.9	12.2	12.5	12.9	13.2	13.5	13.8	14.2	14.5
9.0	9.3	9.6	9.9	10.2	10.5	10.8	11.1	11.4	11.7	12.0	12.3	12.6	12.9	13.2
10.1	10.5	10.8	11.2	11.5	11.8	12.2	12.5	12.9	13.2	13.5	13.9	14.2	14.6	14.9
11.5	11.9	12.3	12.7	13.1	13.5	13.9	14.3	14.7	15.0	15.4	15.8	16.2	16.6	17.0
3.8	3.9	4.0	4.2	4.3	4.4	4.5	4.7	4.8	4.9	5.1	5.2	5.3	5.4	5.6
5.3	5.5	5.6	5.8	6.0	6.2	6.4	6.5	6.7	6.9	7.1	7.2	7.4	7.6	7.8
6.8	7.0	7.3	7.5	7.7	7.9	8.2	8.4	8.6	8.9	9.1	9.3	9.5	9.8	10.0
8.3	8.6	8.9	9.2	9.4	9.7	10.0	10.3	10.6	10.8	11.1	11.4	11.7	12.0	12.2
4.8	4.9	5.1	5.3	5.4	5.6	5.7	5.9	6.0	6.2	6.4	6.5	6.7	6.9	7.0
7.1	7.4	7.6	7.9	8.1	8.3	8.6	8.8	9.1	9.3	9.5	9.8	10.0	10.3	10.5
9.6	9.9	10.2	10.5	10.9	11.2	11.5	11.9	12.2	12.5	12.8	13.1	13.5	13.8	14.1

Continued

Table 4-1

Caloric Expenditure for Various Physical Activities—cont'd

Body Weight (kcal $\cdot$ min^{-1} $\cdot$ kg^{-1})

Kg		45	48	50	52	55	57	59	61	64	66
Pounds		100	105	110	115	120	125	130	135	140	145
Front crawl											
20		3.1	3.3	3.5	3.6	3.8	4.0	4.1	4.3	4.5	4.6
25		4.0	4.2	4.4	4.6	4.8	5.0	5.2	5.4	5.6	5.8
35		4.8	5.1	5.4	5.6	5.9	6.1	6.4	6.6	6.8	7.0
45		5.7	6.0	6.3	6.6	6.9	7.2	7.5	7.8	8.1	8.4
50		7.0	7.4	7.7	8.1	8.5	8.8	9.2	9.5	9.9	10.3
Table tennis		3.4	3.6	3.8	4.0	4.1	4.3	4.5	4.7	4.8	5.0
Tennis											
Singles, recreational		5.0	5.2	5.5	5.7	6.0	6.2	6.5	6.7	7.0	7.2
Doubles, recreational		3.4	3.6	3.8	4.0	4.1	4.3	4.5	4.7	4.8	5.0
Competition		6.4	6.7	7.1	7.4	7.7	8.1	8.4	8.7	9.1	9.4
Volleyball											
Moderate, recreational		2.9	3.0	3.2	3.3	3.5	3.6	3.8	3.9	4.1	4.2
Vigorous, competition		6.5	6.8	7.1	7.5	7.8	8.1	8.4	8.8	9.1	9.4
Walking											
(mph)	(min/mile)										
1.0	60:00	1.5	1.6	1.7	1.8	1.8	1.9	2.0	2.1	2.2	2.3
2.0	30:00	2.1	2.2	2.3	2.4	2.5	2.6	2.8	2.9	3.0	3.1
2.3	26:00	2.3	2.4	2.5	2.7	2.8	2.9	3.0	3.1	3.2	3.4
3.0	20:00	2.7	2.9	3.0	3.1	3.3	3.4	3.5	3.7	3.8	3.9
3.2	18:45	3.1	3.3	3.4	3.6	3.8	4.0	4.1	4.3	4.4	4.5
3.5	17:10	3.3	3.5	3.7	3.9	4.0	4.2	4.4	4.6	4.7	4.9
4.0	15:00	4.2	4.4	4.6	4.8	5.1	5.3	5.5	5.7	5.9	6.1
4.5	13:20	4.7	5.0	5.2	5.4	5.7	5.9	6.2	6.4	6.7	6.9
5.0	12:00	5.4	5.7	6.0	6.3	6.5	6.8	7.1	7.4	7.7	7.9
5.4	11:10	6.2	6.6	6.9	7.2	7.5	7.9	8.2	8.5	8.8	9.2
5.8	10:20	7.7	8.0	8.4	8.8	9.2	9.6	10.0	10.4	10.8	11.1
Water skiing		5.0	5.2	5.5	5.7	6.0	6.2	6.5	6.7	7.0	7.2
Weight training		5.2	5.4	5.7	6.0	6.2	6.5	6.8	7.0	7.3	7.6
Wrestling		8.5	8.9	9.3	9.8	10.2	10.6	11.0	11.5	11.9	12.3

| 68 | 70 | 73 | 75 | 77 | 80 | 82 | 84 | 86 | 89 | 91 | 93 | 95 | 98 | 100 |
150	155	160	165	170	175	180	185	190	195	200	205	210	215	220
4.8	4.9	5.1	5.3	5.4	5.6	5.7	5.9	6.0	6.2	6.4	6.5	6.7	6.9	7.0
6.0	6.2	6.4	6.6	6.8	7.0	7.2	7.4	7.6	7.8	8.0	8.2	8.4	8.6	8.8
7.3	7.5	7.8	8.0	8.3	8.5	8.8	9.0	9.2	9.4	9.7	9.9	10.2	10.4	10.7
8.7	9.0	9.3	9.5	9.8	10.1	10.4	10.7	11.0	11.3	11.6	11.9	12.2	12.5	12.8
10.6	11.0	11.3	11.7	12.0	12.4	12.8	13.1	13.5	13.8	14.2	14.5	14.9	15.2	15.6
5.2	5.4	5.5	5.7	5.9	6.1	6.3	6.4	6.6	6.8	7.0	7.1	7.3	7.5	7.7
7.5	7.8	8.0	8.3	8.5	8.8	9.0	9.3	9.5	9.8	10.0	10.3	10.6	10.8	11.1
5.2	5.4	5.5	5.7	5.9	6.1	6.3	6.4	6.6	6.8	7.0	7.1	7.3	7.5	7.7
9.8	10.1	10.4	10.8	11.1	11.4	11.8	12.1	12.4	12.8	13.1	13.4	13.7	14.1	14.4
4.4	4.5	4.7	4.8	5.0	5.1	5.3	5.4	5.6	5.7	5.9	6.0	6.1	6.3	6.4
9.8	10.1	10.4	10.7	11.1	11.4	11.7	12.0	12.4	12.7	13.0	13.4	13.7	14.0	14.4
2.3	2.4	2.4	2.5	2.6	2.7	2.8	2.9	2.9	3.0	3.1	3.2	3.2	3.3	3.4
3.2	3.3	3.4	3.5	3.6	3.7	3.9	4.0	4.1	4.2	4.3	4.4	4.5	4.6	4.7
3.5	3.6	3.7	3.8	4.0	4.1	4.2	4.3	4.4	4.5	4.7	4.8	4.9	5.0	5.1
4.1	4.2	4.4	4.5	4.6	4.8	4.9	5.0	5.2	5.3	5.4	5.6	5.7	5.9	6.0
4.7	4.8	5.0	5.2	5.3	5.5	5.6	5.8	5.9	6.1	6.3	6.4	6.6	6.8	6.9
5.1	5.3	5.4	5.6	5.8	6.0	6.2	6.3	6.5	6.7	6.9	7.0	7.2	7.4	7.6
6.4	6.6	6.8	7.0	7.2	7.4	7.6	7.9	8.1	8.3	8.5	8.7	8.9	9.1	9.4
7.1	7.4	7.6	7.9	8.1	8.3	8.6	8.8	9.1	9.3	9.5	9.8	10.0	10.3	10.5
8.2	8.4	8.7	9.0	9.2	9.5	9.8	10.1	10.4	10.6	10.9	11.2	11.5	11.8	12.0
9.5	9.8	10.1	10.4	10.8	11.1	11.4	11.8	12.1	12.4	12.7	13.0	13.4	13.7	14.0
11.5	11.9	12.3	12.7	13.1	13.5	13.9	14.3	14.7	15.0	15.4	15.8	16.2	16.6	17.0
7.5	7.8	8.0	8.3	8.5	8.8	9.0	9.3	9.5	9.8	10.0	10.3	10.6	10.8	11.1
7.8	8.1	8.3	8.6	8.9	9.1	9.4	9.7	9.9	10.2	10.5	10.7	11.0	11.2	11.5
12.8	13.2	13.6	14.1	14.5	14.9	15.4	15.8	16.2	16.6	17.1	17.5	17.9	18.4	18.8

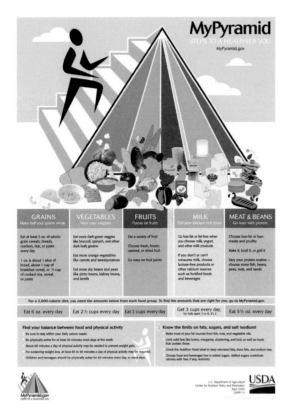

Figure 4-1

Food pyramid. (From United States Department of Agriculture: *MyPyramid Food Guidance System,* 2005, U.S. Department of Agriculture Center for Nutrition Policy and Promotion. Available at www.mypyramid.gov.)

Unfortunately, some limitations with computer and internet programs do exist. These limitations may include lack of frequent database updates, inadequate portion size equivalents between what is reported by the individual and what is available within the computer program, as well as foods that people eat not being listed. To decrease these limitations, one may consider using a combination of computer program and Internet sources.

Additional Resources

Other resources for data analysis include food value tables. One of the most popular hard copy food value tables is *Bowe's and Church Food Values of Portions Commonly Used.*[5] This book contains food values and macro- and micronutrient information of both generic and brand name foods within multiple food categories. This makes for a useful reference, especially for those times when Internet access may not be available. Limitations include interpretation and conversion of portion sizes to meet the needs of the athlete's data, and the number of brand name foods available.

Standard Tables of Recommended Intake

Most methods of evaluating intake involve comparisons with tables of recommended nutrient intake. Dietary reference intakes (DRIs) are reference values established by the National Academy of Sciences (Tables 4-2 to 4-10) that are quantitative estimates of nutrient intakes that also include the recommended dietary allowances (RDAs), adequate intakes, estimated average requirements, and tolerable upper intake levels (ULs).[6] The RDAs are recommended intakes (not requirements) set to meet the nutrient needs for healthy people, and the evaluation of groups rather than individuals. For example, if a healthy individual consumes two-thirds of the RDA, he or she is considered to be meeting the nutrient requirement because the RDA is set on the high side to meet population needs. The nutrient needs of athletes are discussed later in this chapter.

The evaluation of nutrient intake is an estimate that depends on the accuracy of the methods used for dietary assessment and analysis. To identify specific nutrient deficiencies, biochemical and clinical assessments should be considered, along with the dietary assessment.

The Dietary Interview

Because limitations exist with dietary assessment and analysis methods, and people tend to underestimate their food intake (especially those with a weight management issue), a dietary interview is also warranted to further assess general eating patterns and develop rapport with the individual athlete. Questions should address where most meals are eaten; who prepares the food; any foods the athlete avoids; snacking patterns and choices; the athlete's ethnic or cultural practices; what, if any, vitamins, minerals, or other nutritional supplements are used; and the individual's perception of good nutrition: "In your opinion, what constitutes a poor eating day?" "What constitutes a good eating day?" "How often does each occur?" "What are your most difficult challenges in eating a 'healthy' diet?"

The dietary interview should also include questions regarding training and competition schedules. It is important to know the amount of time spent in training as well as the intensity and duration of the individual's activity to calculate caloric needs. Specific questions regarding eating and drinking patterns before, during, and after an event are equally important.

Motivation and Readiness for Behavioral Change

The step after evaluating an athlete's intake and determining needs is to make recommendations for change and assist the athlete in setting individualized goals. One of the most common errors made by health professionals advocating behavior change is to tell the individual what to do and expect that a behavior change will occur. Attention should be given to whether the individual is ready, motivated, and willing to make the changes. Experts in the area of health promotion are suggesting that a shift from an action to a stage paradigm is occurring. The stage paradigm is a proactive and interactive model for behavior change and can be used to assess an individual's readiness in regard to making changes; it also provides guidelines for professional intervention.[7] The stages of change are shown in Table 4-11. During the assessment, it is useful to determine the athlete's stage to determine an appropriate intervention strategy. An example is the athlete who has no idea that his or her diet is nutritionally inadequate and therefore may not be ready to take action and start goal setting.

Information regarding nutrition and exercise is first needed to move the athlete to the next stage: contemplation. Once the athlete has contemplated making the dietary changes, it is time to clarify any preconceived notions and to provide additional information regarding the benefits of the change. The athlete may then be ready to move to the preparation stage. During this stage, the athlete is able to identify a motivation for taking action and begins to investigate strategies for change. A list of action strategies for the athlete ready to implement changes is shown in Box 4-1. Learning whether the individual is ready to make changes requires good listening skills on the part of the interviewer. The interviewer can learn what motivates the athlete and where to start in the process of making behavior changes.

Nutrient Recommendations

The body requires at least 40 nutrients, which are classified into six groups: macronutrients (carbohydrates, fat, and protein), micronutrients (vitamins and minerals), and water. These nutrients are classified as essential because they cannot be made in the body; therefore, they must be supplied from the diet. There are three categories of macronutrients: carbohydrates, fat, and protein; and two categories of micronutrients: vitamins and minerals. The macronutrients, in addition to alcohol, provide energy in the form of calories (Table 4-12). Vitamins, minerals, and water have no calories and therefore are not a source of energy.

Groups of Nutrients

• Carbohydrates	
• Fat	Macronutrients
• Protein	
• Vitamins	Micronutrients
• Minerals	
• Water	

Macronutrients
Carbohydrates

Carbohydrates are the body's preferred source of energy, used to spare protein for body growth and repair. However, storage space for carbohydrates is limited within the body. The predominant method of storage is in the form of glycogen and intracellular polysaccharide. Muscle glycogen represents the major source of carbohydrate in the body (1200 to 1600 kcal or 300 to 400 g), followed by liver glycogen (300 to 400 kcal or 75 to 100 g), and, lastly, blood glucose (100 kcal or 25 g).[8] The liver's glycogen storage is used to maintain blood glucose levels, whereas muscle glycogen is used by the muscles for energy. An athlete's performance (i.e., greater endurance and delayed fatigue) can be maximized by ensuring greater energy reserve in the form of muscle glycogen for endurance and strength activities. During endurance activities requiring 65% maximum oxygen consumption (VO_2 max), our bodies prefer carbohydrate as the primary fuel source.[8-10]

High-intensity, short-duration exercise (sprinting) relies on the anaerobic pathway for the production of energy. Only glucose derived primarily from the breakdown of muscle glycogen can be used as fuel. Muscle glycogen is used about 18 times faster when glucose is broken down anaerobically than when glucose is broken down aerobically. During high-intensity exercise (i.e., more than 70% of aerobic capacity) and in extended mixed anaerobic and aerobic sports (such as soccer, basketball, football drills, and interval running or swimming) the aerobic pathway is also used. A more rapid rate of muscle glycogen breakdown occurs in these events.

Exercise of low-to-moderate intensity is fueled almost entirely aerobically. Increased epinephrine, norepinephrine, growth hormone, and decreased insulin promote the release of fatty acids from the adipose tissue into the bloodstream. Half of the energy is supplied by these fatty acids, whereas muscle glycogen and blood glucose supply the rest for this type of event. However, muscle glycogen is the predominant fuel for most types of exercise.

It is extremely important that endurance athletes (e.g., cyclists, long-distance runners, triathletes) consume a high-carbohydrate diet because one of the limiting factors in prolonged performance is glycogen depletion. Recent debate has been focused around the two primary fuel sources of the body (carbohydrates and fat) during the recovery phase. Burke and colleagues conducted a literature review that focused on successful day-to-day refueling methods and recovery between daily sessions or multiple workouts.[11] Although fat consumption remains an important part of an athlete's overall diet, Burke and colleagues concluded that foods rich in carbohydrate with a moderate-to-high glycemic index value provided a readily available source of carbohydrate for muscle glycogen synthesis, and should be the major carbohydrate choice in recovery meals.[11] They also concluded that even though new interest revolves around the recovery of intramuscular triglyceride stores, at the present time, no evidence supports advantages of high-fat, restricted carbohydrate diets to enhance training.[11]

Recommended carbohydrate intakes for athletes varies, depending on current training needs and other factors such as current body mass and nutrition goals. Generally speaking, most athletes require 6 to 10 g/kg/day.[8] For example, a 65-kg marathon runner would require 455 to 650 g of carbohydrate per day (using 7- to 10-g carbohydrate/day), whereas a 65-kg basketball player may only require 390 to 455 g of carbohydrate per day.

text cont'd on page 77

Table 4-2

Dietary Reference Intakes (DRIs): Recommended Intakes for Individuals, Vitamins (Food and Nutrition Board, Institute of Medicine, National Academies)

Life Stage Group	Vit A (μg/day)^a	Vit C (mg/day)	Vit D (μg/day)^{b,c}	Vit E (mg/day)^d	Vit K (μg/day)	Thiamin (mg/day)
Infants						
0–6 mo	400*	40*	5*	4*	2.0*	0.2*
7–12 mo	500*	50*	5*	5*	2.5*	0.3*
Children						
1–3 y	300	15	5*	6	30*	0.5
4–8 y	400	25	5*	7	55*	0.6
Males						
9–13 y	600	45	5*	11	60*	0.9
14–18 y	900	75	5*	15	75*	1.2
19–30 y	900	90	5*	15	120*	1.2
31–50 y	900	90	5*	15	120*	1.2
51–70 y	900	90	10*	15	120*	1.2
> 70 y	900	90	15*	15	120*	1.2
Females						
9–13 y	600	45	5*	11	60*	0.9
14–18 y	700	65	5*	15	75*	1.0
19–30 y	700	75	5*	15	90*	1.1
31–50 y	700	75	5*	15	90*	1.1
51–70 y	700	75	10*	15	90*	1.1
> 70 y	700	75	15*	15	90*	1.1
Pregnancy						
14–18 y	750	80	5*	15	75*	1.4
19–30 y	770	85	5*	15	90*	1.4
31–50 y	770	85	5*	15	90*	1.4
Lactation						
14–18 y	1,200	115	5*	19	75*	1.4
19–30 y	1,300	120	5*	19	90*	1.4
31–50 y	1,300	120	5*	19	90*	1.4

NOTE: This table (taken from the DRI reports, see www.nap.edu) presents Recommended Dietary Allowances (RDAs) in **bold type** and Adequate Intakes (AIs) in ordinary type followed by an asterisk (*). RDAs and AIs may both be used as goals for Individual intake. RDAs are set to meet the needs of almost all (97 to 98 percent) individuals in a group. For healthy breastfed infants, the AI is the mean intake. The AI for other life stage and gender groups is believed to cover needs of all individuals in the group, but lack of data or uncertainty in the data prevent being able to specify with confidence the percentage of individuals covered by this intake.

^{a} As retinol activity equivalents (RAEs). 1 RAE = 1 μg retinol, 12 μg β-carotene, 24 μg α-carotene, or 24 μg β-cryptoxanthin. The RAE for dietary provitamin A carotenoids is twofold greater than retinol equivalents (RE), whereas the RAE for preformed vitamin A is the same as RE.

^{b} As cholecalciferol. 1 μg cholecalciferol = 40 IU vitamin D.

^{c} In the absence of adequate exposure to sunlight.

^{d} As α-tocopherol. α-Tocopherol includes *RRR*-α-tocopherol, the only form of α-tocopherol that occurs naturally in foods, and the 2*R*-stereoisomeric forms of α-tocopherol (*RRR*-, *RSR*-, *RRS*-, and *RSS*-α-tocopherol) that occur in fortified foods and supplements. It does not include the 2*S*-stereoisomeric forms of α-tocopherol (*SRR*-, *SSR*-, *SRS*-, and *SSS*-α-tocopherol), also found in fortified foods and supplements.

^{e} As niacin equivalents (NE). 1 mg of niacin = 60 mg of tryptophan; 0–6 months = preformed niacin (not NE).

^{f} As dietary folate equivalents (DFE). 1 DFE = 1 μg food folate = 0.6 μg of folic acid from fortified food or as a supplement consumed with food = 0.5 μg of a supplement taken on an empty stomach.

^{g} Although AIs have been set for choline, there are few data to assess whether a dietary supply of choline is needed at all stages of the life cycle, and it may be that the choline requirement can be met by endogenous synthesis at some of these stages.

^{h} Because 10 to 30 percent of older people may malabsorb food-bound B_{12}, it is advisable for those older than 50 years to meet their RDA mainly by consuming foods fortified with B_{12} or a supplement containing B_{12}.

^{i} In view of evidence linking folate intake with neural tube defects in the fetus, it is recommended that all women capable of becoming pregnant consume 400 μg from supplements or fortified foods in addition to intake of food folate from a varied diet.

^{j} It is assumed that women will continue consuming 400 μg from supplements or fortified food until their pregnancy is confirmed and they enter prenatal care, which ordinarily occurs after the end of the periconceptional period—the critical time for formation of the neural tube.

Riboflavin (mg/day)	Niacin (mg/day)[e]	Vit B$_6$ (mg/day)	Folate (μg/day)[f]	Vit B$_{12}$ (μg/day)	Pantothenic Acid (mg/day)	Biotin (μg/day)	Choline (mg/day)[g]
0.3*	2*	0.1*	65*	0.4*	1.7*	5*	125*
0.4*	4*	0.3*	80*	0.5*	1.8*	6*	150*
0.5	6	0.5	150	0.9	2*	8*	200*
0.6	8	0.6	200	1.2	3*	12*	250*
0.9	12	1.0	300	1.8	4*	20*	375*
1.3	16	1.3	400	2.4	5*	25*	550*
1.3	16	1.3	400	2.4	5*	30*	550*
1.3	16	1.3	400	2.4	5*	30*	550*
1.3	16	1.7	400	2.4[i]	5*	30*	550*
1.3	16	1.7	400	2.4[i]	5*	30*	550*
0.9	12	1.0	300	1.8	4*	20*	375*
1.0	14	1.2	400[i]	2.4	5*	25*	400*
1.1	14	1.3	400[i]	2.4	5*	30*	425*
1.1	14	1.3	400[i]	2.4	5*	30*	425*
1.1	14	1.5	400	2.4[h]	5*	30*	425*
1.1	14	1.5	400	2.4[h]	5*	30*	425*
1.4	18	1.9	600[j]	2.6	6*	30*	450*
1.4	18	1.9	600[j]	2.6	6*	30*	450*
1.4	18	1.9	600[j]	2.6	6*	30*	450*
1.6	17	2.0	500	2.8	7*	35*	550*
1.6	17	2.0	500	2.8	7*	35*	550*
1.6	17	2.0	500	2.8	7*	35*	550*

Table 4-3

Dietary Reference Intakes (DRIs): Recommended Intakes for Individuals, Elements (Food and Nutrition Board, Institute of Medicine, National Academies)

Life Stage Group	Calcium (mg/day)	Chromium (µg/day)	Copper (µg/day)	Fluoride (mg/day)	Iodine (µg/day)	Iron (mg/day)	Magnesium (mg/day)
Infants							
0-6 mo	210*	0.2*	200*	0.01*	110*	0.27*	30*
7-12 mo	270*	5.5*	220*	0.5*	130*	**11**	75*
Children							
1-3 y	500*	11*	340	0.7*	90	7	80
4-8 y	800*	15*	440	1*	90	10	130
Males							
9-13 y	1300*	25*	700	2*	120	8	240
14-18 y	1300*	35*	890	3*	150	11	410
19-30 y	1000*	35*	900	4*	150	8	400
31-50 y	1000*	35*	900	4*	150	8	420
51-70 y	1200*	30*	900	4*	150	8	420
> 70 y	1200*	30*	900	4*	150	8	420
Females							
9-13 y	1300*	21*	700	2*	120	8	240
14-18 y	1300*	24*	890	3*	150	15	360
19-30 y	1000*	25*	900	3*	150	18	310
31-50 y	1000*	25*	900	3*	150	18	320
51-70 y	1200*	20*	900	3*	150	8	320
> 70 y	1200*	20*	900	3*	150	8	320
Pregnancy							
14-18 y	1300*	29*	1000	3*	220	27	400
19-30 y	1000*	30*	1000	3*	220	27	350
31-50 y	1000*	30*	1000	3*	220	27	360
Lactation							
14-18 y	1300*	44*	1300	3*	290	10	360
19-30 y	1000*	45*	1300	3*	290	9	310
31-50 y	1000*	45*	1300	3*	290	9	320

NOTE: This table presents Recommended Dietary Allowances (RDAs) in **bold type** and Adequate Intakes (AIs) in ordinary type followed by an asterisk (*). RDAs and AIs may both be used as goals for individual intake. RDAs are set to meet the needs of almost all (97% to 98%) individuals in a group. For healthy breastfed infants, the AI is the mean intake. The AI for other life stage and gender groups is believed to cover needs of all individuals in the group, but lack of data or uncertainty in the data prevent being able to specify with confidence the percentage of individuals covered by this intake.

SOURCES: *Dietary Reference Intakes for Calcium, Phosphorous, Magnesium, Vitamin D, and Fluoride* (1997); *Dietary Reference Intakes for Thiamin, Riboflavin, Niacin, Vitamin B_6, Folate, Vitamin B_{12}, Pantothenic Acid, Biotin, and Choline* (1998); *Dietary Reference Intakes for Vitamin C, Vitamin E, Selenium, and Carotenoids* (2000); *Dietary Reference Intakes for Vitamin A, Vitamin K, Arsenic, Boron, Chromium, Copper, Iodine, Iron, Manganese, Molybdenum, Nickel, Silicon, Vanadium, and Zinc* (2001); and *Dietary Reference Intakes for Water, Potassium, Sodium, Chloride, and Sulfate* (2004). These reports may be accessed via http:www.nap.edu. Copyright 2004 by the National Academy of Sciences. All rights reserved.

Manganese (mg/day)	Molybdenum (μg/day)	Phosphorus (mg/day)	Selenium (μg/day)	Zinc (mg/day)	Potassium (g/day)	Sodium (g/day)	Chloride (g/day)
0.003*	2*	100*	15*	2*	0.4*	0.12*	0.18*
0.6*	3*	275*	20*	3	0.7*	0.37*	0.57*
1.2*	17	460	20	3	3.0*	1.0*	1.5*
1.5*	22	500	30	5	3.8*	1.2*	1.9*
1.9*	34	1250	40	8	4.5*	1.5*	2.3*
2.2*	43	1250	55	11	4.7*	1.5*	2.3*
2.3*	45	700	55	11	4.7*	1.5*	2.3*
2.3*	45	700	55	11	4.7*	1.5*	2.3*
2.3*	45	700	55	11	4.7*	1.3*	2.0*
2.3*	45	700	55	11	4.7*	1.2*	1.8*
1.6*	34	1250	40	8	4.5*	1.5*	2.3*
1.6*	43	1250	55	9	4.7*	1.5*	2.3*
1.8*	45	700	55	8	4.7*	1.5*	2.3*
1.8*	45	700	55	8	4.7*	1.5*	2.3*
1.8*	45	700	55	8	4.7*	1.3*	2.0*
1.8*	45	700	55	8	4.7*	1.2*	1.8*
2.0*	50	1250	60	12	4.7*	1.5*	2.3*
2.0*	50	700	60	11	4.7*	1.5*	2.3*
2.0*	50	700	60	11	4.7*	1.5*	2.3*
2.6*	50	1250	70	13	5.1*	1.5*	2.3*
2.6*	50	700	70	12	5.1*	1.5*	2.3*
2.6*	50	700	70	12	5.1*	1.5*	2.3*

Table 4-4

Dietary Reference Intakes (DRIs): Tolerable Upper Intake Levels (UL^a), Vitamins (Food and Nutrition Board, Institute of Medicine, National Academies)

Life Stage Group	Vitamin A (mg/day)^b	Vitamin C (mg/day)	Vitamin D (μg/day)	Vitamin E (mg/day)^{c,d}	Vitamin K	Thiamin	Riboflavin
Infants							
0-6 mo	600	ND^f	25	ND	ND	ND	ND
7-12 mo	600	ND	25	ND	ND	ND	ND
Children							
1-3 y	600	400	50	200	ND	ND	ND
4-8 y	900	650	50	300	ND	ND	ND
Males,							
Females							
9-13 y	1700	1200	50	600	ND	ND	ND
14-18 y	2800	1800	50	800	ND	ND	ND
19-70 y	3000	2000	50	1000	ND	ND	ND
> 70 y	3000	2000	50	1000	ND	ND	ND
Pregnancy							
14-18 y	2800	1800	50	800	ND	ND	ND
19-50 y	3000	2000	50	1000	ND	ND	ND
Lactation							
14-18 y	2800	1800	50	800	ND	ND	ND
19-50 y	3000	2000	50	1000	ND	ND	ND

^{a}UL = The maximum level of daily nutrient intake that is likely to pose no risk of adverse effects. Unless otherwise specified, the UL represents total intake from food, water, and supplements. Due to lack of suitable data, ULs could not be established for vitamin K, thiamin, riboflavin, vitamin B_{12}, pantothenic acid, biotin, carotenoids. In the absence of ULs, extra caution may be warranted in consuming levels above recommended intakes.

^{b}As preformed vitamin A only.

^{c}As α-tocopherol; applies to any form of supplemental α-tocopherol.

^{d}The ULs for vitamin E, niacin, and folate apply to synthetic forms obtained from supplements, fortified foods, or a combination of the two.

^{e}β-Carotene supplements are advised only to serve as a provitamin A source for individuals at risk of vitamin A deficiency.

^{f}ND = Not determinable due to lack of data of adverse effects in this age group and concern with regard to lack of ability to handle excess amounts. Source of intake should be from food only to prevent high levels of intake.

SOURCES: *Dietary Reference Intakes for Calcium, Phosphorous, Magnesium, Vitamin D, and Fluoride* (1997); *Dietary Reference Intakes for Thiamin, Riboflavin, Niacin, Vitamin B$_6$, Folate, Vitamin B$_{12}$, Pantothenic Acid, Biotin, and Choline* (1998); *Dietary Reference Intakes for Vitamin C, Vitamin E, Selenium, and Carotenoids* (2000); and *Dietary Reference Intakes for Vitamin A, Vitamin K, Arsenic, Boron, Chromium, Copper, Iodine, Iron, Manganese, Molybdenum, Nickel, Silicon, Vanadium, and Zinc* (2001). These reports may be accessed via. http://www.nap.edu. Copyright 2004 by the National Academy of Sciences. All rights reserved.

Niacin (mg/day)[d]	Vitamin B_6 (mg/day)	Folate (μg/day)[d]	Vitamin B_{12}	Pantothenic Acid	Biotin	Choline (g/day)	Carotenoids[e]
ND	ND	ND	ND	ND	ND	ND	ND
ND	ND	ND	ND	ND	ND	ND	ND
10	30	300	ND	ND	ND	1.0	ND
15	40	400	ND	ND	ND	1.0	ND
20	60	600	ND	ND	ND	2.0	ND
30	80	800	ND	ND	ND	3.0	ND
35	100	1000	ND	ND	ND	3.5	ND
35	100	1000	ND	ND	ND	3.5	ND
30	80	800	ND	ND	ND	3.0	ND
35	100	1000	ND	ND	ND	3.5	ND
30	80	800	ND	ND	ND	3.0	ND
35	100	1000	ND	ND	ND	3.5	ND

Table 4-5

Dietary Reference Intakes (DRIs): Tolerable Upper Intake Levels (UL[a]), Elements (Food and Nutrition Board, Institute of Medicine, National Academies)

Life Stage Group	Arsenic[b]	Boron (mg/day)	Calcium (g/day)	Chromium	Copper (µg/day)	Fluoride (mg/day)	Iodine (µg/day)	Iron (mg/day)	Magnesium (mg/day)[c]	Manganese (mg/day)
Infants										
0-6 mo	ND[f]	ND	ND	ND	ND	0.7	ND	40	ND	ND
7-12 mo	ND	ND	ND	ND	ND	0.9	ND	40	ND	ND
Children										
1-3 y	ND	3	2.5	ND	1000	1.3	200	40	65	2
4-8 y	ND	6	2.5	ND	3000	2.2	300	40	110	3
Males, Females										
9-13 y	ND	11	2.5	ND	5000	10	600	40	350	6
14-18 y	ND	17	2.5	ND	8000	10	900	45	350	9
19-70 y	ND	20	2.5	ND	10000	10	1100	45	350	11
>70 y	ND	20	2.5	ND	10000	10	1100	45	350	11
Pregnancy										
14-18 y	ND	17	2.5	ND	8000	10	900	45	350	9
19-50 y	ND	20	2.5	ND	10000	10	1100	45	350	11
Lactation										
14-18 y	ND	17	2.5	ND	8000	10	900	45	350	9
19-50 y	ND	20	2.5	ND	10000	10	1100	45	350	11

[a]UL = The maximum level of daily nutrient intake that is likely to pose no risk of adverse effects. Unless otherwise specified, the UL represents total intake from food, water, and supplements. Due to lack of suitable data, ULs could not be established for arsenic, chromium, silicon, potassium, and sulfate. In the absence of ULs, extra caution may be warranted in consuming levels above recommended intakes.

[b]Although the UL was not determined for arsenic, there is no justification for adding arsenic to food or supplements.

[c]The ULs for magnesium represent intake from a pharmacological agent only and do not include intake from food and water.

[d]Although silicon has not been shown to cause adverse effects in humans, there is no justification for adding silicon to supplements.

[e]Although vanadium in food has not been shown to cause adverse effects in humans, there is no justification for adding vanadium to food and vanadium supplements should be used with caution. The UL is based on adverse effects in laboratory animals and this data could be used to set a UL for adults but not children and adolescents.

[f]ND = Not determinate due to lack of data of adverse effects in this age group and concern with regard to lack of ability to handle excess amounts. Source of intake should be from food only to prevent high levels of intake.

SOURCES: *Dietary Reference Intakes for Calcium, Phosphorous, Magnesium, Vitamin D, and Fluoride* (1997); *Dietary Reference Intakes for Thiamin, Riboflavin, Niacin, Vitamin B₆, Folate, Vitamin B₁₂, Pantothenic Acid, Biotin, and Choline* (1998); *Dietary Reference Intakes for Vitamin C, Vitamin E, Selenium, and Carotenoids* (2000); *Dietary Reference Intakes for Vitamin A, Vitamin K, Arsenic, Boron, Chromium, Copper, Iodine, Iron, Manganese, Molybdenum, Nickel, Silicon, Vanadium, and Zinc* (2001); and *Dietary Reference Intakes for Water, Potassium, Sodium, Chloride, and Sulfate* (2004). These reports may be accessed via.http:www.nap.edu. Copyright 2004 by the National Academy of Sciences. All rights reserved.

Molybdenum (mg/day)	Nickel (mg/day)	Phosphorus (g/day)	Potassium	Selenium (μg/day)	Silicon[d]	Sulfate	Vanadium (mg/day)[e]	Zinc (mg/day)	Sodium (g/day)	Chloride (g/day)
ND	ND	ND	ND	45	ND	ND	ND	4	ND	ND
ND	ND	ND	ND	60	ND	ND	ND	5	ND	ND
300	0.2	3	ND	90	ND	ND	ND	7	1.5	2.3
600	0.3	3	ND	150	ND	ND	ND	12	1.9	2.9
1100	0.6	4	ND	280	ND	ND	ND	23	2.2	3.4
1700	1.0	4	ND	400	ND	ND	ND	34	2.3	3.6
2000	1.0	4	ND	400	ND	ND	1.8	40	2.3	3.6
2000	1.0	3	ND	400	ND	ND	1.8	40	2.3	3.6
1700	1.0	3.5	ND	400	ND	ND	ND	34	2.3	3.6
2000	1.0	3.5	ND	400	ND	ND	ND	40	2.3	3.6
1700	1.0	4	ND	400	ND	ND	ND	34	2.3	3.6
2000	1.0	4	ND	400	ND	ND	ND	40	2.3	3.6

Table 4-6

Dietary Reference Intakes (DRIs): Estimated Energy Requirements (EER) for Men and Women 30 Years of Age^a (Food and Nutrition Board, Institute of Medicine, National Academies)

Height (m [in])	PAL^b	EER, Men* (kcal/day)				EER, Women* (kcal/day)	
		Weight for BMI^c of 18.5 kg/m^2 (kg [lb])	Weight for BMI of 24.99 kg/m^2 (kg [lb])	BMI of 18.5 kg/m^2	BMI of 24.99 kg/m^2	BMI of 18.5 kg/m^2	BMI of 24.99 kg/m^2
1.50 (59)	Sedentary	41.6 (92)	56.2 (124)	1848	2080	1625	1762
	Low active			2009	2267	1803	1956
	Active			2215	2506	2025	2198
	Very active			2554	2898	2291	2489
1.65 (65)	Sedentary	50.4 (111)	68.0 (150)	2068	2349	1816	1982
	Low active			2254	2566	2016	2202
	Active			2490	2842	2267	2477
	Very active			2880	3296	2567	2807
1.80 (71)	Sedentary	59.9 (132)	81.0 (178)	2301	2635	2015	2211
	Low active			2513	2884	2239	2459
	Active			2782	3200	2519	2769
	Very active			3225	3720	2855	3141

^{a}For each year below 30, add 7 kcal/day for women and 10 kcal/day for men. For each year above 30, subtract 7 kcal/day for women and 10 kcal/day for men.
^{b}PAL = physical activity level.
^{c}BMI = body mass index.
*Derived from the following regression equations based on doubly labeled water data:
Adult man: EER = 662 − 9.53 × age (y) + PA × (15.91 × wt [kg] + 539.6 × ht [m])
Adult woman: EER = 354 − 6.91 × age (y) + PA × (9.36 × wt [kg] + 726 × ht [m])
Where PA refers to coefficient for PAL.
PAL = total energy expenditure √ basal energy expenditure
  PA = 1.0 if PAL ≥ 1.0 < 1.4 (sedentary)
  PA = 1.12 if PAL ≥ 1.4 < 1.6 (low active)
  PA = 1.27 if PAL ≥ 1.6 < 1.9 (active)
  PA = 1.45 if PAL ≥ 1.9 < 2.5 (very active)

Table 4-7

Dietary Reference Intakes (DRIs): Acceptable Macronutrient Distribution Ranges (Food and Nutrition Board, Institute of Medicine, National Academies)

Macronutrient	Range (percent of energy)		
	Children, 1-3 year	Children, 4-18 year	Adults
Fat	30-40	25-35	20-35
n-6 polyunsaturated fatty acids[a] (linoleic acid)	5-10	5-10	5-10
n-3 polyunsaturated fatty acids[a] (α-linolenic acid)	0.6-1.2	0.6-1.2	0.6-1.2
Carbohydrate	45-65	45-65	45-65
Protein	5-20	10-30	10-35

[a]Approximately 10% of the total can come from longer-chain *n*-3 or *n*-6 fatty acids.
SOURCE: *Dietary Reference Intakes for Energy, Carbohydrate, Fiber, Fat, Fatty Acids, Cholesterol, Protein, and Amino Acids* (2002). Copyright 2004 by the National Academy of Sciences. All rights reserved.

Daily Recommendations for Carbohydrate Intake[8]

- 4 to 5 g/kg/day for general population with physical activity of low-intensity
- 6 to 7 g/kg/day for general training needs
- 7 to 10 g/day for endurance athletes
- > 10 g/day for ultra endurance athletes

To maximize overall performance during and after an event, athletes who engage in continuous, intense endurance training (i.e., 90 minutes or more) may combine a specific training schedule and dietary regimen termed *carbohydrate loading* or *glycogen super compensation*. Normally, each 100 g of muscle contains about 1.7 g of glycogen; carbohydrate loading packs up to 5 g of glycogen per 100 g of skeletal muscle.[12] Because of the extreme demands of the classic carbohydrate loading method, most athletes resort to a *modified carbohydrate loading* method, which has been an accepted carbohydrate loading method since the early 1980s. Using this method, athletes taper their training, following a more realistic exercise preparation during the week before an important event.[13] As depicted in Figure 4-2, during the first 3 days of the week, exercise duration is longer, carbohydrates are limited to approximately 50% of overall caloric intake for the day (or about 5 g/kg/day), and fat and protein make up the other 50%. As exercise decreases on days 4 and 5, carbohydrates are increased to 70% or more of overall daily caloric intake (7 to 10 g/kg/day), and fat and protein are decreased. Day 6 results in a complete rest day from exercise and maximal carbohydrate uptake, stimulating muscle glycogen storage. The modified carbohydrate loading method results in nearly as much of a gain in muscle glycogen synthesis when compared with the classic method, without all of the struggles of exhaustive exercise and a rigorous carbohydrate diet regimen.

This dietary protocol maintains high glycogen stores and may be followed numerous times throughout the year without health risk.[14] If an athlete adheres to a high-carbohydrate diet, but does not train to develop muscle strength and endurance, there will be a limited capacity to store glycogen. However, reducing exercise 2 days before the event and resting the day before allows the muscles the opportunity to replace depleted glycogen stores. Rest is an essential part of carbohydrate loading to promote muscle glycogen storage for optimal endurance performance.[13]

Protein

Requirements for protein are actually requirements for amino acids, the building blocks of protein. Protein can be compared with a chain-link fence, the links representing amino acids. There are 20 amino acids in which our bodies require and are involved in multiple tasks such as protein turnover, membrane transport, immune function, acid-base regulation, and intermediary metabolism. Amino acids are divided into two categories, nonessential and essential. Essential amino acids are ones the body cannot synthesize and that therefore must be ingested into the body through diets. The term *nonessential* does not mean they are unimportant; rather, they must be synthesized from other compounds already in the body at a rate to meet demands for normal growth and tissue repair.[15]

Protein, the component of many hormones, is a constituent of antibodies for the body's immune system and is part of every enzyme in the body. Approximately 45% of the human body is protein; second only to water, it makes up the largest percentage of material in the human body. Although carbohydrate is the body's most-used source of energy, in aerobic sports amino acids may supply up to 15% of the total energy used.[16]

Evaluation of protein needs should consider the energy content of the diet. Although protein requirements are based on degree and intensity of training, energy intake is the most important factor affecting protein requirements. When energy intake is less than that required by the body, protein breakdown occurs to provide the energy needed. Therefore, sports that require specific body weight such as wrestling, dancing, and gymnastics may lead to insufficient energy intake, and protein needs may exceed the RDA.

Table 4-8

Dietary Reference Intakes (DRIs): Recommended Intakes for Individuals, Macronutrients (Food and Nutrition Board, Institute of Medicine, National Academies)

Life Stage Group	Total Water[a] (L/day)	Carbohydrate (g/day)	Total Fiber (g/day)	Fat (g/day)	Linoleic Acid (g/day)	α-Linolenic Acid (g/day)	Protein[b] (g/day)
Infants							
0-6 mo	0.7*	60*	ND	31*	4.4*	0.5*	9.1*
7-12 mo	0.8*	95*	ND	30*	4.6*	0.5*	11.0[c]
Children							
1-3 y	1.3*	130	19*	ND	7*	0.7*	13
4-8 y	1.7*	130	25*	ND	10*	0.9*	19
Males							
9-13 y	2.4*	130	31*	ND	12*	1.2*	34
14-18 y	3.3*	130	38*	ND	16*	1.6*	52
19-30 y	3.7*	130	38*	ND	17*	1.6*	56
31-50 y	3.7*	130	38*	ND	17*	1.6*	56
51-70 y	3.7*	130	30*	ND	14*	1.6*	56
> 70 y	3.7*	130	30*	ND	14*	1.6*	56
Females							
9-13 y	2.1*	130	26*	ND	10*	1.0*	34
14-18 y	2.3*	130	26*	ND	11*	1.1*	46
19-30 y	2.7*	130	25*	ND	12*	1.1*	46
31-50 y	2.7*	130	25*	ND	12*	1.1*	46
51-70 y	2.7*	130	21*	ND	11*	1.1*	46
> 70 y	2.7*	130	21*	ND	11*	1.1*	46
Pregnancy							
14-18 y	3.0*	175	28*	ND	13*	1.4*	71
19-30 y	3.0*	175	28*	ND	13*	1.4*	71
31-50 y	3.0*	175	28*	ND	13*	1.4*	71
Lactation							
14-18 y	3.8*	210	29*	ND	13*	1.3*	71
19-30 y	3.8*	210	29*	ND	13*	1.3*	71
31-50 y	3.8*	210	29*	ND	13*	1.3*	71

NOTE: This table presents Recommended Dietary Allowances (RDAs) in **bold** type and Adequate Intakes (AIs) in ordinary type followed by an asterisk (*). RDAs and AIs may both be used as goals for individual intake. RDAs are set to meet the needs of almost all (97% to 98%) individuals in a group. For healthy infants fed human milk, the AI is the mean intake. The AI for other life stage and gender groups is believed to cover the needs of all individuals in the group, but lack of data or uncertainty in the data prevent being able to specify with confidence the percentage of individuals covered by this intake.

[a] *Total* water includes all water contained in food, beverages, and drinking water.

[b] Based on 0.8 g/kg body weight for the reference body weight.

[c] Change from 13.5 in prepublication copy due to calculation error.

Copyright 2004 by the National Academy of Sciences. All rights reserved.

Table 4-9

Dietary Reference Intakes (DRIs): Additional Macronutrient Recommendations (Food and Nutrition Board, Institute of Medicine, National Academies)

Macronutrient	Recommendation
Dietary cholesterol	As low as possible while consuming a nutritionally adequate diet
Trans fatty acids	As low as possible while consuming a nutritionally adequate diet
Saturated fatty acids	As low as possible while consuming a nutritionally adequate diet
Added sugars	Limit to no more than 25% of total energy

SOURCE: *Dietary Reference Intakes for Energy, Carbohydrate, Fiber, Fat, Fatty Acids, Cholesterol, Protein, and Amino Acids* (2002). Copyright 2004 by the National Academy of Sciences. All rights reserved.

For years, health professionals have agreed that the RDA for protein "represents a margin of safety to account for amino acids catabolized during exercise and amino acids required for protein synthesis following exercise."[12] Protein's limited capacity for use as a fuel source has been thought to result from its primary role of tissue synthesis, minimal protein breakdown during endurance exercise,[17] and resistance training demands for muscle tissue synthesis. According to recent research, however, protein may have an increased role as a source of fuel for energy. Following endurance or resistance exercise, muscle protein synthesis is increased. Thus, two factors justify re-examining protein intake recommendations for those involved in exercise training: (1) increased protein breakdown during long-term exercise and heavy training and (2) increased protein synthesis in recovery from exercise.[12]

Branched-Chain Amino Acids. Three amino acids, leucine, valine, and isoleucine, are branched-chain amino acids. These amino acids are predominantly oxidized during exercise and are essential amino acids. Increased use of branched-chain amino acids and increased breakdown of protein are two factors contributing to the increased protein requirement in endurance athletes.[18] Protein intakes range from 1.2 to 1.4 g/kg/day for endurance athletes and from 1.6 to 1.7 g/kg/day for resistance-training athletes.[3]

It is unlikely that amino acid oxidation plays an important role in providing energy for strength training because, although it may be intense, each bout is brief. Also, weight training may actually improve the efficiency of protein use.[19] Carbohydrate in the form of glycogen is the major fuel for strength activities.

Most research on the actual protein intake of athletes in developed countries reveals that the average athlete consumes protein in the highest recommended range.[20] Those at highest risk of consuming inadequate protein are individuals who already have elevated protein requirements for reasons other than sports, those who consume inadequate calories, and those who participate in multiple daily training sessions. Protein needs can be calculated both as a percentage of the total energy and on a per–kilogram body weight basis. For athletes with exceptionally high energy intakes, providing 12% to 15% of total energy from protein may be excessive. When energy intake is low, as may be observed for many young women or in low–body weight athletes, protein needs calculated as a percentage of energy may be inadequate. In both of these cases, 1.0 to 1.5 g protein per–kilogram body weight may be a more appropriate guide for intake than protein as a percentage of total energy.[14]

Table 4-13 lists dietary sources of proteins. To add 1 pound of muscle per week, an additional 100 g of protein is needed in the diet.[21] One hundred grams of protein in a week is 14 g of protein per day, which is obtained in 2 oz of high-biological-value protein such as lean red meat, poultry, fish, cheese, or two servings of milk or yogurt. Extra protein is not preferentially laid down as muscle mass. Rather, extra protein is used as an energy source if calories and carbohydrates are inadequate, stored as fat if the protein is in excess of calorie needs, or used for its primary and structural roles (i.e., formation of tissues, hormones, and antibodies; maintenance of water and acid-based balance; and control of blood-clotting processes).

Special Considerations Regarding Protein Intake. In women, research has shown one potential problem with consuming excessive protein—increasing dietary protein leads to elevated calcium excretion.[22,23] A high-protein diet combined with a low intake of calcium can over time lead to osteoporosis. Most studies have been done on sedentary women, and more research is needed on athletes to determine the role of exercise, dietary protein, and calcium in the development and prevention of osteoporosis in athletes.

Another special consideration is that the metabolism of protein requires more water than carbohydrate or fat metabolism. As dietary protein increases, increased water intake is recommended to minimize dehydration.

Vegetarian Diets and Protein. Vegetarian diets are divided into six categories: In the semi category, dairy products, eggs, poultry, and fish are allowed, but red meat (i.e., beef and pork) is not. In the *pesco* category, no beef pork or poultry is allowed. In the *lacto-ovo* category, dairy products and eggs are allowed. In the *lacto* category, plant and dairy products are allowed. In the *ovo* category, only eggs are allowed as a protein source. In the *vegan* category, no animal products or derivatives are allowed.

Table 4-10

Dietary Reference Intakes (DRIs): Estimated Average Requirements for Groups (Food and Nutrition Board, Institute of Medicine, National Academies)

Life Stage Group	CHO (g/day)	Protein (g/day)[a]	Vit A (μg/day)[b]	Vit C (mg/day)	Vit E (mg/day)[c]	Thiamin (mg/day)	Riboflavin (mg/day)	Niacin (mg/day)[d]	Vit B$_6$ (mg/day)
Infants									
7-12 mo		9*							
Children									
1-3 y	100	11	210	13	5	0.4	0.4	5	0.4
4-8 y	100	15	275	22	6	0.5	0.5	6	0.5
Males									
9-13 y	100	27	445	39	9	0.7	0.8	9	0.8
14-18 y	100	44	630	63	12	1.0	1.1	12	1.1
19-30 y	100	46	625	75	11	1.0	1.1	12	1.1
31-50 y	100	46	625	75	12	1.0	1.1	12	1.1
51-70 y	100	46	625	75	12	1.0	1.1	12	1.4
> 70 y	100	46	625	75	12	1.0	1.1	12	1.4
Females									
9-13 y	100	28	420	39	9	0.7	0.8	9	0.8
14-18 y	100	38	485	56	12	0.9	0.9	11	1.0
19-30 y	100	38	500	60	12	0.9	0.9	11	1.1
31-50 y	100	38	500	60	12	0.9	0.9	11	1.1
51-70 y	100	38	500	60	12	0.9	0.9	11	1.3
> 70 y	100	38	500	60	12	0.9	0.9	11	1.3
Pregnancy									
14-18 y	135	50	530	66	12	1.2	1.2	14	1.6
19-30 y	135	50	550	70	12	1.2	1.2	14	1.6
31-50 y	135	50	550	70	12	1.2	1.2	14	1.6
Lactation									
14-18 y	160	60	885	96	16	1.2	1.3	13	1.7
19-30 y	160	60	900	100	16	1.2	1.3	13	1.7
31-50 y	160	60	900	100	16	1.2	1.3	13	1.7

NOTE: This table presents Estimated Average Requirements (EARs), which serve two purposes: for assessing adequacy of population intakes, and as the basis for calculating Recommended Dietary Allowances (RDAs) for individuals for those nutrients. EARs have not been established for vitamin D, vitamin K, pantothenic acid, biotin, choline, calcium, chromium, fluoride, manganese, or other nutrients not yet evaluated via the DRI process.

[a]For individual at reference weight (Table 1-1). *Indicates change from prepublication copy due to calculation error.

[b]As retinol activity equivalents (RAEs). 1 RAE = 1 μg retinol, 12 μg β-carotene, 24 μg α-carotene, or 24 μg β-cryptoxanthin. The RAE for dietary provitamin A carotenoids is two-fold greater than retinol equivalents (RE), whereas the RAE for preformed vitamin A is the same as RE.

[c]As α-tocopherol. α-Tocopherol includes *RRR*-α-tocopherol, the only form of α-tocopherol that occurs naturally in foods, and the 2*R*-stereoisomeric forms of α-tocopherol (*RRR*-, *RSR*-, *RRS*-, and *RSS*-α-tocopherol) that occur in fortified foods and supplements. It does not include the 2*S*-stereoisomeric forms of α-tocopherol (*SRR*-, *SSR*-, *SRS*-, and *SSS*-α-tocopherol), also found in fortified foods and supplements.

[d]As niacin equivalents (NE). 1 mg of niacin = 60 mg of tryptophan.

[e]As dietary folate equivalents (DFE). 1 DFE = 1 μg food folate = 0.6 μg of folic acid from fortified food or as a supplement consumed with food = 0.5 μg of a supplement taken on an empty stomach.

SOURCES: *Dietary Reference Intakes for Calcium, Phosphorous, Magnesium, Vitamin D, and Fluoride* (1997); *Dietary Reference Intakes for Thiamin, Riboflavin, Niacin, Vitamin B$_{12}$*, Folate, Vitamin B$_{12}$, Pantothenic Acid, Biotin, and Choline (1998); *Dietary Reference Intakes for Vitamin C, Vitamin E, Selenium, and Carotenoids* (2000); *Dietary Reference Intakes for Vitamin A, Vitamin K, Arsenic, Boron, Chromium, Copper, Iodine, Iron, Manganese, Molybdenum, Nickel, Silicon, Vanadium, and Zinc* (2001), and *Dietary Reference Intakes for Energy, Carbohydrate, Fiber, Fat, Fatty Acids, Cholesterol, Protein, and Amino Acids* (2002). These reports may be accessed via.www.nap.edu. Copyright 2002 by the National Academy of Sciences. All rights reserved.

Folate (μg/day)[b]	Vit B$_{12}$ (μg/day)	Copper (μg/day)	Iodine (μg/day)	Iron (mg/day)	Magnesium (mg/day)	Molybdenura (μg/day)	Phosphorus (mg/day)	Selenium (μg/day)	Zinc (mg/day)
				6.9					2.5
120	0.7	260	65	3.0	65	13	380	17	2.5
160	1.0	340	65	4.1	110	17	405	23	4.0
250	1.5	540	73	5.9	200	26	1055	35	7.0
330	2.0	685	95	7.7	340	33	1055	45	8.5
320	2.0	700	95	6	330	34	580	45	9.4
320	2.0	700	95	6	350	34	580	45	9.4
320	2.0	700	95	6	350	34	580	45	9.4
320	2.0	700	95	6	350	34	580	45	9.4
250	1.5	540	73	5.7	200	26	1055	35	7.0
330	2.0	685	95	7.9	300	33	1055	45	7.3
320	2.0	700	95	8.1	255	34	580	45	6.8
320	2.0	700	95	8.1	265	34	580	45	6.8
320	2.0	700	95	5	265	34	580	45	6.8
320	2.0	700	95	5	265	34	580	45	6.8
520	2.2	785	160	23	335	40	1055	49	10.5
520	2.2	800	160	22	290	40	580	49	9.5
520	2.2	800	160	22	300	40	580	49	9.5
450	2.4	985	209	7	300	35	1055	59	10.9
450	2.4	1000	209	6.5	255	36	580	59	10.4
450	2.4	1000	209	6.5	265	36	580	59	10.4

Table 4-11

Stages of Change

Stage	Description	Intervention at this Stage
Precontemplation	Athlete unaware of, denies, or minimizes the problem or need to make a change	Provide personalized information, allow athlete to express emotions or feelings
Contemplation	Aware of the problem but weighing costs/benefits of change	Encourage support networks; give positive feedback about athlete's abilities to make the change; clarify notions, misconceptions (e.g., carbohydrates are *not* fattening); emphasize expected benefits
Preparation/motivation	Has made decision to make change, plans to do so within the next month	Encourage athlete to set specific, achievable goals; reinforce small changes that athlete may have already achieved
Action	Plan is in progress, attitudinal and behavioral changes have begun	Refer to an education program for behavioral skill training and to learn tools and techniques to implement goals; set, implement, and evaluate goals
Maintenance/relapse	Action plan maintained for 6 consecutive months; high rate of relapse before 6 months	Encourage athlete to anticipate and plan for potential difficulties; if a lapse or relapse occurs, go back to previous stages; do not assume that initial action means permanent change; do not be discouraged or judgmental about a lapse or relapse

Nutrients to Focus on for Vegetarians

- *Protein* has many important functions in the body and is essential for growth and maintenance. Protein needs can easily be met by eating a variety of plant-based foods. Combining different protein sources in the same meal is not necessary. Sources of protein for vegetarians include beans, nuts, nut butters, peas, and soy products (tofu, tempeh, veggie burgers). Milk products and eggs are also good protein sources for lacto-ovo vegetarians.
- *Iron* functions primarily as a carrier of oxygen in the blood. Iron sources for vegetarians include iron-fortified breakfast cereals, spinach, kidney beans, black-eyed peas, lentils, turnip greens, molasses, whole wheat breads, peas, and some dried fruits (dried apricots, prunes, raisins).
- *Calcium* is used for building bones and teeth and in maintaining bone strength. Sources of calcium for vegetarians include fortified breakfast cereals, soy products (tofu, soy-based beverages), calcium-fortified orange juice, and some dark green leafy vegetables (collard greens, turnip greens, bok choy, mustard greens). Milk products are excellent calcium sources for lacto vegetarians.
- *Zinc* is necessary for many biochemical reactions and also helps the immune system function properly. Sources of zinc for vegetarians include many types of beans (white beans, kidney beans, and chickpeas), zinc-fortified breakfast cereals, wheat germ, and pumpkin seeds. Milk products are a zinc source for lacto vegetarians.
- *Vitamin B$_{12}$* is found in animal products and some fortified foods. Sources of vitamin B$_{12}$ for vegetarians include milk products, eggs, and foods that have been fortified with vitamin B$_{12}$. These include breakfast cereals, soy-based beverages, veggie burgers, and nutritional yeast.

From the United States Department of Agriculture: *Tips and Resources—Vegetarian Diets*, U.S. Department of Agriculture Center for Nutrition Policy and Promotion. Available at http://www.mypyramid.gov/tips_resources/vegetarian_diets_print.html.

Plant sources of protein alone can provide adequate amounts of essential amino acids. Whole grains, legumes, vegetables, seeds, and nuts all contain essential amino acids. It was once thought that vegetarian sources of protein needed to be consciously combined for the vegetarian to meet his or her protein needs; for example, legumes are low in the amino acid methionine but are also low in lysine. But most vegetarian diets provide adequate protein without conscious food combining.[24] Athletes who are striving for a high carbohydrate (60% to 70%), low fat, and moderate protein diet can benefit from a well-planned vegetarian diet. Figure 4-3 provides a daily food guide for planning a vegetarian diet, and Figure 4-4 is a sample lacto-vegetarian menu.

Fat

Dietary fat provides essential fatty acids and is necessary for absorption of fat-soluble vitamins. It is an energy source that provides flavor and meal satiety (feeling satisfyingly full), and converts more efficiently to body fat than other macronutrients.

The degree to which fats are used as fuel during exercise is determined by exercise intensity and duration, diet, endurance training history, and altered metabolic state.[25] Fatty acid metabolism requires more oxygen than carbohydrate metabolism. Low-intensity exercise ($< 50\%$ VO$_2$ max) may rely extensively on free fatty acids for fuel. As exercise intensity increases, there is a greater requirement for glucose as fuel. Blood glucose, muscle, and liver glycogen are the primary fuels when rapid energy is needed.

Box 4-1 Action Strategies

Common Profile Of Many Athletes
1. Skipping meals, most commonly the pre-workout meal
2. Consuming 50% to 70% of total calories in the evening
3. Consuming greater than 30% of calories from fat

Guidelines
1. Redistributing calories throughout the day:

To keep blood glucose even and prevent hypoglycemia, which results in fatigue, shakiness, or irritability, the athlete should eat small, frequent meals or snacks every 3 to 4 hours. If this is not possible, fruit, fruit juice, or a 6% to 8% carbohydrate solution should be consumed during workout sessions to avoid hypoglycemia.

Example

Breakfast	7:00 am
Snack	10:30 am
Lunch	1:00 pm
Snack	4:00 pm
Dinner	7:00 pm
Snack	Optional

Morning Workout
- Encourage a small snack (e.g., granola bar, yogurt, fruit, foods that do not cause discomfort) before or during the workout or 100% fruit juice if the athlete prefers to workout on an empty stomach.

Afternoon Workout
- Encourage consumption of a full breakfast that includes a lean protein source; a low-fat, moderate-protein lunch; a carbohydrate-based mid-afternoon snack prior to exercise; a high-carbohydrate, low-protein snack within 1 to 2 hours after a workout; and a high-carbohydrate dinner with moderate protein.

Evening Workout (After 7:00 pm)
- Lunch should be the main meal of the day, providing daily protein, carbohydrate, and a healthy source of fat. A high-carbohydrate, low-fat dinner should be consumed about 2 hours before working out and a small, carbohydrate-based snack within 1 to 2 hours after the evening workout.

2. Self-monitoring

Eating is often subjective and is regulated by external forces such as time of day, mood, stress, social activities, workout schedule. Maintenance of a food diary will assist athletes in observation of their habits to assess the value of their food intake. From the diary, actions can be planned, goals set, and changes implemented. The diary may then be used by a registered dietitian for analysis of food intake.

Date	Time	Food	Amount	Fat	Carbohydrate	Protein	Beverage	Workout

Table 4-12
Balancing the Sports Diet*

Nutrient	Calories†	Sports Diet (%)
Carbohydrate	4 calories	60-70
Protein	4 calories	15-20
Fat	9 calories	15-20

*Recommended distribution of macronutrients for an athlete.
†Calories per gram of nutrient.

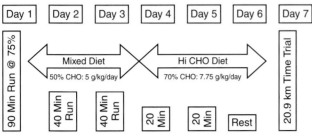

Figure 4-2

Modified carbohydrate loading. (From Doyle JA, Papadopoulos C, Green MS: Utilization of carbohydrates in energy production. In Wolinsky I, Driskell JA, editors: *Sports nutrition, energy, metabolism and exercise*, p 34, Boca Raton, 2008, CRC Press, Taylor and Frances Group. Adapted from Sherman WM, Costill DL, Fink WJ, Miller JM: Effect of exercise-diet manipulation on muscle glycogen and its subsequent utilization during performance, *Int J Sports Med* 2: 114–118, 1981.)

Aerobic training increases the cell's number of mitochondria and enzymes involved in fatty acid oxidation, thereby enhancing the athlete's ability to burn fat as fuel efficiently. This increased ability is demonstrated in four distinct ways:[25] (1) a more efficient use of oxygen; (2) more oxygen can be used at a given work load; (3) less glycogen and more fat used to meet energy needs; and (4) lower lactate production, representing more complete oxidation and improved oxygen use of energy substrates. Training increases the rate of fat use by changing the oxidative potential of the muscle.

National surveys show that total fat consumption (i.e., percentage of overall caloric intake) as well as saturated fat intake of the general public has decreased during the past two decades. However, these reductions in the percentage of energy from total fat and saturated fat are attributed to an increase in total energy intake rather than an actual decline in total amount of fat intake.[6] Although no RDA exists for total fat intake, the American Heart Association suggests total fat intake as a percentage of total energy should be 30% or less. The National Cholesterol Education Program also suggests total energy from fat intake should be 30% or less, and recommends that 10% come from polyunsaturated, 10% from monounsaturated, and a range of 7% to 10% from saturated fats per day.

When discussing fat intake for athletes, these guidelines may not be appropriate unless the athlete suffers from high cholesterol or other implications that require a more strict dietary fat intake. In general, fat intake among athletes varies depending on the sport in which they participate. For instance, long-distance runners tend to consume lower fat diets than short-distance runners and sprinters. Regardless, the position of the American Dietetic Association states that athletes should not restrict their dietary fat intake because there is no performance benefit of very low fat diets (<15% total energy intake) when compared with moderate fat diets

Table 4-13
Protein Sources

Type	Nutritional Breakdown	Food Sources
Lean sources, serving size 1 oz	55 cal, 0 g CHO, 7 g protein, 3 g fat	Lean beef and pork Fish Poultry without skin
Medium-fat sources, serving size 1 oz (or otherwise noted)	75 cal, 0 g CHO, 7 g protein, 5 g fat	Ground beef Skim/part skim mozzarella, ricotta 4 oz tofu 1 egg
High-fat sources, serving size 1 oz (or otherwise noted)	100 cal, 0 g CHO, 7 g protein, 8 g fat	Corned beef, spare ribs, cheese (cheddar, Swiss), cold cuts 1 hot dog 1 tbsp peanut butter
Dairy, nonfat	90-150 cal, 12 g CHO, 8 g protein, 0 g fat	8 oz skim milk Nonfat yogurt
Dairy, low fat, 1%-2%	90-150 cal, 12 g CHO, 8 g protein, 3-5 g fat	8 oz 1%-2% milk Plain low fat yogurt, 1%-2%
Dairy, high fat	90-150 cal, 12 g CHO, 8 g protein, 8 g fat	8 oz whole milk
Vegetables Fruit and fat contain no protein	25 cal, 5 g CHO, 2 g protein, 0 g fat	½ c cooked or 1 c raw

Cal, Calories; *CHO*, carbohydrate; *c*, cup; *g*, gram; *oz*, ounce; *tbsp*, tablespoon.
Data from: American Diabetic Association.

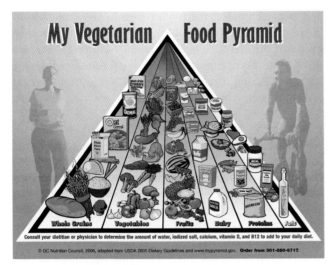

Figure 4-3

Vegetarian food pyramid. (Adapted from the U.S. Department of Agriculture and U.S. Department of Health and Human Services: Nutrition and your health: Dietary guidelines for Americans, Washington, DC, 2005, U.S. Government Printing Office; www.mypyramid.gov; and General Conference [of Seventh-day Adventists] Nutrition Council: My vegetarian food pyramid, Silver Spring, MD, 2006.)

(20% to 25% total energy intake).[3] Athletes should be encouraged to consume a diet that consists of 20% to 35% of total energy from fat and limit saturated fat intake to 10% or less, but discouraged from very low fat diets (15% or less of total energy), given the importance of fat within the body and fat energy use during exercise.

Dietary sources of fat include added fats and hidden fat sources (Table 4-14). Examples of added fats are butter, margarine, oils, mayonnaise, and salad dressings. Fat found in meat, the skin of poultry, nuts, seeds, and baked products are examples of hidden fats. Because fat consumed in amounts in excess of body needs is most likely to be stored in the form of adipose tissue, reducing total fat intake is one way to reduce total calories. Alcohol promotes fat storage;[26] therefore, it may be beneficial to count alcohol calories as part of the athlete's total fat allowance if the athlete consumes alcohol regularly.

Alcohol

Although alcohol has a high caloric content (7 kcal/g), it has limited food value. Alcohol acts on the brain by depressing its ability to reason and make judgments. Information-related processes are slowed; fine-motor skills are decreased; reaction time is reduced; coordination, balance, and visual perception are altered; and muscular reflexes are impaired.

Alcohol can weaken myocardial contractility and diminish sprinting, middle distance,[27] and endurance performance.[28] One of the most harmful effects of alcohol in an athletic event is evident in prolonged endurance contests. The liver is the primary organ for the detoxification of alcohol. Once alcohol is present in the blood, the metabolism

A SAMPLE MENU	YOUR SAMPLE MENU
Breakfast	**Breakfast**
4 oz. orange juice 1 cup hot cereal 1 piece fresh fruit 1 tsp. margarine 4 oz. low-fat milk	
Lunch	**Lunch**
4 oz. apple juice 1 cup vegetarian chili 1 cup tossed salad 1 tbsp. Italian dressing 1 slice whole-grain bread 1 tsp. margarine	
Snack	**Snack**
1 piece fresh fruit	
Dinner	**Dinner**

1 cup pasta entree with
   vegetables (with 1 tbsp. oil)
4 oz. sauteed tofu
   or
1 cup bean soup
1 slice whole-grain bread
8 oz. low-fat milk	

Snack	**Snack**
1 sesame roll 1 tbsp. peanut butter 4 oz. low-fat milk	

Figure 4-4

Sample lactovegetarian menu. (From the Massachusetts General Hospital Department of Dietetics.)

Table 4-14
Dietary Sources of Fats

Type*	Source
Saturated	Animal fats Butter fat Cocoa butter Palm and coconut oils Hydrogenated oils
Polyunsaturated	Most vegetable oils (corn, safflower, sunflower, etc.) Soybean oil Fish oils
Monounsaturated	Canola oil Olive oil

*All fats contain 9 kcal per gram.

of alcohol takes priority over other liver functions. An elevated level of blood alcohol may block the biochemical pathway that supplies extra glucose to the body. A drop in blood glucose during an endurance event could lead to early fatigue.

Peak concentration of alcohol in the blood occurs within 1 hour of consumption, depending on whether or not food is in the stomach. Because the absorbed alcohol is distributed within the water compartments of cells, it can disturb the water balance in muscle cells and consequently alter the cellular enzymatic activity producing adenosine triphosphate, the substrate that provides fuel for muscle contraction, active transport, and biosynthesis within the body.[29] Body size and composition alters dose response; a small, lean athlete is likely to experience fatigue sooner than a larger person with more body fat.

Micronutrients

Micronutrients are vitamins (Table 4-15) and minerals. Vitamins are complex organic compounds and exist in very small quantities in foods. The role of vitamins is in the action of several hundred enzymes that serve as catalysts to body function such as muscle contraction, digestion, absorption, and metabolism. The findings of studies evaluating the effectiveness of high-level vitamin or mineral supplementation on athletic performance lead to the conclusion that large therapeutic doses of vitamins and minerals are not useful in improving athletic performance.[30] However, focusing on the quality of the athlete's caloric intake to ensure that the vitamins and minerals necessary for optimal functioning of energy metabolic process are present is of primary importance. Physical activity increases the need for some vitamins and minerals; however, the increased need can be met by a diet that provides a variety of foods and is high in complex carbohydrates, moderate in protein, and low in fat. Individuals who consume a low-calorie diet are at risk for low vitamin and mineral intake.

Water-Soluble Vitamins

The classification of vitamins is based on their solubility within the body. Water-soluble vitamins are those that do not require fat for their absorption. Vitamins within this category include vitamin C and the B complex vitamins. These vitamins act as co-enzymes or co-factors in metabolic reactions involved in the oxidation of food and the production of energy. Water soluble vitamins are not stored, and therefore need to be consumed on a daily basis.

The B complex vitamins thiamin, riboflavin, niacin, pyridoxine, cyanocobalamin (B_{12}), pantothenic acid, folacin, and biotin, work together to ensure proper digestion, muscle contraction, and energy release.

Through the years, there has been speculation as to whether or not supplementations of the B complex vitamins enhance energy release, thus enhancing overall performance. The latest research fails to show significant performance improvement with vitamin and mineral supplementation in either aerobic or anaerobic exercise within nutritionally adequate healthy people. However, because there have been reports of toxic effects of pyridoxine (vitamin B_6) and niacin, supplementation in large doses is not recommended. Table 4-15 lists food sources for these vitamins.

Vitamin C, also known as *ascorbic acid*, is used in the synthesis of collagen, oxidation of fatty acids, epinephrine, and anti-inflammatory corticoids of the adrenal gland. It also aids in healing, facilitates iron absorption, and is considered an antioxidant. Vitamin C also serves as a protector against oxidative stress within endurance athletes, including upper respiratory infections. Supplementing vitamin C is popular among athletes, possibly as a result of its role in the healing process and the expectation that high doses of vitamin C will improve physical performance, which appears to be unfounded.[31] Well-controlled studies have reported no benefits of vitamin C supplementation on strength, maximum oxygen consumption, or aerobic capacity.[32-36] Athletes should be encouraged not to exceed the UL for vitamin C—adequate diet will supply enough vitamin C without supplementation.

Fat-Soluble Vitamins

The fat-soluble vitamins are A, D, E, and K (see Table 4-15), which are stored in the body in fat. Because these vitamins are stored in the body, excess intake can lead to toxicity. There are few studies on the relation of vitamins A, D, and K regarding physical performance. Vitamin E, an antioxidant, is well known for its role within immune function and prevention of cell membrane free radical damage.[13] As with vitamins A, D, and K, no reports have shown improved exercise performance with supplemental vitamin E. Table 4-15 lists food sources of fat-soluble vitamins.

Minerals

When it comes to exercise metabolism, minerals are equally as important as vitamins. Minerals serve multiple roles within the body. More specifically, minerals help regulate metabolism; provide structure for bone formation, and play functional roles within the cardiac and neural systems.[12] As with vitamins, minerals can be classified into two categories: trace or major.

Trace Minerals. Trace minerals include iron, zinc, copper, selenium, iodide, fluoride, chromium, manganese, molybdenum, boron, and vanadium. They are called *trace minerals* simply because they are found in smaller amounts within the body. Of all of the trace minerals, iron is the only one for which exercise may increase an athlete's required intake, especially if they suffer from iron-deficiency anemia or become iron depleted.

Iron. Iron is a component of hemoglobin and myoglobin, and plays a key role in making oxidative metabolism possible. Problematic factors related to iron associated with exercise are hemolysis of erythrocytes, alterations in iron metabolism, hematuria, increase in erythrocyte osmotic fragility resulting in decreased red blood cell survival time, and a possible shift in the oxygen dissociation curve.[37]

Athletes, especially endurance athletes, tend to have lower hemoglobin concentrations than nonathletes, placing them at greater risk for iron-deficiency anemia. *Sports anemia,* a condition in which hemoglobin levels tend to be at the low end of the normal range when all other blood parameters remain normal, is not a true anemia. This can occur in all athletes initiating a period of intense exercise, as well as the general public just starting an exercise program, and is caused by the quick increase in blood volume. Blood concentration becomes diluted as a result of this rapid change, and causes hemoglobin to show up relatively low during a blood test. After 1 to 2 months of consistent training, blood concentration returns to normal and the sports anemia is remedied.[38]

The most common cause of true anemia in athletes is iron deficiency anemia. Research suggests that female athletes, distance runners, and vegetarian athletes are at greatest risk to become iron-deficient. However, they are not the only athletes at risk of iron-deficiency anemia. Factors that lead to increased risk of iron deficiency anemia include (1) decreased dietary intake of foods rich in iron; (2) high demand for myoglobin, hemoglobin, and energy-producing enzymes; (3) demands of the sport; and (4) loss of iron through sweat.[38] Supplemental iron should only be advised for those athletes in whom true iron deficiency has been diagnosed. Normalizing iron levels improves endurance and performance in the iron-deficient athlete. On the flip side, supplementation of iron by athletes whose iron stores are normal and dietary intake of iron (Table 4-16) is adequate will probably not see any increase in performance and the supplementation may be harmful to the athletes. If an athlete is supplementing iron based on a physician's recommendation, is taking a daily multiple vitamin with iron to meet the RDA for iron, or is consuming dietary sources of iron, the following are recommendations to enhance absorption: (1) include a source of vitamin C at the same time and (2) do not consume iron within 1 hour of having coffee or tea, because these interfere with iron absorption.

Clinical Note

Sports anemia is a condition in which hemoglobin levels tend to be at the lower end of normal range *and* all other blood parameters are normal.

Major Minerals. Calcium, phosphorus, magnesium, sulfur, potassium, sodium, and chloride are classified as *major minerals,* or minerals that are essential to life.[12,13] Like trace minerals, most major minerals occur naturally within our environment. As with vitamins, if an adequate diet is maintained, no supplementation is required. However, if medical evaluation determines that supplementation

is warranted, the DRI should be taken into consideration before supplementing.

Calcium. Many athletes who have low body weight do not consume enough calories or choose low-nutritional-quality foods and, therefore, do not consume adequate calcium. Calcium is necessary for the contractile ability of muscles, the maintenance of healthy bones and teeth, blood clotting, and nerve transmission. Because bone formation and dissolution is a continuous process, calcium must be supplied to the cells on demand. When dietary calcium is low, the body draws from its own reserves in bone, which reduces bone density and can lead to stress fractures. Women are at higher risk because, overall, they have thinner bones (bones that are not as dense) and as they mature, they lose bone density at a faster rate. Amenorrhea, found in many female athletes, is also associated with decreased spinal bone mass.[39]

Osteoporosis is a major health concern for women. Calcium intake; estrogen level; alcohol, caffeine, and protein intake; family history; and the type and amount of physical activity are all related to the development of osteoporosis. Ninety-nine percent of dietary calcium is deposited in the bone. Increased physical activity improves the efficiency of calcium use and is important for the maintenance of optimal bone mass and strength.

The DRIs for calcium are listed in Tables 4-3 and 4-5. Athletes at risk for early osteoporosis, amenorrhea, or have disordered eating may require up to 1500 mg/day of elemental calcium and a recommended 400 to 800 IU per day of Vitamin D.[3] Table 4-17 lists dietary and supplemental sources of calcium.

Sodium. Sodium is an essential mineral needed to regulate water balance in the cells and to maintain blood volume and normal nerve and muscle activity. Sodium increases the absorption of fluids in the small intestine and helps to maintain the osmotic drive for drinking and reduces water clearance associated with reduced serum electrolyte concentration that results from electrolyte losses during exercise. In athletes who train daily at high intensity or in high temperatures, a prolonged state of hypohydration can occur. Rehydration occurs when a dilute solution of sodium rather than plain water is consumed under these conditions.[40]

Sodium makes up as much as 40% of common table salt (chloride constitutes the remaining approximately 60%). Requirements for sodium vary with age, environmental conditions, and level of activity. However, it is recommended that a healthy, sedentary adult consume 1500 to 2400 mg per day, which can be achieved by consuming a typical American diet. During prolonged exercise in hot weather, sodium losses in sweat and urine may exceed 10 g per day. The sodium concentration of sweat is approximately 50 mEq/L; the average daily urine sodium loss is 120 mEq/L.[41] Therefore, an athlete working out 4 hours per day and losing sweat at a moderate rate of 1.5 L per hour may benefit from an electrolyte replacement drink containing 0.5 to 0.7 g/L of sodium or a slightly

Table 4-15
Vitamins: Food Sources and Recommended Amounts

Vitamin	Adult DRI* (AI if no DRI)	Major Food Sources	What it Does	Potential Benefits	Supplementation
A	Males: 900 mcg/day Females: 700 mcg/day	Carrots, broccoli, tomatoes	Promotes good vision; helps form and maintain skin, teeth, bones, and mucous membranes Deficiency can increase susceptibility to infectious disease	May inhibit the development of certain tumors; may increase resistance to infection in children	Not recommended because it is toxic in high doses
C	Males: 90 mg/day Females: 75 mg/day	Citrus fruits and juices, strawberries, tomatoes, peppers (especially red), broccoli, potatoes, kale, cauliflower, cantaloupe, brussel sprouts	Helps promote healthy gums and teeth; aids in iron absorption; maintains normal connective tissue; helps in healing of wounds As an antioxidant, it combats the adverse effects of free radicals	May reduce the risk of certain cancers, as well as coronary artery disease; may prevent or delay cataracts	250-500 mg a day for anyone not consuming several fruits or vegetables rich in C daily and for smokers Larger doses may cause diarrhea
D	Males and females: 5 mcg/day (AI)	Milk, fish oil, fortified margarine; also produced by the body in response to sunlight	Promotes strong bones and teeth by aiding the absorption of calcium Helps maintain blood levels of calcium and phosphorus	May reduce the risk of osteoporosis	400 IU for people who do not drink milk or get sun exposure, especially strict vegetarians and elderly Toxic in high doses
E	Males and females: 15 mg/day	Vegetable oil, nuts, margarine, wheat germ, leafy greens, seeds, almonds, olives, asparagus	Helps in the formation of red blood cells and the use of vitamin K As an antioxidant, it combats the adverse effects of free radicals	May reduce the risk of certain cancers, as well as coronary artery disease; may prevent or delay cataracts; may improve immune function in the elderly	200 to 800 IU advised for everybody; you cannot get that much from food, especially on a low-fat diet No serious side effects at that level, although diarrhea and headaches have been reported
K	Males: 120 mcg (AI) Females: 90 mcg (AI)	Intestinal bacteria produce most of the K needed by the body The rest is supplied by leafy greens, cauliflower, broccoli, cabbage, milk, soybeans, and eggs	Essential for normal blood clotting	May help maintain strong bones in the elderly	Not necessary, not recommended

Nutrient	Amount	Food Sources	Function	Benefit	Supplement Recommendation
Thiamin	Males: 1.2 mcg/day Females: 1-1.1 mcg/day	Whole grains, enriched grain products, beef liver, oysters, peanuts, green peas, raisins, collard greens, brewer's yeast	Helps cells convert carbohydrate into energy Necessary for healthy brain, nerve cells, and heart function	Unknown	Not necessary, not recommended
Riboflavin	Males: 1.3 mg/day Females: 1-1.1 mg/day	Dairy products, liver, meat, chicken, fish, enriched grain products, leafy greens, beans, nuts, eggs, almonds	Helps cells convert carbohydrate into energy Essential for growth, production of red blood cells, and health of skin and eyes	Unknown	Not necessary, not recommended
Niacin (B₃)	Males: 16 mg/day Females: 14 mg/day	Nuts, meat, fish, chicken, liver, enriched grain products, dairy products, peanut butter, brewer's yeast	Aids in the release of energy from foods Helps maintain healthy skin, nerves, and digestive system	Large doses lower elevated blood cholesterol	Megadoses may be prescribed by doctor to lower blood cholesterol May cause flushing, liver damage, and irregular heartbeat
B₆	Males: 1.3-1.7 mg/day Females: 1.2-1.5 mg/day	Whole grains, bananas, meat, beans, nuts, wheat germ, brewer's yeast, chicken, fish, liver	Vital in chemical reactions of proteins and amino acids Helps maintain brain function and form red blood cells	May boost immunity in the elderly	Megadoses can cause numbness and other neurological disorders
B₁₂	Males and females: 2.4 mcg	Liver, beef, pork, poultry, eggs, milk, cheese, yogurt, shellfish, fortified cereals, fortified soy products	Necessary for development of red blood cells. Maintains normal functioning of nervous system	Unknown	Strict vegetarians may need supplements Despite claims, no benefits from megadoses
Folacin (also known as *folate* or *folic acid*)	Males and females: 400 mcg	Dark leafy greens, wheat germ, liver, beans, whole grains, broccoli, asparagus, citrus fruit and juices	Important in the synthesis of DNA, in normal growth, and in protein metabolism AI reduces the risk of certain birth defects, notably spina bifida	May reduce the risk of cervical cancer	400 mcg, from food or pills, for all women who may become pregnant to help prevent birth defects
Biotin	Males and females: 25-30 mg (AI)	Eggs, milk, liver, brewer's yeast, mushrooms, bananas, tomatoes, whole grains	Important in metabolism of protein, carbohydrate, and fats	Unknown	Not necessary, not recommended

Continued

Table 4-15

Vitamins: Food Sources and Recommended Amounts—cont'd

Vitamin	Adult DRI* (AI if no DRI)	Major Food Sources	What it Does	Potential Benefits	Supplementation
Pantothenic	Males and females: 5 mg (AI)	Whole grains, beans, milk, eggs, liver	Vital for metabolism of food and production of essential body chemicals	Unknown	Not necessary, not recommended. May cause diarrhea

AI, Adequate intake; *DNA,* deoxyribonucleic acid; *DRI:* dietary reference intake.

*DRI values adopted from the National Academy of Science.

Among the achievements for which this century will surely be remembered is the discovery of vitamins, a scientific advance truly beneficial to humanity. For hundreds of years, of course, people had noticed that certain foods seemed to prevent diseases—most famously, the limes and lemons that British sailors ate to ward off scurvy—but the first vitamin was isolated in the laboratory only in 1911. That was thiamin, a B vitamin. Now 13 vitamins are known. In the past, vitamins were discussed in terms of preventing deficiency diseases (beriberi, caused by a lack of thiamin, for instance; or scurvy, caused by a lack of vitamin C). The recommended dietary allowances, devised by scientists in the United States and revised and updated over the years, were designed partly to prevent such deficiency diseases and partly to meet the needs, as they were understood, of healthy people.

But we still have much to learn about the functions of these powerful chemicals. Indeed, in the last decade alone, hundreds of scientific studies have found that vitamins play a much larger role in health than was dreamed of even 20 years ago.

What Is a Vitamin?

Vitamins are organic substances required to regulate the functioning of cells. They are essential to life. They take part in myriad biological processes, among them promoting good vision, forming normal blood cells, creating strong bones and teeth, and ensuring the proper function of the heart and nervous system. Although vitamins supply no energy, they do aid in the conversion of foods into energy. The 13 vitamins fall into two categories: fat-soluble (A and its precursor betacarotene, D, E, and K) and water-soluble (the B vitamins and C). This distinction is important because the body stores fat-soluble vitamins in the liver and fatty tissue for relatively long periods (many months), but it stores the water-soluble vitamins for only a short time (up to a few weeks). In general, you have to consume vitamins: the body cannot manufacture them (though it does synthesize some vitamin K, D, and B_{12} and convert betacarotene into vitamin A). For a description of the specific functions of each vitamin, consult the chart.

Who Needs Supplements?

If you follow the government's dietary recommendations, you may not need supplements to meet the DRIs. Still, we think it's wise for adults to consume extra amounts of antioxidants (vitamin E and C and betacarotene), and for premenopausal women to eat a folacin-rich diet or take supplements (see chart for recommended amounts). Most people *do not* need a daily multivitamin and mineral supplement, although millions of Americans take one. It can't be said too often that a pill a day won't turn poor diet into a healthy one. However, elderly people, especially those who may have reduced their food intake for any reason, may benefit from a daily multivitamin. So may frequent aspirin takers, heavy drinkers, smokers, and those with impaired immune systems. Pregnant women have special needs and should follow professional advice. Taking huge doses of most vitamins is not wise. Some vitamins—A and D, specifically—are toxic in large doses. Others, like niacin, have serious side effects in the large doses described on the chart.

Modified from the University of California at Berkeley Wellness Letter. Health Letter Associates, 1994.

Table 4-16
Dietary Sources of Iron

Nonvegetarian Sources of Iron	Vegetarian Sources of Iron
> 5 mg/Serving	4-9 mg/Serving
Liver (high in choles-terol), 3 oz	Fortified cooked cereal, ¾ cup
Oysters ½ cup	Fortified dry cereal, 1 oz
3-5 mg/Serving	6-7 mg/Serving
Most beef, lean	½ cup tofu
1-3 mg/Serving	3-4 mg/Serving
Fish, chicken	Soybeans, ½ cup
	Lentils, ½ cup
	Pumpkin/squash seeds, 1 oz

Table 4-17
Dietary Sources of Calcium

Food	Calcium (mg)
Calcium-enriched bread, 2 slices	580
8 oz lactose-free, calcium-fortified nonfat milk	500
8 oz yogurt, plain, nonfat	452
8 oz yogurt, low fat	415
8 oz milk, skim	352
8 oz yogurt, fruit	314
Calcium-enriched orange juice, 8 oz	293
Swiss cheese, 1 oz	272
Dry cereal, ¾ cup (variable amount)	250
Cheddar cheese, 1 oz	204
Sardines, canned in water with bones, 2 oz	185*
Mozzarella, 1 oz	183
Tofu with calcium sulfate, 3 oz	150†
Almonds, ¼ cup	94
Broccoli, turnip greens, ½ cup	36

*Average of major brands.
†Estimates of brands.
Supplements: calcium carbonate (e.g., Tums) is better absorbed with meals; calcium citrate (e.g., enriched orange juice, tablets) is better absorbed on an empty stomach.

more liberal use of sodium with meals. Concentrated salt tablets are generally not recommended and may actually be harmful. Acclimatization to heat or exercise can compensate for some, but not all, sodium loss.[42] Heat-acclimated subjects lose considerably less salt at a given sweat rate than their unacclimated counterparts. The amount of sodium lost increases as sweat rate increases. During exercise bouts lasting more than 3 hours, sodium losses can result in hyponatremia, a plasma sodium content of less than 130 mEq sodium/L, a potentially fatal condition that can be prevented.[40]

Fluids

When it comes to optimal performance, adequate hydration plays a leading role. To prevent dehydration, athletes should be encouraged to hydrate before, during, and after exercise.[3] Dehydration adversely affects muscle strength, endurance, and coordination. It also increases the risk of cramps, heat exhaustion, and life-threatening heat stroke.[43,44] During exercise, heat produced within working skeletal muscle is carried by the convective flow of blood to the body core, elevating its temperature and stimulating warm receptors located in the anterior hypothalamus. In response to the rise in temperature, sweating is initiated. Sweat loss means the loss of vital body fluids, which can result in circulatory and thermal impairments if these fluids are not replaced. Fluid, electrolyte, and energy supplementation are desirable during exercise to support circulatory, metabolic, and thermoregulatory functions and to maintain plasma volume.

To monitor fluid lost during training and exercise sessions, the athlete should weigh before and after each session. For each pound (0.45 kg) lost, 16 to 24 oz of fluid should be consumed.[3] Sufficient fluids should ideally be consumed during exercise so that weight remains constant before and after activity. It is important to drink fluids before becoming thirsty. Work capacity can be reduced by 10% to 15% due to body fluid loss.

Clinical Note

To monitor fluid loss during activity, the athlete should be weighed before and after each session. For each pound lost, 16 to 24 oz of fluid should be consumed.

The process of rehydration depends on both gastric emptying and intestinal absorption. For exercise longer than 60 to 90 minutes, using a 6% to 8% carbohydrate solution (e.g., diluted fruit juice, Gatorade) during the event optimizes stamina and endurance, because the carbohydrate helps to maintain normal blood glucose levels and to provide energy for muscle.[45] Highly concentrated sweets (i.e., greater than 8%) tend to empty more slowly from the stomach than diluted fluids and impair fluid absorption. Therefore, it is not recommended that high-concentrate sweets be taken during the event.[46] Cold fluids help cool core body temperature and leave the stomach more rapidly than warm fluids.

Once the gastric contents empty into the small intestine, this solution must be absorbed before any benefit of hydration is realized. Absorption from the small intestine is accelerated by the combination of glucose and sodium.[47] It has been reported that the most effective glucose-to-sodium ratio promoting water absorption is 2:1.[40,48]

Caffeine

Caffeine is a central nervous system stimulant, naturally occurring in coffee beans, cocoa beans, cola nuts, and other foods. It can, and is, added to food items such as most carbonated beverages, energy bars, as well as some over-the-counter medications. Some research has shown that caffeine may facilitate the use of fats stored in the muscle as an energy source during exercise.[12] However, most investigators suggest that caffeine's effect is an enhanced psychological function leading to greater work output and increased tolerance to fatigue.[12] Response to the effect of caffeine is variable. In some athletes, performance is hindered because of adverse effects such as anxiety, nervousness, and upset stomach, whereas in others, there may be an increase in time to fatigue during intense aerobic activities, which is considered an ergogenic aid.[12,27,32] Contrary to earlier studies, the latest evidence suggests that caffeine does lead to dehydration or an imbalance in electrolytes.[3] Caffeine does remain a poor hydration choice for those desiring rapid rehydration after exercise.

The National Collegiate Athletics Association has placed caffeine on its list as a restricted substance; levels of more than 15 micrograms/mL^{-1} found within the urine may cause an athlete to experience a positive drug test. This level may be reached by testing within 2 to 3 hours after consuming six to eight cups of coffee in one sitting.[49] The World Anti-Doping Agency, which provides governance for international sports with a vision for sports free of doping, includes caffeine within their monitoring program, but it is not banned.[50]

Food Intake Before, During, and After Exercise

Before exercise, it is most important that the athlete have adequate carbohydrate and fluid intake. Foods eaten prior to an event should be familiar and comforting. Depending on individual preference, the pre-event meal should be consumed 2 to 4 hours before activity and include at least 200 to 300 grams of carbohydrate.[3] The meal should be relatively low in fat and fiber, include moderate protein sources, and be high in carbohydrate. It should be kept in mind that, generally, the athlete knows his or her body the best. Pre-exercise meals should be sure to address the athlete's individual need, rather than suggested needs for the overall population. Table 4-18 lists the carbohydrate contents of various food and beverages. Pre-exercise meal guidelines are presented in Box 4-2. Liquid meals may be consumed closest to exercise time because of shorter gastric emptying time, low stool residue, and they provide an alternative to solid meals for day-long competitions and multiple events. Athletes should experiment with food-and-beverage combinations during preseason or practice sessions to determine what works best for them, and to ensure that they will have access to these items during the time of need.

Many high school and college coaches try to set guidelines for an entire team for safe pre-exercise eating. Because each athlete is unique, this "entire team approach" is not effective. Each individual must discover the best pre-exercise foods for his or her own body. This is based solely on trial and error.

Adverse gut reactions occur in 30% to 50% of endurance athletes. Complaints include stomach and upper gastrointestinal problems such as heartburn, vomiting, bloating, and stomach pain; and lower gastrointestinal problems such as gas, intestinal cramping, urge to defecate, loose stools, and diarrhea. Sports performed in a relatively stable position such as cycling, swimming, and cross-country skiing seem to cause fewer gastrointestinal problems compared with sports that jostle the intestines such as track events, running, football, and basketball.

Untrained individuals just beginning an exercise program report more gastrointestinal problems than do well-trained individuals who may have gradually built up tolerance to

Table 4-18
Carbohydrate Content of Food and Beverages

Food	CHO (grams)	Beverages	CHO (grams/8 oz)
Apple	21	Gatorade	14
Banana, large	40	Apple juice	30
Baked potato, large	51	Powerade	19
Yogurt, fruited (1 cup)	40	Orange juice	26
Bread, whole wheat (2 slices)	22	Cranapple juice	43
Bagel, medium	50	G^2	18
Raisins (⅔ cup)	79	Low-fat chocolate milk (1 cup)	26
Rice (1 cup)	50	All Sport	20
Spaghetti with sauce (1 cup)	37	Propel	3
Tortilla, flour (6")	15	Endurox R^4	35
Waffles, buttermilk (2 waffles)	29		

CHO, Carbohydrates.

Box 4-2 Pre-Exercise Meal Guidelines

- During exercise, athletes rely primarily on their pre-existing glycogen and fat stores.
- Effects of a pre-exercise meal should be tested during training, not before an event.
- Carbohydrate feedings before exercise can help restore suboptimal liver glycogen stores.

How Much Carbohydrate Pre-Exercise:

1 to 4.5 g/kg body weight consumed 1 to 4 hours before exercise. Guidelines: high carbohydrate, low fat, moderate protein, extra fluid, appropriate portions.

Large to moderate meal:	4 to 6 hours prior
Lighter meal:	2 to 3 hours prior
Snack:	0.5 to 1.0 hour prior

Timing of meals and amounts of food varies with duration, intensity, and individual needs and preferences.

Caution: Simple sugar pre-exercise may cause hyperglycemia, lightheadedness, as well as gastrointestinal distress.

Modified from Cummings S, Rewinski MJ: Nutritional Concerns in Athletes. In Zachazewski JE, Magee DJ, Quillen WS, editors: *Athletic injuries and rehabilitation,* p 891, Philadelphia, 1996, WB Saunders.

Box 4-3 Fluid Guidelines

Before Exercise
1. Initiate prehydration at least 4 hours prior to the event.
2. Begin with 5 to 7 mL/kg body weight of water or sports beverage with 6% to 8% carbohydrate solution.
3. Consider sodium-containing beverages to help with retention of needed fluids.
4. If urine output is low or the urine is dark in color, an additional 3 to 5 mL/kg body weight for fluid should be consumed within 2 hours of the event.

During Exercise
1. Intent of fluid consumption during exercise is to prevent water loss of $\geq$ 2% baseline body weight.
2. Customized fluid replacement plans, using pre- and postexercise body weights to determine sweat rates, are key.
3. To enhance electrolyte balance throughout competition, consider beverages containing 6% to 8% carbohydrate and electrolytes.

After Exercise
1. Consume at least 16 to 24 oz of fluid for every pound of body weight lost during exercise.
2. Salty foods and electrolyte-containing beverages should be consumed to increase fluid retention and thirst.

Data from Rodriguez NR, DiMarco NM, Langley S: Position of the American Dietetic Association, Dietitians of Canada, and the American College of Sports Medicine: Nutrition and athletic performance, *Med Sci Sports Exerc* 41(3):709–731, 2009; and, Sawka MN, Burke LM, Eichner ER et al: American College of Sports Medicine position stand: Exercise and fluid replacement, *Med Sci Sport Exerc* 39:377–390, 2007.

exercise and who have discovered their tried-and-true pre-exercise foods. Gastrointestinal problems also occur more frequently in younger athletes who may have less nutrition knowledge and experience with precompetition foods. Women may experience more problems than men, particularly during menstruation. Hormonal shifts during menstruation may contribute to looser bowel movements. During easy and moderately high exercise, the body can simultaneously digest food and comfortably exercise. During intense exercise, the shift of blood flow from the stomach to the working muscles may cause gastrointestinal problems. High-fat foods eaten shortly before exercise can cause problems. Low-fat, high-carbohydrate foods that are tried-and-true favorites are recommended before exercise.

During endurance exercise of more than 1 hour, consuming approximately 15 to 30 grams of carbohydrate every 30 minutes (i.e., 30 to 60 grams per hour) is recommended to maintain endurance performance.[8] Because gastric emptying and absorption time is faster with carbohydrate-containing sports beverages, they are often better tolerated by athletes during activity. These also have the added advantage of replacing fluids. Consuming highly concentrated sugar drinks such as fruit juice and soda during exercise may cause stomach distress; therefore a 6% to 8% carbohydrate solution is recommended during exercise (Box 4-3).

The fastest glycogen replacement occurs within the first 2 hours following exercise. Blood glucose, insulin, and glycogen synthetase levels remain high to promote glycogen synthesis and replete muscle reserves.[51] Muscle will replete glycogen to a higher degree when as much as

600 g of easily digestible carbohydrate is consumed within the first 1 to 3 hours following exercise. Immediately following exercise, it is recommended that 1.0 to 1.5 g of carbohydrate per kilogram body weight be consumed, followed by an additional 1.0 to 1.5 g carbohydrate per kilogram body weight 2 hours later.[3] A protein source may also be included along with carbohydrates after exercise to help repair and rebuild muscle tissues. Many athletes are not ready to eat within an hour after the event; therefore, high-carbohydrate juices immediately after the event are an excellent way to restore glycogen, followed by a high-carbohydrate meal within 2 hours. Alcohol is not recommended as either a fluid or glycogen replacement for all of the reasons already discussed previously and because it is low in carbohydrate and has a diuretic effect.

Fluid Guidelines

As with food consumption, fluid consumption before, during, and after exercise should be individualized. Some basic guidelines are listed in Box 4-3, but athletes should experiment with fluid needs for one's own body during training sessions prior to their event or competitive season.

Weight Management

The diet industry is approximately a $31 billion per year business, which encompasses commercial diet programs, book sales, weight-loss products, and modified diet foods and drinks. Fad diets are popular because of the promise of quick and easy weight loss. Fad diets may be particularly attractive to athletes because of claims to alter body composition. The truth of the matter is that if it sounds too good to be true, it probably is. Ketogenic diets are not appropriate for athletes because of problems with secondary dehydration and hyponatremia (low serum sodium). Most fad diets are nutritionally inadequate, and because hypo caloric diets cannot meet the energy needs of athletes in training, they may promote depletion of glycogen stores and loss of lean body mass.

Appropriate weight-loss programs begin with a complete assessment[52] of the athlete, as discussed in the beginning of this chapter. The assessment includes anthropometric measurements: height, weight, and body composition; weight and diet history; 24-hour recall and food frequency assessment; and information regarding activity, including duration, intensity, and stage of change should also be assessed.

Basal metabolic rate (BMR) can be estimated using height, weight, age, and gender—women's BMR tends to be 5% to 10% lower than their male counterparts. It is considered a reflection of the minimal energy requirement for vital functions in a resting state.[12] One method to estimate caloric needs for maintaining current weight is the Harris-Benedict formula (see the following text). To estimate caloric needs for maintaining current weight, add an activity factor of 1.3 for normal activities of daily living and 1.5 for the very active individual; or calculate up the amount of calories expended during activities of an average day (including exercise), using the activity list in Table 4-1, and add them. Decreasing the maintenance calories by 500 kcal per day promotes a weight loss of approximately 1 lb (0.45 kg) a week; doing additional exercise to use an additional 500 kcal promotes a 2 lb- (0.9 kg-) per-week weight loss. A weight loss of 1 to 2 lb (0.45 to 0.9 kg) per week is a realistic, appropriate goal. With well-trained athletes, measuring body composition using skin calipers, an air-displacement plethysmograph, dual-energy x-ray absorptiometry, or bioelectrical impedance for an analysis of body composition is a better determinant of fat loss than using the scale. The scale weighs water, muscles, and fat, and therefore does not distinguish whether fat was lost or muscle (which is heavier than fat) was gained. The goal is to decrease body fat and preserve lean body mass.

The athlete should be referred to a registered dietitian with knowledge in sports nutrition or a board certified specialist in sports dietetics (CSSD), who will develop an individualized meal plan based on the athlete's likes, dislikes, lifestyle, ethnic food practices, and socioeconomic factors. The diet should be a high to moderate carbohydrate sports diet, limiting fats to 20% of total calories. Box 4-1 and

---

Explanation of Normal Metabolism and Consequences of Abnormal Eating[53-55]

1. Define metabolism and regulation of body weight
2. Estimate caloric requirements at normal metabolic rate:
   Calculate Harris-Benedict equation[56] to predict normal resting energy expenditure
   Women: 655 + (4.4 × weight in pounds) + (4.3 × height in inches) − (6.8 × age in years)
   Men: 66 + (6.2 × weight in pounds) + (12.7 × height in inches) − (6.8 × age in years)
   Multiply the resting energy expenditure × 1.3 for sedentary activity
   Add caloric requirements for exercise or sports event
3. Estimate current caloric and nutrient intake from a 24-hour recall
4. Describe compensatory mechanism of decreased metabolic rate to restricted food intake[55]
5. Relate the connection between abnormal eating and obsessional thinking about food, weight, and hunger
6. Discuss steps in normalizing metabolic rate

Modified from Cummings S, Rewinski MJ: Nutritional concerns in athletes.

Table 4-11 list guidelines for recommending behavioral changes to accomplish the weight-loss goal.

Weight goals should be appropriate and based on both genetic and environmental factors affecting the athlete's weight status. Emphasis should be placed on realistic goals, long-term weight management, and a healthy lifestyle, which includes healthful eating and physical activity. Behavioral-cognitive therapy is an important adjunct to any diet program. Factors associated with successful weight loss are self-monitoring (e.g., food records), goal setting, social support, and length of treatment. Factors associated with successful maintenance are physical activity, self-monitoring, and continued contact with the weight management therapist or counselor. Those factors associated with weight regain are restrictive dieting, life stresses, negative coping style, and emotional or binge eating patterns.[57] It is extremely important to assess the presence or potential risk of eating disorders, particularly in sports in which thinness is stressed.

Nutritional Requirements for Health and Athletic Performance

The nutritional requirements to promote health and ensure optimal athletic performance are presented at the beginning of this chapter. These guidelines provide a critical foundation for the athlete to begin to identify goals for change in food intake and eating patterns. To cover any micronutrient deficiencies caused by inadequate food intake, a multivitamin with minerals containing 100% DRI is recommended.[53,54]

Body Fat and Weight Ranges

In a given sport, body fat, not body weight, is the most important factor influencing performance. Although it is generally true that the leaner the athlete, the better the performance, it is also extremely important for the athlete to recognize that driving body weight too low can have major repercussions.[58] Table 4-19 provides a reference of values of relative body fat for, in most cases, elite athletes in selected sports. There are two important concerns regarding body fat recommendations.[58] First, there are inherent errors in existing techniques for measuring body composition that must be considered. Second, individual variability is a factor. Some athletes are able to achieve slightly lower values and improve performance, whereas others find it impossible or undesirable.

Table 4-19
Ranges of Relative Body Fat for Men and Women

Sport	Men	Women
Baseball, softball	8-14	12-18
Basketball	6-12	10-16
Body building	5-8	6-12
Canoeing and kayaking	6-12	10-16
Cycling	5-11	8-15
Fencing	8-12	10-16
Football	6-18	—
Golf	10-16	12-20
Gymnastics	5-12	8-16
Horse racing	6-12	10-16
Ice and field hockey	8-16	12-18
Orienteering	5-12	8-16
Pentathlon	—	8-15
Racquetball	6-14	10-18
Rowing	6-14	8-16
Rugby	6-16	—
Skating	5-12	8-16
Skiing	7-15	10-18
Ski jumping	7-15	10-18
Soccer	6-14	10-18
Swimming	6-12	10-18
Synchronized swimming	—	10-18
Tennis	6-14	10-20
Track and field		
Running events	5-12	8-15
Field events	8-18	12-20
Triathlon	5-12	8-15
Volleyball	7-15	10-18
Weight lifting	5-12	10-18
Wrestling	5-16	—

From Wilmore JH: Body weight standards and athletic performance. In Brownell KD, Rodin J, Wilmore JH, editors: *Eating, body weight and performance in athletes: Disorders of modern society*, p 326, Philadelphia, 1992, Lea & Febiger.

When athletes are educated about body composition and body fat percentages for their sport, they may be willing to increase food intake and allow for some weight gain. Ranges of body fat and body weight are important to allow for individual variability and normal fluctuations. In the event that lower body fat is desirable and reasonable, the athlete with an eating disorder must first work toward normalizing eating and metabolism and must be carefully guided by the dietitian.

Conclusion

To determine an athlete's nutritional needs and whether they are being met, a complete assessment is necessary. The assessment consist of subjective data: what the athlete has to say about his or her nutritional status; objective data, including anthropometric indices (height, weight, body composition); laboratory data (complete blood count, lipid profile), vitamin and mineral intake (both food and supplemental form); and percentage of total calories contributed by carbohydrate, fat, and protein. An interview is an important component of the assessment and a good time for the practitioner to build a rapport with the athlete, learn about his or her eating and training practices, and determine the athlete's motivation and readiness to make dietary changes.

The recommended sports diet consists of 6 to 10 g/kg/day from carbohydrate sources, 1.2 to 1.7 g/kg/day from protein, and 20% to 35% of overall calories from healthy fat sources—all of which depend on the demands of the athlete's sport. Most nutritional requirements can be met with a balanced diet. Protein needs are best met through dietary sources. Complex carbohydrates are the body's most efficient source of energy and abundant source of vitamins and minerals. Dietary fats are the most energy-dense of the macronutrients and are needed in limited amounts in the diet, but remain an important piece of the overall diet. Because individual needs for calories and nutrients may vary, individual needs should be assessed.

Water-soluble vitamins are the vitamin B complex and vitamin C. Based on their use in the body, these vitamins may play a role in athletic performance. All of these vitamins are readily available in the diet, primarily from grains, fruits, and vegetables. The role of fat-soluble vitamins and athletic performance is not well-studied, and their role in athletic performance is unclear.

The timing of meals and snacks may have a great effect on an athlete's level of energy and physical status. Consumption of pre-exercise and competition foods should be based on the duration and intensity of the activity and the athlete's individual preferences and tolerances.

As technology improves and research continues to expand, the science of nutrition provides us with information that, if implemented, will increase quality of life and optimize an athlete's performance. Because it truly is a science of interest to our population, the popular press will continue to sensationalize information regarding nutrition. Because of the lack of governance over the diet and supplement industry, athletes, health care providers, and the general public are encouraged to seek out registered dietitians (the nutrition experts) for accurate nutrition information, as well as to develop optimal nutrition plans for individualized performance enhancement.

References

1. Manore MM: Health screening and dietary assessment. In Dunford M, editor: *Sports nutrition—A practice manual for professionals*, ed 4, Chicago, 2006, American Dietetic Association.
2. McArdle WD, Katch FI, Katch UL: *Exercise physiology: Energy, nutrition and human performance*, ed 2, Philadelphia, 1986, Lea & Febiger.
3. American College of Sports Medicine, American Dietetic Association, Dietitians of Canada: Nutrition and athletic performance, *Med Sci Sport Exer* 41(3):709–731, 2009.
4. Brown J: *Nutrition through the life cycle*, Belmont, 2002, Wadsworth/Thomas Learning.
5. Pennington JAT, Spungen DB: *Bowe's and Church food values of portions commonly used*, ed 18, Baltimore, 2005, Lippincott Williams & Wilkins.
6. Jonnalagadda SS: Dietary fat and exercise. In Dunford M, editor: *Sports nutrition—A practice manual for professionals*, ed 4, Chicago, 2006, American Dietetic Association.
7. Prochaskas J, DiClemente C, Morcross J: In search of how people change: Applications to addictive behaviors, *Am Psychol* 47(9):1102–1114, 1992.
8. Coleman EJ: Carbohydrate and exercise. In Dunford M, editor: *Sports nutrition—A practice manual for professionals*, ed 4, Chicago, 2006, American Dietetic Association.
9. Sherman WM, Lamb DR: Nutrition and prolonged exercise. In Lamb DR, Murray R, editors: *Perspectives in exercise science and sports medicine: Prolonged exercise*, Indianapolis, 1988, Benchmark Press.
10. Roberts KM, Noble EG, Hayden DB, et al: Simple and complex carbohydrate-rich diets and muscle glycogen content of marathon runners, *J Appl Physiol* 57:70–74, 1988.
11. Burke LM, Kiens B, Ivy JL: Carbohydrates and fat for training and recovery, *J Sports Sciences* 22:15–30, 2004.
12. McArdle WD, Katch FI, Katch VL: *Sports and exercise nutrition*, ed 3, Baltimore, 2008, Lippincott Williams & Wilkins.
13. Doyle JA, Papadopoulos C, Green MS: Utilization of carbohydrates in energy production. In Wolinsky I, Driskell JA, editors: *Sports nutrition energy metabolism and exercise*, Boca Raton, 2008, CRC Press, Taylor and Francis Group.
14. Position of the American Dietetic Association and the Canadian Dietetic Association: Nutrition for physical fitness and athletic performance for adults, *J Am Diet Assoc* 93(6):691–696, 1993.
15. Volpe SL: Vitamins, mineral, and exercise. In Dunford M, editor: *Sports nutrition—A practice manual for professionals*, ed 4, Chicago, 2006, American Dietetic Association.
16. Berning J, McKibben G, Bernardot D, et al: Fuel supplies for exercise. In Bernardoe D, editor: *Sports nutrition: A guide for the professional working with active people*, ed 2, Chicago, 1992, The American Dietetic Association, Chicago.
17. Otten JJ, Hellwig JP, Meyers LD. *Dietary reference intakes: The essential guide to nutrient requirements*, Washington, 2006, National Academies Press.
18. Tarnopolsky M, MacDougall D, Atkinson S: Influence of protein intake and training status on nitrogen balance and lean body mass, *J Appl Physiol* 64:187–193, 1988.
19. Marable NL, Hickson JF, Korslund M, et al: Urinary nitrogen excretion as influenced by a muscle-building exercise program and protein intake variation, *Nutr Rep Int* 19:795–805, 1979.
20. Burke L, Read R: Diet Patterns of elite Australian male triathletes, *Phys Sports Med* 15:140–145, 1987.
21. Williams MH: The role of protein in physical activity. In William MH, editor: *Nutritional aspects of human physical and athletic performance*, Springfield, IL, 1985, Charles C Thomas.
22. Heaney RP: Protein intake and the calcium economy, *J Am Diet Assoc* 93:1261–1262, 1993.
23. Nordin BEC, Need AG, Morris HA, et al: Sodium, calcium and osteoporosis. In Burckhardt P, Heane RP, editors: *Nutritional aspects of osteoporosis*, New York, 1991, Raven Press.
24. Position of the American Dietetic Association: Vegetarian diets, *J Am Diet Assoc* 93(11):1317–1319, 1993.
25. Wright ED, Paige DM: Lipid metabolism and exercise, *J Clin Nutr* 7:28–32, 1988.
26. Berg FM: *Alcohol promotes fat storage*. Obesity Health Nov/Dec 107–108, 1993.
27. McNaughton L, Preece D: Alcohol and its effects on sprint and middle distance running, *Br J Sports Med* 20:56–59, 1986.
28. Houmard JA, Langenfeld ME, Wiley RL, et al: Effects of the acute ingestion of small amounts of alcohol on 5-mile run times, *J Sports Med* 27:253–257, 1987.
29. Berning J, McKibben G, Benardot D, et al: Fuel supplies for exercise in sports nutrition. In Benardot D, editor: *Sports nutrition: A guide for the professional working with active people*, ed 2, Chicago, 1992, American Dietetic Association.
30. Keith RE: Vitamins in sports and exercise. In Wolinsky I, Hickson JF, editors: *Nutrition, exercise and sport*, Boca Raton, FL, 1989, CRC Press.
31. Gerster H: The role of vitamin C in athletic performance, *J Am Coll Nutr* 8:636–643, 1989.
32. Baily D, Carron AV, Teece RD: Effect of vitamin C supplementation upon the physiological response to exercise in trained and untrained runners, *Int Z Vitaminforsch* 40:435–441, 1979.
33. Henschel A, Taylor H, Brozek J, et al: Vitamin C and ability to work in hot environments, *Am J Trop Med Hyg* 24:259–265, 1944.
34. Howald H, Segesser B: Ascorbic acid and athletic performance, *Ann NY Acad Sci* 258:458–464, 1975.
35. Keren G: The effect of high dosage vitamin C intake on aerobic and anaerobic capacity, *J Sports Med Phys Fitness* 20:145–148, 1980.
36. Rasch P, Arnheim D, Klafs C: Effects of vitamin C supplementation on cross-country runners, *Sportsartzliche Prax* 5:10–13, 1962.
37. Clement DB, Sawchuk LL: Iron status and sports performance, *Sports Med* 1:65, 1984.
38. Fink HH, Burgoon LA, Mikesky AE: *Practical applications in sports nutrition*, Sudbury, MA, 2006, Jones and Bartlett.
39. Drinkwater BL, Nilson K, Chestnut CH, et al: Bone mineral content of amenorrheic and eumenorrheic athletes, *N Engl J Med* 311:277–281, 1984.
40. Gisolfi CV, Duchman SM: Guidelines for optimal replacement beverages for different athletic events, *Med Sci Sports Exerc* 24(6):679–687, 1992.
41. Hiller WDB: Dehydration and hyponatremia during triathlons, *Med Sci Sports Exerc* 21:S219–S221, 1989.
42. Morimoto T, Miki K, Nose H, et al: Changes in body fluid and its composition during heavy sweating and effect of fluid electrolyte replacement, *Jon J Biometeorol* 18:31–39, 1981.

43. Nadel ER: Limits imposed on exercise in a hot environment, *Sports Sci Exchange* 3:27, 1990.

44. Sawka MN, Pandolf KB: Effects of body water loss on physiological function and exercise performance. In Gisolfi CV, Lamb DR, editors: *Perspectives in exercise science and sports medicine*, Vol 3: Fluid homeostatis during exercise, Indianapolis, 1990, Benchmark Press.

45. Coggan AR, Coyle EF: Carbohydrate ingestion during prolonged exercise: Effects on metabolism and performance, *Exerc Sports Sci Rev* 19:1–40, 1991.

46. Coyle EF, Montain SJ: Benefits of fluid replacement with carbohydrate during exercise, *Med Sci Sports Exerc* 24(Supplement 9): S324–S330, 1992.

47. Leiper JB, Maughan RJ: Comparison of absorption rates from two hypotonic and two isotonic rehydration solutions in the intact human jejunum, *Clin Sci* 75(Supplement 19):22P, 1988.

48. Lifshitz F, Wapnir RA: Oral hydration solutions: Experimental optimization of water and sodium absorption, *J Pediatr* 106: 383–389, 1984.

49. US Olympic Committee: *Drug Control Program*, Committee on Substance Abuse Research and Education, 1986.

50. World Anti-Doping Agency accessed at www.wada-ama.org.

51. Coyle EF: Carbohydrates and athletic performance, *Sports Sci Exchange* 1(7):October, 1988.

52. Cummings S: Obesity management. In Carlson KM, Eisenstat S, editors: *Primary care of women*, Chicago, 1995, Mosby Year Book.

53. Luder E, Schebendach J: Nutrition management of eating disorders, *Top Clin Nutr* 8:48–63, 1993.

54. Rock CL, Yager J: Nutrition and eating disorders: A primer for clinicians, *Int J Eat Disord* 6:267–280, 1987.

55. Reiff DW, Reiff KKL: *Eating disorders: Nutrition therapy in the recovery process*, Gaithersburg, MD, 1992, Aspen.

56. American Psychiatric Association: *Diagnostic and statistical manual of mental disorders*, ed 4, Washington, DC, 1994, American Psychiatric Association.

57. Foreyt JP, Goodrick GK: Factors common to successful therapy for the obese patient, *Med Sci Sports Exerc* 23:292–297, 1991.

58. Wilmore JH: Body weight standards and athletic performance. In Brownell KD, Rodin J, Wilmore JH, editors: *Eating, body weight and performance in athletes: Disorders of modern society*, Philadelphia, 1992, Lea & Febiger.

CHAPTER

5

ENVIRONMENTAL CONSIDERATIONS FOR SPORTS

Travis L. Francis and Rich Bomgardner

Introduction

Exercise testing and physical training are integral components in the physical rehabilitation process. Regular physical exercise is also an essential component in any preventive medicine program. The stress imposed by the exercise intensity, however, is only one consideration in the exercise testing and prescription process. An equally important stress to consider is that imposed by the environment (i.e., heat, cold, altitude, and air quality). The environment can alter the physiological responses of the muscular, cardiovascular, and thermoregulatory systems and, either singly or in combination with exercise, induce potentially hazardous health conditions.

The purpose of this chapter is to provide the reader with information on the physiological responses that occur when humans are exposed to heat, cold, altitude, and air pollution. The chapter focuses on the effect that each environmental extreme has on the physiological responses to exercise, exercise performance, and exercise prescription. In each section, special considerations are discussed that can modify the physiological responses to the environment, as well as effective ways to prevent, recognize, and treat illnesses arising from environmental exposure.

Note: This chapter includes content from previous contributions by Scott J. Montain, PhD, and Beau J. Freund, PhD, as it appeared in the predecessor of this book: Zachazewski JE, Magee DJ, Quillen WS, editors: *Athletic Injuries and Rehabilitation,* Philadelphia, 1996, WB Saunders.

Temperature Regulation and Energy Balance

Humans, like other homeothermic animals, must maintain body temperature within a relatively narrow range to function optimally and survive. Deviations in body temperature of approximately 4°C (7.2°F) from 37°C (98.6°F) (normal resting core temperature) are known to reduce physical and cognitive performance, and increases of 6°C (10.8°F) or decreases of 12°C (21.6°F) are usually lethal.[1]

Body Temperature

- Normal core body temperature is 37°C (98.6°F).
- Deviations of ±4°C (7.2°F) can reduce physical and cognitive performance.
- Deviations of +6°C (10.8°F) or −12°C (−21.6°F) can cause death.

Body temperature is physiologically regulated by integrating both thermal and nonthermal information within the anterior and preoptic areas of the hypothalamus and sending the appropriate efferent signals to alter heat loss and gain. Thermal signals include afferent input from temperature-sensitive nerve endings located in the brain, body core, and skin. Nonthermal signals include afferent information from the cardiopulmonary and arterial baroreceptors and osmoreceptors. Passive heat transfer properties also affect heat movement within the body. These passive properties include body mass, body mass/surface area ratio, and body composition.

Despite its complex nature, body temperature regulation can be viewed simply as the process of balancing heat production with heat loss. This is accomplished by physiological processes that control the rate of heat production, the transfer of metabolic heat from the body core to the skin surface, and the transfer of heat from the skin surface to the surrounding environment. Deep body (core) temperature remains stable whenever body heat production equals body heat loss. Core temperature increases when heat production exceeds heat loss and falls when heat losses exceed heat production.

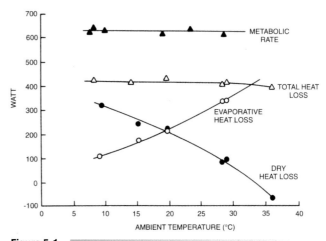

Figure 5-1

Avenues of heat exchange during exercise over a wide range of ambient air temperature. (Modified from Nielsen M: Die Regulation der Körpertemperatur bei Muskelarbeit, *Skand Arch Physiol* 79:193, 1938.)

Body Temperature is Maintained by:

- Controlling the rate of heat production
- Transferring metabolic heat from body core to skin surface via circulation
- Transferring heat from skin surface to surrounding environment by radiation, convection, and evaporation

During exercise, metabolic substrates are broken down to provide energy for cellular metabolism. However, only 20% to 23% of the substrate's energy is used to accomplish work. The remaining 77% to 80% becomes heat that must be dissipated to prevent dangerous elevations in core temperature. Heat production, which can increase 20 times the basal rate, can be conveniently estimated from the measured oxygen uptake and the useful work that is accomplished. The magnitude of heat storage (i.e., increase in body core temperature) depends on the magnitude of heat production, the ability to transfer the heat to the skin surface, and the capacity of the environment to accept heat from the skin surface. In hot environments, the heat produced during exercise may be compounded by heat gained from the environment and further raise core temperature. In cold environments, the heat produced by exercise or involuntary rhythmic contractions of skeletal muscle (shivering) may be needed to attenuate reductions in body temperature.

The majority of heat generated within the body is convected from the inner core to the skin's surface via the circulation. Heat is then dissipated to the environment by three primary means: radiation, convection, and evaporation. The relative contribution of each pathway depends on the environmental conditions, as summarized in Figure 5-1. Any imbalance between the rate of heat dissipation and the rate of heat production results in a change in heat storage or heat debt. To better understand the different pathways for heat loss, a brief description of each is provided.

Radiation is the heat gained or lost at the skin surface because of the arrival or release of energy in the infrared and related portions of the electromagnetic energy spectrum from or to the surrounding radiant surfaces. Radiant heat exchange is independent of ambient air temperature, depending on the temperature gradient between the emitting and receiving surfaces.

Convection is the heat lost or gained because of the mass transfer or conduction of heat at the boundary layer of air (or water) moving past the skin's surface. In thermoneutral conditions and still air, convection accounts for 12% to 15% of total heat loss. However, convective heat loss increases rapidly with air movement. Water is approximately 40 times more effective in convecting heat from the body than is air. As a consequence, cold exposure combined with a wet body surface causes substantial heat loss and is more likely to result in hypothermia than is cold air alone.

Evaporation is the heat lost by vaporization of water from the skin surface. Evaporation is the most effective means of heat loss in terms of absolute quantities of heat, and it is the most important route of heat loss during exercise-heat stress. Evaporation depends on the water vapor pressure gradient between the skin and the air and the air velocity moving over the skin surface. It does not require a positive skin–to–ambient air temperature gradient.

Clinical Point

Under conditions in which there is a positive water vapor pressure gradient between the skin and the ambient air, secreted sweat will evaporate, removing heat from the body. In high ambient humidity conditions however, the evaporative capacity is reduced, and secreted sweat will drip from the skin surface without dissipating body heat.

Heat Exposure

Core Temperature Responses to Exercise-Heat Stress

During physical exercise in ambient conditions that allow steady-state heat balance, core temperature initially increases rapidly and then increases more slowly until heat loss equals heat production (Figure 5-2). The initial increase in core temperature is due to a lag in the activation of the heat dissipation mechanisms (i.e., sweating, cutaneous vasodilatation). The magnitude of increase in core temperature is proportional to the metabolic rate (e.g., the exercise intensity) and is nearly independent of environmental conditions within a range of climatic conditions termed the *prescriptive zone* (Figure 5-3).[2-6] The prescriptive zone refers to a range of ambient air conditions in which there is little or no difference in steady-state exercise core temperature despite varying ambient air conditions. During exercise in climatic conditions above the prescriptive zone, the steady-state core temperature is elevated in proportion to the climatic conditions. Therefore, steady-state body core temperature will be similar during exercise in a temperate (20°C to 28°C/68°F to 82.5°F) environment, but will be elevated when performing the same exercise in hot environments. Equally important, Figure 5-3 illustrates that the upper end of the prescriptive zone is shifted to a lower ambient temperature condition with increasing exercise intensity. This means that core temperature will begin to be affected by environmental conditions at a lower ambient temperature when performing high-intensity exercise than during moderate- or low-intensity exercise.

The core temperature increase during endurance exercise does not reflect a failure of the temperature control system. On the contrary, core temperature is finely regulated even under extremes of exercise and environmental temperature. Under conditions in which skin blood flow is compromised (e.g., dehydration, high exercise intensity),

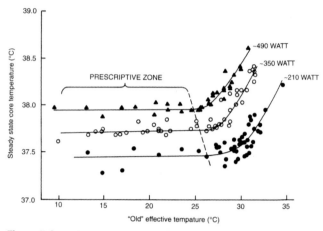

Figure 5-3

Relationship of steady-state core temperature responses and the "old" effective air temperature at three metabolic rates. Effective air temperature derived from dry and wet bulb temperature, and wind speed. (Modified from Lind AR: A physiological criterion for setting thermal environmental limits for everyday work, *J Appl Physiol* 18:51, 1963.)

the core temperature increase widens the temperature gradient between the body core and the skin, preserving heat transport to the peripheral circulation despite lower skin blood flow.

Clinical Point

During exercise, the core temperature increase is the result of integrated physiological responses that optimize skeletal muscle perfusion and heat transport without compromising arterial blood pressure.

There are climatic conditions, however, in which steady-state core temperature values cannot be attained. Whenever heat production exceeds the environment's capacity to accept heat, core temperature progressively increases, and individuals are at increased risk for heat exhaustion and heatstroke. Athletes, race organizers, and trainers must evaluate the ambient weather conditions prior to beginning exercise and modify the exercise intensity and duration, as well as fluid requirements, to reduce the risk of heat injury.

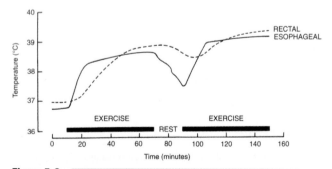

Figure 5-2

Esophageal and rectal temperature responses to rest and exercise during compensable heat stress. (From Sawka MN, Wenger CB: Physiological responses to acute exercise-heat stress. In Pandolf KB, Sawka MN, Gonzalez RR, editors: *Human performance physiology and environmental medicine at terrestrial extremes,* p 110, Indianapolis, 1988, Benchmark Press.)

Clinical Point

The American College of Sports Medicine has recommended that endurance athletic events be rescheduled when the ambient wet bulb globe temperature exceeds 28°C (82.4°F) (WBGT = $0.7 \times T_{wb}$ + $0.2 \times T_g$ + $0.1 \times T_{db}$).

T_{db}, Dry bulb temperature; T_g, black globe temperature; T_{wb}, wet bulb temperature.[7]

Cardiovascular Responses to Exercise-Heat Stress

When exercising is done in warm or hot ambient temperatures, the cardiovascular system is challenged with simultaneously delivering sufficient muscle blood flow to support metabolism and sufficient cutaneous blood flow to support heat loss from the body while still maintaining blood pressure. Because the blood flow demand to these vascular beds can exceed the cardiovascular system's capacity, reductions in blood flow to the skin and muscle may be necessary to preserve cardiovascular stability.

Several adjustments occur during exercise-heat stress to optimize the balance between cutaneous and skeletal muscle blood flow. First, blood flow to the splanchnic organs and kidneys is reduced, with the magnitude of reduction proportional to the exercise intensity and environmental heat stress.[8] The lower blood flow to these organs reduces their blood volume, helping to maintain central blood volume, cardiac filling pressure, and arterial blood pressure. Second, at the onset of exercise, a generalized venoconstriction occurs in proportion to the severity of exercise.[9,10] The venoconstriction acts to reduce skin blood volume, enhancing central blood volume and cardiac filling.[8]

The cardiovascular system has finite limits to its ability to distribute blood volume during exercise-heat stress. The redistribution of blood into the cutaneous circulation during heat stress can compromise cardiac filling, cardiac output, and blood pressure. Figure 5-4 illustrates the cardiovascular responses of six subjects during graded exercise in a neutral (25.6°C/[78.1°F]) and hot (43.3°C/[109.9°F]) environment.[8] When exercising in the hot environment, the subjects had higher heart rates but lower central blood and stroke volumes, compared with the neutral environment. Although the subjects' cardiac output was similar in the hot and neutral environments during the two lower exercise intensities, cardiac output was lower in the hot environment at the two higher exercise intensities. The lack of ability to redistribute sufficient blood volume to preserve cardiac output during heat stress is further evidenced by the 5% to 8% lower maximal oxygen uptake during exercise in hot environments.[11-15] The greater cardiovascular strain can reduce exercise tolerance and impair endurance exercise performance.

Cerebral Response to Exercise-Heat Stress

Cerebral blood flow increases as heart rate elevates with exercise. Temperature in the brain remains stable at approximately 37°C (98.7°F), which seems to lead to the conclusion that heat removal from the brain is consistent with cerebral metabolic heat.[16] However, as core body temperature rises, cerebral temperature also rises. This is because, during physical activity, heat production by the muscles evaluates core temperature. Core temperature increases result in an increase in arterial blood temperature, which subsequently alters cerebral heat balance. Initially, this temperature increases rapidly during exercise. During the first 10 to 15 minutes, the venous-to-arterial temperature difference is limited, which results in storage of heat in the brain. Therefore, during this period, the temperature of the brain increases approximately 1°C (1.8°F) before it stabilizes.[16]

During exercise and heat strain, the core and arterial temperatures keep increasing. Heat removed by venous blood flow is reduced during exercise and hyperthermia. Therefore, there is a constant parallel between the rise in core body and cerebral temperature. In addition, the rise in metabolic heat production in the brain combines with impaired heat removal and results in continuous storage of heat in the brain.

Increases in cerebral heat have been associated with decreases in muscular activity during hot environments. Studies have yielded results demonstrating that elevated core body temperature weakens muscular activity and force production, which in turn produces a relative fatigue factor.[17] In addition, supporting investigations using the Borg Scale of 6 through 20 or a rating of perceived exertion (RPE) yielded similar results of increased fatigue during exercise. These studies support the conclusion that when brain temperatures increase, fatigue elevates and participation level decreases even with continued blood flow and muscular activity in hot environments when compared with cool environments. Therefore, it could be concluded that athletes can exercise longer in cooler environments at the same level of intensity than hot environments. It stands to reason for medical personnel that increases in core temperature should sound an alarm as to the severity of a heat emergency.

Metabolic Responses to Exercise-Heat Stress

Whether heat stress increases the caloric requirement to perform a specific task remains unclear. Although several investigators have reported elevated metabolic rates with exercise-heat stress,[18-22] others have reported no change or lower metabolic rates.[23-26] One explanation for the discrepancy may be contributions of anaerobic metabolism to total energy cost, as the investigations reporting similar or lower metabolic rates during exercise-heat stress also reported increased plasma or blood lactate concentration.[24-26]

The effect of exercise-heat stress on muscle blood flow and metabolism has been examined in several studies. Exercise-heat stress does not appear to impair either blood flow or oxygen delivery to the working muscle. Two studies reported similar leg blood flow and leg oxygen uptake during moderately intense exercise in hot (40°7C/104°F) and temperate (20.5°C to 23°C/69°F to 73.4°F) climates.[22,27] Exercise-heat stress also appears to have little effect on muscle glycogen use.[22,26,28] Therefore, there is little evidence to suggest that hot ambient air temperatures impair oxygen delivery to skeletal muscle or increase skeletal muscle glycogenolysis during exercise.

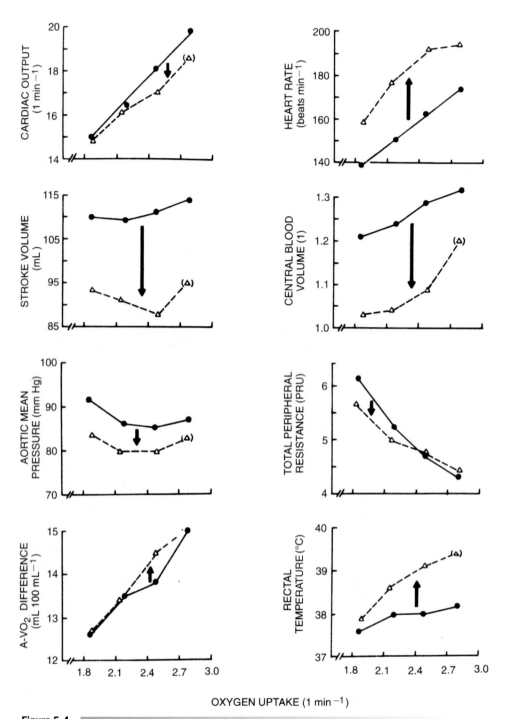

Figure 5-4

Summary of cardiovascular responses to graded upright exercise in neutral (25.6°C, *solid circles*) and hot (43.3°C, *open triangles*) environments. Heat stress–reduced cardiac output at the two higher workloads and depressed stroke volume and central blood volume at all levels of exercise. Each data point is the average of multiple measurements during each 15-minute exercise period from six men. The data points in parentheses show where data from one subject are missing. (From Rowell LB: *Human circulation: Regulation during physical stress,* p 379, New York, 1986, Oxford University Press.)

Special Considerations

Acclimatization

Physical tasks that are relatively easy to perform in cool weather can become extremely difficult to complete during initial exposures to hot weather. Depending on the exercise intensity and accompanying physiological strain, heat exposure may result in higher core temperature, a more rapid heart rate, narrowed pulse pressure, headache, dizziness, cramps, dependent edema, flushing of face and neck, and orthostatic hypotension.[29-31] In addition, these symptoms may be accompanied by a feeling of lassitude and increased fatigue. Fortunately, repeated exposure to hot environments produces adaptations that improve an individual's work capacity during subsequent heat exposures. The physiological adjustments that improve work capacity in the heat are collectively termed *heat acclimatization.*

As depicted in Figure 5-5, most heat acclimatization occurs during the first week of heat exposure, and acclimatization to a given environmental condition is virtually complete after 10 days of exposure. Heat acclimatization leads to marked reductions in exercise heart rate, core temperature, skin temperature, and the core temperature at which cutaneous vasodilatation and sweating begin.[32] There appears to be little change in cardiac output, mean arterial pressure, pulse pressure, or total vascular conductance with acclimatization.[32]

Heat Acclimatization Leads to a Decrease in:

- Exercise heart rate
- Core temperature
- Skin temperature
- Core temperature at which sweating and cutaneous vasodilation begins

The reductions in heart rate and core temperature are greater and occur more quickly with the combination of exercise and heat stress as opposed to heat stress alone.[33] Furthermore, heat acclimatization occurs only when an individual is "stressed" by the environment. Little acclimatization to the hot midday weather occurs if an individual trains in the cool hours of the morning or evening and spends the rest of the day in an air-conditioned room.

Clinical Point

Heat acclimatization occurs in first week of heat exposure, is complete after 10 days of exposure, and occurs best when heat stress and exercise are combined.

Regular exercise in a cool environment has been shown to improve one's ability to thermoregulate during exercise-heat stress.[34,35] The exercise-induced "internal" heat stress (e.g., increased core temperature) stimulates adaptation of the peripheral circulation and evaporative capacity, similar to what occurs with heat exposure. As a result, aerobically trained persons store less body heat during exercise than untrained persons. However, regular exercise in a cool environment does not fully acclimatize an individual to exercise in a hot environment, as regular training in a hot environment can further reduce the thermal and cardiovascular strain associated with exercise in a hot environment.[36-39] Therefore, if exercise is to be performed in hot weather, it is optimal to acclimatize to that climate.

Dehydration

Dehydration, or body-water deficits, occurs during exercise-heat stress if sufficient fluids are not ingested to offset sweat losses. Dehydration results in elevated body core temperature and heart rate during exercise,[35,40-42] with the magnitude of these increases graded in proportion to the amount of dehydration (Figure 5-6).[35,41] Dehydration

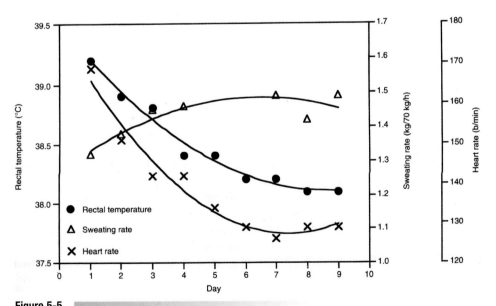

Figure 5-5

Rectal temperature, sweating rate, and heart rate responses over 9 consecutive days of exercise-heat stress. Each data point is the average response of three men after 100 minutes of exercise in a desert climate (49°C$_{db}$, 17% rh). (Modified from Lind AR, Bass DE: Optimal exposure time for development of acclimatization to heat, *Fed Proc* 22:704, 1963.)

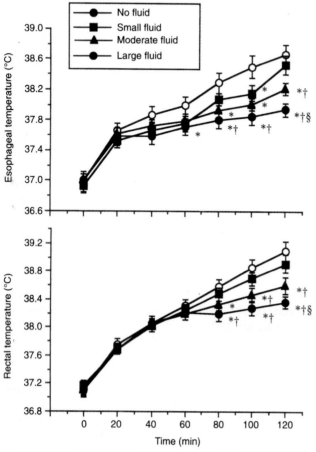

Figure 5-6

Influence of dehydration on esophageal and rectal temperature during 2 hours of moderately intense exercise. (From Montain SM, Coyle EF: Influence of graded dehydration on hyperthermia and cardiovascular drift during exercise, *J Appl Physiol* 73:1340, 1992.)

negates the thermoregulatory advantage of heat acclimatization and aerobic training.[43,44] Dehydration also increases the perception of effort[41] and reduces endurance exercise performance.[35,40,45] In addition, a recent study showed that dehydrated subjects incurred exhaustion from heat strain at lower core temperatures than did normally hydrated subjects during uncompensable heat stress, suggesting that dehydrated persons have a reduced tolerance to exercise-heat strain.[46]

To minimize dehydration, fluids should be ingested during prolonged exercise. The increase in core temperature during

---

Dehydration Leads to:

- Elevated core body temperature
- Elevated heart rate
- Increases perception of effort
- Negates heat acclimatization
- Reduces endurance
- Reduced tolerance to exercise heat strain

---

exercise is smallest when fluid intake most closely matches sweat loss and no dehydration occurs.[41,47] In hot climates, this may require persons to drink 1.0 to 1.5 liters (0.2 to 0.6 gallons) of fluid per hour. The timing of rehydration during exercise is not critical to thermoregulation if the volume of fluid intake is adjusted accordingly; the rise in core temperature depends on the magnitude of fluid loss and not the timing of fluid intake.[48] The composition of the fluid replacement solution can vary as well. Commercial carbohydrate-electrolyte solutions with up to 8% carbohydrate appear to be equally effective as water for attenuating increases in core temperature and heart rate during prolonged exercise.[49]

Although dehydration produces graded increments in core temperature during exercise-heat stress and can impair endurance performance, it remains unclear whether drinking large volumes of fluid to prevent dehydration actually improves athletic performance. Drinking large volumes of fluid during prolonged exercise may force athletes to slow their running pace to enable consumption. Additionally, this may compromise pace because of gastric bloating and discomfort.[50] Each athlete needs to determine whether the time lost as a result of drinking larger volumes of fluid is compensated for by the physiological benefits obtained by attenuating dehydration during prolonged exercise.

Aging

Studies have documented that older populations have a greater incidence of heat intolerance compared with younger adults.[51] The elderly also exhibit a larger-than-normal basal body temperature fluctuation compared with younger adults.[52] This latter liability appears to be largely due to a reduced circulatory effectiveness in controlling heat transport between the body core and the cutaneous circulation. Research suggests, however, that aging per se is not responsible for the greater incidence of heat intolerance in the elderly.[53,54] When matched for activity and aerobic fitness, and when exercise is performed at the same relative percentage of maximal aerobic capacity, older and younger adults have similar increases in core temperature. In addition, aging per se does not impair the ability to acclimatize to hot environments.[53,54] The greater incidence of heat intolerance observed in the elderly is now thought to result from functional changes accompanying a more sedentary lifestyle, obesity, a reduced sweating response, cardiovascular insufficiency, and the effects of medication.[51]

Gender

Both men and women have similar thermoregulatory responses during exercise and moderate heat stress when matched for fitness and training.[55-57] Yet differences between genders do exist. Women appear to sweat more efficiently than men in humid climates, because more of their secreted sweat is evaporated and less sweat drips from the body prior to evaporation.[57,58] The menstrual cycle produces regular fluctuations in basal body temperature. During the luteal phase of the menstrual cycle, basal body temperature is roughly 0.4°C (0.72°F) higher than during the follicular phase.[59] Whether the phase of the menstrual cycle alters the ability to regulate body temperature remains unresolved. Although several investigations reported that the luteal phase simply produces a graded increase in steady-state core temperature during exercise, compared with exercise during the follicular phase,[59,60] a separate investigation found that women were unable to achieve a steady-state core temperature during the luteal phase.[61] The ability of women to effectively train and compete throughout the menstrual cycle, however, suggests that body temperature is adequately regulated during the luteal phase, albeit at a higher core temperature.

To Reduce Heat Stress

- Drink fluids before and during exercise (check body weight before and after exercise).
- Wear proper clothing.
- Modify exercise intensity (check heart rate).

Clothing

Clothing impairs the ability to dissipate heat during exercise-heat stress, because it creates a barrier for the transfer of heat between the skin and the environment. The properties of the clothing, such as its insulation properties and air and vapor permeability, as well as the proportion of the body surface covered, determine the effect of clothing on body temperature regulation and exercise-heat tolerance. Warm-weather clothing should be loose-fitting to permit free circulation of air between the skin and the environment. Furthermore, it should be light colored to reflect radiant light and minimize radiant heat gain in sunny weather. The protective clothing worn by fire-fighters and soldiers on the chemical-biological battlefield greatly increases the thermal and cardiovascular strain of exercise and reduces physiological tolerance to heat strain.[62,63]

Exercise Training in Hot Environments

Exercise training can be conducted safely in hot environments if precautions are taken to minimize the risk of heat illness. Persons exercising in hot environments should attempt to attenuate dehydration by drinking fluids before and during exercise. Individual fluid requirements can be estimated from body weight lost during exercise. Proper clothing should be worn to minimize added heat stress during the exercise bout. Finally, persons exercising in the heat should adjust the exercise intensity to accommodate circulatory strain accompanying exercise in hot environments.

Heart rate remains a reliable indicator of cardiovascular strain during exercise-heat stress. Using the exercise heart rate to set the exercise intensity is a good method for reducing thermal strain in hot climates. However, it should be realized that this method reduces the training stimulus placed on skeletal muscle.

Populations Susceptible to Heat Intolerance

Although the causal factors of heat intolerance are poorly understood, there are a number of congenital and acquired risk factors that have been associated with reduced heat tolerance (Box 5-1). The identification of susceptible persons is important for reducing the risk of heat injury during work in hot weather.

Congenital anomalies underlying heat intolerance usually impair the ability to produce and secrete sweat onto the skin surface. Ectodermal dysplasia is the most common form of congenital anhidrosis (inadequate perspiration). It is attributed to an autosomal-dominant or X-linked recessive trait and therefore affects only males.[64] The sweat glands of those afflicted are either absent, functionally impaired, or histologically present but not innervated. Patients with cystic fibrosis and Parkinson disease have altered neural sweat gland

Box 5-1 Factors Associated with Heat Intolerance

Functional-Physiological Factors
- Dehydration
- Low physical fitness/activity
- Lack of acclimatization
- Surface area/mass ratio
- Age
- Fatigue

Concurrent Disease
- Central nervous system lesions
- Cardiovascular disease
- Sweat gland dysfunction
- Infectious diseases
- Psychiatric illness
- Diabetes mellitus
- Extensive skin burns
- Hyperthyroidism
- Parkinsonism
- Pheochromocytoma (vascular tumor of adrenal medulla or sympathetic paraganglia characterized by hypersecretion of epinephrine and norepinephrine causing hypertension)

Congenital Abnormalities
- Ectodermal dysplasia
- Linear skin dystrophy
- Idiopathic anhidrosis
- Cystic fibrosis
- Scleroderma

Drugs
- Drug abuse
- Medications
- Alcohol

Other
- Clothing
- Previous heatstroke

Data from Epstein Y: Heat intolerance: predisposing factor or residual injury? *Med Sci Sports Exerc* 22:29, 1990.

regulation, which may predispose them to heat intolerance during environmental heat stress.[65-67]

Several skin disorders, such as miliaria rubra (heat rash), impede heat transfer, increase heat storage, and impair performance.[68-70] Psoriatic patients have been shown to have reduced sweating and elevated core temperatures during heat stress.[70] Burn victims have an impaired ability to sweat, and heat tolerance is negatively correlated with the burnt skin area.[51] Conversely, mild sunburn does not seem to increase the thermal strain accompanying exercise in hot climates.[71]

Obese individuals appear to be less tolerant to heat stress.[72,73] The lower heat tolerance in this population may be due to their lower cardiovascular fitness compared with lean individuals (as evidenced by a higher heart rate at rest and during exercise) as well as their lower surface area/body mass ratio.[51]

Spinal cord–injured persons cannot dissipate body heat as effectively as able-bodied persons during exercise-heat stress. They cannot redistribute blood flow as effectively as able-bodied persons, and their maximal whole-body sweat rate is impaired because of insensate skin. The magnitude of this impairment depends on the level of the spinal lesion.

Patients with multiple sclerosis typically demonstrate adverse reactions to heat exposure. External heat, in the form of either climatic conditions or therapeutic modalities, may exacerbate clinical symptoms and induce fatigue.[74]

Various pharmaceutical agents impair heat transfer to the environment.[75-77] For example, anticholinergic drugs, such as atropine, increase core temperature and reduce exercise tolerance time when working in hot environments.[78] Acute amphetamine poisoning commonly leads to hyperpyrexia and fatal heat stroke.[51] Neuroleptic drugs such as chlorpromazine can also impair heat transfer.[75]

Heat Illness

There are several illnesses that may occur during exercise-heat stress (Table 5-1). The clinical features and treatment of these illnesses have been discussed in detail elsewhere.[79,80]

Heat Cramps

Heat cramps can arise after heavy and prolonged sweating. The causal factors are unknown, but are associated with low serum electrolyte concentration. Heat cramps are characterized by skeletal muscle twitching, cramps, and spasm. They generally occur in the arms, legs, and abdomen. The incidence of heat cramps can be minimized by ensuring acclimatization and including salt supplementation at mealtime.

Heat Exhaustion

Heat exhaustion is the most common form of heat illness. It is a "functional" illness and is not associated with organ damage. Heat exhaustion arises when the cardiovascular system is unable to meet the competing demands of thermoregulatory skin blood flow and skeletal muscle and vital organ blood flow. Individuals become fatigued, with orthostatic dizziness and ataxia. Common features include dyspnea and tingling in hands and feet. Persons may be disconsolate, uncoordinated, and mentally dull. Acute management should be focused on reducing cardiovascular demand and reversing water and salt deficits.

Heatstroke

Heatstroke is an inherent risk during any outdoor physical activity and becomes prominent when the ambient temperature and humidity elevates. Heatstroke is the most severe form of the heat-related illnesses and can be associated with neurological dysfunction. There have been two types of heatstroke identified: classic heatstroke (CHS) and exertional heatstroke (EHS).[81] CHS more commonly affects sedentary elderly individuals, persons who are chronically ill, and very young persons. It also occurs during environmental heat waves and is more common in areas that have not experienced a heat wave in many years. The main factor of CHS is the inability of the body to dissipate heat in the hot environment. EHS generally occurs in young individuals who engage in strenuous physical activity for a prolonged period in a hot environment.[81] EHS is one of the most serious conditions that occur when excess heat, generated by muscular exercise, exceeds the body's heat-dissipation rate. The consequent elevated body core temperature causes damage to the body's tissues, resulting in a characteristic multiorgan failure syndrome, which is occasionally fatal. EHS is defined by core temperature of more than 40°C (104°F).[81-83] EHS is a potentially lethal outcome for any athlete, laborer, soldier, or other individual who participates in physical activity in warm or hot conditions. The incidence of EHS varies depending on the event and increases with rising ambient temperature and humidity.

Although heatstroke is relatively rare, its incidence rate is as high as 1 in 1000 at some athletic endurance events because these events often include 10,000 or more participants.[84] Early recognition is critical to the survival of athletes

Signs and Symptoms of Heat Stroke
• Disorientation
• Confusion
• Dizziness
• Unusual behavior
• Headache
• Loss of balance
• Inability to walk
• Vomiting
• Diarrhea
• Seizures
• Syncope
• Coma

Table 5-1

Diagnosis and Treatment of Heat Disorders

Disorder	Cause/Predisposing Factor	Clinical Features and Diagnosis	Treatment	Prevention
Heat cramps	Heavy and prolonged sweating Inadequate salt intake	Low serum and chloride Muscle twitching, cramps, and spasms in arms, legs, and abdomen	Severe cramps: Administer intravenous saline infusion. Mild cramps: Orally administer 0.1% salt solution. Rest in cool environment. Eat salty foods.	Ensure acclimatization. Provide extra salt at meals and with fluids.
Heat exhaustion	Inability of the cardiovascular system to meet demands of thermoregulatory, muscular and visceral blood flow Water or salt depletion caused by heavy, prolonged sweating Inadequate fluid or salt intake Polyuria or diarrhea Vomiting Inadequate acclimatization Heat production exceeds environmental heat-loss capacity	Fatigue, orthostatic dizziness, ataxia, hypotension Syncope Nausea and vomiting Tingling in hands and feet Wrist or ankle spasm Dyspnea Elevated skin and core temperatures High hematocrit, serous protein, and sodium Dry tongue and mouth Excessive thirst Weak, disconsolate, uncoordinated, and mentally dull	Rest supine in cool environment. Provide intravenous saline infusion. Sponge with cool water. Provide small quantities of semiliquid food. Keep record of body weight, water and salt intake, and body temperature. Avoid exercise-heat stress for 24 to 48 hours.	Provide adequate fluids. Ensure acclimatization. Provide opportunity for intermittent cooling and adequate rest. Reduce work rate when exercising in hot temperatures and high-humidity climates.
Heat stroke	Distinguished from heat exhaustion by presence of tissue injury Two types: Classic heatstroke Exertional heatstroke	Collapse Severe encephalopathy and hyperthermia Dehydration Rhabdomyolysis Myoglobinuria Diarrhea and vomiting	Provide active cooling. Administer IV dextrose-saline infusion. Administer isoproterenol, dopamine, or dobutamine as needed. Maintain airway. Monitor and treat hyperkalemia. Monitor and treat acute renal injury. Keep record of core temperature. Treat secondary disorders. Avoid exercise-heat stress until clinical recovery is complete.	Provide adequate fluids. Ensure acclimatization. Provide opportunity for intermittent cooling and adequate rest. Reduce work rate when exercising in hot temperatures and high-humidity climates.

Continued

Table 5-1
Diagnosis and Treatment of Heat Disorders—cont'd

Disorder	Cause/Predisposing Factor	Clinical Features and Diagnosis	Treatment	Prevention
Heat syncope	Inability to maintain blood pressure Peripheral vasodilatation and pooling of blood Circulatory instability and loss of vasomotor tone Hyperventilation Inadequate acclimatization Infection	Weakness and fatigue Hypotension Increased venous compliance Blurred vision Pallor Syncope Elevated skin and core temperatures	Place supine and elevate legs. Rest in cool environment. Provide oral saline if conscious and resting. Keep record of blood pressure and body temperature.	Ensure acclimatization. Avoid sustained upright static work.
Miliaria rubra, miliaria profunda	Local inflammation caused by occlusion of the sweat gland	Pruritic, inflamed papulovesicular skin eruptions High ambient humidity	Cool and dry affected skin Avoid re-exposure until lesions have healed. Control for infection.	Wear loose-fitting clothing. Practice good hygiene.
Hyponatremia	Too low concentration of sodium in bloodstream causes cells to swell Swelling in brain especially dangerous	Nausea, vomiting, headache, fatigue, lethargy, loss of appetite, restlessness and irritability, muscle weakness, muscle cramps and spasm, seizures	Administer IV sodium if severe. Prescribe medications. Prescribe hormone therapy if cause is adrenal insufficiency.	Watch water intake and only drink as much as you lose because of sweating. Consider using sports beverage that contains electrolytes.

IV, Intravenous.

with EHS. Signs and symptoms are often disorientation, confusion, dizziness, unusual behavior, headache, loss of balance, inability to walk, vomiting, diarrhea, seizures, syncope, and possible coma. A body core temperature is essential to establish for an accurate diagnosis. Rectal temperature is the most reliable method and is preferred over other standard measurements. Although oral, tympanic, and axillary methods are often used, these methods are affected by swallowing of cold liquids, hypoventilation, or facilities with air conditioning.[81,83]

> **Clinical Point**
>
> Rectal temperature is the most accurate method of determining core body temperature.

EHS requires immediate attention as a life-threatening medical emergency. The first hour after the athlete collapses has proven to be the most challenging and critical to survival. The best management protocol appears to be total body cooling, which is usually necessary to achieve a positive outcome. The quickest rates of cooling have been reported in therapy using cold-water and ice-water immersion. Secondarily, simultaneously using ice-water towels over the head, trunk, and extremities and ice packs over the axillary, groin, and neck has been demonstrated to be effective in reducing body core temperature.[83] Advanced preparation is critical to minimize delays in reduction of core temperature. Athletes should be placed in a cooling tub so that as much surface area is submerged as possible. Constant supervision and reassessment of blood pressure, heart rate, and rectal temperature are monitored every 5 to 10 minutes. The athlete can be removed from the cooling tub when the rectal temperature reaches 38°C to 39°C (100.4°F to 102°F).[85] However, it is extremely important in event management that personnel are trained and equipped to handle these emergencies.

Recommendations for returning to competition after an EHS episode are undefined; however, the following protocol has been recommended[85]: (1) no activity for 7 days after hospital dismissal, (2) physician consultation after dismissal and a heat tolerance test to be administered within 3 to 4 weeks, (3) gradual acclimation to exercise and heat for 7 to 14 days at the beginning of training with particular attention being paid to intensity and duration, and (4) physician clearance to full participation after the 7- to 14-day trial period of exercise. Medical staff should be trained and prepared to handle EHS conditions, particularly when the event has large groups of athletes competing.

Miliaria Rubra and Miliaria Profunda

Miliaria rubra (heat rash or prickly heat) is a papulovesicular skin eruption that can arise when active eccrine sweat glands become occluded by organic debris. It generally occurs in humid climates or to skin that is sufficiently encapsulated by clothing to produce high-humidity conditions. It is treated by cooling and drying the skin, treating itching symptoms, and controlling for infection. Exercise-heat exposure should be avoided until the rash has disappeared.

Miliaria that becomes generalized and prolonged is termed *miliaria profunda*. It can lead to anhidrotic heat exhaustion, because the occluded sweat glands no longer produce sweat for evaporation. The lesions are truncal, noninflamed, and papular. They are also asymptomatic. Persons with miliaria profunda are less heat tolerant compared with the general population.

Hyponatremia

Hyponatremia is an abnormally low concentration of sodium in the blood. Normal ranges of sodium range are from 135 to 55 mEq/L.[86] Too little sodium can cause cells to malfunction and extremely low sodium can be fatal. Hyponatremia occurs over time if the hypertonic sweat is being replaced by hypotonic fluid (water) leading to a decrease in serum sodium.[87] In other words, as the athlete sweats out water and sodium, water is being replaced, but the sodium is not. Drinking appropriate electrolyte solutions can allow replacement of water and sodium as well as other needed electrolytes. When significant amounts of fluid are lost through high-intensity exercise, replacement with water alone can lead to a chemical imbalance in the body and deficiencies in electrolytes, which are nutrients critical for organ functioning. Sodium circulates in the body fluids outside the cells. It is very important for maintaining blood pressure. Sodium is also needed for nerves and muscles to function properly. Adequate sodium balance is necessary for transmitting nerve impulses and proper muscle function, and even a slight depletion of this concentration can cause problems.

When sodium levels drop in the fluids outside the cells, water seeps into the cells to balance the salt levels. The cells swell as a result of the excess water. Although most cells can handle this swelling, brain cells cannot because the skull confines them. Brain swelling causes most of the symptoms of hyponatremia. Cerebral edema causes elevated intracranial pressure, which can progress to pulmonary edema through either increased alveolar and interstitial fluid or through pulmonary vasoconstriction with increase capillary hydrostatic pressure.[88] At the same time, central nervous system alterations can begin to appear. In hyponatremia, the imbalance of water to salt is caused by one of three conditions:[85]

1. Hypervolemic hyponatremia: Both sodium and water content in the body increase, but water gain is greater
2. Euvolemic hyponatremia: Excess of total body water with either normal or slightly reduced whole-body sodium
3. Hypovolemic hyponatremia: Water and sodium are both lost from the body, but the sodium loss is greater

Reports indicate most hyponatremia events take place during military training, long hikes, marathons, and Ironman or other triathlons.[86,87] Generally, events lasting longer than 7 to 17 hours are more likely to cause hyponatremia. However, depending on the health of the individual, climate, ambient temperature, or humidity, a hyponatremia episode could occur in as little as 4 hours. Besides event duration, individuals who drink water excessively and slower runners are predisposed to hyponatremia. In addition, other common physical predisposing factors include being female, having small or thin stature, sweating excessively, and having a low body mass index of 20 or less.

The severity of hyponatremia depends on how much sodium levels are decreased to produce typical signs and symptoms. These results range from:[87]

1. Mild (sodium = 131-134 mEq/L): Generally no symptoms
2. Moderate (sodium = 126-130 mEq/L): Nausea, vomiting, headache, disorientation, confusion, abnormal behavior, loss of coordination, and muscle weakness
3. Severe (sodium = < 126 mEq/L): Altered mental capacity, coma and potential death

There is some variability in the signs and symptoms; therefore, it is critical for medical personnel to be aware of event participation, predisposing factors, and identification of lowered sodium levels.

Cold Exposure

Thermoregulation in Cold Climates

Cold weather need not be a deterrent for outdoor exercise. Physical exercise can be performed safely in extremely cold conditions if sufficient clothing is worn to maintain body core temperature and protect the skin from cold injury. It does require special consideration for the exercise participant, however, as inadequate clothing can lead to rapid reductions in body temperature and commensurate impairment of exercise performance.

Behavioral thermoregulation (e.g., seeking shelter and wearing warm clothing) is the most effective means of tolerating cold exposure. Cold-weather clothing adds an insulation layer between the body core and the ambient air or water, enabling persons to tolerate extremely cold ambient temperatures without becoming cold. The amount of clothing necessary to maintain thermal balance is inversely related to metabolic rate.

Humans have two primary physiological responses to cold exposure, both of which attempt to prevent or minimize a fall in body core temperature. The initial response is cutaneous vasoconstriction. This reduces blood flow to the periphery and increases insulation. The second response is to increase metabolic heat production by shivering or physical activity.

Physiological Responses to Cold Exposure

- Cutaneous vasoconstriction
- Increased metabolic heat production (shivering)

Peripheral Vasoconstriction

Cutaneous vasoconstriction is sympathetically mediated. It reduces heat transfer from the core to the periphery and adds an insulative layer between the body core and the environment. Depending on the magnitude of cold and the duration of exposure, cold exposure can also induce limb skeletal muscle vasoconstriction.[89] Peripheral vasoconstriction is initiated with the onset of skin cooling, but muscle blood flow is maintained until cold strain is severe enough to compromise the core temperature.[89]

In many individuals, the hands and feet demonstrate cyclic blood flow when exposed to cold. This phenomenon, sometimes referred to as the *hunting reflex* or *hunting response,* is now more commonly termed *cold-induced vasodilatation (CIVD).* It occurs as a result of rhythmic cycling of sympathetic vasoconstrictor stimulation. The cyclic warming and cooling of these peripheral tissues is generally thought to be beneficial in preventing peripheral cold injuries and improving manual dexterity. It is not observed in all persons, however, and can be highly variable within an individual.

Exercise can modify peripheral vasoconstriction. If exercise heat production exceeds the rate of heat loss, peripheral vasoconstriction attenuates, and cutaneous blood flow increases. During moderate cold stress, exercise can completely abolish the peripheral vasoconstriction. However, the peripheral vasoconstrictor drive will persist if the heat produced during exercise is lower than the rate of heat loss.

Thermogenesis

At rest, humans increase heat production primarily through shivering, which is the involuntary contraction of skeletal muscle. Shivering is stimulated when cold stress reduces skin or core temperature. The magnitude of shivering depends on the relative intensity of the cold stress, as shivering is proportional to the decrement in body temperature.[90,91] To support shivering, oxygen uptake increases up to a value of about 1.51 min^{-1} as body temperature declines.[89-91] Some heat may also be released from other metabolic but nonshivering sources, such as digestion, although the contribution appears to be limited.[92]

Physical exercise can produce substantial heat and offset heat loss in cold weather. As discussed, physical activity can increase metabolic heat production 15-fold. During competition, endurance-trained athletes may exercise for several hours at metabolic intensities that produce 700 to 800 watts of heat.[41,48] This rate of heat production enables these individuals to exercise comfortably with minimal clothing in cold air temperatures.

Cardiovascular and Metabolic Responses to Exercise During Cold Stress

The peripheral vasoconstriction induced by cold exposure redistributes blood from the periphery to the body core. As a result of this redistribution of blood, end-diastolic volume and stroke volume are elevated during cold exposure. Cardiac output at a given oxygen uptake remains unchanged, however, as heart rate is reduced during cold exposure.[93] Diastolic blood pressure is increased approximately10 torr (a unit of pressure) as a consequence of peripheral vasoconstriction.[89]

Cold exposure can increase caloric expenditure during submaximal exercise. However, the effect of cold exposure on metabolic rate depends on exercise intensity and the effect of cold exposure on core temperature. At rest and during low-intensity exercise, it is not uncommon for oxygen uptake to be elevated compared with oxygen uptake under temperate conditions.[93-95] During more intense exercise, oxygen uptake is generally similar in cold and temperate conditions. This relationship is likely due to the additive energy cost imposed by shivering during low-intensity exercise.

Cold-weather clothing and winter terrain (e.g., snow and slush) increase caloric expenditure during exercise or other activity. Bulky and heavy cold-weather clothing can increase the energy cost of exercise from 10% to 20%,[96,97] depending on the number of clothing layers and the exercise task. Similarly, walking or running through snow increases the caloric cost compared with exercise on a smooth, firm surface.[98] As illustrated in Figure 5-7, walking in moderately deep snow at 2.5 mph increases the energy cost approximately threefold compared with walking on pavement.

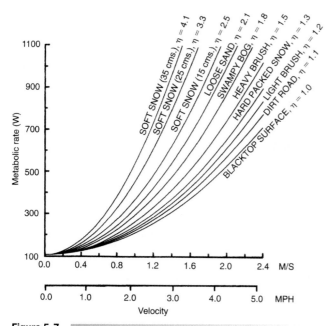

Figure 5-7

Effect of terrain on energy expenditure at various walking speeds. (Modified from Pandolf KB: Predicting energy expenditure with loads while standing or walking very slowly, *J Appl Physiol: Respir Environ Exerc Physiol* 43:577, 1977.)

Effect of Body Cooling on Physical Performance

Some studies report no reduction in physical performance during cold exposure, but it should be noted that the individuals tested often were not cold. It is only when body core or muscle temperatures are reduced that decrements in physical performance occur.

Whole-body cooling can reduce maximal oxygen uptake.[95,99-102] Experiments that have lowered core temperature 0.5°C to 2.0°C (0.9°F to 3.6°F) have reported 10% to 20% reductions in maximal oxygen uptake. The reduction may result from reduced maximal cardiac output,[80] as maximal heart rate is 10 to 30 beats-per-minute lower after body cooling.[89,93] In addition, blood temperature reductions shift the oxygen dissociation curve to the right, reducing oxygen delivery to the cells.

Body cooling has been shown to reduce endurance exercise performance.[99,103,104] This may be due to increased metabolic strain, as blood lactate begins to accumulate at lower workloads and the rate of accumulation is greater during incremental exercise in the cold.[101,102] In addition, because maximal oxygen consumption is reduced in the cold, any given submaximal intensity represents a higher percentage of maximal oxygen consumption and, therefore, a greater relative exercise intensity.

The discomfort of severe cold stress may be, in part, responsible for reduced tolerance to exercise-cold stress. Adolph and Molnar[105] found that their subjects became confused and stuporous when resting or working in the cold. They speculated that the pain and discomfort accompanying cold exposure were important causes for termination. Similarly, Doubt[106] reported that 5 of 63 trials in which subjects were immersed for 6 hours in 5°C (41°F) water were terminated prematurely because of the intolerable discomfort associated with low finger and toe temperatures.

Cold exposure can impair muscle strength, power, and fatigability. Investigations have found that peak power output, sprint performance, and jumping ability are lowered by muscle cooling.[107,108] Similarly, during the initial minutes of recovery from sustained cold-water immersion, there is a reduction in maximal isometric strength and faster time to fatigue during submaximal isometric contractions[109-111] Cooling might reduce muscle strength and endurance by interfering with muscle relaxation.[111] However, there is also evidence that cooling impairs muscle excitation coupling, as supramaximal stimulation of motor nerves produces no muscle action potential when skin temperatures are reduced to less than 6°C (42.8°F).[112,113] Regardless of the mechanisms, muscle performance may be impaired immediately following cold exposure if it has lowered muscle temperature.

During recovery from muscle cooling, strength can be higher compared with that in temperate conditions. Johnson and Leider[114] examined the effect of cold exposure on muscle strength by measuring maximal handgrip strength prior to immersing the forearm in 10°C to 15°C (50°F to 59°F) water for 30 minutes and during a 3-hour recovery period. They reported a significant reduction in maximal handgrip strength immediately following cold exposure. However, maximal handgrip strength was 17% to 21% higher than control measures 100 to 180 minutes into recovery. In similar experiments, Oliver and colleagues[115] observed an acute reduction in plantar flexion strength after precooling the calf in 10°C (50°F) water for 30 minutes. During a 3-hour recovery period, plantar flexion strength became 33% to 40% higher than control measures 120 to 180 minutes into recovery. This muscle strength increase occurred despite the fact that muscle temperature remained below baseline levels during recovery. The mechanisms responsible for these strength gains remain unclear. Limb cooling is known to decrease muscle spindle discharge and the monosynaptic reflex.[116,117] Possibly, the sensitivity of the spindles is suppressed by limb cooling, enabling potentiation of muscle force production during recovery and rewarming.

Special Considerations
Ambient Weather Conditions

The magnitude of environmental cold stress is determined by the ambient temperature, wind velocity, and wetness. The rate of body cooling is inversely related to the air temperature at temperatures below the critical temperature at which heat production cannot balance heat loss. The addition of air motion accelerates body cooling, as the movement of air past the skin surface replaces the warmer insulating air surrounding the body with colder air. As a consequence of air movement, body cooling can occur rapidly in relatively mild ambient air temperatures. The wind-chill index (Table 5-2) provides a useful index for the combined effects of ambient temperature and air velocity on subjective comfort and the potential for peripheral cold injury. Skin wetness increases the effective wind-chill and the rate of body heat loss.

The Magnitude of Environmental Cold Stress is Determined by:

- Ambient temperature
- Wind velocity
- Wetness

Water immersion increases the rate of body cooling compared with ambient air exposure. Water has a 25-fold greater heat transfer coefficient compared with air. As a consequence, body cooling occurs much more quickly and begins at a higher absolute temperature in water than in air. Low-intensity exercise in water can actually speed the

development of hypothermia, as physical movement increases conductive heat transfer from the active limb muscles to the water, with little metabolic heat left to warm the body core.[118] However, moderate-intensity exercise (heat production approximately 400 watts) can retard or prevent the reduction in core temperature that occurs when resting in 20°C to 26°C (68°F to 78.8°F) water.[119]

Clothing

Clothing is an effective method for attenuating body heat loss during cold exposure. By choosing clothing with high insulation, humans can remain comfortably warm even in extreme cold conditions. For optimal effectiveness, the insulative value of the clothing should be balanced with metabolic heat production. It is important not to wear too much clothing during cold exposure, as this can lead to increases in core body temperature and the stimulation of sweating. Profuse sweating is not advisable in cold climates, as many clothing materials lose their insulative properties when wet, and peripheral cold injury is more likely when skin is wet. Similarly, if too little clothing is worn, hypothermia and its consequences can occur. It is generally recommended that individuals wear several layers of clothing during cold exposure. This method of dressing enables the individual to add or remove clothing as exercise intensity and weather conditions dictate.

As discussed, the energy cost of exercise can be 10% to 20% higher when wearing cold-weather clothing. The

---

Table 5-2
Windchill Chart*

| Wind Speed (mph) | Actual Temperature (°F) | | | | | | | | | | | |
| | 50 | 40 | 30 | 20 | 10 | 0 | −10 | −20 | −30 | −40 | −50 | −60 |
	EQUIVALENT CHILL TEMPERATURE (°F)											
Calm	50	40	30	20	10	0	−10	−20	−30	−40	−50	−60
5	48	37	27	16	6	−5	−15	−26	−36	−47	−57	−68
10	40	28	16	3	−9	−21	−33	−46	−58	−70	−83	−95
15	36	22	9	−5	−18	−32	−45	−58	−72	−85	−99	−112
20	32	18	4	−10	−25	−39	−53	−67	−82	−96	−110	−124
25	30	15	0	−15	−29	−44	−59	−74	−89	−104	−118	−133
30	28	13	−2	−18	−33	−48	−63	−79	−94	−109	−125	−140
35	27	11	−4	−20	−35	−51	−67	−82	−98	−113	−129	−145
40	26	10	−6	−22	−37	−53	−69	−85	−101	−117	−132	−148

(Wind speeds greater than 40 mph have little additional effect)

Little danger (Exposed dry skin may freeze in less than 5 hr, greatest hazards from false sense of security)

Increasing danger (Exposed flesh may freeze within 1 min)

Great danger (Exposed skin may freeze within 30 s)

* To determine the windchill temperature, enter the chart at the row corresponding to the wind speed and read right until reaching the column corresponding to the actual air temperature.

greater energy cost means that exercise at the same work rate requires a greater percentage of an individual's maximal oxygen uptake. The greater relative exercise stress may shorten time to fatigue.

Body Morphology

Both body morphology (e.g., mass, surface area) and composition affect the body cooling rate during cold stress. Individuals with small body mass or high surface area/mass ratios cool faster than larger persons with similar body morphology.[119,120] Similarly, persons with thicker layers of subcutaneous fat, and therefore greater peripheral insulation, cool more slowly than those with less fat.[93,94,121,122] A thick subcutaneous fat layer also enables individuals to tolerate lower ambient temperatures before initiating shivering.[123] Differences in body size and composition are considered to be largely responsible for much of the interindividual variability in physiological responses to cold exposure.

Gender

Whether gender alters the ability to defend body temperature during cold stress remains unresolved. Although there are well-documented differences between men and women during cold stress, these differences may not be due to differences between the genders per se but rather due to differences in body mass, body composition, surface area, and aerobic power. To date, no study examining the physiological responses to cold exposure has matched men and women for weight, fitness, body surface area, and fatness.

During cold-water immersion, women generally lose heat at a faster rate than men.[94] This can be explained, in part, because women have a smaller body mass and a greater surface area/body mass ratio. However, women show less increase in metabolic rate for the same magnitude of body cooling,[124] suggesting that they have a blunted response to reductions in core temperature.

During cold-air exposure, women generally maintain body core temperature as effectively as men.[124] They accomplish this by maintaining a lower skin temperature compared with men during cold stress.[124] The lower skin temperature not only reduces heat transfer to the periphery but also serves to increase the insulative barrier between the body core and the environment.

Aerobic Fitness and Training

The physiological adaptations that occur with regular physical activity can improve tolerance to cold environments. Because endurance exercise training increases maximal aerobic power and endurance performance, trained individuals can sustain relatively high exercise intensities for prolonged periods. This ability is of great value when high rates of heat production are necessary to prevent hypothermia during cold exposure.

It is controversial whether exercise training produces adaptations that improve thermoregulatory responses during cold exposure. There is evidence that endurance-trained individuals have a reduced sensitivity to cold stress, as suggested by a delayed onset of shivering during body cooling.[125] However, Bittel and colleagues[126] found that aerobically fit individuals had greater metabolic heat production during cold exposure as well as an increased shivering sensitivity; that is, the onset of shivering began at warmer skin temperatures. Similarly, skin temperatures during cold exposure have been reported to both increase[118,127] and decrease[128] after physical training. Young and colleagues[129] recently showed that aerobic training improves the vasoconstrictor response to cold exposure. Obviously, more study is needed to clarify the role of fitness and training on the physiological responses to cold exposure.

Aging

The risk of hypothermia is widely considered to be greater in older compared with younger adults, and hypothermia is thought to contribute to the increased winter mortality rate in the elderly.[130-132] Studies have found that older persons are less able than younger adults to defend body temperature during cold stress.[133] This has been attributed to a reduced ability to vasoconstrict peripheral arterioles during cold exposure[134,135] and a smaller rise in heat production during cold stress.[136] Older persons have also been reported to have less CIVD response than younger persons.[137] The difference between the older and younger adults in these studies may not have been the result of aging per se, but to other factors such as differences in body morphology, fitness, and health. When these confounding variables are experimentally controlled, the rate of body cooling appears to be similar between old and young adults in some[138,139] but not all studies.[140]

Nutritional Status

Persons who become hypoglycemic during cold exposure have a reduced tolerance to cold stress and are more susceptible to cold injury.[141-143] Those with hypoglycemia exhibit either attenuated shivering or no shivering during cold stress,[142-144] and they therefore have lower rates of heat production. Interestingly, Gale and colleagues[144] demonstrated that intravenous glucose infusion restored shivering within seconds after euglycemia (i.e., normal sugar in blood) was restored in persons rendered hypoglycemic during cold stress. The restoration of shivering occurred even in a limb removed from circulation by arterial occlusion. These findings suggest that hypoglycemia affects temperature regulation through a central rather than peripheral mechanism. Regardless of the mechanism, hypoglycemia can have traumatic consequences for persons working in cold environments and should be prevented whenever possible.

Both carbohydrate and fat are oxidized to meet the metabolic cost of shivering. The increase in plasma catecholamine concentration that typically occurs with cold exposure facilitates the mobilization of both glycogen and triglyceride stores.[145] Debate exists, however, whether muscle glycogen is an important substrate during shivering; some studies[146-148] report reductions in muscle glycogen concentration after cold exposure, but others do not.[149]

Acclimatization

Cold acclimatization has been examined in a variety of populations. Studies of individuals who have a lifetime of repeated cold exposure indicate that cold acclimatization can occur in humans. For example, Australian aborigines, African Bushmen, and women breath-holding divers of Korea have different whole-body thermoregulatory responses during cold stress compared with persons unaccustomed to cold climates.[92,150,151] Similarly, persons whose occupations require repeated limb exposure to cold temperatures have made peripheral adjustments (e.g., enhanced CIVD response) to attenuate the effect of cold during exposure.[152,153] The magnitude of physiologic adaptation to cold exposure appears to be modest, however, when compared with the marked physiological adaptations associated with heat acclimatization.

Chronic Disease or Disability

Individuals with chronic diseases and disabilities may be at more risk for cold-induced injury. Spinal cord–injured persons cannot vasoconstrict peripheral arterioles in the insensate skin and have a blunted shivering response during cold exposure. Both of these factors cause their core temperature to decline during even moderate cold stress.[154] Therefore, care must be taken to ensure that these people wear adequate clothing during cold exposure to protect against cold injury and hypothermia.

Persons with cardiovascular disease are at more risk of having angina during cold exposure, because cold increases blood pressure and myocardial oxygen demand. The positive relationship between the incidence of stroke and myocardial infarction and sudden reductions in air temperature is well recognized.[155]

Cold exposure can elicit asthmalike symptoms. It was generally thought that cold exposure increased respiratory resistance because of intrathoracic airway cooling. Evidence now suggests that the increased pulmonary resistance is due to respiratory tract dehydration.[156] Medication can prevent the asthmalike symptoms in most sufferers.[156]

Persons with multiple sclerosis have improved motor coordination after moderate levels of body cooling. Therefore, cold exposure may be an effective method of temporarily reducing spasticity in this population. Cold appears to exert its effects on motor control by reducing muscle spindle firing and gamma spasticity.[116,117] These cold-induced effects decrease the strength of the stretch reflex and reduce resistance to passive movement. The improvements in motor control may persist for several hours following cold exposure.

Drugs

Pharmaceutical agents and alcohol can predispose persons to cold injury.[141,157,158] Alcoholic beverages, for example, can induce hypoglycemia, which in turn suppresses shivering.[141-143,157] Several prescription medications, such as barbiturates, phenothiazines, reserpine, and narcotics, act directly on the hypothalamus and interfere with normal temperature control.[159]

Cold Disorders

Accidental Hypothermia

Body heat is both required and produced at the cellular level. The environment acts as either a heating or a cooling force on the body. The body must be able to generate heat, retain heat, and discharge heat depending on the body activity and ambient external temperature. Body temperature is a measure of the metabolism (i.e., the general level of chemical activity) within the body. The optimum temperature for chemical reactions to take place in the body is 37°C (98.6°F). At temperatures greater than 40.6°C (105°F), many body enzymes become denatured and chemical reactions cannot take place, leading to death. Below 37°C (98.6°F), chemical reactions slow down with various complications, which can lead to death.[160] Hypothermia occurs in different stages and is determined by the body's core temperature (Table 5-3). The *core* encompasses the internal organs, such as the heart, lungs, and brain, whereas the *periphery* encompasses the appendages, skin, and muscle tissue. Hypothermia is a progressive disorder or injury in that once the body's core temperature begins to drop, the individual will continue down the cascade of hypothermic stages until he or she is able to reverse or stop the factors that are causing or predisposing him or her to this disorder or injury. There are certain predisposing factors that lead to hypothermia such as cold temperatures, inadequate clothing, fatigue and exhaustion, wetness, dehydration, poor food intake, and alcohol consumption. These factors cause vasodilation, leading to increased heat loss.[161]

Clinical Point

Hypothermia is defined as a decrease in the body core temperature to a level at which normal muscular and cerebral functions are impaired.[160]

Hypothermic temperatures are those less than freezing, but can be any temperature less than 37°C (98.6°F) in elderly individuals and individuals with poor peripheral

Table 5-3

Hypothermia Core Temperature, Signs and Symptoms

Stage	Core Temperature	Signs and Symptoms
Mild hypothermia	37.2°C to 36.1°C 99°F to 97°F	Normal, shivering can begin.
	36.1°C to 35.1°C 97°F to 95°F	Individual experiences cold sensation, goose bumps, and is unable to perform complex tasks with hands; shiver can be mild to severe, and hands are numb.
Moderate hypothermia	35°C to 33.9°C 95°F to 93°F	Shivering is intense, muscle incoordination becomes apparent, movements are slow and labored, pace is stumbling, individual experiences mild confusion although he or she may appear alert; use sobriety test: if unable to walk a 30-foot straight line, the individual is hypothermic.
	33.9°C to 32.2°C 93°F to 90°F	Violent shivering persists, individual experiences difficulty speaking and sluggish thinking, and amnesia starts to appear; gross muscle movements are sluggish, is unable to use hands, stumbles frequently, has difficulty speaking, exhibits signs of depression, is withdrawn.
Severe hypothermia	32.2°C to 30°C 90°F to 86°F	Shivering stops, exposed skin appears blue or puffy, muscle coordination is very poor, individual is unable to walk, exhibits confusion and incoherent/irrational behavior, but may be able to maintain posture and appearance of awareness.
	30°C to 27.8°C 86°F to 82°F	Individual experiences muscle rigidity; is semiconscious and in a stupor; and exhibits loss of awareness of others, decreased pulse and respiration rate, and possible heart fibrillation.
	27.8°C to 25.6°C 82°F to 78°F	Individual is unconscious, heart beat and respiration are erratic, pulse may not be palpable.
	25.6°C to 23.9°C 78°F to 75°F	Individual experiences pulmonary edema, cardiac and respiratory failure, and death. Death may occur before this temperature is reached.

Modified from Curtis R: *Outdoor action guide to hypothermia and cold weather injuries.* Rick Curtis, Outdoor Action Program, The Trustees of Princeton University. Retrieved November 18, 2008 from http://www.princeton.edu/~oa/safety/hypocold.shtml.

circulation or disorders.[161] Clinical signs and symptoms of hypothermia often begin before an individual is aware that he or she needs help. The first sign or symptom is shivering. Shivering is the body's first attempt to produce more heat by muscle activity.[160,162] Often, the next sign or symptom is altered motor coordination and changes in consciousness noted when the individual mumbles and stumbles and has slurred speech, an abnormally slow rate of breathing, cold pale skin, and fatigue.[162] To treat an individual with hypothermia, one must rewarm the individual, but this process depends on the stage of hypothermia the individual is experiencing. Individuals with mild hypothermia are often rewarmed passively. Passive rewarming relies of the individual's own body metabolism.[163] All wet clothing must be removed and the skin dried. All other predisposing factors must be remedied, such as removal from an outdoor environment into a shelter and covering the individual in blankets to aid his or her own body to increase core body temperature. The goal is to increase core temperature by 0.5°C to 2°C (0.9°F to 3.6°F) per hour.[163] Moderate hypothermia is best treated with active external rewarming techniques followed by passive techniques. Active external rewarming techniques involve applying heat to the skin by such methods as friction massage over the skin, placing the individual in a warm bath or covering him or her with an electric blanket. With severe hypothermia and some advanced cases of moderate hypothermia, internal rewarming is indicated. Cardiopulmonary bypass, in which the patient's blood is circulated through a rewarming device and then returned to the body, is considered the best, and can raise body temperature by 0.5°C to 1°C (1°F to 2°F) every 3 to 5 minutes. However, many hospitals are not equipped to offer this treatment. The alternative is to introduce warm oxygen or fluids into the body.[163]

Frostbite (Freezing Injury)

Frostbite occurs when skin tissue freezes and is defined as a medical condition in which damage is caused to the skin and other tissues as a result of extreme cold.[164] It primarily affects the digits, ears, and exposed facial tissue. Initially, the frozen tissue is cold, hard, and bloodless. The severity of frostbite is classified by the depth of the injury. *First-degree frostbite* affects the epidermal tissue. After thawing, the skin may become wheal-like, red, and painful, and it may become edematous but does not blister. *Second-degree frostbite* affects the superficial dermis and is characterized by blister formation. *Third-degree frostbite* extends to the reticular layer. It is characterized by edema with hemorrhagic bullae. Permanent tissue loss is possible. *Fourth-degree frostbite* involves the full thickness of skin. Thawing does not restore muscle function, and the affected area shows early necrotic change. There will be permanent tissue and functional loss. The affected area should be warmed gradually (temperatures greater than 39°C [102.2°F] can aggravate injury). During initial treatment, affected areas should be protected from physical injury and excessive cold or heat exposure. The tissue should be elevated to reduce swelling. The risk of frostbite can be minimized by wearing proper clothing, ensuring adequate diet and hydration, and avoiding unduly prolonged cold exposure.

Nonfreezing Injuries

Sustained exposure to cold and wet conditions can induce skin injury. *Chilblain* is a skin condition that primarily affects the hands and feet. Patients present with red, swollen, tender areas on the dorsum of the extremities between the joints. The affected area should be warmed and carefully dried. Persons should be treated for infection, and re-exposure should be avoided until the affected region is healed. *Trench foot* can occur with prolonged exposure to wet, cold conditions when circulation is restricted. The tissue becomes pale,

anesthetic, pulseless, and immobile. The skin is frequently macerated and slightly edematous. After warming, there is marked hyperemia, pain, and blister formation. *Immersion foot* can occur after prolonged immersion in cold water. The clinical features are similar to trench foot. Acute treatment for both trench foot and immersion foot is directed at passively warming the affected feet, protecting the area from physical injury, controlling for infection, and treating concomitant hypothermia and dehydration. Nonfreezing injuries can be reduced by frequent hand and foot inspection and by regularly warming and drying exposed limbs. Table 5-4 summarizes the diagnosis and treatment of cold disorders.

High Terrestrial Altitude

Improved access to mountainous areas has increased the number of people visiting and living at high altitude. It is now possible for travelers to fly to a major airport and quickly drive to a high-altitude destination. In the mountain states of Utah, Colorado, Wyoming, and New Mexico, for example, major roads reach 12,000 feet (3650 meters), some towns are located above 10,000 feet (3050 meters), and lodges are at 9000 feet (2750 meters) and higher. In these states, approximately 7 million people ascend to altitudes above 8500 feet (2590 meters) each year.[165]

Table 5-4
Diagnosis and Treatment of Cold Disorders

Disorder	Cause/Predisposing Factor	Clinical Features and Diagnosis	Treatment	Prevention
Accidental hypothermia	Body heat loss exceeds body heat production Insufficient clothing Inadequate nutrition and fluid intake Alcohol and drug use Infection	Mild hypothermia (core temperature 32°C to 35°C): ability to spontaneously rewarm; no cardiac arrhythmias Severe hypothermia (core temperature < 28°C): active rewarming required, high risk of ventricular fibrillation In conscious victim: Persistent shivering Cool, pale skin Withdrawal and irritability Confusion, lethargy, and obtundation Bradycardia and hypotension Weak peripheral pulse Hypopnea	Measure core temperature. Warm afflicted individual; remove wet clothing. Mild hypothermia: warm, sweet oral fluids. Moderate to severe hypothermia: IV fluid for dehydration and hypovolemia. Maintain airway. Medical management if hypoglycemia is suspected, alcohol or opiate intoxication. Manage secondary complications (e.g., pneumonia, pancreatis, rhabdomyolysis, and renal failure).	Wear proper clothing for weather conditions. Ensure adequate nutritional and hydration state. Seek warm shelter at the earliest suspicion of hypothermia.

Table 5-4
Diagnosis and Treatment of Cold Disorders—cont'd

Disorder	Cause/Predisposing Factor	Clinical Features and Diagnosis	Treatment	Prevention
Freezing injury (frostbite)	Freezing of skin tissue Predominantly afflicts digits, ears, and exposed facial skin	Frozen tissue is cold, hard, and bloodless Classified by depth of injury (see below)	Warm affected areas; temperatures > 39°C will aggravate injury. Protect affected areas from physical injury and excessive cold or heat exposure. Treat coincident medical problems—hypothermia, dehydration. Elevate tissue to reduce swelling. Prescribe prophylactic antibiotics for postinjury infection. Whirlpool debridement for second- to fourth-degree injuries.	Wear proper clothing. Ensure adequate diet and hydration. Avoid unduly prolonged cold exposure.
First-degree frostbite	Epidermal injury Post-thawing is wheal-like, red, and painful Affected area may become edematous but has no blister formation			
Second-degree frostbite	Affects superficial dermis Some initial limits on range of motion Edema with blister formation			
Third-degree frostbite	Affects dermis to reticular layer Edema with hemorrhagic bullae Swelling restricts range of motion Permanent tissue and functional loss			
Fourth-degree frostbite	Involves full thickness of skin Thawing does not restore muscle function, and skin reperfusion is poor Affected area shows early necrotic change Permanent tissue and functional loss			
Nonfreezing injuries Trench foot Immersion foot	Prolonged exposure of extremities to wet, cold conditions Restricted circulation Prolonged immersion in cold water	Initially, afflicted area is pale, anesthetic, pulseless, and immobile Skin is frequently macerated and lightly edematous After warming, marked hyperemia, proximal burning pain, and blister formation appear Classified by degree of severity	Warm (passively) and dry feet. Protect affected area from physical injury. Treat for infection and pain. Treat concomitant hypothermia and dehydration. Avoid weight-bearing activity until healing is complete.	Perform frequent foot inspection. Perform regular warming and drying of feet during exposure. Boots and socks should not be replaced until feet are warm, with normal feeling.
Chilblain	Sustained exposure to cold, wet conditions Primarily afflicts hands and feet	Red, swollen, tender areas on dorsum of extremities between joints Itching Chronic lesions may be turgid, with blister formation	Warm and dry afflicted skin areas. Treat for infection. Avoid re-exposure until affected region is healed.	Perform frequent foot and hand inspection. Take frequent breaks to warm and dry feet and hands. Boots, socks, and gloves should not be replaced until limbs are warm, with normal feeling.

IV, Intravenous.

Most people who ascend to high altitude are unaware of the physiological effect that altitude exposure can have on exercise performance and health. Altitude exposure impairs exercise performance and can produce debilitating illness and death. It has been estimated that 25% of travelers to altitudes greater than 8200 feet (2500 meters) develop acute mountain sickness,[166] a short-duration, debilitating illness that can ruin a long-planned vacation. Fortunately, the human body can adapt to the stress of high altitude, and preventive measures are available for many of the altitude-induced illnesses.

Physical Effect of Altitude Exposure

Ascent to high altitude impairs the ability to transport oxygen to the cell. With ascent from sea level to altitude, the partial oxygen pressure (P_{O_2}) declines proportionately to the reduction in barometric pressure. The lower atmospheric P_{O_2} not only reduces the volume of oxygen inspired at a specific pulmonary ventilation, but also reduces the P_{O_2} at each step of the oxygen transport chain. The result is an impaired ability to transport oxygen to the cell and the development of hypoxia. Typical reductions in P_{O_2} at several steps of the oxygen transport chain are presented in Table 5-5. Secondary problems accompanying altitude exposure are the reduction in air temperature and humidity, decreased ability to sleep, reduced appetite, dehydration, and increased exposure to ultraviolet (UV) radiation.

> **Physiological Responses to Hypoxia**
>
> - Increased pulmonary ventilation
> - Increased respiratory rate

Pulmonary Ventilation at High Altitude

One of the first observable physiological responses to hypoxia (i.e., inadequate O_2 at a cellular level) is an increase in pulmonary ventilation. The increased ventilation serves to increase alveolar P_{O_2} and reduce the alveolar partial carbon dioxide pressure (P_{CO_2}), thereby improving arterial oxygen saturation. The increased ventilatory volume is achieved through an increased tidal volume, but the respiratory rate may also increase. The increase in ventilation can be detected when the inspired P_{O_2} drops below 110 mm Hg or the arterial P_{O_2} is less than 60 mm Hg.[167,168] The increase in pulmonary ventilation is considered by many to be the most important response to hypoxia.[165]

The magnitude of hyperventilation depends on competing signals. The initial increase in ventilation is stimulated by peripheral chemoreceptors within the aortic and carotid bodies, because total denervation of the carotid and aortic bodies significantly attenuates or abolishes the ventilatory response to acute hypoxia.[167] The increase in ventilation, however, produces hypocapnia (i.e., abnormally low arterial CO_2 level) and arterial alkalosis (i.e., pH greater than 7.45), which act to brake further elevations in ventilation.

Altitude acclimatization produces additional increases in minute ventilation, reaching maximum after 4 to 7 days at the same altitude (Figure 5-8).[169] One mechanism facilitating this adaptation is the elimination of excess bicarbonate by the kidneys during the initial days at altitude. By removing excess bicarbonate, the kidneys attenuate the arterial alkalosis and the accompanying hypoventilatory drive. It has also been suggested that there may be an increased sensitivity to hypoxia during the initial weeks at altitude.[170]

Hyperventilation not only improves arterial oxygen saturation but also facilitates transport of oxygen to the peripheral tissues. The systemic alkalosis accompanying hypocapnia increases oxygen affinity to hemoglobin,

Table 5-5

Typical Acute Reduction in Arterial Oxygen Partial Pressure and Saturation with Increasing Altitude for Unacclimatized Men

| Elevation | | P_B | $P_{I}O_2$ | $P_{A}O_2$ | $P_{a}O_2$ | $P_{A}CO_2$ | $S_{a}O_2$ |
m	ft	(torr)	(torr)	(torr)	(torr)	(torr)	(%)
0	0	760	149	104	96	40	96
1600	5248	627	122	82	69	36	94
3100	10,169	522	100	62	57	33	89
4300	14,104	448	84	53	40	30	84
5500	18,000	379	70	38	35	27	75

$P_{A}O_2$, Alveolar oxygen partial pressure; $P_{a}O_2$, arterial oxygen partial pressure; $P_{A}CO_2$, alveolar carbon dioxide partial pressure; P_B, barometric pressure; $P_{I}O_2$, inspired oxygen partial pressure; $S_{a}O_2$, arterial oxygen saturation.
Modified from Fulco CS, Cymerman A: Human performance and acute hypoxia. In Pandolf KB, Sawka MN, Gonzalez RR, editors: *Human performance physiology and environmental medicine at terrestrial extremes*, p 471, Indianapolis, 1988, Benchmark Press.

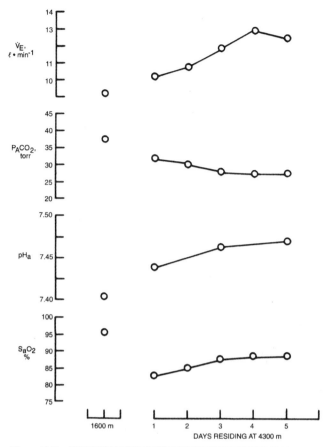

Figure 5-8

Changes in resting minute ventilation (V_E), alveolar P_{CO_2} (P_ACO_2) arterial pH (pH_a) and arterial saturation of hemoglobin (S_aO_2) in 12 low-land residents during the first 5 days at 14,000 feet (4300 m). (Modified from Huang SY, Alexander JK, Grover JT et al: Hypocapnia and sustained hypoxia blunt ventilation on arrival at high altitude, *J Appl Physiol* 56:602, 1984.)

promoting binding of oxygen at the lung. In addition, hypoxia and alkalosis activate the glycolytic enzyme phosphofructokinase, leading to an increased synthesis of 2,3-diphosphoglycerate (2,3-DPG). 2,3-DPG helps oxygen dissociate at the tissue level by decreasing hemoglobin's affinity to oxygen.

Circulatory Responses at High Altitude

Hypoxia alters the cardiovascular responses both at rest and during exercise. Acute exposure to altitude produces a mild increase in blood pressure, moderate increase in heart rate and cardiac output, and increased venous tone.[165] Heart rate at rest may initially rise 20% or more.[166] Initially, cardiac output is elevated secondary to tachycardia, with normal stroke volume, but cardiac output becomes similar to or lower than control values after approximately 1 week of exposure. The decline in cardiac output occurs because of reductions in stroke volume.[171-174] The pulmonary circulation is also affected by hypoxia, because pulmonary vascular

resistance and pulmonary arterial pressure are elevated with acute altitude exposure.[175]

During acclimatization, two additional circulatory adaptations occur to enhance oxygen transport. The first adaptation is an increase in hemoglobin concentration secondary to reduced plasma volume. The hemoconcentration is apparent within 1 to 2 days of exposure and persists for several weeks. It arises as a consequence of the diuresis of excess bicarbonate,[176] and plasma volume may be reduced as much as 10% to 20% (300 to 600 mL).[170] The trade-off to this mechanism, however, is that the lower blood volume reduces stroke volume, increasing circulatory and thermoregulatory strain during exercise.[177] A later adaptation is an increase in red cell volume. Within 2 hours of hypoxemia, plasma erythropoietin concentration is elevated, stimulating red blood cell production in the bone marrow. Within 4 to 5 days of stimulation, new red blood cells are in the circulation.[165] During a period of weeks to months, red cell mass increases.[170,178]

Acclimatization to Altitude Leads to:

- Restoration of cardiac output to normal
- Increased pulmonary arterial pressure
- Decreased plasma volume
- Increased hemoglobin concentration
- Increased red cell volume
- Improved time to exhaustion (endurance)
- Less reliance on anaerobic energy metabolism

Maximal oxygen uptake is not measurably altered between sea level and 4900 feet (1500 meters). Above 4900 feet (1500 meters), however, there is a linear decline in maximal oxygen uptake at a rate of 10% per 1000 meters.[179] At 5100 feet (4300 meters), maximal oxygen uptake is reduced approximately 27% to 28%.[180] There appears to be no gender influence on this response.[181] Although there is evidence that individuals with a high aerobic capacity have larger decrements in maximal oxygen uptake with altitude,[180] there is large interindividual variability in response to hypoxia. Acute hypoxia appears to reduce maximal oxygen uptake by impairing maximal oxygen carrying capacity, as maximal values for heart rate, stroke volume, cardiac output, venous oxygen content, and ventilation are not reduced from sea-level values.[173,182-184] The magnitude of reduction in maximal oxygen uptake is similar to the reduction in arterial oxygen content.[182,184]

Altitude acclimatization has little effect on maximal oxygen uptake. Studies generally report either no change in maximal oxygen uptake or only modest increases (3% to 5%) following short-term altitude acclimatization.[170,174,185-189] The modest results may be due, in part, to detraining, because training time and intensity are reduced as a result of acute mountain sickness and hypoxia. It may also be due to a lower maximal cardiac output, as maximal heart rate is reduced following acclimatization to high altitude,[190,191] and this is not completely reversed either by breathing normoxic air or with atropine infusion.[190]

The reduced oxygen-carrying capacity at high altitude also affects the physiological responses during submaximal exercise. At high altitude, the same absolute power output elicits a greater percentage of maximal oxygen uptake than at sea level (Figure 5-9). As a consequence of the lower maximal oxygen uptake at altitude, heart rate, ventilation, and lactate concentration are higher during hypoxia than at sea level at the same power output.[183,184] During exercise at the same percentage of environment-specific maximal oxygen uptake, however, heart rate, ventilation, and lactate concentration are similar under hypoxia and sea-level conditions.[192-195]

Exercise Performance at High Altitude

Acute exposure to hypoxia impairs endurance performance. Hypoxia reduces the time to exhaustion during exercise at a given absolute power output, with the magnitude of decrement proportional to the magnitude of hypoxia. Reducing the workload to elicit the same percentage of environment-specific maximal oxygen uptake results in similar time to exhaustion during high-altitude and sea-level exercise.[174,195]

Acclimatization to high altitude can dramatically improve time to exhaustion during submaximal exercise[174,195,196] as

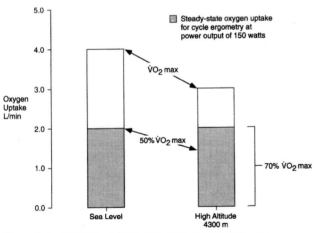

Figure 5-9

Effect of high altitude on the relationship between absolute power output, oxygen uptake *(VO₂)* and relative exercise intensity (% maximal oxygen uptake, % VO₂ max). (Modified from Young AJ, Young PM: Human acclimatization to high terrestrial altitude. In Pandolf KB, Sawka MN, Gonzalez RR, editors: *Human performance physiology and environmental medicine at terrestrial extremes,* p 510, Indianapolis, 1988, Benchmark Press.)

well as athletic performance during sporting events.[187] For example, Maher and colleagues[195] reported a 45% increase in time to exhaustion during cycle exercise between the second and twelfth day at 4300 meters (14,108 feet), and Horstman and colleagues[174] found a 60% increase in treadmill running time between the second and sixteenth day of acclimatization at the same altitude.

The improved endurance performance appears to be due, at least in part, to altered substrate use and less disturbance of cellular homeostasis. Following high-altitude acclimatization, there is less reliance on anaerobic energy metabolism, as evidenced by lower plasma ammonia and lactate concentrations,[195,197,198] less glycogen use,[197] and reduced lactate production.[198] There is also less disturbance of cellular homeostasis, because the adenosine triphosphate/adenosine diphosphate ratio is higher and the inorganic phosphate concentration lower after high-altitude acclimatization.[199] Because intracellular acidosis (which accompanies lactic acid formation) and elevations in inorganic phosphate concentration have been shown to induce fatigue in skeletal muscle,[200] less reliance on anaerobic metabolism should enhance endurance performance.

An improved intracellular buffering capacity may be another possible mechanism for the improved endurance performance following high-altitude acclimatization. Mizuno and colleagues[196] reported that 2 weeks of exercise training at altitude (8850 feet; 2700 meters) produced a 6% increase in in-vitro skeletal muscle buffer capacity. In addition, they reported a strong relationship (r = 0.83) between improved skeletal muscle buffer capacity and short-duration (range 240 to 380 seconds) running endurance time (average improvement of 17%) after high-altitude acclimatization.

Ascent to high altitude does not impair skeletal muscle strength, but does increase fatigability of skeletal muscle during small muscle mass activity.[181,201] Acclimatization to high altitude, however, improves skeletal muscle endurance capacity,[201] presumably as a result of improved oxygen delivery and less disturbance of intracellular homeostasis.

Neuropsychological Behavior at High Altitude

Acute hypoxia exposure can impair neuropsychological function. Relatively small reductions in arterial oxygen saturation significantly impair mental and motor coordination, personality, and judgment.[202] The ability to do mathematical calculations, make decisions, and perform coding and conceptual reasoning tasks is reduced when inspired PO_2 is reduced below 110 torr. Short-term memory begins to be affected at inspired PO_2 below 118 to 127 torr, declining progressively with further reductions in oxygen saturation.

Several of the perceptual and motor decrements associated with acute altitude exposure are lessened with acclimatization. Decrements in ability to perform simple mental tasks, such as coding, are attenuated with as little as 4 days of exposure.

Perception of effort during exercise at a given percentage of maximal oxygen uptake is lower following acclimatization to altitude. However, it has been suggested that the improvements may be related to recovering from mountain sickness rather than acclimatization per se.[170]

Special Considerations at High Altitude

Exercise Training

Because high altitude reduces maximal oxygen uptake and results in elevated heart rate at a given oxygen uptake, exercise prescriptions based on tests at sea level need modification. Heart rate remains a reliable indicator of cardiovascular stress during exercise, but exercise at a given heart rate provides less absolute stress to skeletal muscle. Therefore, to provide the same overload to skeletal muscle, exercise must be performed at a greater absolute heart rate.

Optimal training for improving athletic performance at altitude depends on the altitude of residence and the athletic event. For aerobic activities (events lasting longer than 3 to 4 minutes) at altitudes above 2000 meters (6562 feet) acclimatization for 10 to 20 days is necessary for maximal performance.[165] Highly anaerobic activities at intermediate altitudes require only arrival at the time of the event.[165]

The effects of high-altitude training on sea-level athletic performance remain controversial.[203] Studies have suggested that sea-level performance can be improved by living and training at altitude.[185,189,196,204] These studies, however, often lacked a control group performing similar training at sea level. Studies containing the proper control groups have not found altitude training to be superior to sea-level training with regard to sea-level performance.[186,188,205] Regardless, any benefit appears to depend on choosing an altitude that maximizes physiological stress but minimizes the detraining that is inevitable when maximal oxygen uptake is limited (altitudes greater than 4900 to 6550 feet [1500 to 2000 meters]). Levine and Stray-Gundersen[203] reported that athletes train faster and at greater oxygen uptakes at low altitude (3900 feet; 1200 meters) than at higher altitude (9150 feet; 2800 meters), suggesting that altitude exposure may compromise training overload. They also found that athletes who lived at altitude but trained near sea level had improved maximal aerobic power (5%) and 5000-meter running time (30 seconds) compared with a control group who lived and trained near sea level. Levine and Stray-Gundersen[203] suggested that living at altitude stimulates beneficial changes for athletic performance, and training near sea level provides optimal exercise training.

Chronic Diseases

There is little information on the effect of altitude on the health of people with chronic diseases, nor is much known about the effect of medicines during hypoxia. The first 5 to 10 days at altitude are the most dangerous period for those with cardiovascular disease. It is known that patients with coronary artery disease have decreased exercise tolerance and earlier onset of angina and ST-segment changes during exercise at altitude.[206-208] Those who can achieve 9 minutes on the Bruce protocol without anginal symptoms will probably be safe at altitude.[166] Those with severe angina and limitation of effort at sea level should not go to altitude, as hypoxia will increase cardiac energy demand and precipitate anginal episodes. Those afflicted should choose an itinerary with access to easy descent and medical help. A good suggestion is to simulate the activity at moderate altitudes before attempting a specific activity at higher altitudes.

Individuals with mild to moderate lung disease may tolerate modest altitudes but have a higher incidence of acute mountain sickness.[209] Patients with primary pulmonary hypertension do not do well at altitude. Diabetics may experience problems regulating their insulin doses because of varying energy expenditure and food intake. More frequent insulin dosing may be needed, as well as more frequent blood glucose determinations. The presence of sickle cell disease is a contraindication for ascent to altitude, as ascent to altitudes as low as 6320 feet (1925 meters) is associated with an increased incidence of clinical symptoms.[166]

High-Altitude Illness

Acute Mountain Sickness

Acute mountain sickness is a common illness that arises after rapid ascent (< 24 hours) to altitudes above 8200 feet (2500 meters), with symptoms beginning within hours to days after exposure. Individuals often present with headache, anorexia (loss of appetite), insomnia, nausea, and malaise.[165,166,210] In moderate forms, there may be vomiting, unrelieved headache, and decreased urine production. Severe mountain sickness produces altered consciousness, localized rales (abnormal respiratory sound), cyanosis, and ataxia (uncoordinated movement). It is most common among those who ascend quickly and those who have a past history of acute mountain sickness. Vigorous physical activity during ascent or within 24 hours of ascent increases the incidence and severity of symptoms. Whether physical fitness attenuates the symptoms remains questionable. Mountain sickness is most likely to occur in those who retain fluid at altitude and have a blunted ventilatory response.[176,211] The symptoms typically improve over a few days if hypobaric stress is not increased.

High-Altitude Pulmonary Edema

This illness occurs in 5% to 10% of those with acute mountain sickness and has a high mortality rate.[166] It often occurs the second night after ascent to altitude and is thought to be due to hypoxia-induced pulmonary hypertension and increased permeability of the pulmonary capillary endothelium. It is characterized by elevated pulmonary artery pressures and marked ventilation-perfusion mismatch; a patchy edema is typically seen on chest roentgenograms. The bronchoalveolar fluid has a high protein content and contains increased numbers of macrophages and leukotrienes and evidence of complement activation. Features include decreased exercise performance, dry cough, fatigue, tachycardia, rales in the middle right lobe, and tachypnea (abnormally rapid breathing). Later, cyanosis, extreme weakness, productive cough, and dyspnea (uncomfortable breathing) may be present at rest. Mental confusion, irrational behavior, and coma can also occur. It is most common in people who ascend rapidly, perform strenuous exercise upon arrival, are obese, are male, and have a previous history of pulmonary edema. Acute treatment should be directed at increasing oxygen availability and decreasing pulmonary artery pressure.

Clinical Point

High-altitude pulmonary edema and cerebral edema are medical emergencies requiring rapid descent and medical attention.

High-Altitude Cerebral Edema

This illness usually occurs several days after the onset of mild acute mountain sickness and arises as a result of increased brain cell volume. Symptoms include impaired judgment, inability to make decisions, irrational behavior, severe headache, nausea and vomiting, truncal ataxia (inability to maintain normal posture), severe lassitude, and progression to coma. Cerebral edema is most common in people who ascend rapidly to significant altitudes; it rarely occurs at altitudes below 10,000 feet (3048 meters). High-altitude cerebral edema is a medical emergency requiring rapid descent and medical attention. Acute treatment should be directed at increasing oxygen availability and reducing cerebral edema.

High-Altitude Peripheral Edema

Altitude-related edema of the hands and face may occur in up to one-third of travelers to high altitude.[210] It is thought to be due to hypoxia-induced retention of sodium and water. The condition is benign but may cause enough discomfort to degrade physical performance. It occurs most often in women and in those with a previous history of high-altitude peripheral edema. The condition can be treated successfully with diuretic therapy. Descent is the definitive treatment.

Table 5-6 summarizes the diagnosis and treatment of high-altitude illnesses.

Table 5-6
Diagnosis and Treatment of High-Altitude Illnesses

Disorder	Cause/Predisposing Factor	Clinical Features and Diagnosis	Treatment	Prevention
Acute mountain sickness	Hypoxia-induced subclinical cerebral edema Lack of acclimatization to high altitude Rapid ascent (< 24 hr) to altitudes greater than 6000 ft	Symptoms typically begin 3 to 24 hr after ascent Headache and nausea Anorexia, vomiting, and general malaise Dizziness and oliguria	Descend to lower elevation Supplemental oxygen Acetazolamide therapy Analgesic for headache symptoms Condition self-limited	Ascend in stages or graded manner Acetazolamide prophylaxis High-carbohydrate diet (> 70% of total Kcal)
High-altitude pulmonary edema	Combination of hypoxia-induced hypertension and increased permeability of pulmonary capillaries Lack of acclimatization to high altitude Rapid ascent (< 24 hr) to high altitude	Symptoms typically begin within 2 to 4 days after ascent Early: nonproductive cough and a few rales; as edema progresses, cough becomes productive and rales become numerous Dyspnea on exertion; fatigue and weakness Resting tachycardia and tachypnea Cyanosis	Immediate passive descent Supplemental oxygen Nifedipine Transport to medical facility	Ascend in stages or graded manner Nifedipine prophylaxis Acetazolamide prophylaxis

Table 5-6
Diagnosis and Treatment of High-Altitude Illnesses—cont'd

Disorder	Cause/Predisposing Factor	Clinical Features and Diagnosis	Treatment	Prevention
High-altitude cerebral edema	Edema of the brain associated with high altitude Increased permeability of the blood-brain barrier or alteration of cell fluid regulation Lack of acclimatization to high altitude Rapid ascent (< 24 hr) to altitudes greater than 12,000 ft Acute mountain sickness Prior history	Time of symptom onset is highly variable; generally several days after ascent Severe headache, nausea, vomiting, and lassitude Truncal ataxia Ataxic gait Mental confusion, disorientation, drowsiness Social withdrawal Cyanosis	Immediate passive descent Supplemental oxygen Portable hyperbaric chamber Dexamethasone Transport to medical facility	Staged or graded ascent High-carbohydrate diet Acetazolamide prophylaxis
High-altitude peripheral edema	Hypoxia-induced retention of sodium and water More frequent in females	Primarily afflicts hands and periorbital areas of the face Associated with decreased urine output and weight gain More evident upon awakening	Descent to lower altitudes Diuretic therapy	Salt prophylaxis Acetazolamide prophylaxis

Chronic Disease and Air Pollutants

Air Pollution

There are several chemical compounds present in the atmosphere that can directly affect our health. These compounds, collectively termed *air pollutants,* have been classified as either primary or secondary pollutants. Primary pollutants are those emitted directly into the environment. They are produced primarily from the combustion of petroleum-based fuels and include carbon monoxide, sulfur oxides, nitrogen oxides, hydrocarbons, and particulates. Secondary pollutants are those that develop from the interaction of the primary pollutants with the environment and include ozone, peroxyacetyl nitrate, sulfuric acid, aldehydes, and sulfates. The smog or brown cloud associated with large metropolitan areas usually contains both primary and secondary pollutants.

The quantity of air pollution inhaled during exercise is determined by several factors. The concentration of both primary and secondary air pollutants is influenced by the season, the ambient weather conditions, and the topography of the region. Ozone typically reaches peak concentration in the late morning and early afternoon in summer and is lowest at night during the winter months. The highest carbon monoxide concentrations are typically during peak traffic periods. The geography of the region also affects the dispersion of air pollutants. The relatively high ozone concentrations in the inland valleys of Los Angeles, for example, are the result of prevailing sea breezes pushing the pollutants inland against the mountain ranges that surround the city. Additional factors that determine whether air pollutants will affect our health are whether breathing is done nasally or orally and the quantity of air inspired. Oral ventilation removes fewer air pollutants than nasal breathing, resulting in greater exposure to air pollutants per unit time. Because physical exercise increases the rate and depth of inspiration, more air pollutants are inspired during exercise than at rest.

Certain individuals are more susceptible to the adverse effects of air pollutants. It is well documented that subthreshold concentrations of air pollutants for healthy adults can compromise respiratory and cardiovascular function in children and the elderly, persons with respiratory disorders (e.g., those with asthma or chronic obstructive pulmonary disease), and persons with ischemic heart disease.[212-215]

In many regions of the country, the air quality meets the national air quality standards (Table 5-7). However, in many areas of southern California, the concentration of air pollutants often exceeds national air quality standards. For example, in Los Angeles County, California, each of the 16 Environmental Protection Agency testing stations exceeded the national standard for ozone (0.12 ppm for 1 hour) on one or more occasions during a 2-year period spanning 1991 through 1993, with several locations exceeding the national standard 50 days or more during the calendar year. Similar results have been reported for the other counties along the coast of southern California.

Table 5-7

National Ambient Air Quality Standards

Pollutant	Primary Standards Level	Primary Standards Averaging Time	Secondary Standards Level	Secondary Standards Averaging Time
Carbon monoxide	9 ppm (10 mg/m^3)	8 hr[a]	None	
	35 ppm (40 mg/m^3)	1 hr[a]		
Lead	0.15 μg/m^3 [b]	Rolling 3-month average	Same as primary	
	1.5 μg/m^3	Quarterly average	Same as primary	
Nitrogen dioxide	0.053 ppm (100 μg/m^3)	Annual (arithmetic mean)	Same as primary	
Particulate matter (PM$_{10}$)	150 μg/m^3	24 hr[c]	Same as primary	
Particulate matter (PM$_{2.5}$)	15.0 μg/m^3	Annual[d] (arithmetic mean)	Same as primary	
	35 μg/m^3	24 hr[e]	Same as primary	
Ozone	0.075 ppm (2008 std)	8 hr[f]	Same as primary	
	0.08 ppm (1997 std)	8 hr[g]	Same as primary	
	0.12 ppm	1 hr[h]	Same as primary	
Sulfur dioxide	0.03 ppm	Annual (arithmetic mean)	0.5 ppm	3 hour[a]
	0.14 ppm	24 hr[a]	(1300 μg/m^3)	

From United States Environmental Protection Agency: *National ambient air quality standards.* Retrieved September 1, 2009 from http://www. epa.gov/air/criteria.html.
EPA, Environmental protection agency; *PM,* particulate matter; *STD,* standard.
[a]Not to be exceeded more than once per year.
[b]Final rule signed October 15, 2008.
[c]Not to be exceeded more than once per year on average over 3 years.
[d]To attain this standard, the 3-year average of the weighted annual mean PM2.5 concentrations from single or multiple community-oriented monitors must not exceed 15.0 μg/m^3.
[e]To attain this standard, the 3-year average of the 98th percentile of 24-hour concentrations at each population-oriented monitor within an area must not exceed 35 μg/m^3 (effective December 17, 2006).
[f]To attain this standard, the 3-year average of the fourth-highest daily maximum 8-hour average ozone concentrations measured at each monitor within an area over each year must not exceed 0.075 ppm (effective May 27, 2008).
[g](1) To attain this standard, the 3-year average of the fourth-highest daily maximum 8-hour average ozone concentrations measured at each monitor within an area over each year must not exceed 0.08 ppm.
(2) The 1997 standard—and the implementation rules for that standard—will remain in place for implementation purposes as EPA undertakes rule-making to address the transition from the 1997 ozone standard to the 2008 ozone standard.
[h](1) The standard is attained when the expected number of days per calendar year with maximum hourly average concentrations greater than 0.12 ppm is ≤ 1.
(2) As of June 15, 2005, the EPA has revoked the 1-hour ozone standard in all areas except the 14 8-hour ozone nonattainment early action compact (EAC) areas. For one of the 14 EAC areas (Denver, CO), the 1-hour standard was revoked on November 20, 2008. For the other 13 EAC areas, the 1-hour standard was revoked on April 15, 2009.

Unfortunately, although there has been a great deal of research on the effect of individual air pollutants on pulmonary function and the ability to tolerate the stress of exercise, relatively few studies have investigated the interaction of these pollutants with exercise performance. There is even less information addressing the effect of air pollutants and other environmental stressors (e.g., heat, cold, altitude) on pulmonary function and exercise performance. The goal of this section is to discuss the physiological effect of several major air pollutants, both alone and in combination.

Asthma

Asthma is a disease that affects the respiratory system of individuals of all ages, both sedentary and active, and can be affected by many intrinsic as well as extrinsic environmental factors (Table 5-8). This disease is caused by hyperresponsiveness of the trachea and bronchi to various stimuli resulting in recurrent episodes of reversible airway narrowing, separated by periods of relative normal ventilations.[216] Attacks vary greatly from occasional periods of wheezing and slight dyspnea to severe attacks that almost cause suffocation.[217] Asthma is commonly divided into two types: *allergic* (extrinsic) asthma and *nonallergic* (intrinsic) asthma.[218] Asthma can be triggered by both internal and external factors and stimuli. In general, once the asthma has been triggered by one or more internal or external factors, the airway begins to swell and fill with mucus, causing the individual to wheeze or have a dyspneic attack. Furthermore, the muscles within the airway contract causing further narrowing and restriction of the airway. This process decreases the ability of the individual to exhale from the lungs effectively. This decreased ability to exhale causes the typical symptoms of an asthma attack. Asthma is categorized depending on the body systems affected, or by the stimuli or "trigger" that causes the dyspnea, or even by the time of day.[219]

Table 5-8
Asthma Types and Definitions

Type	Definition
Baker	Reactive disease to inhaled wheat proteins in occupational settings
Bronchial	Allergic reaction or hypersensitivity to an allergen
Cardiac	Wheezing that results from heart disease or failure
Exercise-induced	Asthmatic reaction during physical activity
Extrinsic	Reactive hypersensitivity to an antigen
Intrinsic	Asthma assumed by some endogenous cause
Nocturnal	Asthma symptoms occurring at night
Occupational	Asthma symptoms occurring from exposures at work
Stable	Asthma with no increase in symptoms for at least 4 weeks
Unstable	Asthma with increase in symptoms during the last 4 weeks

From *Taber's Cyclopedic Medical Dictionary*, ed 20, Philadelphia, 2001, FA Davis.

Clinical Point

Asthma is defined as a condition marked by recurrent attacks of dyspnea with airway inflammation caused by spasmodic constriction of the bronchi.

Asthma triggers are things in the environment that worsen or cause asthma symptoms. This process may begin with one or a combination of two or more triggers (Box 5-2). These triggers are specific to each individual, in that one trigger may affect one individual yet may not affect another individual.[219]

Asthma is a treatable condition with the removal or attempt to remove the triggers that cause the episodes. Asthma can also be treated by various medications once the triggers are identified. Generally, people with asthma are

Box 5-2 Common Asthma Triggers

Allergen Triggers	Irritant Triggers	Other Triggers
Animal dander	Cigarette smoke	Medications
Dust mites	Outdoor and indoor air pollution	Sulfites
Cockroaches	Strong odors	Infections or allergens
Pollen	Scented products	Gastroesophageal reflux disease
Mold	Stress	

Data from About.com: *Asthma triggers—Causes of asthma, 2006.* Retrieved November 6, 2008, from http://www.nhlbi.nih.gov/health/dci/Diseases/Asthma/Asthma_SignsAndSymptoms.html.

treated with a combination of long-term control medications, quick-relief medications (usually taken by a hand-held inhaler), and medications used to control allergy-induced asthma symptoms. If the individual's asthma is triggered by an airborne allergen, often the individual is treated with an allergy medication as well. Asthma can change over time, which in turn affects the medications one uses to control the symptoms of asthma. With the help of a physician, each individual must continually monitor and assess which triggers are affecting the asthma symptoms. Long-term medications are those the individual takes daily to help control the symptoms of asthma. Quick-relief medications, or rescue medications, are those used for rapid, short-term relief of asthma symptoms. Quick-relief medications are often used during an asthmatic attack to reduce the symptoms as well as by athletes prior to athletic participation if recommended by their physician. The quick-relief medications should only be used as necessary, and, if used too often, the individual's physician most likely will adjust the long-term medications. Medications for allergy-induced asthma are used to decrease or prevent the sensitivity of the body's immune system from reacting to allergens (Table 5-9).[220] It is important to realize that many medications used to treat asthma are on the banned list of medications. It is important that the athlete and clinician be aware of this and ensure that proper authorization to use the drugs is obtained before competition (see Chapter 7, "Sports Drug Testing").

Clinical Point

For athletes with asthma, knowledge of the workout environment or trigger is critical in understanding the method of treatment.

Typically, asthma is diagnosed by using different types of testing: pulmonary function test and spirometry, methacholine challenge, allergy testing, and x-ray examinations. A pulmonary function test measures the amount of air that can be inhaled with one breath and how quickly it can be exhaled from the lungs with a forceful exhalation.[221] Tests are quantified by the age, height, sex, and ethnicity of the individual and are represented in a percentage. Generally, an individual must achieve at least 80% of the predicted value to be "normal." Individuals with less than 80% of the predicted value are "abnormal."[222] Spirometry is a test of lung function. It determines how much a person can exhale, how fast a person can exhale, and how much air a person can exhale.[221] Spirometry is the most basic and frequently performed test of pulmonary lung function. A spirometer is a device used to determine how much air the lungs can hold and how well the respiratory system can move air in and out of the lungs.[222] The accuracy of this test depends on the individual's understanding of the test, the individual's cooperation, and his or her willingness to put forth a best effort.

Table 5-9

Medications Used to Treat Asthma

Medication	Type
Long-term control medications Taken every day in most cases	Inhaled corticosteroids: Fluticasone propionate (Flovent Diskus), budesonide (Pulmicort), triamcinolone acetonide (Azmacort), flunisolide (Aerobid), beclomethasone dipropionate HFA (Qvar). These medications reduce the airway inflammation and are the most commonly used long-term asthma medications. They are considered to have low risk for long-term corticosteroid side effects. May have to use these medications for several days or weeks to obtain maximal benefit. Long-acting beta-2 agonists: Salmeterol xinafoate (Serevent Diskus), formoterol fumarate inhalation powder (Foradil Aerolizer). These are inhaled medications, called *long-acting bronchodilators,* which open the airways and reduce inflammation. Often used to treat persistent asthma in combination with inhaled corticosteroids. These should *not* be used for quick relief of asthma symptoms. Leukotriene modifiers: Montelukast sodium (Singulair), zafirlukast (Accolate), zileuton extended release tablets (Zyflo CR). These inhaled medications work by opening airways, reducing inflammation, and decreasing mucus production. Cromolyn (Intal) and nedocromil (Tilade): These inhaled medications reduce asthma signs and symptoms by decreasing allergic reactions. They are considered second choice to inhaled corticosteroids. Usually taken three to four times a day. Theophylline (Theolair): A daily pill that opens the airways (bronchodilator). It relaxes the muscles around the airways.
Quick-relief medications, also called *rescue medications* Used for rapid, short-term relief of asthma symptoms. Can be used before exercise. Only use as directed. If used too often, then long-term medications need to be adjusted.	Short-acting beta-2 agonists: albuterol. Inhaled medications, called *bronchodilators,* ease breathing by temporarily relaxing airway muscles. They act within minutes and effects last for up to 6 hours. Ipratropium: Ipratropium (Atrovent). Inhaled anticholinergic for immediate relief of asthma symptoms. Like other bronchodilators, it relaxes the airways, making it easier to breathe. Mostly used for treatment of emphysema and chronic bronchitis. Oral and intravenous corticosteroids: Prednisone, methylprednisolone. Used to treat acute or very severe asthma attacks. These medications relieve airway inflammation. They may cause serious side effects when used long-term.
Allergy-induced medications Decrease body's sensitivity to a particular allergen or prevent immune system from reacting to allergens.	Immunotherapy: Allergy desensitization shots are generally given once a week for a few months, then once a month for a period of 3 to 5 years. Over time, they gradually reduce immune system reaction to specific allergens. Anti-IgE monoclonal antibodies: Omalizumab (Xolair). Medications reduce your immune system's reaction to allergens. Delivered by injection every 2 to 4 weeks.

Data from Mayo Clinic: *Asthma—Treatments and Drugs, 2008.* Retrieved November 6, 2008, from http://www.mayoclinic.com/health/asthma/DS00021/DSECTION=treatments-and-drugs.
IgE, Immunoglobulin E.

A methacholine challenge is a test in which the individual "challenges" his or her bronchial airways with one of the following: methacholine, histamine, cold air, or exercise.[223] The test is used to determine if the bronchial airways are hyper-responsive to a particular stimuli. If the bronchial airways are hyper-responsive, then they will narrow in response to the specific stimuli. If the methacholine challenge does not reproduce hyper-responsiveness, then asthma is unlikely. Generally, the methacholine challenge test is only used if a spirometry test is inconclusive, but asthma is still considered a possibility.[223] Allergy testing may be used for people who have been diagnosed with asthma because certain allergies may play a significant role in exacerbating asthma symptoms. The most common and effective way to determine if allergies play a role in asthma symptoms is by doing skin and blood tests or by eliminating foods in the diet.[224] Chest x-ray examinations are typically not useful in diagnosing asthma, but they are useful in determining if other conditions of the lungs, chest, and heart are present.[223]

An estimated 20 million Americans suffer from asthma (1 in 15 Americans), and 50% of asthma cases are "allergic asthma."[218] Asthma is the most common chronic condition in children and it affects 1 in 20 children, with a higher incidence in male children than female children (3:2 ratio), but it is more common in older women than older men.[225] Ethnic differences in asthma prevalence, morbidity, and mortality are highly correlated with poverty, urban air quality, indoor allergens, and lack of patient education and inadequate medical care (Table 5-10).[226]

Table 5-10

Estimated Average Annual Prevalence Percents for Self-Reported Current Asthma, by Age, Sex, Race, Ethnicity, Region and Poverty Level—National Health Interview Survey, United States, 2001-2003

Characteristic	Total	Age (yrs)									
		< 18	≥ 18	0-4	5-14	15-34	15-19	20-24	25-34	35-64	≥ 65
Sex											
Male	6.2	9.6	4.9	6.8	11.1	6.3	8.9	6.4	4.7	4.5	4.6
Female	8.1	7.4	8.4	5.0	7.8	8.9	10.0	9.4	8.0	8.7	6.8
Race*											
White	6.9	7.7	6.7	4.4	8.8	7.5	9.2	8.0	6.3	6.6	5.8
Male	5.8	8.6	4.8	5.2	10.1	6.1	8.5	6.6	4.5	4.5	4.6
Female	8.0	6.8	8.4	3.6	7.5	8.9	9.8	9.4	8.1	8.7	6.7
Black	9.2	12.5	7.6	12.4	12.8	9.0	11.2	9.7	7.2	7.4	6.1
Male	8.2	14.0	5.2	12.8	15.4	7.3	10.5	6.9	5.2	4.6	3.8
Female	10.0	11.0	9.5	12.0	10.2	10.4	12.0	11.8	8.8	9.7	7.6
Other races NTA	6.8	8.9	5.7	7.1	9.5	6.6	9.4	5.5	5.8	5.4	6.7
Male	6.9	11.2	4.7	9.1	12.1	6.2	10.0	—	5.1	4.1	6.4†
Female	6.7	6.5	6.7	5.0	6.9	7.0	8.7	6.2	6.6	6.7	7.0
Ethnicity‡											
Hispanic or Latino	5.4	7.0	4.6	5.2	7.7	4.9	7.3	4.2	4.0	4.8	5.2
Male	4.8	7.6	3.2	5.7	8.4	3.9	7.2	3.0	2.8	3.1	4.5
Female	6.1	6.3	6.0	4.7	6.9	5.9	7.4	5.4	5.4	6.5	5.7
Puerto Rican	14.5	18.7	12.4	10.7	21.5	14.4	21.0	13.2	11.6	12.1	13.0
Male	12.4	18.7	8.8	10.2	23.1	10.1	16.1	11.5†	5.7	9.3	—
Female	16.6	18.7	15.7	11.2†	19.8	18.9	26.6	14.9	17.2	14.6	15.8
Mexican	3.9	4.8	3.3	3.8	5.4	3.3	4.6	2.9	2.9	3.5	3.9
Male	3.4	5.4	2.2	4.3	5.8	2.8	4.5	2.7	2.0†	2.2	3.0†
Female	4.4	4.2	4.5	3.3	4.9	3.9	4.8	3.2	3.9	4.8	4.7
Not Hispanic or Latino	7.4	8.9	7.0	6.1	9.9	8.1	9.9	8.7	6.8	6.8	5.9
Male	6.4	10.1	5.1	7.0	11.7	6.7	9.3	7.2	5.1	4.6	4.6
Female	8.4	7.6	8.7	5.0	8.0	9.4	10.5	10.2	8.5	8.9	6.9
Region											
Northeast	8.1	10.2	7.4	7.1	11.3	8.4	10.8	9.3	6.6	7.6	6.0
Midwest	7.5	8.7	7.1	6.7	9.5	8.3	9.8	9.0	7.0	6.7	6.3
South	6.7	8.3	6.2	6.0	9.4	7.0	8.9	7.0	6.0	6.1	5.4
West	6.8	7.3	6.6	3.9	8.3	7.1	9.0	7.1	6.1	6.6	6.2
Ratio of family income to poverty threshold§											
0-.99	10.3	11.1	9.8	10.2	11.1	9.5	11.6	9.5	7.8	11.2	8.8
1.00-2.49	7.9	8.5	7.6	6.9	9.1	7.9	9.0	8.2	7.1	7.9	7.1
2.50-4.49	6.8	7.7	6.5	3.9	9.2	7.4	8.9	8.0	6.4	6.3	5.2
≥ 4.50	6.4	8.0	6.0	3.8	9.5	6.9	9.1	7.4	5.9	6.1	4.3
Total	7.2	8.5	6.7	5.9	9.5	7.6	9.5	8.0	6.4	6.6	5.9

Race categorized according to the 1997 revision of Statistical Policy Directive No. 15. Race Ethnic Standards for Federal Statistics and Administrative Reporting. Race categories "white" and "black" are comprised persons who indicated only a single race group. "Other races NTA (not tabulated above) Includes Asian, American Indian and Alaskan Native, Native Hawaiian and Other Pacific Islander, persons reporting more than one race, and persons reporting their race as something other than those listed here or above.

†The estimate is unreliable because the relative standard error of the estimate is 30%-50%. For missing estimate, the relative standard error of the estimate exceeded 50% and the estimate was suppressed. All other relative standard errors are < 30%.

‡The 1997 revision of Statistical Policy Directive No. 15. Race and Ethnic Standards for Federal Statistics and Administrative Reporting changed the ethnicity category name for "Hispanic or Latino," but the definition of persons in that category remained the same. "Puerto Rican" and "Mexican" are a subset of "Hispanic or Latino"; Mexican includes responses of Mexican and Mexican American.

§Missing income responses were not imputed or included.

From Moorman JE, Rudd RA, Johnson CA et al: National Surveillance for Asthma—United States, 1980-2004, *Morb Mortal Wkly Rep* 56(S S08);1-14, 18-54, 2007. Retrieved November 7, 2008, from http://www.cdc.gov/mmwr/preview/mmwrhtml/ss5608a1.htm#tab1.

Vocal Cord Dysfunction

Vocal cord dysfunction (VCD) is a common yet hidden and usually unsuspected cause of throat closure or a choking sensation that can affect any individuals of any age.[227,228] VCD is a respiratory tract disorder characterized by paradoxic closing of the vocal cords during the inspiratory and occasionally the expiratory phase of the respiratory system and may be confused with an asthma attack.[229] Presently, it is not known what causes VCD, although several speculated causes include stress and anxiety. VCD's signs and symptoms are very similar in nature to asthma and anaphylaxis: wheezing, high-pitched grasping sounds, and hysteria from loss of breath. Typically, VCD patients present with shortness of breath, difficulty moving air, chest tightness, choking or coughing profusely, which routinely resolves with rest of approximately 5 minutes.[229] VCD may be triggered in various ways. Exercise seems to be the most common trigger. The amount of exercise needed to trigger VCD depends on the individual. Although environment does not appear to be a trigger, environmental contaminants, including pollution, strong odors, and perfumes, may cause VCD.

Clinical Point

Vocal cord dysfunction can sound like exercise-induced asthma and be caused by environmental allergens or pollutants.

Causes of Vocal Cord Dysfunction

- Gastroesophageal reflux disease, laryngopharyngeal reflux
- Sinusitis
- Postnasal drip
- Occupational exposure to irritant fumes
- Environmental allergens and pollutants
- Psychogenic causes; stress or anxiety

It can be difficult to determine whether one is experiencing an asthma attack or if one is experiencing VCD. Understanding that the symptoms are similar between the two conditions, there are a few ways to help determine which it is; duration of symptoms, recovery period, gender and age, and onset of symptoms when beginning exercise are just a few characteristics. With asthma, the duration of symptoms lasts longer because of the constriction or hyper-responsiveness of the bronchi. VCD duration of symptoms will subside more quickly with rest as the adduction or spasm of the vocal cords are allowed to relax. With asthma, the recovery period is approximately 15 to 60 minutes; VCD's recovery period is approximately 5 to 10 minutes.

Generally, VCD affects young females more than any other population, whereas asthma has a higher prevalence with young males and has many more triggers such as allergies and air quality.[229] The onset of symptoms after beginning exercise with asthma is approximately 5 to 10 minutes, as opposed to VCD, which is typically less than 5 minutes. Many more factors are detailed in Table 5-11 to help determine VCD versus asthma.

Because their signs and symptoms are often similar, testing becomes a very important aspect for determining whether a patient has VCD or asthma. The clinical examination must be thorough and specific to each individual with a good understanding of the history of symptoms. Breathing tests can be used to help with the diagnosis, but to get a true positive test, they must be done while the individual is having symptoms. If a breathing test is done while the patient is asymptomatic, the test could be negative for VCD but may be positive for asthma.[228] The most specific test for VCD is laryngoscopy. This is a procedure that uses a flexible fiberoptic tube with a tiny camera affixed to the end. It is inserted into the back of the throat so the physician can visualize the vocal cords as they open and close.[228] As with spirometry and other breathing tests, the test must be done while the patient is having symptoms because the vocal cords will function properly in the absence of symptoms. With a positive test, the physician visualizes the vocal cords as they spasm or adduct, making it more difficult to move air through them.

The prevalence of VCD in the general population is largely unknown.[229] However, among adult patients referred to a tertiary care facility with what was thought to be intractable asthma, VCD was the sole diagnosis in 10% and was diagnosed with asthma in an additional 30% of patients.[229] Other studies suggest prevalence among the adult population to be approximately 2.5%.[229] Studies regarding the prevalence in athletes are lacking. The evidence reported

Table 5-11

Features of Vocal Cord Dysfunction and Exercise-Induced Asthma Compared

Feature	VCD	EIA
Female preponderance	+	−
Chest tightness	+/−	+
Throat tightness	+	−
Stridor	+	−
Usual onset of symptoms after beginning exercise (min)	< 5	> 5-10
Recovery period (min)	5-10	15-60
Refractory period	−	+
Late-phase response	−	+
Response to beta-agonist	−	+

From Brugman SM, Simons MD, Stephen M: Vocal cord dysfunction: Don't mistake it for asthma, *Phys Sportsmed* 26(5):63–85, 1998.
EIA, Exercise-induced asthma; *VCD*, vocal cord dysfunction.

suggests that VCD may occur in approximately 3% of athletes who have a history of exercise-induced asthma. If VCD is the only diagnosis with no asthma involvement, then speech language therapy is beneficial.[229] Speech language therapy encompasses exercises to increase the patient's awareness of abdominal breathing and relaxing of the throat muscles. This allows the patient to have more control of the vocal cords and throat.[228] Also, learning cough suppression and throat clearing techniques can also be extremely beneficial. Practicing these techniques while asymptomatic is the key to overcoming abnormal vocal cord spasms and controlling the vocal cords to allow for proper airflow.[228]

Carbon Monoxide

Carbon monoxide is the most frequently occurring air pollutant in urban environments. It is released primarily from auto emissions, but is also a byproduct of industrial combustion and cigarette smoke. Carbon monoxide affects our health and physiological function by reducing the oxygen-carrying capacity of the blood, as hemoglobin has a 200-times greater affinity for carbon monoxide than for oxygen. Thus, when the carboxyhemoglobin (COHb) concentration is elevated, there is less hemoglobin available to transport oxygen for cell respiration.

Normal resting COHb concentration is approximately 1%, but many behaviors can significantly increase COHb concentration. Driving with an open window during peak traffic hours, for example, can raise the COHb concentration to 5%.[214] Aerobic exercise under similar conditions can further increase COHb, as the greater minute ventilation increases the amount of carbon monoxide inhaled per unit time. Nicholson and Case[230] reported that 30 minutes of running in New York City resulted in COHb concentrations of 4% to 5%. Smoking three cigarettes over a short time can increase COHb to approximately 5%.[39]

During light- to moderate-intensity aerobic exercise (30% to 75% maximal oxygen uptake), healthy individuals can tolerate COHb concentrations of up to 20% with no reduction in physical performance.[231-233] However, during exercise at 70% to 75% maximal oxygen uptake, individuals with elevated COHb have increased heart rates, greater respiratory distress, and higher blood lactate concentrations compared with control conditions.[231,234] In addition, there is evidence that high COHb (25% to 35%) concentrations may result in higher core temperatures during prolonged exercise.[235]

Carbon monoxide exposure appears to have little effect on maximal oxygen uptake up to 4% COHb.[236] Beyond this apparent threshold, however, maximal oxygen uptake declines approximately 0.9% with every 1% increase in COHb up to 35% COHb.[237] Carbon monoxide appears to reduce maximal oxygen uptake by reducing blood oxygen transport capacity. Maximal cardiac output is unaffected by carbon monoxide exposure.[236]

Persons with cardiovascular or pulmonary disease have a reduced ability to perform exercise when COHb is acutely elevated. Several investigators have reported that patients with angina have a decreased exercise time to angina onset; systolic blood pressure and heart rate are lower at the onset of angina, suggesting that angina occurs at a lower myocardial oxygen uptake.[214,215,238-240] Carbon monoxide exposure has also been shown to reduce the exercise tolerance of persons with chronic bronchitis, emphysema,[241] and anemia.[242]

Sulfur Oxides

Sulfur oxides are products of fossil fuel combustion and are upper respiratory tract irritants that can cause reversible bronchoconstriction and increased airway resistance. The dominant forms of sulfur oxides are sulfur dioxide, sulfuric acid, and sulfate, with 98% of the sulfur released into the atmosphere in the form of sulfur dioxide.[212]

In healthy adults, sulfur dioxide does not impair pulmonary function until the concentration exceeds 1 to 3 ppm.[243] However, in asthmatics and others with pulmonary hyperactivity, the threshold for airway restriction is less than 1 ppm,[244-247] with one study reporting progressive bronchoconstriction with exposure to 0.1 to 0.5 ppm sulfur dioxide.[246] To these authors' knowledge, no study has evaluated whether sulfur dioxide exposure impairs either endurance exercise performance or maximal oxygen uptake.

Repeated exposure to sulfur dioxide does induce adaptation. Industrial workers routinely exposed to 10 ppm sulfur dioxide retain normal pulmonary function when exposed to 5 ppm sulfur dioxide.[248] Andersen and colleagues[249] conducted studies investigating the physiological responses that occur when subjects breathe 1, 5, or 25 ppm sulfur dioxide for 6 hours. They reported that the subjects tolerated each concentration of sulfur dioxide "very well," but investigators who occasionally entered the climatic chamber reported that the 25-ppm sulfur dioxide concentrations were "almost intolerable." These adaptations to sulfur dioxide occur in both healthy and asthmatic individuals.[250]

Nitrogen Oxides

Nitrogen oxides develop from high-temperature combustive processes involving nitrogen and oxygen. The concentration of nitrogen oxides is elevated during peak traffic periods, at airports, and in the smoke accompanying cigarette smoking and fire fighting. There are several forms of nitrogen oxides, including nitrous oxide, nitric oxide, nitrogen dioxide, dinitrogen dioxide, dinitrogen pentoxide, and nitrate ions. Nitrogen dioxide is known to be harmful to health; acute exposure to high nitrogen dioxide levels (200 to 4000 ppm) can cause severe pulmonary edema and death.[251] At lower concentrations (2 to 5 ppm), nitrogen dioxide increases airway resistance and reduces pulmonary diffusion capacity.[252,253] Fortunately, the ambient air concentration of nitrogen dioxide is generally less than 1 ppm.

For healthy persons, nitrogen dioxide concentrations of less than 0.7 ppm appear to have no adverse affects on pulmonary function or exercise performance.[243,254] Aging does not appear to reduce tolerance to nitrogen dioxide.[255] However, people with chronic obstructive pulmonary disease and, presumably, other respiratory diseases have reduced pulmonary function when exposed for 4 hours to 0.3 ppm nitrogen dioxide.[255]

Primary Particulates

Primary particulates include dust, soot, and smoke.[212,256] These pollutants are of physiological importance because they can impair pulmonary function after they are inhaled into the lungs. The fine dust from charcoal[257] and cigarette smoke[258] has been shown to increase airway resistance and reduce forced expiratory volume. The lung depth reached by the dust is determined by the particle size. The dispersion of dust within the lung is influenced by the tidal volume, frequency of breathing, and whether the particle was inhaled nasally or orally.[243] Because aerobic exercise increases ventilation and oral inhalation, it is likely that exercise increases the effective dose of this pollutant.

Unfortunately, there is little information on the physiological consequences of particulate inhalation during exercise. Klausen and colleagues[259] suggested that inhalation of particulates may reduce endurance exercise time. In their study, subjects performed a maximal exercise test under control conditions after inhalation of the smoke of three cigarettes and after sufficient carbon monoxide inhalation to raise their COHb concentration to the same magnitude as when they smoked three cigarettes. Interestingly, Klausen and colleagues found that raising the COHb concentration produced a 7% reduction in maximal oxygen uptake in both treatment groups, but endurance time during the maximal oxygen uptake test was reduced 20% after smoking and only 10% after carbon monoxide inhalation. They interpreted the results to suggest that the decrease in maximal oxygen uptake after smoking or carbon monoxide inhalation was due to reduced oxygen carrying capacity of the blood, whereas the decrease in endurance time was a combined effect of the carbon monoxide concentration and the increased cost of breathing caused by the smoke particulates.

Ozone

Ozone is produced in oxygen-containing atmospheres primarily from the interaction of hydrocarbons and nitrogen dioxide in the presence of solar ultraviolet (UV) radiation. As a consequence, ozone is most prevalent in urban areas and reaches its highest concentration during the midday hours.

Ozone is a potent airway irritant, causing reflex broncho-constriction in upper airways. The most common subjective symptoms are a cough, substernal soreness, and dryness of the upper respiratory passages. These symptoms can occur after brief exposures to low concentrations of ozone (0.05 to 0.10 ppm) and can persist for several hours after exposure.[212] Furthermore, there may be heightened sensitivity to ozone during the initial hours following ozone exposure.[260]

During light- to moderate-intensity exercise, exposure to ozone in the range of 0.2 to 0.4 ppm reduces pulmonary function and enhances subjective discomfort,[261] but does not appear to impair exercise performance. These ozone concentrations can produce cough, substernal pain, wheezing, and malaise during exercise,[262] with the incidence of symptoms increasing in proportion to the ozone concentration.[263,264]

During high-intensity aerobic exercise (75% to 85% maximal oxygen uptake), ozone inhalation can impair endurance exercise performance. Schelegle and Adams[265] evaluated the effect of 0, 0.12, 0.18, or 0.24 ppm ozone exposure on the endurance performance of 10 highly trained athletes during 60 minutes of simulated competition (the last 30 minutes were at 86% of maximal oxygen uptake). All subjects completed the protocol when breathing 0 ppm ozone, whereas one, five, and seven subjects did not complete the exercise when exposed to 0.12, 0.18, and 0.24 ppm ozone, respectively. Folinsbee and colleagues[266] reported that inhalation of 0.21 ppm ozone during 60 minutes of exercise at 75% of maximal oxygen uptake induced significant reductions in pulmonary function, and six of seven subjects developed subjective distress (symptoms included tracheal irritation, substernal soreness, chest tightness, and shortness of breath). Adams and Schelegle[267] also documented decrements in pulmonary function and subjective discomfort. In addition, they reported that 4 of 10 subjects could not complete the exercise trials when breathing 0.35 ppm ozone. Similarly, Gibbons and Adams[268] reported that 3 of 10 subjects discontinued exercise prematurely when exposed to 0.3 ppm ozone during 60 minutes of moderate-intensity (66% maximal oxygen uptake) exercise in a 35°C (95°F) environment.

Ozone inhalation can reduce maximal oxygen uptake. Folinsbee and colleagues[269] reported a 10% reduction in maximal oxygen uptake in those exposed to 0.75 ppm ozone. Similarly, Gong and colleagues[264] reported that 0.20 ppm ozone reduced maximal oxygen uptake (−16%), maximal ventilation (−18%), and exercise tolerance time (−30%) during a graded exercise test following 1 hour of exercise. Not all investigators have reported reductions in maximal oxygen uptake after ozone exposure.[270,271] One explanation for these divergent findings may be the duration of ozone exposure prior to initiating the maximal exercise test, as the studies reporting no change in maximal oxygen uptake exposed the subjects to ozone only during the exercise test.

There is evidence that repeated ozone exposure produces adaptations that attenuate ozone-induced reductions in pulmonary function[261,272-280] and decrements in maximal oxygen uptake and exercise time to exhaustion.[281] This adaptation generally occurs within 2 to 5 days of repeated exposure[261,275-280,282] and persists for 7 to 20 days upon discontinuation of exposure,[280,282] with the least persistent adaptation occurring in persons sensitive to ozone. However, acclimatization to ozone does not attenuate decrements in pulmonary function when subjects are exposed to higher ozone concentrations.[278] The time course of adaptation is similar between genders.[261]

Interactions Between Various Air Pollutants

Because polluted atmospheres contain many contaminants, it is important to investigate whether combinations of various pollutants interact to affect pulmonary function and exercise performance in an additive, synergistic, or subtractive manner. The majority of research has focused on the interaction of various air pollutants with ozone. Although the early work of Hazucha and Bates[283] suggested that exposure to 0.37 ppm ozone and 0.37 ppm sulfur dioxide resulted in synergistic reductions in pulmonary function, subsequent investigations found only additive effects.[272,284-286] Koenig and colleagues[287] reported that asthmatic patients who received prior exposure to ozone had a greater decrement in pulmonary function during subsequent exposure to sulfur dioxide at dosages that were subthreshold for normal subjects. They concluded that ozone exposure made the asthmatic subjects more susceptible to low concentrations of sulfur dioxide.

Experiments that have evaluated the interaction of nitrogen dioxide and ozone suggest that there is no interaction between the two compounds; the effects of the combination produced no greater effects than exposure to ozone alone.[262,263,288] The combination of nitrogen dioxide and sulfur dioxide appears to produce only additive effects. Pulmonary resistance is increased abruptly after sulfur dioxide exposure, with no persistent effects; nitrogen dioxide has a more delayed and persistent effect.[289] Combining subthreshold doses of nitrogen dioxide (0.5 ppm) and sulfur dioxide (0.3 to 0.5 ppm) during 2 hours of light-intensity exercise does not induce deficits in pulmonary function in either healthy or asthmatic subjects.[245]

Particulates interact with carbon monoxide to produce greater reductions in endurance time than carbon monoxide alone.[39] However, particulates do not appear to accentuate the effects of ozone on pulmonary function in either normal subjects or asthmatics.[290-292]

Interactions Between Environmental Stressors

Cold and Altitude

Ascent to high altitude is typically accompanied by reductions in ambient temperature and humidity and increased wind velocity. These added environmental stressors exacerbate the physiological stress of hypoxia, potentially compromising exercise performance and health. Because temperature typically falls approximately 10°C with every 1500-meter (4921 feet) rise in elevation, even moderate increases in elevation can significantly magnify the degree of cold stress.[293] Therefore, individuals traveling to high altitudes should bring adequate clothing to protect themselves against environmental cold stress.

The combined effects of cold and hypoxia on injury and exercise performance remain poorly understood because of a lack of experimental information. However, it is likely that the combined stress of cold and altitude exposure predisposes individuals to injury and premature fatigue because (1) both body cooling and hypoxia impair mental function and decision-making ability; (2) the lower maximal oxygen uptake at altitude reduces an individual's ability to increase heat production and defend core temperature; (3) both cold and hypoxic stress are associated with hemoconcentration and peripheral vasoconstriction, which may contribute to peripheral cold injury; and (4) because both cold and hypoxia increase blood lactic acid concentration at a given exercise intensity, premature fatigue may occur during exercise.

Air Pollution and Heat

Because elevated concentrations of air pollutants are often associated with excessive heat and humidity,[294] which are known to impair exercise performance, it is likely that the combined stresses of excessive heat, humidity, and poor air quality further impair exercise performance. Gibbons and Adams[268] found that subjective symptoms increased when ambient temperature was 35°C (95°F) rather than 25°C (77°F) and subjects were exposed to either 0.15 or 0.30 ppm ozone during 60 minutes of moderately intense exercise. Furthermore, they reported that 3 of 10 subjects were unable to complete the 1-hour exercise bout (66% maximal oxygen uptake) when heat or ozone was present. Similarly, Folinsbee and colleagues[295] reported greater reductions in pulmonary function when subjects were exposed to 0.5 ppm ozone during exercise in a hot climate compared with a cool climate. However, the same primary investigator subsequently found no temperature interaction when subjects were exposed to 0.5 ppm ozone and 0.5 ppm nitrogen dioxide.[288]

Rather surprisingly, there is no evidence that hot ambient temperatures and carbon monoxide produce either additive or synergistic effects on maximal oxygen uptake or performance. Because both hot ambient conditions and increased COHb have individually been shown to reduce maximal oxygen uptake, it would be expected that the combination would produce additive reductions on maximal oxygen uptake and performance. The only studies to date, however, reported no additive effect on maximal oxygen uptake when heat and carbon monoxide were combined.[296-298]

Air Pollution and Cold or Altitude

Exercise in cold environments can induce reflex broncho-constriction and cold-induced asthma in approximately 12% of the population.[299,300] Unfortunately, no studies have evaluated the interaction of cold temperatures and pollution exposure on exercise performance in this population.

Several studies have examined the effect of carbon monoxide at high altitude.[243,301,302] Carbon monoxide exposure at altitude further lowers oxygen transport capacity. The effect appears to be additive, however, as a given COHb at altitude and sea level produces a similar decrement in endurance tolerance time and maximal oxygen uptake at both altitudes.[302] But because it takes a smaller concentration of carbon monoxide at high altitude to elicit the same COHb concentration,[243] persons at high altitude are more sensitive to the effects of carbon monoxide.

Other Environmental Factors

Lightning

Lightning strikes are rare during athletic events, but pose great danger for the athletes and spectators. The National Weather Service estimates that more than 25 million lightning flashes occur per year. From 1978 through 2007, lightning was the fourth leading cause of weather deaths per year.[303] The highest number of flashes occurs in central Florida and along the coasts of Louisiana, Mississippi, and Alabama. However, the majority of the southeastern and midwestern states have lightning storms every year. Lightning occurs mostly in the afternoons during the summer months when outside activities and sporting events are peaking.[304]

There are three main mechanisms of injury for victims struck by lightning; these are a direct strike, contact, and splash.[305] The *direct strike* usually hits the victim in open areas. All athletic fields are considered open areas. Even with this type of strike, death rarely occurs. A *contact strike* occurs when a person is in contact with an object while the strike occurs. The occurrence rate of contact strikes is less than 2%. *Splash strikes* are flashes of lightning that hit an object, usually a tree, and the current travels or "jumps" to hit someone. Golf courses and lakes are typical locations where splash strikes are more likely to occur because people take shelter under trees during storms. Splash strikes have the highest rate of occurrence at 35%. The National Athletic Trainers' Association position statement on lightning also lists two other possible mechanisms of injury. These include *step voltage,* in which a victim is injured by ground current, and a *blunt strike injury,* in which the victim is thrown several feet from the strike point because of violent muscular contractions.[306] The National Severe Storms Laboratory stresses two factors of importance for athletes faced with lightning situations.[307] These involve determining distance from the storm to the location of activity and determining when to return to participation.

Flash-to-Bang Time

The "flash-to-bang" calculation determines the distance from the storm. This process is established by counting the time from the flash of the lightning to the bang of the thunder. Every 5 seconds equals 1 mile. Count the seconds between the lightning flash and the bang, and then divide by 5 to identify the distance in miles from the lightning.

30-30 Rule

If you count to 30 or less (i.e., seconds) between the flash and the bang, there is still imminent danger. When 30 minutes have elapsed since the last flash or thunder, an "all clear" can be established and safe play can resume.

The National Collegiate Athletic Association has also recommended the guideline that if thunder is heard, preparation for evacuation should begin. In addition, if lightning is seen, consider suspending activities and heading for a designated safe location. Specific lightning safety guidelines should be implemented before activities and protective locations should be identified to ensure the safety of athletes and spectators.

Ultraviolet Light

Athletes who participate in outdoor activities potentially have a higher risk of UV light exposure from the sun than the general public. Recent studies have documented UV light exposure in professional cyclists, triathletes, alpine skiers, and mountaineers.[308,309] Excessive or prolonged UV light exposure can present acutely with sunburn and later with the development of melanoma and other skin cancers.[310] Body areas that are routinely left exposed to the UV light such as the face, legs, arms, neck, and feet are also the areas with the highest risk of developing manifestations of prolonged or excessive UV light. Studies have indicated that a history of multiple, severe sunburns in childhood and adolescence is a strong risk factor for the development of melanoma and basal cell carcinoma.[311-314]

Sunburn is defined as an inflammation of the skin (an actual burn) caused by UV rays from the sun. Depending on the severity of the burn, the skin may simply redden or it may become blistered or sore; in more severe cases, a fever may be present.[217] Initial erythema results from vasodilation of the dermis. Vasodilation coupled with an increase in vascular permeability leads to edema.[315] Vesicles and bullae may form in more severe cases. Initial erythema becomes evident in typically 3 to 5 hours after exposure. It reaches a maximum severity at 12 to 24 hours and gradually decreases over the next 72 hours.[315] In addition to these acute effects, UV light can irreversibly damage deoxyribonucleic acid and lead to mutations and pyrimidine dimmer formation in the dermis and epidermis.[310] This sequence of events may lead to the development of skin carcinoma.[316]

Athletes participating in outdoor activities should be mindful of UV light and the negative effects on the skin (also see Chapter 19, "Dermatologic Considerations in Athletics"). Athletes should train during times of low UV light exposure; wear appropriate clothing to adequately cover the skin, especially those areas identified as areas of high risk (neck, legs, arms); and use a sunscreen for areas of the skin that cannot effectively be covered by clothing. A recent study noted high rates of sunburn and low rates of sun-protective behavior in high school and collegiate athletes despite their knowledge of the risks of excessive, unprotected sun exposure.[317] Constant education from the health care team and coaches on appropriate UV light protection from the sun is a critical component to ensure safe and healthy training during outdoor activities.

References

1. Hardy JD: Physiology of temperature regulation, *Physiol Rev* 41:521–606, 1961.
2. Gonzalez RR, Berglund LG, Gagge AP: Indices of thermoregulatory strain for moderate exercise in the heat, *J Appl Physiol* 44:889–899, 1978.
3. Lind AR: A physiological criterion for setting thermal environmental limits for everyday work, *J Appl Physiol* 18:51–56, 1963.
4. Nielsen M: Die Regulation der Körpertemperatur bei Muskelarbeit, *Skand Arch Physiol* 79:193–230, 1938.
5. Nielsen M: Heat production and body temperature during rest and work. In Hardy JD, Gagge AP, Stolwijk JAJ, editors: *Physiological and behavioral temperature regulation*, Springfield, IL, 1970, Charles C. Thomas.
6. Stolwijk JAJ, Saltin B, Gagge AP: Physiological factors associated with sweating during exercise, *Aerospace Med* 1968; 39:1101.
7. American College of Sports Medicine: The prevention of thermal injuries during distance running, *Med Sci Sports Exerc* 19:529–533, 1987.
8. Rowell LB: *Human circulation: Regulation during physical stress*, New York, 1986, Oxford University Press.
9. Bevegård BS, Shepherd JT: Reaction in man of resistance and capacity vessels in forearm and hand to leg exercise, *J Appl Physiol* 21:123–132, 1966.
10. Hanke D, Schlepper M, Westermann K, et al: Venentonus, hut- und mskeldurchblutung an uterarm und hand bei beinarbeit, *Pflugers Arch* 309:115–127, 1969.
11. Klausen K, Dill DB, Phillips EE Jr, et al: Metabolic reactions to work in the desert, *J Appl Physiol* 22:292–296, 1967.
12. Rowell LB, Murray JA, Brengelmann GL, et al: Human cardiovascular adjustments to rapid changes in skin temperature during exercise, *Circ Res* 24:711–724, 1969.
13. Saltin B, Gagge AP, Stolwijk JAJ: Body temperatures and sweating during thermal transients caused by exercise, *J Appl Physiol* 28:318–327, 1970.
14. Sawka MN, Young AJ, Cadarette BS, et al: Influence of heat stress and acclimation on maximal aerobic power, *Eur J Appl Physiol* 53:294–298, 1985.
15. Saltin B, Gagge AP, Bergh U, et al: Body temperatures and sweating during exhaustive exercise, *J Appl Physiol* 32:635–643, 1972.
16. Nybo L: Exercise and heat stress: Cerebral challenges and consequences, *Prog Brain Res* 162:29–43, 2007.
17. Nielsen B, Nybo L: Cerebral changes during exercise in the heat, *Sports Med* 33(1):1–11, 2003.
18. Consolazio CF, Matoush LO, Nelson RA, et al: Environmental temperature and energy expenditure, *J Appl Physiol* 18:65–68, 1963.
19. Consolazio CF, Shapiro R, Masterson JE, et al: Energy requirements of men in extreme heat, *J Nutr* 73:126–134, 1961.
20. Dimri GP, Malhotra MS, Sen Gupta J, et al: Alterations in aerobic-anaerobic proportions of metabolism during work in heat, *Eur J Appl Physiol* 45:43–50, 1980.
21. Fink WJ, Costill DL, Van Handel WJ: Leg muscle metabolism during exercise in the heat and cold, *Eur J Appl Physiol* 34:183–190, 1975.
22. Nielsen B, Savard G, Richter EA, et al: Muscle blood flow and muscle metabolism during exercise and heat stress, *J Appl Physiol* 69:1040–1046, 1990.
23. Brouha L, Smith PE Jr, De Lanne R, et al: Physiological reactions of men and women during muscular activity and recovery in various environments, *J Appl Physiol* 16:133–140, 1960.
24. Petersen ES, Vejby-Christensen H: Effect of body temperature on steady-state ventilation and metabolism in exercise, *Acta Physiol Scand* 89:342–351, 1973.
25. Williams CG, Bredell GAG, Wyndham CH, et al: Circulatory and metabolic reactions to work in heat, *J Appl Physiol* 17:625–638, 1962.
26. Young AJ, Sawka MN, Levine L, et al: Skeletal muscle metabolism during exercise is influenced by heat acclimation, *J Appl Physiol* 59:1929–1935, 1985.
27. Savard G, Nielsen B, Laszczynska I, et al: Muscle blood flow is not reduced in humans during moderate exercise and heat stress, *J Appl Physiol* 64:649–657, 1988.
28. Yaspelkis BB III, Scroop GC, Wilmore KM, et al: Carbohydrate metabolism during exercise in hot and thermoneutral environments, *Int J Sports Med* 14:13–19, 1993.
29. Bean WB, Eichna LW: Performance in relation to environmental temperature: Reactions of normal young men to simulated desert environment, *Fed Proc* 2:144–158, 1993.
30. Eichna LW, Bean WB, Ashe WF, et al: Performance in relation to environmental temperature: Reactions of normal young men to hot, humid (simulated jungle) environment, *Bull Johns Hopkins Hosp* 76:25–58, 1945.
31. Machle W, Hatch TF: Heat: Man's exchanges and physiological responses, *Physiol Rev* 27:200–227, 1947.
32. Wenger CB: Human heat acclimatization. In Pandolf KB, Sawka MN, Gonzalez RR, editors: *Human performance physiology and environmental medicine at terrestrial extremes*, Indianapolis, 1988, Benchmark Press.
33. Armstrong LE, Maresh CM: The induction and decay of heat acclimatization in trained athletes, *Sports Med* 12:302–312, 1991.
34. Gisolfi CV, Wilson NC, Claxton B: Work-heat tolerance of distance runners. In Milvy P, editor: *The marathon: Physiological, medical, epidemiological, and psychological studies*, New York, 1977, New York Academy of Sciences.
35. Armstrong LE, Pandolf KB: Physical training, cardiorespiratory physical fitness and exercise-heat tolerance. In Pandolf KB, Sawka MN, Gonzalez RR, editors: *Human performance physiology and environmental medicine at terrestrial extremes*, Indianapolis, 1988, Benchmark Press.
36. Avellini BA, Shapiro Y, Fortney SM, et al: Effects on heat tolerance of physical training in water and on land, *J Appl Physiol* 53:1291–1298, 1982.
37. Adams WC, Fox RH, Fry AJ, et al: Thermoregulation during marathon running in cool, moderate, and hot environments, *J Appl Physiol* 38:1030–1037, 1975.
38. Piwonka RW, Robinson S, Gay VL, et al: Preacclimatization of men to heat by training, *J Appl Physiol* 20:379–384, 1965.

39. Piwonka RW, Robinson S: Acclimatization of highly trained men to work in severe heat, *J Appl Physiol* 22:9–12, 1967.

40. Ladell WSS: The effects of water and salt intake upon the performance of men working in hot and humid environments, *J Physiol* 127:11–46, 1955.

41. Montain SJ, Coyle EF: Influence of graded dehydration on hyperthermia and cardiovascular drift during exercise, *J Appl Physiol* 73:1340–1350, 1992.

42. Sawka MN, Young AJ, Francesconi RP, et al: Thermoregulatory and blood responses during exercise at graded hypohydration levels, *J Appl Physiol* 59:1394–1401, 1985.

43. Buskirk ER, Iampietro PF, Bass DE: Work performance after dehydration: Effects of physical conditioning and heat acclimatization, *J Appl Physiol* 12:189–194, 1958.

44. Sawka MN, Toner MM, Francesconi RP, et al: Hypohydration and exercise: Effects of heat acclimation, gender, and environment, *J Appl Physiol* 55:1147–1153, 1983.

45. Below PR, Coyle EF: Fluid and carbohydrate ingestion individually benefit intense exercise lasting one-hour, *Med Sci Sports Exerc* 27:200–210, 1995.

46. Sawka MN, Young AJ, Latzka WA, et al: Human tolerance to heat strain during exercise: Influence of hydration, *J Appl Physiol* 73:368–375, 1992.

47. Rothstein A, Towbin EJ: Blood circulation and temperature of men dehydrating in the heat. In Adolph EF, editor: *Physiology of man in the desert*, New York, 1947, Interscience.

48. Montain SJ, Coyle EF: Influence of the timing of fluid ingestion on temperature regulation during exercise, *J Appl Physiol* 75:688–695, 1993.

49. Coyle EF, Montain SJ: Carbohydrate and fluid ingestion during exercise: Are there tradeoffs? *Med Sci Sports Exerc* 24:671–678, 1992.

50. Mitchell JB, Voss KW: The influence of volume on gastric emptying and fluid balance during prolonged exercise, *Med Sci Sports Exerc* 23:314–319, 1991.

51. Epstein Y: Heat intolerance: Predisposing factor or residual injury? *Med Sci Sports Exerc* 22:29–35, 1990.

52. Exton-Smith AN: Accidental hypothermia, *Br Med J* 4:727–729, 1973.

53. Pandolf KB, Cadarette BS, Sawka MN, et al: Thermoregulatory responses of matched middle-aged and young men during dry-heat acclimation, *J Appl Physiol* 65:65–71, 1988.

54. Seals DR: Influence of aging on autonomic-circulatory control at rest and during exercise in humans. In Gisolfi CV, Lamb DR, Nadel ER, editors: *Perspectives in exercise science and sports medicine, Vol 6: Exercise, heat, and thermoregulation*, Dubuque, 1993, Wm. C. Brown.

55. Kolka MA, Stephenson LA, Gonzalez RR: Depressed sweating during exercise at altitude, *J Thermal Biol* 14:167–170, 1989.

56. Kolka MA, Stephenson LA, Rock PB, et al: Local sweating and cutaneous blood flow during exercise in hypoxic environments, *J Appl Physiol* 62:2224–2229, 1987.

57. Frye AJ, Kamon E: Responses to dry heat of men and women with similar aerobic capacities, *J Appl Physiol* 50:65–70, 1981.

58. Avellini BA, Kamon E, Krajewski JT: Physiological responses of physically fit men and women to acclimation to humid heat, *J Appl Physiol* 49:254–261, 1980.

59. Stephenson LA, Kolka MA: Thermoregulation in women, *Exerc Sport Sci Rev* 21:231–262, 1992.

60. Carpenter AJ, Nunneley SA: Endogenous hormones subtly alter women's response to heat stress, *J Appl Physiol* 65:2313–2317, 1988.

61. Pivarnik JM, Marichal CJ, Spillman T, et al: Menstrual cycle phase affects temperature regulation during endurance exercise, *J Appl Physiol* 72:543–548, 1992.

62. Montain SJ, Sawka MN, Quigley MD, et al: Physiological tolerance to uncompensable heat stress: Effect of exercise intensity, protective clothing and climate, *J Appl Physiol* 77:216–222, 1994.

63. Speckman KL, Allan AE, Sawka MN, et al: Perspectives in microclimate cooling involving protective clothing in hot environments, *Int J Ind Ergonomics* 3:121–147, 1988.

64. Cage GW, Sato K, Schwachman N: Eccrine glands. In Fitzpatrick TB, Eisen AZ, Wolff K, et al, editors: *Dermatology in general medicine*, New York, 1987, McGraw–Hill.

65. Davis PB, di Sant'Agnese PA: Diagnosis and treatment of cystic fibrosis: An update, *Chest* 85:802–809, 1984.

66. Matthews LW, Drotar D: Cystic fibrosis—A challenging long-term chronic disease, *Pediatr Clin North Am* 31:133–151, 1984.

67. De Marinis M, Stocchi F, Testa SR, et al: Alterations in thermoregulation in Parkinson's disease, *Funct Neurol* 6:279–283, 1991.

68. Pandolf KB, Griffin TB, Munro EH, et al: Persistence of impaired heat tolerance from artificially induced miliaria rubra, *Am J Physiol* 239:R226–R232, 1980.

69. Pandolf KB, Griffin TB, Munro EH, et al: Heat intolerance as a function of percent of body surface involved with miliaria rubra, *Am J Physiol* 239:R233–R240, 1980.

70. Leibowitz E, Seidman DS, Laor A, et al: Are psoriatic patients at risk of heat intolerance? *Br J Dermatol* 124:439–442, 1991.

71. Pandolf KB, Gange RW, Latzka WA, et al: Human thermoregulatory responses during heat exposure after artificially induced sunburn, *Am J Physiol* 262:R610–R616, 1992.

72. Bar-Or O, Lundegren H, Buskirk ER: Heat tolerance of exercising obese and lean women, *J Appl Physiol* 26:403–409, 1969.

73. Buskirk ER, Lundegren H, Magnusson L: Heat acclimation patterns in obese and lean individuals, *Ann N Y Acad Sci* 131:637–653, 1965.

74. O'Sullivan SB, Schmitz TJ: *Physical rehabilitation: Assessment and treatment*, Philadelphia, 1988, FA Davis.

75. Clark WG, Lipton JM: Drug-related heatstroke. In Schönbaum E, Lomax P, editors: *Thermoregulation: Pathology, pharmacology, and therapy*, New York, 1991, Pergamon Press.

76. Lomax P: Drug induced changes in the thermoregulatory system. In Khogali M, Hales JRS, editors: *Heat stroke and temperature regulation*, New York, 1983, Academic Press.

77. Lomax P: Drug abuse and heatstroke. In Lomax P, Schönbaum E, editors: *Thermoregulation: Research and clinical applications*, Basel, 1988, Karger.

78. Levine L, Cadarette BS, Gonzalez RR, et al: *Atropine and thermoregulation in man (a report of three studies)*, Technical Report T12/85, Natick, MA, 1985, US Army Research Institute of Environmental Medicine.

79. Burr RE: *Heat illness: A handbook for medical officers*, Technical Report 91–3, Natick, MA, 1991, US Army Research Institute of Environmental Medicine.

80. Haymes EM, Wells CL: *Environment and human performance*, Champaign, IL, 1986, Human Kinetics.

81. Howe AS, Boden BP: Heat-related illness in athletes, *Am J Sports Med* 35(8):1384–1395, 2007.

82. Binkley HM, Beckett J, Casa DJ, et al: National Athletic Trainers' Association position statement: Exertional heat illnesses, *J Athl Training* 37(3):329–343, 2002.

83. Armstrong LE, Casa DJ, Millard-Stafford M, et al: Exertional heat illness during training and competition, *Med Sci Sports Exerc* 39(3):556–572, 2007.

84. Roberts WO: A 12-yr profile of medical injury and illness for the Twin Cities Marathon, *Med Sci Sports Exerc* 32:1549–1555, 2000.

85. Casa DJ, Armstrong LE: Exertional heatstroke: A medical emergency. In Armstrong LE, editor: *Exertional heat illnesses*, Champaign, 2003, Human Kinetics.

86. Armstrong LE, Casa DJ, Watson G: Exertional hyponatremia, *Curr Sports Med Rep* 5(5):221–222, 2006.

87. Salis RE: Fluid balance and dysnatremias in athletes, *Curr Sports Med Rep* 7(4):S14–S19, 2008.

88. Mortiz ML, Ayus JC: Exercise-associated hyponatremia: Why are athletes still dying? *Clin J Sports Med* 18(5):379–381, 2008.

89. Pendergast DR: The effect of body cooling on oxygen transport during exercise, *Med Sci Sports Exerc* 20:S171–S176, 1988.

90. Hong SI, Nadel ER: Thermogenic control during exercise in a cold environment, *J Appl Physiol* 47:1084–1089, 1979.

91. Nielsen B: Metabolic reactions to changes in core and skin temperature in man, *Acta Physiol Scand* 97:129–138, 1976.

92. Young AJ: Human adaptation to cold. In Pandolf KB, Sawka MN, Gonzalez RR, editors: *Human performance physiology and environmental medicine at terrestrial extremes*, Indianapolis, 1988, Benchmark Press.

93. McArdle WD, Magel JR, Lesmes GR, et al: Metabolic and cardiovascular adjustments to work in air and water at 18, 25 and 33°C, *J Appl Physiol* 40:85–90, 1976.

94. McArdle WD, Magel JR, Gergley TJ, et al: Thermal adjustment to cold water exposure in exercising men and women, *J Appl Physiol* 56:1572–1577, 1984.

95. Nadel ER, Homer I, Bergh U, et al: Energy exchanges of swimming man, *J Appl Physiol* 36:465–471, 1974.

96. Amor AF, Vogel JA, Worsley DE: *The energy cost of wearing multilayer clothing*, Technical Report 18/73, Farnborough, England, 1973, Royal Aircraft Establishment.

97. Teitlebaum A, Goldman RF: Increased energy cost with multiple clothing layers, *J Appl Physiol* 32:743–744, 1972.

98. Pandolf KB, Givoni B, Goldman RF: Predicting energy expenditure with loads while standing or walking very slowly, *J Appl Physiol* 43:577–581, 1977.

99. Bergh U, Ekblom B: Physical performance and peak aerobic power at different body temperatures, *J Appl Physiol* 46:885–889, 1979.

100. Davies M, Ekblom B, Bergh U, et al: The effects of hypothermia on submaximal and maximal work performance, *Acta Physiol Scand* 95:201–202, 1975.

101. Dressendorfer RH, Morlock JF, Baker DG, et al: Effect of head-out water immersion on cardiorespiratory responses to maximal cycling exercise, *Undersea Biomed Res* 3:177–187, 1976.

102. Holmér I, Bergh U: Metabolic and thermal response to swimming in water at varying temperatures, *J Appl Physiol* 37:702–705, 1974.

103. Patton JF, Vogel JA: Effects of acute cold exposure on submaximal endurance performance, *Med Sci Sports Exerc* 16:494–497, 1984.

104. Faulkner JA, White TP, Markley JM: The 1979 Canadian ski marathon: A natural experiment in hypothermia. In Nagle FJ, Montoye HJ, editors: *Exercise in health and disease—Balke Symposium*, Springfield, IL, 1981, Charles C. Thomas.

105. Adolph EF, Molnar GW: Exchanges of heat and tolerances to cold in men exposed to outdoor weather, *Am J Physiol* 146:507–537, 1946.

106. Doubt TJ: Physiology of exercise in the cold, *Sports Med* 11:367–381, 1991.

107. Bergh U, Ekblom B: Influence of muscle temperature on maximal muscle strength and power output in human skeletal muscles, *Acta Physiol Scand* 107:33–37, 1979.

108. Asmussen E, Bonde-Peterson F, Jorgensen K: Mechano-elastic properties of human muscles at different temperatures, *Acta Physiol Scand* 96:83–93, 1976.

109. Petrofsky JS: *Isometric exercise and its clinical implications*, Springfield, IL, 1982, Charles C Thomas.

110. Edwards RHT, Harris RC, Hultman E, et al: Effect of temperature on muscle energy metabolism and endurance during successive isometric contractions, sustained to fatigue, of the quadriceps muscle in man, *J Physiol* 220:335–352, 1972.

111. Bigland-Ritchie B, Thomas CK, Rice CL, et al: Muscle temperature, contractile speed, and motoneuron firing rates during human voluntary contractions, *J Appl Physiol* 73:2457–2461, 1992.

112. Marshall HC: The effects of cold exposure and exercise upon peripheral function, *Arch Environ Health* 24:325–330, 1972.

113. Vanggaard L: Physiological reactions to wet-cold, *Aviat Space Environ Med* 46:33–36, 1975.

114. Johnson DJ, Leider FE: Influence of cold bath on maximum handgrip strength, *Percept Mot Skills* 44:323–326, 1977.

115. Oliver RA, Johnson DJ, Wheelhouse WW, et al: Isometric muscle contraction response during recovery from reduced intramuscular temperature, *Arch Phys Med Rehabil* 60:126–129, 1979.

116. Michalski WJ, Séguin JJ: The effects of muscle cooling and stretch on muscle spindle secondary endings in the cat, *J Physiol* 253:341–356, 1975.

117. Eldred E, Lindsley DF, Buchwald JS: The effect of cooling on mammalian muscle spindles, *Exp Neurol* 2:144–157, 1960.

118. Keatinge WR: The effect of work and clothing on the maintenance of body temperature, *Q J Exp Physiol* 46:69–82, 1961.

119. Toner MM, McArdle WD: Physiological adjustments of man to the cold. In Pandolf KB, Sawka MN, Gonzalez RR, editors: *Human performance physiology and environmental medicine at terrestrial extremes*, Indianapolis, 1988, Benchmark Press.

120. Toner MM, Sawka MN, Pandolf KB: Thermal responses during arm and leg and combined arm-leg exercise in water, *J Appl Physiol* 56:1355–1360, 1984.

121. Park VS, Pendergast DR, Rennie DW: Decreases in body insulation with exercise in cold water, *Undersea Biomed Res* 11:159–168, 1984.

122. Veicsteinas A, Ferretti GT, Rennie DW: Superficial shell insulation in resting and exercising man in cold, *J Appl Physiol* 52:1557–1564, 1982.

123. Smith RM, Hanna JM: Skinfolds and resting heat loss in cold air and water: Temperature equivalence, *J Appl Physiol* 39:93–102, 1975.

124. Graham TE: Thermal, metabolic, and cardiovascular changes in men and women during cold stress, *Med Sci Sports Exerc* 20:S185–S192, 1988.

125. Baum E, Bruck K, Schwennicke HP: Adaptive modifications in the thermoregulatory system of long-distance runners, *J Appl Physiol* 40:404–410, 1976.

126. Bittel JHM, Nonotte-Varly C, Livecchi-Gonnot GH, et al: Physical fitness and thermoregulatory reactions in a cold environment in men, *J Appl Physiol* 65:1984–1989, 1988.

127. Kollias J, Boileau R, Buskirk ER: Effects of physical conditioning in man on thermal responses to cold air, *Int J Biometeorol* 16:389–402, 1994.

128. Adams T, Heberling EJ: Human physiological responses to a standardized cold stress as modified by physical fitness, *J Appl Physiol* 13:226–230, 1958.

129. Young AJ, Sawka MN, Latzka WA, et al: Effect of aerobic fitness on thermoregulation, *Med Sci Sports Exerc* 25:S62, 1993.

130. Vaisrub S: Accidental hypothermia in the elderly, *J Am Med Soc* 239:1888, 1978.

131. Taylor G: The problem of hypothermia in the elderly, *Practitioner* 193:761–767, 1964.

132. Horvath SM, Rochelle RD: Hypothermia in the aged, *Environ Health Perspect* 20:127–130, 1977.

133. Young AJ: Effects of aging on human cold tolerance, *Exp Aging Res* 17:205–213, 1991.

134. Collins KJ, Dore C, Exton-Smith AN, et al: Accidental hypothermia and impaired temperature control homeostasis in the elderly, *Br Med J* 1:353–356, 1977.

135. Collins KJ, Easton JC, Exton-Smith AN: Shivering thermogenesis and vasomotor responses with convective cooling in the elderly, *J Physiol* 320:76, 1981.

136. Horvath SM, Radcliffe CE, Hutt BK, et al: Metabolic responses of old people to a cold environment, *J Appl Physiol* 8:145–148, 1955.

137. Spurr GB, Hutt BK, Horvath SM: The effects of age on finger temperature responses to local cooling, *Am Heart J* 50:551–555, 1955.

138. Mathew L, Purkayastha SS, Singh R, et al: Influence of aging in the thermoregulatory efficiency of man, *Int J Biometeorol* 30:137–145, 1986.

139. Wagner JA, Robinson S, Marino RP: Age and temperature regulation of humans in neutral and cold environments, *J Appl Physiol* 37:562–565, 1974.

140. Falk B, Bar-Or O, Smolander J, et al: Response to rest and exercise in the cold: Effects of age and aerobic fitness, *J Appl Physiol* 76:72–78, 1994.

141. Freund BJ, O'Brien C, Young AJ: Alcohol ingestion and temperature regulation during cold exposure, *Wildern Med* 5:88–98, 1994.

142. Haight JSJ, Keatinge WR: Failure of thermoregulation in the cold during hypoglycemia induced by exercise and ethanol, *J Physiol* 229:87–97, 1973.

143. Graham T, Dalton J: Effect of alcohol on man's response to mild physical activity in a cold environment, *Aviat Space Environ Med* 51:793–796, 1980.

144. Gale EAM, Bennett T, Green JH, et al: Hypoglycaemia, hypothermia and shivering in man, *Clin Sci* 61:463–469, 1981.

145. Wagner JA, Horvath SM: Influences of age and gender on human thermoregulatory responses to cold exposure, *J Appl Physiol* 58:180–186, 1985.

146. Jacobs I, Tiit T, Kerrigan-Brown D: Muscle glycogen depletion during exercise at 9°C and 21°C, *Eur J Appl Physiol* 54:35–39, 1985.

147. Martineau L, Jacobs I: Muscle glycogen utilization during shivering thermogenesis in humans, *J Appl Physiol* 65:2046–2050, 1988.

148. Blomstrand E, Essén-Gustavsson B: Influence of reduced muscle temperature on metabolism in type I and type II human muscle fibres during intensive exercise, *Acta Physiol Scand* 131:569–574, 1987.

149. Young AJ, Sawka MN, Neufer PD, et al: Thermoregulation during cold water immersion is unimpaired by low muscle glycogen levels, *J Appl Physiol* 66:1809–1816, 1989.

150. Hong SK, Rennie DW, Park YS: Cold acclimatization and deacclimatization of Korean woman divers, *Exerc Sport Sci Rev* 14:231–268, 1986.

151. LeBlanc J: *Man in the cold*, Springfield, IL, 1975, Charles C. Thomas.

152. Nelms JD, Soper DJG: Cold vasodilation and cold acclimatization in the hands of British fish filleters, *J Appl Physiol* 17:444–448, 1962.

153. LeBlanc J: Local adaptation to cold of the Gaspé fishermen, *J Appl Physiol* 17:950–952, 1962.

154. Claus-Walker J, Halstead LS, Carter RE, et al: Physiological responses to cold stress in healthy subjects and in subjects with cervical cord injuries, *Arch Phys Med Rehabil* 55:485–490, 1974.

155. Teng HC, Heyer HE: The relationship between sudden changes in weather and the occurrence of acute myocardial infarction, *Am Heart J* 49:9–20, 1955.

156. Anderson SD: Issues in exercise-induced asthma, *J Allergy Clin Immunol* 76:763–772, 1985.

157. Kalant H, Le AD: Effects of ethanol on thermoregulation, *Pharmacol Ther* 23:313–364, 1984.

158. Kortelainen MJ: Drugs and alcohol in hypothermia and hyperthermia related deaths: A retrospective study, *J Forensic Sci* 32:1704–1712, 1987.

159. Paton BC: Accidental hypothermia. In Schönbaum E, Lomax P, editors: *Thermoregulation: Pathology, pharmacology and therapy*, New York, 1991, Pergamon Press.

160. Curtis R: *Outdoor action guide to hypothermia and cold weather injuries*, Outdoor Action Program, The Trustees of Princeton University. Accessed November 18, 2008.from http://www.princeton.edu/~oa/safety/hypocold.shtml.

161. Wilkerson JA, editor: *Medicine for mountaineering and other wilderness activities*, Seattle, WA, 1992, The Mountaineers Books.

162. Mayo Clinic: *Hypothermia*, Mayo Foundation for Medical Education and Research (MFMER), 2008. Accessed November 18, 2008 from www.MayoClinic.com.

163. Health A to Z: Hypothermia, August 2006. Accessed November 18, 2008 from www.healthatoz.com/healthatoz/Atoz/common/standard/transform.jsp?requestURI5/healthatoz/Atoz/ency/hypothermia.jsp.

164. Wikipedia The Free Encyclopedia: *Frostbite*, Wikimedia Foundation Inc, 2008. Accessed November 18, 2008 from http://en.wikipedia.org/wiki/Frostbite.

165. Hackett PH, Roach RC, Sutton JR: High altitude medicine. In Auerbach PS, Geehr EC, editors: *Management of wilderness and environmental emergencies*, St Louis, 1989, Mosby.

166. Bezruchka S: High altitude medicine, *Med Clin North Am* 76:1481–1497, 1992.

167. Dempsey JA, Forester HV: Mediation of ventilatory adaptations, *Physiol Rev* 62:262–346, 1982.

168. Laciga P, Koller EA: Respiratory, circulatory, and ECG changes during acute exposure to high altitude, *J Appl Physiol* 41:159–167, 1976.

169. Huang SY, Alexander JK, Grover RF, et al: Hypocapnia and sustained hypoxia blunt ventilation on arrival at high altitude, *J Appl Physiol* 56:602–606, 1984.

170. Young AJ, Young PM: Human acclimatization to high terrestrial altitude. In Pandolf KB, Sawka MN, Gonzalez RR, editors: *Human performance physiology and environmental medicine at terrestrial extremes*, Indianapolis, 1988, Benchmark Press.

171. Alexander JK, Hartley LH, Modelski M, et al: Reduction of stroke volume in man following ascent to 3,100 m altitude, *J Appl Physiol* 23:849–858, 1967.

172. Vogel JA, Hansen JE, Harris CW: Cardiovascular responses in man during exhaustive work at sea level and high altitude, *J Appl Physiol* 23:531–539, 1967.

173. Vogel JA, Hartley LH, Cruz JC, et al: Cardiac output during exercise in sea level residents at sea level and high altitude, *J Appl Physiol* 36:169–172, 1974.

174. Horstman D, Weiskopf R, Jackson RE: Work capacity during 3-week sojourn at 4300 m: Effects of relative polycythemia, *J Appl Physiol* 49:311–318, 1980.

175. Lockhart A, Saiag B: Altitude and the human pulmonary circulation, *Clin Sci* 60:599–605, 1981.

176. Milledge JS: Salt and water control at altitude, *Int J Sports Med* 13(suppl 1):S61–S63, 1992.

177. Fortney SM, Nadel ER, Wenger CB, et al: Effect of blood volume on sweating rate and body fluids in exercising humans, *J Appl Physiol* 51:1594–1600, 1981.

178. Hannon JP: Comparative altitude adaptability in young men and women. In Folinsbee LJ, Wagner JA, et al, editors: *Environmental stress*, New York, 1978, Academic Press.

179. Buskirk ER: Decrease in physical work capacity at high altitude. In Hegnauer AH, editor: *Biomedicine of high terrestrial elevations*, Natick, MA, 1969, US Army Research Institute of Environmental Medicine.

180. Young AJ, Cymerman A, Burse RL: The influence of cardiorespiratory fitness on the decrement in maximal aerobic power at high altitude, *Eur J Appl Physiol* 54:12–15, 1985.

181. Fulco CS, Cymerman A: Human performance and acute hypoxia. In Pandolf KB, Sawka MN, Gonzalez RR, editors: *Human performance physiology and environmental medicine at terrestrial extremes*, Indianapolis, 1988, Benchmark Press.

182. Gleser MA: Effects of hypoxia and physical training on hemodynamic adjustments to one-legged cycling, *J Appl Physiol* 34:655–659, 1973.

183. Grover RF, Weil JV, Reeves JT: Cardiovascular adaptation to exercise at high altitude, *Exerc Sport Sci Rev* 14:269–302, 1986.

184. Stenberg J, Ekblom B, Messin R: Hemodynamic response to work at simulated altitude, 4000m, *J Appl Physiol* 21:1589–1594, 1966.

185. Faulkner JA, Daniels JT, Balke B: Effects of training at moderate altitude on physical performance capacity, *J Appl Physiol* 23:85–89, 1967.

186. Hansen JR, Vogel JA, Stelter GP, et al: Oxygen uptake in man during exhaustive work at sea level and high altitude, *J Appl Physiol* 26:511–522, 1967.

187. Buskirk ER, Kollias J, Akers RF, et al: Maximal performance at altitude and on return from altitude in conditioned runners, *J Appl Physiol* 23:259–266, 1967.

188. Adams WC, Bernauer EM, Dill DB, et al: Effects of equivalent sea level and altitude training on VO2 max and running performance, *J Appl Physiol* 39:262–266, 1975.

189. Dill DB, Adams WC: Maximal O2 uptake at sea level and at 3,090 m altitude in high school champion runners, *J Appl Physiol* 30:854–859, 1971.

190. Saltin B: Limitations to performance at altitude. In Sutton JR, Houston CS, Coates G, editors: *Hypoxia: The tolerable limits*, Indianapolis, 1988, Benchmark Press.

191. Reeves JT, Groves BM, Sutton JR, et al: Cardiac function with prolonged hypoxia. In Sutton JR, Houston CS, Coates G, editors: *Hypoxia: The tolerable limits*, Indianapolis, 1988, Benchmark Press.

192. Bouissou P, Peronnet F, Brisson G, et al: Metabolic and endocrine responses to graded exercise under acute hypoxia, *Eur J Appl Physiol* 55:290–294, 1986.

193. Escourrou P, Johnson DG, Rowell LB: Hypoxemia increases plasma catecholamine concentrations in exercising humans, *J Appl Physiol* 57:1507–1511, 1984.

194. Knuttgen HG, Saltin B: Oxygen uptake, muscle high-energy phosphates, and lactate in exercise under acute hypoxic conditions in man, *Acta Physiol Scand* 87:368–376, 1973.

195. Maher JT, Jones LG, Hartley LH: Effects of high altitude exposure on submaximal endurance capacity of man, *J Appl Physiol* 37:895–898, 1974.

196. Mizuno M, Juel C, Bro-Rasmussen T, et al: Limb skeletal muscle adaptation in athletes after training at altitude, *J Appl Physiol* 68:496–502, 1990.

197. Young AJ, Evans WJ, Cymerman A, et al: Sparing effect of chronic high-altitude exposure on muscle glycogen utilization, *J Appl Physiol* 52:857–862, 1982.

198. Brooks GA, Butterfield GE, Wolfe RR, et al: Decreased reliance on lactate during exercise after acclimatization to 4,300 m, *J Appl Physiol* 71:333–341, 1991.

199. Green HJ, Sutton JR, Wolfel EE, et al: Altitude acclimatization and energy metabolic adaptations in skeletal muscle during exercise, *J Appl Physiol* 73:2701–2708, 1992.

200. Cooke R, Pate E: The effects of ADP and phosphate on the contraction of muscle fibers, *Biophys J* 48:789–798, 1985.

201. Fulco CS, Cymerman A, Muza SR, et al: Adductor pollicis muscle fatigue during acute and chronic altitude exposure and return to sea level, *J Appl Physiol* 77:179–183, 1994.

202. Crow TJ, Kelman GR: Psychological effects of mild acute hypoxia, *Br J Anaesth* 45:335–337, 1973.

203. Levine BD, Stray-Gundersen J: A practical approach to altitude training: Where to live and train for optimal performance enhancement, *Int J Sports Med* 13(suppl 1):S209–S212, 1992.

204. Daniels J, Oldridge N: The effects of alternated exposure to altitude and sea level on world-class middle-distance runners, *Med Sci Sports Exerc* 2:107–112, 1970.

205. Levine BD, Engfred K, Friedman DB, et al: High altitude endurance training: Effect on aerobic capacity and work performance, *Med Sci Sports Exerc* 22:S35, 1990.

206. Brammell H, Morgan B, Niccoli S, et al: Exercise tolerance is reduced at high altitude in patients with coronary artery disease, *Circulation* 55(suppl 2):371, 1988.

207. Neill W, Hallenhauer M: Impairment of myocardial O2 supply due to hyperventilation, *Circulation* 52:854–858, 1975.

208. Ziolkowski L, Wojcik-Ziolkowska E: Ischemic alterations in electrocardiogram and hemodynamic insufficiency during physical exercise in the mountain environment in patients after myocardial infarction, *Przegl Lek* 44:400–406, 1987.

209. Graham WG, Houston CS: Short-term adaptation to moderate altitude—Patients with chronic obstructive pulmonary disease, *JAMA* 240:1491–1494, 1978.

210. Cymerman A, Rock PB: *Medical problems in high mountain environments: A handbook for medical officers*, Technical Report TN 94-2, Natick, MA, 1994, US Army Research Institute of Environmental Medicine.

211. Rathat C, Richalet JP, Herry JP, et al: Detection of high-risk subjects for high altitude diseases, *Int J Sports Med* 13(suppl 1):S76–S78, 1992.

212. McCafferty WB: *Air pollution and athletic performance*, Springfield, IL, 1981, Charles C. Thomas.

213. Raven PB: Heat and air pollution: The cardiac patient. In Pollock ML, Schmidt DH, editors: *Heart disease and rehabilitation*, Boston, 1979, Houghton Mifflin.

214. Aronow WS, Harris CN, Isbell MW, et al: Effect of freeway travel on angina pectoris, *Ann Intern Med* 77:669–676, 1972.

215. Aronow WS, Isbell MW: Carbon monoxide effect on exercise-induced angina pectoris, *Ann Intern Med* 79:392–395, 1973.

216. Turcotte H, Langdeau JB, Thibault G, et al: Prevalence of respiratory symptoms in an athlete, *Respir Med* 97(8):955–963, 2003.

217. *Dorland's Illustrated Medical Dictionary*, ed 31, Philadelphia, 2007, Saunders.

218. Allergy and Asthma Foundation of America: *Asthma Overview*, 2008. Accessed November 7, 2008 from http://www.aafa.org/display.cfm?id=8.

219. About.com: *Asthma triggers—Causes of asthma*, 2006. Accessed November 6, 2008 from http://lungdiseases.about.com/od/asthma/a/asthma_causes.htm.

220. Mayo Clinic: *Asthma—Treatments and drugs*, 2008. Accessed November 6, 2008 from http://www.mayoclinic.com/health/asthma/DS00021/DSECTION=treatments-and-drugs.

221. Discovery Health: *Allergies and asthma—Diagnosing allergy and asthma*, 2007. Accessed November 7, 2008 from http://health.discovery.com/centers/allergyasthma/treatment/testing.html.

222. Health A to Z: *Spirometry*, June 2007. Accessed November 7, 2008 from http://www.myoptumhealth.com/portal/Information/item/Spirometry?archiveChannel=Home%2FArticle&clicked=true.

223. About.com: *Methacholine challenge for asthma testing—Bronchoprovation*, May 2008. Accessed November 7, 2008 from http://asthma.about.com/od/asthmatesting/p/methchallenge.htm.

224. About.com: *Allergy testing for asthma. Diagnosing asthma*, December 2007. Accessed November 7, 2008 from http://asthma.about.com/lw/Health-Medicine/Conditions-and-diseases/Allergy-Testing-and-Asthma.htm.

225. Morton AR, Fitch KD: Asthma. In Skinner JS: *Exercise testing and exercise prescription for special cases,* ed 3, Baltimore, 2005, Lippincott Williams & Wilkins.

226. Moorman JE, Rudd RA, Johnson CA, et al: National Surveillance for Asthma –United States, 1980-2009, Morb Mortal Wkly Rep 56(s508):1–4, 18–54, 2007. Accessed 11/7/2008 from http://www.cdc.gov/ mmwr/preview/mmwrhtml/ss5608/al.htm

227. Sidofsky C: *Can't breathe? Suspect vocal cord dysfunction!* 2001. Accessed at http://www.cantbreathesuspectvcd.com/.

228. National Jewish *Health: Management and treatment of vocal cord dysfunction,* July 2006. Accessed November 7, 2008 from http://www.nationaljewish.org/disease-info/diseases/vcd/management.aspx.

229. Brugman SM, Simons MD, Stephen M: Vocal cord dysfunction: Don't mistake it for asthma, *Phys Sportsmed* 26(5):63–85, 1998.

230. Nicholson JP, Case DB: Carboxyhemoglobin levels in New York City runners, *Phys Sportsmed* 11:135–138, 1983.

231. Ekblom B, Huot R: Response to submaximal and maximal exercise at different levels of carboxyhemoglobin, *Acta Physiol Scand* 86:474–482, 1972.

232. Gliner JA, Raven PB, Horvath SM, et al: Man's physiological response to long-term work during thermal and pollutant stress, *J Appl Physiol* 39:628–632, 1975.

233. Pirnay F, Dujardin J, Deroanne R, et al: Muscular exercise during intoxication by carbon monoxide, *J Appl Physiol* 31:573–575, 1971.

234. Vogel JA, Gleser MA: Effect of carbon monoxide on oxygen transport during exercise, *J Appl Physiol* 32:234–239, 1972.

235. Nielsen B: Exercise temperature plateau shifted by a moderate carbon monoxide poisoning, *J Physiol* (Paris) 63:362–365, 1971.

236. Horvath SM, Raven PB, Dahms TE, et al: Maximal aerobic capacity at different levels of carboxyhemoglobin, *J Appl Physiol* 38:300–303, 1975.

237. Horvath SM: Impact of air quality in exercise performance, *Exerc Sport Sci Rev* 9:265–296, 1981.

238. Anderson EW, Andelman RJ, Strauch JM, et al: Effect of low-level carbon monoxide exposure on onset and duration of angina pectoris: A study in ten patients with ischemic heart disease, *Ann Intern Med* 79:46–50, 1973.

239. Allred EN, Bleecker ER, Chaitman BR, et al: Short-term effects of carbon monoxide exposure on the exercise performance of subjects with coronary artery disease, *N Engl J Med* 321:1426–1432, 1989.

240. Adams KF, Koch G, Chatterjee B, et al: Acute elevation of blood carboxyhemoglobin to 6% impairs exercise performance and aggravates symptoms in patients with ischemic heart disease, *J Am Coll Cardiol* 12:900–909, 1988.

241. Calverley PM, Leggett RJ, Flenley DC: Carbon monoxide and exercise tolerance in chronic bronchitis and emphysema, *Br Med J* 283:878–880, 1981.

242. Aronow WS, Schlueter WJ, Williams MA, et al: Aggravation of exercise performance in patients with anemia by 3% carboxyhemoglobin, *Environ Res* 35:394–398, 1984.

243. Pandolf KB: Air quality and human performance. In Pandolf KB, Sawka MN, Gonzalez RR, editors: *Human performance physiology and environmental medicine at terrestrial extremes,* Indianapolis, 1988, Benchmark Press.

244. Kirkpatrick MB, Sheppard D, Nadel JA, et al: Effect of the oronasal breathing route on sulfur-dioxide-induced bronchoconstriction in exercising asthmatic subjects, *Am Rev Respir Dis* 125:627–631, 1982.

245. Linn WS, Jones MP, Bailey RM, et al: Respiratory effects of mixed nitrogen dioxide and sulfur dioxide in human volunteers under simulated ambient exposure conditions, *Environ Res* 22:431–438, 1980.

246. Sheppard D, Saisho A, Nadel JA, et al: Exercise increases sulfur dioxide–induced bronchoconstriction in asthmatic subjects, *Am Rev Respir Dis* 123:486–491, 1981.

247. Sheppard D, Wong WS, Uehara CF, et al: Lower threshold and greater bronchomotor responsiveness of asthmatic subjects to sulfur dioxide, *Am Rev Respir Dis* 122:873–878, 1980.

248. Amdur MO, Melvin WW Jr, Drinker P: Effects of inhalation of sulfur dioxide in man, *Lancet* 265:758–759, 1953.

249. Andersen I, Lundqvist GR, Jensen PL, et al: Human response to controlled levels of sulfur dioxide, *Arch Environ Health* 28:31–39, 1974.

250. Sheppard D, Epstein J, Bethel RA, et al: Tolerance to sulfur dioxide–induced bronchoconstriction in subjects with asthma, *Environ Res* 30:412–419, *1983.*

251. Lowry T, Schuman LM: "Silo-filler's disease"—A syndrome caused by nitrogen dioxide, *JAMA* 162:153–160, 1956.

252. Von Nieding G, Krekeler G, Fuchs H, et al: Studies of the acute effects of NO_2 on lung function: Influence of diffusion, perfusion, and ventilation in the lungs, *Int Arch Arbeitsmed* 31:61–72, 1973.

253. Von Nieding G, Wagner M, Krekeler G, et al: Minimum concentrations of NO_2 causing acute effects on the respiratory gas exchange and airway resistance in patients with chronic bronchitis, *Int Arch Arbeitsmed* 27:338–348, 1971.

254. Horvath SM, Folinsbee LJ: *The effect of nitrogen dioxide on lung function in normal subjects,* Research Triangle Park, NC, 1978, US Environmental Protection Agency.

255. Morrow PE, Utell MJ, Bauer MA, et al: Pulmonary performance of elderly normal subjects and subjects with chronic obstructive pulmonary disease exposed to 0.3 ppm nitrogen dioxide, *Am Rev Respir Dis* 145:291–300, 1992.

256. Pierson WE, Covert DS, Koenig JQ: Air pollutants, bronchial hyperreactivity, and exercise, *J Allergy Clin Immunol* 73:717–721, 1984.

257. Widdicombe JG, Kent DC, Nadel JA: Mechanism of bronchoconstriction during inhalation of dust, *J Appl Physiol* 17:613–616, 1962.

258. Nadel JA, Comroe JH Jr: Acute effects of inhalation of cigarette smoke on airway conductance, *J Appl Physiol* 16:713–716, 1961.

259. Klausen K, Andersen C, Nandrop S: Acute effects of cigarette smoking and inhalation of carbon monoxide during maximal exercise, *Eur J Appl Physiol* 51:371–379, 1983.

260. Schonfeld BR, Adams WC, Schelegle ES: Duration of enhanced responsiveness upon re-exposure to ozone, *Arch Environ Health* 44:229–236, 1989.

261. Dimeo MJ, Glenn MG, Holtzman MJ, et al: Threshold concentration of ozone causing an increase in bronchial reactivity in humans and adaptation with repeated exposures, *Am Rev Respir Dis* 124:245–248, 1981.

262. Hackney JD, Linn WS, Mohler JG, et al: Experimental studies on human health effects of air pollutants II: Four-hour exposure to ozone alone and in combination with other pollutant gases, *Arch Environ Health* 30:379–384, 1975.

263. Hackney JD, Linn WS, Law DC, et al: Experimental studies on human health effects of air pollutants III: Two-hour exposure to ozone alone and in combination with other pollutant gases, *Arch Environ Health* 30:385–390, 1975.

264. Gong H, Brandley PW, Simmons MS, et al: Impaired exercise performance and pulmonary function in elite cyclists during low-level ozone exposure in a hot environment, *Am Rev Respir Dis* 134:726–733, 1986.

265. Schelegle ES, Adams WC: Reduced exercise time in competitive simulations consequent to low level ozone exposure, *Med Sci Sports Exerc* 18:408–414, 1986.

266. Folinsbee LJ, Bedi JF, Horvath SM: Pulmonary function changes after 1 h continuous heavy exercise in 0.21 ppm ozone, *J Appl Physiol* 57:984–988, 1984.

267. Adams WC, Schelegle ES: Ozone and high ventilation effects on pulmonary function and endurance performance, *J Appl Physiol* 55:805–812, 1983.

268. Gibbons SI, Adams WC: Combined effects of ozone exposure and ambient heat on exercising females, *J Appl Physiol* 57:450–456, 1984.

269. Folinsbee LJ, Silverman F, Shephard RJ: Decrease of maximum work performance following ozone exposure, *J Appl Physiol* 42:531–536, 1977.

270. Savin WM, Adams WC: Effects of ozone inhalation on work performance and VO$_2$ max, *J Appl Physiol* 46:309–314, 1979.

271. Horvath SM, Gliner JA, Matsen-Twisdale JA: Pulmonary function and maximum exercise responses following acute ozone exposure, *Aviat Space Environ Med* 50:901–905, 1979.

272. Bell KA, Linn WS, Hazucha M, et al: Respiratory effects of exposure to ozone plus sulfur dioxide in southern Californians and eastern Canadians, *Am Ind Hyg Assoc J* 38:696–706, 1977.

273. Hackney JD, Linn WS, Karuza SK, et al: Effects of ozone exposure in Canadians and southern Californians: Evidence for adaptation? *Arch Environ Health* 32:110–116, 1977.

274. Hackney JD, Linn WS, Mohler JG, et al: Adaptation to short-term respiratory effects of ozone in men exposed repeatedly, *J Appl Physiol* 43:82–85, 1977.

275. Folinsbee LJ: Effects of ozone exposure on lung function in man: A review, *Rev Environ Health* 3:211–240, 1981.

276. Folinsbee LJ, Bedi JF, Gliner JA, et al: Concentration dependence of pulmonary function adaptation to ozone. In Mehlman MA, Lee SD, Mustafa MG, editors: *The biomedical effects of ozone and related photochemical oxidants*, Princeton Junction, NJ, 1983, Princeton Scientific Publishers.

277. Folinsbee LJ, Bedi JF, Horvath SM: Respiratory responses in humans repeatedly exposed to low concentrations of ozone, *Am Rev Respir Dis* 121:431–439, 1980.

278. Gliner JA, Horvath SM, Folinsbee LJ: Preexposure to low ozone concentrations does not diminish the pulmonary function response on exposure to higher ozone concentrations, *Am Rev Respir Dis* 127:51–55, 1983.

279. Horvath SM, Gliner JA, Folinsbee LJ: Adaptation to ozone: Duration of effect, *Am Rev Respir Dis* 123:496–499, 1981.

280. Farrell BP, Kerr HD, Kulle TJ, et al: Adaptation in human subjects to the effects of inhaled ozone after repeated exposure, *Am Rev Respir Dis* 119:725–730, 1979.

281. Foxcroft WJ, Adams WC: Effects of ozone exposure on four consecutive days on work performance and VO$_2$ max, *J Appl Physiol* 61:960–966, 1986.

282. Linn WS, Medway DA, Anzar UT, et al: Persistence of adaptation to ozone in volunteers exposed repeatedly for six weeks, *Am Rev Respir Dis* 125:491–495, 1982.

283. Hazucha M, Bates DV: Combined effect of ozone and sulphur dioxide on human pulmonary function, *Nature* 257:50–51, 1975.

284. Bedi JF, Folinsbee LJ, Horvath SM, et al: Human exposure to sulfur dioxide and ozone: Absence of a synergistic effect, *Arch Environ Health* 34:233–239, 1979.

285. Bedi JF, Horvath SM, Folinsbee LJ: Human exposure to sulfur dioxide and ozone in a high temperature-humidity environment, *Am Ind Hyg Assoc J* 43:26–30, 1982.

286. Folinsbee LJ, Bedi JF, Horvath SM: Pulmonary response to threshold levels of sulfur dioxide (1.0 ppm) and ozone (0.3 ppm), *J Appl Physiol* 58:1783–1787, 1985.

287. Koenig JQ, Covert DS, Hanley QS, et al: Prior exposure to ozone potentiates subsequent response to sulfur dioxide in adolescent asthmatic subjects, *Am Rev Respir Dis* 141:377–380, 1990.

288. Folinsbee LJ, Bedi JF, Gliner JA, et al: Combined effects of ozone and nitrogen dioxide on respiratory function in man, *Am Ind Hyg Assoc J* 42:534–541, 1981.

289. Abe M: Effects of mixed NO$_2$-SO$_2$ gas on human pulmonary functions, *Bull Tokyo Med Dent Univ* 14:415–433, 1967.

290. Avol EL, Linn WS, Shamoo DA, et al: Acute respiratory effects of Los Angeles smog in continuously exercising adults, *J Air Pollut Control Assoc* 33:1055–1060, 1983.

291. Avol EL, Linn WS, Venet TG, et al: Comparative respiratory effects of ozone and ambient oxidant pollution exposure during heavy exercise, *J Air Pollut Control Assoc* 34:804–809, 1984.

292. Linn WS, Jones MP, Bachmayer EA, et al: Short-term respiratory effects of polluted ambient air: A laboratory study of volunteers in a high-oxidant community, *Am Rev Respir Dis* 121:243–252, 1980.

293. Ward M: *Mountain medicine: A clinical study of cold and high altitude*, London, 1975, Crosby Lockwood Staples.

294. Ellis FP: Mortality from heat illness and heat-aggravated illness in the United States, *Environ Res* 5:1–58, 1972.

295. Folinsbee LJ, Horvath SM, Raven PB, et al: Influence of exercise and heat stress on pulmonary function during ozone exposure, *J Appl Physiol* 43:409–413, 1977.

296. Raven PB, Drinkwater BL, Horvath SM, et al: Age, smoking habits, heat stress, and their interactive effects with carbon monoxide and peroxyacetylnitrate on man's aerobic power, *Int J Biometeorol* 18:222–232, 1974.

297. Drinkwater BL, Raven PB, Horvath SM, et al: Air pollution, exercise and heat stress, *Arch Environ Health* 28:177–181, 1974.

298. Raven PB, Drinkwater BL, Ruhling RO, et al: Effect of carbon monoxide and peroxyacetyl nitrate on man's maximal aerobic capacity, *J Appl Physiol* 36:288–293, 1974.

299. Katz RM: Prevention with and without the use of medications for exercise-induced asthma, *Med Sci Sports Exerc* 18:331–333, 1986.

300. Strauss RH, McFadden ER, Ingram RH Jr, et al: Enhancement of exercise-induced asthma by cold air, *N Engl J Med* 297:743–747, 1977.

301. Wagner JA, Horvath SM, Andrew GM, et al: Hypoxia, smoking history, and exercise, *Aviat Space Environ Med* 49:785–791, 1978.

302. Weiser PC, Morrill CG, Dickey DW, et al: Effects of low-level carbon monoxide exposure on the adaptation of healthy young men to aerobic work at an altitude of 1,610 meters. In Folinsbee LJ, Wagner JA, Borgia JF, et al, editors: *Environmental stress: Individual human adaptations*, New York, 1978, Academic Press.

303. *National Weather Service*: http://www.lightningsafety.noaa.gov/overview.htm. Accessed April 10, 2009.

304. DeFranco MJ, Baker CL, DaSilva JJ, et al: Environmental issues for team physicians, *Am J Sports Med* 36(11):2226–2237, 2008.

305. Fish R: Lightning injuries. In Tintinalli JE, Kelen GD, Stapczynski JS, editors: *Emergency medicine: A comprehensive study guide*, New York, 2004, McGraw Hill.

306. Walsh KM, Bennett B, Cooper MA, et al: National Athletic Trainers' Association position statement: Lightning safety for athletics and recreation, *J Athl Training* 35(4):471–477, 2000.

307. National Severe Storms Laboratory: Accessed April 19, 2009 from http://www.nssl.noaa.gov/primer/lightning/ltg_damage.html.

308. Moehrle M: Ultraviolet exposure in the Ironman triathalon, *Med Sci Sports Exerc* 33:1385–1386, 2001.

309. Moehrle M, Heinrich L, Schmid A, et al: Extreme UV exposure of professional cyclists, *Dermatology* 201:44–45, 2000.

310. DeFranco MJ, Baker CL III, DaSilva JJ, et al: Environmental issues for team physicians, *Am J Sports Med* 36:2226–2237, 2008.

311. Cho E, Rosner BA, Feskanich D, et al: Risk factors and individual probabilities of melanoma for whites, *J Clin Oncol* 23: 2669–2675, 2005.

312. Elwood JM, Jopson J: Melanoma and sun exposure: An overview of published studies, *Int J Cancer* 73:198–203, 1997.

313. Gallagher RP, Hill GB, Bajdik CD, et al: Sunlight exposure, pigmentary factors, and risk of nonmelanocytic skin cancer. I Basal cell carcinoma, *Arch Dermatol* 131:157–163, 1995.

314. Kricker A, Armstrong BK, English DR, et al: Does intermittent sun exposure cause basal cell carcinoma? A case-control study in Western Australia, *Int J Cancer* 60:489–494, 1995.

315. Han A, Maibach HI: Management of acute sunburn, *Am J Clin Dermatol* 5:39–47, 2004.

316. Katiyar SK, Matsui MS, Mukhtar H: Kinetics of UV light-induced cyclobutane pyrimidine dimers in human skin in vivo: An immunohistochemical analysis of both epidermis and dermis, *Photochem Photobiol* 72:788–793, 2000.

317. Cohen PH, Tsai H, Puffer JC: Sun-protective behavior among high school and collegiate athletes in Los Angeles, CA, *Clin J Sport Med* 16:253–260, 2006.

USE OF ERGOGENIC AIDS IN SPORT*

Jeffrey J. Zachwieja, Elizabeth A. Mooradian, and Kimberly M. White

Introduction

The term *ergogenic* literally means increasing body energy for physical or mental work. To an athlete, coach, or athletic care professional, an *ergogenic aid* is often thought of as a procedure or agent that improves performance beyond that normally obtained through sound training principals and good nutrition. This chapter discusses a broad range of ergogenic aids that have been used to improve endurance, speed, strength, and power and to improve body composition in response to training. Some discussion of potential ergogenic aids for bone and connective tissue has also been included, but the literature in this regard is far less developed for exercise training and healthy athletes. Furthermore, we have limited our discussion to nutritional ergogenic aids (caffeine and anabolic steroids are the exception) that are safe, legal, and appear to be reasonably effective. We have not addressed mechanical, biomechanical, psychological, or pharmacologic factors as was done in a previous edition of this book, *Athletic Injuries and Rehabilitation*. Our goal in this chapter is to provide greater depth of information on a small number of nutritional ergogenic aids that likely work. Each section starts with an overview of the physiological responses and biochemical pathways important for performance or adaptation. Then efficacy of each ergogenic aid is evaluated within the context of (1) the mechanism of action, (2) existing research, (3) practical application, and (4) potential for adverse effects.

---

* The information contained within this publication reflects the views of the authors and do not represent the official views of PepsiCo.

Ergogenic Aids for Physical Endurance and Perceptual Energy

Activities that Require Physical Endurance

Endurance can be defined as the ability to physically exert oneself aerobically or anaerobically for relatively long periods. Running, cycling, and triathlon are traditionally considered endurance sports, although each also has competitive distances that are classified as "sprint" and require shorter duration, high-intensity efforts for successful completion. Similarly, sports such as tennis, football, basketball, soccer, and hockey involve short-duration, high-intensity bursts of activity that must be maintained for a prolonged period. Thus these sports also contain an element of endurance. For the purpose of this discussion, physical endurance is defined as the ability to maintain repetitive muscle contractions lasting more than several minutes. In this way, we are casting a large net to broaden the applicability of the various nutritional ergogenic aids evaluated in this portion of the chapter.

Physiology and Physiological Consequences of Energy Generation for Endurance Activity

The primary energy substrate for muscle contraction is adenosine triphosphate (ATP). Because there is not enough ATP stored in muscle to support prolonged contraction, it must be constantly resynthesized. Breakdown of glucose in the glycolytic pathway and liberation of reducing equivalents via the citric acid cycle provides the oxygen-consuming electron transport chain in muscle mitochondria with the necessary electrons to generate ATP. Glucose is made available for this process either by the breakdown of muscle glycogen (glycogenolysis) or uptake of blood glucose, which for a time remains relatively constant because liver glucose output is able to keep pace with muscle glucose extraction. Likewise, fatty acids liberated from peripheral adipose tissue or intramuscular triglyceride stores can provide substrate for the citric acid cycle and subsequent ATP production by the electron transport chain. This so-called fatty acid oxidation is fundamentally important, especially during endurance activity, because it lessens the demand on the limited supply of glucose for ATP production. Lastly, amino acids generated from protein breakdown can provide carbon backbone for citric acid cycle intermediates and thereby contribute to reducing equivalent generation during exercise. Furthermore, amino acids such as alanine and glutamine are gluconeogenic precursors in the liver and thus support liver glucose output.

The cardiovascular system is also an integral part of the response to endurance exercise. Heart rate, stroke volume, and blood pressure increase to provide effective delivery of blood throughout the vascular system. Vasodilation and vasoconstrictive processes direct blood flow to and permit adequate perfusion of contracting skeletal muscle, and tissues that are less metabolically active such as the gut, spleen, and kidney are perfused to a smaller extent. Adequate blood perfusion of contracting skeletal muscle is necessary to meet the need for augmented oxygen and nutrient (i.e., glucose, fatty acids, and amino acids) uptake as well as removal of metabolic wastes such as carbon dioxide (CO_2), lactate, and amino nitrogen from amino acid transamination and deamination processes. Metabolic processes within skeletal muscle are not 100% efficient. Therefore, heat is generated and this too must be removed to ensure effective operating temperatures within skeletal muscle. The dissipation of metabolic heat is achieved primarily by vascular adjustments that redirect a portion of the blood flow to the skin. Vasodilatation of blood vessels in the skin allow for heat loss through conductive and convective processes. However, the largest portion of heat loss comes from evaporative cooling. Heat-activated sweat glands secrete large quantities of water and salts (sweat). When this sweat comes in contact with and evaporates from the skin surface, a cooling effect occurs. The cooled skin reduces the temperature of blood that is shunted to it and in turn mitigates an excessive rise in core temperature. Although effective for cooling, sweat evaporation during prolonged exercise can significantly reduce the body's water and electrolyte reserves and induce a state of hypohydration. This can compromise cardiovascular function and impede further heat dissipation.

Adaptation of Physiological Systems to Chronic Endurance Training

Cardiovascular and metabolic adaptations in skeletal muscle occur in response to chronic endurance exercise training. These adaptations allow for an increase in maximum aerobic capacity (i.e., maximum oxygen consumption [VO_2 max]), but, more importantly, also improve an athlete's ability to tolerate a higher percentage of aerobic capacity during prolonged exercise. This equates to a faster pace and hence a reduced time to cover a competitive distance.

Left ventricular hypertrophy accounts for a substantial portion of the increase in heart size that results from endurance exercise training. Left ventricular hypertrophy contributes to an increased stroke volume and greater maximal cardiac output in trained individuals. Submaximal heart rate is decreased during exercise because of a greater stroke volume and expanded plasma volume allowing for a greater venous return in the trained state. Together with an increased hemoglobin concentration and greater capillarization of skeletal muscle, these cardiovascular adaptations allow for a greater oxygen delivery to skeletal muscle during maximal exercise.

Cardiovascular Endurance Adaptations with Training

- Hypertrophy of left ventricle
- Increased stroke volume
- Submaximal heart rate decreases
- Expanded plasma volume
- Greater venous return
- Increased hemoglobin concentration
- Increased capillarization of skeletal muscle

Regular endurance training also stimulates adaptations within skeletal muscle. The most prominent is an increase in mitochondrial biogenesis, which leads to more mitochondria and an expanded reticulum of mitochondria that resides amid the muscle cell architecture. This allows for more efficient oxygen use during submaximal exercise and the ability to consume more of the oxygen delivered to muscle during maximal exercise. The activity of each mitochondria is also enhanced in the trained state, exemplified by elevations in key enzymes responsible for the Krebs cycle and electron-transport activity (i.e., citrate synthase and cytochrome C oxidase, respectively). In the trained state, skeletal muscle has an increased capacity to oxidize fatty acids as a fuel and this helps to conserve carbohydrate during prolonged exercise. Paradoxically, endurance exercise training results in increased intramuscular stores of triglycerides. Muscle glycogen content is also increased, most likely because of greater insulin sensitivity. Lactate production during submaximal exercise is decreased in endurance-trained muscle in addition to a greater capacity for lactate clearance and oxidation. This is exemplified by lower blood lactate levels for any given level of submaximal exercise in the trained state. Lastly, endurance exercise training up-regulates key endogenous antioxidant enzymes and systems most likely to deal with elevated production of reactive oxygen species (ROS) (i.e., free radicals).

Muscle Endurance Adaptations with Training

- Increased mitochondrial biogenesis
- Increased key enzymes
- Increased capacity to oxidize fatty acids
- Increased stores of intramuscular triglycerides
- Increased muscle glycogen
- Decreased lactate production

These training adaptations serve as the base for improvements in exercise performance. There are no nutritional paradigms or ergogenic aids that can induce the types and extent of adaptation described previously. Therefore, ergogenic aids do not have the potential to "make up" for a poor commitment to sound training. Rather, they are most effective when used to maximize adaptation and performance in athletes committed to sound training routines and principles.

Neural Control of Muscle Contraction and Physiological Response

The movement associated with endurance exercise is initiated and regulated by neural pathways linked together in the central nervous system (CNS). Central command theory[1] suggests that signals originating in brain nuclei in the motor cortex lead to activation of motor nerves and subsequent muscle contraction. Importantly, central command signals also activate areas of the brain responsible for autonomic nervous system (ANS) outflow. Therefore, in response to the intent to exercise, central command generates signals that excite spinal motor units as well as ANS effector responses so physiological systems are prepared to take on the challenge of exercise. Peripheral feedback and reflexes are important features to this system because they act to fine-tune central command signals and ANS outflow to maintain the appropriate level of motor activation and overall physiological homeostasis for a given level of exercise.

ANS outflow is particularly important for cardiovascular, thermoregulatory, and metabolic adjustments needed to sustain exercise. The ANS influences these body systems in two primary ways: (1) activity of autonomic nerves and their release of neurotransmitters and (2) responsiveness of peripheral tissues to neurohormonal factors released into circulation. For example, withdrawal of vagal nerve activity at the onset of exercise increases heart rate and cardiac output. With increasing intensity of exercise, further increases in heart rate and ventricular contractility are achieved via activation of sympathetic nerves to cardiac tissue as well as beta-adrenergic stimulation from epinephrine released by the adrenal medulla. Increased cardiac output during exercise provides blood flow to muscles and supports blood pressure in the face of massive vasodilation in muscle, which is a threat for an overall reduction in blood pressure and drop in perfusion capacity. Fortunately,

sympathoadrenal activation also produces constriction in blood vessels to redirect blood away from less metabolically active tissue and sends more to active muscle for oxygen and nutrient delivery and to skin for heat dissipation. Metabolic adjustments achieved as a consequence of sympathoadrenal activity includes epinephrine-induced elevations in peripheral adipose tissue lipolysis and glycogenolysis in the liver. Elevated epinephrine levels also reduce insulin secretion allowing for greater activation of lipolysis and release of glucagon, which contributes to accelerated rates of liver glycogenolysis. Clearly, the CNS and ANS play a key role in physiological initiation and adjustments to go from rest to exercise.

Autonomic Nervous System Influence

- Controls many neurotransmitters
- Responds to release of neurohormones

Perceptual and Brain Metabolic Responses to Physical Work

Under normal circumstances, most endurance athletes do not make objective assessments of power or work output during competition or training (although with the advent of bike computer systems and power cranks, it is becoming more commonplace for cyclists). Thus, during prolonged exercise adjustments in effort to speed up, slow down, or completely stop are usually made based on subjective sensations. What is interesting is that this most basic and familiar aspect of exercise is the least understood. Whether these subjective feelings originate in the CNS, come about as a result of peripheral feedback, or are some integration of the two manifested through intricate neurological feedforward and feedback systems is not known. What is known, however, is that perception of physical effort and actual exercise intensity are well related.[2] Various psychological factors such as mood, drive, motivation, and arousal undoubtedly play a role in subjective sensation of effort. Thus, how an athlete feels, the athlete's previous experiences, and the athlete's expectations are all an integral part of the exercise response. This was cleverly identified by Friedman and Elliot[3] who recently showed that simply exposing subjects to a sports drink (i.e., no consumption) prior to a physical task resulted in that task being viewed as more of a positive challenge and this subsequently led to a greater persistence of physical effort.

Clinical Point

Perception of physical effort and actual exercise intensity are closely related.

The brain is indeed a metabolically active organ and its metabolism is in response to heightened neurological activity and helps to drive such activity. For example, when the brain is activated in response to a mental task, global blood flow to the brain is increased to supply oxygen and nutrients. However, during exercise, global blood flow to the brain is similar to blood flow to the brain at rest because it seems to be under the influence of arterial CO_2 tension rather than changes in the metabolic state related to motor activation.[4] With increasing exercise intensity, arterial CO_2 tension is reduced (as a result of hyperventilation) and this results in a constriction of cerebral arterioles leading to reduced blood flow even though brain metabolic activity is elevated. Fortunately, increased oxygen extraction can compensate for lower perfusion under these circumstances. Regional blood flow in the brain may be the more important dynamic at the onset and with continued exercise.[5,6] During exercise, blood flow to cortical motor areas in the brain increase, as does flow to sensorimotor cortex areas presumably for adjustment of central command or fatigue-related feedback. In addition, exercise increases flow to areas of the brain related to cardiovascular, respiratory, and thermoregulatory control.

Increases in regional blood flow in the brain are important not only for oxygen delivery but also for glucose delivery. Glucose is the main energy source for brain cells and a continuous systemic supply is necessary because there is very little glycogen storage in neuronal tissue. Under conditions of demanding exercise, glucose metabolism in the brain can limit performance in two main ways. First, if neuronal activity exceeds the capacity for aerobic and anaerobic metabolism of glucose, brain cell function will deteriorate, lessening the effectiveness of central command and homeostatic regulation. Second, the energy generated as the result of oxidation of glucose in brain cells will end up entirely as heat because no mechanical work is performed in these cells. Although under normal circumstances this heat is adequately removed by the cerebral circulation, during exercise, especially under conditions of environmental heat stress, heat removal from the brain is impaired and heat storage can occur.

Clinical Point

Elevation of brain temperature above a critical level can reduce activity of motor neurons and thus central drive.

The most popular and well-studied brain biochemical pathway as it relates to exercise is the serotonergic system. Serotonergic neurotransmission depends on the synthesis, storage, release, and re-uptake of serotonin from neuronal projections. Serotonergic neurons play a key role in various autonomic and behavioral functions; elevations in brain serotonin levels have been linked to feeding behavior, temperature regulation, sleep, lethargy, drowsiness, and loss of motivation. The latter behavioral effects of serotonin have been used to form the basis of an exercise central fatigue hypothesis.[7] The amino acid tryptophan is the precursor for serotonin synthesis. During exercise, free tryptophan levels in the blood increase because an elevation in free fatty acids (FFAs) displaces albumin-bound tryptophan. This, in combination with a reduction in circulating branched amino acid concentration, increases the transport of tryptophan across the blood-brain barrier, resulting in an elevated rate of serotonin synthesis and the resultant behavioral effects of lethargy and loss of motivation, leading to a decline in physical effort. Indeed, exercise in humans elevates free tryptophan levels in blood as well as prolactin levels, a hormone secreted from the pituitary gland and under the influence of serotonin stimulation. Thus, an elevation in blood prolactin concentration has been used as a "biomarker" of central serotonergic activity. However, serotonin is one of many neurotransmitters in the brain and it seems extremely unlikely that it could be the sole source of fatigue induction during exercise. For example, dopamine is known to play an important role in motor activation and its metabolism is enhanced during exercise. An emerging variation on the central fatigue hypothesis states the ratio of serotonin-to-dopamine may be an important determinant of fatigue development rather than either one alone.[8]

Clinical Point

Neurotransmitters and its production play a major role in autonomic and behavioral functions.

Causes of Fatigue During Endurance Activity

There are likely two contributing factors to the onset of fatigue during prolonged exercise, one that is centrally mediated and another that is peripherally mediated. Environmental conditions (e.g., hot, humid, cold, altitude) and the level of physical training can have an influence on how and when these site-specific fatigue mechanisms are expressed. Classic literature reduction tells us that peripheral fatigue likely results from substrate depletion (i.e., low muscle glycogen and blood glucose) or accumulation of metabolic byproducts, including the possibility of free-radical mediated oxidative damage to contractile proteins and those proteins responsible for initiating and maintaining calcium fluxes important for contractile activity. Hypohydration and hyperthermia are common during prolonged exercise and can influence centrally mediated mechanisms (e.g., CNS and cardiovascular) that precipitate fatigue. In what seems to be the ultimate central fatigue hypothesis, Noakes and colleagues[9] have proposed the central governor model. Essentially, this model proposes that the brain regulates motor unit recruitment during exercise with a *modus operandi* of preventing complete physiological failure. Nonetheless, exercise-induced fatigue and fatigue processes remain a very controversial topic. The exact mechanism or combinations of mechanisms have not been completely defined and to add to the complexity, no one definition for fatigue during exercise can be agreed upon. For example, does fatigue occur at a specific point in time or are there small, incremental reductions in muscle force production that begin with the onset of exercise that are not detectable (mentally or physiologically) until later?

Clinical Point

Fatigue during endurance exercise may be centrally or peripherally mediated.

What does seem to be clear is that fatigue during prolonged exercise is simply not the result of substrate depletion (i.e., muscle and liver glycogen). Results of research conducted by Coggan and Coyle[10] eloquently support this point. They had cyclists pedal a stationary bicycle to a point of volitional fatigue. Thereafter, three randomized, double-blind treatments were administered in a repeated measures design: (1) placebo, (2) oral glucose, and (3) glucose infusion. During the placebo and oral glucose trials, saline infusions were conducted to achieve complete blinding, as was oral ingestion of a placebo during glucose infusion. Time to volitional fatigue during a second stationary cycling bout was longer during both glucose trials relative to placebo and longest during glucose infusion. Glucose was infused at a rate to match carbohydrate oxidation during exercise and to maintain blood glucose. Thus, glucose substrate supply was not limiting, yet the subjects still became fatigued approximately 40 minutes after initiating the second bout of exercise. This indicates that factors in addition to substrate supply contribute to fatigue during prolonged exercise.

Sorting Out the Pros and Cons for Nutritional Ergogenic Aids

The basic tenet of a nutritional ergogenic aid for endurance exercise is that consumption of a particular ingredient or combination of ingredients will enhance performance, presumably by delaying the onset of fatigue. Often, such aids derive from a focus on single metabolic pathways thought to be integral for muscle energy metabolism or central mediated processes. Given the complexity of the underlying physiological mechanisms contributing to the onset of fatigue, it is not surprising that there is a long list of so-called ergogenic aids that have proven to be ineffective for preventing fatigue during prolonged exercise. In fact, nutritional approaches beyond simple hydration and carbohydrate feeding paradigms often fall short on relative effectiveness scales.

That said, there are some emerging data for protein, various amino acids, antioxidants, and carnitine that make these ingredients increasingly attractive as ergogenic aids. Scientific support and practical application principals for these ingredients are reviewed in the next section.

Ergogenic Aids for Endurance that Have Little Scientific Support, Lack Investigation or Are Illegal

- Aspartate
- Asparagine
- Bee Pollen
- Calcium
- Choline
- Coenzyme Q10
- Dimethylglycine (B_{15})
- Folic acid
- Ginseng
- Inosine
- Citrulline-malate
- Medium chain triglycerides
- Niacin
- Phosphates
- *Rhodiola rosea*
- Riboflavin (B_2)
- Ribose
- Taurine
- Thiamine

Although scientific support is often used as a guiding light for effectiveness, the statistical methodologies used to determine if an experimental result is "significant" may be too stringent for practical use. For example, most exercise and nutrition science research uses hypothesis-testing approaches that deem results significant when there is a probability of 1 out of 20 responses showing a false-positive effect. Most athletes would be far more lenient in their evaluation of the chance to receiving a positive benefit from a nutritional ergogenic aid. Furthermore, such objective measures as power output and time are used as dependent variables in ergogenic aid research. But consideration must be given to mood, sensation, and emotional domains, because they may be more powerful indicators of a positive effect and future success.

Ultimately it comes down to calculating a favorable risk/benefit ratio when athletes and their advisors are deciding whether to use an ergogenic aid. They should develop ergogenic routines rooted in scientific support but also proven within the realm of personal experience.

Clinical Point

If an athlete has a preconceived notion or believes something will work, there is a good chance that a positive performance outcome will be derived from the ergogenic tactic he or she believes in.

Ergogenic Aids for Endurance Activities
Water and Electrolytes

Action. Water and electrolyte intake before and during exercise offset losses caused by sweating and thereby slows the rate of dehydration and limits the amount of hypohydration (decrease in body water levels from normal). Guarding against hypohydration preserves exercise performance and limits the risk for developing a heat illness, especially under conditions of high environmental heat stress.

Research. Prolonged training and competition can elicit substantial water and electrolyte loss through sweating. For example, sweat rates typically exceed 1 L/hr and at times exceed 2.5 L/hr in hot and humid conditions. Other factors that affect sweat rate are intensity of exercise, clothing or protective equipment, fitness level, and acclimation to a hot environment. Although the electrolyte content of sweat is fairly diluted, large absolute volumes of sweat loss can result in large electrolyte losses. For example, an average sweat sodium concentration is approximately 900 mg/L. Thus, for a training session that elicits a total sweat loss of 3 L, 2.7 g ([900 × 3]/1000) of sodium is lost. This amount of sodium loss, which could easily accumulate during a 2-hour training session, is close to the recommended total daily sodium intake (3 g) for an average, nonathletic person.

It goes without saying that it is important to replace water and electrolyte losses. Water is a major constituent of the fluid inside and outside of cells as well as a major component of blood within the vascular system. Electrolyte concentrations and gradients ensure proper distribution of water inside and outside of cells and the vascular space. From a cellular and vascular point of view, no amount of water loss can be tolerated without physiological strain. Hence, whenever athletes train or compete, their physiologic systems are compromised, especially when sweat rate exceeds the rate at which water is voluntarily consumed or the gastric emptying rate. This leads to progressive dehydration and ultimately a state of hypohydration. Hypohydration during exercise results in an abnormally high core temperature, reduced blood volume, decreased stroke volume, increased heart rate, and reduced skin blood flow.[11] Furthermore, hypohydration is known to accelerate glycogen use and increases perception of effort.[11] Many, if not all of these negative physiologic consequences of hypohydration can be reversed or prevented by an appropriate amount of water intake prior to and during exercise.[12] The risk of developing hypohydration and the manifestation of impaired physiologic function is increased when training or competing in hot versus temperate environments. Furthermore, hypohydrated athletes are at increased risk for developing heat-related illnesses such as heat exhaustion and heat stroke.[13]

Hypohydration impairs prolonged exercise performance, especially in hot and humid environments. This is likely caused by elevated core temperature and cardiovascular strain.[14] Hypohydration (as well as hyperthermia) can also negatively affect cellular function in the CNS such that cognitive and mental performance declines.[15] This is relevant for sports that rely on concentration and cognition to drive skill- or tactical-oriented tasks for performance. Indeed, recent data shows that hypohydration of between −2% and −4% initial body mass impaired basketball shooting and movement skill performance.[16] The exact amount of hypohydration needed to elicit impaired physical, cognitive, and skill performance is not really known, although many would suggest that performance drops off considerably at a hypohydration of −2% or more. What does seem to be clear is that performance worsens with progressing dehydration. However, it is important to know what the critical water deficit is for impairment in exercise performance because this helps establish more practical fluid replacement routines that are focused on minimizing hypohydration rather than completely preventing it. The benefits of fluid ingestion while exercising in the heat are likely delayed. Data from Montain and Coyle[17] suggest that it takes 40 to 60 minutes for ingested fluid to be absorbed and distributed throughout the body before it can influence cardiovascular function and thermoregulation. Thus, it may be best to ingest larger volumes early in exercise and continue to ingest throughout to offset absorption and distribution delays on body-water balance and resultant physiological function.

> **Clinical Point**
>
> Dehydration adversely affects exercise, cognitive and mental performance, and thermoregulation.

It is often assumed that athletes are well-hydrated prior to training and competition. In fact, this is not the case. Several studies have documented through urine specific gravity measurements that many athletes show up to train or compete in a hypohydrated state.[18-20] This happens more frequently when multiple training or competitive sessions occur over a short period (e.g., two-a-days, multigame tournaments, or invitationals). In this circumstance, it has been shown that providing high school football players with fluid and drinking instructions after one practice, coupled with fluid intake approximately 1 hour prior to a subsequent practice improved markers of hydration status that were obtained just before taking the field.[18] In some situations in which there is the need to rehydrate even more quickly between training or competitive bouts, intravenous (IV) rehydration has been used to ensure quick delivery of fluid to central circulation. However, research has shown that when rehydrating with equal amounts of IV rehydration and oral fluids, IV rehydration is not superior for restoring plasma volume from a state of hypohydration.[21,22]

Most exercise scientists and practitioners recommend water and electrolyte intake for hydration purposes during prolonged exercise. Sodium is the major electrolyte lost in sweat and its replacement seems to be the most critical for performance and health. Consuming pure water during prolonged exercise at a rate that completely replaces sweat loss results in a progressive decline in plasma sodium, whereas consumption of an equal volume of water with sodium added maintained plasma sodium concentration.[23] Maintenance of plasma sodium during prolonged exercise keeps cells and the vasculature in proper fluid balance for optimal functioning. In addition, consumption of sodium in water appears to increase voluntary drinking through an osmotic stimulus[24] and can result in better replacement of the fluid lost through sweat.[25] In general, the causes of muscle cramping are complex, but there appears to be a subset of muscle cramps that are brought on by large fluid and electrolyte losses during intense exercise in the heat. For example, there is a high incidence of exercise-induced muscle cramping in tennis players,[26] American football players,[27] and military personnel deployed to hot environments.[28] In particular, it has been shown that those football players with a history of muscle cramping exhibit higher sweat rates and sweat sodium concentrations than those who do not.[27] Likewise, Bergeron[26] described a tennis player who suffered from frequent muscle cramping as having a sweat rate of 2.5 L/hr and a sweat sodium concentration of 1.9 g/L (a normal value is approximately 0.9 g/L). Thus, it appears prudent to supplement these players with extra sodium, which is often the recommendation, but to date there is no empirical data to support this approach for preventing or reversing muscle cramps.

On the surface, prevention of hypohydration seems to be as simple as water in versus water out, as can be surmised from the previous discussion; however, there are numerous scientific-, practical-, performance-, and health-related considerations when assessing the effect of exercise-induced water and electrolyte loss and rehydration practices and principles. Many of these topics have been discussed and debated at scientific conferences, in the literature, and in the media. A complete recounting of these topics is not possible within this brief review. Thus, if readers are keen to learn more, the authors point them to several review articles,[29-32] position stands,[33,34] and a recent debate[35] for greater depth and breadth of information.

Application. Because athletes differ in body size, sweat rates, and training regimens, it is difficult to recommend one hydration approach that suits all athletes. Therefore, individual athletes (or those working with the athlete) need to know how much they sweat during prolonged exercise so they can best understand how much fluid they need to replace. Monitoring the change in body weight before and after exercise is a good way to gauge sweat loss and thus fluid needs. For example, if an athlete loses 1.5 pounds (0.7 kg) while consuming 12 ounces of fluid during 1 hour

of exercise, he or she should try to drink an additional 24 ounces for a total of 36 ounces (12 + 24) to keep pace with sweat loss during that hour of exercise. It is important to note, however, the goal is to replace what has been lost without drinking too much. A weight gain after exercise indicates that too much fluid has been consumed. Other practical tips include drinking small volumes of fluid more frequently rather than a large bolus once feeling parched and drinking fluids that are lightly flavored, slightly salty, and somewhat sweet as this will help encourage drinking behavior that better offsets sweat loss, and, whenever possible, drink fluids that are cool (i.e., refrigerator temperature) rather than room temperature or warmer.

Clinical Point

Monitoring body weight before and after exercise is a good way to monitor sweat loss and fluid needs.

Adverse Effects. The only adverse effect associated with hydration practices during prolonged exercise is the development of hyponatremia. Hyponatremia is a complication caused by low plasma sodium levels. A strict definition of hyponatremia is a plasma sodium level less than 130 mEq/L, but symptoms and serious complications generally occur when plasma sodium decreases to less than 125 mEq/L. The cause of hyponatremia is likely associated with multiple factors, but overdrinking fluid has been identified as the greatest risk factor for developing hyponatremia, particularly when overdrinking pure water. This is because the excess water has the potential to dilute the plasma-sodium concentration. Therefore, as indicated previously, one should ingest fluid during prolonged exercise at a rate that closely matches fluid loss and does not result in weight gain after the training or competitive session has ended. Consuming fluids with electrolytes, particularly sodium, has the potential to maintain plasma sodium levels throughout the course of prolonged exercise. Some have suggested that allowing hypohydration would guard against hyponatremia because of a contraction of the extracellular fluid space and consequent rise in plasma sodium. However, the increased risk of heat illness associated with hypohydration does not warrant this approach.

Glycerol

Action. Ingestion of glycerol in a water-based solution prior to exercise promotes fluid retention and increases total body water. This so-called hyperhydration effect could effectively delay the amount of time it takes to reach a level of hypohydration that increases cardiovascular strain, disrupts thermoregulation, and leads to a decrement in exercise performance.

Research. Rapid clearance of excess fluid intake makes it difficult to hyperhydrate with common water-based drinks. However, it has been reported that solutions with a very high sodium and citrate concentration can increase fluid retention and expand plasma volume.[36] The problem is that the palatability of such drinks is quite low. Orally ingested glycerol can also create an osmotic stimulus for hyperhydration, especially when subsequent water intake approaches 20 mL/kg/body weight (bw).[37] The usefulness of this approach to delay the point at which an athlete becomes hypohydrated during exercise has been debated for more than 20 years. Although generally it is agreed that hyperhydration likely provides no clear physiological or performance advantage over normal hydration, involuntary dehydration during exercise is more common than not,[38] even in the presence of readily accessible fluid. Furthermore, there are often logistical issues that preclude accessibility to fluid intake during certain endurance events or team sport competitions. For these reasons, hyperhydration methodologies should not be discounted as means to prevent or delay hypohydration during prolonged exercise.

Glycerol-induced hyperhydration has the potential to increase total body water and expand plasma volume, and thereby improve or maintain cardiovascular function, thermoregulation, and performance during prolonged exercise. There is some evidence to support an increase in plasma volume following glycerol-induced hyperhydration,[39] but the significance of these data should be judged in light of the fact that the changes have been small (75-100 mL) and mostly determined from a commonly used calculation method based on changes in hematocrit and hemoglobin concentration[40] that only predicts percent change in plasma volume. Nonetheless, if plasma volume is truly expanded by hyperhydration, then venous return will be improved and this will increase stroke volume and lower heart rate compared with control conditions. Although some studies do report a reduction in heart rate with glycerol-induced hyperhydration,[41] others report no change.[39] The effect on stroke volume and cardiac output has been equally inconsistent.[42,43] Such equivocal results may derive from a reduction in plasma glycerol concentration during exercise caused by metabolism and discontinued glycerol intake. Consequently, a pre-exercise expansion of plasma volume will not be maintained during exercise. Some have found that glycerol-induced hyperhydration attenuates the rise in rectal temperature during exercise,[44] and in some cases this was related to an increased sweat rate[44,45] and skin blood flow[41] relative to control. Conversely, other studies have found that glycerol intake does not improve thermoregulation.[46,47]

Glycerol-induced hyperhydration has also been investigated for its effects on exercise performance. Endurance times during constant load cycle ergometry exercise have been found to be increased relative to control, but, as with cardiovascular and thermoregulatory variables, other studies have not found improvement in endurance time to

exhaustion following glycerol ingestion.[48,49] Despite this, results from Coutts and colleagues[47] are rather intriguing. They had well-trained triathletes ingest a placebo or a glycerol-containing solution 2 hours prior to competing in an Olympic distance triathlon in a high-temperature environment. Times during the final leg of the triathlon, a 10-km run, were significantly faster after having ingested glycerol. Furthermore, reduced urine output and increased fluid retention suggested that a hyperhydration state had been achieved after glycerol ingestion. This data set offers high ecological value and indicates that more work needs to be done to elucidate the environmental and exercise conditions in which glycerol-induced hyperhydration may impart physiological or performance benefits.

Application. Despite significant knowledge and education on the importance of consuming fluid during exercise evoking a high rate of sweat loss, most athletes and active people still voluntarily dehydrate because they consciously or subconsciously choose not to drink sufficient quantities of fluid. Pre-exercise hyperhydration has the potential to delay the onset of significant hypohydration, especially when combined with a minimal amount of fluid intake during exercise. Furthermore, there are certain athletic situations in which it is extremely difficult to ingest fluid during competition, and those athletes may benefit from a modest level of hyperhydration prior to competition. To this end, Siegler and colleagues[50] have recently shown that consuming a glycerol-containing drink 30 minutes before and at half-time of a soccer simulation resulted in better overall hydration status than when consuming a beverage without glycerol. It is important to note that the hydrating effects of glycerol can wear off after 4 or more hours, so the use of glycerol needs to be properly timed such that the kidneys will not begin excreting excess water just prior to or during a competitive or training session. If a modest level of hyperhydration prior to competition or training is desirable, glycerol (approximately 1 g/kg/bw) in a sufficient quantity of water (20-25 mL/kg/bw) appears to be reasonably effective.

Adverse Effects. Glycerol appears fairly safe, especially when consumed orally at doses less than 5 g/kg/bw. Some investigators have reported side effects such as nausea, vomiting, and headache[46,49] that others have not observed.[48] Incidence of side effects may be particularly related to the ingestion of highly concentrated (i.e., 10% or greater) glycerol solutions. One potential side effect that has not been studied is reduction in plasma sodium (hyponatremia; discussed previously) caused by excess fluid retention, especially when a glycerol solution without sodium is consumed.

Carbohydrate

Action. Carbohydrate intake before and during exercise prolongs time to exhaustion and improves exercise performance (e.g., time to complete a set distance or work accumulation for a set amount of time) by preventing hypo-glycemia, sparing liver glycogen, maintaining a high level of carbohydrate oxidation, or through neuromuscular effects.

Research. A high-carbohydrate diet during periods of intensified training or coupled with reduced training (i.e., taper) helps to maintain or elevate muscle glycogen to higher-than-normal levels.[51,52] This is important because studies dating back to the late 1960s and early 1970s documented a strong correlation between pre-exercise muscle glycogen levels and endurance performance.[53-55] Carbohydrate intake during the 3 to 5 hours prior to training or competition may also elevate muscle glycogen levels[56] and thereby improve performance,[57] but more likely will help to restore liver glycogen levels, especially if the athlete has fasted overnight, and this should lead to better maintenance of blood glucose during subsequent exercise. It has been debated whether carbohydrate should be consumed within the hour that precedes training or completion because early studies showed that the combined stimulatory effects of hyperinsulinemia and contractile activity on glucose uptake resulted in a rapid decline in blood glucose, a reduction in fat use, and an accelerated muscle glycogen use, all of which could predispose to poor performance.[58,59] However, subsequent research has shown that performance is either unchanged or improved when consuming carbohydrate in the hour before exercise.[60-62] Nonetheless, there are some individuals who seem to be particularly sensitive to the "hypoglycemic" effects of pre-exercise carbohydrate feeding, so the usefulness of this practice may have to be based on individual experiences. That said, what seems to be clear is that when carbohydrate is consumed before exercise, it has little or no negative effect on metabolism and performance when ingestion of carbohydrate is continued during exercise.[63]

Clinical Point

Carbohydrate intake improves exercise performance, delays fatigue, and improves motor skill ability and mood state.

Early research indicated that the addition of glucose to water slowed the gastric emptying rate.[64] These authors concluded that their data demonstrated the importance of "minimizing the glucose content of solutions ingested in order to obtain an optimal rate of fluid replacement." This, in combination with other research at the time suggesting that ingested glucose contributed very little to total energy expenditure during exercise,[65] underpinned the thinking that the physiological benefits of fluid replacement during exercise were far greater than energy replacement and there was little need to strike a balance between the two. That consensus began to change in the early 1980s with the publication of a classic article by Coyle and co-workers.[66] In this study, subjects exercised on a stationary bicycle ergometer at an exercise intensity of approximately 74% of VO_2 max. During one test, subjects consumed a glucose polymer solution, and in another test, they received an artificially sweetened placebo. Ingesting the glucose polymer delayed fatigue by approximately 23 minutes. This set off a flurry of research activity and now it is generally accepted that carbohydrate intake during exercise can improve endurance capacity (i.e., time to exhaustion) and performance (time trial) that is prolonged in nature.[67] Furthermore, more recent studies have shown that appropriate mixtures of simple sugars (glucose, polymers of glucose, fructose, sucrose) at an osmolality of less than 400 mOsm results in gastric emptying and intestinal water absorption rates similar to that of water.[68-70] The use of stable (^{13}C) and radioactive (^{14}C) isotopes of glucose and fructose along with advanced mathematical modeling techniques has also yielded strong data to show mixtures of simple sugars ingested during exercise can account for a rather large percentage of the total carbohydrate oxidized, especially late in exercise when endogenous carbohydrate stores are low.[71-73] Taken together, it is indeed possible to strike a balance between fluid availability and carbohydrate delivery during exercise and the benefits of such are well recognized, as reflected in the latest American College of Sports Medicine (ACSM) position stand on exercise and fluid replacement.[34]

Carbohydrate ingestion also seems to be ergogenic during repeated bouts of intermittent shuttle running meant to mimic the physical demands of team sports such as football, basketball, and soccer.[74,75] In addition to a physical performance benefit in this scenario, better maintenance of motor skill ability and improved mood state, including feelings of less fatigue in the later stages of the protocol, were observed.[76,77] This is in line with field research that has shown carbohydrate ingestion during activity is associated with improved stroke quality during the latter part of prolonged tennis play[78] and a trend for reduced ratings of perceived exertion during the final 4 km of a marathon run.[79] Regarding the marathon research, a more substantial finding was that when ingesting carbohydrate relative to placebo, the subjects ran at a higher intensity (i.e., higher heart rate) despite statistically similar overall ratings of perceived exertion. These observations suggest that carbohydrate ingestion affects CNS function and processing, likely by preventing hypoglycemia. Direct evidence of this comes from Nybo.[80] He tested CNS activation of skeletal muscle before and after 3 hours of cycling during two randomized trials, one with and another without (placebo) glucose ingestion. During the placebo trial blood glucose declined to hypoglycemic levels and the level of CNS activation was reduced compared with baseline. Glucose ingestion maintained both blood glucose and CNS activation relative to baseline. An alternative explanation is that glucose ingestion could activate receptors in the mouth or gastrointestinal (GI) track that leads to central activation to improve motor drive or motivation. To this end, Carter and colleagues[81] have shown that simply rinsing the mouth with a glucose polymer solution during a laboratory cycling time trial lasting approximately 1 hour improved performance by 3% versus a placebo. Finally, expectations or a preconceived notion that carbohydrate ingestion during exercise will improve performance must be considered when trying to understand the potential for a true physiological benefit. For example, Clark and colleagues[82] reported that during a 1-hour laboratory cycling time trial, the effect of telling subjects they were receiving a carbohydrate drink although they were in fact receiving a placebo was greater than the "real" physiological effect of carbohydrate when participants were told they were receiving a placebo.

Regardless of the mechanisms, central or peripheral, sufficient evidence exists to recommend carbohydrate intake before and during continuous exercise (running and cycling) and intermittent exercise (team and club sports).

Application. Athletes should maintain a high carbohydrate diet to keep muscle and liver glycogen stores full, consume carbohydrate approximately 1 hour before training and competition to top off fuel stores, and consume diluted carbohydrate solutions during training and competition to prevent fatigue and maximize performance. A high-carbohydrate diet consists of approximately 7 g/kg/bw /day; pre-exercise ingestion of carbohydrate should be equivalent to approximately 1 g/kg/bw. It is recommend that during prolonged exercise, athletes consume 60 to 70 g/hr of simple carbohydrates such as glucose, sucrose, and fructose. This can be accomplished by taking small feedings every 10 to 20 minutes.

Adverse Effects. A typical practical mistake is consuming too much carbohydrate during exercise. Ingesting carbohydrate in a concentration that is too high (> than 8% in solution) or at rates greater than can be absorbed from the GI system (> 100 g/hr) can produce GI discomfort such as bloating, cramping, or nausea. Furthermore, it is important to note that during high-intensity exercise (i.e., ≥ 80% VO_2 max) blood flow to the GI tract is reduced, limiting the absorption of substrate and water and, hence, increasing the likelihood of GI distress even when consuming recommended amounts of fluid and carbohydrate. It is not advisable to start carbohydrate intake before or early within the onset of training and competition and then discontinue its use. All this does is prepare the biological systems to use carbohydrate and then deprive them of the fuel they have been primed to use. Similarly, some individuals are overly sensitive to carbohydrate intake close to the onset of exercise and experience large swings in blood glucose and insulin that could produce symptoms of hypoglycemia (i.e., dizziness, nausea, reduced mental awareness, disorientation), although these symptoms typically reverse as exercise progresses. It is not easy to predict who will respond in this fashion, so it is important to recognize the limitations and use systematic trial and error to identify those that could be susceptible.

Protein

Action. Consumption of a small amount of protein (in addition to carbohydrate) during exercise provides amino acid substrates that can fuel oxidative metabolism, support gluconeogenesis, provide for a greater insulin-stimulated glucose uptake by muscle, and reduce muscle damage for improved recovery from training or competition—all of which should lead to improved endurance and performance versus when not consuming protein during exercise.

Research. One of the first reports on the effects of protein ingestion during prolonged exercise was made by Colombani and colleagues.[83] They compared the ingestion of a carbohydrate drink (65 g/L) to a drink containing carbohydrate and protein (65 g/L and 30 g/L, respectively) during marathon running using an independent group design. Their conclusion was that amino acids liberated from digested protein were absorbed during exercise, these amino acids were partially oxidized, and this had no negative metabolic effects. Interestingly, they also observed no statistical difference in time to complete the marathon race between the two groups. More recently, Koopman and colleagues[84] reported on an experiment that used sophisticated stable isotope tracer techniques to assess amino acid oxidation, protein synthesis and protein breakdown when consuming carbohydrate and carbohydrate-protein drinks during prolonged (6-hour) cycling exercise. Their results indicated that carbohydrate and protein ingestion improved whole-body protein balance during prolonged exercise. However, the significance of this, particularly in terms of exercise performance and recovery, is not clear.

One of the first laboratory experiments to assess the effects of carbohydrate-protein ingestion on exercise performance was conducted by Williams and colleagues.[85] Their findings indicated that consumption of a carbohydrate-protein drink after prolonged glycogen-depleting exercise resulted in greater exercise time to exhaustion in a subsequent exercise endurance test 4 hours later as compared with a carbohydrate-only drink. However, a major limitation to this study was that the test drinks were not matched for carbohydrate content and in fact, the carbohydrate-protein drink contained significantly more carbohydrate. So it was not clear whether protein or the additional carbohydrate was responsible for the performance benefit. This same group has also reported on the ingestion of a carbohydrate-protein drink versus carbohydrate alone during prolonged intermittent cycling.[86] Results from this placebo-controlled experiment suggested that carbohydrate intake increased exercise time to exhaustion, but addition of protein enhanced this effect by an additional 36%. A similar study that has received a great deal of attention took the experimentation one step further. Saunders and colleagues[87] also reported that consuming carbohydrate and protein during exercise extended cycling time to exhaustion when compared with carbohydrate alone. Furthermore, in a subsequent endurance test 12 to 15 hours later, subjects rode 40% longer after having consumed carbohydrate and protein the prior day, and at the onset of this additional exercise blood levels of creatine phosphokinase (a marker for muscle damage) were significantly reduced. There are several concerns that should be noted about this research. First, the experiment was not placebo-controlled and the amount of carbohydrate consumed (approximately 37 g/hr) during both treatments was less than what is normally considered as optimal for enhancing exercise endurance. Second, total energy intake was not matched between the carbohydrate and carbohydrate-protein conditions. Thus, it is difficult to know whether protein intake was driving the response or whether total calorie intake was primarily responsible for the endurance benefit. Indeed, this latter point seems to bear significance because subsequent research by the Saunders group that has controlled for total calorie intake has not provided evidence for a specific carbohydrate-protein benefit.[88,89]

Another issue that has been debated is the significance of a time-to-exhaustion benefit when consuming carbohydrate-protein for endurance athletes. Most competitions require covering a certain distance in the shortest time possible (e.g., cycling time-trial, 10-km running race). To this end, Van Essen and Gibala[90] have reported that ingesting a carbohydrate drink during a simulated 80-km cycling time-trial in a laboratory setting improved performance relative to placebo, but consuming a carbohydrate-protein beverage provided no additional benefit. Osterberg and colleagues recently published data[91] that supports the work of Van Essen and Gibala. Her results indicated that relative to placebo, carbohydrate and carbohydrate-protein intake during 2 hours of stationary laboratory cycling improved subsequent time-trial performance to a similar extent. Thus, it appears carbohydrate-protein ingestion during prolonged exercise may improve time to exhaustion, especially when carbohydrate intake is less than optimal, but when performance is tested in a manner in which endurance athletes normally compete, a protein benefit is not observed. It is also important to note that the Van Essen and Osterberg studies delivered carbohydrate at a rate believed to elicit a significant exogenous carbohydrate oxidation, endogenous carbohydrate sparing, and therefore improvement in performance (i.e., ~ 60g/hr). Thus, an alternative explanation is that when carbohydrate is consumed in sufficient amounts during exercise, protein does not provide any additional performance or endurance advantage. Finally, a limitation to the studies indicating that protein ingestion provides an endurance capacity advantage has been that there is little to no evidence for a biological mechanism through which the benefit is derived.

There is a developing literature on the effect of carbohydrate-protein ingestion after prolonged exercise with the intent to maximize performance during additional exercise 4 to 6 hours later (e.g., two-a-day practices, multi-game and multievent tournaments). In part, the initial observations by Williams and colleagues[85] and Saunders and colleagues[87] has guided these efforts, emanating especially from the observation that protein ingestion reduced circulating markers of muscle damage.[87,89] Nonetheless, this research[92-97] has been equivocal at best and there are no additional studies that have confirmed or denied the observation that carbohydrate-protein ingestion during an initial prolonged exercise bout improves (or maintains) performance in a subsequent bout 12 or more hours later. Additional research on these topics would be useful.

Application. Existing literature could be interpreted to suggest that consuming a combination of carbohydrate and protein during prolonged exercise may be effective for improving performance under certain circumstances. First, when consuming carbohydrate at a low rate (< 60 g/hr) during prolonged exercise, a small amount of protein intake (15–20 g/hr) may be ergogenic, although data to date suggest this is no more effective than consuming carbohydrate at a higher rate.[89] Second, protein may be ergogenic in situations in which training or competition requires prolonged extension of activity or play versus completing a certain amount of work or covering a set distance in the quickest time possible. Examples are "overtime" in team sports or extra sets in a tennis match. As with carbohydrate intake prior to or during exercise, there may be certain individuals who are particularly sensitive to positive or negative effects of consuming protein during exercise. Because protein intake during prolonged exercise has gone through less extensive experimentation, it is advisable when working with athletes to use systematic trial and error to identify whether protein ingestion during prolonged exercise works for them, given their particular training or competitive scenarios. Lastly, protein intake (again, in small amounts— 15-20 g) during or shortly after prolonged training or competition may be an effective recovery nutrition approach, particularly from the standpoint of protein balance and especially when multiple training or competitive events are held within a 24-hour period.

Adverse Effects. When adding protein to the fluids consumed or nutritional strategy employed during prolonged exercise, the biggest risk is a slowed gastric emptying rate resulting from increased energy density.[98] Furthermore, gram for gram, protein in solution may impart a slower gastric emptying rate than a simple carbohydrate.[99] A slowed gastric emptying rate during exercise could lead to feelings of stomach fullness, nausea, and cramping, as well as a delayed water absorption rate from the small intestine and thus a less effective offset of sweating-induced dehydration. Gastric emptying rates vary widely among individuals. Thus, an athlete with a high sweat rate and a low gastric emptying rate may not be a good candidate for consuming a carbohydrate-protein mixture during exercise. Another potential concern for protein consumption during exercise is a reduction in fat metabolism. Maintenance of a high rate of fat metabolism during prolonged exercise is beneficial in that it slows carbohydrate use and, indeed, is a hallmark of a very effectively and highly trained endurance athlete (refer back to "Adaptation of Physiological Systems"). In some studies, protein along with carbohydrate consumption during exercise elevates plasma insulin to a greater extent than when consuming carbohydrate alone. An elevated insulin level acts to depress fat metabolism. More studies are needed to better understand the effect of protein intake during exercise on the interplay of carbohydrate and fat metabolism.

Branched-Chain Amino Acids

Action. Branched-chain amino acid (BCAA) ingestion during prolonged exercise may enhance endurance performance by providing fuel in addition to carbohydrate and fat, reducing net protein breakdown in muscle and by delaying the onset of central fatigue. The efficacy for BCAA to prevent central fatigue has been the most frequently studied topic because it is well known that BCAA competes with tryptophan for transport across the blood-brain barrier. Tryptophan, the direct precursor for serotonin synthesis, is the linchpin of the central fatigue hypothesis as mentioned previously.

Research. As indicated earlier, prolonged exercise lowers muscle glycogen. This sets up a scenario by which BCCA could be taken up and oxidized by muscle to maintain a high rate of energy production late in exercise.[100] Unfortunately, the activities of enzymes involved in the oxidation of BCAA in muscle are too low to allow for a major contribution of BCAA to total energy expenditure during exercise.[101] Thus, consumption of BCCA during exercise does not make sense from the standpoint of energy provision and this is why it has been so surprising that a combination of low carbohydrate-protein intake during exercise has been shown to extend exercise time to exhaustion (see previous discussion on protein). However, ingesting BCCA during prolonged exercise prevents a decline in its blood concentration. This reduces the ratio of total tryptophan to BCCA, which favors a reduced-tryptophan transport across the blood-brain barrier. Thus, this nutritional intervention could potentially enhance prolonged exercise performance by reducing serotonin mediated central fatigue.

Following an initial positive field study,[102] the literature has been mixed on whether BCAA consumption during prolonged exercise delays fatigue or improves performance. Blomstrand and colleagues[102] reported that marathon running performance was improved in "slower" runners when BCAAs were taken throughout the race. However, this study has been criticized for lack of a control group and a creative statistical analysis that included retrospectively dividing the subject population into "slower" and "faster" runners. In a well-designed and controlled laboratory study, Madsen and colleagues[103] compared the effects of placebo, glucose, and glucose-BCAA ingestion on 100-km cycling time-trial performance. Despite an elevation in blood BCAA levels (and a reduced tryptophan/BCAA ratio) by the end of exercise, there was no difference in time to complete the time-trial among the three treatments. Curiously, glucose ingestion alone did not improve performance relative to the placebo. Still, if central fatigue was truly a manipulatable factor as a result of BCAA ingestion, it is likely this would have occurred independent of a glucose effect on performance. That said, other experiments have shown improvements in exercise performance with carbohydrate intake but no further benefit from the addition of BCAA.[104] All of the experiments mentioned to this point were conducted in a reasonably temperate environment. There is reason to believe that heat stress may heighten susceptibility to central fatigue. In this regard, Mittleman and colleagues[105] reported that BCAA supplementation extended exercise time to exhaustion in a hot environment. Watson and colleagues[106] also determined the effect of BCAA ingestion during exercise in a hot environment. Although they reported no significant difference in time to exhaustion for BCAA and placebo, five out of nine subjects had at least a 5% improvement in endurance when consuming BCAA. However, other data seems to indicate that under conditions of greater thermal strain (i.e., higher rectal temperature than that achieved in the Mittleman and Watson studies) and hypohydration, BCAA ingestion does not improve performance.[107]

Much like consumption of protein during exercise, there are reports on how BCAA ingestion before and during prolonged exercise suppresses muscle protein breakdown,[108] attenuates markers of muscle damage,[109,110] and reduces the amount of delayed onset muscle soreness.[110] To some extent, the applicability of these findings should be interpreted with caution because only one of the three studies experimented on reasonably trained subjects. It might be that the effects are more likely to occur in untrained muscle. For example, it is well known that although a single bout of eccentric exercise in a novice exerciser can cause significant muscle damage, a subsequent bout or bouts results in less damage (i.e., the so-called repeated bout effect[111]). Nonetheless, BCAA ingestion during exercise may have particular merits for recovery after exercise. However, as was indicated in the previous section on protein, much more work needs to be done to understand whether reduction in markers of muscle damage lead to a preferred muscle performance outcome.

Application. Fatigue during exercise likely results from a complex array biological and biochemical factors and there is little doubt that limitations in CNS functioning plays a role. Attempts at nutritional manipulations of brain neurotransmission have been equivocal in terms of their ability to offset central fatigue, at least when tested using prolonged exercise protocols characteristic of the demands of running and cycling. Other sports can be prolonged in nature and rely on successful execution of motor skills and tactics that have a high level of dependability on cognitive functioning. Although not tested in this regard, BCAA ingestion during prolonged sports competitions may alter neurotransmission processes such that during the later stages of a game, cognitive functioning for skill and tactical outcomes is better maintained or enhanced despite limited effects on endurance capacity. For this reason, BCAA still should be considered as having ergogenic properties but athletes will need to go through trial and error routines as well as make assessments of personal tolerance in a dose range of between 10 and 20 g per prolonged exercise bout until science catches up with the practical nature of sport. Lastly, consideration should be given to obtaining BCAA through ingestion of small amounts of protein during training or competition. This may result in a more balanced influence over the body's amino acid systems as discussed next in the section about "Adverse Effects."

Adverse Effects. There are few, if any, reports on adverse effects associated with BCAA supplementation. From a metabolic standpoint, however, what should be considered is the potential for excess ammonia production associated with high intakes of BCAA during prolonged exercise. MacLean and colleagues[108] showed that relative to a placebo, contracting skeletal muscle produced much more ammonia when BCAA were consumed before exercise. The amount of BCAA intake was approximately 5 g and enough to double arterial levels of BCAA before and during exercise. Excess ammonia can cross the blood-brain barrier and enter the CNS, where it can have detrimental effects on cerebral function that could lead to the manifestation of central fatigue. In fact, it has been shown that with an increasing arterial concentration of ammonia during prolonged exercise, there is an increased cerebral ammonia uptake.[112] In part, this may be why it has been difficult to demonstrate a robust effect of BCAA ingestion on the mitigation of central fatigue during prolonged exercise. Furthermore, it is interesting to note that protein ingestion during prolonged exercise does not result in excess ammonia accumulation. One reason for this may be that when ingesting protein, both ammonia-producing and ammonia-reducing amino acids are consumed, providing for a more balanced amino acid metabolism. Therefore, consumption of protein during exercise may be a better way to derive a BCAA preventative effect on central fatigue.

Tyrosine

Action. Ingestion of tyrosine before or during prolonged exercise increases central dopamine levels, decreases the ratio of central serotonin to dopamine, and thereby delays the onset of central fatigue.

Research. Tyrosine is a precursor to the synthesis of norepinephrine and dopamine in the brain. During acute mental and physical stress, large amounts of these neurotransmitters are released and a depletion can occur, resulting in a loss of ability to cope with stress-related behaviors. Tyrosine depletion via short-term reduction in dietary tyrosine intake is possible and manifests as low brain levels of dopamine.[113] It then follows that increasing tyrosine intake should elevate brain dopamine and norepinephrine levels. Although there is little direct evidence for this in humans, some studies report the expected behavioral effects associated with an elevation in central catecholamines.[114]

Tyrosine also competes for the same transport mechanism across the blood-brain barrier as tryptophan. Thus, by elevating free tyrosine in blood through supplemental intake, it may be possible to not only reduce central serotoninergic actively but to decrease the ratio of serotonin to dopamine, which has been proposed as key modulator of central fatigue, rather than serotoninergic activity alone.[8] It is also important to note that carbohydrate intake has the potential to reduce central serotoninergic activity. Carbohydrate intake during exercise reduces FFA accumulation in blood, which results in more tryptophan (rather than FFA) being bound to albumin. Thus the free tryptophan levels remain low and less is transported into the brain for serotonin synthesis. Thus a potentially effective way to decrease the serotonin/dopamine ratio during prolonged exercise is to ingest both carbohydrate and tyrosine before and during exercise. Chinevere and colleagues[115] compared the effects of placebo, tyrosine, carbohydrate, and combined carbohydrate and tyrosine on cycling time-trial performance following a 90-minute preload ride at 70% of peak oxygen uptake. Drinks were consumed before (60 and 30 minutes) and every 30 minutes during the 90-minute preload exercise period. Tyrosine was administered each time in an amount of 25 mg/kg/bw for a total intake of approximately 11 g up to the start of the time trial. Results indicated that although carbohydrate intake improved performance, intake of tyrosine did not provide any additional benefit. Likewise, the tyrosine alone and placebo trial were not significantly different. It is interesting to note that numerically, there was slightly more than a 1-minute improvement for carbohydrate-tyrosine versus carbohydrate alone. Likewise, when consuming tyrosine, time to complete the time trial was almost 2 minutes faster than placebo and six of the nine subjects finished faster when on tyrosine than when on the placebo. As can be the case in these types of experiments, the results can inspire a debate about the practical versus statistical benefits. The authors are aware of only one other human study on tyrosine supplementation and prolonged exercise performance. Strüder and colleagues[116] reported no benefit of tyrosine administration when subjects were asked to exercise to exhaustion on a cycle ergometer at an intensity that elicited a blood lactate concentration of approximately 2 mM. However, the amount of tyrosine administered in this experiment may have been too large (20 g), and in fact may have had a negative effect as indicated by hormonal measurements that suggested a decrease rather than an increase in central dopamine levels.

The U.S. military has had a lot of interest in tyrosine supplementation because of its potential to alter mood and enhance cognitive performance under conditions of extreme stress (see reviews by Lieberman[117,118]). In brief, their research has shown that tyrosine administration reduces the psychological stress of military operations,[119] cold stress,[120] combined cold and altitude stress,[121] the negative consequences of sleep deprivation,[122] and stress associated with sustained operations.[123] Although all of these are highly stressful situations, there is some indication that tyrosine can improve cognitive performance under conditions void of significant stress-related biological changes.[124]

Application. It appears that if tyrosine is going to be effective, the ingested dose should be no more than 10 g either as a bolus or spread out over multiple feedings in and around the training or competitive scenario. For possible influence over central fatigue, it makes sense to consume tyrosine along with carbohydrate, but as was discussed previously for BCAA, what still needs to be sorted out is whether effective doses of tyrosine could be ingested as part of protein consumption, especially because as little as 2 to 3 g of tyrosine may provide a benefit. Consideration should be given to tyrosine supplementation under training and competitive conditions at environmental extremes such as altitude and extreme cold and situations in which sleep deprivation has the possibility of contributing to poor performance.

Adverse Effects. Supplemental tyrosine is reasonably safe, especially when consumed in the recommended dose range of 7 to 10 g/day. It should be noted, however, that long-term safety studies in humans consuming supplemental doses have not been conducted. If consumed before bed time, it may result in insomnia. Use should be avoided by those consuming stimulant or antidepressant medications because tyrosine may increase sensitivity to those medications.

Caffeine

Action. Caffeine is a CNS and metabolic stimulant that is known to improve both physical and mental performance. The exact mechanisms behind these effects have not been completely worked out, but more than likely involve three primary modes of action: (1) antagonism of adenosine receptors in the CNS; (2) direct effects of caffeine metabolites on lipolysis, blood vessels, and smooth muscles; and (3) competitive inhibition of cyclic adenosine monophosphate–phosphodiesterase (cAMP).

Research. Caffeine is probably one of the most popular ergogenic aids among endurance athletes, but it is also one of the most controversial. For example, until recently, caffeine was on the list of substances banned by the International Olympic Committee. Caffeine has no nutritive value, yet it is widely available in our food supply. It occurs naturally in coffee beans, tea leaves, kola nuts, and cocoa beans. Endurance athletes have a strong belief that caffeine improves performance. Desbrow and Leveritt[125] recently reported that of 140 triathletes competing in the 2005 Ironman Triathlon World Championships, "73% believed that caffeine is ergogenic" and "84% believe that it improves their concentration." Caffeine intake during triathlon competition was achieved primarily through "flat" cola drinks and caffeinated carbohydrate gels.

Research on caffeine and human endurance exercise performance dates back to the late 1970s. Costill's group at Ball State University examined the effect of ingesting 330 mg of caffeine 1 hour prior to cycling to exhaustion at 80% of VO$_2$ max.[126] They found an improvement in time to exhaustion of 21 minutes compared with a placebo condition. In a subsequent study, 250 mg of caffeine was associated with a 20% increase in the amount of work performed during 2 hours of isokinetic cycling.[127] These observations have held up over the years, especially experiments that have tested caffeine's effect on exercise time to exhaustion. From a series of studies by Graham and Spriet, it was reported that a caffeine dose of 9 mg/kg/bw improved running and cycling time to exhaustion in elite runners and recreational athletes.[128,129] They also tested doses of 3, 6, and 9 mg/kg/bw and found equal improvements for the 3 and 6 mg/kg/bw doses, but no further benefit from the 9 mg/kg/bw dose.[130] This seems to indicate there is a threshold of caffeine intake above which no further ergogenic benefit is derived. Furthermore, they reported that on a habitual basis, "light" caffeine users were least likely to benefit from the highest dose (9 mg/kg/bw), and may even have a negative response. In the most recent time-to-exhaustion research we could find, Hogervosrst and colleagues[131] had their subjects pedal a stationary bike for 2.5 hours at 60% of VO$_2$ max. Thereafter they were required to pedal to exhaustion at 75% of VO$_2$ max. Immediately before exercise they consumed a carbohydrate sports bar, a carbohydrate sports bar with 100 mg of caffeine, or a placebo beverage in a randomized, repeated measures design. Carbohydrate intake improved time to exhaustion, but caffeine intake resulted in an even further increment versus placebo. Thus caffeine appears to have ergogenic benefits in addition to those of carbohydrate. Lastly, it is interesting to note that a majority of caffeine studies have tested the "pure" form of the drug, either in capsule form or incorporated into a processed food or beverage. Ingestion of caffeine as coffee appears to be ineffective for performance as compared with pure caffeine, possibly because there are ingredient components in coffee that modulate caffeine's effect on performance.[132]

As was discussed in the previous section about protein, the significance of time-to-exhaustion protocols within the context of competitive performance has been debated because most endurance competitions are designed to cover a set distance in the shortest time possible. Results from a recent meta-analysis on caffeine and laboratory exercise testing led to the conclusion that caffeine intake improves exercise performance, but time-to-exhaustion protocols are much more likely to reveal this benefit than a time-trial protocol.[133] Thus, if one believes that time to exhaustion is not a relevant performance test for endurance athletes, it seems reasonable to downgrade expectations for a performance benefit from caffeine in "real-world" competitive scenarios. Independent of this comparison, there is fairly robust scientific support for the addition of small amounts of caffeine to carbohydrate-containing drinks to induce improvements in time-trial performance.[134,135] It also appears that consuming a small amount of caffeine (~120 mg) late in exercise is as effective as consuming higher doses of caffeine prior to or during exercise.[135] Regardless, ultimate support for caffeine ergogenicity should derive from field tests of exercise performance. Results from studies in this regard have indicated that consuming 3 and 5 mg/kg/bw of caffeine 1 hour prior to 8- and 5-km running races, respectively, induced small (1%-1.5%) but statistically significant improvements in performance.[136,137] In another controlled field study, caffeine consumption during an 18-km competitive running race did not improve performance relative to placebo; however, total caffeine intake during the race was less than 100 mg.[138] More research concerning the effects of caffeine on performance in ecologically valid race settings seems warranted.

As mentioned earlier, exercise-to-exhaustion type tests may have applicability for individual or team sports in which the game winner is decided in overtime or "sudden-death" scenarios. Although in these sports the type of activity is prolonged, the intensity is high and activity is intermittent in nature. Hence, response to caffeine in time to exhaustion protocols may not necessarily predict performance in this type of physical effort. Thus, Schneiker and colleagues[139] conducted an experiment to test the hypothesis that caffeine consumption improves the performance of intermittent sprints. They had team sport athletes consume caffeine (6 mg/kg/bw) or placebo 1 hour prior to testing. The results revealed that after two bouts of 18 4-second sprints with 2 minutes of active recovery between each sprint, total amount of sprint work accumulated was greater after consuming caffeine. The same amount of caffeine was tested for its ability to improve performance during tests of agility, which is an important component of the athletic skills needed for team sport competition. In this case, measures of agility did not benefit from caffeine consumption.[140] Taken together, it seems caffeine has the potential to improve ability to withstand the high-intensity, intermittent-type activity required in team sports, but a total performance benefit requires a positive effect on skill and agility (positive data lacking) as well as on cognitive function, mental alertness, and concentration.[118]

The "classic" hypothesis for the ergogenic effects of caffeine is that it stimulates epinephrine release, increases peripheral and intramuscular lipolysis, and increases fat oxidation, and thereby spares muscle glycogen use for improved exercise performance. Although there are data to support these various aspects of caffeine's effects,[126,129,141] low doses of caffeine (i.e., < 250 mg) do not always stimulate epinephrine release and fat metabolism, yet performance benefits have been observed.[128,134] Another explanation is that caffeine can have a direct effect on skeletal muscle.[142] For example, caffeine is known to increase the rate of release of calcium from the sarcoplasmic reticulum (SR) and increase the sensitivity of contractile proteins to calcium, both of which could improve excitability for muscle contraction. A third explanation relates to the stimulatory effects of caffeine on the CNS. In this manner, perception of effort may be reduced and signal transduction from the brain to muscle could be improved. It is likely that one or both effects could happen through adenosine metabolism in the brain. Adenosine is believed to be an endogenous inhibitory neurotransmitter. When it binds to functional adenosine receptors brain excitatory activity is reduced. Caffeine is an adenosine receptor antagonist; thus it can compete with adenosine for binding, reduce its effects, and thereby stimulate brain neuronal activity. This is associated with behavioral changes that lead to improvements in mental and physical endurance.[143]

Caffeine is known to maintain brain performance, especially under conditions of sleep deprivation. Furthermore, military research has consistently shown maintenance or improvements in attention, psychomotor skills, memory, concentration, and vigilance under conditions of severe operational stress.[118] Such cognitive, or brain performance, benefits for caffeine have also been identified after prolonged cycling exercise that mimics the intensity and duration of road racing.[131] Such effects combined with the physical performance benefits of caffeine could lead to significant improvement in physically demanding sports that require concentration, quick thinking, and tactical decisions. However, this hypothesis has not been tested in a holistic fashion. Finally, although there are data to show that caffeine consumption reduces perception of effort during exercise,[135] Cole and colleagues[144] used a unique approach to further make this point. They asked test subjects to pedal a stationary cycle ergometer at what they perceived to be a rating of 9, 12, and 15 on a Borg scale for sequential 10-minute bouts of exercise. This was done 1 hour after receiving placebo or caffeine at a dose of 6 mg/kg/bw. Total work performed during the caffeine trial was greater than that of the placebo.

Clinical Point

Caffeine seems to alter neural perception of effort and this either drives or contributes to the physical performance benefits derived after caffeine consumption.

Application. The potential for an ergogenic effect from caffeine is impressive. Nevertheless, caffeine, although prevalent in society, is a drug, and it has been questioned whether athletes should use it for the benefits it can provide or avoid it because it could be considered doping. This ethical dilemma likely will not be solved any time soon. Effective doses appear to be near 100 mg for the mental and cognitive benefits and more than 200 mg for physical performance benefits. Most administration protocols call for pre-exercise dosing to account for absorption and metabolism of caffeine, although there are sufficient data to support benefits from intake during exercise as well as during the latter parts of prolonged exercise. Although data for mental and physical performance benefits derived from caffeine ingestion are largely positive, one must keep in mind that there can be big individual differences in response to caffeine. As with any ergogenic aid, practical experience is as important as science-based decisions for its use. Some of the variability in response to caffeine may be derived from habitual use. Those with a high habitual daily intake of caffeine may have a blunted metabolic response to acute caffeine dosing, but it is debated whether this reduces the performance benefit that can be derived from use. Likewise, it has been hypothesized that a person with a high habitual intake of caffeine may require a larger-than-normal dose to derive a benefit, but there are no data the authors are aware of that supports this. Lastly, it seems unlikely that acute caffeine withdrawal will sensitize body systems for a greater performance effect upon reintroduction of use.

Adverse Effects. The use of caffeine is associated with side effects. First, habitual users who stop using caffeine often experience symptoms of withdrawal such as lethargy and headache. High intakes of caffeine (i.e., > 400 mg) or acute use of a high dose by those who normally avoid caffeine are associated with tachycardia, elevated blood pressure, restlessness, irritability, tremor, and premature ventricular contractions. Caffeine is also considered a diuretic, but the effect this can have on hydration status and performance has recently been challenged.[145] In support of this, it is known that during exercise, the diuretic effect of caffeine is counteracted by an elevation in catecholamines.[146]

Antioxidants

Action. Oral antioxidant supplementation can assist or enhance endogenous antioxidant systems in neutralizing ROS and thereby prevent premature fatigue in contracting skeletal muscle.

Research. There is little doubt that contracting skeletal muscles generate ROS and reactive nitrogen species (RNS). These so-called free radicals can interfere with biological structures and functions within a muscle cell and predispose to early onset fatigue. Although there is reasonably strong evidence that ROS can modify key muscle components and proteins integral to the contractile process, evidence for RNS is less strong. RNS may have particular influence over vascular control, which could be part of the overall fatigue

process, but for simplicity, the authors will limit this discussion to contractile activity per se. Fortunately, skeletal muscle is endowed with a system of antioxidant enzymes that can degrade or "neutralize" ROS. Other molecular structures complement these enzymes and reside both in the aqueous and lipid fractions of the muscle cell. Although there are numerous antioxidant compounds and antioxidant vitamins (A, C, E) available, it is not clear to what extent supplementation complements (or hurts) the endogenous antioxidant systems, especially for the preservation of muscle performance. For example, although supplementation with antioxidant vitamins has been shown to reduce markers of oxidative stress during exercise, they do little to prevent fatigue.[147] Furthermore, numerous phytochemicals (e.g., quercetin, resveratrol, epigallocatechin gallate [EGCG]) in the foods we eat offer antioxidant potential but few have been tested within the context of human muscle fatigue during exercise.[148] To date, it appears that exercise-induced muscle fatigue is most consistently offset by antioxidants or antioxidant systems that target thiol (sulfhydryl groups; RSH) oxidation. Of these, glutathione and the glutathione system seem to be the most important. The thiol moiety of the amino acid cysteine can participate in covalent interactions with muscle-derived ROS. Thiol oxidation is known to occur in important contractile proteins such as actin[149] and myosin[150] and could precipitate the development of fatigue. Glutathione and the glutathione cycle can regulate thiol redox state in muscle and thereby guard against excessive thiol oxidation of important contractile proteins. Glutathione is composed of three amino acids; cysteine, glutamate, and glycine. Availability of cysteine seems to be rate-limiting for glutathione synthesis. Therefore, antioxidant strategies that support glutathione synthesis and the glutathione system have been tested within the context of contraction-induced (exercise) muscle fatigue. For example, *N*-acetylcysteine (NAC) has been used to increase cysteine availability in humans. Administration of NAC has been shown to reduce isolated muscle fatigue in individual muscles[151] or muscle groups[152] subjected to contractile paradigms. Furthermore, NAC has been shown to delay fatigue during prolonged cycling exercise in endurance athletes.[153] Interestingly, α-lipoic acid, also a thiol donor, does not seem to be effective at guarding against muscle fatigue, at least in an animal model.[154] In addition to NAC's ability to stimulate glutathione synthesis, its thiol moiety can interact directly with ROS and may in part explain the difference in effectiveness between NAC and α-lipoic acid. However, muscle performance studies in humans with α-lipoic acid supplementation are lacking. Unfortunately, side effects of NAC administration have limited its experimental and practical use (see following section about "Adverse Effects"). However, experimental evidence from Lands and colleagues[155] is encouraging in that they reported 3 months of supplementation with a cysteine donor protein increased 30-second isokinetic cycling peak power and total work in young, healthy men and women relative to a casein (low cysteine content) control.

Clinical Point

Exercise induced fatigue is offset by antioxidants and their systems.

Application. Antioxidants and antioxidant systems are clearly involved in muscle function and therefore prolonged exercise performance can benefit from their effects. As noted earlier, regular exercise training up-regulates the expression of various antioxidant enzymes and enzyme systems. What remains strongly debated is whether supplementation with various antioxidant compounds is a necessary complement to these up-regulated systems. The most conservative and possibly best approach is to ensure adequate daily fruit and vegetable intake not only for the antioxidant vitamins they provide, but for the various phytochemicals possessing antioxidant potential. There is likely a particular effectiveness of nature's balance and it guards against potential negative effects from over-providing a single antioxidant compound. The acute potential for cysteine donors to up-regulate the glutathione system and thereby improve exercise performance cannot be denied and, although the standard approach to prove this has used a druglike intervention, emerging data suggests that proteins particularly high in cysteine content may provide effective (and safer) glutathione system support.

Adverse Effects. NAC is sold as a nutritional supplement, but strong consideration should be given to the potential for side effects. Dose-dependent side effects of NAC include anaphylactic reactions, hypotension, nausea, lightheadedness, and dysphoria. It appears that only mild side effects occur after oral dosing of 150 mg/kg/bw (~10 g). Nonetheless, the effectiveness and potential harmful effects of chronic low doses of NAC are not known. In this light, what must be considered is that on one hand ROS and RNS create oxidative stress, whereas on the other they can also act as signaling molecules within a cell for various transcription and translation processes leading to cell adaptation. It is possible there is a fine line between complementing and stimulating endogenous antioxidant systems with oral antioxidant compounds for exercise performance benefits and creating potential for deleterious effects on cell messaging systems.

Carnitine

Action. Carnitine is an important molecule that assists in the transport of fatty acids from the cytosol into the mitochondria for subsequent oxidation. Increasing the carnitine content of skeletal muscle should enhance fatty acid uptake and oxidation by mitochondria during exercise and potentially lead to reduced glycogen use and improved endurance capacity.

Research. Carnitine in the body is derived from dietary intake (meat) as well as endogenous synthesis from the amino acids methionine and lysine. Approximately 98% of carnitine in the body is stored in skeletal muscle and heart. Skeletal muscle takes up carnitine against a very large concentration gradient. For example, the concentration of carnitine inside muscle is roughly 100 times that in blood. However, carnitine is actively transported into muscle by a saturable, sodium-dependent, high-affinity, active transport process. The transport protein for carnitine has been identified as the novel organic cation transporter OCTN2.[156] Understanding the regulation of this transport process is key to an effective carnitine supplementation routine.

Carnitine supplementation is effective at enhancing fat metabolism only if it stimulates an increase in muscle total carnitine content. Early research suggested that this was not possible. Barnett and colleagues[157] and Wächter and colleagues[158] reported that both short-term (4 g/day for 2 weeks) and long-term (4 g/day for 3 months) carnitine supplementation did not increase skeletal muscle carnitine content. Furthermore, IV infusion of carnitine for 5 hours did not increase net carnitine uptake across the leg[159] or muscle carnitine content.[160] The latter observation suggests that it is likely transport of carnitine that limits accumulation in muscle. Based on these observations, it is not surprising to find that a majority of well-controlled carnitine supplementation studies have not found an effect on VO_2 max,[161] enhancement of whole-body or muscle-fat metabolism,[159,162,163] muscle glycogen use,[164] or exercise performance.[158] Accordingly, most reviews of ergogenic aids, even recently[165] have concluded that carnitine supplementation is not effective for augmenting muscle fat metabolism during prolonged exercise.

Recent experimentation from Paul Greenhaff's lab at the University of Nottingham Medical School has begun to change opinions on the usefulness of carnitine supplementation for exercise fat metabolism and performance. Understanding that insulin likely stimulates sodium-dependent active transport of carnitine via OCTN2, they hypothesized that simultaneous elevations in plasma insulin and carnitine would stimulate uptake and accumulation of carnitine in muscle. Indeed, Stephens and colleagues[160] have shown that carnitine infusion during a hyperinsulinemic euglycemic clamp procedure resulted in approximately a 15% increase in muscle carnitine content after 5 hours. They have also demonstrated that oral feedings of carnitine (3 g) and carbohydrate, which substantially increased plasma insulin concentration, resulted in an increase in whole-body carnitine retention (versus carnitine supplementation alone) calculated from 24-hour urinary carnitine excretion.[166] Lastly, they have also shown that a combined hyperinsulinemia and hypercarnitinemia resulted in a reduced carbohydrate oxidation in a condition of surfeit carbohydrate availability, possibly resulting from enhanced fat oxidation in muscle.[167] These findings reinvigorate the possibility that carnitine can be used as an effective ergogenic aid to enhance metabolism and possibly performance during prolonged exercise.

Application. The effective dose for elevating muscle carnitine levels seems to be within the range of 2 to 4 g/day when taken with ample carbohydrate to raise circulating insulin levels. Along this line, consuming supplemental carnitine with meals (as would be done with a vitamin pill) may be as effective at getting carnitine into muscle. It is unlikely that acute carnitine ingestion along with carbohydrate will have immediate effects. Thus, carnitine supplementation should be pursued over weeks to months. Because of the potential for elevated fat metabolism when muscle carnitine levels are increased, it is possible that over time, fat loss will be observed. However, carnitine should not be used in the context of a "magic" fat loss remedy.

Adverse Effects. There are no known adverse effects associated with carnitine supplementation. There are reports of poor bioavailability after ingestion, which may indicate slow absorption. This could induce symptoms of GI distress in susceptible individuals; thus individual tolerance needs to be worked out through systematic trial and error.

Ergogenic Aids for High-Intensity Exercise and Physical Strength and Power

Activities that Require Power and Speed

The other two groups by which athletic activities are classified include power and speed. Because the two are often required simultaneously, they are referred to collectively as *high-intensity exercise*. High-intensity exercise is characterized by short-duration, maximal-effort tasks. By definition, high-intensity exercise lasts less than 2 minutes for a given bout. Sprinting, jumping, kicking, wrestling, weightlifting, and throwing are examples of high-intensity activities. Although all sports include some degree of high-intensity exercise, this section of the chapter focuses on those sports or sporting activities that are dominated by intense exercise (i.e., power, speed, or both). The metabolic requirements for high-intensity activities vary greatly from endurance activities and therefore require a different strategy for achieving peak performance.

Physiology and Physiological Consequences of Energy Generation for High-Intensity Activity

Physical activities that primarily consist of high-intensity exercise are often called *anaerobic*. This is because the main energy systems involved do not require oxygen to produce the energy. The ATP produced to fuel high-intensity exercise is primarily generated by immediate energy sources (power) and anaerobic, or fast, glycolysis (speed). Both of these categories of energy production have a much faster rate of energy production than aerobic energy systems, but yield far less total energy.

Power activities, such as shot put or weightlifting, rely heavily on immediate energy sources. There are three main sources for immediate energy production. They include energy production from (1) ATP: hydrolysis (splitting) of ATP yielding adenosine diphosphate (ADP) and an inorganic phosphate, (2) creatine phosphate (CP): combining CP and ADP to produce ATP and creatine, and (3) myokinase: joining two ADP molecules to form ATP and adenosine monophosphate (AMP). All three sources are immediately available to fuel muscle contractions. However, these sources can only sustain activities lasting no longer than 5 to 15 seconds.

Sources of Immediate Energy for Power and Speed (Anaerobic Activity)

- Adenosine triphosphate
- Creatine phospate
- Myokinase reaction

High-intensity exercise with a speed component, such as a 200-meter run or a 50-meter swim, depends most heavily on glycolysis for energy production. This process involves the breakdown of glucose and glycogen stored in the muscle. The breakdown of one glucose molecule results in the production of two ATPs, with the net formation of lactic acid. Anaerobic glycolysis is a rapid process that provides significantly more energy than immediate energy sources. However, even when combined, both sources provide only a small fraction of the energy that can be produced through oxidative means. Therefore, intense exercise lasting more than approximately 30 seconds is supplemented with oxidative energy sources to help sustain the activity. However, oxidative metabolism is much slower to produce energy than nonoxidative energy systems, so it will not play a dominate role in energy production until the exercise exceeds approximately 2 minutes, which is outside the scope of the activities being discussed in this section.

As mentioned, anaerobic or fast glycolysis forms lactate as a byproduct of ATP production. As glucose is broken down, pyruvate is formed. If pyruvate does not enter the mitochondria immediately, it is reduced to lactate. In tissues and cells where there is high glycolytic activity and low mitochondrial density, such as type IIb muscle fibers and red blood cells, lactate accumulation is likely. Therefore, lactate accumulation depends on the glycolytic and mitochondrial activity of the muscle, not the presence of oxygen.

Causes of Fatigue and Optimizing Performance During High-Intensity Exercise

During high-intensity exercise, lactate accumulation occurs because the rate of lactic acid production exceeds the rate at which it is removed. The lactic acid disassociates a hydrogen ion (H^+), leading to a decline in pH. The accumulation of these unbuffered H^+ can have deleterious effects on athletic performance. The three main negative effects of H^+ accumulation (i.e., lower pH) include inhibition of phosphofructokinase, which is the rate-limiting enzyme in glycolysis, causing a slower glycolysis rate; interference of muscular contraction because calcium (Ca^{2+}) is displaced from troponin; and possible stimulation of pain receptors. Therefore, the ability to better buffer the accumulation of H^+ during high-intensity exercise will help optimize performance.

Another means for optimizing high-intensity exercise performance is to increase or better maintain CP levels in the muscle. The ability to sustain muscular contraction depends on the balance between CP use and restoration. During exercise, as ATP levels begin to decline, CP works to maintain them. Because of the relatively small amount of CP stored in the muscle, if there is even a slightly greater rate of CP use versus restoration (as is common during high-intensity exercise), the exercise will not be maintained for long. The rate of CP depletion is directly related to the intensity of exercise (i.e., high intensity exercise leads to faster depletion). Depletion of CP results in muscle fatigue and thereby impaired athletic performance.

Muscle fatigue during high-intensity exercise can also result from a decrease in Ca^{2+} release and responsiveness. It is believed that lactate accumulation plays a role in the impairment in the ability of the ryanodine receptor to release Ca^{2+} in the SR. The resulting lower levels of free Ca^{2+} have been associated with fatigue. Similarly, the decrease in muscle pH that is associated with lactate accumulation during high-intensity exercise, has been linked to a reduction in Ca^{2+} sensitivity. This impairment of Ca^{2+} responsiveness results in a decrement of muscle force. Therefore, preventing declines in Ca^{2+} release and responsiveness is important in preventing fatigue.

The last factor to consider for optimizing speed and power performance is enlargement of the muscle. Muscle hypertrophy allows for an increase in muscular force generation and results primarily from an increase in cellular cross sectional area, not from an increase in the number of muscle fibers (hyperplasia). As the muscle fibers increase in size, there will be an increase in the number of sarcomeres arranged in parallel leading to an increase in force production. Power is also enhanced with muscle hypertrophy because the muscle can move at a faster velocity for a given submaximal workload.

Adaptation of Physiological Systems to High-Intensity Exercise

Physical training is the most effective way to enhance the factors mentioned to improve athletic performance. Using the principle of specificity of training to stress the body systems necessary for the activity, the body will make physiological adaptations to overcome the stress placed on it.

These adaptations lead to an improvement in performance. For example, strength training is important for high-intensity activities. It leads to increased strength and muscle hypertrophy through neural and muscle tissue adaptations. Neural adaptations allow for improved force generation unrelated to muscle hypertrophy. Muscle hypertrophy occurs mainly after the neural adaptations have developed and is due to the muscle tissue adaptations that occur with strength training. Other muscle tissue adaptations that result from strength training are increased cross-sectional area of the muscle, increased myosin heavy chain II_x and II_b isoforms, increased muscle fiber area, decreased muscle fiber mitochondrial density, increased high-energy phosphate pool in the muscle, increased ATP-use rate, increased phosphokinase and myokinase, increased androgen receptor sites, and increased intracellular glycogen and lipids. Beyond increasing the size and strength of the muscle, these adaptations also improve the contractile and energy producing capabilities of the muscle that are beneficial for speed and power. Similar adaptations can result for sprints, plyometrics, and interval exercise.

Neural Adaptations that Occur Early in a Strength Training Program

- Increased electrical activity of the muscle
- Increased rate of motor unit recruitment
- Increased coordination of antagonist muscle groups
- Increased motor unit synchronization
- Improved ability to recruit high-threshold motor units

Taking into account the physiological factors mentioned in this section that can increase high-intensity athletic performance, various ergogenic aids have been proposed to improve high-intensity exercise performance. Others have little scientific support for efficacy or are illegal. Those discussed in the following section have been shown to possibly aid performance, and are safe and legal. However, it should be noted that the best means for improving performance is training. These substances are not meant to be a substitute for a well-designed training program.

Ergogenic Aids for Power and Speed That Have Little Scientific Support, Lack Investigation or Are Illegal

- Amphetamines
- Dehydroepiandrosterone
- Human growth hormone
- Anabolic steroids
- Carnosine

Ergogenic Aids for Speed and Power

Sodium Bicarbonate

Action. A cause of fatigue during high-intensity exercise is the reduction in muscle pH resulting from the accumulation of lactate. Extracellular bicarbonate works to maintain the pH gradient between intra- and extracellular compartments, facilitating the movement of lactate and H^+ out of the cell. It is believed that if additional extracellular bicarbonate were available to buffer H^+, intracellular pH would be better maintained, thereby delaying fatigue.

Research. The literature describing the ergogenic effect of sodium bicarbonate ingestion on high-intensity exercise is conflicted. The discrepancies in studies may be related to the differences in sodium bicarbonate dosage administered, the exercise protocol (e.g., type, intensity, and duration), and the population studied. Studies have shown an increase in plasma pH, bicarbonate, and lactate with the ingestion of sodium bicarbonate. However, in a recent review by Requena and colleagues,[168] only half of the studies showed a benefit of sodium bicarbonate ingestion. The studies reviewed included high-intensity, short-duration (< 120 seconds) running and cycling; high-intensity, long-duration (> 120 seconds) running and cycling; high-intensity intervals; and strength training. The most positive effects were seen in studies lasting 1 to 7 minutes, involving maximal and high-intensity running or cycling, and with a dosage of 0.3 g/kg/bw. The effect of sodium bicarbonate on strength training is inconclusive.

Application. Sodium bicarbonate should be ingested 90 minutes prior to high-intensity activity lasting 1 to 7 minutes. Optimal dosage is 0.3 g/kg/bw. It has been suggested that athletes ingest sodium bicarbonate for 5 to 6 days and then abstain from ingestion 2 days prior to the athletic competition.[169] With this approach, the benefits of supplementation are maintained and the potential for acute side effects that could arise with dosing on the day of competition is eliminated.

Adverse Effects. About half of the subjects who ingested sodium bicarbonate experienced severe GI distress.

Creatine

Action. Ingested creatine is stored mainly in the muscle, thereby increasing muscle creatine phosphate (CP) (also called phosphocreatine [PCr]) stores. Having more CP available can allow for an increase in immediate energy available either through enhanced ATP regeneration (i.e., better maintenance of immediate ATP stores) or increased ATP production by combining with ADP. Creatine can also work as a buffer through the consumption of H^+ during CP dephosphorylation. These actions are thought to delay fatigue and shorten recovery periods after intense exercise.

Research. Much like sodium bicarbonate, the results from creatine studies are mixed. Again, some of the inconsistency in the findings can be explained by methodological

details (e.g., test outcome, exercise protocol, subjects) used in the various studies. Another proposed explanation is the idea of "responders" and "nonresponders." Nonresponders are those who are thought to have already maximized creatine stores through their normal diet. In responders, creatine supplementation can increase CP stores by approximately 20%.[170] The effects of creatine supplementation have been widely studied in various types of athletes with a variety of sport performance outcomes (e.g., speed, maximal force production, endurance capacity, anaerobic capacity, jumping ability, and muscle recovery). A review paper by Bemben and Lamont[171] suggests that creatine supplementation appears to be most effective for repeated-bout, high-intensity, short-duration activities, such as those involving running, cycling, or jumping. With regard to improving power or strength (dynamic or isotonic), creatine supplementation has been shown to increase force production despite sex, age, or sport. However, it has not been shown to be widely effective for isometric or isokinetic force production, aerobic performance, or the prevention of muscle damage.

Application. The most common dosing for creatine supplementation includes a loading phase of 20 g/day for 5 to 7 days, followed by a maintenance phase of 3 to 5 g/day for 1 week to 6 months. The ACSM Roundtable[172] acknowledges that a loading phase of 3 g/day for 30 days will increase creatine stores to the same level as 20 g/day for 5 days, and a maintenance phase of 2 g/day is sufficient to maintain stores. It is recommended that the creatine supplement not be taken immediately before or after exercise because of the possibility of GI distress.

Adverse Effects. Currently, no long-term adverse effects have been reported. It should be noted, however, that there is a lack of detailed studies on the long-term effects of creatine supplementation. A few studies have looked at the effect of creatine supplementation on kidney function and have concluded that creatine supplementation does not impair renal function when taken acutely and chronically (for 5 years). There has been one report of a 25-year-old who experienced renal dysfunction caused by creatine supplementation. However, this man had pre-existing kidney disease. Therefore, creatine supplementation is not recommended for those with pre-existing kidney disease or those at high risk for renal disease.[173] All other reports of adverse effects associated with creatine supplementation (e.g., hypertension, muscle cramping, muscle strains, dehydration, and GI distress) are anecdotal and have not been confirmed with controlled research studies.[172] The ACSM does discourage the use of creatine in athletes younger than 18 years of age because there is not enough evidence to make conclusions about the risk/benefit ratio in this population.

Caffeine

Action. Caffeine stimulates the CNS by stimulating the release of catecholamines and blocking adenosine receptors (adenosine has a calming effect). It increases heart rate and contractility and causes peripheral vasodilation. Studies have also shown caffeine to increase muscle motor unit recruitment and enhance calcium transport through increases in calcium permeability in the SR.

Research. The research on the use of caffeine for improving high-intensity performance is mixed. There does not appear to be a conclusive benefit of caffeine in speed and power activities. The differences in study results might be explained by dosage differences or performance outcome. For example, in a study by Anselme and colleagues,[174] no effect was found with a 200-mg dose of caffeine on consecutive Wingate tests. Yet, with a much higher dose of caffeine (6 mg/kg/bw), Schneiker and colleagues[139] found enhanced intermittent sprint cycle performance with the use of caffeine. The effect of caffeine on strength is also inconclusive. Beck and colleagues[175] studied resistance-trained men and found an improved one-repetition maximum (1-RM) performance on the bench press with caffeine supplementation versus no improvement in the placebo group. Conversely, Astorino and colleagues[176] found no difference in bench press 1-RM performance with caffeine supplementation (6 g/kg/bw) in resistance-trained males. In addition, in a subsequent study, Beck and colleagues[177] were unable to replicate their earlier findings in nonresistance-trained males. This suggests that trained athletes are more likely to display a benefit from caffeine ingestion on strength performance than their untrained counterparts.

Application. Because of the inconsistency in findings, there does not appear to be a recommended efficacious dose for high-intensity exercise. Research studies that have found a beneficial effect of caffeine on high-intensity exercise have used 200 mg—6 mg/kg/bw. The caffeine was ingested 45 to 60 minutes prior to exercise.

Adverse Effects. Caffeine ingestion can cause increased heart rate and blood pressure. It can also lead to insomnia, nervousness, and cardiac arrhythmias. Chronic use can be addictive.

Protein

Action. The timing, type, and amount of protein consumption can enhance high-intensity exercise performance through aiding the development of muscle. The benefits of proper protein intake for muscle development during training are described next.

Ergogenic Aids to Improve Body Composition

Measurement of Body Composition

The composition of an individual's body can be divided into the four compartments of bone, water, muscle, and fat, and analytical techniques have been developed to quantify each. These techniques are expensive and complex. Therefore, measurement of body composition usually quantifies fat mass (FM) and groups bone, water, and muscle together as the fat-free mass (FFM). Common techniques to measure these two components of body composition, FM and FFM, include skinfold measurements, bioelectrical impedance, underwater weighing, air displacement plethysmography (using the Bod Pod), and dual x-ray absorptiometry (DXA). DXA also has the ability to separate out bone mass, resulting in the measurement of lean body mass rather than FFM, an indication of the composition of only water and muscle.

Improving Body Composition Through Nutrition and Exercise

Optimal body composition, achieved via both diet and exercise, is important for both athletic performance and health. Thus, methods to improve body composition, specifically decreasing FM while also increasing FFM, are attractive to athletes.[178] Resistance training is one such method to achieve these alterations in body composition, as well as to increase strength.[178] Various methodologies are used, all involving variations of the types of exercises, amount of resistance, number of repetitions, and number of sets. In addition, athletes often use nutrition and ergogenic aids to maximize the changes in body composition with strength training.

Increased FFM is most often related to an increase in muscle mass. Increased muscle mass with chronic resistance training results from repeated acute positive increments in net muscle protein balance, which is achieved from either an increase in muscle protein synthesis or a decrease in muscle protein breakdown.[179] Muscle protein synthesis is influenced by increases in the hormones insulin, growth hormone, insulin-like growth factor-1, and testosterone, whereas muscle protein breakdown is stimulated by increases in cortisol.[180] These hormones are altered by resistance exercise and nutrition, specifically carbohydrate and protein.[180]

Resistance exercise training is an effective method to increase muscle protein synthesis, and nutrition can influence both muscle protein synthesis (protein and amino acids) and decrease muscle protein breakdown (carbohydrates).[179] For maximal gains in muscle mass with strength training, adequate dietary protein is necessary, in amounts of at least the recommended daily allowance (RDA) of 0.8 g/kg/bw, although slightly more might be necessary for strength athletes (1.2-1.6 g/kg/bw).[181] Dietary protein provides the building blocks for muscle protein synthesis and, particularly when combined with carbohydrate, supports the appropriate balance of hormones. Specifics around supplemental protein, including the timing of ingestion and combination with carbohydrate, is discussed in the following text. Beyond nutrition, a few ergogenic aids, also discussed in the following text, may promote gains in FFM when combined with strength training by stimulating the muscle to contract more forcefully, initiating signaling pathways to stimulate muscle protein synthesis, or decrease muscle protein breakdown.

The most effective method to decrease FM is to expend greater calories than are consumed, which is usually best achieved through a combination of both exercise and calorie restriction. When energy balance is negative, lipolysis (the breakdown of triglycerides stored in adipose tissue) is increased and FFAs are liberated to be used for energy production. Lipolysis is primarily stimulated by the catecholamines (i.e., epinephrine and norepinephrine),[182] which are acutely increased during resistance exercise.[183] Ergogenic aids to alter FM could theoretically work to increase the hormones that signal lipolysis, increase resting metabolic rate and the oxidation of fatty acids for energy, or to decrease fat storage in adipose tissue. To illustrate the relationship between compartments of body composition, increased metabolic rate may be related to the amount of FFM[184]; therefore, one method to decrease FM may be to increase FFM.

Ergogenic Aids to Increase Muscle Mass
Carbohydrate and Protein Supplements

Action. Consumption of protein or amino acids in close proximity to a bout of resistance exercise augments the anabolic response to exercise, resulting in increased muscle mass over the course of a strength training program. The addition of carbohydrate further improves the result, presumably because of the higher insulin response, which helps amino acid uptake into the muscle. The type and timing of protein and carbohydrate supplement consumption are important factors related to the extent of increased muscle hypertrophy.

Research. Acute responses to exercise can be enhanced through appropriate nutrition, which then should translate into chronic adaptations, in this case increased muscle mass.[179] Much of the research conducted on protein and carbohydrate focuses on acute ingestion before or after a bout of resistance exercise to increase muscle protein synthesis and the acute anabolic response.[185] However, the research discussed in this section focuses on the benefit of chronic use of protein and carbohydrate supplements with training to increase muscle mass.

Nutrition in combination with resistance training is more effective than training alone to increase muscle mass. Holm and colleagues[186] conducted a 24-week training program in postmenopausal women who consumed either a supplement containing protein, carbohydrate, calcium, and vitamin D (730 kJ) or a placebo containing minimal energy from carbohydrate (102 kJ) immediately after each training session. Lean body mass was significantly increased in the group provided with nutrition as compared with minimal calories. When comparing the types of nutritional supplement, consumption of a protein supplement around the time of the exercise bout is more effective than a carbohydrate supplement to increase muscle mass with resistance

training programs of 10 to 12 weeks.[187,188] However, the combination of macronutrients appears to be more effective than either alone. During a 6-week resistance training program, consumption of whey or soy protein with sucrose was more effective in increasing lean tissue mass than consumption of the calorie-matched, carbohydrate-only supplement in men and women (n = 27).[189] For each group, the supplement was divided into three equal doses and consumed immediately before and after each training session, as well as before going to bed. No differences were observed between the whey and soy protein groups. Likewise, using fat-free milk as the protein source, Hartman and colleagues[190] observed greater increases in type II muscle fiber area and FFM when compared with calorie-matched carbohydrate or soy protein beverages when consumed immediately following each exercise bout and again 1 hour later. In summary, consumption of a supplement containing both carbohydrate and protein during a strength training program appears to be more effective at increasing muscle mass than providing nutrition to the exercised muscle as carbohydrate or protein alone.

Clinical Point

Protein and carbohydrate supplementation together are more effective at increasing muscle mass during strength training if consumed immediately or within 1 hour of training.

Application. The type, timing, and amount of carbohydrate plus protein supplementation are all important considerations for maximal gains in muscle mass with resistance training. A high-quality protein that provides all of the essential amino acids is the best choice, such as whey, casein, or soy. The benefit of soy protein is equivocal,[189,190] and some concern exists over the relationship between soy protein and testosterone levels. However, Kalman and colleagues[191] found that 12 weeks of supplementation during resistance training with soy protein concentrate or isolate, as compared with a soy isolate and whey blend or whey alone, did not decrease testosterone levels and resulted in similar increases in muscle mass in male subjects (n = 20). Whey and casein have been found to be equally effective in promoting net muscle protein synthesis,[192] as has their combination as found naturally in milk.[190] In general, a high-quality protein supplement, such as whey, casein, or milk-based protein should be the choice as a supplement to resistance training. Any simple carbohydrate source is an effective way to stimulate insulin and maximize the benefit of protein.

Timing of nutrient ingestion in relation to each training session is also an important consideration. Consumption of a carbohydrate and protein supplement either immediately prior or immediately following exercise results in the same effect on net muscle protein synthesis,[193] whereas in elderly subjects a carbohydrate-protein supplement consumed immediately after each session of 12 weeks of resistance training resulted in greater increases in lean body mass as compared with consumption 2 hours following each training bout.[194] In general, carbohydrate with high-quality protein should be consumed immediately or within 1 hour following resistance exercise.[181]

Although most athletes consume adequate protein in a day to support muscle hypertrophy, the timing of a certain amount of protein and carbohydrate in relation to a strength training session may be more important than total daily protein consumption.[181] To stimulate acute net muscle protein synthesis with resistance training, 6 g of essential amino acids plus 35 g of sucrose is sufficient.[195] In terms of whole protein, Tang and colleagues[196] found that 10 g of whey protein with 21 g of fructose was sufficient to significantly increase the rate of muscle protein synthesis in resistance-trained young men when consumed immediately after leg extension exercise, as compared with calorie-matched carbohydrate. The upper limits to the doses of carbohydrate and high-quality protein needed are 35 g and 20 to 25 g, respectively.[181] Protein intake of more than this amount provides no additional stimulation of muscle protein synthesis.[181]

Carbohydrate and protein in the amounts described previously can easily be obtained from whole foods. However, for athletes who need a quick and easy solution, protein and carbohydrate supplements are sold as powders, shakes, and bars. Individuals should check the nutrition labels to make sure the supplement contains a high-quality protein source, does not contain high amounts of fat or other unwanted substances, and the amounts of carbohydrate and protein are reasonable and fit the previously listed guidelines.

Adverse Effects. For individuals with normal renal function, there does not appear to be any adverse effects to consumption of protein plus carbohydrate supplements.[181]

Creatine

Action. CP is the first source of energy the muscle uses for contraction. The creatine found in muscle used to generate CP is synthesized from amino acids (arginine, glycine, and methionine), or consumed in the diet, primarily from meat. Consumption of creatine supplements can add to this creatine pool in the muscle. Although the exact mechanism is not known, creatine supplementation appears to prevent fatigue. Ingestion of creatine itself will not increase muscle mass; however, creatine supplementation in combination with resistance training is effective in increasing muscle mass and strength as compared with training alone.

Research. A large number of studies examining the ergogenic benefit of creatine supplementation have been published, the majority of which find a benefit of increased muscle mass and strength.[197] Branch[198] and Nissen and Sharp[199] have both conducted meta-analyses of the creatine literature, and concluded that creatine supplementation does increase lean body mass and strength. In addition, Rawson and Volek[200]

reviewed 22 studies of creatine supplementation during resistance training, and found 17 to result in an ergogenic benefit. On average, an 8% gain in strength was found with creatine supplementation versus placebo.[200] Although creatine supplementation overall appears to be effective in increasing muscle mass with strength training, individuals may respond differently. Syrotuik and Bell[201] suggest that individuals who respond to creatine supplementation typically begin with a low amount of muscle creatine, have a high percentage of type II muscle fibers, and have the greatest muscle fiber cross-sectional areas and FFM.

Application. Several different protocols are suggested for creatine use; most involve a loading phase followed by a maintenance phase. For example, an effective method is loading with 20 g/day for 5 days, followed by 2 g/day for 30 days.[202] However, loading may not be necessary because supplementation with 3 g/day of creatine for 28 days has been found to result in similar muscle creatine concentrations as the 5-day loading protocol.[202] Addition of carbohydrate alone[203] or with protein[204] may enhance the benefit of creatine supplementation. For example, when combined with a carbohydrate-protein supplement during a 10-week strength training program, creatine supplementation (0.1 g/kg/day) resulted in greater muscle hypertrophy than the carbohydrate-protein supplement alone.[204] A loading phase was not used in this protocol. The use of a carbohydrate-protein-creatine supplement appears to be most effective when consumed immediately before and after the exercise bout.[205]

Adverse Effects. Acute ingestion of creatine does not appear to result in adverse effects in the general population, with clinical studies not reporting significant changes in renal, hepatic, cardiac, or muscle function.[206] Less is known about the long-term side effects of creatine supplementation, but chronic intake of up to 5 g/day for up to 1 year appears to be safe.[207,208]

Beta-Hydroxy-Beta-Methylbutyrate

Action. Beta-hydroxy-methylbutyrate (HMB) supplementation may increase muscle mass when consumed during resistance training. It is hypothesized that the mechanism for this benefit occurs though an inhibition of muscle protein breakdown or by promoting repair of damaged muscle cells.[209] For a detailed description of the mechanism of action, refer to the comprehensive review by Wilson and colleagues.[209]

Research. In individuals without a history of strength training, HMB supplementation during a training program has been found to increase muscle mass[210] and decrease muscle damage,[210,211] although increases in muscle mass have not always been observed even with significant decreases in markers of muscle damage.[212] Regardless of training history or gender, Panton and colleagues[213] found a trend (p = 0.08) to increased muscle mass with HMB supplementation versus placebo (1.4 ± 0.2 versus 0.9 ± 0.2 kg, respectively) during a 4-week strength training study (39 men and

36 women participated in the study). Perhaps a significant difference would have been observed with a longer training program. When examining highly trained athletes, a randomized, double-blind crossover study of collegiate football players (n = 35) did not find a benefit of HMB supplementation on muscle mass or strength versus placebo.[214] More research is needed in trained individuals with training programs designed to induce a greater state of catabolism than needed to see a benefit in untrained individuals. Overall, a meta-analysis conducted by Nissen and Sharp,[199] which included nine studies of HMB supplementation in both trained and untrained individuals, found supplementation with 3 g/day resulted in a 0.28% gain in lean mass and 1.5% increase in strength per week.

Application. HMB is sold as a supplement primarily in the form of calcium HMB monohydrate. The effective dose appears to be 3 g/day, consumed in separate 1-g doses throughout the day, or 38 mg/kg.[209,215] More research is needed to investigate higher doses and define an optimal amount for supplementation.

Adverse Effects. HMB supplementation appears to be safe, with no adverse or side effects reported in the current literature.[209] Eight weeks of supplementation with 0, 38, or 76 mg HMB/kg during resistance training did not alter liver enzyme or renal function, lipid profile, or the immune system.[216]

Ergogenic Aids to Decrease Fat Mass and Increase Fat-Free Mass

Conjugated Linoleic Acid

Action. Conjugated linoleic acid (CLA) is an unsaturated fatty acid, small amounts of which are found naturally in milk and meat. Although there are several isomers of this fatty acid, the most common are c9, t11-CLA and t10, c12-CLA. The supplemental form found to be efficacious contains a 50:50 mixture of these two isomers. The strongest benefit of CLA supplementation appears to be reduction in FM, although some evidence suggests the ability to increase FFM as well when consumed during strength training. The exact mechanism of action is currently unknown.

Research. The ability of CLA to alter body composition has been studied primarily in overweight and obese individuals during routine activities of daily living. Although not all studies have a shown a benefit, a recent meta-analysis indicates consistent-but-modest decreases in FM (average loss of 0.05 kg/wk with 3.2 g CLA/day for 6 months).[217] Applied to an exercising population, it seems CLA may augment the effects of exercise training on body composition. In normal-weight males and females with a moderate strength training history (at least two times per week, n = 85), supplementation with 5 g/day CLA during 7 weeks of resistance training was found to significantly increase lean tissue mass and decrease FM as compared with placebo.[218] When studying resistance-trained athletes (n = 28), CLA supplementation

for 28 days (6 g/day) did not significantly change FFM, FM, or bone mass.[219] However, statistical trends to greater alterations in FFM and FM with moderate to large effect sizes were found. The 28-day study is a very short period to be able to detect any significant changes in body composition associated with training, especially in a highly-trained population; therefore, a longer training period may have resulted in a statistical benefit of CLA.

Application. CLA is sold as a supplement in a 50:50 isomer mixture. The effective dose appears to be approximately 3.2 g/day. More research needs to be conducted to find an ideal effective dose in combination with strength training.

Adverse Effects. In some studies, supplementation with CLA has been found to induce insulin resistance.[220,221] However, this observation has been made in overweight and obese humans, not with exercise training. The majority of studies do not report adverse events with supplementation. The Food and Drug Administration (FDA) has declared CLA to be generally recognized as safe in recommended doses.

The focus of this section is nutritional ergogenic aids that may improve the potential of strength training to increase FFM and decrease FM. There are a few supplements that have limited research relating them to increased FFM (vitamin D in older adults[222-224]) and decreased FM (calcium[225] and alpha-hydroxycitric acid, a plant extract from *Garcinia cambogia*[226]); however, the ability of these supplements to further augment the outcomes of exercise have not been researched. Furthermore, there are various other ergogenic aids that have been proposed to improve body composition but are not discussed in this section because they are illegal or lack scientific support.

Ergogenic Aids for Body Composition that Have Little Scientific Support, Lack Investigation or Are Illegal

- Chromium picolinate
- Pyruvate
- Leucine
- Carnitine
- Anabolic steroids
- Human growth hormone
- Androstenedione

A Note on Anabolic Steroids

Although the focus of this chapter is legal, nutritional ergogenic aids, the media attention and prevalence of anabolic steroid use to increase muscle mass and improve performance warrants a brief discussion. Much of the information for this section was adapted from Chapter 15, "The Use of Ergogenic Aids in Athletics," in *Athletic Injuries and Rehabilitation*.[227]

Anabolic-androgenic steroids are synthetic derivatives of the male hormone testosterone; they were originally developed to hasten tissue repair in debilitating conditions[228] such as human immunodeficiency virus–related muscle wasting, chronic obstructive pulmonary disease, severe burn injuries, and alcoholic hepatitis.[229] The most common anabolic-androgenic steroids approved for therapeutic use by the FDA are nandrolone, decanoate, oxandrolone, oxymetholone, and stanolzolol.[229]

The effects of synthetic steroid derivatives are anabolic (protein building) and androgenic (masculinizing or producing male secondary sex characteristics).[230,231] Similar to endogenous steroid hormones, the synthetic derivatives are thought to have muscle-building properties. The mechanism of action appears to be a combination of muscle cell hypertrophy[5] and formation of new skeletal muscle proteins.[232,233] Published research on the efficacy of synthetic derivatives began to appear in the 1970s, with some of the early studies finding enhancement of muscular mass and strength, and an indication of improved oxygen consumption,[234-237] whereas others yielded conflicting results.[238,239] Overall, the benefit of synthetic steroid use by athletes is to increase strength approximately 5% to 20%[240,241] and lean body mass by 2 to 5 kg.[241] Although androgens may stimulate erythropoesis (increased erythrocyte production),[229] and some athletes report better recovery and the ability to train at a higher capacity, synthetic steroid use does not appear to improve endurance performance.[242]

Anabolic steroids may be taken orally or injected. Athletes frequently use a combination of multiple types of steroids at dosages 10- to 100-fold higher than the recommended therapeutic dosage, a technique called "stacking."[243] An athlete may experiment with different numbers of anabolic steroids and gradually reduce usage as he or she gets closer to competition to avoid detection if drug testing is anticipated.[244]

Although some athletes abusing anabolic-androgenic steroids may experience only minor side effects, according to scientific evidence and personal testimonials from abusers, others may suffer severe and potentially life-threatening effects.[241,245] The potentially harmful medical side effects greatly outweigh any performance-boosting benefits these drugs may offer.

Strong, continuous efforts should be made by sports medicine personnel in every athletic discipline to educate athletes, coaches, the general public, and others associated with athletes about the inconsistent effects of anabolic steroids and their potentially harmful side effects. The potential dangers of taking these substances for long periods in large doses should be made abundantly clear. The use of anabolic-androgenic steroids is considered illegal by sports governing bodies such as the International Olympic Committee and the National Collegiate Athletic Association.[255]

Major Adverse Side Effects of Anabolic-Androgenic Steroid Use[241,245-254]

General
- Liver dysfunction
- Alopecia (hair loss)
- Immune system dysfunction
- Wilms tumor (kidney malignancy)
- Peliosis hepatis (liver cysts filled with blood)
- Decreased high-density lipoproteins
- Increased low-density lipoproteins
- Aggressive behavior (explosive rages)
- Psychiatric problems (depression, suicidal thoughts, psychoses)
- Premature epiphyseal closure in children
- Connective tissue disruption
- Liver and kidney tumors
- Hypercholesterolemia
- Migraine headaches

In Males
- Testicular atrophy
- Prostate gland problems (enlargement, adenocarcinoma)
- Gynecomastia (breast development)
- Increased sexual aggressiveness initially, but impotence with prolonged use
- Acne
- Abnormally low sperm count

In Females
- Enlarged clitoris
- Masculinizing effect
- Menstrual irregularities (dysmenorrhea, amenorrhea)
- Hirsutism (excessive hairiness of face, body)
- Deepening of voice

Ergogenic Aids for Bones and Joints

Bone formation occurs during childhood and adolescence, when bones increase in both length and width.[256] More than 25% of peak bone mineral density is obtained between the ages of 12 to 14 years for girls and 13 to 15 years for boys,[257] with peak bone mass obtained in the early 20s.[256] Once peak bone mass is reached, the bone continues to turn over; however, bone loss occurs continuously and gradually throughout the remainder of the lifespan.[258] Peak bone mass and maintenance, or a slowing of bone loss, are influenced by both proper nutrition and exercise.[256-258]

Calcium and vitamin D are essential nutrients to support healthy bone mass. The RDA for calcium is 1300 mg/day for ages 9 to 18 years, 1000 mg/day for ages 19 to 50, and 1200 mg/day for individuals older than 50 years.[256] The adequate intake of vitamin D is 200 IU/day for individuals younger than 50 years old and 400 IU/day for those older than 50.[256] Other important components of the diet beyond calcium and vitamin D that support bone health are vitamins A, C, and K, magnesium, zinc, copper, iron, fluoride, as well as adequate protein.[256]

Mechanical loading of the bone via weight-bearing exercise is also essential for healthy bone mass both during the formative years and for maintenance.[257-259] Running, walking, strength training, and jumping are all modes of exercise that have positive influence on the bone. When bone is overloaded by exercise, formation is favored over resorption of the bone.[259] Theories as to the mechanism by which the mechanical stimulus from impact exercise enhances bone formation may include prostaglandin release, changes in electrical stimulation, increased bone blood flow, microdamage that leads to the formation of new bone, and alterations in hormones such as testosterone and calcitriol.[259] Exercise appears to enhance the effect of nutrition, particularly calcium, on bone mass.[257,260,261] Additional ergogenic aids beyond the nutrition discussed previously have not been identified to help augment the effect of exercise on bone. However, limited information exists in humans that omega-3 fatty acid consumption may be related to higher bone mass.[262,263]

Joint function and health, particularly the collagen structures linking joints to bone, may also be influenced by supplementation with omega-3 fatty acids. A meta-analysis of 17 randomized, controlled trials conducted by Goldberg and Katz[264] found disease-related joint pain, stiffness, and nonsteroidal anti-inflammatory drug use to be reduced by consumption of omega-3 fatty acids. Greater improvements were observed when the dose was greater than 2.7 g/day. Research has not been conducted on omega-3 fatty acids with athletes suffering from joint pain; however, supplementation with collagen hydrolysate protein (10 g/day for 24 weeks) has been found to decrease joint pain in collegiate athletes suffering from activity- or injury-related pain, but not disease-related joint pain.[265]

A combination of glucosamine and chondroitin is probably the most well-known supplement related to joint health. The evidence for efficacy of these supplements is primarily related to lessening of the symptoms of knee and hip osteoarthritis.[266,267] Osteoarthritis is common several years after joint injuries, particularly injuries to the anterior cruciate ligament;[268] therefore, prevalence in athletes may be high. Also, alleviating symptoms of osteoarthritis may help people stay active. Little information is available on the efficacy of glucosamine and chondroitin for athletes suffering from nonosteoarthritis joint pain or for maintenance of joint health to prevent injury. One published study in athletes investigated glucosamine (1500 mg/day, without chondroitin) use for 4 weeks following knee injury. Significant differences between the glucosamine and placebo groups were not found for swelling or pain during rest or walking. However, at the end of 4 weeks, the glucosamine group had better knee flexion and extension compared with placebo.[269]

Although omega-3 fatty acids, collagen hydrolysate proteins, and glucosamine-chondroitin supplements have not been studied as ergogenic aids to exercise for additive benefits, it can be argued that improved joint functioning or reduced joint pain can lead to better exercise performance.

Conclusion

The information presented in this chapter has focused on nutritional ergogenic aids that are safe, legal, and to date have been shown to be reasonably effective. However, new information on this topic will continue to emerge. The following web resources provide some of the most up-to-date information related to nutritional ergogenic aids: the U.S. Department of Agriculture's website for nutritional supplements and ergogenic aids (fnic.nal.usda.gov), www.ncaa.org (search "nutritional supplements"), www.supplementwatch.com, and www.drugfreesport.com.

References

1. Rowell LB: *Human circulation regulation during human stress*, New York, 1986, Oxford University.
2. Borg G: Simple rating for estimation of perceived exertion. In Borg G, editor: *Physical work and effort*, New York, 1975, Pergamon Press.
3. Friedman R, Elliot AJ: Exploring the influence of sports drink exposure on physical endurance, *Psychol Sport Exerc* 9:749–759, 2008.
4. Nybo L, Nielsen B: Middle cerebral artery blood flow velocity is reduced with hyperthermia during prolonged exercise in humans, *J Physiol* 534:279–286, 2001.
5. Johannsen P, Christensen L, Sinkjaer T, et al: Cerebral functional anatomy of voluntary contractions in ankle muscles in man, *J Physiol* 535:397–406, 2001.
6. Liu JZ, Shan ZY, Zhang LD, et al: Human brain activation during sustained and intermittent submaximal fatigue muscle contractions: An fMRI study, *J Neurophysiol* 90:300–312, 2003.
7. Newsholme EA, Acworth IN, Blomstrand E: Amino acids, brain neurotransmitters and a functional link between muscle and brain that is important in sustained exercise. In Benzi G, editor: *Advances in myochemistry*, London, UK, 1987, John Libby Eurotext.
8. Meeusen R, Watson P, Hasegawa H, et al: Central fatigue: the serotonin hypothesis and beyond, *Sports Med* 36:881–909, 2006.
9. Noakes TD, St. Clair Gibson A, Lambert EV: From catastrophe to complexity: A novel model of integrative central neural regulation of effort and fatigue during exercise in humans, *Br J Sports Med* 38:511–514, 2004.
10. Coggan AR, Coyle EF: Reversal of fatigue during prolonged exercise by carbohydrate infusion or ingestion, *J Appl Physiol* 63:2388–2395, 1987.
11. Cheuvront SN, Carter R, Castellani JW, et al: Fluid balance and endurance exercise performance, *Curr Sports Med Rep* 2:202–208, 2003.
12. Maughan RJ: Physiological responses to fluid intake during exercise. In Maughan RJ, Murray R, editors: *Sports drinks: Basic science and practical aspects*, Boca Raton, FL, 2001, CRC Press.

13. Binkley HM, Beckett J, Casa DJ, et al: National Athletic Trainers' position statement: Exertional heat illness, *J Athl Train* 37: 329–343, 2002.

14. Gonzalez-Alonso J: Separate and combined influences of dehydration and hyperthermia on cardiovascular responses to exercise, *Int J Sports Med* 19:S111–S114, 1998.

15. Lieberman HR: Hydration and cognition: A critical review and recommendations for future research, *J Am Coll Nutr* 26:555S–561S, 2007.

16. Baker LB, Dougherty KA, Chow M, et al: Progressive dehydration causes a progressive decline in basketball skill performance, *Med Sci Sports Exerc* 39:1114–1123, 2007.

17. Montain SJ, Coyle EF: Influence of the timing of fluid ingestion on temperature regulation during exercise, *J Appl Physiol* 75: 688–695, 1993.

18. Stover EA, Zachwieja J, Stofan J, et al: Consistently high urine specific gravity in adolescent American football players and the impact of an acute drinking strategy, *Int J Sports Med* 27: 330–335, 2006.

19. Godek SF, Godek JJ, Bartolozzi AR: Hydration status in college football players during consecutive days of twice-a-day preseason practices, *Am J Sports Med* 33:843–851, 2005.

20. Bergeron MF, Waller JL, Marinik EL: Voluntary fluid intake and core temperature responses in adolescent tennis players: Sports beverage versus water, *Br J Sports Med* 40:406–410, 2006.

21. Castellani JW, Maresh CM, Armstrong LE, et al: Intravenous vs. oral rehydration: Effects on subsequent exercise-heat stress, *J Appl Physiol* 82:799–806, 1997.

22. Casa DJ, Maresh CM, Armstrong LE, et al: Intravenous versus oral rehydration during a brief period: Responses to subsequent exercise in the heat, *Med Sci Sports Exerc* 32:124–133, 2000.

23. Vrijens DMJ, Rehrer NJ: Sodium-free fluid ingestion decreases plasma sodium during exercise in the heat, *J Appl Physiol* 86:1847–1851, 1999.

24. Nose H, Mack GW, Shi XR, Nadel ER: Role of osmolality and plasma volume during rehydration in humans, *J Appl Physiol* 65:325–331, 1988.

25. Wilk B, Bar-Or O: Effect of drink flavor and NaCl on voluntary drinking and hydration in boys exercising in the heat, *J Appl Physiol* 80:1112–1117, 1996.

26. Bergeron MF: Heat cramps during tennis: A case report, *Int J Sports Nutr* 6:62–68, 1996.

27. Stofan JR, Zachwieja JJ, Horswill CA, et al: Sweat and sodium losses in NCAA football players: A precursor to heat cramps? *Int J Sports Nutr* 15:641–652, 2005.

28. Armstrong LE: Considerations for replacement beverages: Fluid –electrolyte balance and heat illness. Marriott BM, editor: *In Fluid replacement and heat stress*, National Academy Press, Washington, DC, 1994.

29. Murray B: Hydration and physical performance, *J Am Coll Nutr* 26:542s–548s, 2007.

30. Coyle EF: Fluid and fuel intake during exercise, *J Sports Sci* 22:39–55, 2004.

31. Maughan RJ, Shirreffs SM, Leiper JB: Errors in the estimation of hydration status from changes in body mass, *J Sports Sci* 25: 797–804, 2007.

32. King RFGJ, Cooke C, Carroll S, O'Hara J: Estimating changes in hydration status from changes in body mass: Considerations regarding metabolic water and glycogen storage, *J Sports Sci* 26(12):1361–1363, 2008.

33. Casa DJ, Armstrong LE, Hillman SK, et al: National Athletic Trainers' Association position statement: Fluid replacement for athletes, *J Athl Train* 35:212–224, 2000.

34. Sawka MN, Burke LM, Eichner ER, et al: American College of Sports Medicine position stand. Exercise and fluid replacement, *Med Sci Sports Exerc* 39:377–390, 2007.

35. Sawka MN, Noakes TD: Does dehydration impair exercise performance? *Med Sci Sports Exerc* 39:1209–1217, 2007.

36. Greenleaf JE, Looft-Wilson R, Wisherd JL, et al: Pre-exercise hypervolemia and cycle ergometer endurance in men, *Biol Sport* 14:103–114, 1997.

37. Riedesel ML, Allen DY, Peake GT, et al: Hyperhydration with glycerol solutions, *J Appl Physiol* 63:2262–2268, 1987.

38. Greenleaf JE: Problem: Thirst, drinking behavior, and involuntary dehydration, *Med Sci Sports Exerc* 24:645–656, 1992.

39. Freund BJ, Montain SJ, Young AJ, et al: Glycerol hyperhydration: Hormonal, renal, and vascular fluid responses, *J Appl Physiol* 79:2069–2077, 1995.

40. Dill DB, Costill DL: Calculation of percentage changes in volumes of blood, plasma, and red cells in dehydration, *J Appl Physiol* 37:247–248, 1974.

41. Anderson MJ, Cotter JD, Garnham AP, et al: Effect of glycerol-induced hyperhydration on thermoregulation and metabolism during exercise in the heat, *Int J Sports Nutr* 11:315–333, 2001.

42. Montner P, Zou Y, Robergs RA, et al: Glycerol hyperhydration alters cardiovascular and renal function, *J Exerc Physiol Online* 2:1–10, 1999.

43. Latzka WA, Sawka MN, Montain SJ, et al: Hyperhydration: Tolerance and cardiovascular effects during uncompensable exercise-heat stress, *J Appl Physiol* 84:1858–1864, 1998.

44. Lyons TP, Riedesel ML, Meuli LE, et al: Effects of glycerol-induced hyperhydration prior to exercise in the heat on sweating and core temperature, *Med Sci Sports Exerc* 22:477–483, 1990.

45. Marino FE, Day D, Cannon J: Glycerol hyperhydration fails to improve endurance performance and thermoregulation in humans in a warm humid environment, *Pflugers Arch* 446:455–462, 2003.

46. Murray R, Eddy DE, Paul GL, et al: Physiological responses to glycerol ingestion during exercise, *J Appl Physiol* 71:144–149, 1991.

47. Coutts A, Reaburn P, Mummery K, et al: The effect of glycerol hyperhydration on Olympic distance triathlon performance in high ambient temperatures, *Int J Sports Nutr* 12:105–119, 2002.

48. Montner P, Stark DM, Riedesel ML, et al: Pre-exercise glycerol hydration improves cycling endurance time, *Int J Sports Med* 17:27–33, 1996.

49. Latzka WA, Sawka MN, Montain SJ, et al: Hyperhydration: Thermoregulatory effects during compensable exercise-heat stress, *J Appl Physiol* 83:860–866, 1997.

50. Siegler JC, Mermier CM, Amorim FT, et al: Hydration, thermoregulation, and performance effects of two sports drinks during soccer training sessions, *J Strength Cond Res* 22:1394–1401, 2008.

51. Sherman WM, Costill DL, Fink WJ, et al: The effect of exercise and diet manipulation on muscle glycogen and its subsequent utilization during performance, *Int J Sports Med* 2:114–118, 1981.

52. Fairchild TJ, Fletcher S, Steele P, et al: Rapid carbohydrate loading after short bout of near maximal intensity exercise, *Med Sci Sports Exerc* 34:980–986, 2002.

53. Bergstrom J, Hultman E: A study of the glycogen metabolism during exercise in man, *Scan J Clin Lab Invest* 19:218–228, 1967.

54. Hultman E: Studies on muscle metabolism of glycogen and active phosphate in man with special reference to exercise and diet, *Scan J Clin Lab Invest* 19:94, 1967.

55. Karlsson J, Saltin B: Diet, muscle glycogen and endurance performance, *J Appl Physiol* 31:203–206, 1971.

56. Coyle EF, Coggan AR, Hemmert MK, et al: Substrate usage during prolonged exercise following a pre-exercise meal, *J Appl Physiol* 59:429–433, 1985.

57. Sherman WM, Brodowicz G, Wright DA, et al: Effects of 4 h preexercise carbohydrate feedings on cycling performance, *Med Sci Sports Exerc* 21:598–604, 1989.

58. Costill DL, Coyle E, Dalsky G, et al: Effects of elevated FFA and insulin on muscle glycogen usage during exercise, *J Appl Physiol* 43:695–699, 1977.

59. Foster C, Costill DL, Fink WJ: Effects of pre-exercise feedings on endurance performance, *Med Sci Sports Exerc* 11:1–5, 1979.

60. Goodpaster BH, Costill DL, Fink WJ, et al.: The effects of pre-exercise starch ingestion on endurance performance, *Int J Sports Med* 17:366–372, 1996.

61. Sherman WM, Peden MC, Wright DA: Carbohydrate feedings 1 h before exercise improves cycling performance, *Am J Clin Nutr* 54:866–870, 1991.

62. Moseley L, Lancaster GI, Jeukendrup AE: Effects of timing of pre-exercise ingestion of carbohydrate on subsequent metabolism and cycling performance, *Eur J Appl Physiol* 88:453–458, 2003.

63. Burke LM, Claassen A, Hawley JA, et al: Carbohydrate intake during prolonged cycling minimizes the effect of glycemic index of pre-exercise meal, *J Appl Physiol* 85:2220–2226, 1998.

64. Costill DL, Saltin B: Factors limiting gastric emptying during rest and exercise, *J Appl Physiol* 37:679–683, 1974.

65. Costill DL, Bennett A, Branam G, et al: Glucose ingestion at rest and during prolonged exercise, *J Appl Physiol* 34:764–769, 1973.

66. Coyle EF, Hagberg JM, Hurley BF, et al: Carbohydrate feeding during prolonged exercise can delay fatigue, *J Appl Physiol* 55:230–235, 1983.

67. Jeukendrup AE: Carbohydrate intake during exercise and performance, *Nutrition* 20:669–677, 2004.

68. Murray R, Bartoli W, Stofan J, et al: A comparison of the gastric emptying characteristics of selected sports drinks, *Int J Sports Nutr* 9:263–274, 1999.

69. Shi X, Summers RW, Schedl HP, et al: Effects of carbohydrate type and concentration and solution osmolality on water absorption, *Med Sci Sports Exerc* 27:1607–1615, 1995.

70. Ryan AJ, Lambert GP, Shi X, et al: Effect of hypohydration on gastric emptying and intestinal absorption during exercise, *J Appl Physiol* 84:1581–1588, 1998.

71. Jentjens RLPG, Moseley L, Waring RH, et al: Oxidation of combined ingestion of glucose and fructose during exercise, *J Appl Physiol* 96:1277–1284, 2004.

72. Jentjens RLPG, Venables MC, Jeukendrup AE: Oxidation of exogenous glucose, sucrose and maltose during prolonged cycling exercise, *J Appl Physiol* 96:1285–1291, 2004.

73. Rowlands DS, Thorburn MS, Thorp RM, et al: Effect of graded fructose coingestion with maltodextrin on exogenous ^{14}C-fructose and ^{13}C-glucose oxidation efficiency and high-intensity cycling performance, *J Appl Physiol* 104:1709–1719, 2008.

74. Nicholas C, Williams C, Lakomy H, et al: Influence of ingesting carbohydrate-electrolyte solution on endurance capacity during intermittent, high-intensity shuttle running, *J Sport Sci* 13:283–290, 1995.

75. Davis JM, Welsh R, Alderson N: Effects of carbohydrate and chromium ingestion during intermittent high-intensity exercise to fatigue, *Int J Sports Nutr* 10:476–485, 2000.

76. Welsh RS, Davis JM, Burke JR, et al: Carbohydrates and physical/mental performance during intermittent exercise to fatigue, *Med Sci Sports Exerc* 34:723–731, 2002.

77. Winnick JJ, Davis JM, Welsh RS, et al: Carbohydrate feedings during team sport exercise preserve physical and CNS function, *Med Sci Sports Exerc* 37:306–315, 2005.

78. Vergauwen L, Brouns F, Hespel P: Carbohydrate supplementation improves stroke performance in tennis, *Med Sci Sports Exerc* 30:1289–1295, 1998.

79. Utter AC, Kang J, Robertson RJ, et al: Effect of carbohydrate ingestion on ratings of perceived exertion during a marathon, *Med Sci Sports Exerc* 34:1779–1784, 2002.

80. Nybo L: CNS fatigue and prolonged exercise: effects of glucose supplementation, *Med Sci Sports Exerc* 35:589–594, 2003.

81. Carter JM, Jeukendrup AE, Jones DA: The effect of carbohydrate mouth rinse in 1-h cycle time trial performance, *Med Sci Sports Exerc* 36:2107–2111, 2004.

82. Clark VR, Hopkins WG, Hawley JA, et al: Placebo effect of carbohydrate feedings during a 40-km cycling time trial, *Med Sci Sports Exerc* 32:1642–1647, 2000.

83. Colombani PC, Kovacs E, Frey-Rindova P, et al: Metabolic effects of protein-supplemented carbohydrate drink in marathon runners, *Int J Sports Med* 9:181–201, 1999.

84. Koopman R, Pannemans DLE, Jeukendrup AE, et al: Combined ingestion of protein and carbohydrate improves protein balance during ultra-endurance exercise, *Am J Physiol* 287:E712–E720, 2004.

85. Williams MB, Raven PB, Fogt DL, et al: Effects of recovery beverages on glycogen restoration and endurance exercise performance, *J Strength Cond Res* 17:12–19, 2003.

86. Ivy JL, Res PT, Sprague RC, Widzer MO: Effect of carbohydrate-protein supplement on endurance performance during exercise of varying intensity, *Int J Sports Nutr* 13:382–395, 2003.

87. Saunders MJ, Kane MD, Todd MK: Effects of carbohydrate-protein beverage on cycling endurance and muscle damage, *Med Sci Sports Exerc* 36:1233–1238, 2004.

88. Romano-Ely BC, Todd MK, Saunders MJ, et al: Effect of an isocaloric carbohydrate-protein-antioxidant drink on cycling performance, *Med Sci Sports Exerc* 38:1608–1616, 2006.

89. Valentine RJ, Saunders MJ, Todd MK, et al: Influence of carbohydrate-protein beverage on cycling endurance and indices of muscle disruption, *Int J Sports Nutr* 18:363–378, 2008.

90. Van Essen M, Gibala MJ: Failure of protein to improve time trial performance when added to a sports drink, *Med Sci Sports Exerc* 38:1476–1483, 2006.

91. Osterberg KL, Zachwieja JJ, Smith JW: Carbohydrate and carbohydrate + protein for cycling time trial performance, *J Sports Sci* 26:227–233, 2008.

92. Betts JA, Stevenson E, Williams C, et al: Recovery of endurance running capacity: Effect of carbohydrate-protein mixtures, *Int J Sports Nutr* 15:590–609, 2005.

93. Betts J, Williams C, Duffy K, et al: The influence of carbohydrate and protein ingestion during recovery from prolonged exercise on subsequent endurance performance, *J Sports Sci* 25:1449–1460, 2007.

94. Millard-Stafford M, Warren GL, Thomas LM, et al: Recovery from run training: Efficacy of a carbohydrate-protein beverage? *Int J Sports Nutr* 15:610–624, 2005.

95. Karp JR, Johnston JD, Tecklenburg S, et al: Chocolate milk as a post-exercise recovery aid, *Int J Sports Nutr* 16:78–91, 2006.

96. Rowlands DS, Rossler K, Thorp RM, et al: Effect of dietary protein content during recovery from high-intensity cycling on subsequent performance and markers of stress, inflammation, and muscle damage in well-trained men, *Appl Physiol Nutr Metab* 33:39–51, 2008.

97. Rowlands DS, Thorp RM, Rossler K, et al: Effect of protein-rich feeding on recovery after intense exercise, *Int J Sports Nutr* 17:521–543, 2007.

98. Hunt JN, Stubbs DF: The volume and energy content of meals as determinants of gastric emptying, *J Physiol* 245:209–225, 1975.

99. Maughan RJ, Leiper JB, Vist GE: Gastric emptying and fluid availability after ingestion of glucose and soy protein hydrolysate solutions in man, *Exp Physiol* 89:101–108, 2004.

100. Blomstrand E, Celsing F, Newsholme EA: Changes in plasma concentrations of aromatic and branched-chain amino acids during sustained exercise in man and their possible role in fatigue, *Acta Physiol Scand* 133:115–121, 1988.

101. Wagenmakers AJM, Beckers EJ, Brouns F, et al: Carbohydrate supplementation, glycogen depletion and amino acid metabolism during exercise, *Am J Physiol* 260:E883–E890, 1991.

102. Blomstrand E, Hassmen P, Ekblom B, et al: Administration of branched chain amino acids during sustained exercise—Effects on performance and on plasma concentration of some amino acids, *Eur J Appl Physiol* 63:83–88, 1991.

103. Madsen K, MacLean DA, Kiens B, et al: Effects of glucose, glucose plus branched-chain amino acids, or placebo on bike performance over 100 km, *J Appl Physiol* 81:2644–2650, 1996.

104. Davis JM, Welsh RS, De Volve KL, et al: Effects of branched-chain amino acids and carbohydrate on fatigue during intermittent, high-intensity running, *Int J Sport Med* 20:309–314, 1999.

105. Mittleman KD, Ricci MR, Bailey SP: Branched-chain amino acids prolong exercise during heat stress in men and women, *Med Sci Sports Exerc* 30:83–91, 1998.

106. Watson P, Shirreffs SM, Maughan RJ: The effect of acute branched-chain amino acid supplementation on prolonged exercise capacity in a warm environment, *Eur J Appl Physiol* 93:306–314, 2004.

107. Cheuvront SN, Carter R, Kolka MA, et al: Branched-chain amino acid supplementation and human performance when hypohydrated in the heat, *J Appl Physiol* 97:1275–1282, 2004.

108. MacLean DA, Graham TE, Saltin B: Branched-chain amino acids augment ammonia metabolism while attenuating protein breakdown during exercise, *Am J Physiol* 267:E1010–E1022, 1994.

109. Koba T, Hamada K, Sakurai M, et al: Branched-chain amino acids supplementation attenuates the accumulation of blood lactate dehydrogenase during distance running, *J Sports Med Phys Fitness* 47:316–322, 2007.

110. Greer BK, Woodard JL, White JP, et al: Branched-chain amino acid supplementation and indicators of muscle damage after endurance exercise, *Int J Sport Nutr* 17:595–607, 2007.

111. Clarkson PM, Hubal MJ: Exercise-induced muscle damage in humans, *Am J Phys Med Rehabil* 81:S52–69, 2002.

112. Nybo L, Dalsgaard MK, Steensberg A, et al: Cerebral ammonia uptake and accumulation during prolonged exercise in humans, *J Physiol* 563:285–290, 2005.

113. Montgomery AJ, McTavish SFB, Cowen PJ, et al: Reduction of brain dopamine concentration with dietary tyrosine plus phenylalanine depletion: An [^{11}C]raclopride PET study, *Am J Psychiatry* 160:1887–1889, 2003.

114. Young SN: Behavioral effects of dietary neurotransmitter precursors: Basic and clinical aspects, *Neurosci Biobehav Rev* 20:313–323, 1996.

115. Chinevere TD, Sawyer RD, Creer AR, et al: Effects of L-tyrosine and carbohydrate ingestion on endurance exercise performance, *J Appl Physiol* 93:1590–1597, 2002.

116. Strüder HK, Hollmann W, Platen P, et al: Influence of paroxetine, branched-chain amino acids and tyrosine on neuroendocrine system responses and fatigue in humans, *Horm Metab Res* 30:188–194, 1998.

117. Lieberman HR: Amino acid and protein requirements: Cognitive performance, stress, and brain function. In The Committee of Military Nutrition, editor: *The role of protein and amino acids in sustaining and enhancing performance*, Washington, DC, 1999, National Academy Press.

118. Lieberman HR: Nutrition, brain function and cognitive performance, *Appetite* 40:245–254, 2003.

119. Deijen JB, Wientjes CJE, Vullinghs HFM, et al: Tyrosine improves cognitive performance and reduces blood pressure in cadets after one week of a combat training course, *Brain Res Bull* 48:203–209, 1999.

120. Shurtleff D, Thomas JR, Schrot J, et al: Tyrosine reverses a cold-induced working memory deficit in humans, *Pharmacol Biochem Behav* 47:935–941, 1994.

121. Banderet LE, Lieberman HR: Treatment with tyrosine, a neurotransmitter precursor, reduces environmental stress in humans, *Brain Res Bull* 22:759–762, 1989.

122. Magill RA, Walters WF, Bray GA, et al: Effects of tyrosine, phentermine, caffeine, D-amphetamine, and placebo on cognitive and motor performance deficits during sleep deprivation, *Nutr Neurosci* 6:237–246, 2003.

123. Neri DF, Wiegmann D, Stanny RR, et al: The effects of tyrosine on cognitive performance during extended wakefulness, *Aviat Space Environ Med* 66:313–319, 1995.

124. Thomas JR, Lockwood PA, Singh A, et al: Tyrosine improves working memory in a multitasking environment, *Pharmacol Biochem Behav* 64:495–500, 1999.

125. Desbrow B, Leveritt M: Well-trained endurance athletes' knowledge, insight and experience of caffeine use, *Int J Sports Nutr* 17:328–339, 2007.

126. Costill DL, Dalsky G, Fink W: Effects of caffeine ingestion on metabolism and exercise performance, *Med Sci Sports Exerc* 10:155–158, 1978.

127. Ivy JL, Costill DL, Fink WJ, et al: Influence of caffeine and carbohydrate feedings on endurance performance, *Med Sci Sports Exerc* 11:6–11, 1979.

128. Graham TE, Spriet LL: Performance and metabolic responses to a high caffeine dose during prolonged exercise, *J Appl Physiol* 71:2292–2298, 1991.

129. Spriet LL, MacLean DA, Dyck DJ, et al: Caffeine ingestion and muscle metabolism during prolonged exercise in humans, *Am J Physiol* 262:E891–E898, 1992.

130. Graham TE, Spriet LL: Metabolic, catecholamine, and exercise performance responses to various doses of caffeine, *J Appl Physiol* 78:867–874, 1995.

131. Hogervorst E, Bandelow S, Schmitt J, et al: Caffeine improves physical and cognitive performance during exhaustive exercise, *Med Sci Sports Exerc* 40:1841–1851, 2008.

132. Graham TE, Hibbert E, Sathasivam P: Metabolic and exercise endurance effects of coffee and caffeine ingestion, *J Appl Physiol* 85:883–889, 1998.

133. Doherty M, Smith PM: Effects of caffeine ingestion on exercise testing: A meta-analysis, *Int J Sports Nutr* 14:626–646, 2004.

134. Kovacs EMR, Stegen JHCH, Brouns F: Effect of caffeinated drinks on substrate metabolism, caffeine excretion, and performance, *J Appl Physiol* 85:709–715, 1998.

135. Cox GR, Desbrow B, Montgomery PG, et al: Effect of different protocols of caffeine intake on metabolism and endurance performance, *J Appl Physiol* 93:990–999, 2002.

136. Bridge CA, Jones MA: The effect of caffeine ingestion on 8 km run performance in a field setting, *J Sports Sci* 24:433–439, 2006.

137. O'Rourke MP, O'Brien BJ, Knez WL, et al: Caffeine has a small effect on 5-km running performance of well-trained and recreational runners, *J Sci Med Sport* 11:231–233, 2008.

138. Van Nieuwenhoven MA, Brouns F, Kovacs EMR: The effect of two sports drinks and water on GI complaints and performance during an 18-km run, *Int J Sports Med* 26:281–285, 2005.

139. Schneiker KT, Bishop D, Dawson B, et al: Effects of caffeine on prolonged intermittent-sprint ability in team-sport athletes, *Med Sci Sports Exerc* 38:578–585, 2006.

140. Lorino AJ, Lloyd LK, Crixell SH, et al: The effects of caffeine on athletic agility, *J Strength Cond Res* 20:851–854, 2006.

141. Essig D, Costill DL, van Handel PJ: Effects of caffeine ingestion on utilization of muscle glycogen and lipid during leg ergometer cycling, *Int J Sports Med* 1:86–90, 1980.

142. Tarnopolsky M, Cupido C: Caffeine potentiates low frequency skeletal muscle force in habitual and nonhabitual caffeine consumers, *J Appl Phsyiol* 89:1719–1724, 2000.

143. Davis JM, Zhao Z, Stock HS, et al: Central nervous system effects of caffeine and adenosine on fatigue, *Am J Physiol* 284: R399–R404, 2002.

144. Cole KJ, Costill DL, Starling RD, et al: Effect of caffeine ingestion on perception of effort and subsequent work production, *Int J Sports Nutr* 6:14–23, 1996.

145. Ganio MS, Casa DJ, Armstrong LE, et al: Evidence-based approach to lingering hydration questions, *Clin Sports Med* 26:1–16, 2007.

146. Wemple RD, Lamb DR, McKeever KH: Caffeine vs. caffeine-free sports drinks: Effects on urine production at rest and during prolonged exercise, *Int J Sports Med* 18:40–46, 1997.

147. Powers SK, Deruisseau KC, Quindry J, et al: Dietary antioxidants and exercise, *J Sports Sci* 22(1):81–94, 2004.

148. Bischoff AC: Quercetin: Potentials in the prevention and therapy of disease, *Curr Opp Clin Nutr Metab Care* 11:733–740, 2008.

149. DalleDonne I, Milzani A, Colombo R: H_2O_2-treated actin: Assembly and polymer interactions with cross-linking proteins, *Biophys J* 69:2710–2719, 1995.

150. Ajtai K, Burghardt TP: Fluorescent modification and orientation of myosin sulfhydryl 2 in skeletal muscle fibers, *Biochemistry* 28:2204–2210, 1989.

151. Matuszczak Y, Farid M, Jones J, et al: Effects of N-acetylcysteine on glutathione oxidation and fatigue during handgrip exercise, *Muscle Nerve* 32:633–638, 2005.

152. Reid MB, Stokic DS, Koch SM, et al: N-acetylcysteine inhibits muscle fatigue in humans, *J Clin Invest* 94:2468–2474, 1994.

153. McKenna MJ, Medved I, Goodman CA, et al: N-acetylcysteine attenuates the decline in muscle Na^+, K^+-pump activity and delays fatigue during prolonged exercise in humans, *J Physiol* 576:279–288, 2006.

154. Coombes JS, Powers SK, Rowell B, et al: Effects of vitamin E α-lipoic acid on skeletal muscle contractile properties, *J Appl Physiol* 90:1424–1430, 2001.

155. Lands LC, Grey VL, Smountas AA: Effect of supplementation with a cysteine donor on muscle performance, *J Appl Physiol* 87:1381–1385, 1999.

156. Tamai I, Ohashi R, Nezu J, et al: Molecular and functional identification of sodium ion-dependent, high affinity human carnitine transporter OCTN2, *J Biol Chem* 273:20378–20382, 1998.

157. Barnett C, Costill DL, Vukovich MD, et al: Effect of L-carnitine supplementation on muscle and blood carnitine content and lactate accumulation during high-intensity sprint cycling, *Int J Sports Nutr* 4:280–288, 1994.

158. Wächter S, Vogt M, Kreis R, et al: Long-term administration of L-carnitine to humans: Effect on skeletal muscle carnitine content and physical performance, *Clin Chim Acta* 318:51–61, 2002.

159. Soop M, Björkman O, Cederblad G, et al: Influence of carnitine supplementation on muscle substrate and carnitine metabolism during exercise, *J Appl Physiol* 64:2394–2399, 1988.

160. Stephens FB, Constantin-Teodosiu D, Laithwaite D, et al: Insulin stimulates L-carnitine accumulation in human skeletal muscle, *FASEB J* 20:377–379, 2006.

161. Greig C, Finch KM, Jones DA, et al: The effect of oral supplementation with L-carnitine on maximum and submaximum exercise capacity, *Eur J Appl Physiol* 56:457–460, 1987.

162. Oyono-Enguelle S, Freund H, Ott C, et al: Prolonged submaximal exercise and L-carnitine in humans, *Eur J Appl Physiol* 58:53–61, 1988.

163. Decombaz J, Deriaz O, Acheson K, et al: Effect of L-carnitine on submaximal exercise metabolism after depletion of muscle glycogen, *Med Sci Sports Exerc* 25:733–740, 1993.

164. Vukovich MD, Costill DL, Fink WJ: Carnitine supplementation: Effect of muscle carnitine and glycogen content during exercise, *Med Sci Sports Exerc* 26:1122–1129, 1994.

165. Spriet LL, Perry CG, Talanian JL: Legal pre-event nutritional supplements to assist energy metabolism, *Essays Biochem* 44: 27–43, 2008.

166. Stephens FB, Evans CE, Constantin-Teodosiu D, et al: Carbohydrate ingestion augments L-carnitine retention in humans, *J Appl Physiol* 102:1065–1070, 2006.

167. Stephens FB, Constantin-Teodosiu D, Laithwaite D, et al: Skeletal muscle carnitine accumulation alters fuel metabolism in resting human skeletal muscle, *J Clin Endocrinol Metab* 91:5013–5018, 2006.

168. Requena B, Zabala M, Padial P, et al: Sodium bicarbonate and sodium citrate: Ergogenic aids? *J Strength Cond Res* 19: 213–224, 2005.

169. McNaughton LR, Backx K, Palmer G, et al: Effects of chronic bicarbonate ingestion on the performance of high-intensity work, *Eur J Appl Physiol* 80:333–336, 1999.

170. Harris RC, Soderlund K, Hultman E: Elevation of creatine in resting and exercised muscle of normal subjects by creatine supplementation, *Clin Sci* 83:367–374, 1992.

171. Bemben MG, Lamont HS: Creatine supplementation and exercise performance: Recent findings, *Sports Med* 35:107–125, 2005.

172. Terjung RL, Clarkson P, Eichner ER, et al: American College of Sports Medicine Roundtable. The physiological and health effects of oral creatine supplementation, *Med Sci Sport Exerc* 32:706–717, 2000.

173. Pritchard NR, Kalra PA: Renal dysfunction accompanying oral creatine supplementation, *Lancet* 351:1252–1253, 1998.

174. Anselme F, Collomp K, Mercier B, et al: Caffeine increases maximal anaerobic power and blood lactate concentration, *Eur J Appl Physiol* 65:188–191, 1992.

175. Beck TW, Housh TJ, Schmidt RJ, et al: The acute effects of a caffeine-containing supplement on strength, muscular endurance, and anaerobic capabilities, *J Strength Cond Res* 20: 506–510, 2006.

176. Astorino TA, Rohmann RL, Firth K: Effect of caffeine ingestion on one-repetition maximum muscular strength, *Eur J Appl Physiol* 102:127–132, 2008.

177. Beck TW, Housh TJ, Malek MH, et al: The acute effects of a caffeine-containing supplement on bench press strength and time to running exhaustion, *J Strength Cond Res* 22:1645–1658, 2008.

178. Winett R, Carpinelli R: Potential health-related benefits of resistance training, *Preventive Medicine* 33:503–513, 2001.

179. Tipton K, Ferrando A: Improving muscle mass: Response of muscle metabolism to exercise, nutrition and anabolic agents, *Essays Biochem* 44:85–98, 2008.

180. Volek J: Influence of nutrition on responses to resistance training, *Med Sci Sports Exerc* 36:689–696, 2004.

181. Phillips S, Moore D, Tang J: A critical examination of dietary protein requirements, benefits, and excesses in athletes, *Int J Sport Nutr Exerc Metab* 17:S58–S76, 2007.

182. Jaworski K, Sarkadi-Nagy S, Duncan R, et al: Regulation of triglyceride metabolism IV. Hormonal regulation of lipolysis in adipose tissue, *Am J Physiol Gastroinest Liver Physiol* 293: G1–G4, 2007.

183. Kraemer W, Ratamess N: Hormonal responses and adaptations to resistance exercise and training, *Sports Med* 35:339–361, 2005.

184. La Forgia J, van der Ploeg G, Withers R, et al: Impact of indexing resting metabolic rate against fat-free mass determined by different body composition models, *Eur J Clin Nutr* 58:1132–1141, 2004.

185. Tipton K, Rasmussen B, Miller S, et al: Timing of amino acid-carbohydrate ingestion alters anabolic response of muscle to resistance exercise, *Am J Physiol Endocrinol Metab* 281:E197–206, 2001.

186. Holm L, Olesen J, Matsumoto K, et al: Protein-containing nutrient supplementation following strength training enhances the effect on muscle mass, strength, and bone formation in postmenopausal women, *J Appl Physiol* 105:274–281, 2008.

187. Willoughby D, Stout J, Wilborn C: Effects of resistance training and protein plus amino acid supplementation on muscle anabolism, mass, and strength, *Amino Acids* 32:467–477, 2007.

188. Kerksick C, Rasmussen C, Lancaster S, et al: The effects of protein and amino acid supplementation on performance and training adaptations during ten weeks of resistance training, *J Strength Cond Res* 20:643–653, 2006.

189. Candow D, Burke N, Smith-Palmer T, et al: Effect of whey and soy protein supplementation combined with resistance training in young adults, *Int J Sport Nutr Exerc Metab* 16:233–244, 2006.

190. Hartman J, Tang J, Wilkinson S, et al: Consumption of fat-free fluid milk after resistance exercise promotes greater lean mass accretion than does consumption of soy or carbohydrate in young, novice, male weightlifters, *Am J Clin Nutr* 86:373–381, 2007.

191. Kalman D, Feldman S, Martinez M, et al: Effect of protein source and resistance training on body composition and sex hormones, *J Int Soc Sports Nutr* 4:4, 2007.

192. Tipton K, Elliott T, Cree M, et al: Ingestion of casein and whey proteins result in muscle anabolism after resistance exercise, *Med Sci Sports Exerc* 36:2073–2081, 2004.

193. Tipton K, Elliott T, Cree M, et al: Stimulation of net muscle protein synthesis by whey protein ingestion before and after exercise, *Am J Physiol Endocrinol Metab* 292:E71–E76, 2007.

194. Esmark B, Anderson S, Olsen E, et al: Timing of post-exercise protein intake is important for muscle hypertrophy with resistance training in elderly humans, *J Physiol* 535:301–311, 2001.

195. Rasmussen B, Tipton K, Miller S, et al: An oral essential amino acid-carbohydrate supplement enhances muscle protein anabolism after resistance exercise, *J Appl Physiol* 88:386–392, 2000.

196. Tang J, Manolakos J, Kujbida G, et al: Minimal whey protein with carbohydrate stimulates muscle protein synthesis following resistance exercise in trained young men, *Appl Physiol Nutr Metab* 32:1132–1138, 2007.

197. Volek J, Rawson E: Scientific basis and practical aspects of creatine supplementation for athletes, *Nutrition* 20:609–617, 2004.

198. Branch JD: Effect of creatine supplementation on body composition and performance: A meta-analysis, *Int J Sport Nutr Exerc Metab* 13:198–226, 2003.

199. Nissen SL, Sharp RL: Effect of dietary supplements on lean mass and strength gains with resistance exercise: A meta-analysis, *J Appl Physiol* 94:651–659, 2003.

200. Rawson E, Volek J: The effects of creatine supplementation and resistance training on muscle strength and weightlifting performance, *J Strength Cond Res* 17:822–831, 2003.

201. Syrotuik D, Bell G: Acute creatine monohydrate supplementation: A descriptive physiological profile of responders and nonresponders, *J Strength Cond Res* 18:610–617, 2004.

202. Hultman E, Soderlund K, Timmons J, et al: Muscle creatine loading in men, *J Appl Physiol* 81:232–237, 1996.

203. Green A, Hultman E, Macdonald I, et al: Carbohydrate ingestion augments skeletal muscle creatine accumulation during creatine supplementation in humans, *Am J Physiol* 271:E821–E826, 1996.

204. Cribb P, Williams A, Hayes A: A creatine-protein-carbohydrate supplement enhances responses to resistance training, *Med Sci Sports Exerc* 39:1960–1968, 2007.

205. Cribb P, Hayes A: Effects of supplement timing and resistance exercise on skeletal muscle hypertrophy, *Med Sci Sports Exerc* 38:1918–1925, 2006.

206. Persky A, Rawson E: Safety of creatine supplementation, *Subcell Biochem* 46:275–289, 2007.

207. Kreider R, Melton C, Rasmussen C, et al: Long-term creatine supplementation does not significantly affect clinical markers of health in athletes, *Mol Cell Biochem* 244:95–104, 2003.

208. Shao A, Hathcock J: Risk assessment for creatine monohydrate, *Regul Toxicol Pharmacol* 45:242–251, 2006.

209. Wilson G, Wilson J, Manninen A: Effects of beta-hydroxy-beta-methylbutyrate (HMB) on exercise performance and body composition across varying levels of age, sex, and training experience: A review, *Nutr Metab* 5:1, 2008.

210. Nissen S, Sharp M, Ray J, et al: Effect of leucine metabolite beta-hydroxy-beta-methylbutyrate on muscle metabolism during resistance-exercise training, *J Appl Physiol* 81:2095–2104, 1996.

211. Van Someren K, Edwards A, Howatson G: Supplementation with beta-hydroxy-beta-methylbutyrate (HMB) and alpha-ketoisocaproic acid (KIC) reduces signs and symptoms of exercise-induced muscle damage in man, *Int J Sport Nutr Exerc Metab* 15:413–424, 2005.

212. Gallagher P, Carrithers J, Godard M, et al: Beta-hydroxy-beta-methylbutyrate ingestion, part I: Effects on strength and fat free mass, *Med Sci Sports Exerc* 32:2109–2115, 2000.

213. Panton L, Rathmacher J, Baier S, et al: Nutritional supplementation of the leucine metabolite beta-hydroxy-beta-methylbutyrate (HMB) during resistance training, *Nutrition* 16:743–749, 2000.

214. Ransone J, Neighbors K, Lefavi R, et al: The effect of beta-hydroxy-beta-methylbutyrate on muscular strength and body composition in collegiate football players, *J Strength Cond Res* 17:34–39, 2003.

215. Crowe M, O'Connor D, Lukins J: The effects of beta-hydroxy-beta-methylbutyrate (HMB) and HMB/creatine supplementation on indices of health in highly trained athletes, *Int J Sport Nutr Exerc Metab* 13:184–197, 2003.

216. Gallagher P, Carrithers J, Godard M, et al: Beta-hydroxy-beta-methylbutyrate ingestion, part II: Effects on hematology, hepatic and renal function, *Med Sci Sports Exerc* 32(12):2116–2119, 2000.

217. Whigham L, Watras A, Schoeller D: Efficacy of conjugated linoleic acid for reducing fat mass: A meta-analysis in humans, *Am J Clin Nutr* 85:1203–1211, 2007.

218. Pinkoski C, Chilibeck P, Candow D, et al: The effects of conjugated linoleic acid supplementation during resistance training, *Med Sci Sports Exerc* 38:339–348, 2006.

219. Kreider R, Ferreira M, Greenwood M, et al: Effects of conjugated linoleic acid supplementation during resistance training on

body composition, bone density, strength, and selected hematological markers, *J Strength Cond Res* 16:325–334, 2002.

220. Thrush A, Chabowski A, Heigenhauser G, et al: Conjugated linoleic acid increases skeletal muscle ceramide content and decreases insulin sensitivity in overweight, non-diabetic humans, *Appl Physiol Nutr Metab* 32:372–382, 2007.

221. Riserus U, Vessby B, Arnlov J, et al: Effects of cis-9, trans-11 conjugated linoleic acid supplementation on insulin sensitivity, lipid peroxidation and proinflammatory markers in obese men, *Am J Clin Nutr* 80:279–283, 2004.

222. Roth S, Zmuda J, Cauley J, et al: Vitamin D receptor phenotype is associated with fat-free mass and sarcopenia in elderly men, *J Geronotol Biol Sci Med Sci* 59:10–15, 2004.

223. Bischoff-Ferrari H, Stahelin H, Dick W, et al: Effects of vitamin D and calcium supplementation on falls: A randomized controlled trial, *J Bone Miner Res* 18:343–351, 2003.

224. Sato Y, Iwamoto J, Kanoko T, et al: Low-dose vitamin D prevents muscular atrophy and reduces falls and hip fractures in women after stroke: A randomized controlled trial, *Cerebrovasc Dis* 20:187–192, 2005.

225. Teegarden D: Calcium intake and reduction in weight or fat mass, *J Nutr* 133:249S–251S, 2003.

226. Downs B, Bagchi M, Subbaraju G, et al: Bioefficacy of a novel calcium-potassium salt of (−)-hydroxycitric acid, *Mutat Res* 579:149–162, 2005.

227. Bell AT: The use of ergogenic aids in athletics. In Zachazewski JE, Magee DJ, Quillen WS: *Athletic injuries and rehabilitation*, Philadelphia, 1996, WB Saunders.

228. Gregg D: Anabolic steroids: The debate builds up, *Clin Update Sports Med* 1:3, 1984.

229. Shahidi N: A review of the chemistry, biological action, and clinical applications of anabolic-androgenic steroids, *Clin Ther* 23:1355–1390, 2001.

230. Prentice B: Pharmacologic considerations for sports medicine. In Malone T, editor: *Physical and occupational therapy: Drug implications for practice*, Philadelphia, 1989, JB Lippincott.

231. Celotti F, Negri Cesi P: Anabolic steroids: A review of their effects on the muscles, of their possible mechanisms of action and of their use in athletics, *J Steroid Biochem Mol Biol* 43:469–477, 1994.

232. Kadi F, Eriksson A, Holmner S, et al: Effects of anabolic steroids on the muscle cells of strength-trained athletes, *Med Sci Sports Exerc* 31:1528–1534, 1999.

233. Rogozkin V: Metabolic effects of anabolic steroids on skeletal muscle, *Med Sci Sports Exerc* 11:160–163, 1979.

234. Stamford B, Moffat R: Anabolic steroid: Effectiveness as an ergogenic aid to experienced weight trainers, *J Sports Med Phys Fitness* 14:191–197, 1974.

235. Ward P: The effect of anabolic steroids on strength and lean body mass, *Med Sci Sports* 5:277–282, 1973.

236. Johnson L, Fisher G, Sylvester L, Hofheins CC: Anabolic steroid: Effects on strength, body weight, oxygen uptake, and spermatogenesis upon mature males, *Med Sci Sports* 4:43–45, 1972.

237. Bowers RW, Reardon JP: Effects of Dianabol on strength development and aerobic capacity, *Med Sci Sports* 4:54, 1972.

238. Golding LJ, Freydinger J, Fishel S: Weight, size, and strength—Unchanged with steroids, *Phys Sports Med* 2:39–45, 1974.

239. Fahey TD, Brown CH: The effects of anabolic steroids on strength, body composition, and endurance of college males when accompanied by a weight training program, *Med Sci Sports* 5:272–276, 1973.

240. Elashoff J, Jacknow A, Shain S, et al: Effects of anabolic-androgenic steroids on muscular strength, *Ann Intern Med* 115:387–393, 1991.

241. Hartgens F, Kuipers H: Effects of androgenic-anabolic steroids in athletes, *Sports Med* 34:513–554, 2004.

242. Baume N, Schumacher Y, Sottas P, et al: Effect of multiple oral doses of androgenic anabolic steroids on endurance performance and serum indices of physical stress in healthy male subjects, *Eur J Appl Physiol* 98:329–340, 2006.

243. Trenton A, Currier G: Behavioural manifestations of anabolic steroid use, *CNS Drugs* 19:571–595, 2005.

244. Graham M, Davies B, Grace F, et al: Anabolic steroid use: Patterns of use and detection of doping, *Sports Med* 38:505–525, 2008.

245. Nieminen M, Ramo M, Viitasalo M, et al: Serious cardiovascular side effects of large doses of anabolic steroids in weight lifters, *Eur Heart* 17:1576–1583, 1996.

246. Bahrke M, Yesalis C, Wright J: Psychological and behavioural effects of endogenous testosterone and anabolic-androgenic steroids. An update, *Sports Med* 22:367–390, 1996.

247. Beaver K, Vaughn M, Delisi M, et al: Anabolic-androgenic steroid use and involvement in violent behavior in a nationally representative sample of young adult males in the United States, *Am J Public Health* 98:2185–2187, 2008.

248. Ebenbichler C, Sturm W, Ganzer H, et al: Flow-mediated, endothelium-dependent vasodilatation is impaired in male body builders taking anabolic-androgenic steroids, *Atherosclerosis* 158:483–490, 2001.

249. Hartgens F, Rietjens G, Keizer H, et al: Effects of androgenic-anabolic steroids on apolipoproteins and lipoprotein (a), *Br J Sports Med* 38:253–259, 2004.

250. Laseter J, Russell J: Anabolic steroid-induced tendon pathology: A review of the literature, *Med Sci Sports Exerc* 23:1–3, 1991.

251. Martin N, Abu Dayyeh B, Chung R: Anabolic steroid abuse causing recurrent hepatic adenomas and hemorrhage, *World J Gastroenterol* 14:4573–4575, 2008.

252. Modlinski R, Fields K: The effect of anabolic steroids on the gastrointestinal system, kidneys, and adrenal glands, *Curr Sports Med Rep* 5:104–109, 2006.

253. Nottin S, Nguyen L, Terbah M, et al: Cardiovascular effects of androgenic anabolic steroids in male bodybuilders determined by tissue Doppler imaging, *Am J Cardiol* 97:912–915, 2006.

254. Pope H, Katz D: Psychiatric and medical effects of anabolic-androgenic steroid use. A controlled study of 160 athletes, *Arch Gen Psychiatry* 51(5)375–382, 1994.

255. Jenkinson D, Harbert A: Supplements and sports, *Am Fam Physician* 78:1039–1046, 2008.

256. Illich J, Kerstetter J: Nutrition in bone health revisited: A story beyond calcium, *J Am Coll Nutr* 19:715–737, 2000.

257. Weaver C: The role of nutrition on optimizing peak bone mass, *Asia Pac J Clin Nutr* 17:135–137, 2008.

258. Bailey C, Brooke-Wavell K: Exercise for optimizing peak bone mass in women, *Proc Nutr Soc* 67:9–18, 2008.

259. Chilibeck P, Sale D, Webber C: Exercise and bone mineral density, *Sports Med* 19:103–122, 1995.

260. Vicente-Rodriguez G, Ezquerra J, Mesana M, et al: Independent and combined effect of nutrition and exercise on bone mass development, *J Bone Miner Metab* 26:416–424, 2008.

261. Borer K: Physical activity in the prevention and amelioration of osteoporosis in women: Interaction of mechanical, hormonal and dietary factors, *Sports Med* 35:779–830, 2005.

262. Griel A, Kris-Etherton P, Hilpert K, et al: An increase in dietary n-3 fatty acids decreases a marker of bone resorption in humans, *Nutr J* 6:2, 2007.

263. Hogstrom M, Nordstrom P, Nordstrom A: n-3 Fatty acids are positively associated with peak bone mineral density and bone accrual in healthy men: The NO2 study, *Am J Clin Nutr* 85:803–807, 2007.

264. Goldberg R, Katz J: A meta-analysis of the analgesic effects of omega-3 polyunsaturated fatty acid supplementation for inflammatory joint pain, *Pain* 129:210–223, 2007.

265. Clark K, Sebastianelli W, Flechsenhar K, et al: 24-Week study on the use of collagen hydrolysate as a dietary supplement in athletes with activity-related joint pain, *Curr Med Res Opin* 24:1485–1496, 2008.

266. McAlindon T, LaValley M, Gulin J, et al: Glucosamine and chondroitin for treatment of osteoarthritis: A systematic quality assessment and meta-analysis, *JAMA* 283:1469–1475, 2000.

267. Poolsup N, Suthisisang C, Channark P, et al: Glucosamine long-term treatment and the progression of knee osteoarthritis: Systematic review of randomized controlled trials, *Ann Pharmacother* 39:1080–1087, 2005.

268. Lohmander L, Englund P, Dahl L, et al: The long-term consequence of anterior cruciate ligament and meniscus injuries: Osteoarthritis, *Am J Sports Med* 35:1756–1769, 2007.

269. Ostojic S, Arsic M, Prodanovic S, et al: Glucosamine administration in athletes: Effects on recovery of acute knee injury, *Res Sports Med* 15:113–124, 2007.

Sports Drug Testing

Gary A. Green

Introduction

Drug testing has become as much a part of sports as grass stains on a uniform and has been accepted by both the public and athletes as a necessary part of the rules of the game. To illustrate the point, when the National Collegiate Athletic Association (NCAA) began drug testing in 1986, several schools went to court to block their athletes from having to comply with the regulations. Contrast that with 2007 when the New Jersey High School Athletic Federation instituted statewide drug testing. Among the thousands of athletes and their families who were asked to sign consent forms for the testing, there were no refusals.[1] Although there is certainly debate regarding the types of drugs that are screened and how drug testing is applied, drug testing has become an accepted part of sports at most levels. It is therefore incumbent on anyone associated with sports to have at least a rudimentary knowledge of the drug testing process.

There are several incorrect assumptions about sports drug testing that need to be explored. The first is that drug testing is like a "black box" in which a sample enters one end and a positive or negative result is returned. In reality, drug testing is fairly complicated and requires a significant amount of interpretation before a result can be determined. This chapter explores how a sample is analyzed before a final determination can be made. The second myth is that drug testing is like a precise surgical scalpel that can deliver detailed information about the sample. In reality, drug testing is more akin to a blunt instrument that has significant limitations. Simply put, sports drug testing is a tool that must be applied correctly to be effective. This chapter discusses the scope and limitations of drug testing to present a realistic assessment of the present science.

Sports Pharmacology

An understanding of sports pharmacology is necessary before delving into the science of sports drug testing. Sports pharmacology, as compared with general medical pharmacology, classifies drugs according to their reason for use. Traditional pharmacology groups drugs according to their chemical structure and mechanisms of action (e.g., stimulants are separated from depressants). In sports pharmacology, drugs are classified as *ergogenic, recreational,* or *therapeutic* depending on the main reason for use.

Sports Pharmacology-Drug Classification
Ergogenic drugs-Performance-enhancing substances
Recreational drugs-Stimulants and depressants
Therapeutic drugs-Treat underlying disease or condition

Ergogenic drugs are defined as substances taken specifically to increase performance. Examples of this include anabolic-androgenic steroid (AAS) use by a weightlifter or erythropoietin (EPO) use by an endurance athlete. Although these drugs may also have therapeutic uses in certain disease states, athletes use them to gain a competitive advantage. *Recreational drugs,* the second category, are essentially used by athletes for the same reasons as nonathletes: to escape, for social reasons, and as stimulants or depressants. Most studies demonstrate that athletes are at the same risk for using recreational drugs as their nonathlete peers and playing sports does not lessen the risk of addiction to these drugs. Examples of recreational drugs include marijuana, cocaine, heroin, and alcohol. These drugs are almost solely used for recreational purposes and tend to have either no effect or a negative effect on performance. *Therapeutic drugs,* the third category, are taken to treat an underlying condition or disease. Although some of these drugs are banned by sports organizations, therapeutic use exemptions (TUEs) are generally allowed if there are no nonprohibited alternatives. An explanation of the TUE process can be found at the end of the chapter. An example of this is an asthmatic athlete that needs to use a beta-2 agonist (e.g., albuterol) inhaler to treat his or her disease while competing.

Under this system, a single drug can be classified in multiple categories depending on usage pattern. One example is a stimulant such as amphetamines. These are sometimes used ergogenically by athletes to ward off fatigue and to achieve a perceived increase in energy. Amphetamine, in the form of a drug like methamphetamine, can also be used recreationally and has a high risk for addiction. Finally, amphetamines can be prescribed as therapy for the treatment of conditions such as attention deficient hyperactivity disorder (ADHD). Although the same drug can be used in three different situations, an understanding of why the athlete used it is imperative to deter its unauthorized use. It is very clear that each of these scenarios need to be addressed quite differently.

Although the abuse of recreational, and to a lesser extent therapeutic, drugs can be a significant issue in sports, this chapter focuses on drug testing for ergogenic drugs. There are several reasons for this approach. The first is that, as mentioned previously, recreational drugs tend to have ergolytic (performance-reducing) effects. Educational and behavioral programs designed to inform athletes about the negative consequences of these drugs on performance can often be very effective at reducing their use. Athletes are goal-oriented by nature and can respond very favorably to these types of educational programs. If an athlete does develop an abuse problem with a recreational drug, then interventions, treatment, and counseling are required to treat serious addiction. In these circumstances, drug testing may become part of the treatment plan, but is rarely used alone. Second, it is unusual to develop significant problems with therapeutic drugs and these situations are typically handled by the TUE process.

Drug testing for ergogenic drugs is the main focus of this chapter. The actual effects of these drugs are addressed in other chapters. Educational programs have had mixed results deterring this type of drug use because the substances often have short-term positive results on athletic performance. Athletes focus on their performance and are often willing to try drugs to improve performance even if they are prohibited by the sport, illegal, or have significant adverse effects. An example of this is an Internet study of 500 AAS users in which 100% of the respondents reported experiencing at least one adverse effect from the drugs, yet continued to use them. The fact that so many would continue to use AAS even in the face of negative health consequences is testimony to both their perceived "positive" effects and addictive potential.[2] For this reason, drug testing is often needed to ensure a fair playing field for all athletes. Indeed, athletes are amongst the biggest proponents of comprehensive and evenly applied drug testing programs. The author's personal experience, as well as NCAA surveys, confirms that the majority of athletes support drug testing programs.

Collection and Chain of Custody Issues

Drug testing begins with an overlooked, but vitally important, first step in the process: sample collection. A drug testing program can have the most comprehensive prohibited list and use the most thorough and expensive laboratory, but unless the process starts with an accurate collection process, it is of limited value. A substandard collection process can render the results worthless and can embolden drug-using athletes and dismay clean athletes. In the author's opinion, a drug testing program that does not employ a stringent collection process is worse than no program at all. Sports drug testing is much different from basic biomedical drug testing or even workplace drug testing, and it is imperative to understand the distinction.

Urine Testing

Most athletic drug testing begins with witnessed urine collection according to a rigorous set of standards that must be adhered to in order to have a valid sample. It is not unusual for athletes to resort to very creative methods of substituting a urine sample. The collection process is the first step in a strict chain of custody. In sports drug testing, chain of custody usually describes any written procedures to ensure that the collection, transportation, and laboratory analysis of urine, blood, or other specimens remain secure from outside tampering, review, or disclosure. Sports drug testing programs publish chain-of-custody protocols to provide athletes with assurance that their specimens' location, possession, and security are known at all times. These procedures should be available for athletes to review before they consent to be tested. Chain of custody usually includes three facets of the testing process: collection, transportation, and laboratory analysis.[3] Any material deviation from the chain of custody procedure typically invalidates the test.

Chain of Custody in Testing Process

- Collection
- Transportation
- Laboratory analysis

The collection of urine specimens in sports drug testing is a sequential process with many steps. Such steps include but are not limited to identification of the athlete to be tested, selection of a collection container by the athlete, completion of the voiding process under the direct observation of a same-sex validator, completion of specimen integrity checks (e.g., specific gravity, pH), completion of specimen numbering and packaging by the athlete or by the collector under the athlete's watch, and the certification by all parties that the published collection process was followed. Once completed, the typical protocol is for the athlete's sample to be divided into "A" and "B" bottles that are both securely sealed. These steps are essential because when athletes challenge the validity of positive drug test results, the integrity of the collection process is often called into question.[4] The increased legal scrutiny of the process has led to the formation of independent companies that serve as "third party administrators" for the drug testing process.

Once the sample has been sealed, it is securely transported to an accredited laboratory. Although there are a variety of commercial laboratories in the United States that perform workplace drug testing and are certified by organizations such as Substance Abuse and Mental Health Services Administration, the World Anti-Doping Agency (WADA) has a rigorous certification process for those laboratories that are qualified to perform Olympic-caliber testing. As of this writing, there are only three WADA-certified laboratories in North American in Los Angeles, Montreal, and Salt Lake City.

Once received by the laboratory, the samples are immediately examined to ensure there has been no break in the chain of custody and the samples are intact. An internal chain of custody is generated to allow tracking of the sample throughout the analytical process and to account for each individual who has access to that particular sample. Initially, only the "A" bottle is unsealed and undergoes screening analysis. If the screening is negative, no further testing takes place and eventually both the "A" and "B" samples are discarded. However, in the event the "A" screening is positive, a confirmation test is performed on a new aliquot from the "A" bottle. Only if the second "A" confirmation test is positive are the results reported to the sports organization. At this point, the athlete is generally entitled to have the "B" sample analyzed and is allowed to either witness the analysis or have a representative present. The "B" sample bottle is then unsealed for the first time and analyzed. If the "B" result does not match the "A" result, it is considered a negative test. In summary, by the time a positive result is reported by a WADA laboratory, there have been at least two and usually three separate analyses performed on the athlete's sample that all yield the same result.

Blood Testing

Although urine testing has typically been the mainstay of sports drug testing, athlete abuse of drugs such as EPO and human growth hormone (hGH) have exposed some of the limitations of urine testing. Owing to this, blood testing on a limited basis has been conducted in Olympic sports. This represents a major change in sports drug testing, and guidelines have been developed for blood testing in sports. The specific tests for these drugs are discussed later in this chapter.

Blood testing requires the same strict chain of custody protocol as urine collection; however, there are several unique aspects of blood collection that require special consideration. The first is the personnel required to perform the testing. Blood testing requires a trained phlebotomist who is in compliance with all of the local regulations regarding blood collection. These requirements vary from state to state and also by country. Next is a proper setting for the blood collection. Although urine testing is typically performed in a bathroom facility, blood collection requires a hygienic environment to reduce the risk of infection. Typically, blood sampling requires 6 to 10 mL of blood from an athlete for the currently available testing, which should not affect an athlete's performance. The present WADA guidelines allow for up to three attempts at venipuncture before terminating the collection.[5] Finally, all blood samples must be handled and stored according to established safety guidelines.

Clinical Point

At the present time, the majority of drug testing is conducted via urine tests, but the proliferation of bioengineered substances and the potential for genetic doping may increase the need for blood testing in sport. Blood testing is currently limited to the Olympics and there are serious practical, legal, and ethical issues that need to be addressed prior to blood testing becoming commonplace in American professional and collegiate sports.

Drug Testing Methodology

The next several sections discuss various specific methods that are frequently used to interpret drug test results. Although not inclusive of all testing, these represent some of the more common performance-enhancing drugs that offer challenges in interpretation. The 2010 WADA list of prohibited substances can be found in Box 7-1.

Anabolic-Androgenic Steroids (AASs)

AASs represent an area of great concern because of their ability to enhance strength and threaten the integrity of sports, and because of their widespread availability. There are two types of AASs that are identified by drug testing: exogenous (xenobiotic) and endogenous compounds. Some of the more common AASs are listed in Table 7-1. The relative popularity of these types of AAS depends to a large degree on the detectability of various drugs, and testing for AASs has been an integral part of doping control since the 1970s. The introduction of gas chromatography–mass spectrometry (GC-MS) to doping control in the 1980s heralded a new era and continued improvement and refinement of technique has allowed for the identification of several designer AASs in the past several years, including tetrahydrogestrinone (THG),

Box 7-1 World Anti-Doping Association 2010 Prohibited List

Substances and Methods Prohibited at All Times (In and Out of Competition)

S1. Anabolic Agents
1. Anabolic-androgenic steroids
   a. Exogenous AAS
   b. Endogenous AAS
2. Other anabolic agents (e.g., clenbuterol, zeranol, zilpaterol), selective androgen receptor modulators (SARMs)

S2. Hormones and Related Substances
1. Erythropoiesis-Stimulating Agents [e.g. EPO, darbepoetin, methoxy glycol-epoetin beta (CERA)]
2. Chorionic gonadotropins, luteinizing hormones in males
3. Insulins
4. Corticotrophins
5. Growth hormone, insulin-like growth factor (IGF-1), mechano growth factors, Platelet-derived growth factor, fibroblast growth factors, vascular-endothelial growth factor and hepatocyte growth factor
6. Platelet-derived preparations (e.g., Platelet Rich Plasma-PRP) by intramuscular route

S3. Beta-2 Agonists

S4. Hormone Antagonists and Modulators
1. Aromatase inhibitors
2. Selective estrogen receptor modulators
3. Other antiestrogenic substances
4. Agents modifying myostatin function

S5. Diuretics and Other Masking Agents

Prohibited Methods
M1. Enhancement of Oxygen Transfer
M2. Chemical and Physical Manipulation
M3. Gene Doping

Substances and Methods Prohibited In Competition
S6. Stimulants
1. Nonspecified stimulants
2. Specified stimulants

S7. Narcotics
S8. Cannabinoids
S9. Glucocorticosteroids

Substances Prohibited in Particular Sports
P1. Alcohol
P2. Beta-blockers

Data from The World Anti-Doping Agency 2010 Prohibited List International Standard. http://www.wada-ama.org/Documents/World_Anti-Doping_Program/WADP-Prohibited-list/WADA_Prohibited_List_2010_EN.pdf. Accessed February 2010

AAS, Anabolic-androgenic steroid.

Table 7-1
List of Common Anabolic Steroids

Generic Name	Trade Name
Testosterone	Depo-testosterone
Nandrolone	Deca-durabolin
Methandienone	Dianabol
Oxandrolone	Oxandrin/Anavar
Oxymetholone	Anadrol
Stanozolol	Winstrol
Trenbolone*	Finaplix
Boldenone*	Equipoise

From Green G: Doping control for the team physician, *Am J Sports Med* 34(10):1-9, 2006.
*Veterinary products.

norbolethone, and desoxymethyltestosterone (Madol), which were developed as part of the Bay Area Laboratory Cooperative (BALCO) scandal.[6-8]

GC-MS testing involves separating the components of a mixture based on chromatographic retention time and fragmenting each component to its characteristic ions. The retention time and fragmentation pattern is then matched against those of reference standards. This allows for a specific "fingerprint" of a compound. Identification is achieved by matching the relative retention times and mass spectra of the parent drug or metabolites with those of known reference standards. The finding of metabolites confirms that the individual had in fact ingested the AAS in question.[9] GC-MS results have been accepted in both the formal legal system as well as sports arbitration.

The assay process involves enzymatic hydrolysis and solid-phase extraction from the urine to prepare the steroids for the analysis. The extract is then derivatized using a trimethylsilyl ether forming reagent before being analyzed by GC-MS. Derivatization protects the more polar groups and increases the molecular weight. This has the effect of assisting the fragmentation process and augmenting the amenability to GC-MS. A GC-MS can be operated in either the full scan or the more sensitive selective ion monitoring (SIM) mode. Typically, steroid screening tests are conducted in the SIM mode. If a banned drug is detected, a confirmation test must be employed for definitive identification. The more specific full-scan mode is used for confirmation when the concentration of an AAS is high.[10] The introduction of high-resolution mass spectrometry in doping control has extended the period of detectability of exogenous AAS as a result of the instrument's greater sensitivity. For example, nandrolone decanoate may be detectable for more than a full year after an intramuscular injection.

The AAS nandrolone, or 19-nortestosterone, deserves special mention as it is one of the most commonly detected exogenous AASs and there is a great deal of confusion regarding positive test results. Some of the reasons for this are the long period of detection following injection of nandrolone decanoate and the relative availability of 19-norandrostenedione, which was previously sold as a dietary supplement. The first clarification is that a "nandrolone"-positive result does not indicate that the AAS nandrolone was found in the urine. In actuality, the laboratory measures two metabolites of nandrolone, 19-norandrosterone (19NA), and 19-noretiocholanolone (19NE) with the former more commonly reported. Further confusing the situation is that 19NA and 19NE can result from the use of either nandrolone, 19-norandrostenedione, or 19-norandrostenediol.[11] Until the passage of the 2004 Anabolic Steroid Control Act, these latter two were available as dietary supplements, creating more uncertainty. Although the Act reclassified 19-norandrostenedione and 19-norandrostenediol as AAS and banned them from being sold as dietary supplements, enforcement of the Act is lax and these substances can still be found in dietary supplements. It was also discovered that microgram amounts of 19-norandrostenedione, which could occur from microcontamination, could result in a positive test.[12] Although it is difficult to determine which of the three substances resulted in a positive test, it is typically a moot point in that all three compounds are banned by most sports organizations

The second area of clarification is that whereas the mere presence in the urine of all other exogenous AASs is reported as a positive result, nandrolone (or more properly 19NA) is the only one reported with a specific concentration level. This is because small amounts of 19NA can occur without ingesting a prohibited substance and WADA has therefore set cut-off levels for 19NA of 2 ng/mL. Pregnant women excrete small amounts of 19NA and consumption of oral contraceptives containing norethisterone may result in the excretion of small amounts of 19NA. The latter case can be resolved by locating specific norethisterone metabolites.[13] It has also been found that some males may naturally produce miniscule amounts of 19NA in the urine, and thus a cut-off level has been established at 2 ng/mL.

Nandrolone-positive results have been involved in additional controversy because of dietary interference or exercise effects. Athletes have claimed that consuming large quantities of uncastrated boar organs resulted in a positive test for nandrolone metabolites.[14] Although highly improbable, a positive test could technically result from consuming more than a half-pound of uncastrated boar testicles, liver, and kidney within 24 hours of a test. Intense exercise was also mentioned as a potential cause of elevated 19NA levels, but studies have refuted this claim.[15,16]

Lastly, the use of injectable nandrolone decanoate has been detected for many months and in some cases more than a year after injection. This creates a quandary for sports authorities to determine if a repeat positive test represents continued use. Many sports organizations require a clean "exit" urine test before allowing an athlete to return from

suspension and others do not make any exception for multiple positives from a single use. The opinion justifying this latter case is based on several reasons: that parenteral use is a more serious offense, that the athlete receives a continued advantage with a long-acting AAS, and that there is no definitive method for determining whether a subsequent positive test represents a residual positive or continued use.

As testing for xenobiotic AAS improved, athletes predictably turned to endogenous compounds (e.g., testosterone) as an ergogenic aid. Testosterone is problematic because pharmaceutical and endogenous testosterone both have identical patterns on mass spectrometry. Since 1983, the accepted approach has been to monitor the testosterone/epitestosterone (T/E) ratio that normally exists in approximately a 1:1 ratio.[17] The use of testosterone, or compounds that increase testosterone (e.g., dehydroepiandrosterone [DHEA], androstenedione, androstenediol), will raise urinary testosterone proportionally much more than epitestosterone. Historically, a level greater than 6:1 was considered an indication of testosterone use. Athletes, however, attempted to subvert the test by taking epitestosterone (a biologically inactive compound) in conjunction with testosterone to maintain a normal T/E. To prevent this, epitestosterone is quantified in a urine test and concentrations of more than 200 ng/mL result in a positive test. Owing to these factors, WADA lowered the threshold in 2005 and decreed that a T/E ratio of greater than 4 requires further investigation. Other organizations, such as the National Football League, quickly followed suit.

An elevated T/E ratio is a common reason for an athlete to be required to undergo additional testing. The main limitation of the T/E ratio is that there are a small percentage of individuals who are naturally in the 4 to 10:1 range, despite not using testosterone or related compounds. Several options exist in these individuals to determine whether they are misusing testosterone or have a "naturally occurring" elevated T/E ratio. The most common method is to perform serial, unannounced drug tests and compare the results. The T/E ratio should be relatively stable and a marked drop in T/E ratio is suggestive of previous use. WADA recommends three unannounced tests in a 3-month period.[18] The T/E test has the disadvantage of requiring a great deal of time and expense and still can be subverted by an athlete carefully monitoring his or her T/E ratio. Media coverage from the United States BALCO affair revealed that athletes were given a cream containing both testosterone and epitestosterone to maintain their T/E ratio. An alternative to serial testing is the ketoconazole challenge in which the drug ketoconazole is orally administered and the T/E ratio measured. Normal males react to ketoconazole by suppressing testosterone and a reducing the T/E ratio, whereas T/E ratio increases in the face of exogenous testosterone administration. In fact, this test is rarely employed. The most reasonable solution is likely to be carbon isotope ratio testing (also called *isotope ratio MS [IRMS]*), which can differentiate exogenous testosterone and epitestosterone from that which is naturally occurring.[9]

Isotope Ratio Mass Spectrometry

One of the WADA-acceptable methods to determine whether an elevated T/E ratio is the result of exogenous testosterone is a new tool called *gas chromatography–combustion–IRMS*. This can detect small differences in the isotopic composition of organic compounds relative to an international conventional reference standard. IRMS is based on the finding that 98.9% of the carbon atoms in nature are ^{12}C, with 1.1% being ^{13}C, an isotope of carbon that contains an additional neutron. The ratio of $^{13}C/^{12}C$ can be measured with high accuracy and precision by an IRMS scan. Accordingly, very small differences in the abundance of ^{13}C can be detected to allow differentiation of carbon sources. IRMS values for steroids are expressed as delta values: $\delta\ ^{13}C\ \permil$. The more negative a delta value, the less ^{13}C the compound contains.

The basis for IRMS is that plants fix atmospheric CO_2 at varying rates and most plants fall into one of two main photosynthetic processes, C_3 or C_4, each of which yields different amounts of ^{13}C content. C_3 plants, such as soybeans, are considered isotopically "light" because they fix relatively less ^{13}C. On the other hand, C_4 plants (e.g., corn) incorporate more ^{13}C and are thus "heavy" with respect to their carbon. Most humans eat both plants and animals containing various amounts of ^{13}C and studies have determined ethnic differences in the IRMS of different populations, depending on their respective diets. IRMS has also been shown to be sensitive to changes in diet and the total amount of ^{13}C consumed. As applied to the detection of anabolic steroids, IRMS has the ability to distinguish exogenous from endogenous testosterone. Pharmaceutical testosterone is manufactured from stigmasterol (a soy compound) that contains relatively less ^{13}C content as compared with endogenously produced testosterone thus yielding significantly different results on IRMS analysis.

IRMS testing can determine much more than the amount of ^{13}C in urinary testosterone and can provide more definitive information as to the source. Following pharmaceutical testosterone administration, the delta values of urinary testosterone metabolites, such as androsterone and etiocholanolone, will be more negative. In contrast, the delta values of testosterone precursors, or endogenous steroids not involved in testosterone metabolism, will not change. These compounds can be used as endogenous references. A significant difference in the delta value between testosterone or its metabolites and an endogenous reference compound indicates an exogenous source of testosterone or of any steroid in its metabolism. Looking for such gaps is a superior approach because the delta value of testosterone alone in a nonuser might be affected by factors such as diet and is difficult to interpret. Taking testosterone levels in comparison with precursors provides strong indication of the use testosterone or its precursors such as androstenedione, androstenediol, or possibly DHEA. The test is frequently used to obtain additional information to consider whether an elevated T/E ratio is consistent with the misuse of male hormones.[19] IRMS has also been used to resolve cases of low levels of 19NA and 19NE in the setting of potentially "unstable" urine samples.[20]

Testing for Erythropoiesis-Stimulating Agents such as Erythropoietin and Darbepoetin

The synthesis of a recombinant human EPO (r-HuEPO) in 1987 dramatically changed the landscape of endurance sports events. Although it had been well known that increasing the red cell mass would improve maximum oxygen consumption, prior to 1987 rapid increases in hemoglobin could only be accomplished through the inconvenient, complicated, and potentially dangerous process of packed red blood cell transfusions. The advent of r-HuEPO meant that a simple subcutaneous injection could increase hematocrit to the desired level. Even more advantageous, r-HuEPO and its long-acting cousin darbepoetin (introduced in 2001), is nearly identical to naturally produced EPO, making detection by conventional means impossible. The only difference is the presence of additional sugar chains on the synthetic compounds. Although banned by the International Olympic Committee in 1990, the lack of an effective test led to reports of rampant use in sports such as long-distance running and cycling. Despite a previous report in the literature, neither GC-MS nor high-performance liquid chromatography can be used to detect r-HuEPO.[21]

The detection of r-HuEPO was attempted through both blood and urine testing. The blood test relies on an index of various markers, such as hematocrit, reticulocytes, and iron parameters, which are known to change following the administration of nonphysiological r-HuEPO.[22] This test is considered "indirect" or "pharmacodynamic" because it measures the effect of the drug, rather than the actual drug or metabolite as in GC-MS testing for AAS. The urine test takes advantage of the additional charges associated with the extra sugar molecules on r-HuEPO and darbepoetin. This glycosylation allows for separation of exogenous and endogenous EPO in an pH gradient electrical field and detection with a very sensitive and selective method. This results in the so-called isoform patterns of EPO in urine[23] and the isoform pattern of rHuEPO is distinctively different from natural EPO. The isoelectric focusing urine test also yields a pattern for darbepoetin that is distinct from both EPO and r-HuEPO.[24]

The urine method provides a direct test for r-HuEPO and has been upheld in court many times since three cross-country skiers tested positive for darbepoetin at the 2002 Salt Lake City Olympics. Although it is unlikely that someone outside a laboratory would be asked to interpret an electropherogram, it is important to understand the process when confronted with a positive finding for these substances.

An example of how medical progress can be co-opted by the athletic community is demonstrated by the new drug methoxy glycol-epoetin beta (CERA). By surrounding the EPO molecule with a very large polyethylene glycol moiety, the EPO is minimally excreted in the urine and thus has an extremely long therapeutic half-life. While this is advantageous for patients, the lack of urinary excretion makes it very difficult to detect by urinary isoelectric focusing. In order to detect it, a modified form of isoelectric focusing can be used on blood samples. Several high-profile athletes have tested positive for this drug and been sanctioned as a result.

Testing for Human Growth Hormone

The validation of a test for r-HuEPO left growth hormone as the major challenge for drug detection in the 21st century. Similar to EPO, the synthesis of a recombinant form of hGH in the late 1980s freed athletes and patients alike from dependence on small supplies of cadaveric GH and its attendant infectious risks. Since its introduction, multiple anecdotal reports have appeared: Ben Johnson's 1988 admission of combining hGH with anabolic steroids, the discovery of large amounts of hGH in a Tour de France support vehicle in 1998, the confiscation of hGH from the baggage of Chinese swimmers prior to the 2000 Sydney Olympics, and the 2008 admission by former world sprint champion Tim Montgomery that he used hGH in addition to AAS.[25]

Naturally occurring GH is a polypeptide hormone of 191 amino acids that is produced in the anterior pituitary at a rate of 0.4 to 1.0 mg/day in healthy adult males. Natural GH is secreted in the form of multiple isomers with the predominant one being a 22–kilodalton (kD) monomer and approximately 10% being the 20-kD form. This is in contrast to hGH, which contains only the 22-kD isomer. Parenteral administration of hGH peaks in 1 to 3 hours and is imperceptible at 24 hours. Administration of hGH stimulates the production of various markers, the most prominent being insulin-like growth factor (IGF-1) or somatomedin-C and others such as procollagen type III and osteocalcin. Although there is some debate about whether substances such as hepatic-produced IGF-1 are markers or mediators, hGH exerts most of its effects through receptors at target cells.

Owing to the lack of glycosylation, the isoelectric focusing method developed for r-HuEPO cannot be applied to hGH. However, there has been some progress in testing for hGH, and blood testing was performed at the Athens, Turin, and Beijing Olympiads in 2004, 2006, and 2008, respectively. The method used at these Games measured the amount of the 20 kD isomer in the serum, which is present in 10% of normal samples but is suppressed when hGH is given. This method has been shown to be capable of detecting hGH within 24 hours of the last dose; however, it requires a blood test and cannot detect cadaveric GH. An alternative method has been explored as well that relies on pharmacodynamics and measures evidence of supraphysiological use of hGH. Studies have revealed that of the many markers of hGH use, IGF-1, and procollagen type III can consistently discriminate hGH users from nonusers.[26,27] It remains to be seen whether this approach to drug testing would survive forensic challenges to a system that has traditionally relied on a "fingerprint" identification of the banned substance. Although testing for growth hormone continues to make strides, hGH remains a significant challenge for doping control at all levels.[28]

Stimulant Testing

Although most of the current media attention of ergogenic drug use in sports is devoted to anabolic steroids and growth hormone, stimulant use by athletes has a much longer history and is still commonly used in sports. Stimulant use by athletes probably dates back thousands of years and the first modern death by an athlete from ergogenic substance abuse was recorded in 1896 when the Welsh Grand National Cycling champion Arthur Linton died of an overdose. The 1960s saw the deaths of cyclists Knud Jensen and Tom Simpson from amphetamines and recently baseball player Steve Bechler and football player Kori Stringer were alleged to have died in part from ingesting large amounts of ephedrine.

Whether it is athletes using stimulant-containing dietary supplements to lose weight or clobenzorex ("greenies") to increase energy, athletes have always been drawn to the use of various stimulants. Most sports organizations ban the use of various stimulants, and drug testing, especially in competition, generally tests for these substances. Indeed, the WADA-prohibited list specifically names more than 60 banned stimulants,[18] not to mention related compounds. Screening for stimulants is accomplished through liquid chromatography–mass spectrometry or GC-MS for screening, and then one of the two is usually used for confirmation testing.

Another type of testing, chiral analysis, is sometimes used for stimulants. Most stimulants have optical isomers, usually referred to as *D*- and *L-isomers*. Chiral analysis can be used to determine the various percentages of the two isomers in a particular compound. This can be useful when an athlete is using a stimulant for the treatment of a medical condition, such as ADHD. Chiral analysis can confirm whether athletes are being compliant with their medication, or supplementing it with other banned stimulants. For example, a drug such as dextroamphetamine (Dexedrine) should result in almost 100% D form, whereas dextroamphetamine mixed salts (Adderall) would produce a D/L ratio of approximately 3:1.

To determine the optical isomers, chiral derivatization for GC-MS is performed.

Lastly, stimulants tend to be very short-acting compounds and an understanding of when they are used is necessary to design the most effective deterrence program for these substances. They generally are most likely to be used just before or in competition and thus testing after an event gives the best chance of detection. Unfortunately, that can often be logistically difficult and a drug testing program needs to balance many competing interests. Although other ergogenic drugs have come and gone over the past years, stimulants apparently will always be part of the landscape of drug use in sports.

Interpretation of Drug Testing Levels

There are two types of results that are encountered in drug testing: (1) the presence of substances for which any amount represents a positive test, and (2) tests that have quantitated detection limits or thresholds of reporting. The former are relatively easy to interpret in that the test is either positive or negative; the reporting laboratory performs semiquantitative tests and exact levels are not necessary. In the latter category, we have discussed examples such as 19NA and testosterone and epitestosterone in conjunction with the T/E ratio. Other substances are not reported as a positive test result unless they exceed certain levels. Examples of this include the stimulants cathine, caffeine, and ephedrine. In addition, many sports organizations set a threshold for tetrahydrocannabinol (THC), the active ingredient in the recreational drug marijuana. A level of 15 ng/mL is high enough to distinguish between passive inhalation of marijuana smoke and actual use. Owing to its half-life of 2 weeks and its popularity, a positive test for THC is frequently encountered in the athletic population. When evaluating an athlete with a positive drug test for THC, it is incumbent on the professional to thoroughly review the athlete's drug history and not merely focus on marijuana use. In the author's experience, athletes with a positive test for THC are more likely to have a problem with drugs other than THC, such as alcohol or cocaine.[29] Substances with reporting thresholds are summarized in Table 7-2.

Genetic Alteration for Performance Enhancement (Gene Doping)

Genetic manipulation for the expressed purpose of enhancing athletic performance once seemed like science fiction, but may soon become a reality for sports. Whether this involves the manipulation of genetic material in a person or embryonic alterations, it has the capacity to redefine drug testing, performance enhancement, and the definition of sports. Although it is still mainly theoretical, WADA specifically banned gene doping in its 2004 Prohibited List in its prohibited methods section. It is defined as the

Table 7-2
Substances with Threshold Reporting Levels

Substance	Reporting Threshold
Caffeine	15 micrograms/mL*
Cathine	5 micrograms/mL
Ephedrine	1.5; 10 micrograms/mL†
Epitestosterone	200 ng/mL
Methylephedrine	10 micrograms/mL
19 Norandrosterone (19NA)	2 ng/mL males
Salbutamol	1 microgram/mL
Tetrahydrocannabinol (THC)	15 ng/mL
Testosterone/epitestosterone ratio	> 4:1; > 6:1‡

From Green G: Doping control for the team physician, *Am J Sports Med* 34(10):1-9, 2006.
*Caffeine is monitored by WADA, but not subject to sanctions, NCAA sanctions at this level.
†WADA and NCAA threshold is 10 micrograms/mL; NFL threshold is 1.5 micrograms/mL.
‡WADA and NFL threshold is 4:1; NCAA threshold is 6:1.
NCAA, National Collegiate Athletic Association; *NFL,* National Football League; *WADA,* World Anti-Doping Agency.

nontherapeutic use of genes, genetic elements, or cells that have the capacity to enhance athletic performance.[18]

Gene transfer technology has focused on inserting genetic sequences to induce synthesis of various substances. It has the potential to correct genetic diseases, such as immunodeficiency states, in a manner that will revolutionize the treatment of many diseases. Once a genetic abnormality is identified, inserting a correct genetic sequence can potentially reverse the disease. However, just as in sports pharmacology, a distinction must be drawn between therapeutic and ergogenic use. An example is of therapeutic use is using gene transfer to treat a child with absolute growth hormone deficiency. An example of ergogenic use is using it to help a child with normal levels achieve a basketball scholarship.

Gene therapy is a difficult issue for a variety of reasons. First, it challenges the notion of a "level playing field" because it offers the opportunity for everyone to have similar genetic endowments with respect to sports (e.g., testosterone, growth hormone, hemoglobin, muscle fiber type). It also speaks to the dichotomy of traditional enjoyment of sports encompassing both the adoration of an ideal, super athlete and the appreciation for the underdog triumphing over adversity.

Second, genetic manipulation would render current testing methods essentially obsolete. The transferred genetic material would turn on the body's own machinery to produce ergogenic substances. This has already been achieved with the experimental drug Repoxygen that induces EPO production in response to lowered oxygen tension. It was developed for patients with anemia and designed to turn off EPO production when normal oxygen tension returns. Although it would be unlikely to be helpful in healthy athletes training at sea level, athletes might try inducing hypoxemia to use Repoxygen. This drug is still in clinical trials, but represents a potential for abuse in athletes.

Genetic manipulation can theoretically be achieved in a variety of ways and may offer potential clues to detection. If genetic material is introduced via a viral vector, detection of the viral genome may be possible. Alternatively, if gene transfer turns on a gene, then identifying the "switch" may provide evidence of genetic doping. Clearly, the best deterrent for genetic manipulation in athletes is the strict control of this technology by scientists, governments, corporations, researchers, and physicians. WADA has called for inclusion of genetic manipulation under banned doping practices and for tight regulation of this technology. However, if the history of ergogenic drug use is a guideline, the lure of money and fame from athletic victory will likely lead to abuse of this new technology. It is not difficult to imagine two sets of Olympiads: one for the genetically enhanced and one for the non-genetically altered.

Therapeutic Use Exemption (TUE)

TUEs recognize that there are some drugs that, although prohibited by sport, have legitimate medical indications. Although this appears obvious, its application is complex. For example, the use of insulin in a type I diabetic would not be debatable. There are well-established criteria for both the diagnosis and the treatment of diabetes with easily measured parameters. However, in other situations, like the use of stimulants in the treatment of ADHD, there is considerable controversy regarding what constitutes the diagnosis, the necessity of treatment, and the types of medications.

To balance medical necessity with providing an unfair advantage, the TUE process has been developed. WADA has adopted an international standard for TUE and the five basic criteria are listed in Box 7-2.[30] It falls to the antidoping agency of each country to recruit qualified physicians to serve on a TUE committee and review individual cases.

The first condition of the TUE is that it must be requested prospectively. The athlete and his or her health care provider must work in concert prior to an event and secure approval. WADA does grant contingencies for emergency treatment of an acute condition or exceptional circumstances, but the majority of TUEs are reviewed and granted in advance. The second tenet ensures that the medication in question is necessary. As mentioned, this can sometimes be ambiguous and the TUE committee must rely on the testimony of the treating physician to fulfill this requirement.

The third requirement is to ensure that the athlete does not receive any additional ergogenic benefit other than the return to normal health. In some conditions, for example, in an asthmatic using a beta-2 agonist, pulmonary function tests can clearly prove this point. However, other diseases do not lend themselves to a quantitative measure and are

> **Box 7-2 2010 World Anti-Doping Code International Standard for Therapeutic Use Exemption Criteria**
>
> I. The athlete should submit an application for a TUE no less than 30 days before he or she needs approval.
> II. The athlete would experience a significant impairment to health if the prohibited substance or prohibited method were to be withheld in the course of treating an acute or chronic medical condition.
> III. The therapeutic use of the prohibited substance or prohibited method would produce no additional enhancement of performance other than that which might be anticipated by a return of normal health following the treatment of a legitimate medical condition. The use of any prohibited substance or prohibited method to increase "low-normal" levels of any endogenous hormone is not considered an acceptable therapeutic intervention.
> IV. There is no reasonable therapeutic alternative to the use of the otherwise prohibited substance or prohibited method.
> V. The necessity for the use of the otherwise prohibited substance or prohibited method cannot be a consequence, wholly or in part, of prior nontherapeutic use of any substance from the prohibited list.
>
> From WADA International Standard for Therapeutic Use Exemptions, 2010. http://www.wada-ama.org/Documents/World_Anti-Doping_Program/ WADP-IS-TUE/WADA_ISTUE_2010_EN.pdf. Accessed February 2010. *TUE,* Therapeutic use exception.

more subjective. Owing to this, WADA specifically states that a TUE cannot be granted for "low-normal" levels of endogenous hormones. Given the wide range and individual variability of hormones such as testosterone and growth hormone, this is a necessary caveat. The fourth principle is that there must be no reasonable therapeutic alternative. Although this criteria is easily demonstrable in diseases such as diabetes in which insulin is the standard treatment, it becomes more problematic in deciding how far an athlete should go to satisfy this condition. For example, in the treatment of ADHD atomoxetine is approved for this condition and is not prohibited. Is it reasonable to require that every athlete with ADHD have a therapeutic trial of atomoxetine before being granted a TUE for methylphenidate? It seems onerous and bordering on medical malpractice to take a patient who is well controlled on a medication and substitute another to satisfy a nonmedical standard. Clearly, this requires medical judgment because if the athlete truly satisfied the second criterion, then it would be contraindicated to apply this requirement.

The final requirement in Box 7-2 is that the TUE cannot be a consequence to any degree of prior nontherapeutic use of a prohibited substance. This is an important restriction for it also closes a potential gambit to circumvent doping control. For example, following the extended use of AAS (particularly long-acting compounds) the pituitary-gonadal axis is impaired, often for several months. An athlete could potentially apply for a TUE to use testosterone on the basis of subnormal testosterone levels. This TUE criterion makes it clear that an athlete could not receive a benefit after such use.

The WADA criteria may not be appropriate for every sports organization and is not an exact science, but it does provide a framework for developing a program. It offers guidelines for ensuring that all athletes adhere to similar principles with respect to using prohibited substances for legitimate therapeutic indications. Physicians and other medical personnel play key roles in reporting accurate information in the TUE application and applying sound medical judgment to their evaluation.

Designing a Drug Testing and Drug Education Program

Institutions and organizations are at times motivated to develop their own sports drug testing programs and may, in fact, consult other health professionals who are associated with their athletic program. Drug testing is often a knee-jerk response to reports of drug use by athletes or a positive test by a supervising agency. In any event, the most important first step is to determine the purpose of the program, because this will shape subsequent decisions. Drug testing is a complicated process and a poorly designed program is usually worse than none at all. There should be adequate resources available for the collection and testing aspects of the program. The use of third-party administrators to collect the samples is preferred over the use of existing institutional personnel, such as certified athletic trainers, sport physical therapists, or ancillary medical staff. Although it is economically tempting to use these personnel, it creates inherent conflicts among the staff and athletes that can ultimately doom a program. This author's recommendation is to use third-party administrators and minimize the involvement of institutional employees. Finally, the highest quality laboratory should be employed, especially if AAS are being tested.

> **Clinical Point**
>
> Third-party administrators should be used to collect samples, not existing medical or paramedical personnel.

Institutional drug testing programs also tend to be more successful if as many "stakeholders" support it as possible. These include administrators, coaches, athletes, certified athletic trainers, sports physical therapists, and physicians. Interestingly, most studies of athletes[31] reveal that athletes are in favor of drug testing programs. In addition to these personnel, it is imperative that legal counsel be involved early in the planning stages. Decisions need to be made concerning which drugs are tested for, how often testing is

performed, how much advance notice is given to athletes, who is informed of the positive tests, counseling options, and penalty structure. Each one of these is an important component of a comprehensive drug testing program and failure to adequately consider them can reduce a program to little more than window dressing.

> **Clinical Point**
>
> Effective drug testing programs for athletes are complex, expensive processes involving many steps and procedures to ensure they are effective and successful.

Lastly, drug education and counseling should be considered a necessary part of any drug testing program. At the very minimum, athletes have the right to be informed about the drug testing program and the prohibited list. In addition, it is useful to place the drug testing program in the larger context of drug use among athletes and educate them regarding adverse effects, consequences of use, and ethics of sports. The latter is often neglected, but the use of banned performance-enhancing drugs is cheating and this should be clearly communicated. There are several comprehensive educational programs available and institutions can access existing materials to develop their programs.[32,33] Another error in many drug education programs is to focus only on the athlete. Education for ancillary personnel, including equipment personnel, sport therapists, coaches, and administrators should not be omitted. All of these groups are in position to influence the athlete and are part of the larger circle of drug use.

> **Clinical Point**
>
> Drug education and counseling are a necessary part of any drug testing program.

Ethical Considerations

Any discussion of sports drug testing is incomplete without mentioning its ethical implications. Drug testing is often described as expensive, time-consuming, and ineffective, and it is argued that athletes should be allowed to do what they wish to improve themselves. There have been several rationales proposed as to why sports drug testing is unethical. These include rebuttals of paternalism, protecting the athlete, and violating the spirit of sport. The most cogent argument in favor of sports drug testing is to consider the alternative sports world where any type of drug use is allowed. Under this scenario, the athlete who wants to compete drug-free faces three obvious choices: (1) compete at a competitive disadvantage, (2) quit the sport, or (3) go against his or her principles and take the drug. This is not a theoretical ethical dilemma. Indeed, an excellent example of the quandary that athletes experience was succinctly stated by the disgraced British sprinter Dwain Chambers. Mr. Chambers tested positive for THG in the BALCO scandal in 2003. In an interview in 2009 explaining why he chose to use banned performance-enhancing drugs, Chambers stated, "I had to make a decision: If I wasn't going to beat them [by not using drugs], I had to join them. The decision ended up ruining me."[34]

This author would argue that all three are poor ethical choices. Some also argue that drug testing is arbitrary and the banned drug list is also arbitrary. In fact, all sports follow arbitrary rules, but it is those rules that define a sport and provides a common framework that allows fair competition. For example, is there any rational reason why a baseball team fields 9 players on defense? It would clearly be unfair if some teams were allowed to use 10 players in the field.

Clinical Point

Ergogenic drug use has the potential to change a sport so dramatically that it renders competition meaningless. What our society has come to value in sports are the expression of natural talents and the virtuous perfection of those talents.[35] There may be legitimate scientific debate as to which drugs violate these principles and should be prohibited, but there is good agreement that there should be a banned drug list in sports.

Legal Challenges to Sports Drug Testing

One of the key components of any sports drug testing program is the ability of the athlete to appeal the results of a positive drug test. This can take many forms, including institutional appeals, arbitration, or a formal legal process. Although legal challenges occur, courts in the United States have consistently upheld the right of sports organizations to conduct athletic drug tests. Although it is beyond the scope of this chapter to provide an in-depth report of the legal process, it is worth noting some of the more common challenges to a positive drug test.

The usual first step in an appeal of a positive result to an "A" sample is to have the "B" bottle tested. The athlete, or his or her representative, is allowed to witness the entire analytical process to ensure that it is correct. As mentioned previously, if the "A" and "B" samples are not identical, the test result is considered negative. Once that is confirmed, the next focus is on the collection process and chain of custody. In most appeals, the laboratory produces a documentation pack that provides a full chain of custody for the sample. The athlete can review this and ensure that there are no discrepancies. Regarding the collection process, most drug testing programs include a form that the athlete signs upon completion of the urine sample stating that all procedures were followed.

Many appeals focus on the actual analysis of the sample. In these cases, the laboratory must produce appropriate documentation to support the result. This usually includes the laboratory standard operating procedure for the test in question, the laboratory accreditation, quality controls, and sample analysis. The athlete, his or her representatives, and experts all have the option to review the laboratory analysis. Any significant breaches are grounds for concern and may lead to a successful appeal.

Although all of the above reasons are legitimate grounds for an appeal, the collection process, chain of custody, and sample analysis are almost always correct during an appeal. The reasons for this are that if these steps have not been conducted properly, the athlete is usually exonerated well before any appeal process. For example, the United States Anti-Doping Agency convenes a review board at the athlete's request that reviews all written documentation. The review board has the ability to set aside a positive result on the basis of a significant discrepancy or protocol violation. By the time an appeal is filed, there have been multiple reviews of the test result.

Many appeals for a positive drug test then typically involve an acceptance of the analytical result and a request to have the result overturned because of extenuating circumstances. These may include failure to be notified that a substance was on the prohibited list, lack of awareness of the drug testing program, or inadvertent ingestion of a banned substance. These are mentioned because it is important when designing a drug testing program to be aware of any potential gaps in the program. For example, it is important to educate athletes with respect to the details of the drug testing program. Athletes need to be fully educated about the prohibited list in their sport and the penalties for use.

Inadvertent ingestion of a banned substance is a common reason given for having a positive test. This has been exacerbated by the wildly unregulated nature of the dietary supplement industry in the United States and elsewhere. Many banned substances can be found, either labeled or unlabeled, in easily available dietary supplements and can obfuscate drug test results. Owing to the fact that it can be very difficult or impossible to sort this out, many sports organizations have adopted a strict liability policy with respect to drug test results. This means that if an athlete has consented to participate in a drug testing program and a drug test confirms the presence of a banned substance, the athlete is guilty regardless of how it entered the body. Under this type of program, the only legitimate appeals are for challenges to the collection, chain of custody, or analytical process. This creates a situation in which the testing authority is responsible for the quality of the program and the athlete is responsible for what he or she puts into his or her body. Although draconian, it does make the program very clear to all involved.

Gender Verification Testing

There is a final form of testing that also attempts to ensure a level playing field regarding the role of gender identification in sports. Although ergogenic drug use has been present in sports since the ancient Olympics, the concept of gender verification testing is relatively new. As opposed to surreptitious drug use in which sophisticated methods of detection are needed, gender verification was unnecessary in ancient Greece because athletes competed in the nude. Gender verification became popular during the Cold War Olympics in the 1960s and1970s when Eastern European countries purportedly tried to disguise male athletes as women to win Olympic medals. In the late 1960s, buccal smears for sex chromatin were used to verify the gender of a contestant. This test was used for more than 20 years despite the fact that it was known to be medically inaccurate. For example, phenotypic women who carried an XY variant and had androgen insensitivity syndromes would be disqualified. Although athletes with the XY variant have a male chromosome, they do not have a competitive advantage because they are resistant to natural androgens. In the 1990s the sex chromatin test was replaced with a more accurate deoxyribonucleic acid–based test.[36] Eventually, chromosomal testing for gender verification was completely abandoned, and currently the International Olympic Committee evaluates suspicious individuals on a case-by-case basis. Given the fact that drug testing now involves witnessed urination, gender verification has come full-circle back to ancient Greece in which the naked eye is the best method of detection.

Conclusion

As history shows, the desire to take performance-enhancing drugs dates back thousands of years. The use of performance-enhancing drugs in sports has unfortunately necessitated that drug testing become an integral part of athletics. Owing to this necessity, it is essential that those involved with athletes have a thorough understanding of drug use among athletes and the drug testing procedure. Although drug testing has grown to encompass lawyers, administrators, and other nonmedical personnel, there are still significant medical aspects to both drug testing and drug use. The one constant in the field of sports pharmacology is the ever-changing nature of the drugs and the methods of detection. Those who work with athletes are often in the position of providing advice, and it is incumbent to render accurate information. Although it appears that cheating through the use of performance-enhancing drugs is centuries old, the idea of clean competition is also thousands of years old. This is captured in a quote from the Greek dramatist Sophocles, who stated 2500 years ago, "Rather fail with honor than succeed by fraud."

References

1. Personal communication with Frank Uryasz, National Center for Drug Free Sport.
2. Parkinson AB, Evans NA: Anabolic androgenic steroids: A survey of 500 users, *Med Sci Sports Exerc* 38(4):644-651, 2006.
3. Uryasz F: Chain of custody issues. In Bartlett R, Gratton C, Rolf CR, editors: *Encyclopedia of international sports studies*, New York, 2006, Routledge.
4. Uryasz F: Collection issues. In Bartlett R, Gratton C, Rolf CR, editors: *Encyclopedia of international sports studies*, New York, 2006, Routledge.
5. WADA Guidelines for Blood Sample Collection. http://www.wada-ama.org/rtecontent/document/2008-06_GuidelinesBloodSample_unmarked.pdf. Accessed January 2009.
6. Catlin DH, Sekera MH, Ahrens BD, et al: Tetrahydrogestrinone: Discovery, synthesis, and detection in urine, *Rapid Commun Mass Spectrom* 18(12):1245–1249, 2004.
7. Catlin DH, Ahrens B, Kucherova Y: Detection of norbolethone, an anabolic steroid never marketed, in athletes' urine, *Rapid Commun Mass Spectrom* 16:1273–1275, 2002.
8. Sekera MH, Ahrens B, Chang YC, et al: Another designer steroid: Discovery, synthesis, and detection of 'madol' in urine, *Rapid Commun Mass Spectrom* 19(6):781–784, 2005.
9. Catlin DH, Hatton CK, Starcevic SH: Issues in detecting abuse of xenobiotic anabolic steroids and testosterone by analysis of athlete's urine, *Clin Chem* 43(7):1280–1288, 1997.
10. Green GA: Anabolic agents. In Bartlett R, Gratton C, Rolf CR, editors: *Encyclopedia of international sports studies*, New York, 2006, Routledge.
11. Green GA, Catlin DH, Starcevic B: Analysis of over-the-counter dietary supplements, *Clin J Sport Med* 11(4):254–259, 2001.
12. Catlin DH, Leder BZ, Ahrens B, et al: Trace contamination of over-the-counter androstenedione and positive urine test results for a nandrolone metabolite, *JAMA* 284(20):2618–2621, 2000.
13. Hatton CK: Nandrolone. In Bartlett R, Gratton C, Rolf CR, editors: *Encyclopedia of international sports studies*, New York, 2006, Routledge.
14. Le Bizec B, Gaudin I, Monteau F, et al: Consequences of boar edible tissue consumption on urinary profiles of nandrolone metabolites, *Rapid Commun Mass Spectrom* 14:1058–1065, 2000.
15. Schmitt N, Flament M, Goubault C, et al: Nandrolone excretion is not increased by exhaustive exercise in trained athletes, *Med Sci Sports Exerc* 34(9):1436–1439, 2002.
16. UK Sport: Nandrolone progress report to the UK Sports Council from the Expert Committee on Nandrolone, 2003. http://www.uksport.gov.uk/assets/File/Generic_Template_Documents/Drug_Free_Sport/Nandrolone_Progress_Report_Feb03.pdf. Accessed 15 January, 2009.
17. Donike M, Barwald KR, Klosterman K, et al: The detection of exogenous testosterone. In Heck H, Hollmann W, Liesen H, Rost R, editors: *Sport: Leistung und Gesundheit, Cologne*, 1983, Deutscher Arzte Verlag.
18. The World Anti-Doping Agency 2010 Prohibited List International Standard http://www.wada-ama.org/Documents/World_Anti-Doping_Program/WADP-Prohibited-list/WADA_Prohibited_List_2010_EN.pdf. Accessed February 2010.
19. Hatton CK: Carbon isotope ratio testing. In Bartlett R, Gratton C, Rolf CR, editors: *Encyclopedia of international sports studies*, New York, 2006, Routledge.
20. *WADA explanatory technical note: Stability of 19-norandrosterone findings in urine*, May 13, 2005. Montreal, Canada, 2005, World Anti-Doping Agency.

21. Tokish JM, Kocher MS, Hawkins RJ: Ergogenic aids: A review of basic science, performance, side effects, and status in sports, *Am J Sports Med* 32(6):1543–1553, 2004.

22. Parisotto R, Wu M, Ashenden MJ, et al: Detection of recombinant human erythropoietin abuse in athletes utilizing markers of altered erythropoiesis, *Haematologica* 86:128–137, 2001.

23. Lasne F, De Ceaurriz J: Recombinant erythropoietin in urine, *Nature* 405:635, 2000.

24. Breidbach A: Erythropoietin (EPO)/darbepoetin. In Bartlett R, Gratton C, Rolf CR, editors: *Encyclopedia of international sports studies*, New York, 2006, Routledge.

25. Green GA: HGH/somatomedins. In Bartlett R, Gratton C, Rolf CR, editors: *Encyclopedia of international sports studies*, New York, 2006, Routledge.

26. Zida W, Bidlingmaier M, Dall R, Strasburger CJ: Detection of doping with human growth hormone, *Lancet* 353:895, 1999.

27. Erotokritou-Mulligan I, Bassett EE, Kniess A, et al: Validation of the growth hormone (GH)-dependent marker method of detecting GH abuse in sport through the use of independent data sets, *Growth Horm IGF Res* 17(5):416–423, 2007.

28. Green GA: Doping control for the team physician: A review of drug testing procedures in sport, *Am J Sports Med* 34(10):1690–1698, 2006.

29. Green GA: Cannabinoids. In Bartlett R, Gratton C, Rolf CR, editors: *Encyclopedia of international sports studies*, New York, 2006, Routledge.

30. *WADA international standard for therapeutic use exemptions.* Accessed February 2010 from http://www.wada-ama.org/Documents/World_Anti-Doping_Program/WADP-IS-TUE/WADA_ISTUE_2010_EN.pdf.

31. National Collegiate Athletic Association: *NCAA 2005 study of substance use habits of collegiate student athletes*, Indianapolis, IN, 2006, NCAA.

32. Goldberg L, Elliot DL, Clarke GN, et al: Effects of a multidimensional anabolic steroid prevention intervention. The Adolescents Training and Learning to Avoid Steroids (ATLAS) Program, *JAMA* 276(19):1555–1562, 1996.

33. Elliot DL, Goldberg L, Moe EL, et al: Preventing substance use and disordered eating: Initial outcomes of the ATHENA (athletes targeting healthy exercise and nutrition alternatives) program, *Arch Pediatr Adolesc Med* 158(11):1043–1049, 2004.

34. *Los Angeles Times*, "Boxer Shane Mosley, sprinter Dwain Chambers take different paths after BALCO allegations." January 22, 2009, p D8.

35. Murray T: Ethical considerations. In Bartlett R, Gratton C, Rolf CR, editors: *Encyclopedia of international sports studies*, New York, 2006, Routledge.

36. Genel M: Gender verification no more? *Medscape Women's Health* 5(3), 2000. Accessed February 5, 2009 from http://womenshealth.medscape.com/Medscape/WomensHealth/journal/2000/v05.n03/wh7218.gene/wh7218.gene.html.

APPLIED BIOMECHANICS OF CYCLING

Robert J. Gregor, Eileen G. Fowler, and W. Lee Childers

Introduction

The cycling task is relevant to several domains in the movement sciences including high-level competition, recreation, exercise regimens used for musculoskeletal and aerobic conditioning, and as a widely used modality for rehabilitation applied to a variety of physiological system disorders (e.g., musculoskeletal injury, neurodegenerative disease, and cardiac rehabilitation). In the competition setting, the primary focus is on performance efficiency; the rider assumes a position on the bicycle designed to minimize wind resistance and maximize energy input to the bicycle. Research on elite competitive cyclists usually focuses on factors such as bicycle components (e.g., frame and pedal design), safety features (e.g., helmet design), aerodynamic positions on the bicycle, aerodynamic clothing, physiological and mechanical response to changes in load, body position, and frame setup. In an aerobic exercise setting, the primary focus is usually on comfort, safety, and the ability to regulate position on the bicycle, resistance, and cadence to accommodate a broad range of individual needs and goals. The stationary bicycle is commonly used as a form of aerobic exercise for weight loss and cardiac rehabilitation. Finally, patients with selected musculoskeletal, cardiorespiratory, or neurodegenerative disease (e.g., Parkinson disease [PD]) use the rhythmic cadence of cycling to attenuate the side effects of the disease (e.g., tremor in PD) and to improve overall health and well-being—a goal common to all populations.

The bicycle uniquely combines lower-extremity strengthening, range of motion (ROM), and cardiovascular conditioning while controlling joint, musculotendinous, and ligament stress. It promotes rhythmic movement patterns in the lower extremities (i.e., cyclic loading) important to ligament, muscle, and tendon repair as well as proprioceptive input to the central nervous system. Adjustments can be made to a stationary bicycle to precisely meet the requirements of individuals at various stages of their conditioning or rehabilitation. The degree of lower-limb loading, which can be regulated through changes in the resistance setting on the bicycle, and the speed of joint movement, which can be regulated by pedaling cadence and seat height changes, offer the potential for objective measurements to document progress and gradually increased exercise intensity. Outdoor cycling is also an option; however, it is difficult to control the amount of muscular effort and stress due, in part, to the high inertial loads that are generated, for example, in propelling the bike up a hill. Despite these limitations, outdoor cycling is less "boring" and more challenging and thus may be a matter of choice for the athlete or patient who has achieved an advanced stage of rehabilitation. A person undergoing rehabilitation, however, should receive careful guidance to ensure that the benefits exceed the risks that may otherwise be introduced.

The purpose of this chapter is to describe how the cycling task has been used in a wide range of applications in exercise and rehabilitation. Being able to *"personalize"* the interface between the rider and the bicycle allows the clinician or trainer to provide the ROM necessary to enhance proprioceptive input in patients with certain neuromuscular disorders. In addition, being able to regulate load to increase strength or to gradually rehabilitate selected tissues in repair allows the clinician or trainer to modify training programs for non-disabled individuals and athletes as well as patients with special needs. Specific emphasis is placed on the lower extremities, because they assume the primary role in the production and transmission of power to the bicycle and, as a consequence, experience the largest loads and the most profound chronic injuries. The authors begin with a review of cycling kinematics and kinetics related to loading of the lower extremity and then describe the mechanics of individual lower extremity muscles used in the cycling task.

Muscles are major force producers as well as sensors that provide both length and force input to the nervous system during movement. Finally, common cycling injuries and cycling used by more challenged populations for rehabilitation, exercise, and elite competition (e.g., amputee athletes) are presented.

> **Cycling Domains**
>
> • High-level competition
> • Recreational activity
> • Aerobic and anaerobic conditioning
> • Rehabilitation of disease and injury
> • Enhancing quality of life

Cycling Kinematics

Most reports on cycling kinematics have been limited to sagittal plane motion: hip and knee flexion and extension and ankle dorsiflexion and plantar flexion. Displacements, velocities, and accelerations of the thigh, shank (tibia), and foot are most affected by cadence and bicycle geometry (e.g., seat height or crank length). *Seat height* is defined as the distance from the top of the pedal to the top of the saddle when the crank is down and in line with the seat tube. The complex interactions between bicycle geometry and rider kinematics and attempts at "optimizing" the bicycle-rider interface have been the subject of many studies that systematically varied rider kinematics by changing bicycle configuration, pedaling cadence, or both.[1] Peak flexion and extension of the lower extremity joints varies depending on the seat height and fore-aft seat adjustments. However, once the rider position is established, the constrained cyclic movement of the lower extremity remains quite consistent.

Kinematic, kinetic, and muscle activity patterns during cycling are most often described relative to the angle of the crank, with 0° or 360° representing top dead center (TDC) and 180° representing bottom dead center (BDC) in upright cycling. The power, or propulsive, phase takes place between TDC and BDC. During this time, the contralateral limb is in the recovery phase between BDC and TDC. A point to remember is that during recumbent cycling the power phase rotates back approximately 90° making the power phase between 270° and 90°. This point is raised again in the "Muscle Mechanics" section later in this chapter.

Kinematic data, for example the ROM at each joint, vary according to bicycle set-up. Although linear and angular displacements, velocities, and accelerations change with bike fit changes, it is useful to present some examples regarding steady-state seated cycling performance. Faria and Cavanagh[2] studied sagittal plane kinematics and reported a

total excursion of 45° for the thigh, 75° for the knee, and 20° for the ankle. These values were measured at a seat height chosen for comfort by the cyclist. Using an angle convention similar to the one employed by Faria and Cavanagh[2] (Figure 8-1), Rugg and Gregor[3] (Figure 8-2) demonstrate the effect of seat height changes on hip and knee ROM as seat height varied from 100% to 115% of pubic symphysis height (i.e., height measured from the pubic symphysis, or crotch, to the floor). This range of seat heights is considered somewhat extreme however, because the comfortable range chosen by most competitive riders usually varies from 106% to 109% of pubic symphysis height.

A striking feature of the hip and knee patterns is the increase in peak knee extension (approximately 30°) coupled with smaller increases in peak hip extension (less than 10°) as seat height increases,. The general shape and timing of each joint's kinematic profile, however, remained fairly

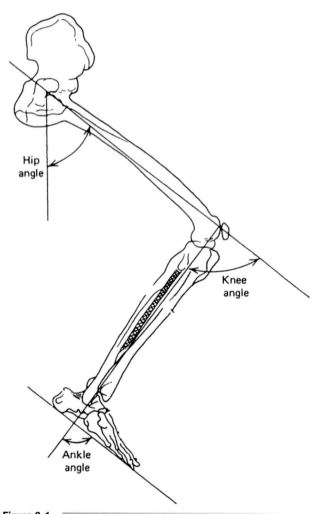

Figure 8-1

Sketch of the right lower extremity showing reference angles for the hip, knee, and ankle. An angle of 0° at the hip is the vertical reference, with a positive angle representing hip flexion; 0° at the knee is full extension, and 0° at the ankle is the anatomic position.

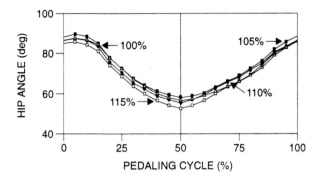

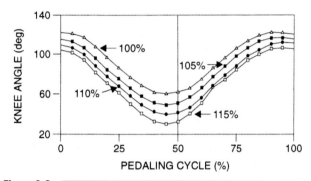

Figure 8-2

Angular displacement of the hip and knee for one pedaling cycle at four different seat heights: 100%, 105%, 110%, and 115% of leg length. Angle convention is presented in Figure 8-1.

suggest this variable may be regulated by the nervous system to maintain single-joint knee extensors within an operational range of their force-length relationships.[8] This is plausible given that the knee joint contributes the most energy to work production at the crank,[9] whereas the ankle is used more for transferring energy[10,11] and thus is less critical for task performance.

While seat height and STA are important considerations when setting up the bicycle for each individual, Sanderson and colleagues[12] reported the effects of cadence on ROM focusing on the knee and ankle joints. It seems when cadence increases from 50 to 110 rpm, the ankle joint becomes 10° more plantar flexed while the knee joint becomes 4° more flexed. These patterns were associated with a decrease in ROM in both joints.[12] These kinematic changes may also result in smaller increases in contraction velocity in the triceps surae group (i.e., gastrocnemius and soleus) and could reflect a strategy to maintain the operation of the muscles in the triceps surae group within a more effective region of their force-velocity relationship. These results should be considered in light of the information discussed in the section on "Muscle Mechanics" later in this chapter.

Fatigue is another important factor to consider because it also affects lower limb kinematics.[13,14] Exact changes vary within subjects, but generally the trunk becomes more horizontal,[14] the thigh becomes more vertical,[13,14] and the ankle becomes more dorsiflexed,[13] while the knee joint showes little change.[13,14] Sanderson and Black[13] showed degradation in the recovery phase effective force (see section on "Kinetics" later in this chapter) with an increase in power phase effective force and suggested these changes were related to joint flexors being the first to fatigue. Dingwell and colleagues[14] presented evidence of localized fatigue in joint flexors more often than joint extensors and concluded that the changes in cycling kinematics could be related to the fatigue within those muscle groups.

Cyclists display different patterns of ankle motion (termed *ankling*) that has created speculation regarding what pattern, if any, may be considered *"optimal"*[1] in terms of cycling efficiency. Also under consideration, aside from the changes in the pattern of ankle motion, was the ROM changes as a result of ankling. Although ankling has not been investigated specifically, several authors have commented on this technique.[1,4,8,11] Pierson-Carey and colleagues,[11] for example, reported that limiting ROM in one or both ankles during cycling reduced the magnitude and effectiveness of resultant pedal forces during the bottom of the pedal stroke. These data suggest that by using an ankling motion the rider may optimize pedaling performance. This also supports the notion that ankling could reflect a strategy by the neuromuscular system to maintain muscles about the ankle[12] and knee joints[8] within an optimal range of muscle performance.

Efforts to more completely describe lower-extremity kinematics involve three-dimensional analyses, (i.e., movements

similar across the four seat height conditions. In all conditions, peak hip flexion and extension occurred at approximately 10° and 180° of the pedaling cycle, respectively, whereas peak knee flexion and extension occurred at approximately 350° and 170° of the pedaling cycle, respectively. More recent data reported by Price and Donne[4] showed similar trends in the knee and ankle following changes in seat height, suggesting that kinematic adaptation to changes in seat height is quite predictable.

Lower limb kinematic patterns seem to be influenced to a lesser degree by changes in seat tube angle (STA).[4-8] STA determines the angular orientation of the body and may affect kinematic patterns and hence the range of length change experienced by individual muscles as the neuromuscular system adjusts to the new orientation of the gravitational vector with respect to the leg.[6] Heil and colleagues[7] examined a range of STAs available for conventional (upright) bicycles as well as positions using aero-bars that allowed the rider to assume a more aerodynamic position. Their findings suggest that knee kinematics were generally unaffected by STA and that hip and ankle angles showed a trend to increase with increases in STA. Reiser and colleagues[8] showed similar results for cycling kinematics over a broader range to include recumbent cycling positions. The immutable kinematic patterns observed at the knee joint over such a broad range of body orientations in the sagittal, transverse and frontal planes). For example, internal and external rotation of the tibia about its long axis, knee translation in the frontal plane, and movement of the lower extremity outside the sagittal plane have all been reported in a study related to knee injury.[15] Movement of the knee in the frontal plane has been reported by several investigators including McCoy,[16] Ruby and colleagues,[17] and Boutin and colleagues,[18] and their data indicate that the joint center can move as much as 6 cm in the mediolateral direction during one pedaling cycle. Beginning at TDC, the femur internally rotates and adducts as the lower extremity proceeds through the power phase. The knee moves medially with respect to the pedal, the tibia inwardly rotates as the foot pronates. Allowing these natural movements to take place with minimal constraint could markedly decrease joint forces and tissue stress in the foot and ankle as well as the entire lower extremity (see section on "Kinetics" later in this chapter).

Addressing another aspect of this issue—that is, how much frontal plane and rotational movement should be allowed to minimize load on muscle and connective tissue structures—Hannaford and colleagues[15] and Bailey and colleagues[19] reported that subjects without knee problems showed less transverse and frontal plane movement than did riders with a history of knee pain. Francis,[20] using qualitative video analysis, reported less knee movement in the frontal plane in elite cyclists. Because these cyclists also used in-shoe orthotics, Francis[20] concluded that foot position did indeed influence knee motion. Finally, Francis,[20] used trial-and-error adjustments in pedal cant and provided video feedback to assist cyclists in their efforts to reduce frontal plane movement. These techniques decreased knee pain in elite cyclists per subjective reports. More recently, Gregersen and colleagues[21] showed that the inversion and eversion angle of the foot altered the varus and valgus moment at the knee joint, and that this moment was minimized by inverting the foot 5° and 10° within the nonsymptomatic cyclists studied. The issue of how much to limit natural movement of lower extremity structures for symptomatic cyclists remains open to discussion.

McCoy[16] investigated the effects of different seat positions on lower extremity kinematics and kinetics in the frontal plane. Seat height was varied from 94% to 106% of leg length, a range comparable to that reported by Rugg and Gregor.[3] Results indicated the knee was medial of the pedal center of pressure throughout the power phase. The greatest magnitude of deviation occurred at approximately 90° of crank rotation in the low seat height condition (94% of pubic symphysis height) and at 150° of crank rotation at the medium and high seat heights (100% and 106% of pubic symphysis height, respectively). Data presented in Figure 8-3 represent average patterns for 150 pedal revolutions from five subjects riding at 200 watts (W) at the three seat-height conditions just

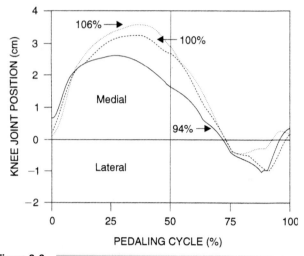

Figure 8-3

Position of the knee, at the mid-knee joint, during the pedaling cycle with respect to the pedal center of pressure at three different seat heights: 94%, 100%, and 106% of leg length. Each curve is an average of 150 pedal revolutions (10 subjects in five trials) at 200 watts W and 80 rpm. (From McCoy RW: *The effect of varying seat position on knee loads during cycling,* unpublished doctoral dissertation, University of Southern California Department of Exercise Science, 1989.)

mentioned. The zero line is corrected for the natural excursion of the pedal center of pressure, with the data showing the knee moving from a position medial to the center of pressure during the power phase to one lateral to the center of pressure during recovery. Similar data have been presented by Ruby and colleagues[22] although their measurements were referenced to the center of the pedal and not the center of pressure. In summary, the lower extremity displays considerable movement in the frontal plane, and variation in seat height has a marked effect on the amount of actual movement.

Clinically, the stationary bike is often used to provide gentle knee ROM exercises during the initial stages of a rehabilitation program. Seat height can be set relatively high if the patient has limited knee flexion and low if knee extension is limited so that the patient can perform a full pedal revolution. In addition, some companies manufacture telescoping cranks that can be adjusted for the involved or injured side. Permanent adjustments can be made to the crank to customize the patient's bicycle for chronic conditions such as arthritis and persons with lower-limb loss. As stated earlier, a minimum knee flexion range of approximately 75° is necessary to permit a complete crank revolution for a normal (106% to 109% of pubic symphysis height) seat height position without adjusting the crank. If the patient has knee pain and is presenting with excessive knee motion in the frontal plane, the shoe–pedal interface could be altered with either a foot orthosis[20] or by inverting or everting the entire foot[21] to better align the patient's knee over the pedal.

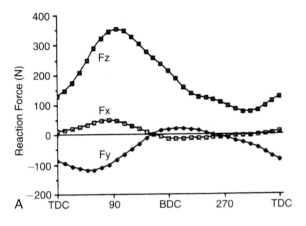

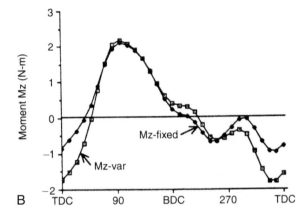

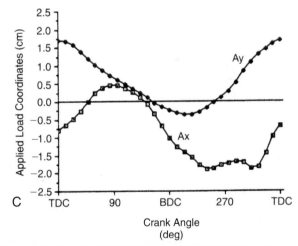

Clinically Relevant Points: Cycling Kinematics

- Limb range of motion on a bicycle can be affected by:
  - Seat height
  - Seat tube angle
  - Foot–pedal interface
- Power phase during cycling generally occurs between 0° and 180° in upright cycling and from 270° to 90° in recumbent cycling
- During upright cycling, joint excursions are approximately 45° for the hip, 75° for the knee and 20° for the ankle
- Localized fatigue may alter lower-limb kinematics
- Mediolateral knee motion of up to 6 cm normally occurs during cycling as the tibia internally rotates and the foot pronates

Cycling Kinetics

Reaction Forces Between the Rider and the Bicycle

A kinetic analysis of lower extremity function requires knowledge of the interactive forces between the rider and the bicycle. Newton's third law of motion states that forces act in pairs that are equal in magnitude and opposite in direction. Therefore, when the foot applies a force to the pedal, it will be met with a reaction force acting on the foot that is equal in magnitude and opposite in direction. These forces, called *pedal reaction forces,* act on the foot during cycling and have been quantified in many laboratories using specially instrumented pedals.[1] All pedal designs are basically similar to the force platforms widely used to measure ground reaction forces during gait. Force components perpendicular to the pedal surface (Fz) and shear forces tangential to the pedal surface, both mediolateral (Fx) and anteroposterior (Fy) (Figure 8-4, *A*) have been widely reported. From these components a center of pressure (Figure 8-4 *C, Ay* and *Ax*), or point-of-force application, can be calculated. In addition, a rotational moment about an axis perpendicular to the surface of the pedal (Figure 8–4 *B, Mz*) and positioned at the center of pressure can be calculated and has been used to monitor cycling performance related to injury.[23] Although pedal reaction forces have been reported for more than 100 years, the complexity of the instrumentation used to make the measurements has had little effect on the overall pedal reaction force profiles in standard seated.[1] The effects of load, cadence, and position on the bicycle on both the magnitude and direction of these force components are discussed later in this section.

In addition to the magnitude of the pedal reaction force, the orientation of the resultant vector (Fr) with respect to the lower extremity is an important factor that will markedly influence how the leg musculature responds to various pedal loading demands. An exemplar pattern of the resultant pedal reaction force measured in the sagittal plane at six intervals during the pedaling cycle is presented in Figure 8-5, together with the relationship between the resultant vector

Figure 8-4

Mean patterns for five pedal revolutions for the pedal reaction force (**A**), applied moment (**B**), and center of pressure patterns (**C**) during one pedaling cycle (top dead center [TDC] at 0 degrees to TDC at 360 degrees). **A,** Fz is the component orthogonal to the pedal surface, Fy is anteroposterior *(AP)* shear, and Fx is the medial-lateral shear. **B,** The applied moment *(Mz)* about an axis orthogonal to the pedal surface when this axis is through the center of pressure *(Mz-var)* or through the center of the pedal *(Mz-fixed).* **C,** Coordinates of the applied load in the x *(Ax)* and y *(Ay)* directions. (From Broker JP, Gregor RJ: A dual piezoelectric element force pedal for kinetic analysis of cycling, *Int J Sport Biomech* 6:394–403, 1990. Copyright 1990 by Human Kinetics Publishers, Inc.)

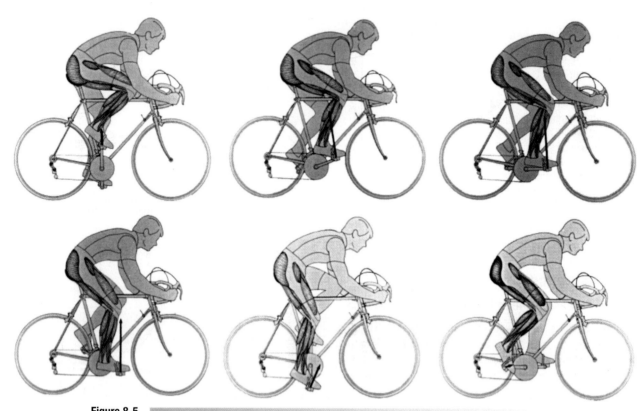

Figure 8-5

Resultant pedal reaction force with respect to the right lower extremity for six separate locations during the pedaling cycle. The length of the arrow indicates increases and decreases in magnitude.

and the right lower extremity. The objective of any training or rehabilitation program is to effectively transmit power to the bicycle; making sure these reactive loads are oriented in a way that utilizes lower extremity musculature in an efficient and effective manner; and in a way that ensures unusually high loads, which may result in overuse injuries to the legs, are kept to a minimum.

The general position of the pedal reaction force with respect to each segment of the lower extremity in the frontal plane (e.g., the knee) is important, and published reports[17,24] indicate that a varus load is applied to the knee during the power phase (Figure 8-6),[2] a phase when the pedal reaction forces are the greatest. This is because the resultant force is passing medial to the knee, despite the fact that the knee appears to be medial to the pedal center. McCoy[16] calculated movement of the center of pressure in the frontal plane during the pedaling cycle and described the position of the resultant force vector acting at the center of pressure with respect to the knee (see Figure 8-6). Three seat height conditions—94%, 100%, and 106% of leg length—were used. These types of data can be very useful visually, but this presentation gives only a general impression of the potential effects of these loads on the segments of the lower extremity. Joint moments

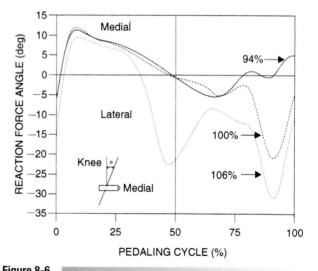

Figure 8-6

Position of the pedal reaction force with respect to the knee center during the pedaling cycle in the frontal plane. Each curve is an average of 150 pedal revolutions (10 subjects in five trials) at 200 W and 80 rpm. Separate patterns are an average at three seat conditions: 94%, 100%, and 106% of leg length. (From McCoy RW: *The effect of varying seat position on knee loads during cycling,* unpublished doctoral dissertation, University of Southern California Department of Exercise Science, 1989.)

and reaction force components must be calculated using either inverse dynamics or forward dynamics simulations[25] to more completely evaluate the effect of these loads on muscle and bone.

Translation of pedal force components to *"effective"* force patterns designed to *"optimize"* crank rotation is of great interest to cyclists, engineers, movement scientists, and physical therapists, and can be calculated using pedal reaction forces and knowledge of pedal and crank position. LaFortune and Cavanagh[26] first presented the concept of pedaling effectiveness by calculating the "effective" force on the crank, that is, the force component perpendicular to the crank doing work to rotate the crank (Figure 8-7). In addition, a component parallel to the crank was calculated and considered to be the *"ineffective force,"* that contributes minimally to crank rotation. An index of effectiveness has also been presented as the ratio between the effective and ineffective force components.

These calculations can be used to enhance training and rehabilitation. Broker and colleagues[27,28] examined the effect of visual feedback, both summary and concurrent, on the ability to produce a more effective pattern of force application during cycling. Additionally, Perell[29] reported the use of an effective force pattern as feedback for stroke patients to enhance lower limb symmetry with carry-over to gait symmetry. More recently, Hasson and colleagues[30] used a force-directing task during cycling to study how the nervous system coordinates one- and two-joint muscles in directing force at the pedal. Using real-time feedback of the force component orthogonal to the crank during constant cadence cycling, their results suggest the subjects were able to learn a complex task by changing the direction of their applied pedal forces through reorganization of joint torques

(see section later in this chapter on joint moments) and one- and two-joint muscle coordination (see section later in this chapter on muscle and EMG patterns during cycling). This latter example may be very useful in the rehabilitation of neurologically impaired patients as well as elite athletes recovering from injury to a single joint in which intervention strategies warrant a redistribution of joint moments to "off-load" an injured joint during the early rehabilitation period.

Although the legs receive the largest loads (i.e., pedal reaction forces), interactive forces also exist at the handlebar–rider and seat–rider interfaces. One of the first reports documenting these loads was presented by Bolourchi and Hull.[31] Varying cadence from 63 to 100 rpm, a fully instrumented bicycle was used to measure reactive and propulsive forces continuously during each successive pedaling cycle. Results suggest seat load profiles were independent of rider and cadence and at all conditions, seat load profiles went through two complete periods for each crank cycle (Figure 8-8).

Although very few reports have emerged since these studies, it is important to realize that there are five points of contact in seated cycling (i.e., two pedals, one seat, and two sides of the handlebar). At each interface, loads vary (e.g., hill climbing in a standing position involves substantial forces at each pedal and the handlebars) and if a complete description of the task is warranted, all loads must be considered. This is also true of course, in the recumbent cycling position in a rehabilitation environment (see "Muscle Mechanics" section on the effect of body position on muscle activity patterns). Anything the body comes in contact with produces reactive loads on the individual that should be considered in any program designed for rehabilitation or training.

Specific to recumbent cycling, one must keep in mind the change in the power and recovery phases in the pedaling cycle (i.e., a rotation of the power phase from vertical TDC to vertical BDC as used often in upright cycling) to a power phase that in some cases ranges from deepest flexion of the lower extremity to full extension and in some cases from the 270° point to the 90° point in the normal upright cycle orientation. It is important to consider the power phase relative to the pedaling cycle convention when interpreting joint reaction forces,[8,32,33] muscle activity patterns,[6,34,35] and unique clinical applications.[36-41]

Pressure Distribution at the Pedal Surface

Forces acting on the bottom of the foot can be quantified by examining pressure (i.e., force per unit area) and such quantification is a useful measure to examine injuries related to the interface between the foot and the pedal. Sanderson and Cavanagh,[42] for example, studied the

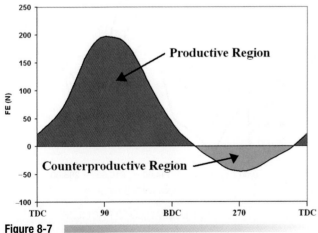

Figure 8-7

Effective force profile during one pedal revolution. The productive region is positive work done to drive the crank; the counterproductive region during recovery represents an extra load that the contralateral limb must work against during its power phase (top dead center to bottom dead center).

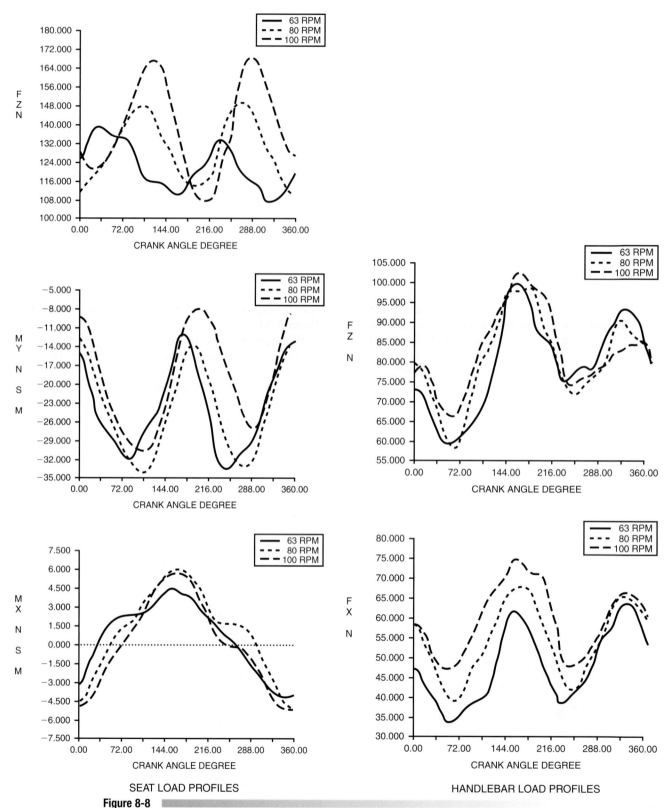

Figure 8-8

Loading patterns for the seat and handlebars at three separate cadences. (From Bolourchi F, Hull ML: Measurement of rider-induced loads during simulated bicycling, *Int J Sports Biomech* 1:325–326, 1985.)

variations in pressure distribution throughout the pedaling cycle using a specially designed insole with 256 discrete force measuring elements (Figure 8-9). Further reports by Sanderson and Hennig,[43] Amoroso and colleagues,[44] and Hennig and Sanderson[45] generally concluded that pressure distribution patterns and magnitudes are affected by the rigidity of the sole of the shoe, increased load, and increased cadence. Implications for injury and rehabilitation focused on chronic foot problems that may lead to injurious load patterns up the skeletal chain (e.g., low back pain). Greater attention should be given to the foot-pedal interface in people with disabilities or injuries, particularly for individuals with diabetes. (See section on "Common Cycling Injuries" later in this chapter.)

Torsion Measurements at the Pedal Surface

Knowledge of torsion, or rotation of segments about a long axis through the center of the segment, is significant to understanding musculoskeletal function and mechanisms of injury. With respect to cycling, the foot naturally moves (e.g., internally and externally rotates, everts and inverts) similar to its function during the stance phase of gait. The amount of constraint imposed on these *"normal"* movements could have significant implications for injury and the effective delivery of energy to the crank. In one of the earlier reports, focusing on function and potential injury, Francis[46] and Sanderson[47] discussed the pathomechanics of tibial internal rotation and valgus knee position during the propulsive phase of cycling and compared this situation to running kinetics during midstance. It is during these phases of cycling and running that the greatest loads are imposed on the lower extremities. Several similarities were found.

Quantification of the applied moment at the pedal surface about an axis perpendicular to the pedal surface (Figure 8-10) is a kinetic parameter that has been suggested by many to be directly related to knee loads and subsequent overuse knee pain.[17,23,48] In an effort to further understand pedal loads, Gregor and Wheeler[48] showed that the center of pressure varied throughout the pedaling cycle and that it influenced the calculated twisting moment, or Mz, at the pedal. In support of this finding, Ruby and colleagues[17] calculated knee loads from force pedal data, sagittal plane kinematics, and frontal plane knee motion and reported that the moment, Mz, about the axis orthogonal to the pedal surface was a significant contributor to Mz at the knee.

Mz at the pedal relates directly to the pedal design and the nature of the "connection" between the foot or shoe and the pedal. One hypothesis is that allowing greater movement at the foot–pedal interface would minimize strain and reduce injury. Initial support for this hypothesis is presented

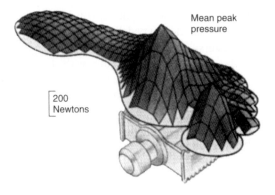

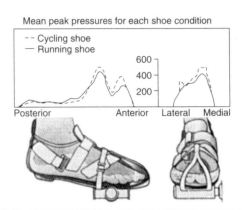

Figure 8-9

Pattern of pressure distribution on the sole of the cycling shoe, including data from a subject using a cycling shoe and a running shoe. (From Sanderson DJ: The biomechanics of cycling shoes, *Cycling Sci* Sept:27–30, 1990.)

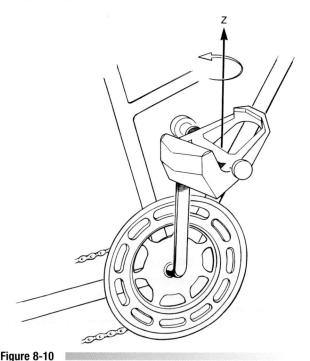

Figure 8-10

Sketch of the applied moment *(Mz)* about an axis orthogonal to the pedal surface.

in Figure 8-11 (i.e., the magnitude of Mz was reduced when using a "float" design pedal). It seems when using this pedal force analysis system the peak internally applied moment (+Mz) increased significantly with load whereas the "clipless" float system decreased both the internally and externally applied moments. Knee pain subjects exhibited distinctly different moment patterns, whereas cyclists with chronic anterior knee pain—the most common type reported by cyclists—demonstrated exaggerated peak internally applied moments, increased rates of loading (dMz/dt), and a longer duration of the applied internal moment during the power phase (0° to 180°).

Although this information seems to be important to function and injury, little is known about what amount of rotation is desirable for the foot at the pedal surface or the shank and thigh during the pedaling cycle. A review of the literature[49] regarding clipless pedal designs concluded that permitting the foot to rotate at the pedal surface markedly attenuates the loads experienced by the joints in the lower extremity, especially the knee joint.

Joint Reaction Forces

Data specific to the loads imposed on each joint in the lower extremity are critical to understanding joint function ranging from elite performance to rehabilitation. Although all segments are of interest, data related to knee joint loads are the most abundant in the literature. Select articles related to these forces and some recent work related to cycling in

anterior cruciate ligament (ACL)–deficient individuals are reviewed.

Vector components in the sagittal plane specific to the knee joint are schematically presented in Figure 8-12, with a positive tensile-compressive component (Fy_k) and positive anteroposterior component (Fx_k); the mediolateral component is orthogonal to this vector, described with respect to the tibial plateau. These three vector components, both magnitude and direction, are affected by load, cadence, rider position relative to the bike (e.g., bike set-up), the type of bicycle, (e.g., recumbent versus upright), and type of shoe–pedal interface.

In a recent investigation,[50] four separate instrumented pedal platforms were used to test the effect of foot position on intersegmental knee loads in three dimension. The multidegree of freedom pedal interface allowed both inversion and eversion and adduction and abduction separately or in combination. There was a general reduction in both coupled knee moments and in the valgus knee moment when using the dual-rotation platform. Consistent with

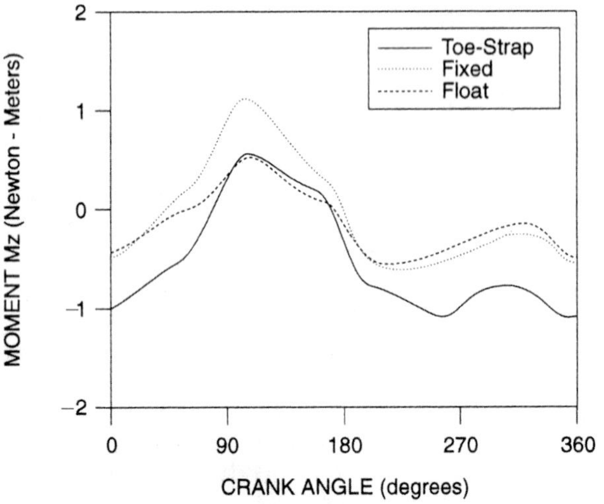

Figure 8-11

The applied moment *(Mz)* pattern during the pedal cycle averaged across 27 subjects using three separate shoe–pedal interface designs: a standard toe-strap and cleat, a clipless fixed design, and a clipless float design. A positive moment indicates an inwardly applied moment against the pedal surface (heel out). (From Wheeler JB, Gregor RJ, Broker JP: The effect of clipless float design on shoe/pedal interface kinetics: Implications for overuse injuries during cycling, *J Appl Biomech* 11:119–141, 1995. Copyright 1995 by Human Kinetics Publishers, Inc.)

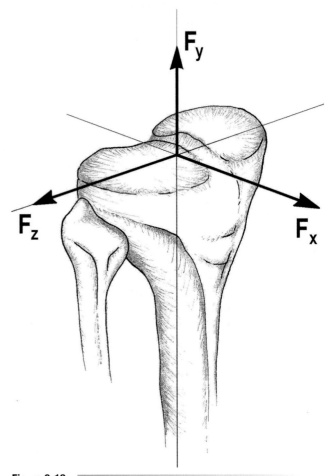

Figure 8-12

Isometric view of the proximal tibia showing orientation and direction of forces with respect to the long axis of the tibia. F_y is the tensile-compressive component, F_x is the anteroposterior component, and F_z is the mediolateral knee reaction force component.

issues raised previously (see section on torsion moments at the pedal and knee injuries), increased movement at the foot–pedal interface resulted in a reduction of knee loads during cycling. Although one might assume that loads at the shoe–pedal interface affect loads up the kinetic chain, differences in methods described in recent reports makes it difficult to come to a clear conclusion. A larger base of evidence, however, continues to be collected supporting the notion that foot movement is desirable. Changing pedal design, foot position, and levels of constraint at the pedal affect the magnitude, direction, and timing of almost all load components up the kinetic chain. The translatable message, then, is to critically evaluate the foot-pedal interface when personalizing the bike to the subject or patient.

Seat height and fore/aft position of the rider on the saddle and foot on the pedal affects knee loads, both in magnitude and timing[51] (Figure 8-13). A large body of evidence supports the hypothesis that changes in seat height can have a marked effect on the direction of the shear force component at the knee. These findings have direct relevance for the rehabilitation of ACL-deficient patients using a cycling task as part of their rehabilitation plan.

In an investigation of ACL-deficient patients, Furumizo[52] studied three patients and three control subjects riding between 70 and 90 rpm at a power output of 250 W on a stationary ergometer. Postoperative time at testing varied from 3 to 9 months. A standard approach in Newtonian mechanics was used to solve for the joint forces and moments correcting for the orientation of the shear component of the knee joint reaction force with an 8° posterior tilt of the tibial plateau. All three control subjects displayed an anteriorly directed shear force (positive values) at the knee during the first 135° of crank rotation, with two of the three subjects continuing this pattern up to at least 230° in the pedaling cycle. Patients who were ACL-deficient displayed essentially the same patterns (anteriorly directed shear forces until at least 135° in the cycle), but considerable differences among the subjects and between the involved and contralateral limbs was observed (Figure 8-14). Axial loads were not reported in this study, because the primary purpose was to study shear loads in ACL-deficient patients.

More recent studies support original contentions that there can be considerable asymmetry between the ACL-deficient limb and the intact limb in power output, creating a situation in which the intact limb "compensates" for the ACL-deficient limb during exercise (i.e., exercise designed to strengthen the ACL-deficient limb)[53,54] (Figure 8-15). Initial ROM therapy is critical to recovery, but great care and vigilance must be given to the portion of the rehabilitation plan in which the loads are increased to strengthen the limb but not further damage already injured tissues. As previously mentioned, the use of instrumented pedals with visual feedback has been used to identify cycling characteristics (e.g., pressure distribution,

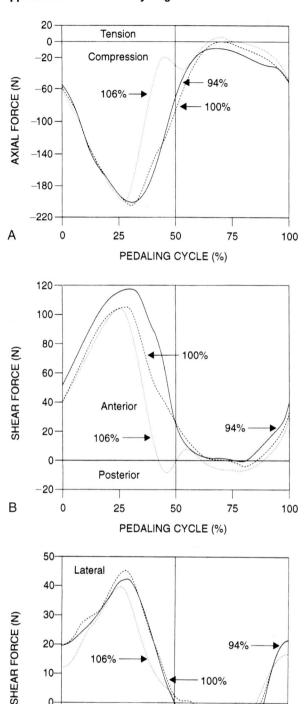

Figure 8-13

Knee joint reaction force components averaged for 150 pedal revolutions (ten subjects in five trials) at 200 W and 80 rpm for three seat height conditions: 94%, 100%, and 106% of leg length. **A,** The axial component along the shaft of the tibia. **B,** The anteroposterior shear force component. **C,** The medial/lateral shear force component. (From McCoy RW: *The effect of varying seat position on knee loads during cycling,* unpublished doctoral dissertation, University of Southern California Department of Exercise Science, 1989.)

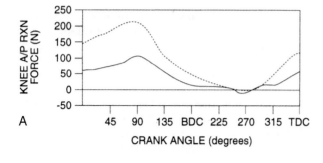

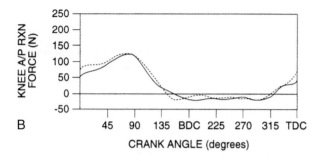

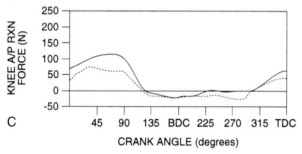

Figure 8-14

Anteroposterior knee joint reaction force profiles for three anterior cruciate ligament (ACL)–deficient patients. The *solid line* represents the ACL-deficient limb, and the *dashed line* represents the contralateral limb. (From Furumizo SH: *A biomechanical analysis of anterior/ posterior shear joint reaction forces in the ACL-deficient knee during stationary cycling,* unpublished master's thesis, UCLA Department of Kinesiology, 1991.)

orientation of the pedal reaction force) that are transferable to patient population to be used during the rehabilitation plan.

Information concerning calculated knee joint reaction force components, when combined with kinematic and electromyographic (EMG) data, indicates that cycling is an excellent form of rehabilitation for patients after ACL injury and surgical repair. Changing seat height, for example, changes the ROM in individual joints; changing shoe–pedal interface mechanics changes the orientation of joint reaction force vectors (i.e., changes ACL loading patterns); changing load modifies loads experienced by the different tissues (e.g., the ACL); and changing cadence modifies loading rates on muscle, ligaments, tendons, and bone.

Knowledge of these factors can assist in the design of an optimal rehabilitation program to enhance recovery from ACL injuries.

Muscle Moments

Muscle moments may be calculated for the cycling task using a linked segment model and equations of motion with kinematic, pedal reaction force, center of pressure, and anthropometry (i.e., mass and moment of inertia of each of the segments) data used as input. Zajac[25] used forward dynamics simulations in analyzing the cycling task and for the most part he and his colleagues focused their efforts on rehabilitation and neural control.

The vast majority of data reported in the literature has focused on moments calculated in the sagittal plane, in particular, the large hip and knee extensor moments, as the primary source of energy used to rotate the crank during propulsion. During recovery, flexor moments may act to unload the pedal (e.g., unload the pedal by pulling up on the pedal during the recovery phase), potentially minimizing resistance to the contralateral propulsive limb. Investigations using a force pedal system to evaluate lower extremity kinetics during cycling have produced a great deal of information on moment patterns during normal, steady-state cycling and recently on cycling mechanics during standing, climbing, and crank acceleration. These data have demonstrated, as first reported by Gregor[55] (Figure 8-16), that the moments at the hip, knee, and ankle have *fairly repeatable patterns,* despite changes in loading conditions, subject population, and bike setup. Magnitudes appear to increase in response to increased load, and timing features seem to be affected by cadence as well as during acceleration cycling. However, in almost all cases, the general patterns remain essentially the same.

As presented in Figure 8-16, the hip and knee perform very different actions during the propulsive phase of cycling (i.e., the hip consistently produces an extensor moment, while the knee produces an extensor and then flexor moment during the power phase). These observations are well documented in the literature.[56-60] Gregor and colleagues[56] for example, discussed the moment reversal at the knee during propulsion with reference to the paradoxical behavior of biarticular muscles, in that a two-joint muscle may act as an extensor of the joint of which it is a flexor.[61] Andrews[57] redefined "paradoxical" muscle action in that any explanation of two-joint muscle function in a kinetic analysis of the lower extremity may depend on the method of classification employed in the study. Van Ingen Schenau[62] concluded that the uniarticular muscles were "power producers" and the biarticular muscles were "power distributors" in the coordinated action of the lower extremity segments during the cycling task. More recently, Kuo[63] argued that any classification of muscles according to the joints they span could be

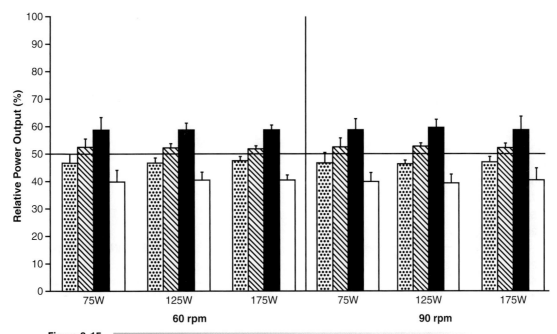

Figure 8-15

Mean percentage of power output (± standard deviation) that each limb contributed to the total power output during cycling at two cadences and three power outputs. Patterns indicate left leg control *(dots)*, right leg control *(diagonal lines)*, anterior cruciate ligament (ACL)–intact limbs *(black)*, and ACL-deficient limbs *(open)*. The horizontal line represents 50% contribution from each limb. (From Hunt MA, Sanderson DJ, Moffet H, Inglis JJ: Interlimb asymmetry in persons with and without an anterior cruciate ligament deficiency during stationary cycling, *Arch Phys Med Rehabil* 85:1475–1478, 2004.)

misleading. The manner and degree to which a muscle contributes to a task such as cycling ultimately depends on the redundant nature of the musculoskeletal system and the synergism of the muscles involved in responding to the specific task. Hence, in cycling, the integrated response of the entire lower extremity needs to be considered when meeting the imposed challenges (e.g., increased load) and not just the output of individual muscles and joints (see "Muscle Mechanics" section later in this chapter).

Moment patterns can be influenced to a limited degree by bike configuration. For example, Browning and colleagues[58] reported that the ankle muscle moment, although almost entirely plantar flexor throughout the pedaling cycle, increased in peak magnitude as seat height decreased. Seat height also affected the magnitude of peak knee moment (i.e., higher peak extensor magnitudes at lower seat heights and higher peak flexor magnitudes at higher seat heights), a finding also supported by McCoy[16] and McCoy and Gregor.[51]

Hip moments, although extensor for almost the entire cycle, can also be affected to some degree by changes in seat height. Greater variability was observed at the hip as opposed to the knee and ankle, and the magnitude of the hip moment tended to increase as seat height increased.[58]

Moments in the frontal plane have also been reported and appear to be affected as well by bike setup, rider position

with respect to the bike, cadence, and load. Because large frontal plane knee moments may result in injury and the bike is commonly employed in the rehabilitation of medial collateral ligament injuries, the greatest amount of data reported has focused on the knee.

For example, McCoy and Gregor[51] reported frontal plane moments at the knee beginning as a valgus moment at TDC, with initial values between 6 and 7 Nm (Newton-meters) across different seat height conditions and pedaling at a modest load[51] (Figure 8-17). Magnitudes increased and peaked near 90° of crank rotation at each seat height condition.[51] Ruby and colleagues[64] suggested that because external loads are applied to the foot during pedaling, variations in foot inversion and eversion may contribute to the loads transmitted to the knee, the potential orientation of these loads and, subsequently, to the potential for knee joint injury. A valgus moment is calculated at the knee during the power phase in response to a medially directed pedal reaction force whereas a varus moment is calculated during recovery in response to a laterally directed pedal reaction force (see Figure 8-6). Collectively, data from these two studies[51,64] suggest that if knee injuries result from varus and valgus loads, then lateral knee structures may be more vulnerable during the power phase, whereas medial knee structures may be more vulnerable during the recovery phase.

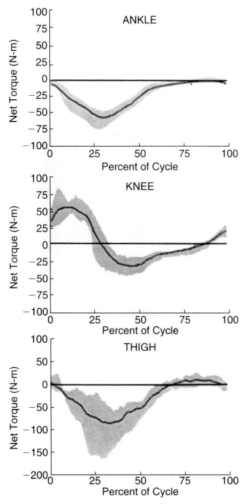

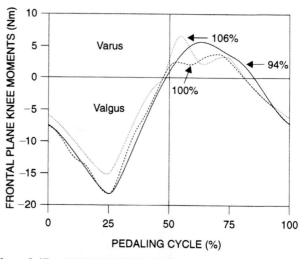

Figure 8-17

Knee moment patterns in the frontal plane averaged for 150 pedal revolutions (10 subjects in five trials) at 200 W and 80 rpm for three seat height conditions: 94%, 100%, and 106% of leg length. (From McCoy RW: *The effect of varying seat position on knee loads during cycling,* unpublished doctoral dissertation, University of Southern California Department of Exercise Science, 1989.)

Figure 8-16

Muscle moment patterns for the ankle, knee, and hip (thigh) during the pedaling cycle. Patterns represent the average of 25 pedaling cycles (five subjects in five trials) at approximately 260 W and 84 rpm. (From Gregor RJ, Cavanagh PR, LaFortune M: Knee flexor moments during propulsion in cycling—A creative solution to Lombardi's paradox, *J Biomech* 18:307–316, 1985.)

Mechanical Work and Power

Ultimately, the lower extremities are responsible for generating and transmitting power to the bicycle. Although this mechanical transmission involves elements on the bicycle (e.g., gear selection, crank length), the focus of this final section is on the human *"machine"* and how effectively it operates within the constraints imposed by the personally established bicycle geometry.

Mechanical work and power are biomechanical variables reported in the literature using two fundamentally different methods (i.e., the fractions approach and the sources approach)[65] that result in strikingly different results, sometimes a nine-fold difference. Combine this with the different methods of estimating caloric equivalencies to determine metabolic cost, and a situation exists in which almost all

measures of efficiency (i.e., output and input) have fundamental inaccuracies in either side of the divider. This section is limited to the general power profiles of each joint in the lower extremity that have been presented in the literature.[61] The reader is cautioned when evaluating literature on this topic to critically evaluate the methods used.

In an effort to address load sharing among the hip, knee, and ankle joints during cycling and the possibility of energy transfer between segments, Broker and Gregor[9] used a clipless pedal design to study the management of mechanical energy in the lower extremities of 12 elite cyclists. Power delivered to the bicycle was calculated from pedal reaction forces and kinematics at 200, 250, and 300W at 90, 100, and 110 rpm. Newtonian equations were used in a sagittal plane model of the right lower extremity to calculate joint powers (i.e., the product of the muscle moment and angular velocity for each joint) (Figure 8-18) and the hip joint force power (i.e., the product of the hip joint reaction force and velocity of the estimated center of rotation of the hip) for all riders at all conditions. It was suggested by Ericson and colleagues[66] and Van Ingen Schenau[62] that more than 80% of the energy generated at the joints in the lower extremity can be delivered to the pedals as useful energy to drive the bicycle. This is in contrast to the results of similar analyses on running and walking, in which the mechanical efficiency of the task is much lower. Broker and Gregor[9] reported the use of three energy models to study the issue of energy production and transmission during cycling. Considering that single-joint muscles such as the vastus lateralis may be energy producers, and biarticular muscles such as the hamstrings may be able to transfer, or distribute, energy from one joint to another, the

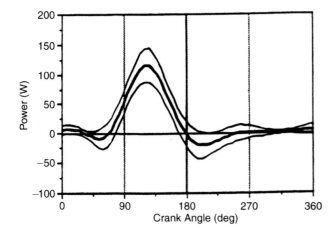

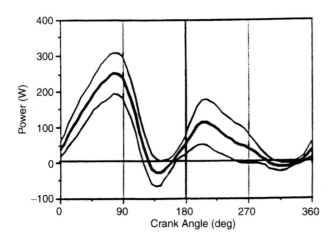

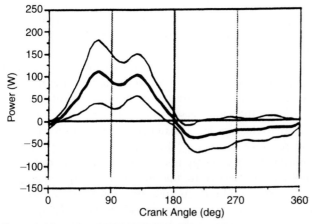

Figure 8-18

Mean (±1 standard deviation) patterns of muscle power (calculated as the product of the muscle moment and angular velocity for each joint) during the pedaling cycle for 12 subjects riding at 250 W and 100 rpm. The top trace is the ankle, the middle trace is the knee, and the bottom trace is the hip. (From Broker JP, Gregor RJ: Mechanical energy management in cycling: Source relations and energy expenditure, *Med Sci Sports Exerc* 26:64–74, 1994.)

three models ranged from one in which only hypothetical single-joint muscles acted (no transfer) to one in which multijoint muscles acted and permitted unlimited transfer. The latter model has no basis in anatomic function and was purely hypothetical. A third model apportioned joint muscle powers to single- and two-joint muscles and muscle groups in accordance with minimum energy expenditure criteria. During the cycling task, the third model—which has a sound basis in anatomic function and is consistent with reported EMG patterns in the lower extremity during cycling (see the "Muscle Mechanics" section)—resulted in the appropriate transfer of energy across two-joint muscles limiting the energy dissipated to nontransferable sources to less than 6 J per limb during cycling. The muscles primarily responsible for the appropriate transfer of energy were the hamstrings, modeled as a group, and the gastrocnemius muscle.

In summary, the cycling task presents a unique opportunity to the lower extremity through the use of appropriate two-joint muscle action to conserve mechanical energy and effectively deliver power to the bicycle. Unlike walking and running, the stretch-shorten cycle of muscle action during cycling is not necessary to reduce mechanical energy expenditure. Finally, knowledge of lower extremity kinetics at the level of intersegmental dynamics and load sharing among all segments (i.e., the thigh, leg, and foot) responsible for the coordination of energy delivery to the crank is important in the clinical setting in which certain areas of the lower extremity are impaired (see section on "Muscle Mechanics" later in this chapter). For example, how does the contralateral leg adapt to the loss of the involved leg when energizing the bicycle during rehabilitation in a unilateral stroke patient? How do the hip and knee adapt in a unilateral below-knee amputee (see section on "Challenged Populations")? How does each lower extremity adapt in a patient after ACL reconstruction? A great deal of work is needed in applying existing biomechanical analysis procedures to clinical problems.

Clinically Relevant Points: Cycling Kinetics

- Patients can learn to redistribute the forces applied through the foot–pedal interface to increase their effectiveness
- When using a bicycle, reactive loads are produced at all locations where the body comes in contact with the bike (e.g., pedals, seat, handlebars)
- In special populations (e.g., diabetics), special attention must be given to how the foot is secured to the pedal
- The advantage of most clipless pedals is that they allow normally occurring foot rotation; thereby reducing rotational forces acting at the knee as well as other lower-extremity joints
- Changes in seat height can affect the amount of shear force at the knee (i.e., higher seat, less shear) and joint range of motion. Hip load increases as seat height increases
- Changing resistance and cadence alters stress and loads on muscle, ligaments, and bone

Lower Extremity Muscle Mechanics

Muscle Activity Patterns in the Lower Extremity

To rehabilitate a patient following injury or appropriately condition an athlete, knowledge of muscle activation patterns (considering intensity, duration, and timing in the pedaling cycle) is paramount. Activation intensity in muscles used to energize the bicycle should be optimized at the proper time during the pedaling cycle with intensity minimized in muscles whose action may be counterproductive to propulsion or may stress healing tissue. Muscle recruitment patterns during cycling have been reported for major lower extremity muscles using both surface and fine-wire EMG.[10,67-70] Activity patterns are most commonly described relative to the angle of the crank and, in general, the greatest activity occurs in the leg that is in the propulsive phase between 0° (TDC) and 180° (BDC) of crank rotation, when almost all of the energy needed to drive the bicycle is imparted from the rider to the bicycle. During this time, the opposite-side limb is in the *recovery phase* between BDC and TDC. During this recovery phase, however, observable muscle activity in the flexors (e.g., hamstring muscles) has been shown to assist net forward propulsion of the crank and observable activity in the extensors (e.g., gluteus maximus) could act to oppose net forward propulsion of the bicycle.

Several reports published over the past twenty years have shown a generally repeatable pattern of muscle activation among the major flexors and extensors in the lower extremity during the pedaling cycle. Representative data published from 18 experienced cyclists riding at 90 rpm and 250 W on their own bicycles are shown in Figure 8-19.[10] During the propulsive phase, power is imparted to the bicycle via forceful hip and knee extension, with the gluteal (e.g., gluteus maximus) and quadriceps muscles heavily recruited during this time. For example, onset of activity for the gluteus maximus occurs just before TDC, with peak activity observed at approximately 55° of crank rotation. Both medial and lateral vasti muscles exhibit a rapid onset and cessation with relatively constant activity in between, while the rectus femoris demonstrates a more gradual rise and decline. Rectus femoris activity onset occurs before the vasti and declines earlier in the power phase, a pattern generally attributed to its biarticular function at the knee and hip. EMG activity ceases shortly after 90° in all three of these quadricep muscles, essentially ending their role as significant contributors to the work necessary to drive the bicycle.

Major ankle extensors are also active during the propulsive phase and, although not considered major power producers, these muscles are important in providing a stable link between the pedal, the foot, and the more proximal joints enabling the energy produced in lower extremity musculature to be transmitted to the pedal. Both the soleus and gastrocnemius are active before TDC. The soleus is recruited just prior to the gastrocnemius with peak activity occurring before 90° in the pedaling cycle. Peak gastrocnemius activity occurred at an average of 107° into the pedal cycle, declining gradually during recovery, and ending at approximately 270° of crank rotation. This phase shift in the gastrocnemius relative to soleus onset may be related to two factors. First, peak stretch occurs later in the gastrocnemius than in the soleus and in both muscles peak EMG activity occurs just prior to peak stretch. Second, a delay in peak gastrocnemius activation would support its contribution to the knee flexor moment consistently observed after 90° in the pedal cycle (see previous section on "Kinetics"). Force enhancement may occur as a result of the presence of active stretch prior to muscle shortening in both the gastrocnemius and the soleus muscles.[71] In addition, the anterior tibial muscle is active during the propulsive phase in many individuals, is coactive with the ankle extensors, and may be used to enhance ankle stability during propulsion and force transmission to the crank.

The hamstring muscles are also active during the power phase of cycling and most likely function to extend the hip during simultaneous knee extension. The semimembranosus and semitendinosus muscles are recruited after TDC, with peak activity occurring at or slightly after 90°, when activity in the gluteal and vasti muscles is rapidly declining. Peak activity in the semitendinous muscle occurs slightly after that of the semimembranous. Biceps femoris activity is the most variable of the hamstring group. In some individuals, timing of the biceps femoris is similar to that in the semimembranous and semitendinous muscles, while in others, the biceps femoris is already maximally active at TDC and declines throughout propulsion.[10] Finally, continued activation of the hamstrings for the remainder of the power phase contributes to the knee flexor moment, especially in the absence of any quadriceps activity after 90° of crank rotation.[54]

While the power phase is of primary interest because of high loads and energy transfer to the bicycle, the recovery phase has been given greater attention in recent years for essentially the same reason (i.e., effective transmission of energy to the bicycle). The fundamental question regarding the recovery phase is, "Does the recovery leg assist or impede effective energy transmission to the bicycle?" Formulating an answer to this question usually requires an understanding of the activation patterns of major lower extremity muscles during this period in the pedaling cycle. Ideally, net flexion of the lower extremity during recovery would require just enough energy to match the acceleration of the crank between 180° and 360° of the cycle. If this were the case, no counter-torques would be present to resist crank rotation or the efforts of the propulsive limb, and the recovery limb would not be "pulling up" on the crank, actively adding to crank rotation. In short, there should be a fine balance of active muscles during recovery to provide just enough energy to lift the limb. More energy would actively lift the

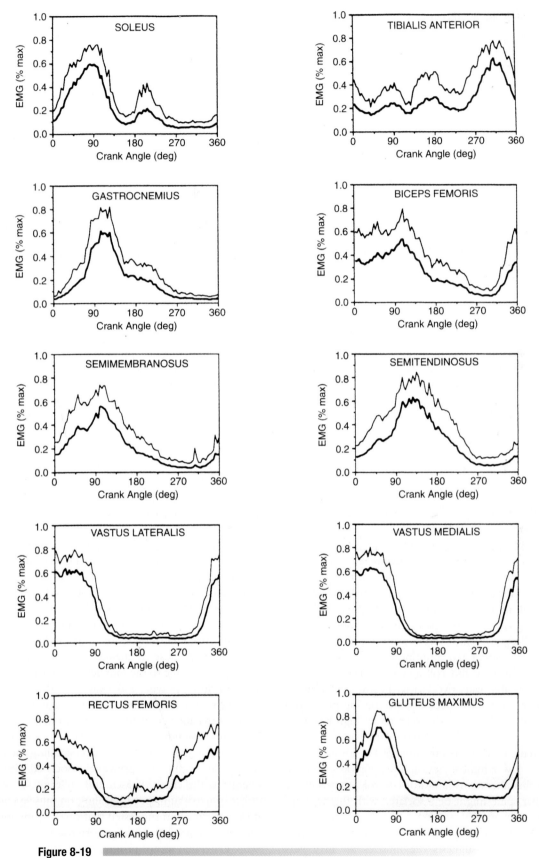

Figure 8-19

Mean patterns of muscle activation during the pedaling cycle for 10 muscles in the lower extremity. The *dark lower curve* is the average pattern from 15 pedaling cycles across 18 subjects (270 cycles), and the *lighter upper curve* is one standard deviation above the mean. Magnitudes are normalized to maximal activation. (From Ryan MM, Gregor RJ: EMG profiles of lower extremity muscles during cycling at constant workload and cadence, *J Electromyogr Kinesiol* 2:69–80, 1992.)

crank and possibly be an efficient contribution to crank rotation, while less energy (i.e., lower magnitude EMG) would be counterproductive and force the propulsive limb to provide excess energy to lift the recovery limb and drive the bicycle forward. In reviewing EMG patterns in the "recovery leg," the representative data in Figure 8-19 show that between 180° and 235° of the pedal cycle, the hamstrings and gastrocnemius, already active, provide a major component to flex the knee. Later in the recovery phase, between 235° and 360°, the tibialis anterior muscle acts to dorsiflex the ankle, and the rectus femoris (also a knee extensor) acts to flex the hip.

Although reports on single-joint hip flexor activity are few, Juker and colleagues[72] presented data on the activity patterns of the lumbar psoas, erector spinae, and three different layers of the abdominal wall muscles during five different styles of cycling. These data are difficult to obtain but valuable to an understanding of hip and low-back function during cycling, and an understanding of lower limb function during the "recovery" phase of the pedaling cycle. The five different stationary cycling positions presented by Juker and colleagues[72] included normal posture (slightly flexed), upright posture, a racing flexed posture, standing, and standing while sprinting. The general conclusion from this novel investigation was that position on the bike influenced the timing and magnitude of the muscles under study. During normal posture the psoas was active, at approximately 14% of maximum voluntary contraction (MVC), and was most active during recovery near TDC. Activity then increased to approximately 30% of MVC during a flexed posture and 60% of MVC during sprinting. Activity in the abdominal wall was very low, with almost no activity during standing and sprinting.

When discussing activity patterns in hip and pelvic muscles during cycling, it should be remembered that cyclists are known to be vulnerable to low back pain. Because of this, interest in the abdominal muscles, internal and external obliques, and in particular the erector spinae function during cycling has recently increased. Data presented by Juker and colleagues[72] show very low erector spinae activity except for the standing and sprinting postures when it was much higher. Burnett and colleagues[73] further suggested one of the possible causative factors in low back pain in cyclists was an overactive erector spinae during prolonged forward flexion and mechanical creep under high mechanical loads. Evaluating key stabilizers of the lumbar spine, they reported loss of co-contraction of the lower lumbar multifidus as lower lumbar flexion and rotation increased, suggesting that alterations in motor control patterns in the lower lumbar spine might be associated with the development of low back pain in cyclists.

Although most of the evidence on muscle activity patterns during cycling suggests the muscles act in a very repeatable manner, data presented by Juker and colleagues[72] suggest these patterns, although generally robust under steady-state conditions, are *changeable* and can be affected by, for example, changes in body position with respect to the bicycle (i.e., "bike fit," cadence, load, and cycling ability). These variables are somewhat interdependent, and the following text is devoted to recent work describing how and under what conditions these patterns may change.

Data from Chapman and colleagues[74] suggest EMG patterns may differ between novice and highly skilled cyclists, and that changes in cadence can affect certain aspects of muscle activation. Fine-wire electrodes were placed in the tibialis anterior, tibialis posterior, peroneus longus, lateral gastrocnemius, and soleus muscles. Using their own bicycles on a magnetically loaded trainer, four ranges of cadence were employed: 55 to 60 rpm, 75 to 80 rpm, 90 to 95 rpm, and each cyclist's own preferred cadence. Novice riders displayed greater variability in their EMG, greater co-activation, and greater EMG magnitudes between the primary bursts of activity within each pedaling cycle. Peak EMG increased with cadence, but lower EMG magnitude was observed at the preferred cadence in all 19 subjects. EMG timing was affected by cadence in novice riders, but not in the elite riders, suggesting some level of neuromuscular adaptation resulting from repeated performance in the elite riders.

Pursuing the effects of cadence on the performance of specific muscles, Sanderson and colleagues[12] reported interesting differences in the way the gastrocnemius and soleus muscles responded to changes in cadence from 50 rpm to 110 rpm. It seems the soleus peak EMG is not affected by cadence, but at the highest cadence of 110 rpm a second smaller peak appeared during early recovery. In contrast, the gastrocnemius muscle increased dramatically as cadence increased and, although there was a second smaller peak in early recovery at lower cadences, this was not observed at the higher cadences. The authors attributed these differences in part to the higher shortening velocities experienced by the gastrocnemius relative to the soleus as cadence increased. This hypothesis was supported by the findings of Wakeling and colleagues[75] showing higher muscle fascicle strains in the gastrocnemius as pedaling cadence increased. In short, although muscles seem to modify their activation patterns in response to changes in cadence, these changes seem to be specific to the muscles themselves with regard to articulation, fiber type, and location in the limb.

Finally, a series of papers have been published using forward dynamic simulation with two major goals being a better understanding of the role played by different muscles in energizing the bicycle and understanding the fundamental muscle coordination principles associated with delivering energy to the crank. Raasch and colleagues,[76] studied the effect of maximum speed pedaling on muscle coordination during cycling and suggested that certain functional muscle groups exhibited alternating patterns representing a centrally generated motor program. The value of reducing the many different muscles in the lower extremity to apparently functional groups lies in their possible relationships to central commands from the nervous system. Maximum speed pedaling was a clearly defined goal, but the theory behind the study is applicable to a variety of circumstances and populations using cycling for exercise and rehabilitation. It seems the uniarticular extensors are important in the down-stroke or power phase and uniarticular flexors in the upstroke or recovery phase. It was reported that dorsiflexors and the rectus femoris were important in the transition through TDC and that the plantar flexors and hamstrings were important in the transition through BDC. Cadence dictates the role certain muscles play in controlling the lower extremities during the cycling task. And although patterns, in general, are fairly robust, timing of muscle activation, even at a constant resistance, appears to be affected by cadence.

Body position is an important consideration that is related to the type of bicycle used (e.g., upright versus recumbent) and the position the rider assumes on the bike. Controlled studies conducted in the laboratory use a range of cycling positions (e.g., upright to an advanced aerodynamic position), similar to the ones used by elite competitors during road and track races. Addressing the issue of upper body position and its potential effect on the rider's performance, Savelberg and colleagues[77] manipulated trunk angle during ergometer cycling and, directing their attention to recumbent cycling, found a dramatic effect of trunk inclination on muscle activity patterns. In a position extended 20° back from an upright trunk position, peak EMG increased in seven of the eight muscles studied. Peak activity only decreased in the gluteus maximus. Gluteus maximus activity, however, did increase in a position 20° forward, more flexed, of the neutral upright trunk position. In opposition to these general findings Chapman and colleagues[78] suggested that upper body position had *no substantial effect* on muscle recruitment (i.e., the main bursts of muscle activity) during cycling but did report greater co-activation and poor EMG modulation (i.e., greater magnitude of EMG) between the primary bursts of EMG in an aerodynamic riding position among novice and elite triathletes. This finding was not present in elite cyclists and supports their contention that elite cyclists have better control over muscle recruitment as a consequence of repeated training performances.

Muscle-Tendon Unit Length and Velocity Measurements

Changes in limb kinematics will naturally affect the length-tension and force-velocity relationship of separate muscle-tendon units (MTUs), as well as the performance of muscle groups (e.g., quadriceps and hamstrings). Therefore, knowledge of muscle length, velocity, previous history (e.g., muscle stretch), muscle architecture, and activation—all variables that affect the muscle's ability to produce force—is important. ROM information is also significant when applied to a situation in which the MTU sustains an injury, because it is important to know what type of length changes

(both active and passive) the rehabilitation program imposes. Following acute injuries, rehabilitation should begin with exercises that minimize muscle length changes, especially in active muscle, because muscle length changes may increase tension on healing structures. Cycling can be an especially gentle exercise following injuries that might occur to two-joint muscles of the lower extremity (e.g., hamstrings, gastrocnemius, and rectus femoris). Angular changes in adjacent joints have an opposing effect on muscle length, for example (increasing versus decreasing), resulting in minimal length change in these two-joint muscles. During cycling, hip extension acts to decrease hamstring length, while knee extension acts to increase it during the propulsive phase. During the recovery phase, hip flexion acts to increase hamstring length, while flexion at the knee acts to decrease it.

Using hip, knee, and ankle joint angular kinematics and lower-extremity anatomy, estimates of length changes for all major lower-extremity MTUs have been developed.[18] Results indicate that changes in seat height have a marked effect on muscle-length patterns and further imply that as seat height increases, MTU shortening and lengthening velocities increase. In addition, for all cases, cyclic patterns of lengthening and subsequent shortening appear in each muscle group during a complete pedaling cycle.

Rugg and Gregor[3] reported that changes in seat height appear to affect the soleus more than the gastrocnemius MTUs. These data were obtained at a constant cadence using seat height conditions of 96% to 108% of pubic symphysis height.[3] The gastrocnemius displays essentially the same pattern at each seat height condition, lengthening markedly during the first 90° of crank rotation (approximately 1.5 cm), then shortening approximately 2 cm, only to lengthen again prior to TDC. In contrast, the soleus MTU displays very different patterns at the separate seat height conditions, lengthening slightly during the early stages of propulsion and then markedly shortening as the crank approaches BDC. The MTU then lengthens again during the second half of the pedaling cycle (180° to 360°). Although the magnitude of initial lengthening is approximately the same for each seat height, the magnitude of shortening dramatically increases from less than 1 cm at the 96% condition to approximately 2.5 cm at the 108% condition. Shortening velocities of the MTU increased as well.

Sanderson and colleagues[12] focused on the effects of cadence on MTU lengths, velocities, and EMG in the gastrocnemius and soleus muscles. These data showed a differential response to changes in cadence between the gastrocnemius and soleus and supported the data of Gregor and colleagues[71,79] and Marsh and Martin.[80] EMG, MTU length, and MTU velocity patterns are different between the two muscles in response to changes in cadence, suggesting the soleus muscle was more involved in generating initial propulsive forces, while the gastrocnemius shifted in phase to peak later in the cycle and made a more prolonged contribution to the ankle extensors in delivering force to the pedal. Data showing the differential response of these two muscles highlighting their individual contributions to delivering energy to the crank at different cadences are presented in Figures 8-20 and 8-21. Sanderson and colleagues[12] continued to focus on differences between the gastrocnemius and soleus manipulating seat height (i.e., a preferred height), 10% below this height and 5% above this height at a constant cadence of 80 rpm at 200 W. Their data suggested recruitment of the soleus to be minimally affected and recruitment of the gastrocnemius to be dramatically affected by seat height changes. MTU lengths were differentially affected and supported the notion that the ranges of MTU length and velocity of the biarticular gastrocnemius were affected by seat height changes as the knee joint angle increased. The single-joint soleus displayed different results, generating discussion on the effects of seat height changes on the force-length and force-velocity properties of the two muscles. These together with different activation patterns support previous notions on why these two muscles make different contributions to propulsion in cycling.

Finally, Wakeling and colleagues[75] investigated muscle recruitment in the gastrocnemius and soleus muscles and its response to changes in the mechanics of muscle contraction. Length and velocity changes in muscle fascicles were quantified using ultrasonography, and MTU length and velocity changes were quantified using a kinematic model.[12,71] EMG patterns were sampled using surface EMG in the soleus, medial, and lateral gastrocnemius. The general conclusions, again focusing on the differential aspects of these two muscles, was that the soleus muscle was used more in the high force–low velocity contractions while the gastrocnemius was used more in the higher velocity contractions. Cadence was varied at a constant load and load was varied at a constant cadence in six male cyclists. Results suggested the selective recruitment of faster motor units in the medial gastrocnemius occurred in response to increasing fascicle strain rates. Collectively, these findings support the fact that faster fibers are used in faster tasks (e.g., higher cadences), and the motor unit recruitment during cycling matches the contractile properties of the fibers to the mechanical demands of the task.

Clinically Relevant Points

- Low back pain in cyclists is due to altered motor control patterns. During prolonged lumbar flexion, overactive erector spinae muscles or a loss of co-activation of the multifundus muscles has been reported for a subset of cyclists and may contribute to low back pain
- Muscle activation patterns are altered with changes in cadence
- Increasing seat height increases shortening and lengthening velocities of individual muscle fibers and the whole muscle-tendon unit

---

Common Cycling Injuries

The injuries associated with road cycling are proportional to the increased popularity of the sport over the past few decades. Serious or fatal injuries may result from collisions and falls. Helmets and other safety features are essential to minimize trauma. Rehabilitation efforts are focused on overuse injuries affecting the musculoskeletal system. Although the incidence and severity are low compared with sports that are associated with greater limb loads, injuries can be painful and often require medical treatment. Most overuse injuries result from a bike that is not properly fit to the rider. Because each pedal revolution is nearly identical and may be repeated hundreds or thousands of times during each training session, minor alignment problems without adequate recovery time may lead to overuse injuries. Consequently, alterations made to the bicycle in an effort to improve performance must be made with caution.

Clinical Point

In the clinical setting, proper adjustments must be made to the stationary bicycle to provide the range of motion necessary to stress all muscles and surrounding connective tissue structures within appropriate limits (i.e., to prevent any further damage to injured tissues targeted by the rehabilitation program), yet "push the envelope" to regain normal range of motion.

Standardized commercial systems, used by most bike dealers, provide guidelines for proper alignment under typical road riding conditions. Additional factors to consider include individual pedaling technique, structural variations among cyclists, and anatomic asymmetry in the same cyclist. These factors may necessitate individual variations in bike setup and selective modifications of equipment components. To obtain a proper fit, a tube and stem combination should consider both torso and leg length. Adjustments should be made to the frame, including the seat height, seat fore and aft position, handlebar height, pedal type, crank length, and selection of gears. To maximize power production while minimizing the risk of knee injury, a seat height should be chosen that results in a knee angle of between 25° and 35° of flexion at BDC.[81]

Certain training regimens may make the rider more vulnerable to overuse injuries. Regimens that incorporate extensive hill climbing can change the bike–rider interface and may necessitate a re-evaluation of bike adjustments. Also, training to the point of fatigue has been shown to have a negative effect on muscle activation patterns and joint kinematics.[14] As with other types of overuse injuries, excessive training is a common factor; therefore, rest and a gradual increase in cycling intensity is essential to prevent the injury from becoming a chronic condition.

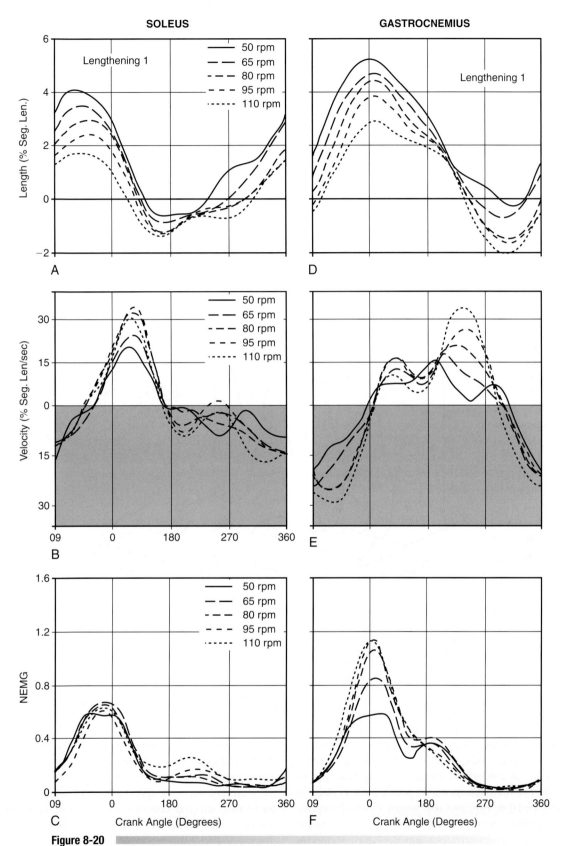

Figure 8-20

Mean length, velocity, and electromyogram (EMG) for the soleus muscle *(left panel)* and the gastrocnemius muscle *(right panel)*. Panels **A** and **D** are length change, **B** and **E** are muscle velocity, and **C** and **F** are the normalized EMG data. In panels *B* and *E* the shaded portion indicates lengthening velocity. (From Sanderson DJ, Martin PE, Honeyman G, Keefer J: Gastrocnemius and soleus muscle length, velocity, and EMG responses to changes in pedaling cadence, *J Electromyogr Kinesiol* 16:642–649, 2006.)

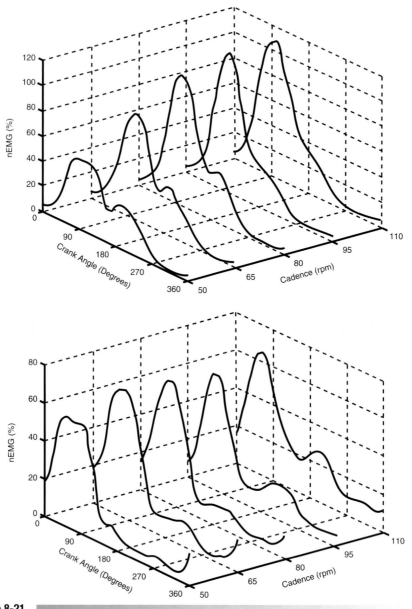

Figure 8-21

Mean normalized electromyographic data plotted in a three-dimensional format to illustrate the appearance of a second bump in soleus *(bottom panel)* and the simultaneous disappearance of the second bump in the gastrocnemius *(top panel)*. (From Sanderson DJ, Martin PE, Honeyman G, Keefer J: Gastrocnemius and soleus muscle length, velocity, and EMG responses to changes in pedaling cadence, *J Electromyogr Kinesiol* 16:642–649, 2006.)

Overuse injuries caused by cycling may affect the foot and ankle, knee, hip, back, or neck. The incidence of overuse injuries to the ankle–foot complex is usually related to the interface between the foot and pedal. Factors such as shoe design, pedal design, and seat height should be examined if discomfort occurs. Shoe design is an important factor and must incorporate foot support and comfort as well as effective transmission of force.[47] Shoes should be sufficiently stiff to distribute pressure, but flexible enough to permit natural foot motion.

The knee is the most common site for sports-related injuries, and cycling is no exception. A recent prospective study examined the number of knee injuries per 1000 hours of exposure across a spectrum of physical activities for a randomly selected cohort (n = 3633).[82] The number of knee injuries caused by cycling as a commuting activity was quite low (0.1), but increased considerably when performed as a recreation or competitive sport activity (0.43). This incidence was similar to the average found for all other recreation or competitive sport activities (0.44), but was considerably lower than that reported for team sports and ball games (1.17). Overuse injuries to the knee during cycling typically result from improper mechanics and the accumulation of insult through repetitive loading. The primary factor influencing knee joint dynamics and subsequent tissue strain is the "fit" between the rider and bicycle. In a report by Holmes and colleagues,[83] cyclists with complaints of chronic knee pain were evaluated over a 5-year period. They found that 64% of the patients in the professional and advanced amateur categories had anterior knee pain, specifically chondromalacia patella and patellar tendonitis, and attributed this problem to intense training loads and high mileage. In a cycling knee pain survey conducted for the U.S. Olympic Committee at the University of California–Los Angeles Biomechanics Laboratory,[48] overuse injuries and shoe- and pedal-type data were collected from 168 experienced racers. Of these respondents, 60% reported anterior knee pain, especially retropatellar pain, followed by lateral and medial knee pain.

Overuse injuries at the hip joint are rare and consequently not well documented in the literature. Mellion[84] stated that trochanteric bursitis and iliopsoas tendonitis can occur when the seat is set too high and may be associated with a bike frame that is too large. It is the authors' experience that very few experienced cyclists are set up with excessively high seat positions for extended periods. This may explain why chronic hip problems are not a major complaint among competitive cyclists.

Neck and back pain are more common problems among cyclists and can be quite debilitating. Because cyclists often maintain the same trunk and neck position for long durations, slight changes in handlebar position may be problematic. Lowering handlebar height to maximize aerodynamic performance can result in excessive neck hyperextension or lumbar lordosis and injury. (See section on Muscle Activity Patterns.) Unilateral neck pain may result from neck positioning while looking in rear view mirrors.[84] Pruitt and Matheny[81] consider leg length inequities to be a common cause of low back pain. They recommend adding shims to the cleat on the short side for inequities as small as 3 mm when back pain is present.

Clinically Relevant Points

- Proper fit of a bicycle includes considering torso and leg length, seat height, seat fore and aft position, handlebar height, pedal type, crank length, shoe design, and gear selection
- For maximum power production, the seat height should result in a knee angle between 25 degrees and 35 degrees of flexion at bottom dead center
- The knee is the most common site for overuse injury in cycling

Table 8-1 lists common cycling injuries along with their predisposing factors and adjustments.[81,84,85]

Cycling in Challenged Populations
Cycling in Persons with Amputation

Cycling has been shown as a viable method to maintain or increase cardiovascular fitness for persons with an amputation.[86] Cycling also provides a medium for locomotion and exercise without exposing either limb to the large impact forces associated with walking or running.[87] Performance of a cyclist with an amputation is different in that the prosthesis introduces an additional mechanical interface that the cyclist must use to effectively apply and direct forces to propel the bicycle. These challenges are different, depending on whether the cyclist has an upper or lower limb amputation, the level of amputation, and secondary complications following the amputation.

Clinically Relevant Points

- Cyclists with a lower limb amputation depend more on their sound limb for work production
- Dynamic response–type prosthetic feet designed for walking are acceptable for low-power outputs used in recreational cycling, but do not have sufficient stiffness for higher outputs used by competitive cyclists
- Joint deformities and excessive joint motion in the frontal and transverse planes may increase stress on the hip and knee joints in individuals with cerebral palsy

A person with an upper-extremity amputation has compromised handlebar control and upper-body support. Thus the design of the prosthesis should reflect a way to help stabilize the torso while allowing for enhanced steering control. The bicycle may be modified to allow some form of attachment and quick disconnect of the prosthesis from the handlebar. The brake and shifting controls can be relocated to the sound limb assuming it has the strength and dexterity to operate the controls.[88] A bilateral upper-extremity involvement imposes additional challenges and may require a bicycle with a foot actuated "coaster" brake and a single speed.

Lower extremity amputation are the most common and pose an interesting challenge to persons engaged in a cycling task.[89] For example, a unilateral transtibial amputee has lost the structure of the ankle joint as well as control and proprioceptive information from that joint and the surrounding musculature. These amputees must now interact with their environment through a prosthetic limb on one side and an intact limb on the other. The obvious structural asymmetries between limbs translate to asymmetries in generating torque to turn the crank.[90] Despite these asymmetries, an unpublished study involving three cyclists with unilateral transtibial amputation (CTA) showed that the metabolic efficiency was the same as 10 control subjects.[91] This may be because the

Table 8-1
Common Cycling Injuries[81,84,85]

Problem	Predisposing Factors	Adjustments
Metatarsalgia	Poor foot position Tight or flat-bottom shoes Unsupported foot varus Small pedals Pes cavus, pes planus Equinus deformity	Adjust foot and cleat position Soft-soled shoes or soft insert Metatarsal pad Pedals with a larger platform Wedges to level foot and distribute pressure Reduce resistance = increase cadence
Foot paresthesia	Tight shoes	Loosen straps Clipless pedals
Achilles tendonitis	Cleat too far forward Low saddle Excessive pronation Tight Achilles tendon	Move both cleats back an equal amount Raise saddle Orthotics or taping to correct pronation Stretching
Medial tibial stress syndrome (shin splints)	Excessive foot pronation Increase in training intensity	Orthotics or wedges to reduce pronation
Patellofemoral pain syndrome	High resistance = low cadence or hill riding in high gear High or lateral patella Weak vastus medialis Tight knee musculature Large quadriceps angle Femoral anteversion External tibial torsion Hyperpronated feet with hindfoot valgus	Raise saddle or move aft Lower gears Patellofemoral taping or bracing Orthoses or wedges to reduce pronation Stretching
Patellar tendonitis	Internal tibial rotation Knee valgus alignment Pronation	Adjust cleat position Raise saddle or move aft Wedges or orthotics
Pes anserine bursitis	Tight hamstrings High saddle Wide stance	Hamstring stretching Lower saddle Adjust pedals to a more narrow stance
Thickened medial knee plica	Valgus knee alignment Internal tibia rotation Foot hyperpronation Low saddle	Adjust cleat position to compensate for alignment problems Orthoses or wedges to reduce pronation
Iliotibial band syndrome	High saddle Tight iliotibial band or gluteus maximus Varus knee alignment Internal tibial rotation Excessive pronation	Lower saddle Move seat forward Increase trunk extension, adjust handlebars Position cleats to allow a wider stance Orthoses or wedges to reduce pronation Iliotibial band and gluteus maximus stretching
Biceps tendonitis Popliteus tendonitis	High saddle Varus knee alignment	Lower saddle
Trochanteric bursitis	High saddle Frame is too large	Lower saddle Smaller frame
Iliopsoas tendonitis	Tight hip flexors High saddle	Stretching for hip flexors Lower saddle
Low back pain	Unequal leg length: actual or functional Weak trunk musculature Low handlebars	Add a shim to the cleat on the short side Move cleat forward for the shorter leg Strengthening and stretching exercises Change position frequently by standing up
Neck pain	Low handlebars Neck hyperextension	Raise handle bars or install longer stem Turn head to the side when looking ahead Adjust helmet mirror to enhance rear view

sound limb was compensating for the amputated limb enough to maintain the same output so that, despite the asymmetry, metabolic efficiency was maintained.

The cycling task provides an excellent method to study asymmetries between limbs because the cranks provide a mechanical coupling between limbs. This coupling holds each limb 180° out of phase while allowing energy from one limb to transfer to the other (presumably deficient) limb. When one limb compensates for the other, an asymmetry develops between the two limbs. Asymmetry between the limbs can be quantified from a force or work perspective and each of these measures tell a slightly different story. Asymmetry in the magnitude of force production is related to geometric (i.e., leg length), inertial, and strength differences between limbs.[92] Work asymmetry combines not just the force magnitude (and thus force asymmetries) but also the direction of those forces to turn the cranks and produce work.[92] Therefore, it is affected by everything related to force production but also everything related to how the body may manipulate the direction of that force. One goal of the neuromuscular system is to generate and direct forces appropriately to turn the crank. If one limb has not only lost the ability to generate forces but also direct those forces, a change within the motor control strategy should occur to compensate for this. Factors that can account for a change in motor control strategy are differences in muscle properties, difficulty in sensorimotor integration, and poor coordination between limbs. Work asymmetries have been well documented in the intact population and are generally low (i.e., less than 10%),[92-94] whereas pedaling asymmetries within CTAs have been documented as higher than the intact population (i.e., approximately 30%).[90,95] Within these cyclists, the sound limb becomes dominant and work asymmetries are three times greater than force asymmetries. These results indicate that strength imbalances documented with unilateral transtibial amputees do not fully explain the work asymmetries between limbs, thus indicating a change in the motor control strategy.[96] More research is necessary to fully understand the underlying causes of the increase in work asymmetries so that better rehabilitation strategies may be developed.

Asymmetries are quantified by comparing forces developed at the foot–pedal interface of each limb.[92] Some commercial power measuring devices claim to quantify asymmetries by measuring the total power output of both limbs. These systems are measuring the sum of both limbs and not each limb individually as is done by placing load cells within each pedal.[97] The clinician should use caution interpreting asymmetry or power fraction data gathered using these commercially available power measuring system.[97]

CTA cycling performance is also influenced by the stiffness of the prosthetic foot. Flexible or dynamic response–type prosthetic feet are designed for walking to deflect and store energy at initial contact, and then decompress and release that energy at toe-off. The demands of cycling are different than walking and use of these feet in cycling may not be the best solution. During cycling, lower limb muscles generate much of the energy necessary to turn the cranks.[98] A lot of this energy is produced during the power phase and then declines during the bottom of the pedal stroke (see Figure 8-18). When a flexible prosthetic foot is used for cycling, some of the energy produced during the power phase is absorbed and stored in the prosthetic foot, only to be returned ineffectively at the bottom of the pedal stroke. This removes energy from the cyclist–pedal system and requires input of additional energy from the sound limb to compensate. The result is a larger dependence on the sound limb and increases in work asymmetries compared with a rigid prosthetic foot.[90] However, the vertical forces in cycling increase with power output[87] and commercially available prosthetic feet are generally stiff enough at lower outputs seen by recreational cyclists. Dynamic response–type prosthetic feet designed for walking are acceptable for low-power outputs used in recreational cycling, but do not have sufficient stiffness for higher outputs used by competitive cyclists.[99]

Muscle coordination is also altered within the CTAs' gastrocnemius.[100] An amputation through the tibia results in the alteration of the gastrocnemius from a two-joint knee flexor/ankle extensor to a single-joint knee flexor. The other, more proximal muscles have not been surgically affected by the amputation and retain their original bony attachment points. Questions about neuromuscular adaptation following a change in muscle function were investigated in a group of six CTAs. Measurements were taken using surface EMG over the gastrocnemius, rectus femoris, biceps femoris, and vastus medialis bilaterally. The results indicated a shift in muscle activation within three of the six CTAs to a later period of the crank cycle (Figure 8-22) when a knee flexion moment is present. This new activation pattern is more appropriate for a single-joint knee flexor and reflects neuromuscular adaptation of the gastrocnemius to its new functional role following amputation.[100] However, data could only be obtained in three of the six CTAs studied. Problems with signal artifact from the electrodes hitting the prosthetic socket caused problems in one subject, and no signal could be gathered in the other two subjects. It is not clear why no signal was collected from these CTAs, but it could be related to excessive scarring of the residual limb and presumably the muscle underneath the skin or possible detachment of the muscle's distal end following surgery. More research needs to be done to determine what factors affect this neuromuscular adaptation and if this also occurs with transfemoral amputees.

Cycling Interventions for Individuals with Cerebral Palsy

The importance of strength and cardiorespiratory exercise to improve and maintain general health in the general population is well known. Individuals with cerebral palsy (CP) have difficulty performing fitness programs because of balance, strength, and motor control deficits. In addition, there are

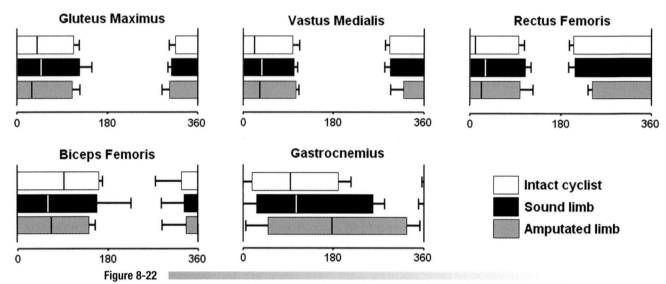

Figure 8-22

Onset, offset, and peak muscle activity for five muscles in the lower limb for intact cyclists *(white)*, the sound limb *(black)*, and amputated limb *(grey)* of cyclist with unilateral transtibial amputation. Peak activation is indicated by a vertical line within the bar. Note the shift in activation of the amputated gastrocnemius muscle.

barriers to accessing equipment and facilities. The promotion of fitness interventions for this population has been a recent focus of the Pediatric Section of the American Physical Therapy Association.[101] Cycling is an excellent exercise mode because there are minimal requirements for balance and coordination. With modifications, both overground and stationary cycles are options. In addition to physiological benefits, road cycling using adapted bicycles or tricycles is a form of mobility and provides opportunities for participation in community recreation and sports programs. Cycling has been recommended as an appropriate exercise for individuals with CP;[102] however, therapeutic evidence is limited.

Available evidence indicates that children with CP can successfully pedal a stationary bicycle, although physical assistance may be required.[103] Assistance may be required initially for forward pedal progression at TDC, prevention of knee hyperextension during recumbent cycling and to prevent excessive hip motion.[104] Recumbent stationary cycling kinematics, EMG, and pedal forces were described for 10 adolescents with CP at 30 and 60 rpm.[105] The foot was positioned on the pedal to accommodate limb deformities and minimize hip and knee movement out of the sagittal plane. Despite this modification, excessive joint excursions were observed in children with CP in the frontal and transverse planes. Greater peak hip flexion, knee extension, and dorsiflexion were found. As previously outlined in this chapter, these anatomic deviations are predisposing factors that contribute to chronic overuse injuries; particularly at the knee joint. Differences in muscle activation patterns were observed. Compared with adolescents without disability, excessive co-activation was found, which was greater at 60 rpm (Figure 8-23). Additional research revealed an increased duration of negative (pulling up) as opposed to positive pedal forces for adolescents with CP.[106]

Less information is available about responses to training protocols. Children with CP exhibiting a wide range of disability were able to improve oxygen uptake, at a given heart rate HR, following an intervention regimen emphasizing stationary cycling.[107,108] In addition, six adolescents with mild CP improved their physical endurance during cycling, as evidenced by VO_2 at the anaerobic threshold, following the first 3 months of a stationary cycling intervention.[109] Benefits also have been reported for children with more severe physical disability. Following a 6-week intervention using an adapted stationary bicycle, eleven nonambulatory adolescents with CP improved their gross motor function (p = .01).[110] A randomized control trial investigating a cycling intervention for children with spastic diplegia was recently completed.[111] Sixty-four children were randomized to either Cycling or Control (no-cycling) groups. This 12-week, 30 session cycling intervention focused on both lower extremity strengthening and cardiorespiratory training. While many children required physical assistance to cycle at the beginning of the program, all became independent with practice. While a significant difference in outcome measures was not found between the two groups, significant baseline to post-intervention improvements were found within the cycling group for gross motor function, walking and running endurance and a subset of isokinetic knee extensor and flexor moments (p < 0.05). Considerable intra-subject variability in performance was observed contributing to this result. Following the intervention, participants were provided with an adapted bicycle and their level of participation and enjoyment is currently being assessed. In summary, cycling is a safe and effective exercise for individuals with CP that promotes muscular strength and cardiorespiratory endurance. More research is needed to examine the potential for long-term health benefits and the prevention of secondary conditions in this population.

Percentage of Co-contraction

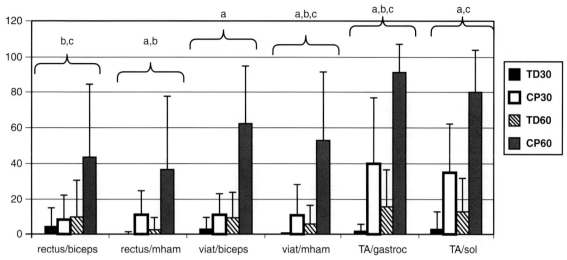

Figure 8-23

Percentage (mean and standard deviation) of the cycling revolution in which co-contraction occurred for each agonist and antagonist pairing around the left knee and ankle for each subject. Subjects with cerebral palsy had increased co-contraction compared with the subjects with typical development (TD), and all subjects displayed increased co-contraction when cycling at 60 rpm compared with 30 rpm. *Rectus,* Rectus femoris muscle; *biceps,* biceps femoris muscle; *vlat,* vastus lateralis muscle; *mham,* medial hamstring muscle; *TA,* anterior tibialis muscle; *gastroc,* gastrocnemius muscle; *sol,* soleus muscle. *a,* Significant main effect of group. *b,* Significant main effect of cadence. *c,* Interaction of group and cadence. Significance defined as *p* < .004 caused by 12 agonist and antagonist pairings being studied (6 per side). *TD30,* Subjects typically developing TD at cadence of 30 rpm; *CP30,* subjects with cerebral palsy (CP) at cadence of 30 rpm, *TD60,* subjects TD at cadence of 60 rpm; *CP60,* subjects with CP at cadence of 60 rpm. (From Johnston TE, Barr AE, Lee SCK: Biomechanics of submaximal recumbent cycling in adolescents with and without cerebral palsy, *Phys Ther* 87:572–585, 2007.)

Conclusion

The cycling task is widely used in the fields of exercise and rehabilitation science primarily because it offers an intervention that can be controlled by the user. Just as elite competitive cyclists match the bicycle to their specific morphological needs and strengths, the clinician, exercise specialist, and physical therapist must "match" the bicycle to the rider or patient to meet the specific objectives of each selected intervention. The rider's physical interface with the bicycle (e.g., "bike fit"), as well as the resistance (i.e., load) can be regulated by the clinician or exercise specialist to selectively meet needs related to, for example, cardiorespiratory exercise, strength training, rehabilitation of the knee post ACL repair or proprioceptive input resulting from the cyclic nature of the task. The objective of this chapter is to convey the idea that cycling is a very useful task with wide-ranging applications in exercise and rehabilitation. The kinematics and kinetics of the task from the level of the muscle fiber to the whole lower extremity have been presented and applications to individuals with special needs discussed. The clinician and exercise specialist can use this information to continue to develop unique applications of this task to improve human performance.

References

1. Gregor RJ, Broker JP, Ryan MM: The biomechanics of cycling, *Exerc Sport Sci Rev* 19:127–169, 1991.
2. Faria E, Cavanagh PR: *The physiology and biomechanics of cycling,* ACSM Series, New York, 1978, John Wiley & Sons.
3. Rugg SG, Gregor RJ: The effect of seat height on muscle lengths, velocities and moment arm lengths during cycling, *J Biomech* 20:899, 1987.
4. Price D, Donne B: Effect of variation in seat tube angle at difference seat heights on submaximal cycling performance in man, *J Sports Sci* 15:395–402, 1997.
5. Too D: The effect of hip position/configuration on anaerobic power and capacity in cycling, *Int J Sport Biomech* 7:359–370, 1991.
6. Brown DA, Kautz SA, Dairaghi CA: Muscle activity patterns altered during pedaling at different body orientations, *J Biomech* 29:1349–1356, 1996.
7. Heil DP, Derrick TR, Whittlesey S: The relationship between preferred and optimal positioning during submaximal cycle ergometry, *Eur J Appl Physiol* 75:160–165, 1997.
8. Reiser RF, Peterson ML, Broker JP: Anaerobic cycling power output with variations in recumbent body configuration, *J Appl Biomech* 17:204–216, 2001.
9. Broker JP, Gregor RJ: Mechanical energy management in cycling: Source relations and energy expenditure, *Med Sci Sport Exerc* 26:64–74, 1994.

10. Ryan MM, Gregor RJ: EMG profiles of lower extremity muscles during cycling at constant workload and cadence, *J Electromyogr Kinesiol* 2:69–80, 1992.

11. Pierson-Carey CD, Brown DA, Dairaghi CA: Changes in resultant pedal reaction forces due to ankle immobilization during pedaling, *J Appl Biomech* 13:334–346, 1997.

12. Sanderson DJ, Martin PE, Honeyman G, Keefer J: Gastrocnemius and soleus muscle length, velocity, and EMG responses to changes in pedaling cadence, *J Electromyogr Kinesiol* 16:642–649, 2006.

13. Sanderson DJ, Black A: The effect of prolonged cycling on pedal forces, *J Sports Sci* 21:191–199, 2003.

14. Dingwell JB, Joubert JE, Diefenthaeler F, Trinity JD: Changes in muscle activity and kinematics of highly trained cyclists during fatigue, *IEEE Trans Biomed Eng* 55:2666–2673, 2008.

15. Hannaford DR, Moran GT, Hlavac HF: Video analysis and treatment of overuse knee injury in cycling: A limited clinical study, *Clin Podiatr Med Surg* 3:671–678, 1986.

16. McCoy RW: *The effect of varying seat position on knee loads during cycling*, unpublished doctoral dissertation, University of Southern California, Department of Exercise Science, 1989.

17. Ruby P, Hull ML, Hawkins D: Three-dimensional knee loading during seated cycling, *J Biomech* 25:41–53, 1992.

18. Boutin RD, Rab GT, Hassan IAG: *Three dimensional kinematics and muscle length changes in bicyclists*, Proceedings 13th Annual Meeting ASB, Burlington, VT, UVM Conferences, 1989.

19. Bailey MP, Maillardet FJ, Messenger N: Kinematics of cycling in relation to anterior knee pain and patellar tendonitis, *J Sports Sci* 21:649–657, 2003.

20. Francis PR: Injury prevention for cyclists: A biomechanical approach. In Burke ER, editor: *Science of cycling*, Champaign, IL, 1986, Human Kinetics.

21. Gregersen CS, Hull ML, Hakansson NA: How changing the inversion/eversion foot angle affects the nondriving intersegmental knee moments and the relative activation of the Vastii muscles in cycling, *J Biomed Eng* 128:391–398, 2006.

22. Ruby P, Hull ML, Kirby KA, Jenkins DW: The effect of lower-limb anatomy on knee loads during seated cycling, *J Biomech* 25:1195–1207, 1992.

23. Wheeler JB, Gregor RJ, Broker JP: A dual piezoelectric bicycle pedal with multiple shoe/pedal interface compatibility, *Int J Sports Biomech* 8:251–258, 1992.

24. Ericson MO, Nisell R, Ekholm J: Varus and valgus loads on the knee joint during ergometer cycling, *Scand J Sports Sci* 6:39–45, 1984.

25. Zajac FE: Understanding muscle coordination of the human leg with dynamical simulations, *J Biomech* 35:1011–1018, 2002.

26. LaFortune MA, Cavanagh PR: Effectiveness and efficiency during bicycle riding. In Matsui H, Kobayashi K, editors: *Biomechanics VIII-B*, Champaign, IL, 1983, Human Kinetics.

27. Broker JP, Browning RC, Gregor RJ, Whiting WC: Effect of seat height on force effectiveness in cycling, *Med Sci Sports Exerc* 20:S83, 1988.

28. Broker JP, Gregor RJ, Schmidt RA: Extrinsic feedback and the learning of kinetic patterns in cycling, *J Appl Biomech* 9:111–123, 1993.

29. Perell KA: *Force summary feedback training on the bicycle in patients with unilateral cerebrovascular accidents*, unpublished doctoral dissertation, UCLA, 1994.

30. Hasson CJ, Caldwell GE, van Emmerik REA: Changes in muscle and joint coordination in learning to direct forces, *Hum Mov Sci* 27:590–609, 2008.

31. Bolourchi F, Hull ML: Measurement of rider-induced loads during simulated bicycling, *Int J Sports Biomech* 1:308–329, 1985.

32. Reiser RF, Peterson ML, Broker JP: Understanding recumbent cycling: Instrumentation design and biomechanical analysis, *Biomed Sci Instrum* 38:209–214, 2002.

33. Reiser RF, Broker JP, Peterson ML: Knee loads in the standard and recumbent cycling positions, *Biomed Sci Instrum* 40:36–42, 2004.

34. Brown DA, Kautz SA: Speed-dependent reductions of force output in people with post-stroke hemiparesis, *Phys Ther* 79:919–930, 1999.

35. Hakansson NA, Hull ML: Functional roles of the leg muscles when pedaling in the recumbent versus the upright position, *J Biomech Eng* 127:301–310, 2005.

36. Gregor SM, Perell KL, Rushatakankovit S, et al: Lower extremity general muscle moment patterns in healthy individuals during recumbent cycling, *Clin Biomech* 17:123–129, 2002.

37. Johnston TE: Biomechanical considerations for cycling interventions in rehabilitation, *Phys Ther* 87:1243–1252, 2007.

38. Perell KL, Gregor RJ, Scremin AME: Lower extremity cycling mechanics in subjects with unilateral CVAs, *J Appl Biomech* 14:158–179, 1998.

39. Perell KL, Gregor RJ, Kim G: Comparison of cycling kinetics during recumbent bicycling in subjects with and without diabetes, *J Rehabil Res Dev* 39:13–20, 2002.

40. Kautz SA, Patton C: Interlimb influences on paretic leg function in post-stroke hemiparesis, *J Neurophysiol* 93:2460–2473, 2005.

41. Kerr A, Rafferty D, Moffat F, Morlan G: Specificity of recumbent cycling as a training modality for the functional movements: Sit-to-stand and step-up, *Clin Biomech* 22:1104–1111, 2007.

42. Sanderson DJ, Cavanagh PR: An investigation of the in-shoe pressure distribution during cycling in conventional cycling shoes or running shoes. In B Jonsson, editor: *Biomechanics X-B*, Champaign, IL, 1987, Human Kinetics.

43. Sanderson DJ, Hennig EM: *In-shoe pressure distribution in cycling and running shoes during steady-rate cycling*, Proceedings of the Second North American Congress on Biomechanics, Chicago, August 24–28, 1992.

44. Amoroso AT, Hennig EM, Sanderson DJ: *In-shoe pressure distribution for cycling at different cadences*, Proceedings of the Second North American Congress on Biomechanics, Chicago, August 24–28, 1992.

45. Hennig EM, Sanderson DJ: *In-shoe pressure distribution for cycling at different power outputs*, Proceedings of the Second North American Congress on Biomechanics, Chicago, August 24–28, 1992.

46. Francis PR: Pathomechanics of the lower extremity in cycling. In Burke E, Newsom B, editors: *Medical and scientific aspects of cycling*, Champaign, IL, 1988, Human Kinetics.

47. Sanderson DJ: The biomechanics of cycling shoes, *Cycling Sci* Sept: 27–30, 1990.

48. Gregor RJ, Wheeler JB: Knee pain: Biomechanical factors associated with shoe/pedal interfaces: Implications for injury, *Sports Med* 17:117–131, 1994.

49. Wheeler JB, Gregor RJ, Broker JP: The effect of clipless float design on shoe/pedal interface kinetics: Implications for overuse injuries during cycling, *J Appl Biomech* 11:119–141, 1995.

50. Boyd TF, Neptune RR, Hull ML: Pedal and knee loads using a multi-degree-of-freedom pedal platform in cycling, *J Biomech* 30:505–511, 1977.

51. McCoy RW, Gregor RJ: The effect of varying seat position on knee loads during cycling, *Med Sci Sports Exerc* 21:S79, 1989.

52. Furumizo SH: *A biomechanical analysis of anterior/posterior shear joint reaction forces in the ACL-deficient knee during stationary cycling*, unpublished Masters thesis, UCLA Department of Kinesiology, 1991.

53. Hunt MA, Sanderson DJ, Moffet H, Inglis JJ: Interlimb asymmetry in persons with and without an anterior cruciate ligament deficiency during stationary cycling, *Arch Phys Med Rehabil* 85:1475–1478, 2004.

54. Hunt MA, Sanderson DJ, Moffet H, Inglis JJ: Biomechanical changes elicited by an anterior cruciate ligament deficiency during steady state cycling, *Clin Biomech* 18:393–400, 2003.

55. Gregor RJ: *A biomechanical analysis of lower limb action during cycling at four different loads, unpublished doctoral dissertation*, The Pennsylvania State University, 1976.

56. Gregor RJ, Cavanagh PR, LaFortune M: Knee flexor moments during propulsion in cycling—A creative solution to Lombard's paradox, *J Biomech* 18:307–316, 1985.

57. Andrews JG: The functional roles of the hamstrings and quadriceps during cycling: Lombard's paradox revisited, *J Biomech* 20:565–575, 1987.

58. Browning RC, Gregor RJ, Broker JP, Whiting WC: Effects of seat height changes on joint force and moment patterns in experienced cyclists, *J Biomech* 21:871, 1988.

59. Jorge M, Hull ML: Biomechanics of bicycle pedaling. In Terauds T, Barthels K, Kreighbaum E, et al, editors: *Sports biomechanics*, Del Mar, CA, 1984, Research Center for Sports.

60. Redfield R, Hull ML: On the relation between joint moments and pedaling rates at constant power in bicycling, *J Biomech* 19:317–329, 1986.

61. Lombard WP: The action of two-joint muscles, *Am Phys Ed Rev* 8:141–145, 1903.

62. Van Ingen Schenau GJ: From rotation to translation: Constraints on multi-joint movements and the unique action of bi-articular muscles, *Hum Mov Sci* 8:301–337, 1989.

63. Kuo AD: The action of two-joint muscles: Legacy of WP Lombard. In Latash ML, Zatsiorsky VM, editors: *Classics in movement science*, Champaign, IL, 2001, Human Kinetics.

64. Ruby P, Hull ML, Kirby KA, Jenkins DW: The effect of lower-limb anatomy on knee loads during seated cycling, *J Biomech* 25:1195–1207, 1992.

65. Zatsiorsky V, Gregor R: Mechanical power and work in human movement. In Sparrow WA, editor: *Metabolic energy expenditure and the learning and control of movement*, Champaign, IL, 2000, Human Kinetics.

66. Ericson MO, Bratt A, Nisell R: Load moments about the hip and knee joints during ergometer cycling, *Scand J Rehabil Med* 18:165–172, 1986.

67. Desipres M: An electromyographic study of competitive road cycling conditions simulated on a treadmill. In Nelson RC, Morehouse CA, editors: *Biomechanics IV*, Champaign, IL, 1974, Human Kinetics.

68. Ericson MO, Nisell R, Arborelius UP: Muscular activity during ergometer cycling, *Scand J Rehabil Med* 17:53–61, 1985.

69. Houtz SJ, Fischer FJ: An analysis of muscle action and joint excursion during exercise on a stationary bicycle, *J Bone Joint Surg Am* 41:123–131, 1959.

70. Jorge M, Hull ML: Analysis of EMG measurement during bicycle pedaling, *J Biomech* 19:683–694, 1986.

71. Gregor RJ, Komi PV, Browning RC, Jarvinen M: Comparison between the triceps surae and residual muscle moments at the ankle during cycling, *J Biomech* 24:287–297, 1991.

72. Juker D, McGill S, Kropf P: Quantitative intramuscular myoelectric activity of lumbar portions of the psoas and abdominal wall during cycling, *J Appl Biomech* 14:428–438, 1998.

73. Burnett AF, Cornelius MW, Dankaerts W, O'Sullivan PB: Spinal kinematics and trunk muscle activity in cyclists: A comparison between healthy controls and non-specific chronic low back pain subjects—A pilot investigation, *Man Ther* 9:211–219, 2004.

74. Chapman AR, Vincenzino B, Blanch P, Hodges PW: Patterns of leg muscle recruitment vary between novice and highly trained cyclists, *J Electromyogr Kinesiol* 18:359–371, 2008.

75. Wakeling JM, Vehli K, Rozitis AI: Muscle fiber recruitment can respond to the mechanics of the muscle contraction, *J Royal Soc Interface* 3:533–544, 2006.

76. Raasch CC, Zajac FE, Ma B, Levine WS: Muscle coordination in maximum speed pedaling, *J Biomech* 30:595–602, 1997.

77. Savelberg H, Van de Port I, Willems P: Body configuration in cycling affects muscle recruitment and movement patterns, *J Appl Biomech* 19:310–324, 2003.

78. Chapman AR, Vincenzino B, Blanch P, et al: Influence of body position on leg kinematics and muscle recruitment during cycling, *J Sci Med Sport* 11:519–526, 2008.

79. Gregor RJ, Komi PV, Jarvinen M: Achilles tendon forces during cycling, *Int J Sports Med* 8:9–14, 1987.

80. Marsh AP, Martin PE: The relationship between cadence and lower extremity EMG in cyclists and non-cyclists, *Med Sci Sport Exerc* 27(2):217–225, 1995.

81. Pruitt AL, Matheny F: *Andy Pruitt's complete medical guide for cyclists*, Boulder, CO, 2006, Velo Press.

82. Haapasalo H, Parkkari J, Kannus P, et al: Knee injuries in leisure-time physical activities: A prospective one-year follow-up of a Finnish population cohort, *Int J Sports Med* 28:72–77, 2007.

83. Holmes JC, Pruitt AL, Whalen NJ: Cycling knee injuries, *Cycling Sci* June:11–14, 1991.

84. Mellion MB: Common cycling injuries: Management and prevention, *Sports Med* 11:52–70, 1991.

85. Wanich T, Hodgkins C, Columbier J, et al: Cycling injuries of the lower extremity, *J Am Acad Orthop Surg* 15:748–756, 2007.

86. Chin T, Sawamura S, Fujita H, et al: Effect of endurance training program based on anaerobic threshold (AT) for lower limb amputees, *J Rehab Res Dev* 38:7–11, 2001.

87. Childers WL, Perell-Gerson KL, Kistenberg R, Gregor RJ: *Pedaling forces normalized to body weight in intact and uni-lateral transtibial amputees during cycling*, Proceedings of the 4th International State-of-the-Art Congress "Rehabilitation: Mobility, Exercise & Sports", Amsterdam, NL, April 7–9, 2009. (in press).

88. Walther V: *MTB Amputee*. Retrieved 2002 from http://www.mtb-amputee.com/.

89. Dillingham TR, Pezzin LE, Mackenzie EJ: Limb amputation and limb deficiency epidemiology and recent trends in the United States, *South Med J* 95:875–883, 2002.

90. Childers WL, Kistenberg R, Gregor RJ: *Pedaling asymmetry in cyclists with uni-lateral transtibial amputation and the effect of prosthetic foot stiffness*, Proceeds of the AAOP 35th Annual Meeting and Scientific Symposium, Atlanta, GA, March 4–7, 2009 (in press).

91. Murray JB: *Efficiency of simulated amputee cycling*, unpublished Master's thesis, UC Boulder, Department of Integrative Physiology, 2003.

92. Sanderson DJ: The influence of cadence and power output on asymmetry of force application during steady-rate cycling, *J Hum Mov Stud* 19:1–9, 1990.

93. Daly DJ, Cavanagh PR: Asymmetry in bicycle ergometer pedaling, *Med Sci Sport* 8:204–208, 1976.

94. Smak W, Neptune RR, Hull ML: The influence of pedaling rate on bilateral asymmetry in cycling, *J Biomech* 32:899–906, 1999.

95. Broker JP, Gregor RJ: Cycling biomechanics. In Burke ER, editor: *High-tech cycling*, ed 1, Champaign, IL, 1996, Human Kinetics.

96. Isakov E, Burger H, Gregoric M, Marincek C: Isokinetic and isometric strength of the thigh muscles in below-knee amputees, *Clin Biomech* 11:233–235, 1996.

97. Broker JP: Cycling biomechanics. In Burke ER, editor: *High-tech cycling*, ed 2, Champaign, IL, 2003, Human Kinetics.

98. Kautz SA, Hull ML: A theoretical basis for interpreting the force applied to the pedal in cycling, *J Biomech* 26:155–165, 1993.

99. Childers WL, Kistenberg R, Gregor RJ: *Clinical guidelines for adapting the bicycle to recreational cyclists with transtibial amputation*, Proceeds of the AAOP 35th Annual Meeting and Scientific Symposium, Atlanta, GA, March 4–7, 2009 (in press).

100. Childers WL, Hudson-Toole EF, Gregor RJ: *Activation changes in the gastrocnemius muscle: Adaptation to a new functional role following amputation*, Proceeds of the ACSM 56th Annual Meeting, Seattle, WA, May 27–30, 2009 (in press).

101. Fowler EG, Kolobe TH, Damiano DL, et al: Promotion of physical fitness and prevention of secondary conditions for children with cerebral palsy, Section on Pediatrics Research Summit Proceedings, *Phys Ther* 87:1495–1510, 2007.

102. Rimmer JH: Physical fitness levels of persons with cerebral palsy, *Dev Med Child Neurol* 43:208–212, 2001.

103. Kaplan SL: Cycling patterns in children with cerebral palsy, *Dev Med Child Neurol* 37:620–630, 1995.

104. Siebert K, DeMuth SK, Knutson LM, Fowler EG: A stationary cycling intervention for children with cerebral palsy: A report on two children, *Phys Occup Ther Pediatr* (in press).

105. Johnston TE, Barr AE, Lee SCK: Biomechanics of submaximal recumbent cycling in adolescents with and without cerebral palsy, *Phys Ther* 87:572–585, 2007.

106. Johnston TE, Prosser LA, Lee SCK: Differences in pedal forces during recumbent cycling in adolescents with and without cerebral palsy, *Clin Biomech* 23:248–251, 2008.

107. Berg K: Effect of physical training of school children with cerebral palsy, *Acta Paediatr Scand* 204:27–33, 1970.

108. Berg K, Bjure J: Methods for evaluation of the physical working capacity of school children with cerebral palsy, *Acta Paediatr Scand* 204:15–26, 1970.

109. Shinohara TA, Suzuki N, Oba M, et al: Effect of exercise at the AT point for children with cerebral palsy, *Bull Hosp Joint Dis* 61:63–67, 2002.

110. Williams H, Pountney T: Effects of a static bicycling programme on the functional ability of young people with cerebral palsy who are non-ambulant, *Dev Med Child Neurol* 49:522–527, 2007.

111. Fowler EG, Knutson LM, DeMuth SK, et al: Pediatric endurance and limb strengthening (PEDALS) for children with cerebral palsy using stationary cycling: a randomized controlled trial, *Phys Ther* (in press).

APPLIED BIOMECHANICS OF GOLF

David Lindsay and Anthony A. Vandervoort

Introduction

Golf is a very popular sport, with approximately 30,000 golf courses and 55 million worldwide participants.[1] The popularity of golf is likely due to a variety of reasons including perceived health benefits.[2] The health benefits from golf are being supported through a number of scientific investigations. For example, Parkkari and colleagues,[3] in their investigation of the benefits of golf among a previously sedentary group of 55 healthy Finnish male subjects aged 48 to 64, observed an increased aerobic performance on a walking treadmill test, as well as improved body composition and high-density lipoprotein serum cholesterol levels. Sell and colleagues[4] reported that the total caloric expenditures during a round of 18 holes of golf while walking with and without carrying golf clubs were 1954 kcal and 1527 kcal, respectively. The authors concluded that walking the golf course provided an amount of physical activity sufficient to improve overall health and well-being, especially for older golfers whose physiological training threshold is lowered by age.[5] Although golf may provide health and fitness benefits, the sport also appears to have certain injury risks.[6]

The effortless appearance of a professional golfer's swing tends to disguise the true force required to generate high clubhead speed. Although not obvious to the "naked eye," many body parts are moving at high velocity and through extreme ranges of motion (ROMs). The magnitude and complexity of these motions has led some to regard the full golf swing as one of the most difficult biomechanical motions to execute.[7] Mastering these motions as demonstrated by elite amateur and touring professionals requires dedicated practice during which these powerful movements may be repeated several hundred times per day. The subsequent and cumulative stresses on the limb and spinal joints associated with such practice may lead to the development of overuse injuries.[8,9] Furthermore, because swing mechanics may contribute to injury susceptibility,[10] the less efficient

and inappropriate movement patterns demonstrated by less skilled recreational golfers may further increase injury susceptibility.

Epidemiological research has shown that golf injuries are quite common. Professional Golf Association (PGA) tour players average two injuries per year, with half of these injuries limiting the ability to play for an average of 5 weeks.[11] Recreational players, on average, lose approximately 4 weeks of playing time per injury.[8] In terms of injury location, the lower back appears to be the most commonly affected body part,[8,9,11,12] followed by a relatively even distribution between the shoulder, elbow, and wrist.[2,8,12] In terms of severity, most golfers regard their injury as minor (52%) compared with moderate (28%) or major (21%) severity.[8] McCarroll[11] reported that 54% of professional golfers and 45% of amateur players categorize their injury as chronic. The prevalence of chronic minor injuries among golfers may partly explain why as many as one-third of elite touring professionals are playing injured at any given time.[13]

As mentioned, the repetitive nature of the asymmetrical (i.e., either left- or right-handed) golf swing, in which emphasis is placed on generating high clubhead speed, are key factors in the causes of golf injuries. Clearly, the best solution to the problem of golf injuries is to avoid them in the first place. Injury prevention requires a combination of good judgment and appropriate preparation before playing, as well as good technique and proper equipment. Although the prevention of injuries is idyllic, the reality is that a proportion of the golfing population will suffer an injury and will seek some form of health care intervention. McNicholas and colleagues[14] found that golfers who sought early medical and physical therapy treatment for their injuries were more likely to make a full recovery. However, "full recovery" does not imply that any biomechanical deficiencies in the golfer's swing that may have contributed to the injury have been identified and corrected. It is reasonable to expect that if a golfer returns in a timely fashion with the same swing as before, and if there were components of that swing that contributed to the injury, then it is only a matter of time before the player will suffer a relapse. In other words, as a health care provider, "the best treatment we can give is to study the biomechanics of a patient's golf swing and try and spot any mechanical flaws that may be causing injury."[15]

General Swing Mechanics

The ultimate goal of the full golf swing is to consistently and predictably hit the golf ball in the desired direction for the proper distance. Although the goal of the golf swing may be consistent across different skill levels, the methods used to execute the swing obviously vary. The following section describes the typical swing mechanics that occur during a full golf swing from predominantly a kinematic and muscle activity perspective. Detailed biomechanical descriptions of key segments of the body during the swing, particularly as they relate to injury susceptibility and rehabilitation, are discussed later in this chapter. The terms *lead* and *trail* are used to identify the different sides of the body, although *left* and *right* designations are occasionally added for clarity and refer to a right-handed player. The lead side is the side closest to the target, which for a right-handed player is the left side.

There are few more contentious issues in the sport of golf than what constitutes the ideal swing. One of the more respected scientific texts dealing with the golf swing was written in 1968 by Alastair Cochran and John Stobbs and titled *The Search for the Perfect Swing*.[16] In their book, they describe the swing as a sequence of body rotations involving the legs, hips, torso, shoulders, arms, and wrists that works together to create movement of the clubhead toward the ball in such a manner that a desirable and efficient transfer of energy is imparted to the ball at impact. These various body parts are essentially like springs that are "wound up" on the backswing until maximum stretch is achieved. The greatest speed of the clubhead on the downswing is created only if the spring tension in each of the various body segments is released in sequence starting from the ground (i.e., legs) up:

> [E]very part of the rotating and swinging system must be pulled around by the part nearer the ground, until that part can no longer apply useful effort. That is, in terms of a human golfer, the legs pull around the hips, the hips the trunk, the trunk the upper chest and shoulders, the shoulders the arms, the arms the hands, the hands the shaft, and the shaft the clubhead.[16]

In essence, the ideal swing pattern allows the golfer to rotate the club away from the start position in a large arc, and then return it to an impact position in such a way that optimal launch conditions are achieved for the distance and

accuracy requirements of the planned shot. Furthermore, the large momentum developed by the various body segments during the downswing must be effectively decelerated during the postimpact phase while still maintaining postural stability and balance. Although the preceding description explains the general elements of an ideal swing, it appears that there is considerable variation in how this is accomplished, even among elite players.[17] This suggests there may not necessarily be one ideal swing for all players. The reader is encouraged to keep this in mind as the general mechanics of the full golf swing are discussed in the following sections. The following descriptions are gathered from a number of scientific sources[5,6,18-21] and refer to a full swing for a right-handed player. The general swing phases, which consist of set-up, backswing, downswing, and follow-through, are illustrated schematically in Figure 9-1.

Phases of Golf Swing

- Setup
- Backswing
- Downswing (forward swing, impact)
- Follow-through

Set-Up

The set-up position, sometimes referred to as *ball address* (see Figure 9-1, *A*), is the starting position for executing the golf swing in proper alignment with an established target. The role of the set-up is to provide an initial stable platform to allow the swing to proceed in a balanced and biomechanically efficient manner. The set-up is influenced by a number of factors, including the club being used and the nature of the intended shot. The following description of the set-up position is based on a typical full shot in which maximal distance is desired.[5] The set-up incorporates a relatively symmetrical weight distribution with the feet approximately shoulder width apart. Both hips are externally rotated approximately 25°, although this is often described as *turning the feet out* rather than *hip motion*. It is worth noting that some golf coaches teach a relatively neutral position of the trail hip. The knees are flexed approximately 25°, which positions the patellae vertically above the balls of the feet. This knee flexion helps maintain the body's center of gravity under the mid-portion of the feet by allowing the weight of the hip and buttock region to offset the weight of the upper body as the trunk leans forward. The forward lean or flexion of the trunk is needed to bring the clubhead down behind the ball. However, this lean should be produced by hip flexion rather than spinal flexion (i.e., the spine maintains a relatively straight or "neutral" position). The spine does demonstrate a slight right side bend and left rotation to compensate for the lower position of the

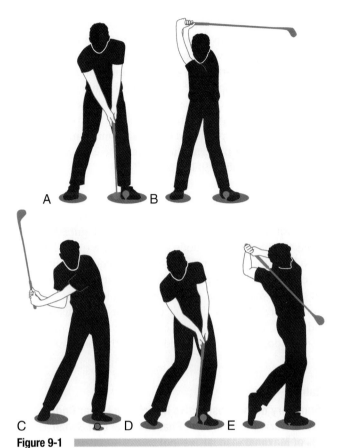

Figure 9-1

Body positions at key moments during the full golf swing. **A,** Set-up. **B,** Top of backswing. **C,** Forward swing. **D,** Impact. **E,** Finish. (Reproduced with permission, Fit Fore Golf, Inc.)

right hand on the grip of the club.[21,22] Both upper limbs hang in a somewhat vertical orientation with the glenohumeral joints in neutral rotation, the elbows extended, and the wrists in slight ulnar deviation.

Backswing

The backswing involves the drawing back of the club using predominantly a rotary motion of the body while maintaining a consistent amount of hip and trunk flexion, as well as a steady position of the head. The rotary motion is initiated with the legs and pelvis, followed by the trunk, shoulders, arms, and club. The typical backswing of an elite player takes approximately 0.8 seconds to complete.[23] The backswing is usually regarded as complete when the club stops moving, which is typically when the club shaft is approximately parallel with the ground. At the top of the backswing the pelvis has turned approximately 40° away from the target while an imaginary line bisecting both shoulder joints has turned more than 100°.[21,24] The difference between the pelvis and shoulder turn is the result of near maximal right rotation of the spine,[25] as well as lead side scapular protraction and trail side retraction.[26] The pelvic turn places the lead or left hip in external rotation, while the

right hip is in internal rotation.[21] Meanwhile, the full shoulder turn to the right while keeping the head facing the ball results in full left cervical rotation ROM (see Figure 9-1B).

During the backswing, both arms and the golf club are progressively moved onto the trail (right) side of the body, resulting in a shift of weight to that same side. At the top of the backswing, approximately 60% to 70% of the body's weight is positioned under the right foot.[21,27] At the top of the backswing, the lead or left glenohumeral joint is in approximately 110° of elevation, 35° of horizontal adduction, and full internal rotation. Meanwhile the trail shoulder demonstrates approximately 60° of elevation (combination of flexion and abduction) and full (i.e., 80° +) external rotation.[28] The wrists of both hands radially deviate during the backswing, producing approximately a 90° angle between the club shaft and lead (i.e., left) arm at the finish of the backswing (see Figure 9-1, *B*).[29]

Downswing

The downswing portion of the golf swing is where the velocity of the clubhead and the angle of contact between the club face and the golf ball are determined. However, the resultant forces produced during this phase also increases injury susceptibility.[30] The downswing includes two subphases; the *forward swing* (see Figure 9-1, *C*) and *ball impact* (see Figure 9-1, *D*). As mentioned previously, the movement of the golf club away from the ball to the top of the backswing takes approximately 0.8 seconds to complete. However, the forward swing actually starts approximately 0.1 seconds *before* the arms and golf club finish the backswing.[23,24] In other words, there is an initial shift of body weight as well as a rotation of the lower body and pelvis toward the target (i.e., left) just before the upper body and golf club finish rotating to the right. This initiation of the downswing with the lower limbs results in the hips and shoulders momentarily rotating in opposite directions, further increasing the amount of trunk rotation stretch at the start of the downswing.[24] This increase in spinal rotation at the initial phase of the downswing has been referred to as the *X-factor stretch*.

Cheetham and colleagues[23] attempted to quantify the X-factor stretch between 10 highly skilled golfers and nine less skilled players (handicap > 14). Results showed that the more-skilled players increased the X-factor stretch (i.e., the amount of spinal rotation) by 19% during the early part of the downswing. This compared with 13% for the less-skilled players. The authors went on to state that the extra stretch on the muscle, along with the active resistance to that stretch, can increase muscular contraction forces, leading to more force production on the downswing and a resultant higher clubhead speed through impact.

Approximately 0.08 seconds after the lower limbs (followed by the trunk) commence the downswing, the shoulder joints start to powerfully rotate toward the left. These shoulder movements occur immediately *before* the golf club reaches the top of the backswing. The lead (left) shoulder abducts and externally rotates while the trail side internally rotates and adducts bringing the arms down and across the torso towards the ball.

The final critical element of the downswing is the "uncocking" or "release" of both wrist joints, which occurs just before impact between the golf club and the ball. The wrist release has two motion components, frontal plane (e.g., radial and ulnar deviation) and axial rotation (supination and pronation)[31] that allow the hands to "turn over" or rotate through impact.[18,21] It is interesting to note that the peak movement of these two components occurs at different stages of the downswing. The peak timing of the frontal plane portion of the wrist release (i.e., ulnar deviation) occurs 0.1 seconds before impact, whereas the axial rotation motion (supination of the left forearm, pronation of the right forearm) peaks less than 0.002 seconds before impact.[31]

For the downswing to proceed with maximum efficiency, the pelvic, spinal, shoulder, and wrist rotations must conform to the segmental rotation pattern identified by Cochran and Stobbs[16] and subsequently described by Burden and colleagues[24] as the *summation of speed principle*. This principle states that to maximize the speed of the distal end of the system (i.e., the clubhead), the swing must start with movements at the more proximal segments (legs) and progress sequentially to faster movements of the more distal segments. The increased velocity of the distal segment often occurs as the velocity of the more proximal segments starts to decrease.[32] The summation of speed principle has also been called the *kinematic sequence* and underlies the importance of initiating the downswing by contraction of the large muscles of the lower limbs and pelvis.

Kinematic Sequence

The swing must start in the legs and progress sequentially and progressively to the more distal segments and finally the club for maximum force and velocity to the ball.

Bechler and colleagues[33] studied the activity patterns of the thigh and hip muscles in competitive golfers and reported that the hip extensors and abductors on the trail side, in conjunction with the lead adductor muscles, initiate pelvic rotation and weight shift toward the target at the beginning of the downswing. The lead vastus lateralis and the hamstrings acted to stabilize the knee joints during this pelvic rotation. Contraction of the large trunk muscles, in particular the abdominal oblique, erector spinae, and latissimus dorsi, follows closely behind the lower limb and hip muscles. Watkins[34] reported that the trail-side abdominal oblique muscles showed the highest relative activity although the authors did not differentiate between the

external and internal oblique muscles. Other authors have found a higher relative contribution from the lead internal oblique compared with the trail external oblique on the downswing,[35,36] with both muscles contracting before the club reached the top of the backswing. High levels of bilateral erector spinae activity on the downswing are thought to help stabilize the spine during the powerful trunk flexion and rotation forces produced by the abdominal muscles.[34,37] Muscle activation patterns throughout the entire swing are summarized in Tables 9-1 and 9-2.[38]

Impact

The position of the body at impact (see Figure 9-1, *D*) results from a shift of the body's center of mass toward the left as well as the rotary motions and subsequent centrifugal forces generated by the powerful muscle contractions throughout the lower limbs, trunk, and shoulders. At impact, approximately 80% of the golfer's weight is situated on the lead foot.[27] The hips and trunk extend slightly from the flexed posture adopted during ball address and the spine side bends

Table 9-1

Summary of the Most Active Muscles in Lower Body/Trunk During the Different Phases of the Golf Swing (% of Maximal Manual Testing)

Phase of Swing	Left Lower Body/Trunk	Right Lower Body/Trunk
Backswing	Erector spinae (26%)	Semimembranosus (28%)
	Abdominal oblique (24%)	Biceps femoris (27%)
Downswing—early	Vastus lateralis (88%)	Gluteus maximus (100%)
	Adductor magnus (63%)	Biceps femoris (78%)
Downswing—late	Biceps femoris (83%)	Abdominal oblique (59%)
	Gluteus maximus (58%)	Gluteus medius (51%)
	Vastus lateralis (58%)	
Follow-through—early	Biceps femoris (79%)	Gluteus medius (59%)
	Vastus lateralis (59%)	Abdominal oblique (51%)
Follow-through—late	Semimembranosus (42%)	Vastus lateralis (40%)
	Vastus lateralis (42%)	Gluteus medius (22%)
	Adductor magnus (35%)	

Modified from McHardy A, Pollard H: Muscle activity during the golf swing, *Br J Sport Med* 39:802, 2005.

Table 9-2

Summary of the Most Active Muscles in Upper Body/Trunk During the Different Phases of the Golf Swing (% of Maximal Manual Testing)

Phase of Swing	Left Upper Body/Trunk	Right Upper Body/Trunk
Backswing	Subscapularis (33%)	Upper trapezius (52%)
	Upper serratus (30%)	Middle trapezius (37%)
Downswing—early	Rhomboid (68%)	Pectoralis major (64%)
	Middle trapezius (51%)	Upper serratus (58%)
Downswing—late	Pectoralis major (93%)	Pectoralis major (93%)
	Levator scapulae (62%)	Upper serratus (69%)
Follow-through—early	Pectoralis major (74%)	Pectoralis major (74%)
	Infraspinatus (61%)	Subscapularis (64%)
Follow-through—late	Infraspinatus (40%)	Subscapularis (56%)
	Pectoralis major (39%)	Upper and lower serratus (40%)

Modified from McHardy A, Pollard H: Muscle activity during the golf swing, *Br J Sport Med* 39:801, 2005.

to the right approximately 25° to 30°.[22,25] This side bend is partially due to the pelvis moving approximately 12 cm laterally toward the target,[19,24] while still keeping the head in the same spatial orientation as that observed at set-up. Localized muscular contraction forces within the upper limbs as well as centrifugal forces on the downswing cause the elbows to extend and the wrists to "release" immediately before and through impact. At impact, both wrists are in ulnar deviation with the left side measured at approximately 23°.[29] The majority of golf injuries occur during the impact phase when the velocities of the various body segments are at or near maximum.[30]

Clinical Point

Most golf injuries occur during the impact phase.

Follow-Through

The follow-through phase (see Figure 9-1, *E*) consists of deceleration of the target-directed movements of the body and golf club. Almost all of the player's body weight finishes on the lead side with the hip in full internal rotation, while just the toes of the trail foot remain in contact with the ground and the hip is in neutral rotation. At the completion of the follow-through, the torso is maximally rotated toward the target (i.e., left). The finish position for the shoulder joints is noteworthy in that it is characterized by a reversal of the shoulder positions seen at the top of the backswing. The lead shoulder finishes in complete external rotation, approximately 70° of horizontal abduction and 60° of elevation. The trail shoulder at follow-through demonstrates approximately 30° of horizontal adduction, 110° of elevation and full or near-full internal rotation.[28] During the follow-through, the lead wrist proceeds into extension and radial deviation while the trail wrist folds into flexion and radial deviation.

According to McCarroll and colleagues,[10] 25% of all golf injuries occur during the follow-though, with the back, shoulder, knees, and wrists most often affected. Also notable are the stresses on the neck and lead-side hip. The neck is subjected to a relatively violent rotation to the right soon after impact because of the rapid rotation of the torso toward the target (left) while the head remains facing the spot on the ground where the ball lay prior to impact.

Clinical Point

Twenty-five percent of golf injuries occur to the back, shoulders, knees, and wrist during follow-through.

Lower Limb Biomechanics and Injury Relationships

The lower limbs, which for the purposes of this chapter include the hip, knee, and ankle joints, are critical for generating clubhead speed during a full golf swing. As a result, injuries to this region do occur, although not to the extent that they occur in the upper limbs or spine.[2,8,11] The contribution of the lower-limb segment to clubhead speed is made possible by the interaction between the golf shoe and the surface on which the golfer is standing. The biomechanical forces associated with this interaction are referred to as *ground reaction forces*. The ground reaction forces that occur under a golfer's feet are influenced by a number of factors, including the club being used and the type of shoe being worn.[39] Worsfold and colleagues[39] found that the rotation torques under the front (i.e., left) foot were typically approximately two to three times higher than those under the trail foot. This increased rotational torque on the lead ankle, knee, and hip joints occurs at the same time as nearly 950 N of compression load is applied to the leg,[40] and thus results in considerable stress to this region.

Lindsay and colleagues,[17] in their review of golf biomechanics, reported that the sole-to-ground interactions vary considerably between groups of elite and less-skilled players. To summarize, less-skilled golfers were found to have greater lateral forces on the feet during the backswing and downswing, delayed weight shift on the downswing, more movement of weight onto the anterior or toe portion of the feet, and a delay in the timing of essential joint actions. These differences likely correspond to reduced efficiency and a reduction in clubhead speed at impact. Overall, highly skilled golfers did a better job harnessing the rotational power from the body through an effective weight shift, better balance, and proper rotational kinematic sequencing.

As can be seen in the previous description, a key difference between the swings of highly skilled and less-skilled players is the nature of the weight transfer and rotational forces as the downswing progresses. The ground reaction forces created by the golfer on the downswing have three important components; a medial-lateral component, an anterior-posterior component, and a torque or rotational component. These components correspond with the relative motions of the lower limbs and pelvis during the golf downswing. In their biomechanical study of baseball swings, Welch and colleagues[41], in a baseball study, describe how linear (i.e., lateral) and rotational motions, associated with ground reaction forces, contribute to the generation of maximum bat speed. In a similar way, the golf swing also produces lateral and rotational motions. The interaction between these two components determines how the proximal segment of the kinetic sequence (i.e., the lower limbs) will be used and ultimately what must happen within the remaining segments, including the upper limbs to square the club face through impact to produce an optimum swing.

As the downswing commences, the lower body powerfully *rotates* toward the target. This rotational motion is the result of the clockwise torque (22 Nm) provided by the trail (right) foot against the ground as well as the anterior (186 N) and posterior (145 N) force couple produced by the lead and trail feet respectively.[40] Lateral movement of

the body toward the target is also being created at the same time as the rotational motion. If the lateral component is exaggerated or occurs too early in the downswing, then significantly greater pressure is carried to the front foot early in the acceleration phase. This results in an effective shear force being produced *only* under the lead foot, thereby reducing the efficiency of the rotational force couple applied to the hip segments.

It appears from the previous description that a balance exists between the amounts of lateral and rotational forces that a golfer uses on the downswing to create optimal clubhead speed. It is very possible that injuries around the lower limbs and in particular the hips may also be affected by how far a golfer's weight shift characteristics vary from the "balance" alluded to previously. Excessive lateral movement toward the target not only tends to diminish the rotary force couple beneath the golfer's feet but may also create increased internal loading of the lead hip joint, which in turn could lead to increased wear and tear on that side. Many factors likely contribute to increased lateral movement on the downswing, including poor trunk stability.[42] It is interesting to note that Jack Nicklaus and Tom Watson, two great players who in their primes employed a fairly aggressive lateral weight shift, required hip replacement surgery only on their lead (left) side. In contrast to the previous description, maintaining excessive weight on the trail foot in the latter part of the downswing and through impact tends to increase the abduction and external rotation forces occurring on the trail (right) hip. Forceful abduction and external rotation has been linked with injury to the hip acetabular labrum.[43] Acetabular labral injuries have affected the right hip of many elite PGA players including Greg Norman.

The hip is not the only part of the lower limb susceptible to injury from the golf swing. The knee issues affecting top professional golfer Tiger Woods have received worldwide media attention. The magnitude of knee joint forces and moments generated during the golf swing are not of sufficient magnitude to categorize golf as high-risk for acute knee trauma.[44] This is supported by the epidemiological literature that shows that knee injuries are relatively uncommon, making up approximately 3% to 6% of the total number of golf injuries.[8,13,45] Although knee injuries occur infrequently from golf, they are common among active individuals and as such many recreational golfers have knee problems that do not originate from golf but are aggravated by golfing activities.[8]

The lead or left knee is more often affected than the trail side, especially among professional players.[11] One of the first studies to quantify the various compressive loads, shear forces, and joint moments affecting the knee joints during the golf swing was performed by Gatt and colleagues.[44] The authors reported that the forces and moments produced in the knee joints were similar in magnitudes to the forces associated with activities such as a side-cutting maneuver while running. The authors cautioned that clinicians should take into account the implication of these forces to the internal structures of the knee when setting return-to-golf activity guidelines after knee injury or surgery.

Lynn and colleagues[46] investigated frontal plane moments affecting the lead knee during the full golf swing. In particular, the authors were interested in how a straight (i.e., neutral hip rotation) versus a turned out (externally rotated) lead foot affected the knee varus (adduction) and valgus (abduction) moments. Results showed that turning the lead foot out significantly decreased the varus moment at impact resulting in less medial compartment stress. The authors postulated that golfers with medial compartment osteoarthritis would likely experience less cartilage wear and pain from adopting a turned-out lead foot. Furthermore, the authors suggested that having the front foot turned out should allow golfers to more easily transfer their weight onto this foot during the downswing, resulting in a more efficient swing. Lynn and colleagues did caution that having the front foot turned out resulted in a nonsignificant increase in the valgus moment, which could reflect an increase in lateral compartment knee stress.

Clinical Relevance Summary – Lower Limb

- Excessive lateral movement of the lower limbs toward the target increases internal loading of the lead hip joint, which in turn could lead to increased wear and tear on that side. Poor trunk stability may contribute to increased lateral movement.
- Maintaining excessive weight on the trail foot in the latter part of the downswing and through impact increases the abduction and external rotation forces on the trail (right) hip and may harm the hip acetabular labrum.
- Forces on the lead (left) knee from the golf swing are similar to those produced during a side-cutting maneuver when running.
- Turning the lead foot out at set-up results in less medial compartment stress and an easier transfer of weight onto this foot, but may increase lateral compartment knee stress.

Spinal Biomechanics and Injury Relationships

Injuries to the spine account for approximately 30% of all golf ailments, with the vast majority of these specifically affecting the lumbar spine.[8,10,14,45] Several factors are likely responsible for the apparent high incidence of lower back injuries among golfers, including the forceful nature of the full golf swing, which clearly incorporates considerable spinal movement. In general terms, the golf swing involves a slow deliberate rotation of the trunk away from the target on the backswing followed by a very powerful rotation of the trunk toward the left (right-handed golfer) on the downswing. Although it is clear that other spinal motions besides rotation occur during a golf swing, aggressive axial twisting has been identified as a significant risk factor for low back disorders in occupational settings.[47]

Clinical Point

Thirty percent of golf injuries primarily occur to the lumbar spine and predominantly on the trail side with compressive leads up to eight times the golfer's body weight being applied.

Hosea and colleagues[48] calculated the compressive, shear, lateral-bending, and rotational loads on the L3-4 segment of the lumbar spine during golf swings using a five iron. Kinetic, kinematic, and surface electromyography (EMG) data were collected from four professional (mean age: 37 yr) and four amateur (mean age: 34 yr) golfers. The authors concluded that, except for compressive load, professional golfers produced less spinal loads than amateur players. The average compressive load for amateurs and professionals was 6100 N and 7584 N, respectively, which represents forces equivalent to approximately 8 times the golfer's body weight. In comparison, running produces spinal compression forces equal to approximately 3 times the runner's body weight.[9] It is worth noting that cadaveric studies have shown disc prolapse to occur with compressive loads of approximately 5500 N.[49] The complex, rapid, and intense nature of the spinal loads associated with the golf swing led Hosea and colleagues[48] to conclude that preparticipation conditioning, reasonable practice habits, and proper warm-up were important for preventing low back pain (LBP) from golf.

It appears the golf swing produces sufficient force to potentially create traumatic injury to the lumbar spine. However, even when the back survives a well-struck golf shot without any apparent ill-effect, it is possible that undetected microtearing of the lumbar structures may still occur. This is referred to as the *cumulative load theory*.[50] The cumulative load theory takes into account the total stress placed on the system over time. Kumar[51] reported that workers who developed LBP were found to have consistently worked for more hours over their lifetimes than their pain-free colleagues, supporting the cumulative load theory. Because many golfers (particularly elite players) identify overuse as the cause of their LBP,[13] the high frequency of swing repetitions combined with large-magnitude spinal forces likely results in lower back injury through the cumulative load process. Lindsay and Horton[52] showed that players who consistently suffered LBP during golfing activities tended to have a higher frequency of swing repetitions (i.e., spent more time playing and practicing) than healthy golfers.

The kinetic results of Hosea and colleagues' study[48] showed that the golf swing produces considerable (and likely cumulative) stress on the lower back. Sugaya and colleagues,[53] in a survey of 283 Japanese professional golfers, reported that LBP predominantly occurred on the trail (i.e., right) side. Furthermore, radiological investigations of elite players revealed a significantly higher rate of trail-side vertebral body and facet joint arthritic change than age-matched control subjects. The authors concluded that both the repetitive and asymmetric nature of the golf swing contributed to LBP and injury in elite golfers. Morgan and colleagues[54] used the term *crunch factor* to describe the instantaneous product of lumbar right side–bend angle and left axial rotation velocity that occurred during the golf downswing. Both axial rotation velocity and side-bending angles reached peak values almost simultaneously and just after ball impact—which coincided when the majority of players in their cohort reported experiencing LBP. They concluded a high crunch factor (i.e., during and after the impact phase) was damaging to the lumbar spine, resulting in injury and pain particularly on the trail side. Maximum right side–bend angles and left rotation velocities on the downswing have been measured at approximately 30° and 200° per second respectively.[22,25]

Research on industrial workers by Marras and colleagues[55] has also shown that only small amounts of side-bending combined with rotation are classified as high-risk for back injury. The combination of side-bending with rotation creates a large amount of intervertebral lateral shear. This shearing motion is potentially harmful because it is resisted primarily by disc strength rather than bony architecture.[55] Furthermore, Tall and DeVault[56] found that the most common cause of disc herniation in a healthy disc was lateral bending combined with compression and torsion. Based on these findings, it is not unexpected that the very nature of the golf swing could lead to disc irritation and subsequent injury.

Lindsay and Horton,[52] in their investigation of spinal kinematics, were unable to show any difference in the "crunch factor" magnitudes between elite golfers with and without LBP. The authors did show that golfers with LBP tended to address the ball with more spinal flexion, used more left side–bend during the backswing, and tended to use considerably more rotation ROM during the follow-through than the maximum rotation ROM that these same players were able to demonstrate in a clinical setting from a neutral posture and controlled speed. The authors suggested that spinal irritation and pain could result from this relative over-rotation of the spine while performing the golf swing. In a single case study design, Grimshaw and Burden[57] reported

successfully eliminating golf-related LBP in a professional golfer by increasing the range of hip turn on the backswing to reduce the relative amount of spinal rotation or torsion. Other coaching changes included reducing the amount of trunk flexion and lateral flexion during the downswing.

Bulbulian and colleagues[58] also postulated that excessive rotation of the trunk during the golf swing could contribute to LBP. These authors investigated using a shortened backswing on ball-contact accuracy, clubhead speed and EMG activity of select trunk and shoulder muscles. Results showed that restricting the backswing by almost 20% had no negative effect on swing performance (e.g., ball-contact accuracy and clubhead speed). Furthermore, there was a significant decrease in EMG root-mean square activity of the right abdominal external oblique muscle on the downswing, which the authors suggested would decrease low back stress. However the shorter swing tended to increase shoulder muscle activation, which could in turn increase shoulder injury susceptibility.

It has been speculated that golfers with LBP may use key trunk muscles such as the abdominals differently during the downswing phase than golfers without LBP.[34] Horton and colleagues[36] attempted to quantify abdominal muscle activity during the golf swings of elite golfers with and without LBP. Results indicated that the magnitude of the muscle activity for the rectus abdominis, external oblique, and internal oblique did not differ significantly between those golfers with LBP and those without. However, the authors found onset times of major bursts of activity from some of the abdominal muscles were delayed in the golfers suffering LBP. In particular, the lead external oblique (left in right-handed golfers) was activated significantly later during the backswing in the golfers with LBP when compared with the asymptomatic controls. Furthermore, lead internal oblique onset times on the downswing were also delayed in the chronic LBP golfers, although this difference did not reach statistical significance. In a related study investigating spinal kinematics, Lindsay and Horton[52] reported that golfers without LBP demonstrated more than twice as much trunk flexion velocity on the downswing compared with the golfers with LBP. They went on to suggest that golfers without LBP may use their anterior trunk muscles (i.e., abdominal muscles) to a greater degree on the downswing than golfers with LBP. However, results from a study by Cole and Grimshaw[59] investigating the magnitude of trunk muscle activity in a small number of golfers with and without LBP showed that, in general, the low-handicap LBP golfers demonstrated reduced erector spinae activity and *increased* external oblique activity during the downswing compared with their asymptomatic counterparts.

The EMG findings of Horton and colleagues[36] plus Cole and Grimshaw[59] do not appear to support the speculation that golfers with LBP do not activate their abdominal muscles to the same magnitude as healthy golfers. However, it is interesting to note that several studies have demonstrated decreased abdominal muscle strength and endurance performance in golfers suffering LBP.[60-62] It is possible the observed deficiencies in abdominal strength and endurance could be a reflection of lower activity levels from these muscles. Furthermore, Archambault and colleagues[63] recommended the use of a *stabilized-spine* golf swing to facilitate the use of the abdominal and other large trunk muscles to control LBP during the swing motion. This technique involves setting up with a "proper" spine angle and initiating the backswing with the hips and shoulders moving together. Kinetic testing showed the stabilized-spine swing significantly increased trunk rotation velocity on the downswing while reducing spinal lateral bending force, shear force, and compression force, as well as axial torsion force compared with a more traditional "modern" golf swing.

Clinical Relevance Summary – The Spine

- Average spinal compressive loads for the golf swing are equivalent to approximately eight times the golfer's body weight which, in cadaveric studies, is sufficient to cause disc prolapse.
- The asymmetrical nature of the golf swing may cause increased trail (right) side vertebral body and facet joint arthritic change, which may relate to increased right side–bend range of motion during and just after impact.
- Golfers with low back pain address the ball with more spinal flexion and tend to over-rotate their spines during the follow-through based on the maximum rotation range of motion these same players were able to demonstrate in a clinical setting.
- Golfers suffering low back pain demonstrate delayed abdominal muscle recruitment. They also show abdominal muscle weakness, which may reflect poor recruitment strategies during the swing.

Upper Limb Biomechanics and Injury Relationships

Biomechanical investigation of the upper limbs in golf is limited to kinematic and muscle activation studies. Kinetics, which describes the resultant joint forces and torques that occur during the golf swing, are typically measured via force transducers or force plates, which is partly why this method of investigation has limited application for the upper limbs. Also, in golf, it is very difficult to separate upper limb moments because both hands grip the club, thus creating a closed kinetic chain linking the movements of the body to the forces ultimately imparted on the golf ball. As a result of the lack of quantifiable data on upper limb forces, the influence of swing technique on upper limb joint loads and hence injury susceptibility is not as clear as it is for the spine and lower body.

Epidemiological data on golf injuries shows some variation among studies, but from a general perspective the upper limbs account for approximately 50% of the injury totals.[2,8,10,12,45] Furthermore, it appears from these studies

that there is a fairly similar distribution of upper limb injuries between the shoulder, elbow, and the wrist and hand. However, there appears to be some regional differences in injury susceptibility depending on the demographic profile of the golfers being studied. For example, elite golfers (i.e., tour professionals) appear more susceptible to wrist problems,[8,13] whereas recreational golfers, particularly men, are more likely to suffer elbow injury.[8,10] Meanwhile, McCarroll and Mallon[64] reported that most shoulder injuries from golf occurred in older players.

Clinical Point

In golf, 50% of the injuries occur to the upper limb.

The following section examines some of the specific biomechanical factors associated with the golf swing that may contribute to injury problems in the various major joints composing the upper limbs.

Shoulder

It has previously been mentioned that both shoulder joints undergo considerable ROM during a full golf swing. However, injury data suggests the lead shoulder is more susceptible to problems compared with the trail side. For example, McCarroll and Gioe[13] reported that injuries to the lead shoulder occurred three times more often than to the trail side among professional players. Other authors have estimated that as many as 90% of all golf-related shoulder injuries occur to the lead side.[65] This suggests that there is something inherent in the technique of the golf swing contributing to increased lead shoulder stress.

McCarroll and Mallon[64] reported that injury to the lead shoulder typically occurred during the transition between the backswing and downswing and often involved the rotator cuff muscles. Injuries to the rotator cuff are especially prevalent among middle-aged and senior golfers.[66,67] Rotator cuff muscles serve to both rotate and stabilize the normally loose glenohumeral joint. Several researchers have studied rotator cuff muscle function during the golf swing.[65,68,69] In all cases, these researchers found relatively low but constant EMG activity from the rotator cuff external rotator muscle groups (i.e., infraspinatus and supraspinatus) during the downswing. However, high levels of EMG activity were noted from the lead side internal rotator subscapularis muscle during the initial downswing even though this shoulder joint was powerfully rotating in the opposite (i.e., external rotation) direction. The range of activity varied from 41% maximum voluntary contraction (MVC) to almost 60% MVC[65,68] at the initiation of the downswing and progressed to even higher levels at the midpoint of the downswing. This level of activity from an antagonistic muscle suggests a high stability or protection function for the lead-side subscapularis muscle.[65] Shoulder injury could result from either a reduction in the stability function (e.g., weakness) of the rotator cuff or from excessive activity (and hence load) from other larger shoulder muscles.

> ### Clinical Point
>
> Most shoulder injuries in golf occur during the transition between the backswing and downswing.

One factor that could cause a detrimental increase in shoulder load is an inappropriate kinematic sequence resulting in overcompensation from the shoulder muscles to produce acceptable clubhead speed.[17,70] It has also been shown that a shortened backswing resulting from a reduction in the amount of trunk rotation caused an increase in EMG activity from the large pectoralis major shoulder muscles.[58] These researchers cautioned that this may lead to increased shoulder injury susceptibility. It is interesting to note that shoulder injuries appear more common among older golfers,[14] and that older golfers use less trunk rotation on the backswing.[71]

Elbow

Elbow injury among golfers is sufficiently recognized that the term *golfer's elbow* is an established medical condition (medial epicondylitis). However, tennis elbow (lateral epicondylitis) from golf reportedly occurs five times more often than golfer's elbow.[10] Although it appears that injury to the elbow from golf-related activities is common, little research of any kind, let alone biomechanical study, has been conducted in this area.

Golf-related lateral epicondylitis occurs most frequently on the lead (left) elbow, whereas medial epicondylitis usually occurs on the trailing elbow.[2] Both conditions may result from a single traumatic incident or overuse creating cumulative load and microtearing of the structures that attach to the respective epicondyles.[2,72] A well-executed full golf shot always involves some form of sudden deceleration at impact as the club makes contact with the ball, ground, or both. These decelerations produce a varus and valgus moment about the lead and trail elbows respectively. These moments are resisted by traction to noncontractile soft-tissue restraints (e.g., joint capsule, ligaments) particularly on the lead side of each elbow and by the dynamic contractile structures overlying the lateral and medial joint surfaces. Varus stress to the lateral aspect of the lead elbow is controlled by contraction of the muscles composing the common extensor mechanism (i.e., radial and ulnar extensors

of the wrist, extensor digitorum, extensor digiti minimi, and the supinator). Valgus stress to the medial side of the trail elbow is resisted by contraction of the common flexor origin muscles (i.e., radial and ulnar flexors of the wrist, flexor digitorum and profundus, as well as pronator teres). Weakness or premature fatigue of these muscles may diminish the ability of these muscles to control the varus and valgus loads and result in injury to the underlying capsular and ligamentous structures.[72]

> ### Clinical Point
>
> Weakness or premature fatigue of the forearm muscles may diminish the ability of these muscles to control the varus and valgus loads on the elbow and result in injury.

Increases in varus and valgus elbow stress may also occur from an especially sudden deceleration of the clubhead such as that encountered when hitting a buried object such as a rock or tree root through impact.[2] Another factor influencing elbow (and wrist) stress is how the hands are positioned on the golf grip. The use of a *neutral* grip (see the next paragraph) is regarded as extremely important for reducing the risk of suffering elbow pain from golf.[21] Positioning the lower (right) hand in a *stronger*, more supinated position on the golf club tends to increase the valgus load to the trail elbow. Likewise, positioning the upper (left) hand in a *weaker*, more supinated position increases the varus load on the lead elbow. See Figure 9-2 for an illustration of lower hand placements.

The *correct* or *neutral* golf grip means both hands, at address, are placed on the club in such a manner that the wrist, elbow, and shoulder joints are in relatively relaxed resting positions. This neutral position allows adequate and

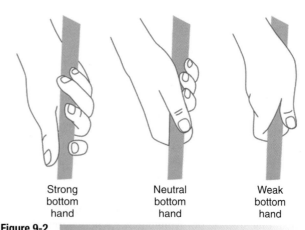

| Strong bottom hand | Neutral bottom hand | Weak bottom hand |

Figure 9-2

Terminologies associated with variations in lower hand positions on the golf club. (Reproduced with permission. Fit Fore Golf Inc.)

synchronous wrist ROM during the backswing and downswing to properly position the club face at impact.[21] Because of individual anatomic variations, the neutral grip does not look exactly the same on every golfer. As each hand is placed on the club, the direction of the line formed between the thumb and proximal portion of the index finger should be noted. This line (on both hands) should be aimed somewhere between the trail-side eye and acromioclavicular joint (Figure 9-3).

In addition to hand position, grip tension is thought to be a very important risk factor for elbow and forearm pain.[18] Gripping the club with excessive tension in the fingers increases the eccentric load on the wrist extensor (lead) and flexor (trail) muscles as the clubhead makes contact with the ball and ground at impact. This potentially excessive muscular loading may result in cumulative microtearing at the common origin of the wrist extensor and flexor muscles (lateral and medial epicondyles respectively) and result in subsequent pain. A preliminary investigation into grip pressures by Broker and Ramey[73] showed that less-skilled amateur golfers tended to grip the golf club with greater force than highly skilled players. This may partially account for the almost sixfold increase in elbow injuries among recreational golfers compared with professional players.[74]

Clinical Point

Lateral epicondylitis is more likely to be seen in the lead elbow, whereas medical epicondylitis is more common in the trailing elbow.

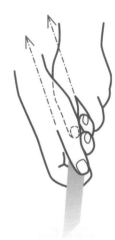

Neutral grip

Figure 9-3
Lines formed between thumb and first finger aligned between eye and shoulder region on trail side. (Reproduced with permission. Fit Fore Golf Inc.)

Another mechanism contributing to additional loading on the lead elbow pertains to the amount the left elbow remains flexed at the top of the backswing. Biomechanical research by Zheng and colleagues[70] found that less-skilled (i.e., recreational) golfers demonstrated increased lead-side elbow flexion compared with elite players. As the downswing proceeds, muscular contraction forces as well as centrifugal forces tend to straighten the elbows (and wrists) through impact. This relatively violent straightening of the lead elbow at impact likely produces considerable joint compression stress and potential microtrauma (Figure 9-4).

Wrist and Hand

The wrist and hand represent the final (i.e., most distal) hinge in the chain of body segments composing the golf swing kinematic sequence,[16,23] and as such are associated with the largest rotational velocities (approximately 1000 m/s).[31,75] Furthermore, the wrist joints are subjected to large-amplitude ROM during the downswing and follow-through. For example, Cahalan and colleagues[29] recorded wrist flexion and extension ROM in a population of healthy golfers of approximately 35 degrees and 103 degrees respectively in the lead (left) and trail sides. Radial and ulnar deviation ROM totals were 36 degrees and 31 degrees respectively for the lead and trail wrist joints.

This combination of large amounts of wrist angle on the downswing and the timing of the wrist release is critical for producing a highly efficient swing. Robinson[76] reported that 60% of the variation in clubhead speed between recreational and elite golfers can be predicted by knowing the magnitude of the angle between the left forearm and the club shaft at the midpoint of the downswing (Figure 9-5). This angle is the result of radial deviation of the wrists. In other words, elite golfers tend to incorporate more radial deviation at the top of the backswing and delay the release of this angle much later in the downswing.[17,21] Excessive repetition of the high-velocity, large-amplitude wrist release likely produces considerable stress on the wrist structures and increases injury susceptibility, particularly among professional

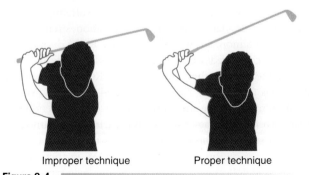

Improper technique   Proper technique

Figure 9-4
Excessive lead elbow flexing can cause tennis elbow. (Reproduced with permission. Fit Fore Golf Inc.)

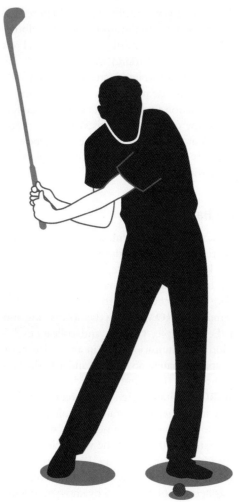

Figure 9-5
Angle between the lead arm and the golf club at the midpoint of the downswing is important for producing clubhead speed. (Reproduced with permission. Fit Fore Golf Inc.)

Other Rehabilitation Considerations

Biomechanical analyses show the golf swing to be a very complex dynamic asymmetrical movement involving powerful muscle contractions and extreme ROMs. Previous sections have discussed the association between certain biomechanical factors and injury susceptibility, but there still remain other factors that may assist health care providers to manage and prevent golf injuries. In particular, the influences of equipment factors on biomechanical risk factors as well as the role of an appropriate warm-up for preventing golf injuries are discussed.

Equipment Considerations

There are at least three equipment factors that health care providers should consider when rehabilitating injured golfers: whether the golf club is properly matched to the golfer, the type of surface used by the golfer to hit balls from when practicing, and the type of footwear used when hitting full shots.

players.[8,13] This stress may be amplified if the player uses an inappropriate grip at the set-up or swings at the ball using an overly steep descending swing path.[77]

In addition to overuse, a lack of wrist strength and flexibility may further predispose a golfer to increased injury risk. Cahalan and colleagues[29] noted that golfers suffering forearm and wrist pain demonstrated less supination strength and actually used more left wrist frontal plane ROM during their swing as compared with healthy golfers (68° versus 36°), despite the fact that they had less passive ROM in these same directions (61° versus 75°). This limited passive ROM and strength may increase stress on the ulnar-carpal junction and triangular fibrocartilage complex as the left wrist ulnarly deviates and supinates through impact. It is interesting to note that the association between wrist ROM restriction and weakness in golfers with wrist pain has also been reported for trunk rotation ROM restriction[52] and weakness[62] in golfers with LBP.

Golf clubs represent the critical link between the human body and the golf ball. When golfers use clubs that are not well-suited to their particular physical dimensions or swing characteristics, the body is forced to compensate. As mentioned, the spine is particularly susceptible to injury from golf and as such needs to be protected during the swing. Golfers who suffer LBP tend to address the ball with more spinal flexion.[52] Increased spinal flexion at set-up may result from not using the hip joints to tilt the trunk forward when addressing the clubhead behind the ball or from using a golf club that is too short. For men, the standard club length is reportedly designed for someone 70 inches (178 cm) in height, whereas for women this number is 64 inches (163 cm). However, these industry standards appear to be based more on tradition than scientific testing. Also, it is interesting to note that most major equipment manufacturers only offer a range of approximately 2.7 to 3.1 inches (7-8 cm) in the length of the shafts when "fitting" golf clubs to new customers. However, the range in overall vertical height of these customers would be more in the vicinity of 12 inches (30 cm). This variation suggests that a golfer who is quite tall will likely receive a proportionately shorter shaft (resulting in increased flexion when setting up to the ball) than a much shorter golfer even though in both instances they were fitted with the shaft length that was "recommended" by the manufacturer for their respective sizes.

There is biomechanical evidence that the length of the club shaft can affect spinal biomechanics. Neal and colleagues[78] reported on the effects of using an inappropriately matched golf club on spinal swing mechanics. The authors found that using a club with a shaft that was 2 inches (5 cm) shorter than the recommended length resulted in approximately 4° less spinal rotation at the top of the backswing, and 8° more flexion at impact. However, these numbers were not part of a specific scientific investigation and were based on a single golfer. Lindsay and colleagues[22] completed an investigation comparing spinal mechanics among elite golfers using a driver and 7-iron. The purpose was to investigate the changes in set-up posture and spinal motion during the swing caused by the different length clubs. The 7-iron is approximately 18 cm shorter than the driver. The address position flexion angles recorded in this study using the 7-iron (35.1° ± 12.8°) were significantly higher than the driver results (28.9° ± 10.9°). During the actual swing, greater maximum flexion and side-bend ROM were observed when using the 7-iron. The explanation for increased side-bending when swinging the 7-iron may relate to the effect of the shorter club on swing plane. *Swing plane* refers to the oblique plane the golf club is moved through during the swing. The shorter-length 7-iron typically requires the ball to be positioned closer to the body and the spine to be more flexed than when using the driver. This combination necessitates a more vertical orientation of the 7-iron shaft during the set-up as well as during the actual swing, compared with the driver. As the club is accelerated, the linear forces associated with a more vertical or steeper swing plane tend to drive the hips and trunk laterally, resulting in an increase in thoracolumbar side-bend motion. Side-bending of the spine during the golf swing has been postulated as a contributing factor to low back injury.[53,71]

These studies appear to show, from a general perspective, that shorter clubs produce additional loading on the lower spine, which may contribute to LBP. However this is the case only if the shorter and longer clubs were swung with similar intensity. A *matching set* of golf clubs includes as many as 14 different clubs, all of which are a different length. The reason is that each club has a unique purpose that varies between how far the club can hit the ball and the desired accuracy of the shot. This is why certain clubs, such as wedges, are referred to as *scoring clubs* if the intention is to be as accurate as possible. In comparison, the driver club is expected to hit the ball the longest distance possible and as such is manufactured with a much longer shaft than the wedge. Results from Neal and colleagues[78] and Lindsay and colleagues[22] might suggest that the shorter length clubs (i.e., wedge) produce more harmful stresses on the lower back. However, these shorter clubs are typically not swung as hard as a "distance club" such as a driver, which in turn would tend to reduce the magnitude of the spinal load. The important message for health care providers is to at least question golfers suffering from LBP on whether their clubs were measured for their particular body dimensions (called *club fitting*). More specifically, golfers with LBP should not use clubs that are shorter than the length recommended by the manufacturer for their particular body dimensions. All golf clubs can relatively easily and inexpensively be adjusted for length by appropriately trained staff at most golf courses or golf retail outlets.

It has been mentioned that repetitive practice is essential for consistent performance. Often such practice involves hitting full golf shots off hard artificial surfaces such as driving range mats. Contact between the golf club and the driving range mat before, during, or after ball impact is another possible contributing factor to upper limb stress and potential injury from golf activity. Repetitive and excessive loading may contribute to injuries such as wrist tendinopathy, elbow epicondylitis, and rotator cuff strain.[9,67] A number of manufacturers produce simulated turf mats, and there are typically two main types installed at practice facilities. One type is a solid mat that incorporates a thin layer of a durable synthetic turf that is implanted or glued onto a 30-mm thick base composed of dense foam. The other common mat consists of a pliable brushlike surface composed of closely packed vertical strands of nylon fibers (approximately 40 mm long) set into a hard polymer base (Figure 9-6). Although there is a lack of kinetic data comparing upper limb impact forces using different artificial mats, Lindsay and colleagues[79] did compare the perceived impact forces, upper limb stress, quality of shots, and similarity to hitting from grass between the two most common

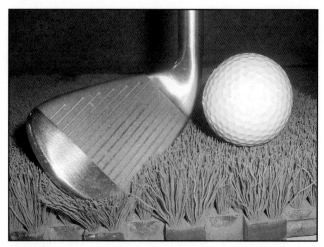

Figure 9-6
Brush fiber mat.

types of hitting mats. Results from this study showed that perceptual differences clearly exist in how different types of practice mats affect upper limb stress and the quality of golf shots. A minimum of 80% of the study participants selected the brush fiber mat over the solid mat in terms of the comfort and quality of the hitting experience. The largest perceived difference between mats pertained to upper limb stress, with almost 91% of subjects stating they felt the brush fiber mat produced the least stress during impact.

The ground reaction forces that occur under a golfer's feet are another source of potential stress from golf, particularly to the lower limbs. These forces are influenced by a number of factors, including the type of shoe being worn. Worsfold and colleagues[39] reported that rotation torques under the front (i.e., left) foot were typically approximately 2 to 3 times higher than those under the trail foot when executing full shots. The peak magnitude of this torque coincides with a rapid shift of weight onto the lead side.[79] This rotational force and weight shift occurs while the front foot remains firmly anchored to the ground, usually with specially designed "spikes" attached to the undersurface of the shoe. Recently, a golf shoe has been designed and marketed in which the upper portion of the lead-side shoe can "release" or rotate farther toward the target than the soleplate portion of the same shoe. An interesting biomechanical case study carried out at the Sports Science Institute of the Eberhard Karls University in Tübingen, Germany, was able to show that the shoe released after impact, and, as such, did not affect the kinematics of the back and downswings. However, at the finish position, the free-release mechanism allowed the left foot to turn approximately 20° to 25° farther toward the target than when the foot was constrained within a standard golf shoe. This release of the shoe decreased the amount of lead-hip internal rotation at the finish position by approximately 10° and decreased spinal rotation by approximately 5°. The manufacturer claims that this results in a considerable decrease in the

force moments about the ankle, knee, hip, and spine, which in turn decreases the risk of injury to these areas (http://www.united-golfers.de/). Further research is needed to substantiate the proposed benefits from this unique shoe design. However, based on this information, it is reasonable for health care providers to caution golfers with lower limb injuries from playing in shoes that excessively anchor their feet to the ground.

Warmup Considerations

The powerful movements making up the typical full golf swing are repeated 100 or more times per practice session or game, resulting in considerable stress being generated and dissipated during each of these sessions. Owing to these stresses, it seems logical that an adequate warmup routine should be performed prior to playing or practicing. However, research suggests that most golfers do not perform an adequate warmup, especially seniors who often contend with both age-related changes in the musculoskeletal system and chronic conditions such as osteoarthritis.[5,80]

The purpose of the warmup is to physiologically and psychologically prepare the body for competition while at the same time reducing the risk of injury. Palmer and colleagues[81] examined the typical warmup habits of a convenience sample of Canadian golfers, both men and women, with an average age of 70 years. Less than 25% of the 100 recreational players surveyed spent more than 5 minutes stretching and warming up prior to playing. Fradkin and colleagues,[82] in a survey of 304 golfers in the United States, found that only 18% of the sample performed an adequate warmup. The authors also reported that golfers who did not adequately warm up were 1.3 times more likely to have suffered a golf-related injury. Gosheger and colleagues[8] also reported that only 19% of golfers surveyed in their European study warmed up appropriately, and that these golfers reported 60% fewer injuries than the golfers who did not warm up.

An appropriate warmup should last a minimum of 10 minutes and can be broken down into four sections.[80,82] The first involves low-intensity activity that uses as many of the large muscle groups as possible. Examples include brisk walking, climbing a flight of stairs, or carefully rotating the trunk from side to side with a golf club held behind the back. One very good tip for golfers is to park at the far end of the parking lot when they arrive at the golf course, thus using the walk to the clubhouse to assist with the warmup process. The next component of the warmup involves stretching the key muscles used in the golf swing (i.e., muscles of the back, hip, neck, shoulders, and forearms). Pregame stretching exercises for golf can be found at www.fitforegolf.com. The third component involves dynamic stretching and may be accomplished by initially swinging a short iron back and forth and progressing by gently swinging two clubs at once. It is important, due to the asymmetrical nature of the full swing, for warmup swings to be performed *both left and right handed* to optimize muscle balance and coordination. The final part of the warmup involves practicing actual shots. This further helps warm up the golf muscles and facilitates timing and consistency. Players should be instructed to start with a short club such as a wedge and begin by hitting only shots that travel approximately 20 yards. The length of the shots should increase progressively, followed by using other clubs that produce different trajectories and distance.

Clinical Relevance Summary - Equipment

- Golf equipment, in particular shaft length, should be matched to the size of the golfer using the equipment.
- Using a set of clubs that are too short causes an increase in spinal flexion throughout the swing. This produces a steeper swing plane, resulting in increased thoracolumbar side-bend motion on the downswing, which increases the risk of suffering an injury to the lower back.
- Hitting golf balls off a brush fiber mat at the practice range is perceived to be more like hitting from grass and produces less stress on the upper limbs compared with a more solid hitting mat.
- Golf shoes that allow the front foot to release or rotate farther toward the target after impact can potentially reduce the range of motion magnitude (and hence stress) on the spine and lead hip at the completion of the swing.
- Most golfers do not perform an adequate warmup prior to playing. A proper warmup should last at least 10 minutes and should include a general body warmup, static stretching, dynamic stretching, and progressive practice shots. An effective warmup routine is particularly important for the senior golfer, whose age-related musculoskeletal changes result in increased stiffness and susceptibility to soft-tissue injuries.

Conclusion

Golf has both real health benefits as well as certain injury risks, particularly to the upper limbs and spine. Many of these injuries occur as a result of overuse in combination with biomechanical swing flaws creating unnecessary stress on certain parts of the body. Therefore, it is important for health care providers treating injured golfers to investigate factors such as swing technique when determining appropriate rehabilitation strategies. Correction of biomechanical deficiencies in a player's swing does not rest exclusively on the health care provider, but often involves collaboration between the health care provider and a certified golf coach. Although the recognition and correction of swing flaws causing excessive stress on a golfer's body are very important, it is also clear that other factors including equipment and appropriate warmup also play a role. Because golf is

often played in a group of four individuals, Figure 9-7 metaphorically represents the "foursome" of management strategies for injured golfers. The effective implementation of a combination of the various elements outlined in Figure 9-7 will not only help the injured player get back on the golf course in the shortest time possible but, just as importantly, will likely prevent the injury from recurring in the future.

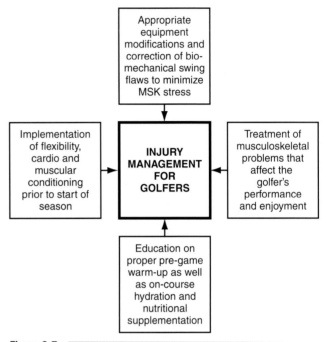

Figure 9-7
The "foursome" of management strategies for injured golfers. (Reproduced with permission. D. Lindsay and A. Vandervoort.)

References

1. Farrally MR, Cochran AJ, Crews DJ, et al: Golf science research at the beginning of the twenty-first century, *J Sports Sci* 21:753–765, 2003.
2. Thériault G, Lachance P: Golf injuries: An overview, *Sports Med* 26:43–57, 1998.
3. Parkkari J, Natri A, Kannus P, et al: A controlled trial of the health benefits of regular walking on a golf course, *Am J Sport Med* 109:102–108, 2000.
4. Sell TC, Abt JP, Lephart SM: Physical activity-related benefits of walking during golf. In Crews DS, Lutz RS, editors: *Science and golf V.* Proceedings of the Fifth World Scientific Congress of Golf, Mesa, AZ, 2008, Energy in Motion.
5. Versteegh TH, Vandervoort AA, Lindsay DM, Lynn SK: Fitness, performance and injury prevention strategies for the senior golfer, *Ann Rev Golf Coach* 2:199–214, 2008.
6. Cann AP, Lindsay DM, Vandervoort AA: Optimizing the benefits versus risks of golf participation by older people, *J Geriatr Phys Ther* 28:85–92, 2005.
7. Nesbit SM, Serrano M: Work and power analysis of the golf swing, *J Sports Sci Med* 4:520–533, 2005.
8. Gosheger G, Liem D, Ludwig K, et al: Injuries and overuse syndromes in golf, *Am J Sports Med* 31:438–443, 2003.

9. McHardy A, Pollard H, Luo K: Golf injuries: A review of the literature, *Sports Med* 36:171–187, 2006.

10. McCarroll JR, Rettig AC, Shelbourne KD: Injuries in the amateur golfer, *Phys Sportsmed* 18:122–126, 1990.

11. McCarroll JR: The frequency of golf injuries, *Clin Sport Med* 15:1–7, 1996.

12. Fradkin AJ, Windley TC, Myers JB, et al: Describing the epidemiology and associated age, gender and handicap comparisons among golfing injuries, *Int J Inj Contr Safety Prom* 14:264–266, 2007.

13. McCarroll JR, Gioe TJ: Professional golfers and the price they pay, *Phys Sportsmed* 10:64–70, 1982.

14. McNicholas MJ, Neilsen A, Knill-Jones RP: Golf injuries in Scotland. In Farrally MR, Cochran AJ, editors: *Science and golf III*: Proceedings of the World Scientific Congress of Golf, Champaign, IL, 1999, Human Kinetics.

15. Duda M: Golf injuries: They really do happen, *Phys Sportsmed* 15:191–196, 1987.

16. Cochran AJ, Stobbs J: *The search for the perfect swing*, Philadelphia, 1968, Lippincott.

17. Lindsay DM, Mantrop S, Vandervoort AA: A review of biomechanical differences between golfers of varied skill levels, *Ann Rev Golf Coaching* 2:187–197, 2008.

18. Adlington GS: Proper swing technique and biomechanics of golf, *Clin Sport Med* 15:9–26, 1996.

19. Mann R, Griffin F, Locum G: *Swing like a pro: The breakthrough method of perfecting your golf swing*, New York, 1998, Broadway Books.

20. Okuda I, Armstrong CW: Biomechanical analysis of professional golfer's swing. In Thain E, editor: *Science and golf IV*: Proceedings of the World Scientific Congress of Golf, London, 2002, Routledge.

21. Hume PA, Keogh J, Reid D: The role of biomechanics in maximizing distance and accuracy of golf shots, *Sports Med* 35:429–449, 2005.

22. Lindsay DM, Horton JF, Paley RD: Trunk motion of male professional golfers using two different golf clubs, *J Appl Biomech* 18:366–373, 2002.

23. Cheetham PJ, Martin PE, Mottram RE, St Laurent BF: The importance of stretching the X-factor in the downswing of golf. In Thomas PR, editor: *Optimizing performance in golf*, Brisbane, 2001, Australian Academic Press.

24. Burden AM, Grimshaw PN, Wallace ES: Hip and shoulder rotations during the golf swing of sub-10 handicap players, *J Sports Sci* 16:165–176, 1998.

25. McTeigue M, Lamb SR, Mottram R, Pirozzolo F: Spine and hip motion analysis during the golf swing. In Cochran AJ, Farrally MR, editors: *Science and golf II*: Proceedings of the World Scientific Congress of Golf, London, 1994, E & FN SPON.

26. Wheat JS, Vernon T, Milner CE: The measurement of upper body alignment during the golf drive, *J Sports Sci* 25:749–755, 2007.

27. Wallace ES, Graham D, Bleakley EW: Foot-to-ground pressure patterns during the golf drive: A case study involving a low handicap player and a high handicap player. In Cochran AJ, editor: *Science and golf*: Proceedings of the First World Scientific Congress of Golf, London, 1990, E & FN SPON.

28. Mitchell K, Banks S, Morgan D, Sugaya H: Shoulder motions during the golf swing in male amateur golfers, *J Orthop Sport Phys Ther* 33:196–203, 2003.

29. Cahalan TD, Cooney WP, Tamai K, Chao EYS: Biomechanics of the golf swing in players with pathological conditions of the forearm, wrist and hand, *Am J Sport Med* 19:288–293, 1991.

30. McCarroll JR: Overuse injuries of the upper extremity in golf, *Clin Sports Med* 20:469–479, 2001.

31. Neal R, Lumsden R, Holland M, Mason M: Body segment sequencing and timing in golf, *Ann Rev Golf Coach* 1:25–36, 2007.

32. Putnam CA: Sequential motions of body segments in striking and throwing skills, *J Biomech* 26:125–135, 1993.

33. Bechler JR, Jobe FW, Pink M, et al: Electromyographic analysis of the hip and knee during the golf swing, *Clin J Sport Med* 5:162–166, 1995.

34. Watkins RG: Dynamic electromyographic analysis of trunk musculature in professional golfers, *Am J Sport Med* 24:535–538, 1996.

35. Lim TY: *Lower trunk muscle activities during the golf swing—Pilot study*, Proceedings of the third North American Congress on Biomechanics, Waterloo, August 14–18, 1998.

36. Horton JF, Lindsay DM, MacIntosh BR: Abdominal muscle characteristics of elite male golfers with and without chronic low back pain, *Med Sci Sports Exerc* 33:1647–1654, 2001.

37. Pink M, Perry J, Jobe FW: Electromyographic analysis of the trunk in golfers, *Am J Sport Med* 21:385–388, 1993.

38. McHardy A, Pollard H: Muscle activity during the golf swing, *Br J Sport Med* 39:799–804, 2005.

39. Worsfold P, Smith NA, Dyson RJ: Low handicap golfers generate more torque at the shoe-natural grass interface when using a driver, *J Sports Sci Med* 7:408–414, 2008.

40. Barrentine SW, Fleisig GS, Johnson H: Ground reaction forces and torques of professional and amateur golfers. In Cochran AJ, Farrally MR, editors: *Science and golf II*: Proceedings of the World Scientific Congress of Golf, London, 1994, E & FN SPON.

41. Welch CM, Banks SA, Cook FF, Draovich P: Hitting a baseball: A biomechanical description, *J Orthop Sports Phys Ther* 22:93–201, 1995.

42. Hellstrom J, Tinmark F: The association between stability and swing kinematics of skilled high school golfers. In Crews DS, Lutz RS, editors: *Science and golf V*: Proceedings of the Fifth World Scientific Congress of Golf, Mesa, AZ, 2008, Energy in Motion.

43. Fitzgerald RH: Acetabular labral tears: Diagnosis and treatment, *Clin Orthop* 311:60–68, 1995.

44. Gatt CJ, Pavol MJ, Parker RD, Grabiner MD: A kinetic analysis of the knees during a golf swing. In Farrally MR, Cochran AJ, editors: *Science and golf III*: Proceedings of the World Scientific Congress of Golf, Champaign, IL, 1999, Human Kinetics.

45. Batt ME: A survey of golf injuries in amateur golfers, *Br J Sport Med* 26:63–65, 1992.

46. Lynn SK, MacKenzie H, Vandervoort AA: Frontal plane knee moments during the golf swing: Effect of target side foot position at address. In Crews DS, Lutz RS, editors: *Science and golf V*: Proceedings of the World Scientific Congress of Golf, Mesa, AZ, 2008, Energy in Motion.

47. Marras WS, Granata KP: A biomechanical assessment and model of axial twisting in the thoracolumbar spine, *Spine* 20:1440–1451, 1995.

48. Hosea TM, Gatt CJ, Galli KM, et al: Biomechanical analysis of the golfer's back. In Cochran AJ, editor: *Science and golf*: Proceedings of the First World Scientific Congress of Golf, London, 1990, E & FN SPON.

49. Adams MA, Hutton WC: Mechanics of the intervertebral disc. In Ghosh P, editor: *The biology of the intervertebral disc*, Boca Raton, FL, 1988, CRC Press.

50. Gluck GS, Bendo JA, Spivak JM: The lumbar spine and low back pain in golf: A literature review of swing biomechanics and injury prevention, *Spine J* 8:778–788, 2008.

51. Kumar S: Theories of musculoskeletal injury causation, *Ergonomics* 44:17–47, 2001.

52. Lindsay DM, Horton JF: Comparison of spine motion in elite golfers with and without low back pain, *J Sports Sci* 20:599–605, 2002.

53. Sugaya H, Tsuchiya A, Moriya H, et al: Low back injury in elite and professional golfers: An epidemiologic and radiographic study. In Farrally MR, Cochran AJ, editors: *Science and golf III*: Proceedings of the World Scientific Congress of Golf, Champaign, IL, 1999, Human Kinetics.

54. Morgan D, Sugaya H, Banks S, et al: *A new twist on golf kinematics and low back injuries*, Proceedings of the 21st Annual Meeting of the American Society of Biomechanics, Sept 24–27, 1997.

55. Marras WS, Lavender SA, Leurgans SE, et al: Biomechanical risk factors for occupationally related low back disorders, *Ergon* 38:377–410, 1995.

56. Tall RL, DeVault W: Spinal injury in sport: Epidemiologic considerations, *Clin Sports Med* 12:441–448, 1993.

57. Grimshaw PN, Burden AM: Case report: Reduction of low back pain in a professional golfer, *Med Sci Sports Exerc* 32:1667–73, 2000.

58. Bulbulian R, Ball K, Seaman D: The short golf backswing: Effects on performance and spinal health implications, *J Manipulative Physiol Ther* 24:569–575, 2001.

59. Cole MH, Grimshaw PN: Electromyography of the trunk and abdominal muscles in golfers with and without low back pain, *J Sci Med Sport* 11:174–81, 2008.

60. Evans C, Oldreive W: A study to investigate whether golfers with a history of low back pain show a reduced endurance of transverse abdominis, *J Man Manip Ther* 8:162–174, 2000.

61. Evans K, Refshauge KM, Adams R, Aliprandi L: Predictors of low back pain in young elite golfers: A preliminary study, *Phys Ther Sport* 6:122–130, 2005.

62. Lindsay DM, Horton JF: Trunk rotation strength and endurance in healthy normals and elite male golfers with and without low back pain, *North Am J Sport Phys Ther* 1:80–91, 2006.

63. Archambault ML, Ling W, Chen B, Gatt C: A kinematic and kinetic analyses of the modern and stabilized-spine golf swings. In Crews DS, Lutz RS, editors: *Science and golf V*: Proceedings of the World Scientific Congress of Golf, Mesa, AZ, 2008, Energy in Motion.

64. McCarroll JR, Mallon WJ: Epidemiology of golf injuries. In Stover CN, McCarroll JR, Mallon WJ, editors: *Feeling up to par: Medicine from tee to green*, Philadelphia, 1994, FA Davis.

65. Lindsay DM, Horton JF, Vandervoort AA: A review of injury characteristics, aging factors and prevention programs for the older golfer, *Sports Med* 30:89–103, 2000.

66. Kim DH, Millett PJ, Warner JJP, Jobe FW: Shoulder injuries in golf, *Am J Sport Med* 32:1324–1330, 2004.

67. Jobe FW, Moynes DR, Antonelli DJ: Rotator cuff function during a golf swing, *Am J Sport Med* 14:388–392, 1986.

68. Jobe FW, Perry J, Pink M: Electromyographic shoulder activity in men and women professional golfers, *Am J Sport Med* 17: 782–787, 1989.

69. Pink M: Electromyographic analysis of the shoulder during the golf swing, *Am J Sport Med* 18:137–140, 1990.

70. Zheng N, Barrentine SW, Fleisig GS, Andrews JR: Kinematic analysis of swing in pro and amateur golfers, *Internat J Sports Med* 29:965–70, 2008.

71. Morgan D, Cook F, Banks S, et al: The influence of age on lumbar mechanics during the golf swing. In Farrally MR, Cochran AJ, editors: *Science and golf III*: Proceedings of the World Scientific Congress of Golf, Champaign, IL, 1999, Human Kinetics.

72. McHardy AJ, Pollard HP: Golf and upper limb injuries: A summary and review of the literature, *Chiropr Osteopathy* 13:1–7, 2005.

73. Broker JP, Ramey MR: Understanding golf club control through grip pressure measurement. In Crews DS, Lutz RS, editors: *Science and golf V*: Proceedings of the World Scientific Congress of Golf, Mesa, AZ, 2008, Energy in Motion.

74. Kohn HS: Prevention and treatment of elbow injuries in golf, *Clin Sports Med* 15:65–83, 1996.

75. Nago M, Sawada Y: A kinematic analysis of the golf swing by means of fast motion picture in connection with wrist action, *J Sports Med* 17:413–418, 1977.

76. Robinson RL: A study of the correlation between swing characteristics and club head velocity. In Cochran AJ, Farrally MR, editors: *Science and golf II*: Proceedings of the World Scientific Congress of Golf, London, 1994, E & FN SPON.

77. Dalgleish MJ, Vicenzino B, Neal RJ: Swing technique change and adjunctive exercises in the treatment of wrist pain in a golfer: A case report. In Thomas PR, editor: *Optimizing performance in golf*, Brisbane, 2001, Australian Academic Press.

78. Neal RJ, Sprigings EJ, Dalgleish MJ: How has research influenced golf teaching and equipment. In Thomas PR, editor: *Optimizing performance in golf*, Brisbane, 2001, Australian Academic Press.

79. Lindsay, DM, Hadi W, Wright I, Vandervoort AA: Comparison of perceived golf shot performance, upper limb stress and ball flight characteristics between solid and brush fiber hitting mats. In Crews DS, Lutz RS, editors: *Science and golf V*: Proceedings of the World Scientific Congress of Golf, Mesa, AZ, 2008, Energy in Motion.

80. Vandervoort AA: Aging of the human neuromuscular system, *Muscle Nerve* 25:17–25, 2002.

81. Palmer JL, Young SD, Fox E, et al: Senior recreational golfers: A survey of musculoskeletal conditions, playing characteristics and warm up patterns, *Physio Can* 55:79–86, 2003.

82. Fradkin AJ, Windley TC, Myers JB, et al: Describing the warm-up habits of recreational golfers and the associated injury risk. In Crews DS, Lutz RS, editors: *Science and golf V*: Proceedings of the World Scientific Congress of Golf, Mesa, AZ, 2008, Energy in Motion.

APPLIED BIOMECHANICS OF JUMPING

Scott A. Riewald

Introduction

Jumping is an important and fundamental component of many athletic activities. Basketball, volleyball, soccer, and track and field are just a few of the sports that include jumping as one of the prerequisite skills needed to achieve optimal performances. Although almost anyone can jump, proper execution that maximizes performance while also minimizing the potential for injury is actually a complicated biomechanical task. Consequently, a great deal of research has gone into trying to understand the biomechanical principles and motor control strategies underlying the proper execution of a jump. When attempting to maximize jump performance, the difficulty of guiding technique is further confounded when sport-specific demands are taken into consideration; jumps come in all "shapes and sizes," and each carries with it specific biomechanical considerations. As it relates to injury, although the takeoff portion of jumping is not commonly linked to any stereotypical injury patterns, the landing often is; numerous scientific studies link the biomechanics of landing to noncontact lower-body injuries. This chapter serves to consolidate information on jumping biomechanics, highlighting what is known about the mechanics behind optimal vertical and horizontal jump performance, its relevance in athlete screening and evaluation, as well as to look at the mechanics of the landing.

Terminology

Jumping incorporates a wide range of activities and investigators frequently have athletes perform various types of jumps, manipulating mechanical variables in the process, in an attempt to gain the insight into the biomechanical and motor control mechanisms that underlie performance. Some of these jumping techniques have direct correlates to what is seen in sport, but others do not. With this in mind,

it is important to lay out some basic definitions and techniques related to jumping, as these terms arise in the remainder of the chapter.

Vertical Jump. *Vertical jumps* are performed with the goal of reaching as high as possible, as in executing a volleyball block, or getting the body's center of mass (COM) as high as possible after the athlete leaves the ground, as in a high jump. The vertical jump is typically performed as either a squat jump or countermovement jump from one or two legs. The vertical jump is also commonly used as a test to estimate lower-body power and as a strength and conditioning exercise.

Squat Jump (SJ). A *squat jump*, shown graphically in Figure 10-1, starts from a static squat position in which the hips, knees, and ankles are initially flexed. From here, the athlete vigorously extends the hips, knees, and ankles to accelerate the COM upward toward take-off.[1]

Countermovement Jump (CMJ). Most individuals rapidly lower the body's COM from a standing position into a squat in preparation for the vertical jump (see Figure 10-1). This lowering of the COM via the coordinated flexion of the hips, knees, and ankles is typically referred to as the *countermovement* because it moves the body in the opposite direction of the eventual jump.[1]

Horizontal Jump (HJ). *Horizontal jumps* are jumps performed with the goal of maximizing the distance covered by the jump. The most common horizontal jumps are the running long jump and the standing broad jump.

Depth Jump (DJ). A *depth jump* or *drop jump* is a type of plyometric exercise used to develop explosiveness and lower-body power. When executing a DJ, the athlete steps off a platform of a specified height, lands with one or both feet, and *immediately* jumps vertically as high as possible. The goal is to minimize ground-contact time, placing an emphasis on the muscles' ability to absorb the energy associated with the landing impact and contract concentrically to execute the subsequent jump.

Countermovement Jump

Squat Jump

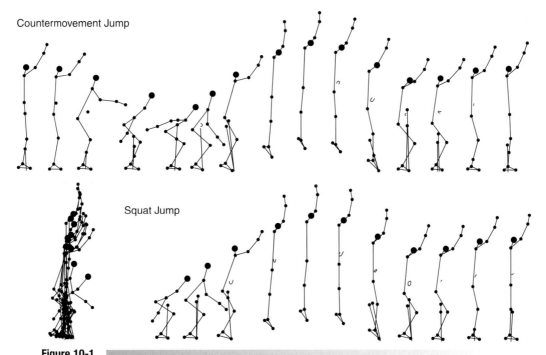

Figure 10-1

Shown are sagittal plane representations of an athlete executing countermovement *(top)* and squat *(bottom)* vertical jumps with an arm swing. Also shown is the magnitude and direction of the ground reaction force produced during each jump. Note that each image represents the position of the jumper at a different point in time—the athlete is not jumping across the page. The image in the *lower left* is what the jump would look like if the images were not spaced apart. (From Reiser R, Rocheford E, Armstrong CJ: Building a better understanding of basic mechanical principles through analysis of the vertical jump, *Strength Cond J* 28[4]:70-80, 2006.)

Biomechanics of Vertical Jumps

Factors Affecting Jump Performance

The vertical jump is probably the most common jump seen in sports, and the goal, in general, is to elevate the COM as high as possible. There are many factors that affect jump performance and the interactions can be complex. Hay and Reid introduced the concept of using a deterministic model to establish the relationships between various factors and how they affect athletic performance.[2] Since that time, numerous authors have used this technique to describe the relationships between the various biomechanical variables contributing to vertical jump performance. An example of a deterministic model for a two-footed vertical jump is provided in Figure 10-2.

At the top level of the model, the ultimate goal is identified—*jump height*. Jump height is directly influenced by the two factors identified in the next level of the model, *takeoff height* and *flight height*. The process of identifying "contributing factors" continues with each subsequent level until ultimately one reaches a "base" level of controllable and uncontrollable factors that affect performance. As the takeoff height is influenced primarily by uncontrollable anthropometric factors (see Figure 10-2), any improvements

to jump height will be mainly determined by the factors contributing to the flight height, specifically the vertical velocity that can be achieved at takeoff. As such, much of the biomechanical research has focused on identifying how flight height can be maximized.

Deterministic Models of Performance

A deterministic model is one of the best ways to identify and establish relationships between variables and factors that affect athletic performance.

Variations of this model have been developed by other investigators for both 2-foot[3] and 1-foot jumps.[4] The model developed by Vint and Hinrichs[3] (Figure 10-3) introduces two additional factors that directly affect jump height: *reach height,* which, like the takeoff height, is largely determined by body size and anthropometric variables; and *loss height* which is related to the timing and coordination necessary to achieve maximum reach at the same time the COM reaches its peak height. This model

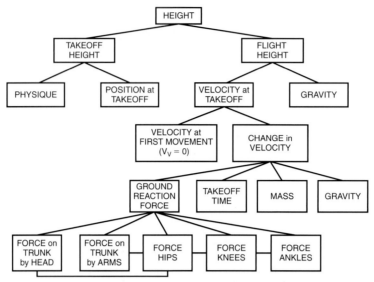

Figure 10-2

The deterministic model establishes relationships between various factors that contribute to vertical jump performance. Variables at one level are "determined" by the variables on the next lower level. Ultimately, one reaches "base factors" that the athlete can, or in some cases cannot, control. (From Feltner ME, Fraschetti DJ, Crisp RJ: Upper extremity augmentation of lower extremity kinetics during countermovement vertical jumps, *J Sport Sci* 17:449-466, 1999.)

has been used successfully to evaluate jump performance in activities such as volleyball in which the elevation of the hands, and not just the COM, is important. In determining the contributions made by each of the four "top-level" factors, it was found that takeoff height, flight height, and reach height accounted for 41%, 17%, and 42% of the total jump height, respectively.[3] The loss height was found to be negligible, accounting for only 0.2% of the overall jump height (see Figure 10-3). Again, although flight height contributes the lowest percentage toward total height, it is the one variable that can be controlled or altered to any degree via technique changes or training.

Factors Contributing to Jump Height

- Takeoff height 41%
- Flight height 17%
- Reach height 42%
- Loss height 0.2%
- Take-off velocity

What Aspects of Vertical Jump Height Can One Control?

Flight height is the only variable that can be modified through technique changes or training.

Full Body Kinematics and Kinetics

Numerous studies have recorded kinematic profiles of SJs and CMJs, tracking the position, velocity, and acceleration of the COM (Figure 10-4). Vertical jump height is noticeably larger when a jump is performed with a countermovement and this is due to the fact that the countermovement allows the individual to produce a greater vertical velocity during the propulsive phase of the jump. The *propulsive phase* is defined as the time between the minimum position of the COM (vertical velocity = 0) and takeoff. Although the propulsive phase starts with the onset of movement in an SJ, it occurs at approximately 67% to 72% of the total movement time[5-7] in a CMJ. In most cases, the COM height is slightly higher at takeoff than what is seen in standing because of the ankle extension that occurs late in the jump.

Jumping is a Ballistic Activity

Jump height is determined entirely by what happens before the feet leave the ground.

Vertical jumping is a ballistic activity, and jump height is completely determined by the vertical takeoff velocity. Vertical takeoff velocity typically ranges from 2.30 to 3.07 m/sec in elite jumpers and physically active individuals,[5,6,8-10] leading to reported flight heights ranging from 0.30 to 0.53 meters.[5-8,11-14] Note that vertical velocity peaks a short time before takeoff and decreases by approximately 6% to

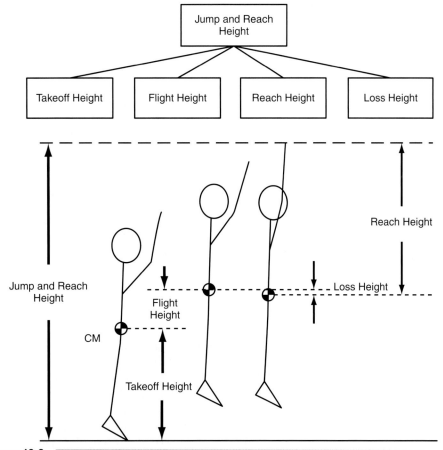

Figure 10-3

Deterministic model for athletic performances in which reach is critical. This deterministic model adds two factors at the top level of the model that affect how high the hand can reach in a vertical jump, compared with the previous model that only deals with the COM trajectory. (From Vint P: Vertical jumping performance: One-foot vs two-foot takeoff techniques. In *Performance and conditioning for volleyball*, vol 3, pp 4-7, Lincoln, NE, 1996, Conditioning Press.)

7% before the feet leave the ground.[5] This is a consistent finding across individuals and has been attributed to the mechanical "disadvantage" faced by many of the shortened extensor muscles as their force producing capabilities are compromised near full extension according to the force-length relationship for muscle as well as the need for the body to dial back activation to protect the joints from hyperextension.

There are two ways of viewing how vertical velocity is produced. The first is through the framework of impulse and momentum and the second is by analyzing the work performed and energy changes in the body. According to the impulse-momentum theorem, the final takeoff velocity is determined by vertical impulse produced during the propulsive phase, or the average net vertical force multiplied by the length of the propulsive phase.

Impulse-momentum theorem:

$$m(v_{v,f} - v_{v,i}) = \sum F_{v,avg} \bullet \Delta t$$

In which v_{vf} and v_{vi} are the final and initial vertical velocity of the COM, respectively, and $\sum F_{vavg}$ and Δt are the sum of the average vertical forces acting on the body and the time during which they act.

Neglecting air resistance, the only forces acting on the body in the vertical direction are body weight (BW) and the vertical *ground reaction force* (GRF). In addition, the vertical velocity at the start of the propulsive phase is zero in both SJs and CMJs.

According to this relationship, jump height can be improved by increasing the magnitude of the vertical GRF or the length of time during which that force acts. However, research has shown that athletes have very little direct control over the amount of time they are in contact with the ground.

It is generally accepted that the best way to maximize jump height is to focus on developing a larger GRF. GRF profiles typical to what is seen in SJs and CMJs are shown in Figure 10-5. The "shape" of the GRF tracing closely resembles that of the acceleration tracing in Figure 10-4, as would be expected according to Newton's second law

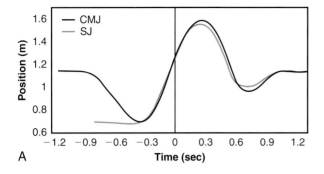

A

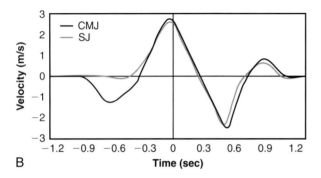

B

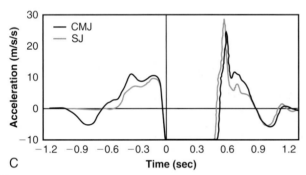

C

Figure 10-4

Vertical position *(A)*, velocity *(B)*, and acceleration *(C)* of subject's center of mass are shown during the course of a countermovement *(black)* and squat *(gray)* jump. Plots are aligned to the point of takeoff (t = 0). Vertical position is defined as positive relative to the ground. Similarly, velocity and acceleration are defined as positive in the upward vertical direction. (From Reiser R, Rocheford E, Armstrong CJ: Building a better understanding of basic mechanical principles through analysis of the vertical jump, *Strength Cond J* 28(4):70-80, 2006.)

(F = mass × acceleration). In the SJ, the force on the plate starts at BW (represented by the horizontal line *W* in the figure) and, as muscular forces are generated, the GRF increases to accelerate the COM upward. In the CMJ tracing, there is an initial unweighting that accompanies the downward acceleration and displacement of the COM. The GRF then becomes larger as the athlete first decelerates the downward descent of the COM and then accelerates the body upward during the propulsive phase. When considering how vertical velocity is generated and why CMJ height is higher than what is seen in SJs, note that although the vertical GRFs are larger with a CMJ, the propulsive phase is shorter; investigators have found propulsion times to be

0.46 to 0.64 seconds and 0.3 to 0.34 seconds for SJs and CMJs respectively.[6,8,13,15] Total movement time for the CMJ is markedly longer than for SJs (0.96 to 1.3 seconds compared with 0.46 to 0.64 seconds).[6,15]

It is important to note the magnitude of the impact force experienced by the body on landing, as the muscles and other structures of the body must be able to effectively dissipate this energy to prevent overload and potential injury.

The second way to analyze jump height is to look at how the work done by the contracting muscles contributes to the final vertical velocity.[16] *Work* is defined as the change in energy of a system, and Stefanyshyn and Nigg have stated that maximum jump height is largely determined by the work performed by the muscles and the mechanical energy input to the "body system" prior to take-off (see the following equation).[17] Mechanical work is performed by the muscles to change the kinetic energy (kinetic energy = $\frac{1}{2}mv^2$) and potential energy (potential energy = mgh, where *m* is the individual's mass, *g* is the acceleration due to gravity, and *h* is the height of the COM) of the body during the propulsive phase of the jump; the more work performed by the muscles, the greater the change in energy and vertical velocity of the COM. Muscles are capable of doing negative work (i.e., energy absorption) during eccentric contractions, and this would be the case while decelerating the COM during a countermovement. However, once an athlete enters the propulsive phase, the muscles typically perform positive work through concentric contractions, resulting in an increase in kinetic energy as well as vertical velocity of the COM. For example, consider a gymnast performing a double back flip with a full twist at the end of tumbling run. Part of the force produced during the jump is used to accelerate the entire body upward. However, because of the orientation of the GRF vector with respect to the COM, the forces will also initiate the rotations necessary to execute the skill. Once the feet leave the ground, energy is mostly conserved and the ultimate height achieved by the COM is determined by

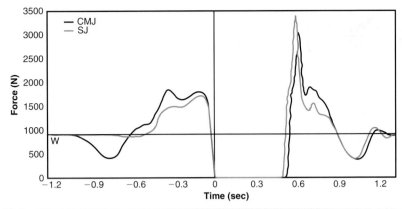

Figure 10-5
Representative vertical ground reaction forces are shown for an athlete performing squat *(gray)* and countermovement *(black)* jumps. The traces are aligned to the point of takeoff (t = 0). For reference, a *horizontal line* indicating the athlete's body weight *(W)* has been added to the force profile. The ground reaction force is defined as positive acting upward. (From Reiser R, Rocheford E, Armstrong CJ: Building a better understanding of basic mechanical principles through analysis of the vertical jump, *Strength Cond J* 28[4]:70-80, 2006.)

the kinetic energy at takeoff. Researchers have reported the total work performed during a vertical jump as 5.1[18] and 8.2[6] J/kg of body mass for SJs and CMJs, respectively.

The total work performed during a jump is equal to the change in energy of the system (ΔE_{system}). In other words the combined change of the system's kinetic and potential energy ($\Delta KE_{system} + \Delta PE_{system}$).

$$\text{Work performed} = \Delta E_{system} = \Delta KE_{system} + \Delta PE_{system}$$

Although most of the work done by the muscles is used to impart potential and kinetic energy to the body's COM as it accelerates upward, some is used to move the COM horizontally and provide rotational energy to the body segments. This is frequently thought of as inefficient energy because it is essentially "lost" and does not contribute to jump height. An efficacy ratio has been computed to relate the effective energy (i.e., energy associated with the vertical movement and position of the COM) to the total energy of the system or work performed by the muscles. This ratio has been found to be approximately 0.86 to 0.87 for maximal vertical jumps (indicating approximately 13% to 14% of the work performed by the muscles was "lost" to horizontal movement or segment rotation) but increases for lower-intensity jumps.[19] Vanrenterghem and colleagues found, in studying jumps of increasing height, the amount of noneffective energy increased from 3% in the lowest-intensity jumps (25% of maximum jump height) to 14% for maximal jumps.[20]

Power is a measure of how quickly work is performed during the propulsive phase (in other words, power equals the work performed divided by the time it took to produce the work, $Power = \dfrac{Work}{\Delta t}$), and peak lower-body power is frequently cited as the variable most tightly correlated with jump height.[5,21,22] Again, considering that propulsion

time essentially remains unchanged across jumps, increased power indicates that an individual is able to produce more work (resulting in greater energy, higher velocity) during the propulsive phase. Figure 10-6 provides a typical profile for the instantaneous power generated during SJs and CMJs.[1] From the graph, it is clear that peak power is higher in CMJs and occurs just prior to takeoff. The power output drop seen immediately before takeoff in Figure 10-6 parallels the drop seen in vertical velocity and is attributed to the inability of the legs to generate high movements as they near full extension. Peak power values have been reported by Harman and colleagues for physically active adults[5] performing various jump types and are presented in Table 10-1. In addition, Cormie and colleagues provide evidence that power production is related to experience, finding that experienced jumpers produced 28% more power compared with inexperienced jumpers (71.74 ± 10.69 W/kg of body mass vs. 55.89 ± 7.96 W/kg).[23] Although it is not immediately apparent from Figure 10-6, average power is also higher in CMJs (see Table 10-1). Keep in mind when evaluating the work and power in a vertical jump that it is important to look at normalized values (e.g., work and power expressed as J/kg and W/kg) as well as absolute values. This allows for more effective comparisons to be made across subjects who may have different body masses.

Clinical Point

Experienced jumpers are able to jump higher than novice jumpers—as much as 28% higher—suggesting practice and training plays a role in how high an individual can jump.

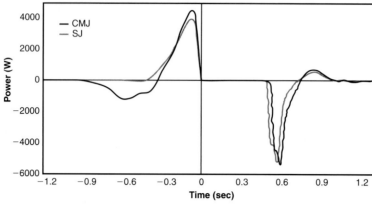

Figure 10-6

The time course of power production (and absorption) is shown for an athlete performing squat *(gray)* and countermovement *(black)* jumps. Positive power indicates that power is being produced, whereas negative power indicates power absorption during eccentric muscle contraction as the COM is decelerated in the countermovement and on landing. The plots are aligned to the point of takeoff at which time equals zero. (From Reiser R, Rocheford E, Armstrong CJ: Building a better understanding of basic mechanical principles through analysis of the vertical jump, *Strength Cond J* 28[4]:70-80, 2006.)

Table 10-1

Peak and Average Power Performed During Maximal Vertical Jump Tasks

Movement	Peak Power (W)	Average Power (W)
CMJ—no arms	3216 ± 607	1470 ± 351
CMJ—with arms	3896 ± 681	1450 ± 436
SJ—no arms	3262 ± 626	1260 ± 371
SJ—with arms	3804 ± 684	1337 ± 339

Data from Harman EA, Rosenstein MT, Frykman PN et al: The effects of the arms and countermovement on vertical jumping, *Med Sci Sport Exerc* 22:825-833, 1990.
CMJ, Countermovement jump; *SJ,* squat jump.

The area between the power curve and the x-axis in Figure 10-6 is the amount of positive (or negative) work done during the various phases of the jump. A great deal of energy is absorbed during the countermovement and some believe that a portion of this energy is stored in the muscles as *elastic strain energy* that is then returned to augment the power delivered during the propulsion phase. This is discussed in greater detail later in the chapter. In addition, one must appreciate the amount of energy that must be absorbed by the muscles on landing from the jump. The inability to effectively dissipate and absorb this energy is thought to contribute to lower limb injuries.

Joint Kinematics and Kinetics

The full body kinematics and kinetics presented for the COM are the result of what happens at the individual joints. The rotational motions of the hip, knee, and ankle are converted into the vertical translational velocity of the COM. Figure 10-7 shows representative hip, knee, and ankle joint angles; angular velocities; joint movements; and joint power for the hips, knees, and ankles during the propulsive phase of one- and two-legged CMJ.[13] Focusing primarily on the kinematics of the two-legged jumps, two key observations can be made from these data:

1. The hips and knees are nearly fully extended at take-off. In this extended posture, muscle force–generating ability is compromised because of shorter muscle lengths, and the body must slow angular velocities to protect the joints at the end ranges of motion. Consequently, joint torques and moments and COM vertical velocity also decrease during this period.

2. Segmental rotations, joint movements, and joint power (computed as the product of joint movement and angular velocity) all are initiated, and subsequently peak, in a proximal to distal sequence (i.e., hips, knees, then ankles).

Clinical Point

The inability of the muscles to effectively absorb the energy produced when landing from a jump is primary contributor to lower-limb injuries during jumping.

Clinical Point

The hip extensors provide 28% to 52% of the total work done by the lower body in maximum effort vertical jumps. The knee extensors contribute 29% to 45% and ankle plantar flexors 16% to 29%.

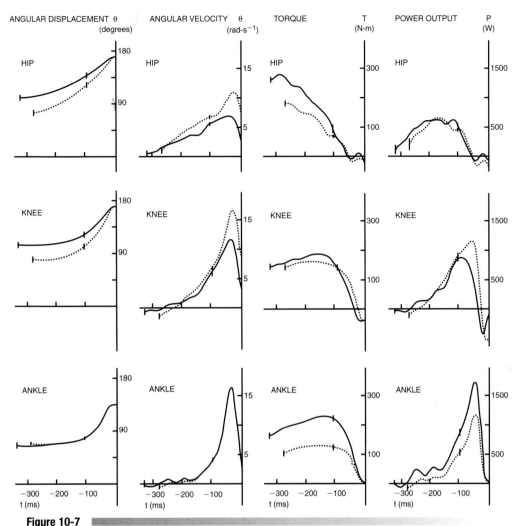

Figure 10-7

Joint angles, angular velocities, joint moments, and instantaneous joint power are shown for the hip, knee, and ankle during the execution of a one-foot *(solid line)* and two-foot *(dashed line)* countermovement jump. The traces represent the average of 10 subjects, beginning with the initiation of the propulsive phase and ending with takeoff (t = 0). (From van Soest AJ, Roebroeck ME, Bobbert MF et al: A comparison of one-legged and two-legged countermovement jumps, *Med Science Sports Exerc* 17[6]:635-639, 1985.)

The movement patterns have been shown to be fairly consistent for a given athlete executing repeated maximal and moderate intensity vertical jumps. As an example, the coefficients of variation (standard deviation/mean) describing the variability in hip, knee, and ankle excursion during vertical jumps achieving 50% or more of an individual's maximum height were 12.1%, 11%, and 20.5%, respectively. Variability was found to increase appreciably, however, for lower-intensity jumps representing only 25% of an individual's maximum.[20]

A number of studies have also examined the kinetics of individual joints and the contributions each of them makes to jump performance, particularly the work and power produced by the muscles acting at the hip, knee, and ankle joints. Figure 10-7 shows the joint movements and power generated at the hip, knee, and ankle during typical one- and two-footed CMJs.[13] The joint movements and power show a proximal-to-distal pattern that parallels the kinematic profile. The greatest movements are typically seen at the hip, whereas the highest power is observed at the ankle. The hip moment decreases during the duration of the propulsive phase, whereas the knee and ankle movement increase during the first part of the propulsive phase before decreasing during the final 150 ms of the jump. Table 10-2 summarizes the peak joint movements, work, and peak power (normalized with respect to body mass) reported for vertical jumps in the literature. Additional data for "un-normalized" peak joint movements[13,15,24]; work performed[13,17]; and peak power[13] at the hip, knee, and ankle can also be found in the literature.

The percentage of the total work performed by each joint is presented in Table 10-3. These data are interesting as they reflect how each joint affects the development of

Table 10-2

Peak Movements, Total Work Performed, and Peak Power Are Reported for Various Jump Styles and Are Normalized with Respect to Body Mass

Normalized Peak Movements (Nm/Kg) at the Hips, Knees, and Ankles During Maximal Vertical Jump Tasks				
Movement	Ankles	Knees	Hips	Study
SJ no arms	1.8 ± 0.24	5.3 ± 0.46	2.3 ± 0.33	Ravn et al.[34]
CMJ no arms	1.3 ± 0.15	5.8 ± 0.41	3.0 ± 0.55	Ravn et al.[34]
CMJ volleyball jump with arms	2.2 ± 1.00	5.8 ± 1.31	5.37 ± 1.19	Ravn et al.[34]
CMJ with arms	2.56 ± 0.33	1.05 ± 0.72	2.73 ± 0.36	Challis[11]
CMJ with arms, good jumpers	3.23 ± 0.53	3.54 ± 0.59	3.45 ± 0.57	Vanezis and Lees[7]
CMJ with arms, poor jumpers	2.89 ± 0.46	3.09 ± 0.59	3.12 ± 0.81	Vanezis and Lees[7]
CMJ no arms, good jumpers	3.06 ± 0.44	3.40 ± 0.81	3.50 ± 0.78	Vanezis and Lees[7]
CMJ no arms, poor jumpers	2.75 ± 0.41	3.13 ± 0.53	3.09 ± 0.74	Vanezis and Lees[7]
CMJ with arms	2.06 ± 0.35	1.94 ± 0.47	3.24 ± 0.60	Lees et al.[6]
CMJ no arms	2.03 ± 0.31	1.94 ± 0.50	2.84 ± 0.78	Lees et al.[12]

Normalized Work (J/Kg) Performed During Maximal Vertical Jump Tasks				
Movement	Ankles	Knees	Hips	Study
SJ no arms	1.39 ± 0.27	1.24 ± 0.38	1.98 ± 0.63	Hara et al.[18]
SJ with arms	1.60 ± 0.30	1.98 ± 0.21	2.34 ± 0.40	Hara et al.[18]
CMJ with arms, good jumpers	2.21 ± 0.15	2.28 ± 0.68	3.16 ± 0.88	Vanezis and Lees[7]
CMJ with arms, poor jumpers	1.82 ± 0.22	2.08 ± 0.55	2.46 ± 0.81	Vanezis and Lees[7]
CMJ no arms, good jumpers	2.21 ± 0.15	2.28 ± 0.68	3.16 ± 0.88	Vanezis and Lees[7]
CMJ no arms, poor jumpers	1.82 ± 0.22	2.08 ± 0.55	2.46 ± 0.81	Vanezis and Lees[7]
CMJ with arms	2.06 ± 0.35	1.94 ± 0.47	3.24 ± 0.60	Lees et al.[6]
CMJ no arms	2.03 ± 0.31	1.94 ± 0.50	2.84 ± 0.78	Lees et al.[12]

Normalized Peak Power (W/Kg) Performed During Maximal Vertical Jump Tasks				
Movement	Ankles	Knees	Hips	Study
SJ no arms	10.8 ± 1.9	35.0 ± 2.2	9.3 ± 2.2	Ravn et al.[34]
CMJ no arms	6.6 ± 0.94	38.1 ± 3.28	9.0 ± 1.87	Ravn et al.[34]
CMJ volleyball jump with arms	12.53 ± 7.07	39.4 ± 12.18	18.6 ± 4.85	Ravn et al.[34]
CMJ with arms, good jumpers	22.39 ± 3.29	19.14 ± 3.12	15.04 ± 3.51	Vanezis and Lees[7]
CMJ with arms, poor jumpers	17.38 ± 3.26	15.79 ± 3.26	12.47 ± 4.34	Vanezis and Lees[7]
CMJ no arms, good jumpers	21.62 ± 2.42	18.47 ± 3.74	15.87 ± 4.64	Vanezis and Lees[7]
CMJ no arms, poor jumpers	17.10 ± 3.78	15.60 ± 3.48	12.57 ± 3.19	Vanezis and Lees[7]

CMJ, Countermovement jump; *SJ*, squat jump.

vertical velocity of the COM. Although there is some variability, the hip extensors generally perform the majority of the work during maximal jumps (range 28% to 52% of the total work). The knee and ankle extensors provide between 29% to 45% and 16% to 29% of the total work, respectively. Interestingly, Vanrenterghem and colleagues[20] and Lees and colleagues[12] both found that in submaximal jumps, the percentage of work performed by the hips decreased, and work output is dominated by the knees and ankles.

Electromyography and Muscle Function

Bobbert and van Ingen Schenau[25] recorded the electromyographic (EMG) activity from selected lower limb muscles of volleyball players while performing a CMJ and

provided a picture of how these muscles are activated in relation to the production of the vertical GRF (Figure 10-8).[25] The authors described a proximal-to-distal activation pattern in the joint extensors with muscles being activated in the following order: semitendinosus, biceps femoris–long head, gluteus maximus, vastus medialis, rectus femoris, soleus, and gastrocnemius. This sequencing follows the proximal-to-distal movement pattern seen in the kinematic data and lends additional support to the idea that extension of the hips and backward rotation of the trunk occurs prior to knee and ankle extension.

Great interest, and much debate, has been centered on the function of the biarticular (two-joint) muscles in the lower limb, specifically the rectus femoris and the gastrocnemius, as

Table 10-3

Percentage of Work Performed at the Hip, Knee, and Ankle During the Propulsive Phase of a Vertical Jump

Movement	Ankles	Knees	Hips	Study
SJ with arms—max jump	19%	38%	43%	Fukashiro and Komir[24]
SJ no arms—max jump	28%	49%	23%	Hubley and Wells[16]
CMJ no arms—max jump	28%	49%	23%	Hubley and Hubley[16]
CMJ no arms—max jump	29%	30%	41%	Vanezis and Lees[7]
CMJ with arms—max jump	28%	29%	43%	Vanezis and Lees[7]
CMJ with arms—max jump	16%	33%	51%	Fukashiro and Komir[24]
CMJ with arms—max jump	23%	25%	52%	Vanrenterghem et al.[20]
CMJ with arms—75% height	34%	32%	34%	Vanrenterghem et al.[20]
CMJ with arms—50% height	47%	37%	16%	Vanrenterghem et al.[20]
CMJ with arms—25% height	78%	16%	6%	Vanrenterghem et al.[20]
CMJ with arms—max height	29%	27%	45%	Lees et al.[12]
CMJ with arms—HIGH jump	35%	32%	33%	Lees et al.[12]
CMJ with arms—LOW jump	40%	36%	23%	Lees et al.[12]

CMJ, Countermovement jump; *SJ*, squat jump.
25%, 50%, 75% and HIGH and LOW represent submaximal jumps.

these muscles have been described as perfectly suited for transferring power and energy from proximal to more distal segments of the lower limb.[26-31] Take the function of the gastrocnemius, a knee flexor and ankle extensor, as an example. Because of its dual function, extension of the knee while the gastrocnemius is active will naturally cause plantar flexion of the ankle (think of the muscle as having a fixed length). In this way, it is believed power can be transferred from proximal segments distally, allowing for a high power output to be generated at the ankle, even when angular velocities are high. An additional benefit arising from the biarticular nature of the gastrocnemius is that it can help decelerate knee extension near the end of its range of motion. If the gastrocnemius was not activated, the knee extensors would have to be "shut down" to reduce knee extension velocity and protect the joint from hyperextension. By activating the gastrocnemius, the knee extensors can remain active until takeoff, producing work that can be used to extend the ankle joint. The trade-off for transferring energy to the ankle is a drop in the knee power near full extension, which is seen to occur approximately 60 ms prior to takeoff in the knee power tracing of Figure 10-4 and the knee moment in Figure 10-9. The rectus femoris would be expected to perform similarly by transferring power from the hip to the knee, making it possible for the hip extensors to contribute to the power generated at the knee and the ankle.

This theory has been supported by several computer simulations of jump performance.[31] However, some investigators have debated the role played by biarticular muscles, and using computer simulations have suggested that humans would jump just as high if the biarticular muscle were replaced with uniarticular muscles.[32,33]

Clinical Point

Two joint muscles are thought to allow power to be transferred from proximal to more distal segments allowing high power output with high angular velocities at the more distal joint (e.g., the ankle) while decelerating the joint motion at the proximal joint (e.g., the knee).

Common Movement Patterns

When performing vertical jumps, individuals tend to use either a sequential or simultaneous movement pattern. This distinction is based on the time course of joint angular velocities; the pattern of muscle activation; and the production of joint movements at hip, knee, and ankle. The simultaneous strategy, as the name suggests, involves the synchronous extension of the hip, knee, and ankle, whereas in the sequential strategy, the hip extensors are activated first to start the rearward rotation of the trunk, followed by the knee and then the ankle extensors.

In a study of six elite volleyball players and professional ballet dancers, Ravn and colleagues[34] found that, although both strategies were used, the sequential strategy was preferred by the majority of athletes when executing SJs and CMJs. In addition, the choice of styles was athlete-specific and not necessarily related to the sport or training background. Figure 10-9 provides a clear example of an SJ performed with a sequential strategy.[34] The athlete shows a distinct proximal-to-distal pattern of joint movement. In addition, analysis of the joint movements found the start and maximum hip extension movement to occur on average 70 ms before the start of knee movement and peak knee extension, respectively,

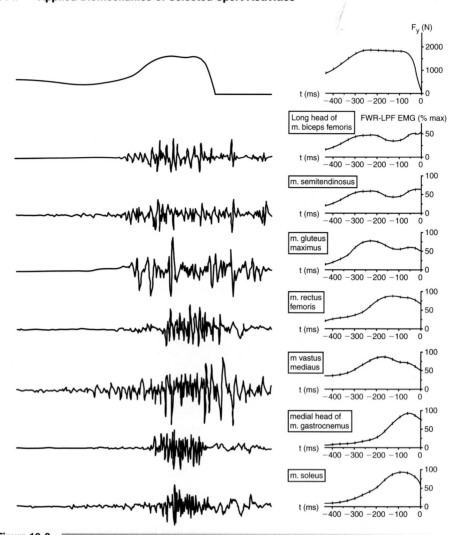

Figure 10-8

Muscle activity recorded from the lower limb during a countermovement jump. The left trace shows the vertical ground reaction force and lower-limb muscle activity for one subject performing a countermovement vertical jump. The right trace shows averages for the same variables across 10 subjects. Electromyography is expressed as a percentage of maximum activation. Trials have been synchronized at takeoff, represented by *time = 0*. Muscles studied include the biceps femoris long head, semitendinosus, gluteus maximus, rectus femoris, vastus lateralis, gastrocnemius-medial head, and the soleus. (From Bobbert M, van Ingen Schenau, GJ: Coordination in vertical jumping, *J Biomech* 21(3):249-262, 1988.)

when performing SJs (this was reduced to 50 ms in CMJs). Extension of the knee, similarly, began prior to extension of the ankle. An example of an athlete using the simultaneous strategy is shown in Figure 10-10. Note how the angular velocities, joint movements, joint powers, and EMG for muscles at the hip, knee, and ankle all start at essentially the same time. Hudson, in a 1986 study of twenty athletic individuals,[14] found most subjects used a simultaneous strategy when performing CMJs and SJs. However, the classification of a simultaneous strategy was based on the criteria that adjacent joints provided "positive contributions" more than 50% of the time. In actuality, although most subjects showed a sequential pattern, the short time delay between the start of successive

joint movements was not sufficient to "officially" classify them as using a sequential pattern.

The proximal-to-distal pattern of activation has been reported as the predominant, and optimal, movement pattern for jumping vertically. This control scheme is thought to (1) restrain the angular velocities of proximal segments, allowing the athlete to stay in contact with the ground for as long as possible and the muscles to produce work over their full shortening range; (2) optimally involve monoarticulate and biarticulate muscles and balance the segmental contributions to the COM vertical velocity; and (3) maximize the efficacy of the work produced.[21] With this pattern of activation, most of the energy is used (productively) to propel the body vertically. Very little

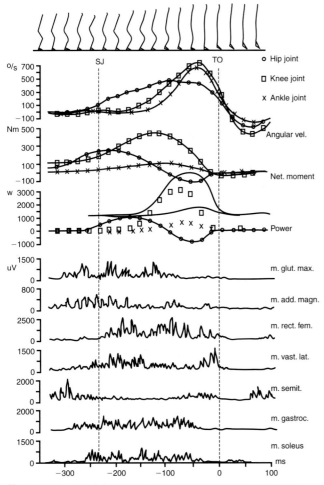

Figure 10-9
Kinematic (joint angular velocities), kinetic (joint movements, power) and muscle activity levels are presented for an athlete performing a squat jump using a sequential movement pattern. Note the proximal-to-distal movement pattern, which is exemplified in the angular velocity, joint movement, and electromyography traces. (From Ravn S, Voigt M, Simonsen EB et al: Choice of jumping strategy in two standard jumps, squat and countermovement jump—effect of training background or inherited preference? *Scand J Med Sci Sports* 9:201-208, 1999.)

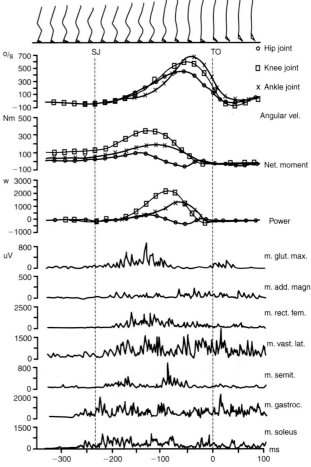

Figure 10-10
Kinematic (joint angular velocities), kinetic (joint movements, power) and muscle activity levels are presented for an athlete performing a squat jump using a simultaneous movement pattern. Note how extension of the hip, knee, and ankle and development of joint movements occur in synchrony along with the mass activation of all the muscles in the lower limb. (From Ravn S, Voigt M, Simonsen EB et al: Choice of jumping strategy in two standard jumps, squat and countermovement jump—effect of training background or inherited preference? *Scand J Med Sci Sports* 9:201-208, 1999.)

energy is "lost" to motions that do not contribute to jump height.

Computer simulations designed to optimize jump performance found the greatest jump heights were achieved when this scheme was followed.[21] However, when the same dynamic optimization schemes were used to reverse the order of muscle activation (e.g., activation of the soleus first), jump height was reduced by 9% and the efficacy ratio dropped from 0.87 to 0.83. The authors estimate that approximately 30% of this reduced jump height was due to the drop in efficacy, whereas the remaining 70% was due to a reduction in the total work performed by the muscles—mainly the hip extensors—simply because the optimal order of activation was altered.

Clinical Point

The activation pattern of proximal-to-distal is the optimal pattern for maximizing vertical jump height.

Submaximal Jumping

Experimental evidence and computer modeling of jump performance both indicate there is an underlying optimal motor control scheme the body employs to achieve maximal jump height and it has been suggested that the scheme serves to optimize "movement effectiveness," or the energy cost of executing the jump. Using submaximal jumping protocols, Lees and colleagues[6] and Vanrenterghem and colleagues[20] have been able to gain important insights into the way the body organizes movement. Figure 10-11 profiles the average joint excursions for a group of 10 male volleyball players executing vertical jumps representing 25%, 50%, 75%, and 100% of their maximums.[20] Jump height was found to correlate with the depth of the countermovement, but the greater depth for the high-intensity jumps was achieved almost exclusively via an increased range of motion at the hip. The ankle joint excursion remained consistent across all jump intensities, whereas the knee angle excursion did not change significantly for jumps of 50% intensity and higher.

Analysis of the joint movements yielded results that paralleled what was seen in the joint motion patterns

(Figure 10-12). Vanrenterghem and colleagues[20] showed that the peak hip extension movement increased systematically with jump height and intensity. The ankle movement was seen to peak during the 50% trials and the knee movement reached its highest values in the 75% trials. Although the ankle movement did not change with increased jump height, the knee movement was been found to decrease significantly as an athlete jumped for maximal height. Similar findings have been provided by other researchers.[6] Qualitative analysis of the EMG shows this drop in knee extensor movement to correspond with increased early activity of the biceps femoris, likely because of the increased forward lean in the maximum jumps and the increased hip extension movement, as well a decreased activity in the vastus lateralis and rectus femoris.

In looking at the work and power performed during the jumps, the total positive work performed increased with each successive increase in jump intensity (Table 10-4). Work output was low for all joints in the 25% condition

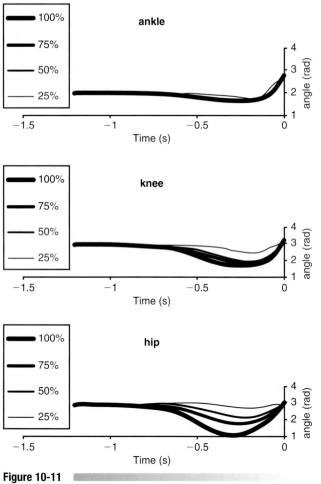

Figure 10-11

Averaged time curves for ankle *(top)*, knee *(middle)*, and hip *(lower)* joint angles recorded during maximal and sub maximal jumps are shown for comparison. Note the progressive increase in hip range of motion with increased intensity while the motion at the ankle remains relatively constant for all jumps. All trials are aligned at takeoff (t = 0). (From Vanrenterghem J, Lees A, Lenoir M, et al: Performing the vertical jump: Movement adaptations for submaximal jumping, *Human Mov Sci* 22:713-727, 2004.)

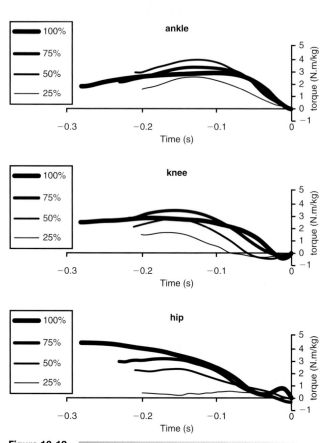

Figure 10-12

Averaged time curves for ankle *(top)*, knee *(middle)*, and hip *(lower)* joint movements produced during the execution of maximal and submaximal jumps. Note the progressive increase in the hip extension movement with jump intensity while the ankle and knee movements peak for lower-intensity jumps. Extension movements are denoted as positive and all trials are aligned at takeoff (t = 0). (From Vanrenterghem J, Lees A, Lenoir M, et al: Performing the vertical jump: Movement adaptations for submaximal jumping, *Human Mov Sci* 22:713-727, 2004.)

with 78% of the total work being performed at the ankle joints. The increased jump height seen in the 50% trials was the result of increased positive work performed at all of the joints. However, the increased jump height in the 75% trials could only be attributed to increased work from the hip and knee, and the further increases seen in the 100% condition were due to increased work at the hip, which contributed more than 52% of the total work. Investigations into submaximal SJs with an arm swing have made similar findings in that the positive work performed at the hip increases with jump intensity and that contributions from the ankle reach maximum levels even in submaximal jumps.

Table 10-4

Work Contributions from Individual Joints During Countermovement Jumps with and without an Arm Swing

Countermovement Jumps with No Arm Swing				
Joint	25%	50%	75%	100%
Ankles	1.23 ± 0.19	1.71 ± 0.20	1.87 ± 0.36	1.80 ± 0.58
Knees	0.26 ± 0.21	1.36 ± 0.36	1.75 ± 0.65	1.90 ± 0.56
Hips	0.09 ± 0.11	0.60 ± 0.38	1.84 ± 1.07	4.05 ± 1.19
Total	1.58	3.67	5.46	7.75

Countermovement Jumps With Arm Swing			
Joint	LOW	HIGH	MAX
Ankles	1.80	1.97	2.06
Knees	1.62	1.77	1.94
Hips	1.03	1.84	3.24
Total	4.45	5.58	7.24

Data from Lees A, Vanrenterghem J, DeClerq D: The energetics and benefit of an arm swing in submaximal and maximal vertical jump performance, *J Sport Sc* 24(1):51–57, 2006; and Vanrenterghem J, Lees A, Lenoir M et al: Performing the vertical jump: Movement adaptations for submaximal jumping, *Human Mov Sci* 22:713–727, 2004.
Mean and standard deviation of the positive work performed at individual joints, expressed in J/ kg of body weight, during the propulsive phase of maximal and submaximal vertical jumps. 25%, 50%, and 75% represent submaximal jump heights in the study by Vanrenterghem et al.,[20] as do the low-and high-intensity tests performed by Lees et al.[6]

Athletes performing submaximal jumps followed a consistent strategy that maximized the contributions from the distal joints (i.e., knee and ankle) and modulated the contributions from the hip to increase jump height. There is a high energy cost to rotating proximal body segments because of their higher movement of inertia. Although rotation of the trunk is necessary to achieve maximum jump heights, the body tends to avoid this by relying primarily on the ankle and knee, with smaller segmental masses and rotational movements of inertia, to perform the necessary work at lower-intensity jumps. The fact that the work done by the ankle was maximized for trials of 50% effort and higher, and knee contributions were maximized for efforts of 75% and greater, lends support to this hypothesis.

Contributions from the Arms

The use of an arm swing when performing a vertical jump is common and has been shown to improve vertical jump performance from 5% to 10% in both SJs[5,18,35-37] and CMJs.[5,9,12] The reason for this is twofold: the arm swing increases the takeoff height (height of the COM) by approximately 3% and also increases the vertical velocity of the COM at takeoff between 6% and 13%. The increased takeoff height is due in large part to the elevation of the arms at takeoff, whereas the increases in vertical velocity likely result from a combination of factors that allow the arms to build up energy early in the jump and transfer it to the trunk during the later stages of the jump. Typically, the arms are swung behind the body at the start of the jump and during the countermovement and then are swung downward, forward, and finally upward during the propulsive phase of the jump (Figure 10-13). Kinematic and kinetic profiles of arm-swing and no-arm-swing CMJs are provided in Figure 10-14 and Figure 10-15.

But what are the specific mechanisms by which the arm swing improves flight height? The improvements seen with the addition of an arm swing seem to result because (1) the upper body musculature actually produces positive work and (2) the arm swing augments the work done by the hip extensors. It has been suggested that the upward acceleration of the arms produces a downward force on the shoulders and the rest of the body. This slows the extension of the hips and knees, allowing the large muscles of the legs to create larger forces (translating to higher GRFs) according to the force-velocity (F-V) profile properties of skeletal muscle. Late in the jump, the energy built up by the arms is then transferred to the torso, essentially pulling it upward into the jump.[5,12] Payne and colleagues[38] reported that the addition of an arm swing altered the GRF profile to contain an "extra" late peak. Feltner and colleagues[9] added support to this hypothesis in finding increased hip and knee movements over the majority of the propulsive phase in athletes executing CMJs with an arm swing. In reviewing the joint movements in Figure 10-15, the arm swing allows for greater movements to be generated at all three lower-limb joints in the later stages of the propulsive phase.

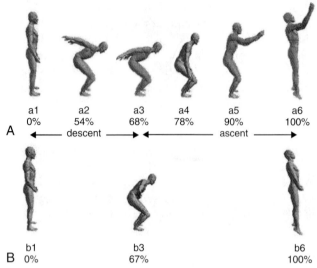

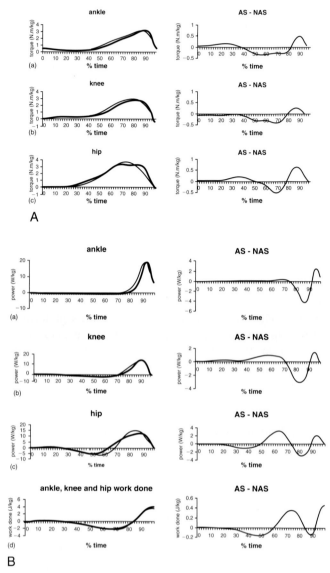

A

Figure 10-13

Positions of the body during the arm swing *(A)* and no-arm swing *(B)* jumps. Position 1 = start, 2 = maximum arm hyperextension, 3 = low point of countermovement, 4 = arms in downward vertical orientation, 5 = arms reach horizontal orientation, 6 = take-off. Positions 2, 4, and 5 are omitted for the no-arms jump. (From Lees A, Vanrenterghem J, DeClerq D: Understanding how an arm swing enhances performance in the vertical jump, *J Biomech* 37:1929-1940, 2004.)

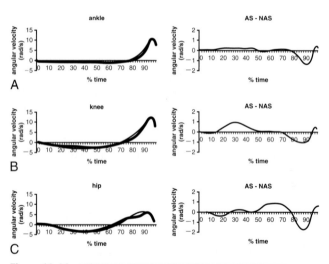

Figure 10-14

Averaged time-normalized angular velocities for the **(A)** ankle, **(B)** knee, and **(C)** hip during the execution of countermovement jumps with an arm swing (AS—*thick line*) and no-arm swing (NAS—*thin line*). The difference between the AS and NAS jumps is shown at the *right*. (From Lees A, Vanrenterghem J, DeClerq D: Understanding how an arm swing enhances performance in the vertical jump, *J Biomech* 37:1929–1940, 2004.)

B

Figure 10-15

Averaged time-normalized joint movement *(A)* and joint power and work *(B)* graphs for the ankles, knees, and hips for arm swing (AS—*thick line*) and no-arm swing (NAS—*thin line*) swing vertical jumps. The difference between the two jump styles (AS-NAS) is shown to the right. (From Lees A, Vanrenterghem J, DeClerq D: Understanding how an arm swing enhances performance in the vertical jump, *J Biomech* 37:1929-1940, 2004.)

Further evidence has been provided by Lees and colleagues[12] who found that the arm swing induces greater forward rotation of the trunk (which has been shown to augment lower-body power) as well as an increase in the positive work done by the joints, 8.15 J/kg compared with 6.81 J/kg for jumps with no arm swing. This observed increase was largely attributable to the work performed by the shoulder and elbow musculature, which produced 0.63 ± 0.26 g and 0.28 ± 0.26 J/kg of work, respectively (accounting for approximately 16% of the total work performed during the arm-swing jumps). The arm swing also augmented the work done at the hip, which increased from 2.84 ± 0.78 J/kg to 3.24 ± 0.62 J/kg. Similar findings were made by Hara and colleagues,[18] who found the arm swing increased the positive work at the hips by 18%, representing 65.9% of the total increase in work when an arm swing was added, and the arm musculature directly contributed the other 34.1% of the observed increases. Interestingly, although Lees and colleagues[12] found no change in the work done by the knee and ankle during CMJs, Hara and colleagues found the work done by the knee decreased whereas the work done by the ankle increased with the addition of the arms.[18] To round things out, it is important to note that the change in vertical velocity is due almost entirely to an increase in the GRF, as both Harman and colleagues[5] and Feltner and colleagues[9] reported no significant changes in the time during which the jump was performed with an arm swing, although Feltner and colleagues[10] reported a trend toward a longer propulsive phase when an arm swing was added.

Effect of a Countermovement

Time after time, a countermovement has been shown to increase vertical jump height from 3% to 12% compared with a conventional SJ.[5,39] This is true even when the body position at the start of the propulsive phase is controlled (i.e., the SJs are initiated from the position achieved at the bottom of the countermovement), suggesting it is the dynamics of the countermovement that led to the increased jump height. Figures 10-9 and 10-10 illustrate the kinematic and kinetic differences between SJs and CMJs.[34] The specific mechanisms underlying the improvements are open for debate, but it is likely that a number of different factors contribute to the improved performance. Several that are discussed in the literature include the following:

Use of "Suboptimal" Control and Coordination Schemes When Performing Squat Jumps

Individuals will naturally perform a countermovement during a vertical jump and the lack of familiarity with performing a "novel task" like the SJ may affect the vertical velocity achieved at takeoff.

Energy Absorption and Return - Stretch Shortening Cycle

During a countermovement, the extensors of the hip, knee, and ankle contract eccentrically to slow the downward descent of the COM before contracting concentrically during the propulsive phase of the jump. It has been theorized that *elastic strain energy* is stored in the muscles during the eccentric contraction, energy that could then be returned during the concentric phase to augment the muscle's "natural" force-generating capability.[40,41] It has been suggested that the storage and release of elastic strain energy can contribute as much as 40% of the total work performed by the lower limb musculature during a vertical jump[26] and that this energy storage increases with the speed and length of the stretch.[41] However, computer simulations and experimental evidence[15,24,32,33] suggest that differences in the storage and release of elastic strain energy may not be as great as initially believed. Computer simulations have shown that the elastic tissues deliver essentially the same amount of energy to the skeleton during the propulsive phase of SJs and CMJs.[32] Nearly the same amount of elastic strain energy is stored in the two jumps, but more energy is lost as heat in the CMJs.

Increased "Active State" in the Hip Extensors

Through experiments and computer simulations, Bobbert and colleagues found that an increased activation in the lower-limb extensors, particularly the hip extensors, could explain the difference seen in SJ and CMJ performances.[42] The increased activation resulted from the need to halt the descent of the body in the countermovement so the extensors are maximally activated (or are near maximal activation) at the start of the propulsive phase. This allows these muscles to produce more force and perform more work during the first 30% of the jump (on average, work at the hip has been show to increase by 10%). In the SJ, muscles must essentially "take up any slack" during the initial part of the contraction before they can produce peak forces. Bobbert and colleagues commented that the enhancement of work in the CMJ can be attributed mainly to the fact that the joint movements are higher during the first part of the propulsive phase compared with the execution of an SJ.[15] Figure 10-16 shows data obtained from an individual subject and highlights the difference in work performed during SJs and CMJs. In this figure, the height of the COM is plotted against the vertical GRF for both an SJ and a CMJ synchronized to the time the athlete left the force plate. The shaded area represents the added energy gained and work performed during the first third of the propulsive phase.

Single-Leg Jumping

In many sports, jumping is not performed from a static position, but involves a running approach and a takeoff from either one or both legs. Athletes achieve higher vertical

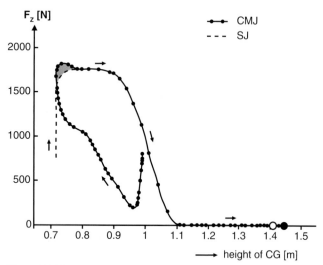

Figure 10-16

The vertical ground reaction force produced during squat and countermovement jumps (CMJ; y-axis) are plotted against the height of the center of mass COM (x-axis). The *shaded area* represents the added work performed by the muscles (added energy to the COM), which contributed to the increased vertical velocity and jump height achieved in the CMJ. (Data from Bobbert MF, Casius LJ, Sijpkens IWT et al: Humans adjust control to initial squat depth in vertical squat jumping, *J Appl Physiol* 105[5]:1428-1440, 2008.)

Table 10-5

Kinematic Differences Between One- and Two-Leg Jumps with an Approach

Variable	One-Leg Jumps	Two-Leg Jumps
Jump height (m)	3.08 ± 0.11	3.07 ± 0.10
Takeoff height (m)	1.34 ± 0.06	1.24 ± 0.05*
Flight height (m)	0.45 ± 0.06	0.54 ± 0.08*
Reach height (m)	1.29 ± 0.05	1.29 ± 0.04
Approach velocity (m/s)	3.77 ± 0.41	3.41 ± 0.55
Horizontal velocity at takeoff (m/s)	1.88 ± 0.10	1.01 ± 0.22
COM drop during contact (m)	0.002 ± 0.003	0.064 ± 0.023

From Vint P, Hinrichs R: Differences between one-foot and two-foot vertical jump performances, *J Appl Biomech* 12:338–358, 1996.
COM, Center of mass.
*Significant difference (p < 0.0042) between one- and two-leg jumps.

jumps when they can enter the jump with a 1½- to 5-step approach for one- and two-foot jumps when compared with stationary jumps. Saunders found in one-foot jumps that vertical velocity and jump height increased with approach speeds up to 60% to 70% of the athlete's maximum sprint speed, and decreased once this "optimal speed" had been surpassed.[43] Similarly, jump heights were maximized in two-foot jumps with approach speeds up to 50% to 60% of an athlete's maximum.[43]

Studying a group of male physical education students, Vint and Hinrichs found that maximum jump height was no different when jumping off one or two feet following a four-step approach.[3] However, the mechanism by which the jump height was achieved differed between the two jump styles (Table 10-5).[3] The one-foot jumps benefitted primarily from an increased takeoff height that was due to the COM of the free "swinging leg" being elevated 0.35 meters at takeoff, and a slightly greater degree of extension in the support leg at takeoff compared with the two-foot jumps.

Greater flight heights were seen in the two-foot jumps, and, although the increase was significant, it amounted to only a 9-cm (17%) increase versus those achieved with one-foot jumps. In both jump styles, the legs made the greatest contributions to jump height with the arms contributing only 7% and 4% to the vertical velocity for the one- and two-foot jumps, respectively.[3] Equally as interesting, although the COM drops after foot contact in the two-foot jumps (see Table 10-5), similar to what is seen in a

countermovement, the COM height remains relatively consistent and does not drop following foot contact during one-foot jumps.[3,44] In addition, research has shown that the COM vertical velocity in one-foot jumps is positive for all but the first 0.01 seconds of foot contact, despite continued flexion of the stance leg through much of the support phase. Similar findings led Dapena and Chung to suggest that the mechanism of loading the stance limb must be different from two-legged jumps.[44] They proposed that loading is due to the unique radial motion of the COM. Vint and Hinrichs found that the radial velocity of the COM was initially negative at foot contact and became positive midway through the contact phase for one-footed and two-footed jumps with an approach.[3] It was suggested that the observed radial kinematics lead to faster eccentric contractions and slower concentric contractions in the lower-limb extensors would contribute to the ability to produce greater muscular forces.

Dapena and Chung also found that vertical velocity in a one-footed takeoff is proportional to the approach velocity.[44] With a higher approach velocity, muscles are able to store more elastic energy and take advantage of the body "pivoting" over the plant foot, which effectively "converts" horizontal to vertical velocity. In a study of 1984 Olympic Trials high jumpers, Dapena found horizontal velocity decreased 48% and 42% for men and women, respectively, during the takeoff, whereas vertical velocity of the COM increased from −0.3 to −0.4 m/s at touchdown to 4.2 and 3.4 m/s, respectively, at takeoff.[45]

Stefanyshyn and Nigg analyzed the hip, knee, and ankle movement profiles for five basketball players during the propulsive phases of a one-footed jump and found them to closely resemble those seen in individuals executing a standing CMJ.[17] They also noted distinct periods of power absorption and generation at each joint. However, these power profiles were not consistent and varied widely among the individuals tested. In several subjects, the hip was a net energy producer, whereas the knee primarily absorbed energy. In others, the knee was a net energy producer and the hip was an energy absorber. In general, the ankle absorbed the most energy on impact and produced the greatest amount of work during the jumps. The researchers also examined the metatarsophalangeal joint, which was found to be strictly an energy absorber and performed no positive work during the jump.

It is well documented that athletes performing two-foot vertical jumps do not jump twice as high as they do when jumping from one leg despite having twice the available muscle mass.[46] The difference is largely attributed to an inhibitory neural mechanism, termed *bilateral deficit,* in which the force produced during a bilateral task effort is less than the sum of the two individual, unilateral efforts. Individuals performing one-foot SJs have been shown to reach heights representing 58.1% and 58.5% of the flight height achieved when executing two-foot CMJs and SJs, respectively, despite using half the muscle mass of two-foot jumps.[13] Van Soest and colleagues reported an 18% greater work output per leg for the one-foot jump along with 15% increased propulsion time (0.328 ± 0.043 s vs. 0.284 ± 0.045 s), compared with the two-foot CMJ.[13] Similarly, Challis found a 30% increase in propulsion time for the one-foot SJs (0.423 ± 0.069 s vs. 0.305 ± 0.064 s), but it accompanied a 22% drop in peak GRF.[11] Challis found that although the hip, knee, and ankle did not exhibit significant range-of-motion differences between jump types, the vertical impulse and joint movements were larger for the one-foot jumps, and the angular velocities were higher for the two-foot jumps, with the greatest angular velocity difference seen at the hip.[11] In addition, Van Soest and colleagues found a trend toward reduced muscle activation in the lower limb for two-footed jumps, although the only significant reduction was seen in the rectus femoris.[13] Analysis of the work performed showed the single leg produced nearly 20% more work compared with the output for the same leg in the two-foot jump (391.6 ± 56.9 J and 329.8 ± 49.9 J per leg for one- and two-foot jumps, respectively).

Several factors are thought to contribute to bilateral deficit and the observed differences in jump height in individuals performing one- and two-foot jumps. Because the angular velocities of the lower limb joints are higher in bilateral efforts, muscle force–generating capacity is likely compromised according to the F-V properties of muscle. In addition, as the weight of the body is distributed over two legs prior to execution of the two-foot jump, the active state of the muscles will also likely be lower during the jump's preparatory phase. This would lead to the extensors contracting over a larger portion of the jump in a submaximal activation state, resulting in a decreased work output.

> **Clinical Points**
>
> - Total jump height for one- and two-legged jumping are very similar, but the mechanisms used in achieving those heights are vastly different. One-legged jumps benefit from the increased height of the leg's center of mass while the two-legged jumps take advantage of the increased work done by the lower body when using both legs.
> - The work performed by a given leg is 20% higher when executing a single-legged jump compared with the work performed by the same limb when both legs are used together.
> - Bilateral deficit implies the net force produced and work performed during a bilateral task is less than the sum of the two, individual, unilateral efforts.

Although it is not possible to directly measure the contributions of these two factors experimentally, computer simulations of jump performance suggest that as much as 75% of the observed bilateral deficit can be explained by higher contraction velocities with the remainder attributed to a lower active state.[47]

Sport Specificity

It is not always possible for athletes to fully engage in a countermovement or use the arms during a jump. A volleyball player, for example, may need to execute a block with the arms extended overhead the entire jump. Or an athlete may not have the time to perform a full countermovement prior to jumping. As such, it is reasonable to expect there will be sport-specific differences in the way athletes execute a jump.

> **Clinical Point**
>
> The physical constraints imposed by certain sports will dictate how a vertical jump can be performed; for example, having to maintain an upright upper body posture while executing a jump will limit jump height.

Ravn and colleagues, studying volleyball players and dancers, found that sport-specific "constraints" can, in fact, dramatically alter vertical jump mechanics.[34] The ballet dancers in their study were instructed to perform a CMJ with the constraints that they keep the feet externally rotated, hold the arms in a static position in front of the body, and maintain an upright torso during the jump (Figure 10-17).[34] The volleyball players, on the other hand, were able to use a three-step approach and use an arm swing when executing their jumps. As might be expected, the kinetic and kinematic profiles differed dramatically. For one,

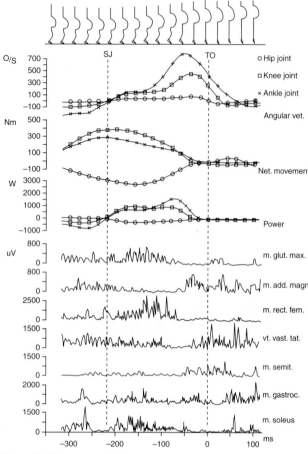

Figure 10-17

In a ballet-specific jump, the dance must maintain an upright upper body posture and externally rotate the legs during the propulsive phase. Consequently, the kinematic, kinetic, and electromyography profiles differ from the countermovement and squat jumps shown in Figures 10-7 and 10-9. Specifically noteworthy is the lack of positive power from the hip. (From Ravn S, Voigt M, Simonsen EB et al: Choice of jumping strategy in two standard jumps, squat and countermovement jump—Effect of training background or inherited preference? *Scand J Med Sci Sports* 9:201-208, 1999.)

the volleyball players consistently achieved higher jump heights and used a sequential movement strategy, whereas the ballet dancers tended toward using a simultaneous strategy. In addition, although the majority of the work was done at the hip and knee in the volleyball jumps, the ankle dominated the work produced in the ballet dancers, whereas the hip actually performed negative work during the jump. This finding is not unexpected, as it has been reported by Vanrenterghem and colleagues that constraining forward lean in a vertical jump decreases vertical jump performance by 10% and leads to a redistribution of power in the lower limb, with the hip contributing 37% less and the knee 13% more power, respectively, compared with unconstrained jumps.[48]

Dapena and colleagues[44,45,49,50] and McEwen[51] have extended the vertical jump research to evaluate performance

in the high jump. The mechanics behind maximizing the height of the COM in the high jump are much the same as when executing a one-footed vertical jump. However, there are some additional considerations that are important in trying to clear a bar. For one, the approach is critical to high-jump performance and the execution of a successful jump. Once the athlete leaves the ground he or she essentially is rotating around all three axes, and this rotation is generated by the GRFs and movement of the body at takeoff[45,49,51]:

1. Rotation about the longitudinal axis occurs as the result of the swing leg being rotated from pointing at the bar to being parallel to the bar during takeoff.
2. Rotation about the transverse axis results from planting the foot in front of the knee and shoulder on the last stride, which produces a forward somersaulting motion with the head lowering and the legs rising.
3. Rotation about the anteroposterior axis is generated from the approach, as the turn at the end of the approach forces the athlete to lean in toward the center of the turn. At the point of take off, the vertical GRF and body movement rotate the body medially.

Once in the air, the athlete's focus is mainly on controlling the rotation. The best jumpers are able to enter the takeoff with a high horizontal velocity and a low COM, allowing the vertical impulse to be developed over a longer period. Although this requires considerable leg strength, energy can be stored via the eccentric contraction of the extensors that can then be returned during the propulsive phase of the jump.

Lending further support to the idea that there are sport-specific strategies for optimizing jump performance, Laffaye and colleagues performed a principal component analysis of one-foot vertical jumps performed by 25 athletes from five different sport backgrounds.[52] They identified two principle components, composed of six variables, that could account for up to 78% of the variance in vertical jump height: a temporal component (i.e., jump height is most strongly influenced by the ability to optimize the timing of the jump), and a force component (e.g., jump height determined mainly by factors related to force production). Interestingly, the authors found the athletes from different sports approached vertical jumping differently (Figure 10-18). Volleyball players relied more heavily on optimizing temporal aspects and timing of the jump, whereas handball, high jump, and basketball players maximized the force component to achieve higher jump heights.

Testing and Training

Because of the relatively straightforward objective (jump as high as you can), the defined relationship with peak power, and the ease of testing with one of several commercially available products, the vertical jump is frequently used as a testing tool to assess total lower-body power. The vertical

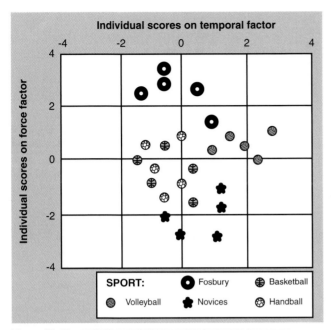

Figure 10-18

Performance of athletes in various sports with respect to the principle components affecting jump performance. The x-axis represents the temporal factor and the y-axis represents the force factor. Vertical-jump athletes emphasize the force factor, whereas volleyball athletes rely more on the temporal factor to increase jump height. (From Laffaye G, Bardy B, Durey A: Principal component structure and sport-specific differences in the running on-leg vertical jump, *Int J Sports Med* 28:420-425, 2007.)

jump has also been shown to improve lower-limb power when used as a strength training exercise. Guidelines and recommendations related to using the vertical jump as a testing and training tool are provided in Box 10-1.

Biomechanics of the Horizontal Jumps

Long Jump Takeoff Biomechanics

Like the vertical jump, numerous investigators have studied the biomechanical factors contributing to horizontal jump performance.[55-64] However, unlike the vertical jump, analyses have been principally based on kinematic data. Hay and colleagues developed a deterministic model (Figure 10-20)[58] identifying the biomechanical factors contributing to jump performance, which has subsequently been adapted by various investigators.[56] This model not only identifies relevant performance factors, but also provides correlations between levels of the model. For example, flight distance is the second level variable that contributes most to jump distance (correlation coefficient = 0.93), accounting for more than 87% of the variability seen in jump distance.[56,58,59,61,62,64] Similarly, flight distance is most influenced by the speed at takeoff. Continuing in this way, one is able to get a feel for the levels of "impact" different variables have on performance.

Box 10-1 Using Vertical Jumps as a Training Tool

Vertical jumps can also be used to build lower-body power and are often used as a strength and conditioning exercises. The points listed here should be considered when determining how to integrate vertical jumps into a training program.

- *Maximal jumps are needed to maximally engage the hip extensors.* The work performed at each joint does not increase proportionally with jump height. Although the work performed by the ankle and knee is maximal even with submaximal jumps, to fully engage the hip extensors, it is necessary to perform maximal effort vertical jumps.[53] Training designed to target the ankles and knees can be performed at submaximal intensities and elicit the same, or greater, effect for these joints.

- *A forward lean (or restricting the amount of forward lean) changes the dynamics of the jump.* Vanrenterghem and colleagues showed decreases in hip power at the hip and reduced jump height when the upper body posture was constrained to be vertical.[48] The common practice of using a barbell across the shoulders and upper back when performing weighted vertical jumps limits the amount of trunk flexion and consequently the degree to which the hip extensors can be engaged. Weight vests or other equipment that will not affect body position to the same degree may be more effective at developing hip power.

- *Plyometric depth jumps engage the knees and ankles primarily.* Depth jumps provide overload to the legs by requiring them to develop greater force, moments, and power to decelerate the center of mass during the landing. However, research by Bobbert and colleagues demonstrated that differences in jumping technique affect how muscles are used.[54] Examining countermovement depth jumps (CDJs) and bounce depth jumps (BDJs) and comparing them kinetically to countermovement jumps (CMJs), they found greater moments about the knee and ankle for the CDJs and BDJs then "standard" CMJs (Figure 10-19).[54] The ankle joint dominated power production in the BDJ and the knee produced the greatest power in the CDJs. In addition, it was found that the role of the ankle musculature increased with jump height. Different jump styles can therefore be used to develop different aspects and components of leg strength.

- *Training to develop lower-body power can lead to improved jump performance.* Cormie and colleagues recently provided evidence that engaging in a strength training protocol designed to improve lower-body power can improve jump performance by an average of 7 cm. They found increased peak power (57.71 ± 6.57 to 70.19 ± 11.46 W/kg) and work (4.67 ± 0.67 to 5.15 ± 1.24 J/kg) that led to an increased peak vertical velocity (3.14 ± 0.31 to 3.66 ± 0.34 m/sec).[23]

Much of the long jump research has focused on the biomechanics and techniques associated with the approach and takeoff. Through the analysis of elite long jumpers, Hay and colleagues[57,58] and others[56,61,62] have identified consistent biomechanical adaptations athletes go through during the final stages of the approach and takeoff to seemingly maximize performance.

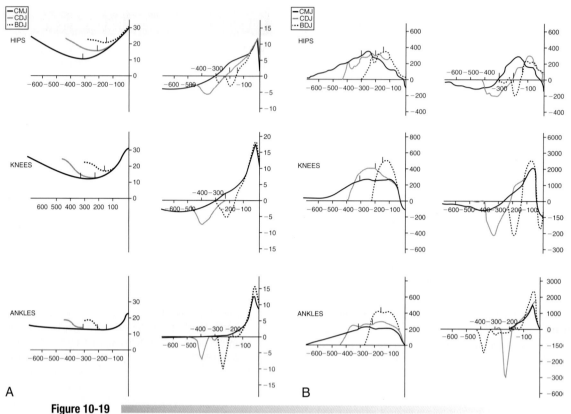

Figure 10-19

Joint kinematics (**A**) and kinetics (**B**) for countermovement jumps *(CMJ)*, countermovement depth jumps *(CDJ)*, and bounce depth jumps *(BDJ)*. *Arrows* indicate the start of the propulsive phase for each jump type. (From Bobbert MF, Huijing P, van Ingen Schenau GJ: Drop jumping I: The influence of jumping technique on the biomechanics of jumping, *Med Sci Sports Exerc* 19[4]:332-338, 1987.)

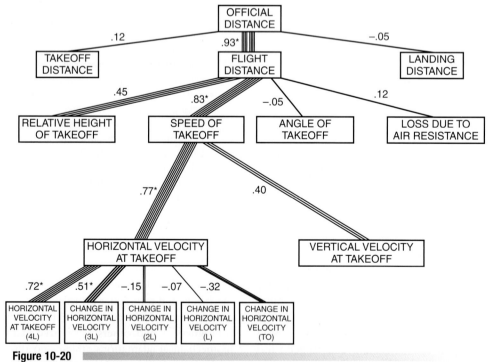

Figure 10-20

The deterministic model of long jump performance correlates various factors to jump performance. (From Hay J, Miller J, Canterna RW: The techniques of elite male long jumpers, *J Biomech* 19[10]: 855-866, 1986.)

Biomechanical Adaptations Athletes Use During Approach and Takeoff to Maximize Long Jump Performance

In reviewing the techniques used by elite long jumpers, it has been found that the best jumpers consistently execute the approach and takeoff as follows by:

- Having an approach that optimizes horizontal velocity, peaking within the last two strides, and places the dominant foot in the proper position at takeoff
- Lowering the center of mass (COM) (approximately 3 cm [1.2 inches]) during ground contact of the last stride, compared with the COM position for the strides immediately preceding it
- Taking a final stride length that is significantly shorter than those preceding it (Figure 10-21)
- Placing the foot, in preparation for the jump, that is significantly farther in front of the COM compared with those strides preceding it (see Figure 10-21)
- Having a significantly shortened horizontal distance between the contact foot and the COM at takeoff compared with the strides preceding it (see Figure 10-21)
- Using an active pawing motion by the plant foot that results in the foot traveling rearward when it hits the ground
- Employing a vigorous upward movement of the swing leg, arms, and torso entering the jump

Although on the surface many of these adjustments may seem to be compensatory movements used to make up for positioning errors accrued during the approach, research indicates these adjustments, in fact, impart a performance advantage to the athletes. Lees and colleagues[61,62] and others have suggested the positioning of the limbs in this way increases contact time, vertical impulse, and work that can be performed by the lower limb. Their analysis of takeoff mechanics broke the final foot contact and subsequent takeoff into two phases; a compression phase, or the time from foot contact to the point of maximal knee flexion, and the lift phase, measured from the point of maximum knee flexion until takeoff. Their findings indicate that 60% to 70% of the vertical velocity is generated during the compression phase via purely mechanical means[56,61,62] as the body essentially pivots over the plant foot much like the inverted pendulum described for one-foot jumping. The remaining 30% to 40% of the vertical velocity is achieved as the result of muscular contraction, return of stored elastic strain energy, and contributions from the upward swing of the free leg, arms, and torso.

The preparatory movements seen during the last stride, specifically the lowering of the COM and the placing of the foot farther in front of the COM, are believed to facilitate the development of this vertical velocity. Alexander believes that an optimal distance exists that will maximize performance[55]

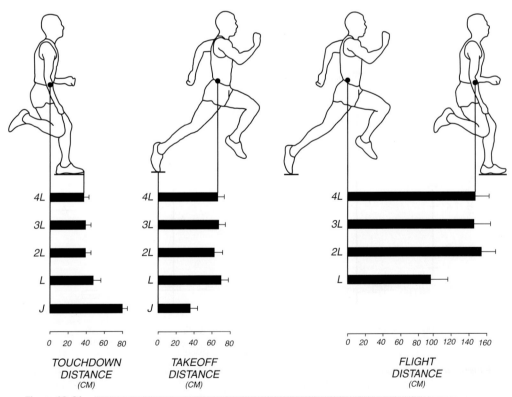

Figure 10-21

Analysis of the stride characteristics in the final strides leading to takeoff in the long jump shows the flight distance is shorter for the final stride, the plant foot is placed down further in front of the center of mass (COM) on the last step, and the position of the COM relative to plant foot is shortened at takeoff. (From Hay J: Citius, altius, fortius (Faster, higher, longer): The biomechanics of jumping for distance, *J Biomech* 26(Suppl 1):7-21, 1993.)

and this concept is supported by Lees and colleagues.[61,62] Critical to generating this vertical velocity is the ability to resist flexion of the stance limb during foot contact.[61-63] As approach speed increases, dynamic leg strength must also increase to be able to withstand the external forces working to flex the limb. Graham-Smith and Lees[56] found that athletes who have greater knee extension at contact generally exhibit less peak knee flexion during the compression phase and attain higher vertical velocities in the jump. These findings have since received additional support from experimental testing[65] and computer simulations that suggest the leg should have at least a minimum level of stiffness to optimize performance.[63,64]

As was seen in vertical jumps, vertical velocity peaks just before takeoff and comes at the expense of a 12% to 14% reduction in horizontal velocity (Figure 10-22). Unfortunately Lees and colleagues[62] were unable to establish definitive relationships between vertical velocity and any of the two-dimensional kinematic variables they examined. However, Graham-Smith and Lees[56] have since used multiple regression techniques to develop regression equations that relate flight distance, vertical velocity, and the loss of horizontal velocity to observed three-dimensional kinematic variables.

Kinetic data for the long jump is lacking in the literature. Kyrolainen and colleagues[60] performed one of the few studies to measure GRFs during competition. They reported average peak vertical forces for five Finnish athletes. The peak vertical

> **Clinical Point**
>
> Of the vertical velocity attained during the long jump takeoff, 60% to 70% is generated by the leg pivoting over the plant foot. The remaining 30% to 40% comes from muscular contraction.

GRF on the final foot contact and takeoff was found to be 8368 ± 1237 N, compared with a peak force of 4111 ± 1011 N on the next to last stride. These results should be interpreted carefully, however, as they are not normalized to body mass and reflect data from a combined pool of male and female athletes. Lees and colleagues[61] have reported the average work done by the muscles of elite female long jumpers as -5.9 ± 2 and 3.3 ± 2.3 J/kg for the compression and lift phases, respectively, indicating a greater amount of energy is absorbed during the compression phase than is produced during the takeoff. They were not able, however, to compute contributions made by individual joints.

Long Jump Flight Biomechanics

It is also important to consider the biomechanics of the long jump flight phase, as this also contributes to overall jump performance. One of the primary goals in the flight phase is to control the angular momentum developed during the

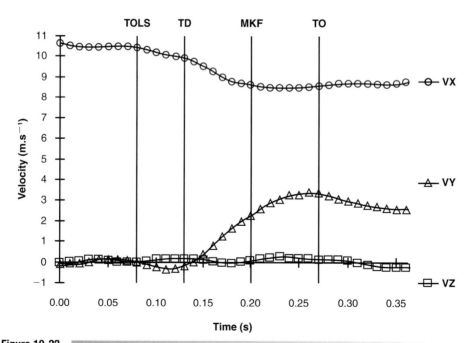

Figure 10-22

Center of mass (COM) velocity profile during the execution of a long jump. The mean velocity of the COM was tracked in three dimensions during the final stride and takeoff during the long jump. V_x, V_y, and V_z are the horizontal, vertical, and mediolateral velocities, respectively. *MKF,* Point of maximum knee flexion; *TD,* touch down; *TO,* takeoff into the jump; *TOLS,* take off from the last stride. (From Graham-Smith P and Lees A: A three-dimensional kinematic analysis of the long jump take-off, *J Sport Sci* 23(9):891-903, 2005.)

approach and takeoff.[58,59] Typically athletes leave the ground with a small amount of angular momentum that, if unchecked, would cause the body to somersault forward in the air. Skilled athletes use one of two techniques to control this angular momentum. Some will raise their arms and extend their legs to increase the body's moment of inertia and slow the forward rotation. More commonly, athletes use a modified running technique in the air, using the motions of the arms and legs to check the forward angular momentum of the body and position the body for landing.

Broad Jump Kinematics and Kinetics

The broad jump is commonly used as a testing tool to assess lower-body power, but also has a place in many sporting activities. Although not studied as extensively as the vertical jump, several investigators have reported kinetic and kinematic data related to performance in the standing broad jumps.[65-67] One of the most comprehensive studies was recently conducted by Hara and colleagues[67] who looked at broad jumping mechanics and specifically the contributions made by the arms. Figure 10-23 shows average joint angles, angular velocities, and joint movements during the performance of three jump "types"[67]: (1) a forward jump with no arm swing, (2) a forward jump with a forward arm swing, and (3) a forward jump with a backward arm swing. Figure 10-24 shows the corresponding joint power and work data. The main findings were that the velocity and jump distance were increased with the addition of an arm swing[65,67] and that the arm swing contributed positive work directly to the jump while also augmenting the work performed by the lower limbs (Table 10-6). The increase in lower-body work was primarily attributable to increases in the hip extension movement as the arm swing loaded the lower limb and slowed the extension velocity of the hip. This mechanism is similar to what was found when an arm swing was added to a vertical jump. Although the peak movement was not higher with the inclusion of an arm swing, the movement was increased in the time surrounding the peak, leading to the observed increase in work and power at this joint.

Landing from a Jump

Overview

Although the mechanics underlying a jump are important for maximizing performance, the mechanics used in landing are more commonly associated with injury and injury prevention. Gray and colleagues[68] and Gerberich and colleagues[69] have found that between 58% and 63% of the noncontact injuries seen in jumping sports are associated with the landing, and between 61% to 72% of those injuries occur at the knee. The high incidence of lower-limb injury is related to the high impact forces that occur with landing and the amount of energy that must be dissipated during a short time (see power curve in Figure 10-6). Peak forces can reach three

to six times an individual's BW when landing from moderate heights on one or two legs,[70,71] and can exceed nine times an individual's BW when landing from a jump height of a meter (3.3 feet) or more.[72] The inability to dissipate the energy associated with landing can lead to acute injuries, such as a tear of the anterior cruciate ligament (ACL), or a chronic, overuse injury like patellar tendinopathy (i.e., jumper's knee). Muscles act as the primary shock absorbers when landing from a jump and the eccentric contractions that occur in many of the limb extensors are important for absorbing much of the energy of the landing.[73] However, other lower-limb structures, including the ACL, bear some of the burden. Consequently, the techniques used when landing are critical to preventing overload to any one structure that could lead to injury either acutely or in time with repetitive jumps.[74,75]

> **Clinical Point**
>
> Of noncontact jumping injuries, 58% to 63% occur during landing and 61% to 72% of those occur to the knee.

> **Clinical Point—Landing Forces Exert**
>
> - Three to six times body weight from moderate heights
> - More than nine times body weight from 1 meter (3.3 feet) or more

Landing Kinetics

Researchers have identified two primary landing "styles"[76,77]: a *toe-heel style* and a *flatfoot style* (although toe-only, heel-only, and heel-toe variations may also be used with lower frequencies). In landing with a toe-heel pattern, an individual typically produces a bimodal GRF profile (Figure 10-25) in which the first peak occurs with toe contact (F1) and the second, larger peak, occurs with heel contact (F2).[78,79] Valiant and Cavanaugh found the first and second peak average 1.3 and 4.1 times an individual's BW, respectively, in individuals landing from a simulated basketball rebound.[77] Flatfoot landings produce a unimodal GRF pattern with peak reaching forces rising in excesses of six times BW.[77] The demands placed on the structures of the leg are closely linked to the type of jump that is performed. Bisseling saw marked differences in landing from a block jump compared with a spike jump in volleyball, for example; the vertical GRF experienced after a spike jump was 64% higher than what was seen in landing from a block jump and 46.7% higher than the landing force experienced when landing from a countermovement vertical jump.[80] The peak joint movements, powers, and loading rates all increased in parallel with the greater GRFs. Interestingly, individuals landing with a

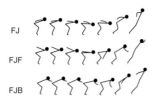

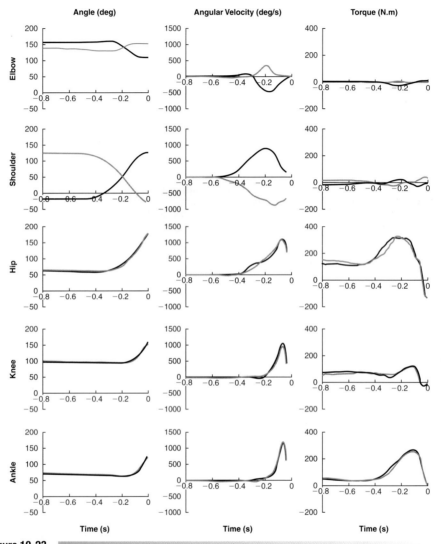

Figure 10-23

Average joint angles, angular velocities, and torques and movements for the elbow, shoulder, hip, knee, and ankle in the performance of forward jumps (FJ) *(thin black line)*, forward jumps with a forward arm swing (FJF) *(thick black line)*, and forward jumps with a backward arm swing (FJB) *(gray line)*. The positive direction represents extension for all joints except the shoulder, which is positive for shoulder flexion. (From Hara M, Shibayama A, Arakawa H et al: Effect of arm swing direction on forward and backward jump performance, *J Biomech* 41:2806-2815, 2008.)

toe-only pattern, in which the heels never touch the ground, have been shown to produce peak GRFs that are 22% lower than in toe-heel jumps.[76]

Looking at specific activities, it is possible to get an idea of how much jumping athletes do during practice and competition and why injuries are so common. Beach volleyball players have been found to perform and land from 219 ± 7.4 jumps in a typical match,[81] whereas indoor volleyball players may perform between 300 and 500 blocks and spikes during a 4-hour practice.[82] Similarly, it is not uncommon for dancers to land 100 jumps in a 90-minute practice session. However, the demands placed on the lower body

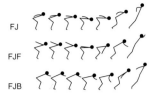

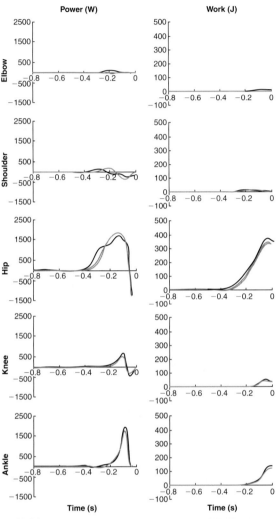

Figure 10-24

Average joint power and work produced during the performance of forward jumps (FJ) *(thin black line)*, forward jumps with a forward arm swing (FJF) *(thick black line)*, and forward jumps with a backward arm swing (FJB) *(gray line)*. The positive direction represents extension for all joints except the shoulder, which is positive for shoulder flexion. (From Hara M, Shibayama A, Arakawa H et al: Effect of arm swing direction on forward and backward jump performance, *J Biomech* 41:2806-2815, 2008.)

Clinical Point—Types of Landing

- Toe-heel
- Flatfoot
- Toe only
- Heel only
- Heel-toe

Table 10-6

Kinematic and Kinetic Comparison of Standing Broad Jumps with and without an Arm Swing

Variable	Forward Jump with No-Arm Swing	Forward Jump with a Forward Arm Swing
Jump distance (m)	2.08 ± 0.29	2.39 ± 0.32
COM velocity at takeoff (m/s)	3.34 ± 0.59	3.60 ± 0.44
Total work (J)	514 ± 77	583 ± 96
Work performed at hips (J)	322 ± 53	361 ± 53
Work performed at knees (J)	47 ± 37	44 ± 31
Work performed at ankles (J)	132 ± 15	140 ± 18
Work performed at shoulders (J)	—	5 ± 19
Work performed at elbows (J)	—	17 ± 12

Modified from Hara M, Shibayama A, Arakawa H et al: Effect of arm swing direction on forward and backward jump performance, *J Biomech* 41:2806-2815, 2008.
COM, Center of mass.

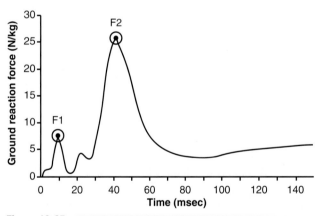

Figure 10-25

Vertical ground reaction forces during a landing from a jump. *F1* and *F2* represent the two ground reaction force peaks associated with a toe-heel landing from a jump. (From Dufek J, Bates B: Biomechanical factors associated with injury during landing in jump sports, *Sports Med* 12(5):326-337, 1991.)

may be quite different in these examples, as landing on a harder or stiffer surface requires the structures in the lower limb to produce higher joint movements and absorb a greater amount of energy. It is also important to note that there is a "performance tradeoff" related to surface stiffness; although a stiffer landing surface places increased demands on the lower limb, it also allows an individual to move more quickly—an important skill in many sports.

Also of interest are situations in which an athlete lands and must immediately run or jump again. Although common in actual athletic practices and competitions, plyometric exercises that emphasize rapidly changing the direction and velocity of the COM after a jump are also a staple in many strength and conditioning programs. Evaluating the forces produced in performing a DJ, the peak GRF experienced when landing is considerably greater than the force produced during takeoff. Chappell and colleagues also found that the shear forces at the knee are also greater when landing compared with what is seen in the propulsive phase of a jump.[83] Bobbert and colleagues[54] found extreme differences in the GRF profiles when studying traditional countermovement vertical jumps, 20-cm countermovement depth jumps (CDJ; goal is to allow some flexion of the limbs and lower-leg stiffness), and 20-cm bounce depth jumps (BDJ; goal is to minimize time on the ground with high-leg stiffness). The peak GRF was found to be 4099 ± 815 N on average for the BDJ—55% higher than what was seen in the CDJ (average 2649 ± 499 N) and 96% higher than the forces produced in a typical CMJ (average 2094 ± 218 N). In a companion study, Bobbert and colleagues examined the kinetics of performing BDJs from heights of 20, 40, and 60 cm, and presented data on the energy absorbed as the COM is decelerated (Table 10-7).[84] As can be imagined, the amount of negative work performed by the muscles during the downward movement phase increased with the DJ height, but no differences were found in the duration of the downward movement time. Consequently, the power produced by the muscles increased, as did the risk of injury.

Landing and Injuries

Although all athletes are required to dissipate large amounts of energy when landing from a jump, females are 1.6 times more likely to experience a knee injury[85] and 4.6 times more likely to suffer a season-ending knee injury compared with males.[86] In large part, the increased risk of injury is related to the motor control and kinematic strategies employed when landing from a jump.[87-91] Research has shown females may experience greater GRFs than males with respect to their BW (males 3.51 ± 0.0.63% of BW, females 4.71 ± 0.71% of BW). This increased force has been attributed to kinematic differences as females tend to land with greater hip and knee extension,[88,89] increased ankle dorsiflexion,[90] and increased foot pronation on landing. It should be noted that other studies have found no differences in joint kinematics at contact, but attribute greater loading of the legs and the increased risk of injury to poor motor planning in preparation for the landing.[91] Females also tend to experience greater ranges of motion in the lower limb joints, presumable to provide a longer time for the muscles to dissipate the energy of landing (greater impulse time).[90]

Table 10-7

Kinematic and Kinetic Differences Between Three Types of Depth Jumps

Variable	Joint	DJ20	DJ40	DJ60
M_{max} (Nm)	Hip	314 ± 70	328 ± 56	361 ± 93
	Knee	399 ± 70	475 ± 122	508 ± 183
	Ankle	337 ± 58	411 ± 90	427 ± 64
P_{max} (W)	Hip	−852 ± 164	−1168 ± 639	−1653 ± 659
	Knee	−1655 ± 287	−2431 ± 876	−4233 ± 2235
	Ankle	−1748 ± 424	−3439 ± 896	−5378 ± 1219
W_{neg} (J)	Hip	−45 ± 17	−59 ± 50	−68 ± 39
	Knee	−124 ± 39	−153 ± 54	−244 ± 86
	Ankle	−115 ± 33	−147 ± 38	−177 ± 53

Modified from Bobbert MF, Huijing P, van Ingen Schenau GJ: Drop jumping II: The influence of drop jump height on the biomechanics of drop jumping, *Med Sci Sports Exerc* 19:339-346, 1987.

DJ20, Drop jump from 20 cm height; *DJ40*, drop jump from 40 cm height; *DJ60*, drop jump from 60 cm height; M_{max}, maximum joint moment; P_{max}, peak joint power; W_{neg}, negative work.

Data represents the average of six subjects.

One primary area of concern is the knee, specifically the varus and valgus movement and movements experienced as an athlete lands.[87,92-94] Females have consistently been shown to experience greater maximum knee valgus as well as a greater valgus range of motion, and this is thought to be a significant risk factor.[87,92] Kernozek and colleagues found that recreationally active females experience maximum knee valgus angles of 24.9° ± 8.5°, whereas the males studied achieved varus angles of 0.7° ± 6.9° when landing from a 60-cm (24-inch) drop.[87] Although the finding that females experience increased knee valgus has been well substantiated in the literature, the extent of the discrepancy between males and females has been disputed. Hughes and colleagues suggest the magnitude of valgus may depend on experience,[92] because a group of collegiate athletes landed with less knee valgus than the recreational athletes in the Kernozek study (Figure 10-26—female average angle 10.4° ± 7.7° of valgus). In addition, Kernozek and colleagues[87] has speculated that the ability to generate an internal varus moment may be insufficient for controlling the valgus position of the knee, particularly at the point of peak valgus, suggesting weakness may be a contributing factor to the motion experienced at the knee. It is unknown whether the increased knee valgus seen in females is a performance effect or due to anatomic differences between males and females. Females tend to have a larger Q-angle, which is often associated with increased valgus loads. Regardless, an increased valgus torque, especially when coupled with anterior shear at the knee, increases the load on the ACL.

Strength imbalances in the lower limb are also thought to contribute to an increased injury risk in females. Of particular interest is the ratio of hamstring-to-quadriceps strength as individuals with a hamstring to quadriceps strength ratio less than 0.75 are thought to be at a

1.6 times increased risk of injury.[95] When the quadriceps muscles contract near full knee extension, they produce an anterior shear force at the knee, which can, in turn, increase ACL strain versus what it would experience from the jump landing alone.[96] Appropriately timed activation of hamstring muscles that are sufficiently strong could reduce the magnitude of anterior shear and reduce the risk of injury.[97] Large strength imbalances have been noted in the upper leg of females, often in conjunction with increased quadriceps activity and decreased hamstrings activity on landing compared with males.[98-100] Bennett and colleagues, however, caution against using peak forces or movements to evaluate strength imbalances as they do not take into consideration the dynamics of an activity nor do they take into account where in the range of motion those peaks occur.[101]

> **Clinical Point**
>
> Individuals with weak hamstrings (relative to the quadriceps) are at an increased risk for knee injury when landing from a jump.

Because of the factors affecting acute injury to the knee, efforts to improve landing mechanics have historically focused on improving the mechanics of the landing, which usually includes manipulating factors such as contact patterns, foot placement, and limb geometries to lower GRFs, and addressing strength imbalances in the leg to mechanically reduce the shear forces experienced at the knee.[102-106] Several studies have, in fact, shown it is possible to affect changes in landing mechanics through neuromuscular training programs. Hewett and colleagues found a 6-week training program designed to improve jumping and landing technique was able to decrease landing forces by 22%, reduce the knee varus and valgus movements by 50%, and increase the hamstring-to-quadriceps strength ratio by 13% and 26% in the dominant and nondominant legs in female athletes, respectively.[102,103] But others have made contrary findings. Programs that have chosen to focus only on addressing the strength imbalance or any singular aspect of landing performance, however, have achieved minimal success in reducing knee injuries in athletes.[104,105] Several authors have also shown that programs designed to provide augmented feedback to an athlete landing from a jump can be effective at reducing GRFs and presumably an athlete's injury risk.[107,108]

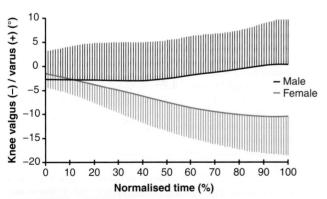

Figure 10-26

Gender differences in varus-valgus range of motion at the knee when landing from a jump. Varus is represented as positive, valgus is shown as negative. The *vertical lines* represent the standard deviation of the data at each point in time. (From Hughes G, Watkins J, Owen N: Gender difference in lower limb frontal plane kinematics during landing, *Sports Biomech* 7(3):333–341, 2008.)

> **Clinical Point**
>
> Jumper's knee (patellar tendinopathy) is one of the most frequently occurring overuse injuries and is seen in approximately 20% of athletes participating in a "jumping sport."

Related to chronic and overuse injuries, patellar tendinopathy (i.e., jumper's knee) occurs most frequently and is seen in approximately 20% of the athletes participating in jumping sports. The highest rates of occurrence are seen in male volleyball, in which 34% to 40% of elite athletes have reported experiencing this injury.[109-111] Rates of occurrence are typically lower in females, affecting approximately 7% of the elite female volleyball players.[110] As with ACL injuries, it is believed that both biomechanical and muscular factors contribute to jumper's knee. Bisseling found that athletes with a history of jumper's knee employ a "stiffer" landing strategy and that GRFs can be reduced when landing with greater knee flexion and ankle plantar flexion.[80] This stiffness, although related to joint configuration, may also have an age dependence as well; older individuals tend to exhibit greater limb stiffness.[112] Other proposed injury mechanisms surrounding jumper's knee have been related to anatomic and muscular factors (e.g., overall upper leg strength, with particular emphasis on the vastus medialis oblique, hamstring and quadriceps flexibility, leg-length discrepancy, foot pronation) although the relative contributions to injury are debated in the literature.[113-115] One additional factor to consider is rest and recovery. As jumper's knee typically presents itself as an overuse injury, lack of recovery between intense workouts is believed to contribute to the injury mechanism as well.[80]

Conclusion

Jumping is a complex biomechanical task and myriad variables can and do affect jump performance and injury risk. In the vertical jump, performance ultimately boils down to producing a high vertical velocity at takeoff and this is, in turn, affected by such variables as muscle strength, power, and rate of force development as well as the coordinated integration of a countermovement and arm swing. In addition, sport-specific constraints affect the technique used and the height attained when executing a vertical jump. Similar factors also play a role in the standing broad jump. In the long jump, the approach mechanics and the kinetics of the takeoff are what largely determine jump distance. When considering injuries, most noncontact leg injuries occur on landing from a jump and an individual's susceptibility to injury depends on the landing technique as well as on lower-limb strength.

References

1. Reiser R, Rocheford E, Armstrong CJ: Building a better understanding of basic mechanical principles through analysis of the vertical jump, *Strength Cond J* 28(4):70–80, 2006.
2. Hay J, Reid JR: *Anatomy, mechanics and human motion*, Englewood Cliffs, 1988, Prentice-Hall.
3. Vint P, Hinrichs R: Differences between one-foot and two-foot vertical jump performances, *J Appl Biomech* 12:338–358, 1996.
4. Ham D, Knez W, Young, WB: A deterministic mode of the vertical jump: Implications for training, *J Strength Cond Res* 21(3):967–972, 2007.
5. Harman EA, Rosenstein MT, Frykman PN, et al: The effects of the arms and countermovement on vertical jumping, *Med Sci Sport Exerc* 22:825–833, 1990.
6. Lees A, Vanrenterghem J, DeClerq D: The energetics and benefit of an arm swing in submaximal and maximal vertical jump performance, *J Sport Sci* 24(1):51–57, 2006.
7. Vanezis A, Lees A: A biomechanical analysis of good and poor performers of the vertical jump, *Ergonomics* 48(11–14): 1594–1603, 2005.
8. Urgrinowitsch C, Tricoli V, Rodacki ALF, et al: Influence of training background on jumping height, *J Strength Cond Res* 21(3):848–852, 2007.
9. Feltner ME, Fraschetti DJ, Crisp RJ: Upper extremity augmentation of lower extremity kinetics during countermovement vertical jumps, *J Sport Sci* 17:449–466, 1999.
10. Feltner ME, Bishop EJ, Perez CM: Segmental and kinetic contributions in vertical jumps performed with and without an arm swing, *Res Q Exerc Sport* 75(3):216–230, 2006.
11. Challis J: An investigation of the influence of bi-lateral deficit on human jumping, *Human Mov Sci* 17:307–325, 1988.
12. Lees A, Vanrenterghem J, DeClerq D: Understanding how an arm swing enhances performance in the vertical jump, *J Biomech* 37:1929–1940, 2004.
13. Van Soest AJ, Roebroeck ME, Bobbert MF, et al: A comparison of one-legged and two-legged countermovement jumps, *Med Sci Sports Exerc* 17(6):635–639, 1985.
14. Hudson J: Coordination of segments in the vertical jump, *Med Sci Sports Exerc* 18(2):242–251, 1986.
15. Bobbert MF, Gerritsen KGM, Litjens MCA, et al: Why is countermovement jump height greater than squat jump height? *Med Sci Sports Exerc* 28(11):1402–1412, 1996.
16. Hubley C, Wells R: A work-energy approach to determine individual joint contributions to vertical jump performance, *Eur J Appl Physiol* 50:247–254, 1983.
17. Stefanyshyn D, Nigg B: Contributions of the lower extremity joints to mechanical energy in running vertical jumps and running long jumps, *J Sport Sci* 16:177–186, 1998.
18. Hara M, Shibayama A, Takeshita D, et al: The effect of arm swing on lower extremities in vertical jumping, *J Biomech* 39:2503–2511, 2006.
19. Bobbert, M, van Soest AJ: Why do people jump the way they do? *Exerc Sport Sci Rev* 29(3):95–102, 2001.
20. Vanrenterghem J, Lees A, Lenoir M, et al: Performing the vertical jump: Movement adaptations for submaximal jumping, *Human Mov Sci* 22:713–727, 2004.
21. Aragon-Vargas L, Gross M: Kinesiological factors in vertical jump performance: Differences among individuals, *J Appl Biomech* 13:24–22, 1997.
22. Aragon-Vargas L, Gross M: Kinesiological factors in vertical jump performance: Differences within individuals, *J Appl Biomech* 13:46–65, 1997.
23. Cormie P, McBride JM, McCaulley GO: Power-time, force-time, and velocity-time curve analysis of the countermovement jump: Impact of training, *J Strength Cond Res* 23(1):177–186, 2009.
24. Fukashiro S, Komi PV: Joint moment and mechanical power flow of the lower limb during vertical jump, *Int J Sports Med* 8(Suppl):15–21, 1987.
25. Bobbert, M, van Ingen Schenau, GJ: Coordination in vertical jumping, *J Biomech* 21(3):249–262, 1988.
26. Bobbert MF, van Soest AJ: Two-joint muscles offer the solution, but what was the problem? *Motor Control* 4:48–52, 2000.

27. Gregoire L, Veeger H, Huijing P, et al: Role of mono- and biarticular muscles in explosive movements, *Int J Sports Med* 5:301–305, 1984.

28. Prilutsky B: Coordination of two- and one-joint muscles: Functional consequences and implications for motor control, *Motor Control* 4:1–44, 2000.

29. Prilutsky B: Muscle coordination: The discussion continues, *Motor Control* 4:97–116, 2000.

30. Van Ingen Schenau GJ, Bobbert M, Rosendal RH: The unique action of bi-articular muscles in complex movements, *J Anat* 155:1–5, 1987.

31. Van Soest AJ, Schwab A, Bobbert MF, et al: The influence of the biarticularity of the gastrocnemius muscle on vertical-jumping achievement, *J Biomech* 26(1):1–8, 1993.

32. Anderson F, Pandy M: Storage and utilization of elastic strain energy during jumping, *J Biomech* 26(12):1413–1427, 1993.

33. Pandy M, Zajac F: Optimal muscular coordination strategies for jumping, *J Biomech* 24(1):1–10, 1991.

34. Ravn S, Voigt M, Simonsen EB, et al: Choice of jumping strategy in two standard jumps, squat and countermovement jump—Effect of training background or inherited preference? *Scand J Med Sci Sports* 9:201–208, 1999.

35. Khalid W, Armin M, Bober T: The influence of the upper extremities movement on take-off in vertical jump. In Tsarouchas VL, Terauds J, Gowitzke B, Holt L, editors: *Biomechanics in sport V*, Athens, Greece, Hellenic Sports Research Institute, 1989.

36. Luhtanen P, Komi PV: Segmental contributions to forces in vertical jumps, *Eur J Appl Physiol Occup Ther* 38:181–188, 1978.

37. Shetty A, Entyre B: Contribution of arm movement to the force components of a maximum vertical jump, *J Orthop Sports Phys Ther* 11:198–201, 1989.

38. Payne A, Slater W, Telford T: The use of a force platform in the study of athletic activities, *Ergonomics* 11:123–143, 1968.

39. Enoka R: *Neuromechanical basis of kinesiology,* Champaign, IL, 1988, Human Kinetics.

40. Bosco C, Komi PV: Influence of countermovement amplitude in potentiation of muscular performance. In Marek A, Fidelis K, Kedzies K, Wit A, editors: *Biomechanics VII-A,* Baltimore, M, University Park Press, 1981.

41. Cavagna G, Dusman B, Margaria R: Positive work done by the previously stretched muscle, *J Appl Physiol* 24:21–32, 1968.

42. Bobbert MF, Casius LJ, Sijpkens IWT, et al: Humans adjust control to initial squat depth in vertical squat jumping, *J Appl Physiol* 105(5):1428–1440, 2008.

43. Saunders H: *A cinematographical study of the relationship between speed of movement and available force,* Dissertation. College Station, Texas A&M University, 1980.

44. Dapena J, Chung: Vertical and radial motions of the body during the takeoff phase of high jumping, *Med Sci Sports Exerc* 20:290–302, 1988.

45. Dapena J: Basic and applied research in the biomechanics of high jumping, *Med Sport Sci* 25:19–33, 1987.

46. Bobbert MF, De Graaf WW, Jonk JN, et al: Explanation of the bilateral deficit in human vertical squat jumping, *J Appl Physiol* 100(2):493–499, 2006.

47. Bobbert MF, Casius LJR: Is the effect of a countermovement on jump height due to active state development? *Med Sci Sports Exerc* 37(3):440–446, 2005.

48. Vanrenterghem J, Lees A, DeClerq D: Effect of forward trunk inclination on joint power output in vertical jumping, *J Strength Cond Res* 22(3):708–714, 2008.

49. Dapena J: How to design the shape of a high jump run-up, *Track Coach* 131:4179–4181, 1995.

50. Dapena J, McDonald J, Cappaert J: A regression analysis of high jumping technique, *Int J Sports Biomech* 6:246–261, 1990.

51. McEwen F: High jump: Teaching the Fosbury Flop, *Modern Athlete & Coach* 45(4):10–14, 2007.

52. Laffaye G, Bardy B, Durey A: Principal component structure and sport-specific differences in the running on-leg vertical jump, *Int J Sports Med* 28:420–425, 2007.

53. Holcomb W, Lander J, Rutland RM, et al: A biomechanical analysis of the vertical jump and three modified plyometric depth jumps, *J Strength Cond Res* 10(2):83–88, 1996.

54. Bobbert MF, Huijing P, van Ingen Schenau GJ: Drop jumping I: The influence of jumping technique on the biomechanics of jumping, *Med Sci Sports Exerc* 19(4):332–338, 1987.

55. Alexander R: Optimum take-off techniques for high and long jumps, *Phil Trans R Soc Lond* B329:3–10, 1990.

56. Graham-Smith P, Lees A: A three-dimensional kinematic analysis of the long jump take-off, *J Sport Sci* 23(9):891–903, 2005.

57. Hay J: Citius, altius, fortius (faster, higher, longer): The biomechanics of jumping for distance, *J Biomech* 26(Suppl 1):7–21, 1993.

58. Hay J, Miller J, Canterna RW: The techniques of elite male long jumpers, *J Biomech* 19(10):855–866, 1986.

59. Hay J, Nohara H: Techniques used by elite long jumpers in preparation for takeoff, *J Biomech* 23(2):229–239, 1990.

60. Kyrolainen H, Avela J, Komi PV, et al: Function of the neuromuscular system during the two last steps in the long jump. In deGroot H, Huijing PA, and van Ingen Schenau GJ: *Biomechanics XI-B,* Amsterdam, 1998, Free University Press.

61. Lees A, Fowler N, Derby D: A biomechanical analysis of the last stride, touch-down and take-off characteristics of the women's long jump, *J Sport Sci* 11:303–314, 1993.

62. Lees A, Graham-Smith P, Fowler N: A biomechanical analysis of the last stride, touchdown, and takeoff characteristics of the men's long jump, *J Appl Biomech* 10:61–78, 1994.

63. Muraki Y, Ae M, Yokozawa T, et al: Mechanical properties of the take-off leg as a support mechanism in the long jump, *Sports Biomech* 4(1):1–16, 2005.

64. Seyfarth A, Friedrichs A, Wank V, et al: Dynamics of the long jump, *J Biomech* 32:1259–1267, 1999.

65. Ashby B, Heegaard J: Role of arm motion in the standing long jump, *J Biomech* 35:1631–1637, 2002.

66. Ashby B, Delp S: Optimal control simulations reveal mechanisms by which arm movement improves standing long jump performance, *J Biomech* 39:1726–1734, 2006.

67. Hara M, Shibayama A, Arakawa H, et al: Effect of arm swing direction on forward and backward jump performance, *J Biomech* 41:2806–2815, 2008.

68. Gray J, Taunton J, Taunton DC, et al: A survey of injuries to the anterior cruciate ligament of the knee in female basketball players, *Int J Sports Med* 6:314–316, 1985.

69. Gerberich SG, Luhmann S, Finke C, et al: Analysis of severe injuries associated with volleyball injuries, *Phys Sports Med* 15(8):75–79, 1987.

70. Adrian M, Laughlin C: Magnitude of ground reaction forces while performing volleyball skills. In Kobayashi MA, editor: *Biomechanics VIII-B,* Champaign, 1983, Human Kinetics.

71. Steele J, Milburn P: Ground reaction forces on landing in netball, *J Human Mov Studies* 13:399–410, 1987.

72. McNitt-Gray J: *The influence of impact speed on joint kinematics and impulse characteristics of drop landings,* 12th International Congress of Biomechanics, Los Angeles, 1989.

73. Devita P, Skelly P: Effect of landing stiffness on joint kinetics and energetics in the lower extremity, *Med Sci Sports Exerc* 24(1):108–115, 1992.

74. Kovacs I, Tihanyi J, Devita P, et al: Foot placement modifies kinematics and kinetics during drop jumping, *Med Sci Sports Exerc* 31(5):708–716.

75. Murphy D, Connolly D, Beynnon BD: Risk factors for lower-extremity injury: A review of the literature, *Br J Sports Med* 37(1):13–29, 2003.

76. Dufek J: *The effect of landing on lower extremity function,* Dissertation from the University of Oregon, 1988.

77. Valiant G, Cavanaugh P: A study of landing from a jump: Implications for the design of a basketball shoe. In Winter DA, Norman RW, Wells RP, et al: *Biomechanics IX-B,* Champaign, 1985, Human Kinetics.

78. Dufek J, Bates B: *The relationship between ground reaction forces and lower extremity extensor joint moments in landing,* Proceedings of the 14th Annual American Society of Biomechanics, Miami, 1990.

79. Dufek J, Bates B: Biomechanical factors associated with injury during landing in jump sports, *Sports Med* 12(5):326–337, 1991.

80. Bisseling R: *Biomechanical determinants of the jumper's knee in volleyball,* Doctoral dissertation, University of Groningen, 2008.

81. Turpin JP, Cortell JM, Chinchilla JJ, et al: Analysis of jump patterns in competition for elite male beach volleyball players, *Int J Performance Anal Sport* 8(2):94–101, 2008.

82. Coleman J, Adrian M, Yamamato H: *The teaching of the mechanics of jump landing,* Second National Symposium on Teaching Kinesiology and Biomechanics in Sport, DeKalb, IL, 1984.

83. Chappell J, Yu B, Kirkendall DT, et al: A comparison of knee kinetics between male and female recreational athletes in stop-jumping, *Am J Sports Med* 30:261–267, 2002.

84. Bobbert MF, Huijing P, van Ingen Schenau GJ: Drop jumping II: The influence of drop jump height on the biomechanics of drop jumping, *Med Sci Sports Exerc* 19:339–346, 1987.

85. Zelisko J, Noble H, Porter MA: A comparison of men's and women's professional basketball injuries, *Am J Sports Med* 10(5):297–299, 1982.

86. Chandy T, Grana W: Secondary school athletic injury in boys and girls: A three-year comparison, *Phys Sportsmed* 13:314–316, 1985.

87. Kernozek TW, Torry MR, van Hoof H, et al: Gender differences in frontal and sagittal plane biomechanics during drop landings, *Med Sci Sports Exerc* 37(6):1003–1012, 2005.

88. Hewett TE, Meyer G, Gregory D, et al: Biomechanical measures of neuromuscular control and valgus loading of the knee predict anterior cruciate ligament injury risk in female athletes: A prospective study, *Am J Sports Med* 33:492–501, 2005.

89. Padua DA, Carcia CR, Arnold BL, et al: Gender differences in leg stiffness and stiffness recruitment strategy during two-legged hopping, *J Motor Behav* 37:111–115, 2005.

90. Decker MJ, Torry MR, Wyland DJ, et al: Gender differences in lower extremity kinematics, kinetics, and energy absorption during landing, *Clin Biomech* 18:662–669, 2003.

91. Cortes N, Onate J, Abrantes J, et al: Effects of gender and foot-landing technique on lower extremity kinematics during drop-jump landings, *J Appl Biomech* 23:289–299, 2007.

92. Hughes G, Watkins J, Owen N: Gender difference in lower limb frontal plane kinematics during landing, *Sports Biomech* 7(3):333–341, 2008.

93. Russell KA, Palmieri RM, Zonder SM, et al: Sex differences in valgus knee angle during a single-leg drop jump, *J Athl Training* 41(2):166–171, 2006.

94. Noyes FR, Barber-Westin SD, Fleckerstein C, et al: The drop-jump screening test, *Am J Sports Med* 33(2):197–207, 2005.

95. Knapick JJ, Bauman CL, Jones BH, et al: Preseason strength and flexibility imbalances associated with athletic injuries in female collegiate athletes, *Am J Sports Med* 19:76–81, 1991.

96. Withrow TJ, Huston, Wojtys EM, et al: The relationship between quadriceps muscle force, knee flexion, and anterior cruciate ligament strain in an in-vivo simulated jump landing, *Am J Sports Med* 34:269–274, 2006.

97. Withrow TJ, Huston LJ, Wojtys EM, et al: *A lengthening hamstring contraction condition reduces ACL strain in and in-vitro jump landing model: An ACL protective mechanism,* 52nd Annual Meeting of the Orthopaedic Research Society, Chicago, 2006.

98. Colby S, Francisco A, Yu B, et al: Electromyographic and kinematic analysis of cutting maneuvers, *Am J Sports Med* 28:234–240, 2000.

99. Lephart SM, Ferris CM, Reimann BL, et al: Gender differences in strength and lower extremity kinematics during landing, *Clin Orthop Relat Res* 401:162–169, 2002.

100. Malinak RA, Colby SM, Kirkendall DT, et al: A comparison of knee joint motion patterns between men and women in selected athletic tasks, *Clin Biomech* 16:438–445, 2001.

101. Bennett DR, Blackburn JT, Boling MC, et al: The relationship between anterior tibial shear force during a jump landing and quadriceps and hamstring strength, *Clin Biomech* 23:1165–1171, 2008.

102. Hewett TE, Stroupe AL, Nance TA, et al: Plyometric training in female athletes: Decreased impact force and increased hamstring torques, *Am J Sports Med* 24(6):765–773, 1996.

103. Hewett TE, Lindenfeld TN, Riccobene JV, et al: The effect of neuromuscular training on the incidence of knee injury in female athletes, *Am J Sports Med* 27:699–706, 1999.

104. Hewett TE, Ford K, Myer GD: Anterior cruciate ligament injuries in female athletes: Part 2, a meta-analysis of neuromuscular interventions aimed at injury prevention, *Am J Sports Med* 34:490–498, 2006.

105. Irmischer BS, Harris C, Pfeiffer RP, et al: Effects of a knee ligament injury prevention exercise program on impact forces in women, *J Strength Cond Res* 18(4):703–707, 2004.

106. Padua D, Marshall S: Evidence supporting ACL-injury prevention exercise programs: A review of the literature, *Athletic Therapy Today* 11:11–23, 2006.

107. Cronin J, Bressel E, Finn L: Augmented feedback reduces ground reaction forces in the landing phase of the volleyball spike jump, *J Sports Rehabil* 17:148–159, 2008.

108. Prapavessis H, McNair PJ: Effects of instruction in jumping technique and experience jumping on ground reaction forces, *J Orthop Sports Phys Ther* 29(6):352–356, 1999.

109. Ferretti A, Papandrea P, Conteduca F: Knee injuries in volleyball, *Sports Med* 10:132–138, 1990.

110. Gisslen K, Gyulai C, Soderman K: High prevalence of jumper's knee and sonographic changes in Swedish elite junior volleyball players compared to matched controls, *Br J Sports Med* 39: 298–301, 2005.

111. Lian O, Engebresten K, Bahr R: Prevalence of jumper's knee among elite athletes from different sports: A cross-sectional study, *Am J Sports Med* 33:561–567, 2005.

112. Wang L, Lin D, Huang C: Age effects on jumping techniques and lower limb stiffness during vertical jump, *Res Sports Med* 12:209–219, 2004.

113. Blazina ME, Kerlan RK, Jobe FW: Jumper's knee, *Orthop Clin North Am* 4:665–678, 1973.

114. Cook J, Kiss ZS, Khan KM: Anthropometry, physical performance, and ultrasound patellar tendon abnormality in elite junior basketball players: A cross-sectional study, *Br J Sports Med* 38:206–209, 2004.

115. Witvrouw E, Bellemans J, Lysens R: Intrinsic risk factors for the development of patellar tendinitis in an athletic population, *Am J Sports Med* 29:190–195, 2001.

APPLIED BIOMECHANICS OF TENNIS

Todd S. Ellenbecker, E. Paul Roetert, W. Ben Kibler, and Mark S. Kovacs

Introduction

The modern game of tennis is characterized by specific inherent movement patterns that use sequential segmental rotations that ultimately result in powerful ground strokes and serves and precise, accurate volleys. These characteristic movement patterns use the body's entire kinetic chain to produce power and optimize functional performance. Analysis of the patterns of play in elite players identifies that 75% or more of the shots hit in tennis involve the serve and forehand ground stroke,[1] which use extremely powerful concentric shoulder internal rotation muscular work that can lead to traditional muscular imbalances and predispose the player to overuse injury. Although the primary scope of this chapter is tennis, these muscular imbalances and characteristic concentric internal shoulder rotation use do apply to nearly all racquet sports and overhead activities involving spiking, serving, and throwing. The primary purpose of this chapter is to provide a detailed review of the biomechanics of tennis strokes and movement patterns to give the clinician an appreciation of the demands of the game of tennis on the human body. This information has particular relevance for understanding injury patterns, and anatomical adaptations and maladaptations in the tennis player's musculoskeletal system.

Overview of Tennis Ground Strokes, Volley, and Serve

The forehand and backhand strokes, collectively referred to as *ground strokes* in tennis, are characterized and studied using three primary phases. As a matter of definition, ground strokes in tennis typically involve hitting the ball after it bounces. These include the preparation phase, acceleration phase, and follow-through phase. Ball contact separates the acceleration and follow-through phases in

both the forehand and backhand. Similar stages are used to describe the volley and half-volley strokes, with the former characterized with ball contact prior to the ball striking the court surface on the player's side of the court and the latter pertaining to ball contact nearly immediately following the bounce, typically from a mid-court location.

The serve is studied and analyzed in a similar fashion to the throwing motion in many studies.[2-4] It contains a wind-up or preparation phase, arm-cocking phase, acceleration phase, and follow-though phase (Figure 11-1). The separation between the preparation and arm-cocking phases includes the initiation of the ball toss with the contralateral extremity with the initiation of the acceleration phase occurring following maximal external rotation of the glenohumeral (GH) joint. Ball contact again separates the acceleration and follow-through phases as opposed to ball release separating the same phases in the throwing motion.

Phases of a Tennis Serve
• Wind-up (preparation) phase
• Arm-cocking phase
• Acceleration phase
• Follow-through phase

Muscular Activity Patterns

The high-velocity dynamic muscular contractions present in the tennis serve and ground strokes have been studied in minimally skilled and elite-level tennis players. Yoshizawa and colleagues[5] recorded the peak and median muscular activity patterns of the shoulder and forearm muscles during the serve and ground strokes. They found significantly

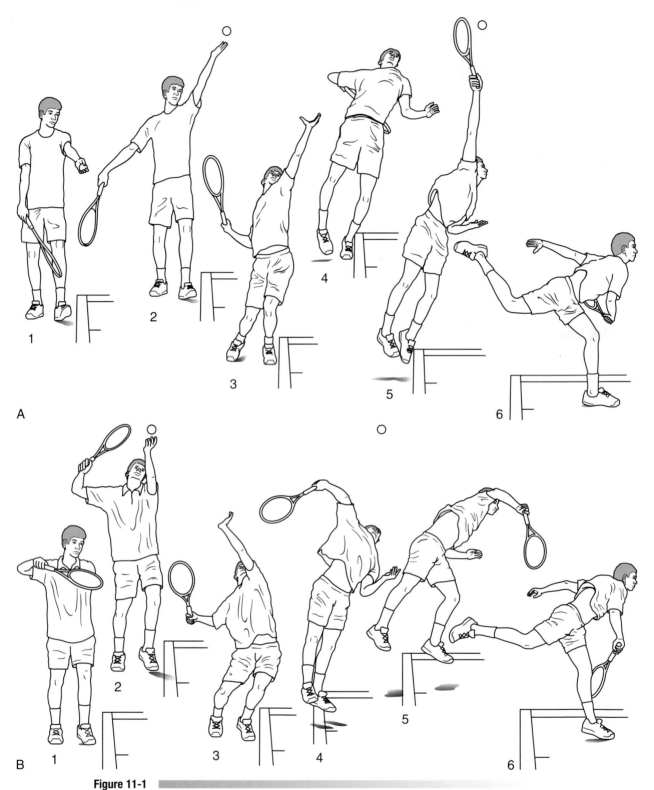

Figure 11-1

A, Traditional tennis serve. *1.* Preparation phase; *2.* Preparation phase; *3.* Cocking phase (max external rotation); *4.* Early acceleration phase; *5.* Late acceleration phase near ball contact; *6.* Follow-through phase. **B,** Abbreviated tennis serve. *1.* Preparation phase; *2.* Preparation phase; *3.* Cocking phase (max external rotation); *4.* Acceleration phase; *5.* Early follow-through phase; *6.* Late follow-though phase.

higher muscular activity levels during the serve, indicating that it is the most strenuous stroke in tennis from an upper-extremity muscular standpoint.

The serve is broken down into the four previously mentioned phases. The *windup phase* is characterized by the initiation of the serving stance to the toss of the ball by the contralateral extremity. There is very low electromyographic (EMG) activity during this phase in the muscles surrounding the shoulder.[2] The second phase of the serving motion is the *cocking phase*, which begins after the ball toss and terminates at the point of maximal external rotation of the GH joint of the racquet arm. Muscular activity during this phase is moderately high in the supraspinatus, infraspinatus, subscapularis, biceps brachii, and serratus anterior. Muscular activity levels expressed as a percentage of the maximum voluntary isometric contraction (MVC) were 53%, 41%, 25%, 39%, and 70%, respectively.[2] The stabilizing and approximating role of the rotator cuff identified by Inman and colleagues[6] is clearly shown in the cocking phase of the tennis serve.[7] The moderately high activity during this phase shows the importance of both anterior and posterior rotator cuff strength, as well as scapular stabilization for proper execution of the required mechanics for the cocking phase.[8]

Clinical Point

Anterior (subscapularis) and posterior (infraspinatus and teres minor) rotator cuff muscles and scapular stabilizers (primarily trapezius and serratus anterior) play a key role in the cocking phase.

The third phase of the tennis serve is *acceleration*. This phase begins at maximal external rotation and terminates at ball impact. Consistent with EMG recordings during the acceleration phase of throwing,[4] high muscular activity was found in the pectoralis major, subscapularis, latissimus dorsi, and serratus anterior during the forceful concentric internal rotation of the humerus.[2] EMG research published by VanGheluwe and Hebbelinck[9] using intermediate tennis players and by Miyashita and colleagues[10] using skilled and unskilled tennis players also found high activity levels of the pectoralis major, as well as the deltoid, trapezius, and triceps, during the acceleration phase. Both reports showed a relative silence of electrical activity in the accelerating musculature during impact with peak levels of muscular activity occurring just before impact. One exception is the stabilizing contribution of the infraspinatus, which remained active during impact.[9]

The fourth and final phase occurs after impact and is termed the *follow-through*. This phase is characterized by moderately high activity of the posterior rotator cuff, serratus anterior, biceps brachii, deltoid, and latissimus dorsi.

After the electrical silence of the shoulder musculature during impact or collision,[9,10] forceful eccentric muscular contraction is necessary to decelerate the humerus and maintain GH joint congruity.

A relatively consistent pattern of muscular activity is reported for skilled tennis players. The presence of increased, as well as overlapping, muscular activity patterns across the outlined stages in the tennis serve has been reported by untrained[5] and less skilled[10] tennis players. This increase in the muscular contribution during the serving motion in less-skilled players is a perfect example of how nonoptimal timing and a lack of whole-body contributions to force generation and deceleration subject an individual's shoulder to overuse injury. The contribution of the larger muscle groups in the lower extremities and trunk via proper biomechanical energy transfer during the tennis serve protect the player from injury and optimize performance.[11-14]

Inherent Demands of Tennis on the Shoulder

The shoulder faces high loads in those playing tennis. Elite players reach rotational velocities of up to 1700 deg/sec, resulting in arm velocities of up to 72 miles per hour (115.2 kph) on the serve.[15] The one-hand backhand stroke generates rotational velocities up to 900 deg/sec (arm velocities of 34 miles per hour [54.4 kph]), and the open-stance forehand generates 280 deg/sec, which, with trunk rotation through the kinetic chain, created arm velocities of up to 46 miles per hour (73.6 kph).[15] Ranges of motion were found to be correspondingly large. Total arc of rotational motion (internal + external rotation) was between 160° and 180°.[15]

Torques generated in the serve by these loads and motions were found to be high at two critical times—maximum external rotation (MER) during cocking and acceleration to ball impact (ABI). At MER, men recorded 65 Nm and women 46 Nm. At ABI, men recorded 70 Nm and women 50 Nm. Torques greater than 50 Nm are considered a significant and potentially injurious factor in loading of the upper extremity, so those inherent loads have the potential to create overload injury.[16]

The deceleration force between the trunk and the arm at ball impact and follow-through can be as high as 300 Nm. This is required to stabilize and support the shoulder against the distraction forces that equal 0.5 to 0.75 times body weight.

These loads are placed on the shoulder with every stroke. The numbers of strokes per match vary greatly, depending on the type of match, skill level, opponent, and playing surface. The average elite tennis match involves at least 100 repetitions of "game" serves and 250 repetitions of "game" ground-strokes.[17] In junior tennis tournaments in scholastic or collegiate tennis, these numbers are larger, because two to three matches may be played per day. These numbers do not include the number of "practice" strokes, which in most estimates is four to five times higher.

Application of the Kinetic Chain Concept in Serving Biomechanics

The role of other body segments and their effect on the shoulder and elbow during the tennis serve was studied by Elliott and colleagues.[18] They measured kinetic and kinematic variables of the serve in professional tennis players and characterized them as having either an effective "leg drive" (front knee flexion angle greater than 14.7°) or an ineffective "leg drive" (maximal front knee flexion less than 14.7°). Most important from an injury prevention standpoint was the finding of significantly greater medial elbow loading (varus elbow torque 3.9% versus 5.3%) when comparing the group with greater knee flexion with the group with less knee flexion respectively.[18] In addition, the group with a more effective leg drive showed reduced shoulder internal rotation torques when the shoulder was placed in maximal external rotation than the group of elite players who had less leg drive during their serving motion.[18] This study shows the importance of the use of the entire kinetic chain to produce power during the tennis serve and highlights the ramifications of using a pattern of serving biomechanics for the shoulder elbow when the lower extremity and trunk are not optimally integrated.

Clinical Point

An effective leg drive to decrease injuries involves a front knee flexion angle of greater than 14.7°.[17]

The thought behind the use of elastic energy is to stretch the muscle followed by a shortening of the muscle. For example, in the backswing phase of the serve, the shoulders are rotated more than the hips, stretching the muscles across the upper trunk and shoulder area.[19,20] This stored energy can then provide force in the forward phase of the swing. If not prepared through proper training, these forces could put significant stress on the shoulder joint. Proper strength exercises, particularly of the rotator cuff and scapular stabilizers, are critical for the protection of the shoulder joint. Although it makes logical sense to increase the distance the racquet travels to increase the production of force, only recently have researchers and tennis teaching professionals begun to focus on the distance between the racquet head and the trunk in the backswing. The old "backscratch" position is counterproductive in the production of force. As Elliott and colleagues[18] have pointed out, leg drive forces the racquet in a downward motion and away from the back. This energy will be recovered to assist in generating racquet velocity during internal rotation of the upper arm. This increase in the distance of the racquet path in the swing, use of elastic energy, and coordinated use of the kinetic link principle (i.e., proper use of the sequencing of body segments initiated by a ground reaction force [GRF]) will aid in the protection of the shoulder joint during repeated services actions.

Research has recently compared the traditional service motion in which the racquet arm is brought downward below the waist as the hands separate in the preparation phase to the "abbreviated" backswing motion in which the racquet is not brought into the downward position in an abbreviated movement pattern. Elliott and colleagues[18] and Seeley and colleagues[21] have both shown no significant differences in either shoulder or elbow loads comparing the traditional backswing with the abbreviated backswing in players who use proper leg drive. It must be emphasized that use of the abbreviated technique in the absence of proper kinetic chain involvement may subject the upper limb to abnormal physiological loads leading to potential shoulder and upper-extremity injury.

Biomechanics of Force Production and Force Control—The Kinetic Chain

Schonbrun[22] has calculated that the advanced tennis player is required to generate approximately 4000 watts of energy to hit a strong, forcing shot. This amount of energy is equivalent to running up a 10-step flight of stairs in 2 seconds. This high energy output is one more of the inherent demands of the sport. The kinetic chain is the biomechanical system by which the body meets the inherent demands of tennis. It generates the required forces and helps to regulate and modify loads seen at the joints, especially the high loads at the shoulder.[23]

Clinical Point

Stroke power is maximized by using the whole kinetic chain.

In the normally operating kinetic chain, the legs and trunk segments are the engine for the development of force and the stable proximal base for distal mobility.[15,24,25] This link develops 51% to 55% of the kinetic energy and force delivered to the hand[24]; creates the back leg–to–front leg angular momentum to drive the arm forward[9,11]; and, because of its high cross-sectional area, large mass, and high moment of inertia, creates an anchor that allows centripetal motion to occur.[16,26]

Clinical Point

- The trunk and legs deliver 51% to 55% of the kinetic energy to the hand
- The shoulder delivers 13% of the kinetic energy

The functional result of this stable base is considered to represent core stability.[27] In addition to generating force in the trunk and leg segments, kinetic chain activation through the core also generates force in the distal segments through the creation of interactive movements, or forces generated at joints by the position and motion of adjacent segments.[28] At the shoulder, the interactive movement produced by trunk rotation around a vertical axis is the most important factor in generating forward arm motion, and the interactive movement produced by trunk rotation around a horizontal axis from front to back is the most important factor in generating arm abduction.[17]

The remaining kinetic chain segments play smaller roles in intrinsic force generation, mainly because of their smaller cross-sectional area and the production of interactive movements. The shoulder produces only 13% of the total kinetic energy for the entire service motion. The high velocities and forces seen at the shoulder are predominantly produced through sequential kinetic chain activation.

The shoulder functions in the kinetic chain primarily as a funnel, transferring the forces developed in the engine of the core to the delivery mechanism of the hand.[24] Efficient activation of the segments within the kinetic chain regulates the loads seen at distal joints.[23] In addition, the kinetic chain can modify loads at the shoulder by aligning the bones of the GH articulation so that ball-and-socket kinematics that produce concavity compression and stabilize the joint may be maximized through the majority of the range of motion (ROM) of the shoulder. Coordinated coupled motions of the humerus and the scapula (scapulohumeral rhythm) keep the GH angle within 30° of the plane of the scapula. This angle minimizes muscle activations required for joint stability,[29] keeps the compression forces directed into the concavity of the glenoid,[30] and minimizes strain of the GH ligaments.[31] These actions maximize the shoulder's role as a funnel for transfer of forces and motion of the adjacent segments. Studies using baseball players have demonstrated that at the moment of ball release, which is equivalent to ball contact in tennis, only four body segments are responsible for forward movement of the arm. They are trunk forward flexion, shoulder internal rotation, elbow extension, and wrist flexion. Half of the force produced at the shoulder, 70% of the force produced at the elbow, and more than 80% of the force produced at the wrist is generated through the interactive moments.[32,33]

Kinetic Chain Activation and Nodes

Kinetic chain activation is required to generate the forces and motions at the shoulder to produce the two most important individual biomechanical functions in the tennis serve. The first is long-axis rotation, which couples shoulder internal rotation and forearm pronation and produces the most force at ball impact.[25] The second is maximum shoulder abduction, which decreases shoulder impingement in acceleration and allows the hand to go up and through the ball in follow-through to create topspin.

Because the kinetic chain is composed of multiple segments, there are multiple (up to 244) degrees of freedom within the system.[34] Preprogrammed muscle activations can temporarily stabilize several links of the kinetic chain in "coordinative structures" that convert multiple degrees of freedom into one or two degrees of freedom.[34] The task-specific linkages have the effect of decreasing the degrees of freedom within a linked system, creating maximal torques with minimal force development throughout the kinetic chain. The result of these linkages is to create "nodes"—specific body segment positions and motions that are fundamental for efficiency and maximal sequencing of multiple segment activations within a linked kinetic chain.[34] Because of the task specific requirements of the nodes, each sport or activity within a sport can have a unique set of nodes for that activity. From data compiled from a variety of scientific studies[16-18,25,35-38] and from discussions with tennis coaches,[37,39] it has been determined that five specific nodes appear to be required in the tennis serve. These nodes are observable in the tennis serve. In sequential order from the ground up, they are (1) adequate knee flexion in cocking progressing to knee extension at ball impact, (2) hip and trunk counter-rotation away from the court in cocking, (3) coupled scapular retraction and arm rotation to achieve cocking in the scapular plane, (4) back leg–to–front leg motion to create a "shoulder over shoulder" motion at ball impact, and (5) long-axis rotation into ball impact and follow-through (Figure 11-2).

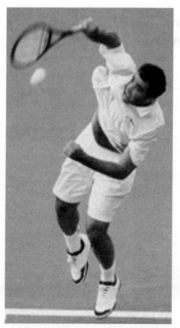

Figure 11-2

Example of long-axis rotation. (From Herbst R, McEnroe P: The interplay of tactics and techniques. In Roetert P, Groppel J, editors: *World-class tennis technique,* Champaign, IL, 2001, Human Kinetics.)

Specific Body Segment Positions and Motions (Nodes) Required for Tennis Serve

- Adequate knee flexion (cocking) and extension (ball impact)
- Hip and trunk counter rotation (cocking)
- Coupled scapular retraction and arm rotation (cocking)
- Back-to-front leg motion (ball impact)
- Long-axis rotation (ball impact to follow through)

Achievement of the proper sequencing of the nodes implies the most efficient use of the kinetic chain,[23,37] which will minimize the stresses on the shoulder. This has the capability to maximize force through kinetic chain activation and interactive moments, and minimize injury risk by controlling joint positions and forces, and eliminating kinetic chain breakage.

Kinetic Chain Break Down and "Catch-Up" During the Service Motion

Because of the importance of the proximal kinetic chain in developing force and protecting the distal joints, deficits in the proximal chain result in either decreased force delivered to the hand and racquet,[24] resulting in decreased ball velocity, altered interactive movements at the distal joints with increased forces at the joints,[18,28] or increased activation of distal segments to develop maximal forces at the hand.[24] There are multiple methods by which the deficits may be developed, including poor stroke techniques,[40] previous injury, muscle inflexibility,[41-43] or muscle weakness or imbalance.[27,36,44] The most common anatomical areas involved are the hip (inflexibility and decreased strength), trunk (inflexibility and altered strength balance), scapula (scapular dyskinesis), and shoulder rotation (glenohumeral internal rotation deficiency), but any injured area in the proximal kinetic chain (e.g., sprained ankle, knee meniscal tear) may be involved.

Development of Kinetic Chain Deficits

- Loss of lower kinetic chain force
- Poor stroke techniques
- Injury
- Inflexibility
- Muscle weakness or force couple imbalance

Most Common Kinetic Chain Deficit Areas

- Hip (inflexibility and decreased strength)
- Trunk (inflexibility and strength imbalance)
- Scapula (dyskinesia)
- Shoulder (GIRD — glenohumeral internal rotation deficit)

"Catch-up" occurs when the athlete tries to compensate for the kinetic chain breakage by increasing distal segment activation to maintain maximal force production. Deficiencies in energy or force production in one segment require more energy or force from other more distal segments to develop the same force to the end segment and maintain athletic performance. This means the mass of the distal segments, which is usually less than the proximal segments, must significantly increase, or the velocity of the segment, which is already high, must increase even more. Neither increase in mass nor velocity is easy to achieve. In the mathematical model of the kinetic chain of the tennis player,[24] a 20% reduction in kinetic energy from the trunk requires a 34% increase in velocity or a 70% increase in mass to achieve the same kinetic energy to the hand. Alteration of normal activation sequencing can also place extra loads on distal joints. Inadequate flexion of the knee less than 10° at MER in cocking in the service motion, breaking the kinetic chain push-through activation sequencing, significantly increases shoulder internal rotation torque at MER by 17.6% and at ABI by 18.2% in athletes who do maintain the same serve velocity.[18]

Analysis of two specific kinetic chain patterns in the serve will show the effect of kinetic chain activation on the loads, performance, and consequences for injury risk at the shoulder. The two serve sequences are "push-through/pull-through" kinetic chains, and traditional versus abbreviated service motions.

Push-Through/Pull-Through Kinetic Chains During the Service Motion

The "push-through" activation sequence uses knee flexion and back-leg drive to maximize GRFs that push the body upward from the cocking position into ball impact and create long-axis rotation in the arm. Push-through uses the large leg muscles to provide the majority of the power,[23] decreases the internal rotation torques at the shoulder,[8] produces greater muscle forces at the shoulder,[23] allows higher degrees of shoulder abduction to produce top spin and decrease impingement,[34] and generates greater ball velocities.[17,45] This type of activation is the most efficient and is seen more frequently in elite male players. Figure 11-3, Figure 11-4, and Figure 11-5 demonstrate EMG activation patterns in the lower extremity that are characteristic of the push-through pattern. Figure 11-3 (elite player) demonstrates the back leg–to–front leg progression of activation in the gastrocnemius and quadriceps muscles before ball impact,[45] and Figures 11-4 and 11-5 demonstrate back-leg hamstring and gluteus medius activation prior to ball impact. Figure 11-6 demonstrates observational characteristics of push-through activations.

"Pull-through" activation uses trunk muscles to pull the trunk and arm from cocking into ball impact and create long-axis rotation in the arm. Knee flexion and use of the

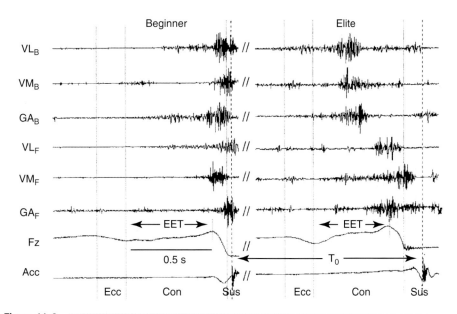

Figure 11-3

Differences between beginner and elite tennis players in lower extremity muscle activation during the tennis serve. VL_B, back vastus lateralis; VM_B, back vastus medialis; GA_B, back gastrocnemius lateralis; VL_F, front vastus lateralis; VM_F, front vastus medialis; GN_F, front gastrocnemius lateralis; F_Z, vertical ground reaction force; Acc, accelerometer; Ecc, eccentric phase; Con, concentric phase; Sus, suspension phase. (From Girard O, Micallef JP, Millet GP: Lower-limb activity during the power serve in tennis: Effects of performance level, *Med Sci Sports Exerc* 37([6]):1021-1029, 2005.)

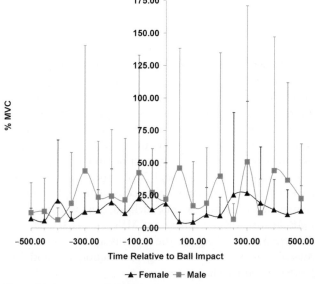

Figure 11-4

Hamstring activation of nondominant leg during tennis serve.

legs is minimized. This activation increases internal rotation torques at the shoulder,[23] creates increased scapular protraction and GH "hyperangulation,"[46] decreases shoulder abduction and the ability to hit topspin,[35] and is associated with lower ball velocities.[45] This type of activation results from lack of full use of the proximal kinetic chain segments

and occurs more frequently in female elite players and recreational players. Figure 11-7 demonstrates nondominant external oblique activation to pull the trunk and arm into ball impact. Figure 11-8 and Figure 11-9 demonstrate observational characteristics of pull-through.

Clinical Point

Push-through kinetic chain patterns of serve produce more stroke power than pull-through patterns.

Pull-through activation patterns are shown to develop less stable kinematic patterns and higher force loads at the shoulder. No epidemiological studies have looked at the correlations of shoulder injury with the type of service motion. However, the kinematic pattern of GH hyperangulation and increased scapular protraction has been implicated in the generation of shoulder injury,[36,46] and the pattern of increased abduction angle is known to relate to impingement.[42] The inefficiency of the motion is shown by higher force loads but lower ball velocities.

Finally, research has recently compared the traditional service motion in which the racquet arm is brought downward below the waist as the hands separate in the preparation phase with the "abbreviated" backswing

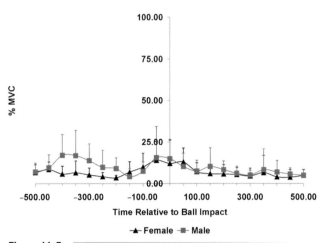

Figure 11-5
Gluteus medius activation of dominant leg during tennis serve.

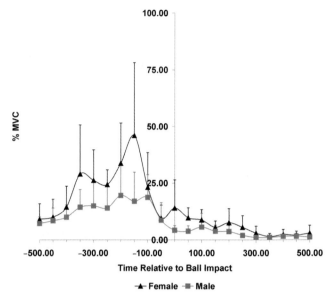

Figure 11-7
Nondominant external oblique activation during tennis serve.

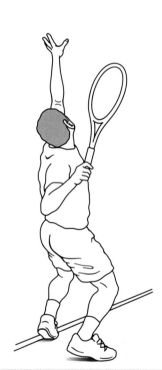

Figure 11-6
Observable characteristics of the "push-through" serve are scapular retraction and large degrees of knee flexion during cocking.

motion that the player in Figure 11-1 uses in which the racquet is not brought into the downward position in an abbreviated movement pattern. Elliott and colleagues[18] and Seeley and colleagues[21] have both shown no significant differences in either shoulder or elbow loads comparing the traditional backswing to the abbreviated backswing in players who use proper leg drive. It must be emphasized, that use of the abbreviated technique in the absence of proper kinetic chain involvement may subject the upper limb to abnormal physiological loads leading to potential shoulder and upper extremity injury.

Ground Strokes

The forehand and backhand ground strokes can be broken down into three phases: *preparation, acceleration,* and *follow-through* (Figures 11-10 to 11-13). EMG activity during the preparation phases of both the forehand and backhand is relatively low. Acceleration during the forehand involves very high activity in the subscapularis, biceps brachii, pectoralis major, and serratus anterior with a percentage of MVC of 102%, 86%, 85%, and 76%, respectively.[2] Acceleration during the backhand stroke consists of high muscular activity levels in the middle deltoid, supraspinatus, and infraspinatus with percentage of MVC of 118%, 73%, and 78%, respectively.[2] Again, the serratus anterior and biceps musculature was active during acceleration for both the forehand and backhand strokes.

Phases of Tennis Forehand and Backhand Ground Strokes

- Preparation
- Acceleration
- Follow through

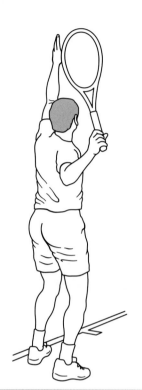

Figure 11-8

Observable characteristic of the "pull-through" serve is the lack of knee flexion during cocking.

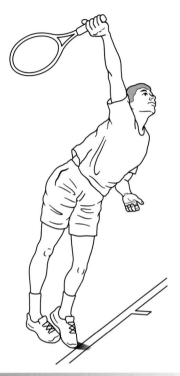

Figure 11-9

The "hip-back" position during a pull-through serve.

The follow-through phase of the forehand ground stroke produced moderately high activity of the serratus anterior, subscapularis, infraspinatus, and biceps musculature.[2] The continued activity of the infraspinatus was evident during impact and continued into the follow-through phase of the forehand ground stroke.[9] Follow-through activity during the backhand was moderately high in the biceps, middle deltoid, supraspinatus, and infraspinatus, but this level of activity was significantly lower than during the acceleration phase.

One of the primary changes in the modern game of tennis is the use of open stances with the lower extremities.[19] An open stance forehand is depicted in Figure 11-10 and shows how it contrasts with more traditional closed or square stances in which the entire body is perpendicular or sideways to the net. The open stance is characterized by the feet being essentially parallel to the net or baseline.[19,20] Despite the placement of the feet parallel to the baseline, the shoulders remain rotated such that the degree of separation between the hips and shoulders is optimized. This position enables the player to use greater levels of angular momentum during the stroke and facilitates the rotation during the execution of the stroke. This segmental rotation, however, can be a liability when premature opening of the pelvis and early rotation of the shoulders leads to arm lag and hyperangulation at the shoulder joint.[19,20,47,48] This premature opening, which is similar to that seen in baseball pitchers, can lead to shoulder injury and requires biomechanical intervention to prevent more serious injury and optimize technique.

Joint Kinematics

To further understand the demands placed on the upper extremity, analysis of shoulder joint angular velocities and ranges of motion incurred during tennis play are indicated. Angular velocities incurred during the serving motion necessitate high-velocity muscular stabilization outlined previously. Biomechanical study of the tennis serve has produced data measuring the speed of internal rotation of the humerus during acceleration. Shapiro and Stine[14] filmed 14 highly skilled male tennis players and reported a maximum internal rotation velocity of 1074 to 1514 deg/sec. Slightly faster velocities were reported by Dillman[49] in a pilot study of professional tennis players with maximal internal rotation velocities up to 2300 deg/sec. Comparable velocities of internal rotation during the acceleration phase of throwing have been reported to exceed 7000 deg/sec.[50]

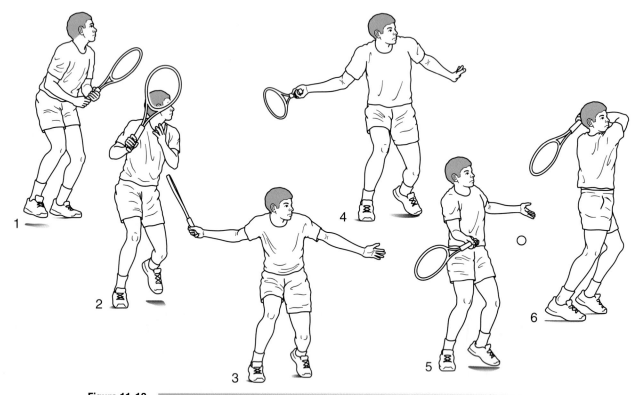

Figure 11-10
Forehand ground stroke. *1-3.* Preparation phase of the forehand. *4-5.* Acceleration phase of the forehand. *6.* Follow-through phase of the forehand.

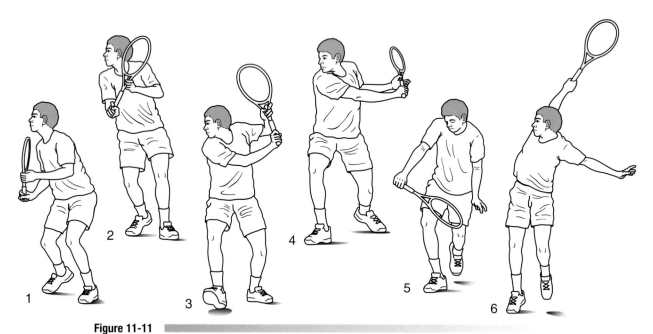

Figure 11-11
One-handed backhand ground stroke. *1-3.* Preparation phase of the backhand. *4-5.* Acceleration phase of the backhand. *6.* Follow-through phase of the backhand.

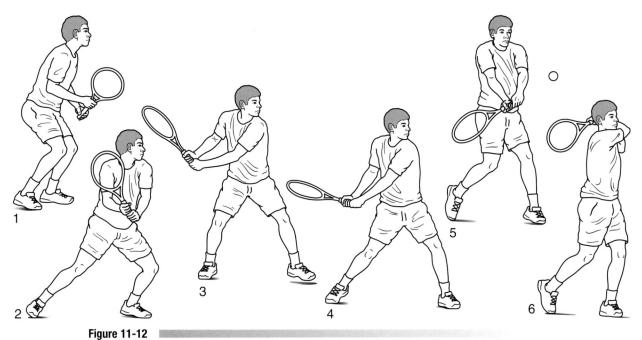

Figure 11-12

Two-handed backhand ground stroke. *1.* Ready position. *2-4.* Preparation phase of the two-handed backhand. *5.* Acceleration phase of the two-handed backhand ground stroke. *6.* Follow-through phase of the two-handed backhand ground stroke. Note, player is left-handed in this illustration.

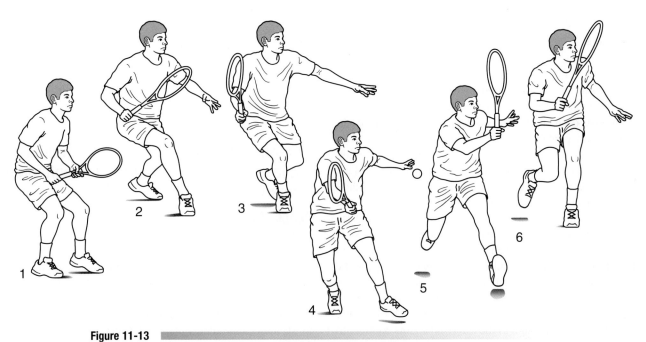

Figure 11-13

Forehand volley. *1.* Starting phase of the split step. *2.* Initial lateral step of split step. *3.* Preparation phase of the forehand volley. *4.* Acceleration phase (forward phase) of the volley. *5-6.* Follow-through phase of the forehand volley.

Demands placed on the dominant shoulder during the tennis serve are also high with respect to ROM. Dillman[49] reported maximal external rotation values of 154°. Abduction angles at the shoulder in elite Australian players were reported to average 83° during the cocking phase at the time of 90° of elbow flexion.[3]

These ROM characteristics have definite implications for overuse shoulder injury. Repeated maximal external rotation during the cocking phase of the tennis serve produces adaptations of the GH joint ROM on the dominant arm.[51-53] Greater external rotation of the GH joint may come at the expense of anterior capsular attenuation and is similar to the ROM and anterior laxity patterns found in highly skilled baseball players.[54]

The degree of GH joint abduction during cocking and acceleration is of prime importance in proper mechanical serve execution. Increases in GH joint abduction can lead to the shoulder being placed in a position of subacromial impingement. Initial observation of a highly skilled player's service motion shows an apparent vertical orientation of the arm to contact the ball overhead. Closer observation reveals that highly skilled players have significant contributions from contralateral trunk lateral flexion and scapular abduction. These components allow for a midrange of GH joint abduction throughout the four phases of the tennis serve.

Analysis of joint angular velocities during forehand ground strokes shows maximum internal rotation at the shoulder to be between 364 and 746 deg/sec.[14] This finding again has implications in determining appropriate exercises for prevention and rehabilitation of shoulder injuries. Groppel,[11,55] outlined the rationale and methodology for generation of topspin to the forehand ground stroke. Topspin is a desired characteristic used to improve both velocity and control of a shot and has been taught by coaches emphasizing a low backswing during preparation and a high follow-through. This creates a low-to-high stroke path that requires proper timing and body segment positioning and preparation.[13] Many unskilled and intermediate players use a method of "rolling over" the ball to achieve topspin. This effect increases the pronation influence of the distal upper extremity and also increases internal rotation acceleration during the stroke.[12] The close association between pronation of the forearm and internal rotation of the shoulder has been reported during the serve.[56] Distal upper extremity acceleration of pronation and internal rotation compensation to incorrectly produce topspin increase the demand on the posterior rotator cuff musculature during the follow-through as the external rotators contract to counteract the internally rotating humerus after impact.

Angular velocities of external rotation during the backhand stroke in highly skilled tennis players range between 328 and 1640 deg/sec.[14] Rotation of the shoulders into a position perpendicular to the net is of vital importance to optimize the contribution of torso rotation and lower-extremity input to force generation.[55] Use of a two-handed backhand has been recommended for players with upper extremity injury, particularly tennis elbow, because of bilateral upper extremity force generation and load sharing.[57]

Implications for Evaluation of Stroke Mechanics

Review of the athlete's stroke mechanics by video or direct observation is very helpful to check on poor techniques. The "nodes" model gives a framework for the evaluation. Observation of multiple repetitions of the motion and focusing on one node per serve repetition can demonstrate if any of the nodes are not being used. The most commonly deficient nodes are lack of knee flexion and hip counter-rotation, which results in the "pull-through" service motion, and lack of cocking, which results in GH hyperangulation. The observable characteristics include minimal knee flexion upon ball toss, limited hip counter rotation away from the court, prominence of the back hip as the player moves to ball impact (the "hip back" position) (see Figure 11-9), and arm position behind the scapular plane at cocking. The Sony Ericsson Women's Tennis Association tour has started a program of evaluation of the nodes in the serve in professional players. Players are observed by both direct visualization and by video for the presence or absence of progression through the nodes in multiple successful serves in actual game play. The preliminary data shows that the predominant nodes that are not consistently being used in this group of players are hip counter-rotation and coordinated arm cocking in the maximum back scratch position. Specific coaching techniques can be developed to modify these positions once they are observed.[37,39,40] Also, specific physical examination for musculoskeletal-limiting factors such as knee injury, hip weakness or rotational inflexibility, trunk inflexibility, or scapular dyskinesis should be performed.

Anatomical Adaptations of Elite Tennis Players in Response to the Biomechanical Demands of Tennis

Range of Motion

The kinematic analysis presented earlier in this chapter showed the large arcs of humeral rotation required for highly skilled tennis players' stroke execution. Several clinical studies have presented active ROM measures of the shoulder in elite tennis players. Chandler and colleagues[51] measured active ROM of the shoulder internal and external rotators in 90° of abduction in 86 junior elite tennis players between the ages of 12 and 21 years. They found significantly less mean internal rotation range in the dominant arm compared with the nondominant arm (65° versus 76°). The dominant shoulder had only slightly greater external rotation active ROM (100° versus 103°). Similar findings were reported by Ellenbecker[52] in an earlier study of 26 elite junior players aged 11 to 14 years measured at 90° of abduction with scapular stabilization. Significantly greater external rotation was found on the dominant arm of male tennis players only, with both male and female players showing less internal rotation active ROM on the dominant arm in players as young as 11 years of age.

Another study by Ellenbecker and colleagues[53] measured humeral rotation with scapular stabilization in elite junior tennis players and professional baseball pitchers. This study also compared humeral rotation using the total rotation ROM concept. The total rotation ROM value is obtained by summing the external and internal rotation measures together to obtain a combined or composite total of humeral rotation. The findings of this study showed the professional baseball pitchers to have greater dominant arm external rotation and significantly less dominant arm internal rotation, when compared with the contralateral nondominant or nonthrowing side. The total rotation ROM, however, was not significantly different between extremities in the professional baseball pitchers (145° dominant arm, 146° nondominant arm). This research showed that despite bilateral differences in the actual internal and external rotation ROM in the GH joints of baseball pitchers, the total arc of rotational motion remained the same.[53]

In contrast, Ellenbecker and colleagues[53] tested 117 elite male junior tennis players. In the elite junior tennis players, significantly less internal rotation ROM was found in the dominant arm (45° versus 56°), as well as significantly less total rotation ROM in the dominant arm (149° versus 158°) The total rotation ROM did differ between extremities. Approximately 10° less total rotation ROM can be expected in the dominant arm of the uninjured elite junior tennis player, as compared with the nondominant extremity; however, differences of greater than 10° should be cautiously monitored as healthy, uninjured elite players from this study had total rotation ROM bilateral comparisons within the 10° range of their contralateral side. Humeral rotation measured with scapular stabilization is an important part of the evaluation of the elite tennis player both during rehabilitation as well as during preventative screening evaluation.[47,48]

The loss of internal rotation ROM is significant for several reasons. The relationship between internal rotation ROM loss (i.e., tightness in the posterior capsule of the shoulder) and increased anterior humeral head translation has been scientifically identified.[58,59] The increase in anterior humeral shear force reported by Harryman and colleagues[60] was manifested by a horizontal adduction cross-body maneuver, similar to that incurred during the follow-through of the throwing motion or tennis serve. Tightness of the posterior capsule has also been linked to increased superior migration of the humeral head during shoulder elevation.[61] Koffler and colleagues[62] studied the effects of posterior capsular tightness in a functional position of 90° of abduction and 90° or more of external rotation in cadaveric specimens. They found, with imbrication (building a surface of overlapping layers) of either the inferior aspect of the posterior capsule or imbrication

of the entire posterior capsule, that humeral head kinematics were changed or altered. In the presence of posterior capsular tightness, the humeral head will shift in an anterior superior direction, as compared with a normal shoulder with normal capsular relationships.[62] With more extensive amounts of posterior capsular tightness, the humeral head was found to shift posterosuperiorly. These effects of altered posterior capsular tensions experimentally representing in vivo posterior GH joint capsular tightness highlight the clinical importance of using a reliable and effective measurement methodology, to assess internal rotation ROM during examination of the shoulder. In addition, Burkhart and colleagues[36] have clinically demonstrated the concept of posterior-superior humeral head shear in the GH joint, in which the inherent abducted externally rotated position along with posterior capsular tightness has been hypothesized to lead to superior labral and rotator cuff injury.

A Tight Posterior Capsule of the Shoulder Causes:

- Loss of internal rotation
- Anterosuperior translation of humeral head
- Superior migration of humeral head during abduction

Muscular Strength

Objective measurement of shoulder strength has been performed in elite and recreational tennis players.[52,63-66] Concomitant with ROM, specific relationships in shoulder strength have been identified in the tennis player that has implications for the development of preventative and rehabilitative exercise programs.

Ellenbecker[64] used a Cybex II isokinetic dynamometer to measure both shoulder internal and external rotation and flexion and extension in 22 highly skilled men tennis players. He found significantly greater dominant-arm internal rotation, extension, and flexion compared with the nondominant extremity. No difference between extremities was found in shoulder external rotation. Significantly lower external and internal rotation unilateral strength ratios were reported for the dominant arm, showing a relative external rotation strength deficit on the tennis playing shoulder. Similar research by Ellenbecker,[52,66] Chandler and colleagues,[51] and Koziris and colleagues[65] found similar results of greater internal rotation muscular strength on the dominant extremity with no significant difference between extremities in external rotation strength. In addition, Ellenbecker and Roetert[67] identified significantly lower absolute and relative fatigue indexes in the external rotators when compared with the internal rotators in the dominant arm of elite junior tennis players, highlighting the importance of endurance-based strengthening of the posterior rotator cuff to prevent shoulder injury.

Ellenbecker[64] measured significantly greater wrist flexion and extension strength and forearm pronation strength on the dominant arm compared with the nondominant extremity using and isokinetic dynamometer in elite tennis players. Ellenbecker and Roetert[68] found similar patterns of distal strength in elite junior tennis players with greater wrist flexion and extension and forearm pronation strength on the dominant extremity. One final upper-extremity study measured elbow extension and flexion strength in elite junior tennis player.[69] Greater dominant arm elbow extension strength was found compared with the nondominant extremity. These strength adaptations closely reflect the sport-specific demands identified in the earlier part of this chapter based on the biomechanics inherent in tennis and the repetitive activation elite players endure during practice and competition.

Biomechanics of Tennis Movement

Tennis movement is highly situation-specific and is performed in a reactive environment.[70] This irregularity of movement and the need to continually respond to situations requires a fine understanding of the athlete's game style, strategy, and movement strengths and weakness. Movement biomechanics for tennis is a complex area both from a practical coaching standpoint, but especially from a research environment. Tennis stroke biomechanics has been a fertile area of study, yet little information has been researched on tennis-specific movement biomechanics. This limited research may be due to the nature of the sport and the inconsistency of movement patterns. Although tennis movement has some consistent traits among all athletes, it is highly specific to the athlete's position on the court and the type of shot his or her opponent has just made. The movement biomechanics of tennis play has some movement mechanics that are similar to other sports, but many of tennis's movements require a different movement pattern, motor unit requirement continuum, and overall muscular strength profile than is needed to be a successful track sprinter or football wide receiver. Therefore, the data that is available in some other high-profile sports may not be appropriate to use as a guide for tennis. To understand the biomechanical requirement of tennis movement, an analysis of movement demands needs to first be discussed.

Typical Movement Demands

In competitive tennis, the average point length is less than 10 seconds,[71,72] with the recovery between points usually between 20 to 25 seconds depending on certain rules. Tennis players make an average of four directional changes per point,[73,74] but a given point can range from a single movement to more than 15 directional changes during a long rally. In a competitive match, it is common for players to have more than 1000 direction changes. At the French Open (one of the four Grand Slam professional tournaments), which is played on a clay surface, a study was undertaken on 1540 strokes to determine the typical distances covered. It was found that 80% of all strokes were played with less than 2.5 meters (8.2 feet) and fewer than 5% of strokes were played requiring more than 4.5 meters (14.8 feet) between strokes.[75] Other similar studies have found movement distances on average to cover less than 4 meters (13.1 feet) per change of direction.[76] Ferrauti and Weber[75] have revealed that approximately 80% of all strokes are played within less than 3 meters (9.8 feet) from the baseline ready position. Relatively short distances that a player covers on each stroke is typically less than 2 meters (6.6 feet), yet under higher time-pressure (increased running demand) athletes can run on average approximately 4 meters (13.1 feet) (maximum of between 8 to 12 meters [26.2 to 39.4 feet]).[77] It is interesting to note that tennis players can cover approximately 0.25 to 0.50 meters (0.8 to 1.6 feet) more on their forehand side than their backhand side.[77] This piece of information is very helpful when devising movement training programs for tennis, as slightly longer distances may need to be trained to an athlete's right side (i.e., right-handed forehand) than the athlete's left side. These are important findings, as most speed and quickness programs for other sports focus on distances that are longer in which a full traditional acceleration position may be reached. In tennis, it is rare that distances are achieved in which a traditional acceleration technique will be experienced by the athlete, and a maximum velocity running stride is never experienced during the confines of a tennis match.

Furthermore, the majority of tennis movements are in a lateral direction. In a study of professional players' movement, it was found that more than 70% of movements were side-to-side with less than 20% of movements in forward linear direction and less than 8% of movements in a backward linear direction.[77] This is a vitally important statistic, because the development of lateral acceleration and deceleration in the distances described previously are the major determining factors in great tennis movement. It is known that linear acceleration, linear maximum velocity, and agility are all separate and distinct motor skills that need to be trained separately,[78] as training one motor skill will not directly affect the improvement of the other. Therefore, preferred training recommendations for tennis should be to focus training time between 60% to 80% on lateral movements, 10% to 30% on linear forward movements, and only approximately 10% on linear backward movement.

Preferred Training Recommendations for Tennis

- 60% to 80% lateral movements
- 10% to 30% linear forward movement
- 10% linear backward movement

Tennis Surfaces and How They Influence Movement

Tennis is the only sport that is played on a number of different playing surfaces, even at the professional level. Although there are dozens of different surfaces around the world, for sake of discussion, there are three major groups of surfaces that players typically compete on: hard courts, clay courts, and grass courts. These different court surfaces result in different movement requirements because of the speed, cushioning, and friction of the court. Brody has found that the horizontal frictional force greatly affects ball speed and is a determining factor in court speed.[79] There can be as much as a 15% difference in ball speed after the bounce, depending on the court surface. Typically, a clay court is slower than a hard court. This reduction in ball speed allows athletes more time to reach the ball, therefore lengthening the duration of points played on clay courts. A computerized notational analysis of 252 professional singles matches found that rallies from women's singles matches (average 7.1 seconds) were significantly longer than rallies from men's singles matches (5.2 seconds). Rallies on clay courts at the professional level were significantly longer than any other surface.[80] At four Grand Slam events, O'Donoghue and Ingram found the following percentages for baseline rallies: (1) French Open (clay court): 51%; (2) Australian Open (hard court): 46%; (3) US Open (hard court), 35%; and (4) Wimbledon (grass) 19%.[80]

Another interesting difference between surfaces is that on hard courts, professional players are under increased time-pressure 45% of the time, whereas it is only 29% on clay courts.[76] Therefore, court surfaces do play a role in the movement requirements of tennis athletes and training needs to be adapted based on these differences.

More research is required before surfaces can be assessed using mechanical testing alone, especially in terms of the effect that such mechanical test results have on human movement on the tennis court.[81]

Tennis players have been shown to subjectively rate cushioning of tennis surfaces that correlate highly with mechanical testing. Peak and mean loading rates of vertical GRF, peak horizontal force, peak heel pressure, and rates of loading demonstrate significant correlations ($p < 0.05$) with the participant's perceived levels of cushioning between four different tennis court surfaces (acrylic, rubber, thin foam, and thick foam) (Figure 11-14).[81] Kinematic data for a running forehand has not been shown to provide significantly different responses based on these four surfaces.[81]

Lateral Movement in Tennis

Because tennis movements are predominantly lateral in focus, the muscle recruitment patterns and mechanics of lateral movements are discussed.

With lateral-focused agility training, the spinal reflex times of the following muscles improve (vastus medialis and lateralis medialis because of anterior tibialis translation) and the

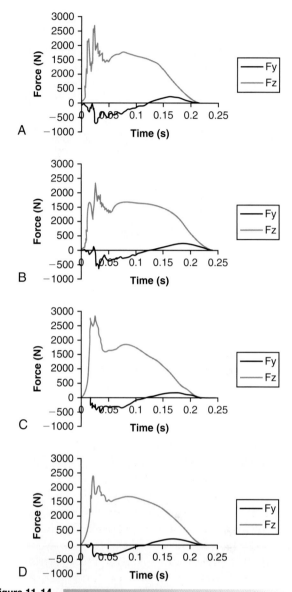

Figure 11-14

Typical vertical *(Fz)* and horizontal *(Fy)* ground reaction force profiles for the four surface conditions: **A**, baseline acrylic; **B**, rubber; **C**, thin foam; **D**, thick foam. (From Stiles V, Dixon S: Biomechanical response to systematic changes in impact interface cushioning properties while performing a tennis-specific movement, *J Sport Sci* 25[11]: 1229-1239, 2007.)

cortical response time improved in the gastrocnemius and medial hamstring (semimembranosus, semitendinosus).[82] This is helpful when designing training programs in the gym, as it should help to focus training on the specific muscle (listed previously) along with movements that are performed on court.

To aid in the understanding of tennis-distinct movements during lateral displacement on court, there are three initiating movements that are usually used by players during baseline movement—jab step, pivot step, and the gravity step (Figure 11-15, Figure 11-16, and Figure 11-17).

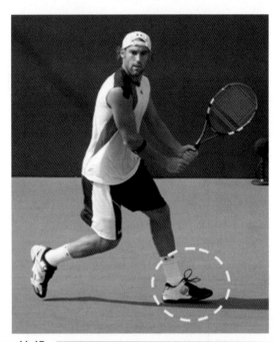

Figure 11-15
Jab step. (From Kovacs MS: Movement for tennis: The importance of lateral training, *Strength Cond J* 31[4]:79, 2009.)

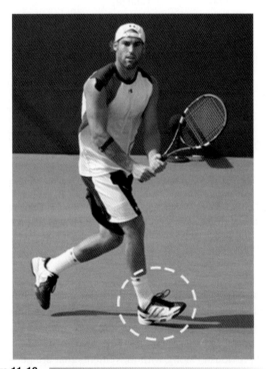

Figure 11-16
Pivot step. (From Kovacs MS: Movement for tennis: The importance of lateral training, *Strength Cond J* 31[4]:79, 2009.)

> ## Initiating Steps Used during Tennis Baseline Movement
>
> - The jab step has been defined as stepping first with the lead foot in the direction of the oncoming ball (see Figure 11-15).
> - The pivot step involves pivoting on the lead foot while turning the hips toward the ball and making the first step actually toward the ball with the opposite leg (see Figure 11-16).
> - The gravity step involves bringing the lead foot in toward the body and away from the direction of the oncoming ball and ultimately away from the direction of the intended movement (see Figure 11-17). This small step (unweighting) actually moves the center of gravity outside the base of support.

In a study that compared the jab, pivot, and gravity step on tennis movement, it was found that the fastest method to move laterally was by using the gravity step.[83] The authors speculated that the greater speed to the ball and greater control was due to the fact that the gravity step produces an overall movement toward the ball after the initial movement of the lead leg in a direction away from the ball. Unlike the jab step (in which the center of gravity remains between the base of support), the gravity step creates a "dynamic imbalance."[83] This movement of the center of gravity outside the base of support actually assists in moving the body laterally to the ball. This is a similar principle to the back step (or drop step) seen when athletes attempt to break inertia in a forward direction.[84]

Recovery Movement

Recovery movement occurs immediately after the athlete has completed his or her stroke and is attempting to return to a position that will allow for efficient movement toward the next stroke. There are two typical movement patterns used during the recovery after a stroke—the lateral crossover (Figure 11-18) or the lateral shuffle (Figure 11-19). The lateral crossover is more appropriate for movements that require quicker responses and greater distances. The lateral shuffle is more common when the athlete has a little extra time to get back into position before having to explosively move to the next shot.

> ## Types of Recovery Movement in Tennis
>
> - Lateral crossover (for quicker responses and greater distances)
> - Lateral shuffle

Split Step Misconception

Because of the evolution of tennis and the reliance on speed and power in today's game, the movement patterns of players have adapted. Early descriptions of the split step reported both feet landing on the court simultaneously, and

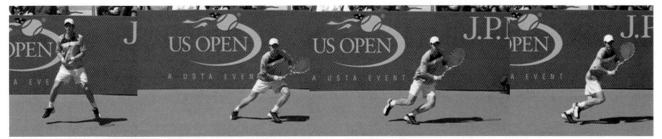

Figure 11-17
Gravity step. (From Kovacs MS: Movement for tennis: The importance of lateral training, *Strength Cond J* 31[4]:79, 2009.)

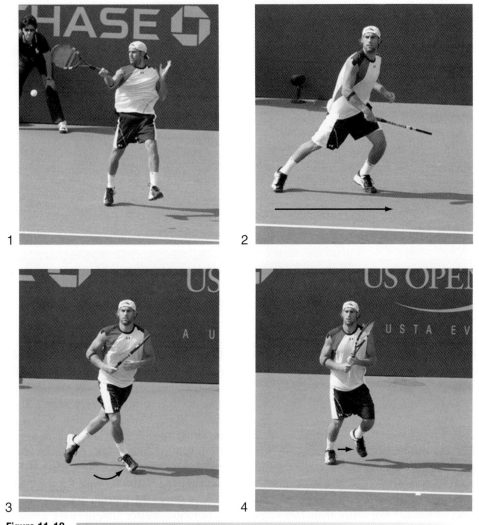

Figure 11-18
Lateral cross-over step. (Modified from Kovacs MS: Movement for tennis: The importance of lateral training, *Strength Cond J* 31[4]:79, 2009.)

then the athlete would react left, right, forward, or backward depending on the flight path, speed, direction, or spin of the oncoming ball. However, because of advances in the speed of the sport and the technological advances available to analyze athletes using high-speed video, it has emerged that elite players actually react in the air during the split and land on the foot furthest from their intended target a split second ahead of the other foot. An example is that a right-handed athlete preparing to hit a forehand would land on the left foot first (Figure 11-20). Before the right foot touches the ground, the athlete subtly rotates the hip externally toward the intended movement of the ball. In the right-handed player, this results in the right foot landing pointing outwards (see Figure 11-20). The movement pattern described

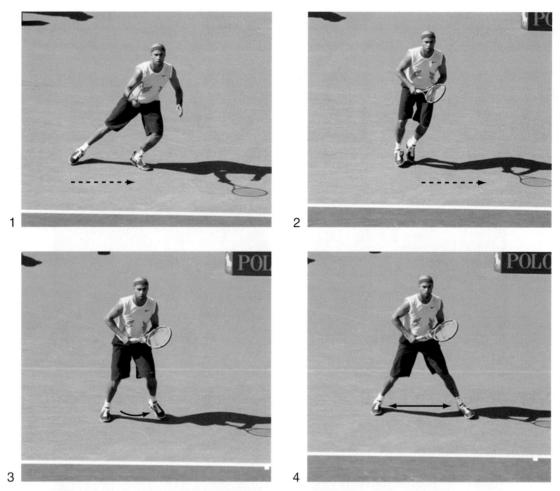

Figure 11-19
Lateral shuffle step. (Modified from Kovacs MS: Movement for tennis: The importance of lateral training, *Strength Cond J* 31[4]:80, 2009.)

previously has been a natural evolution to improve an athlete's ability to react to the incoming ball and maximize the movement/time ratio.

Reaction Time

One other area that can have an immediate effect on how fast an athlete *appears* in short distances is the athlete's reaction time. *Reaction time* is defined as the time from a stimulus (visual awareness of the opponent's stroke or ball) until the production of force.[85] For more than 100 years, the accepted figures for simple reaction times for college-age individuals has been approximately 190 ms (0.19 s) for light stimuli and approximately 160 ms (0.16 s) for sound stimuli.[86,87] However, the fastest athletes in the world consistently have reaction times less than 0.15 seconds.[88,89] In identical events, women have been shown to have longer reaction times than men.[90] However, reaction time does not correlate well with sprints lasting longer than a few seconds,[89] yet it does correlate very well with distances typically seen in tennis play.[89] Therefore, training an athlete

to improve reaction time should be a component of training tennis movement, alongside technique, strength, and power. In the training drills, a visual stimulus needs to be used to help develop visual reaction time. An auditory stimulus (e.g., whistle, voice, hand clap) is less tennis-specific than the visual cue. A study looking at average reaction times (from ball machine release to initial racquet movement) in skilled tennis players' volleys were 0.226 seconds for the forehand and 0.205 seconds for the backhand.[91]

After breaking inertia, the athlete's aim is to increase acceleration. Faster athletes have greater force production and horizontal velocity than the slower athletes during the last contact points on the ground.[90] This means that the power output at the last stage of ground contact is higher in faster athletes and this is an area that coaches should focus on during training sessions. Developing this increased power output at ground contact will directly increase GRFs, translating to quicker responses. Professional track sprinters running the 100 meter have movement velocities from a standard block start of between 4.65 to 5.16 ms^{-1} for the first ground contact and approximately 5.7 ms^{-1} at toe-off

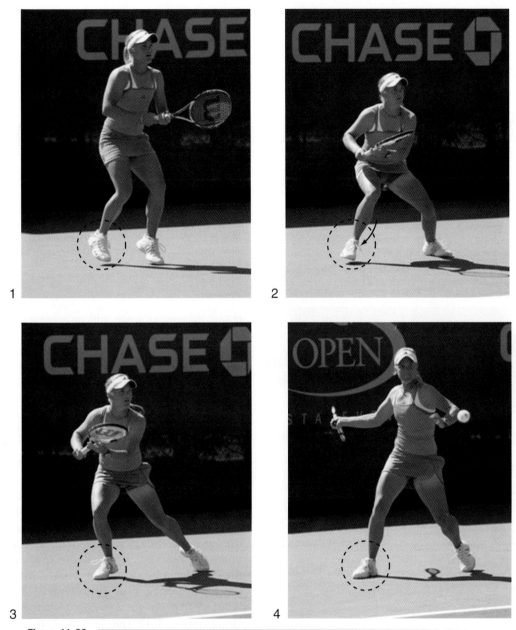

Figure 11-20
Split step. (Modified from Kovacs MS: Movement for tennis: The importance of lateral training, *Strength Cond J* 31[4]:80, 2009.)

for the second step from a block start.[89,92,93] It is interesting to compare this information with professional tennis players who have movement velocities that range substantially during any given point (Figure 11-21).

Sprinting technique during an athlete's acceleration is vastly different than that of an athlete who is running at or near maximum velocity (Figure 11-22).[94,95] Most competitive athletes do not reach maximum velocity until 40 to 60 meters (131 to 197 feet) (depending on training level and genetic ability). As mentioned previously, tennis athletes typically move less than 2.5 meters (8.2 feet) and rarely exceed 5 meters (16.4 feet) (Figure 11-23 provides an

example of a movement pattern during a long point) and less than 30% of movements are linear (forward and backward).[77] It is imperative that the majority of training programs are structured appropriately to train specifically for the movements experienced during tennis.

Kinetic and Kinematic Data

Although extensive kinetic and kinematic data have been presented analyzing tennis strokes in this chapter, currently there is limited published kinetic and kinematic data on ennis-specific movement. However, there is some information that

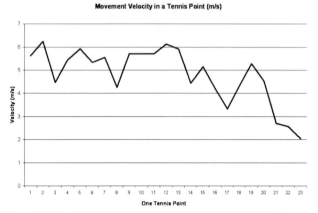

Figure 11-21

Movement velocities in a tennis point. (Data from Strauss D: *Biomechanical analysis of the impact characteristics of an open stance forehand drive in tennis,* Key Biscayne, FL, 2005, USTA Sport Science.)

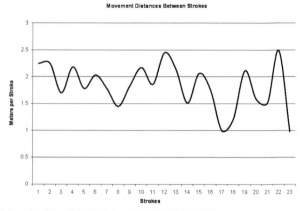

Figure 11-23

Movement distances between tennis strokes. (Data from Strauss D: *Biomechanical analysis of the impact characteristics of an open stance forehand drive in tennis,* Key Biscayne, FL, 2005, USTA Sport Science.)

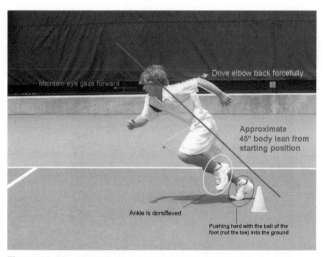

Figure 11-22

Acceleration. (From Kovacs M, Chandler WB, Chandler TJ: *Tennis training: Enhancing on-court performance,* p 23, Vista, CA, 2007, Racquet Tech Publishing.)

has been performed in tennis, but more commonly in other sports, that can have direct representation to tennis specific movement from a biomechanical perspective. During a laboratory-based movement analysis of tennis movement toward a forehand stroke, it was found that approximately 16% of total foot contact time is spent during the braking phase of the forehand drive,[96] with peak breaking magnitudes occurring at between 8% to 10% of total time spent in ground contact. It has been shown that the maximum breaking peak for distance running occurs at approximately 22% of the contact phase.[97] This information is helpful in showcasing the different requirements of tennis movement compared with distance running.

The demands of tennis movement are vastly different from that of other sports and appropriate training programs should take into account the biomechanical uniqueness of

tennis movement while still incorporating the traditional laws of motion that guide efficient and effective movement patterns and muscle recruitment principles. The majority of tennis movements are lateral in nature. Therefore, preferred training recommendations for tennis should be to focus training between 60% to 80% of the time on lateral movements, 10% to 30% of the time on linear forward movements, and only approximately 10% of the time on linear backward movement.

As mentioned previously, the three distinct initiating movements that are frequently used by players during baseline movement are (1) the jab step, (2) the pivot step, and (3) the gravity step (see Figures 11-15 to 11-17). In addition, there are two typical movements used during the recovery: the lateral crossover, which is more appropriate for quicker responses and greater distances, and the lateral shuffle, when the athlete has more time and shorter distances. It is important to incorporate all of these actions when structuring tennis movement sessions (see Figures 11-18 and 11-19). Training (such as plyometric programs with a lateral focus) accomplishes the goal of increasing motoneuron excitability to improve the speed and force of the muscle contraction to improve movement.

Conclusion

This chapter has provided an overview of the biomechanics of tennis strokes and movement patterns that highlight the demands on the entire body during repetitive play. The clinical ramifications of these biomechanical forces and movement patterns have been discussed and include primarily overuse injury risk. Knowledge of the forces and movement characteristics inherent in tennis allows the clinician to design both preventative conditioning and optimal rehabilitation programs for players.

References

1. Johnson CD, McHugh MP: Performance demands of professional male tennis players, *Br J Sports Med* 40:696-699, 2006.

2. Rhu KN, McCormick J, Jobe FW, et al: An electromyographic analysis of shoulder function in tennis players, *Am J Sports Med* 16:481–485, 1988.

3. Elliot B, Marsh T, Blanksby B: A three dimensional cinematographic analysis of the tennis serve, *Int J Sport Biomech* 2:260–271, 1986.

4. Fleisig GS, Andrews JR, Dillman CJ, et al: Kinetics of baseball pitching with implications about injury mechanisms, *Am J Sports Med* 23:233–239, 1995.

5. Yoshizawa M, Itani T, Jonsson B: Muscular load in shoulder and forearm muscles in tennis players with different levels of skill. In Jonsson B, editor: *Biomechanics X-B*, Champaign, IL, 1987, Human Kinetics.

6. Inman VT, Saunders JB de CM, Abbot LC: Observations on the function of the shoulder joint, *J Bone Joint Surg Am* 26:1–30, 1944.

7. Van der Hoeven H, Kibler WB: Shoulder injuries in tennis players, *Br J Sports Med* 40(5):435–440. 2006.

8. Bradley JP, Tibone JE: Electromyographic analysis of muscle action about the shoulder, *Clin Sports Med* 10:789–805, 1991.

9. VanGheluwe B, Hebbelinck M: Muscle actions and ground reaction forces in tennis, *Int J Sport Biomech* 2:88–99, 1986.

10. Miyashita M, Tsunoda T, Sakurai S, et al: Muscular activities in the tennis serve and overhand throwing, *Scand J Sports Sci* 2:52–58, 1980.

11. Groppel JL: *Tennis for advanced players: and those who would like to be*, Champaign, IL, 1984, Human Kinetics.

12. Groppel JL: The utilization of proper racket sport mechanics to avoid upper extremity injury, In Pettrone FA, editor: *Proceedings of the Symposium on Upper Extremity Injuries: Sponsored by the Academy of Orthopaedic Surgeons*, St Louis, 1986, Mosby.

13. Groppel JL: *High tech tennis*, Champaign, IL, 1992, Human Kinetics.

14. Shapiro R, Stine RL: *Shoulder rotation velocities*. Technical report submitted to the Lexington Clinic, Lexington, KY, 1992.

15. Elliott BC. The development of racquet speed, In Elliott BC, Reid M, Crespo M, editors: *Biomechanics of advanced tennis*, London, 2003, International Tennis Federation.

16. Zattara M, Bouisset S: Posturo-kinetic organization during the early phase of voluntary upper limb movement, *J Neurol Neurosurg Psychol* 51:956–965, 1988.

17. Bahamonde R: Changes in angular momentum during the tennis serve, *J Sport Sci* 18:579–592, 2000.

18. Elliott B, Fleisig G, Nicholls R, Escamillia R: Technique effects on upper limb loading in the tennis serve, *J Sci Med Sport* 6(1):76–87, 2003.

19. Roetert EP, Groppel J: *World class tennis technique*, Champaign, IL, 2001, Human Kinetics.

20. Segal DK: *Tenis Sistema Biodinamico*, Buenos Aires Argentina, 2002, Tenis Club Argentino.

21. Seeley MK, Uhl TL, McCrory J, et al: A comparison of muscle activations during traditional and abbreviated tennis serves, *Sports Biomech* 7(2):248–259, 2008.

22. Schonbrun R: *Advanced techniques for competitive tennis*, Aachen, Germany, 1999, Meyer and Meyer.

23. Fleisig GS, Nicholls R, Elliott BC, Escamilla RF: Kinematics used by world class tennis players to produce high-velocity serves, *Sports Biomech* 2:51–71, 2002.

24. Kibler WB: Biomechanical analysis of the shoulder during tennis activities, *Clin Sports Med* 14(1):79–85, 1995.

25. Elliott BC, Marshall R, Noffal G: Contributions of upper limb segment rotations during the power serve in tennis, *J Appl Biomech* 11:443–447, 1995.

26. Cordo PJ, Nasher LM: Properties of postural adjustments associated with rapid arm movements, *J Neurophysiol* 47:287–308, 1982.

27. Kibler WB, Press J, Sciascia A: The role of core stability in athletic function, *Sports Med* 36(3):189–198, 2006.

28. Putnam CA: Sequential motions of body segments in striking and throwing skills: Descriptions and explanations, *J Biomech* 26:125–135, 1993.

29. Nieminen H, Niemi J, Takala EP: Load sharing patterns in the shoulder during isometric flexion tasks, *J Biomech* 28:555–566, 1995.

30. Lippitt SB, Vanderhooft JE, Harris SL, et al: Glenohumeral stability from concavity-compression: A quantitative analysis, *J Shoulder Elbow Surg* 2:27–35, 1993.

31. Weiser WM, Lee TQ, McMaster WC, McMahon PJ: Effects of simulated scapular protraction on anterior glenohumeral stability, *Am J Sports Med* 27:801–805, 1999.

32. Hirashima M, Kudo K, Watarai K, Ohtsuki T: Control of 3D limb dynamics in unconstrained overarm throws of different speeds performed by skilled baseball players, *J Neurophysiol* 97:680–691, 2007.

33. Hirashima M, Yamane K, Nakamura Y, Ohtsuki T: Kinetic chain of overarm throwing in terms of joint rotations revealed by induced acceleration analysis, *J Biomech* 41(13):2874–2883, 2008.

34. Davids K, Glazier P, Araujo D: Movement systems as dynamical systems, *Sports Med* 33:246–260, 2003.

35. Bahamonde R, Knudson D: Linear and angular momentum in stroke production. In Elliott BC, Reid M, Crespo M, editors: *Biomechanics of advanced tennis*, London, 2003, International Tennis Federation.

36. Burkhart SS, Morgan CD, Kibler WB: The disabled throwing shoulder: Spectrum of pathology. Part I: Pathoanatomy and biomechanics, *Arthroscopy* 19(4):404–420, 2003.

37. Elliott BC, Mester J, Kleinoder H, Yue Z: Loading and stroke production, In Elliott BC, Reid M, Crespo M, editors: *Biomechanics of advanced tennis*, London, 2003, International Tennis Federation.

38. Marshall R, Elliott BC: Long axis rotation: The missing link in proximal to distal segmental sequencing, *J Sport Sci* 18:247–254, 2000.

39. Kibler WB, Van Der Meer D: Mastering the kinetic chain. In Roetert EP, Groppel J, editors: *World class tennis technique*, Champaign, IL, 2001, Human Kinetics.

40. Kibler WB, Brody H, Knudson D, Stroia K: *Tennis technique, tennis play, and injury prevention. USTA Sports Science Committee White Paper*, New York, 2005, United States Tennis Association.

41. Kibler WB, Safran MR: Musculoskeletal injuries in the young tennis player, *Clin Sports Med* 19(4):781–792, 2000.

42. Lukasiewicz AC, McClure P, Michener L: Comparison of three dimensional scapular position and orientation between subjects with and without shoulder impingement, *J Orthop Sports Phys Ther* 29:574–586, 1999.

43. Vad VJ, Gebeh A, Dines D, et al: Hip and shoulder internal rotation range of motion deficits in professional tennis players, *J Sci Med Sport* 6(1):71–75, 2003.

44. Kibler WB, McMullen J: Scapular dyskinesis and its relation to shoulder pain, *J Am Acad Orthop Surg* 11:142–151, 2003.

45. Girard O, Micallef JP, Millet GP: Lower-limb activity during the power serve in tennis: Effects of performance level, *Med Sci Sports Exerc* 37(6):1021–1029, 2005.

46. Pink MM, Perry J: Biomechanics of the shoulder. In Jobe FW, editor: *Operative techniques in upper extremity sports injuries*, St. Louis, 1996, Mosby.

47. Ellenbecker TS: *Clinical examination of the shoulder*, Philadelphia, 2004, Elsevier Saunders.

48. Ellenbecker TS: *Non-operative rehabilitation of the shoulder*, New York, 2006, Theime Publishers.

49. Dillman CJ: *Presentation on the upper extremity in tennis and throwing athletes*, United States Tennis Association National Meeting, Tucson, Arizona, March 1991.

50. Andrews JR, Kupferman SP, Dillman CJ: Labral tears in throwing and racquet sports, *Clin Sports Med* 10:901–911, 1991.

51. Chandler TJ, Kibler WB, Uhl TL, et al: Flexibility comparisons of junior elite tennis players to other athletes, *Am J Sports Med* 18:134–136, 1990.

52. Ellenbecker TS: Shoulder internal and external rotation strength and range of motion of highly skilled junior tennis players, *Isokinetics Exerc Sci* 2:1–8, 1992.

53. Ellenbecker TS, Roetert EP, Bailie DS, et al: Glenohumeral joint total rotation range of motion in elite tennis players and baseball pitchers, *Med Sci Sports Exerc* 34(12):2052–2056, 2002.

54. Jobe FW, Bradley JP: The diagnosis and nonoperative treatment of shoulder injuries in athletes, *Clin Sports Med* 8:419–439, 1989.

55. Groppel JL: The biomechanics of tennis: An overview, *Int J Sport Biomech* 2:141–155, 1986.

56. VanGheluwe B, DeRuysscher I, Craenhals J: Pronation and endorotation of the racket arm in a tennis serve, In Jonsson B, editor: *Biomechanics X-B*, Champaign, IL, 1987, Human Kinetics.

57. Nirschl RP: Tennis elbow, *Prim Care* 4:367–382, 1977.

58. Tyler TF, Nicholas SJ, Roy T, Gleim GW: Quantification of posterior capsular tightness and motion loss in patients with shoulder impingement, *Am J Sports Med* 28(5):668–673, 2000.

59. Gerber C, Werner CML, Macy JC, et al: Effect of selective capsulorraphy on the passive range of motion of the glenohumeral joint, *J Bone Joint Surg Am* 85(1):48–55, 2003.

60. Harryman DT, Sidles JA, Clark JM, et al: Translation of the humeral head on the glenoid with passive glenohumeral motion, *J Bone Joint Surg Am* 72:1334–1343, 1990.

61. Matsen FA III, Arntz CT: Subacromial impingement. In Rockwood CA Jr, Matsen FA III, editors: *The shoulder*, ed 1, Philadelphia, 1990, WB Saunders.

62. Koffler KM, Bader D, Eager M, et al: *The effect of posterior capsular tightness on glenohumeral translation in the late-cocking phase of pitching: A cadaveric study*, Abstract (SS-15) presented at Arthroscopy Association of North America Annual Meeting, Washington, DC, 2001.

63. Ellenbecker TS, Davies GJ, Rowinski MJ: Concentric versus eccentric isokinetic strengthening of the rotator cuff: Objective data versus functional test, *Am J Sports Med* 16:64–69, 1988.

64. Ellenbecker TS: A total arm strength isokinetic profile of highly skilled tennis players, *Isokinetics Exerc Sci* 1:9–21, 1991.

65. Koziris LP, Kraemer WJ, Triplett NT, et al: Strength imbalances in women in tennis players (abstr), *Med Sci Sports Exerc* 23:253, 1991.

66. Ellenbecker TS, Roetert EP: Age specific isokinetic glenohumeral internal and external rotation strength in elite junior tennis players, *J Sci Med Sport* 6(1):63–70, 2003.

67. Ellenbecker TS, Roetert EP: Isokinetic muscular fatigue of the shoulder internal and external rotators, *J Orthop Sports Phys Ther* 29(5):275–281, 1999.

68. Ellenbecker TS, Roetert EP: Isokinetic profile of wrist and forearm strength in elite junior tennis players, *Br J Sports Med* 40(5): 411–414, 2006.

69. Ellenbecker TS, Roetert EP: Isokinetic profile of elbow flexion and extension strength in elite junior tennis players, *J Orthop Sports Phys Ther* 33(2):79–84, 2003.

70. Kovacs MS: Tennis physiology: Training the competitive athlete, *Sports Med* 37(3):1–11, 2007.

71. Kovacs MS: A comparison of work/rest intervals in men's professional tennis, *Med Sci Tennis* 9(3):10–11, 2004.

72. Kovacs MS: Applied physiology of tennis performance, *Br J Sports Med* 40(5):381–386, 2006.

73. Roetert EP, Ellenbecker TS: *Complete conditioning for tennis*, ed 2, Champaign, IL, 2007, Human Kinetics.

74. Kovacs M, Chandler WB, Chandler TJ: *Tennis training: Enhancing on-court performance*, Vista, CA, 2007, Racquet Tech Publishing.

75. Ferrauti A, Weber K: *Stroke situations in claycourt tennis*, Unpublished data, 2001.

76. Pieper S, Exler T, Weber K: Running speed loads on clay and hard courts in world class tennis, *Med Sci Tennis* 12(2):14–17, 2007.

77. Weber K, Pieper S, Exler T: Characteristics and significance of running speed at the Australian Open 2006 for training and injury prevention, *Med Sci Tennis* 12(1):14–17, 2007.

78. Young WB, McDowell MH, Scarlett BJ: Specificity of sprint and agility training methods, *J Strength Cond Res* 15(3):315–319, 2001.

79. Brody H: *Fast courts—slow courts*, New York, 1995, United States Tennis Association.

80. O'Donoghue P, Ingram B: A notational analysis of elite tennis strategy, *J Sports Sci* 19:107–115, 2001.

81. Stiles V, Dixon S: Biomechanical response to systematic changes in impact interface cushioning properties while performing a tennis-specific movement, *J Sport Sci* 25(11):1229–1239, 2007.

82. Wojtys EM, Huston LJ, Taylor PD, Bastian SD: Neuromuscular adaptations in isokinetic, isotonic, and agility training programs, *Am J Sports Med* 24(2):187–192, 1996.

83. Bragg RW, Andriacchi TP: *The lateral reaction step in tennis footwork*, XIX International Symposium on Biomechanics in Sports, San Francisco, 2001.

84. Kraan GA, van Veen J, Snijders CJ, Storm J: Starting from standing: Why step backwards, *J Biomech* 34:211–215, 2001.

85. Schmidt RA, Lee TD: *Motor control and learning: A behavioral emphasis*, ed 3, Champaign, IL, 1999, Human Kinetics.

86. Galton F: On instruments for (1) testing perception of differences of tint and for (2) determining reaction time, *J Anthropol Inst* 19:27–29, 1899.

87. Brebner JT, Welford AT: Introduction and historical background sketch. In Welford AT, editor: *Reaction times*, New York, NY, 1980, Academic Press.

88. Gambetta V, Winckler G: *Sport specific speed: The 3S system*, Sarasota, FL, 2001, Gambetta Sports Training Systems.

89. Mero A, Komi PV: Reaction time and electromyographic activity during a sprint start, *Eur J Appl Physiol* 61:73–80, 1990.

90. Mero A, Komi PV, Gregor RJ: Biomechanics of sprint running, *Sports Med* 13(6):376–392, 1992.

91. Chow JW, Carlton LG, Chae WS, et al: Movement characteristics of the tennis volley, *Med Sci Sports Exerc* 31(6):855–863, 1999.

92. Mero A: Force-time characteristics and running velocity of male sprinters during the acceleration phase of sprinting, *Res Q Exerc Sport* 59(2):94–98, 1988.

93. Schot P, Knutzen K: A biomechanical analysis of four sprint start positions, *Res Q Exerc Sport* 2:137–147, 1992.

94. USA Track and Field (USATF): *Sprints and Hurdles*, Starkville, MS, 2004, United States Track and Field Level II Coaching School.

95. Kyröläinen H, Komi PV, Belli A: Changes in muscle activity patterns and kinetics with increasing running speed, *J Strength Cond Res* 13(4):400–406, 1999.

96. Strauss D: *Biomechanical analysis of the impact characteristics of an open stance forehand drive in tennis*, Key Biscayne, FL, 2005, USTA Sport Science.

97. Cavanagh PR, Lafortune MA: Ground reaction forces in distance running, *J Biomech* 13:397–406, 1980.

APPLIED BIOMECHANICS OF SOCCER

Sérgio T. Fonseca, Thales R. Souza, Juliana M. Ocarino, Gabriela P. Gonçalves, and Natália F. Bittencourt

Introduction

According to a 2006 survey, soccer, or *football*, as it is called everywhere other than North America, is the world's most popular sport in number of participants.[1] Currently, with 208 countries affiliated to its main association and around 265 million participating players worldwide, soccer is played in all continents. In addition, this sport continues to grow among youngsters and women, especially in North America and Asia.[1] Despite its popularity, soccer has a high injury incidence among players.[2-4] Therefore, the number of injuries is increasing as the number of new players grows. According to Arnason and colleagues,[2] soccer is responsible for between one-fourth and one-half of all sports-related injuries. Considering the financial and personal costs of injuries and delays in returning to competition, there is a growing interest in the prevention of soccer-related injuries, as well as in the development of rehabilitative measures to promote a safe return to competition of the injured athlete. However, the complexity of the sport makes the establishment of these measures a difficult task to accomplish.

Soccer is a sport composed of many athletic components and requires different physical attributes and skills from the individual. For example, a soccer player has to be able to run, sprint, dribble, pivot, cut, jump, land, and head and kick a ball. In addition, as a contact sport, tackling and collisions are frequent during matches and practices.[3] This complex demand of soccer poses a real challenge to the musculoskeletal system of the athlete and may be related to the high incidence of soccer-related injuries. Because many of these athletic components are related among themselves or overlap in occurrence during a soccer match, there is the need to consider the biomechanics of the whole kinetic chain to be able to understand the main factors related to performance and injury prevention in soccer. As a player performs any of these tasks, the whole body is submitted to internal and external forces that have to be dissipated or transferred appropriately to improve performance or to protect the different biological tissues from injury. The involvement of the whole body in the process of dealing with internal and external forces during the performance of any activity, defines the kinetic chain. Thus, even when describing a single component of the sport, such as kicking, the contribution of the kinetic chain to the task performance has to be considered. In summary, any analysis of the processes related to injury prevention and performance in soccer has to be performed in a comprehensive manner.

The understanding of the complex biomechanics of soccer is crucial to allow the implementation of effective preventive and rehabilitation approaches. In addition, the performance of soccer players requires a musculoskeletal system that is capable of dealing with the demands originated by the sport. Thus, this chapter is organized in three main sections. The first section describes the biomechanics of soccer. This section is intended to review the biomechanics of the main activities and skills related to soccer practice. The demands that soccer places on the musculoskeletal system are established. The second section illustrates some common soccer-related injuries. In this section, the demands of soccer that can lead to typical soccer injuries are discussed, together with the players' capacities required to prevent these injuries or to return to sport safely following an injury. The final section focuses on the implication of soccer biomechanics to prevention, rehabilitation, and performance. This section is intended to demonstrate to the reader how the understanding of the biomechanical demands of soccer, and the player's capacities required to deal with them (Table 12-1), can be used to plan effective programs for the rehabilitation and prevention of soccer injuries.

Table 12-1

Capability and Demand Definitions

Parameter	Definition
Capability	Ability (potential) of the musculoskeletal system to generate, dissipate, and transfer mechanical energy
Demand	Amount of stress applied to the musculoskeletal system during a given activity

Biomechanics of Soccer

Although soccer is composed of many skills, this section focuses only on the specific components that place the most stress on the musculoskeletal system or are fundamental components of the sport. Thus, this section concentrates on describing the biomechanics of kicking, heading, and cutting. For each of these tasks, subtasks or components are appropriately addressed when needed. For example, heading a ball requires jumping and landing, whereas cutting is embedded in pivoting, dribbling, and running. The selection of only kicking, heading, and cutting was made based on the fact that these components are crucial for soccer practice. The focus on only these components facilitates a deeper understanding of their biomechanics and the demands that they place on the musculoskeletal system. However, it is worth remembering that, during a soccer match, these activities occur in an overlapping manner and thus pose an even greater challenge to the musculoskeletal system.

Classical analyses of the biomechanics of a given sport frequently separate the kinematic and kinetic aspects of that sport. In this section, a different approach is taken. Initially, the components and their subphases are described, observing the differences among existing styles. For example, in this section, different types of kicking and cutting are described. Finally, the biomechanical description of each of the soccer components introduced will focus on a global analysis of the demands and requirements of the task, considering simultaneously the kinematic and kinetic aspects of the soccer component. In this case, whenever possible, the energetics of the task (i.e., energy flow in the kinetic chain) will be emphasized to allow a better understanding of the musculoskeletal demands imposed from soccer practice.

Biomechanics of Kicking

Kicking is the playing action of soccer used to shoot the ball to a desired direction, either to pass the ball to a teammate or in an attempt to score a goal. This task is accomplished by hitting the ball with the foot of the swing limb while the support limb sustains the body. Kicking involves complex motions and large demands on the musculoskeletal system, as it is one of the soccer components most related to noncontact injuries.[2] The main techniques of kicking are the side-foot kick and the instep

kick (Table 12-2).[5] The side-foot kick is more frequently used for short, precise passes and shooting, whereas the instep kick is often used to propel the ball with high velocity.[5] Although such techniques have distinct goals, they are generally performed with similar biomechanical strategies, in which the key function of the musculoskeletal system in kicking is to efficiently transfer mechanical energy to the ball by imparting a force to it with precise power and direction.

Descriptions of the biomechanics of kicking have focused on the behavior of the lower swing limb in the sagittal plane and have divided this action into four consecutive phases: backswing, leg cocking, leg acceleration, and follow-through (Figure 12-1, A).[5-7] The backswing phase lasts from toe-off (which takes place just before the contact of the support limb with the surface) to the time of maximum hip extension.[5] The swing limb is displaced backward in relation to the rest of the body, and there is hip extension and knee flexion.[6] The leg-cocking phase begins with maximum hip extension and ends with maximum knee flexion of the swing limb and, subsequently, the leg acceleration phase lasts until the contact of the swing foot with the ball.[5] These last two phases are characterized by the predominant anterior displacement and acceleration of the swing limb, in the direction of the ball.[6] During the leg-cocking phase, hip flexion and knee flexion continue to occur.[7] During the leg-acceleration phase, the hip continues to flex and the knee begins to extend.[7] Finally, the follow-through phase lasts from ball contact to the end of the anterior displacement of the foot and is characterized by the final deceleration of hip flexion and knee extension.[5] The displacements at the ankle joint are minimal in comparison with hip and knee, because the foot accompanies shank linear and angular motions.

Clinical Relevance Summary - Kicking

- Analyses of the kicking action should include transverse and sagittal plane motions of the upper body, in addition to sagittal plane motions of the lower swing limb.
- The contractile and passive properties of the myofascial structures that interconnect the lower swing limb, pelvis, trunk, and nonkicking-side lower and upper limbs are crucial for kicking performance, because the patterns of energy flow depend on the mechanical interactions between these segments.

Table 12-2

Types of Kicking

Type of Kicking	Definition
Side-foot kick	Kick executed by striking the ball with the medial aspect of the swing-limb midfoot
Instep kick	Kick executed by striking the ball with the dorsum of the swing-limb foot

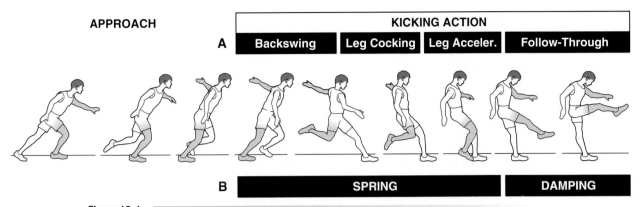

Figure 12-1

Sagittal view of the kicking kinematics. Limbs in *gray color* are the kicking-side lower limb (swing limb) and the nonkicking-side upper limb. **A,** Kicking phases related to the sagittal plane kinematics of the swing limb. **B,** Kicking phases related to the main functions of the kinetic chain. (Redrawn from Shan G, Westerhoff P: Full-body kinematic characteristics of the maximal instep soccer kick by male soccer players and parameters related to kick quality, *Sports Biomech* 4(1):59-72, 2005.)

The musculoskeletal system may be understood as having two major functions during kicking: the spring function and the damping function (see Figure 12-1, *B*).[8] According to these functions, the kicking action can be divided into three main stages: an initial stage when potential energy is stored (backswing), a second stage when the kinetic energy involved in the anterior acceleration of the swing limb is resultant from the conversion of the potential energy previously stored and from energy generation (i.e., leg cocking and leg acceleration), and a final stage when this energy is absorbed and mostly dissipated with limb deceleration (i.e., follow-through). During the two initial stages, the system works as a spring and during the third stage the damping (braking) function is predominant. Joint kinetics of the lower swing limb, estimated from inverse dynamics, reinforces such roles.[5] During backswing, there is energy absorption and deceleration of hip extension and knee flexion. During leg cocking and leg acceleration, there is energy generation and acceleration of hip flexion and knee extension. Finally, during the follow-through, there is energy absorption and deceleration of hip flexion and knee extension. This dynamic action is due to predominant hip flexor and knee extensor net torques during backswing, leg cocking, and leg acceleration, and due to hip extensor and knee flexor net torques during the follow-through. At the ankle, the predominant net torque is dorsiflexion.[5] It is important to recognize that inverse dynamics methods estimate only the joint torques necessary to generate the observed kinematics of an action, regardless of the structures and interactions that produce them.[9] Thus, the torques and energetic changes described may be influenced by interactions with other joints and segments within the chain.

The muscles of the swing and support limbs are active during the entire kicking cycle[7] so that muscles that are agonist and antagonist to the occurring motion are co-contracted. This co-contraction allows the maintenance of a certain amount of joint stiffness and stability and allows for adequate energy dissipation and transfer among segments.[10] The differences between soccer players and nonplayers (i.e., between individuals who have, by practice, exploited extensively their neuromusculoskeletal resources in the performance of kicking and those who have not) help clarify the kicking demands. In soccer players, the antagonist muscles are more active than the agonist, whereas in nonplayers, the opposite is true.[11] Such differences indicate that eccentric contractions have essential roles in the spring function[12,13] by absorbing and storing energy during the backswing and by releasing it back to the system (energy return) during swing limb anterior acceleration. In the swing limb, the flexors, adductors, and anterior external rotators of the hip and extensors of the knee are mostly responsible for this function. Concentric contractions of these muscles are also required, mainly during the anterior acceleration of the swing limb, to add energy to the segments.[14] Limb anterior acceleration is enhanced by the muscles' previous eccentric contractions and myofascial stretching.[15] Eccentric contractions during the follow-through are also essential for the kicking-damping function[16] by dissipating mechanical energy for limb deceleration. This action has a crucial involvement of hip extensors and knee flexors in the swing limb.

Another difference between players and nonplayers is that, in general, players show less swing-limb muscle activation (although they produce greater ball velocity) than nonplayers.[11] This demonstrates that, in experienced players, the demands of kicking are also met by efficiently using the passive properties of the musculoskeletal system. The passive tension of myofascial structures and their resulting passive stiffness can be used for energy transfer among segments, energy storage and return (stretching and shortening, respectively), and energy dissipation (tissue viscosity), with minimal metabolic cost.[17,18]

Segments other than the lower swing limb are also part of the kicking kinetic chain. The pelvis, trunk, contralateral upper limb and the support limb are involved in the function of transferring mechanical energy to the ball. Skilled players, compared to novice players, clearly show greater motions of the upper body segments[19] to take advantage of the great kinetic energy produced by the large masses of these segments. In preparation for kicking, soccer players often prefer to walk or run toward the ball with a diagonal approach angle close to 45°.[20] Such approach requires transverse plane rotations of the body to shoot the ball forward. These rotations take place at the hip joint of the support limb and at the trunk. During the backswing, the pelvis is rotated backward (toward the kicking side) (Table 12-3), with hip external rotation at the support limb, while the swing limb is displaced backwards.[21] The upper trunk is rotated in the opposite direction, toward the nonkicking side, and there is trunk extension. The shoulder contralateral to the swing lower limb is abducted and extended.[19,22] During the leg-cocking and acceleration phases, the pelvis rotates forward (toward the nonkicking side) (see Table 12-3), with internal hip rotation at the support limb, accelerating the swing limb forward.[21] The upper trunk is rotated toward the kicking side and there is trunk flexion. The nonkicking side shoulder is adducted and flexed during the acceleration and follow-through phases.[19,22]

The spring function of the system is also influenced by structures of the upper body that are stretched during the backswing. During a kick, anterior muscles connected by fascia are stretched by the rotation of the upper trunk toward the nonkicking side, extension of the trunk, extension and abduction of the nonkicking side shoulder, and backward rotation of the pelvis. These muscles function as an anterior force propagation line constituted by the rectus abdominis, the kicking-side external obliquus abdominis, and the nonkicking-side internal obliquus abdominis and pectoralis major.[23] These muscles are functionally continuous with hip flexors and adductors and knee extensors of

the swing limb during kicking execution. Pelvic backward rotation stretches the internal hip rotators of the support limb, which also participate in this force propagation pattern. Eccentric contractions of all of these muscles improve energy absorption and storage.[12] The motion of the nonkicking-side upper limb increases the angular momentum of the upper body,[22] enhancing the superior inertial anchoring of this ventral force propagation line and the transfer of energy from the upper body to the swing lower limb. During leg cocking and leg acceleration, the potential energy stored in these structures is returned, with great energy transfer to the swing limb. Concurrently, concentric contractions of the involved muscles, enhanced by their previous stretching,[15] reverse motion directions and add energy to the chain.

At ball contact, the stiffness of all tissues and joints involved in this mechanism must be high, from the kicking ankle to the nonkicking-side shoulder. Appropriate stiffness, provided both passively by tissue tension and actively through eccentric contractions and co-contractions, may produce a "sum of masses" of the segments involved in kicking, allowing for greater energy transfer from the musculoskeletal system to the ball. The capability of using this whole kinetic chain may explain the greater ball velocity produced by the angled approach (45°) in comparison with less angled approaches, even with similar anterior foot velocities before ball contact.[24] It may also explain why individuals who can kick the ball significantly farther do not necessarily have greater muscle strength in the lower swing limb.[25]

After ball contact, upper body structures also participate in the damping function of the system. During the follow-through, rotation of the upper trunk toward the kicking side, flexion of the trunk, flexion and adduction of the nonkicking-side shoulder, and forward rotation of the pelvis[19,21,22] stretch dorsal myofascial structures whose fiber alignments make them capable of decelerating such motions. The nonkicking-side latissimus dorsi, the thoracolumbar fascia, and the erector spinae muscles and the kicking-side gluteus maximus, iliotibial band, and hamstrings constitute such a functional force propagation line.[26] Pelvic forward rotation also stretches the external hip rotators of the support limb. The passive tension and viscosity of all of these structures and the eccentric contractions of the muscles involved allow for the damping function of the system, with motion deceleration and energy absorption and dissipation.[16,17]

Biomechanics of Cutting

Cutting occurs frequently in sports activities such as soccer, basketball, North American football, and handball. Specifically in soccer, cutting is observed during dribbling maneuvers. These maneuvers occur during offensive or defensive strategies.[27] During dribbling maneuvers in a game situation,

Table 12-3
Pelvic Rotations in the Transverse Plane of Motion

Pelvic Motion in the Transverse Plane	Definition
Forward rotation	The anterior face of the pelvic ring (pubis) rotates toward the nonkicking side (kicking) or support-limb side (cutting)
Backward rotation	The anterior face of the pelvic ring (pubis) rotates toward the kicking side (kicking) or swing-limb side (cutting)

the athlete has to be able to run with the ball and abruptly change direction, so cutting is an effective strategy used to beat the opponent. Because of its relevance in different situations, the biomechanics of cutting has received much attention in scientific literature. In addition, cutting in soccer games has a great potential to result in ligament injuries,[28-31] which reinforces the importance of studying this motion. However, most studies on cutting focus only on the biomechanics of the knee joint and neglect the contribution of the whole kinetic chain to the execution of this maneuver.

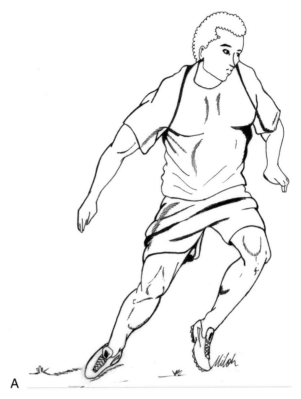

Clinical Relevance Summary - Cutting

- Cutting involves planting the feet to decelerate and an abrupt change of direction with subsequent acceleration.
- There are great demands of absorption and generation of energy to musculoskeletal system during cutting.
- The efficiency of the cutting maneuvers depends on proper energy transfer through trunk, pelvis, and lower limbs.

Cutting maneuvers are accomplished in two ways: sidestep (outside) cutting and crossover (inside) cutting (Table 12-4). The sidestep cut occurs when the direction change proceeds away from the support limb side.[32] For example, a soccer player executes a sidestep cut when the right foot is planted and the athlete cuts to the left, away from the support foot (Figure 12-2, A).[33] A crossover cut is executed when, during running, the player plants one foot and then crosses the contralateral lower extremity anteriorly to provide acceleration to run in a new direction.[31] For example, when the player plants the left foot, the right foot crosses over the left foot to change direction (see Figure 12-2, B).[33] Thus, in a crossover cutting, the direction change

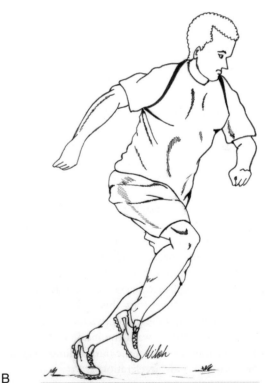

Figure 12-2

Cutting maneuvers. **A,** A sidestep cut with direction change to the left. The right limb represents the support limb. **B,** A crossover cut with direction change to the left. The left limb represents the support limb. (Redrawn from Queen RM, Haynes BB, Hardaker WM, et al: Forefoot loading during 3 athletic tasks, *Am J Sports Med* 35(4):630-636, 2007.)

Table 12-4
Sidestep and Crossover Cutting Definitions

Type of Cutting	Definition
Sidestep	Sidestep cutting occurs when the athlete turns to the opposite side of the support limb. For example, a sidestep cut to the left occurs when the soccer player plants the right foot and cuts to the left, away from the support limb
Crossover	Crossover cutting occurs when the athlete turns to the same side of the support limb. For example, a crossover cut to the left occurs when the soccer player plants the left foot and crosses the right foot over the support limb

occurs toward the support-limb side.[32] In general, both types of cutting are characterized by an abrupt direction change named the *plant-and-cut phase*. This phase involves deceleration during the initial ground contact and acceleration during propulsion in a new direction.[31] The mechanisms involved in body deceleration are very similar in both sidestep and crossover cutting. However, the biomechanical patterns during direction change and acceleration phases have marked differences between the two types of cutting. In this section, the biomechanical mechanisms involved in deceleration, direction change, and acceleration phases during cutting maneuvers are discussed in detail.

The fast deceleration and subsequent acceleration observed in the cut-and-plant phase of both cutting maneuvers impose great demands of absorption and generation of energy on the musculoskeletal system. In both cutting maneuvers, during deceleration following ground–foot contact, there is a kinematic pattern in the sagittal plane of hip, knee, and ankle flexion movements. During this phase, the impact forces at initial ground contact are absorbed through eccentric contraction of the hip, knee, and ankle extensor muscles of the support leg.[34] This energy stored is eventually released during the acceleration phase to add the mechanical energy necessary for the player to change direction. This mechanism of storing and recovering energy in the support limb is similar to a simple mass-spring system.[35] According to this view, the support limb behaves as a longitudinal spring, storing energy during the deceleration phase (kinematic pattern of hip, knee, and ankle flexion with eccentric action of the opposing muscles)[34,36] and returning the stored energy to provide a propulsive force in a new direction (kinematic pattern of hip, knee, and ankle extension).[36] The capability of the biological tissues to absorb and to return energy depends on interaction between muscle activation and the viscoelastic properties of the muscle and connective tissues, which determine tissue and joint stiffness. Thus, soccer players with an adequate level of lower limb stiffness take advantage of the properties of their systems to efficiently exploit the elastic energy stored in the support leg and reduce the muscle work necessary to change direction during cutting maneuvers. This role of the support limb in generating part of the propulsive force in cutting maneuvers is also observed during running on a nonlinear (curved) pathway. In this activity, the ground reaction force (GRF) and the propulsive force in the outside limb accelerate the body toward the inside curve, suggesting a role of the musculature of the outside limb to generate energy necessary to body acceleration.[37]

Sidestep Cutting

After terminal deceleration, the directional change in cutting maneuvers and subsequent propulsion involve coordinated movements of body segments. However, the dynamics involved in the kinetic chain during this phase differ for the two types of cutting. The direction change during

sidestep cut movement is characterized by kinematic patterns of subtalar joint pronation, internal rotation of the tibia and abduction of the knee joint, internal rotation of the femur (segment motion with respect to external reference–global coordinate system) and rotation of the trunk and pelvis toward the new direction.[28,36] The magnitudes of adduction and internal rotation torques on the knee joint during sidestep cutting are greater than during movements such as running and landing.[38] This fact suggests that cutting generates a great stability demand to the knee joint. Besier and colleagues[38] demonstrated that, during a sidestep cut, the torque on the knee joint is approximately 150 Nm for an athlete with a body mass of 75 kg. In addition, sidestep cutting produces the highest overall pressure on the foot with the peak pressure observed in the medial forefoot and hallux.[33]

The propulsive force necessary to accelerate the body into a new direction during sidestep cutting is obtained by the energy storing and recovering mechanisms of the support limb.[36] However, the movement efficiency and stability observed in this phase also depends on the energy generated by trunk and pelvic motions. Because these segments are attachment sites for the largest muscles of the body, they generate a great portion of the mechanical energy necessary to accelerate the body in the new direction. During sidestep cutting, the trunk and pelvis rotate toward the swing limb to change direction. This backward pelvic rotation produces external hip rotation (relative motion between two adjacent body segments) of the support limb. Classical analysis of this motion indicates that the torque to rotate the pelvis and trunk is generated by external hip rotator muscles.[36] However, a complex pattern of force transmission is observed, because of the coupling between different anatomical structures.[26,39] According to this view, the gluteus maximus "couples" with the contralateral latissimus dorsi via superficial thoracolumbar fascia and the iliotibial band, transferring the kinetic energy of the trunk to the supporting limb. Rotational force transmission is an effective way of providing the mechanical energy necessary to rotate the pelvis and trunk and, consequently, to change the athlete's direction during sidestep cutting. This energy transfer mechanism is only possible as a result of fascial organization of the tissues around the lower back.[26] Thus the effect of a given muscle is not limited to moving the joint or joints it crosses. In addition, eccentric contractions of the adductor muscles decelerate the pelvic rotation and hip abduction on the support limb. This mechanism helps to explain the high rate of adductor muscle strains in activities that involve running with abrupt direction change.[40]

The efficiency of the mechanisms related to generation and transference of energy through trunk and pelvis rotation depend not only on the rotational force transmission capacity, but also on the kinetic chain global stiffness. An adequate level of hip joint stiffness, for example, allows the necessary force transmission through the kinetic chain to promote appropriate movement patterns and consequently decrease the stress demand on the lower limb joints. On the other hand, diminished hip or subtalar joint stiffness can promote altered movement patterns that may increase stress demand on some joints of the lower limb. This excessive energy flow through the kinetic chain (i.e., stress demand) is among the main factors responsible for injury production.[10] The role of stress demand in injury production during cutting maneuvers is discussed in more detail in the "Biomechanics of Soccer-Related Injuries" section in this chapter.

Crossover Cutting

Similar to the sidestep cutting, in crossover cutting, the direction change with subsequent body propulsion is accomplished by energy storing-and-recovering mechanisms in the support limb, trunk, and pelvis. However, during crossover cutting, trunk and forward pelvis rotation toward the support limb are observed, which cause internal hip rotation on this limb. This trunk and pelvis rotation allow the contralateral limb to swing forward in the direction of the new pathway. The mechanism related to directional change during crossover cutting also involves rotational force transmission. In this case, force is transmitted between internal hip rotator muscles and obliquus abdominis muscles to provide the mechanical energy necessary to rotate the trunk and pelvis and accelerate the body in the new direction. This rotational force transmission mechanism increases the efficiency of the movement and diminishes demand on the joints of the lower limb. As explained previously, this energy transference throughout the kinetic chain depends on an adequate level of hip joint stiffness. For example, if the hip joint has low stiffness, the energy generated by the trunk and pelvis motions is, in great part, absorbed at the hip, which decreases the energy transference to the support limb. This altered energy flow allows potentially injury-producing motions to occur, such as excessive internal hip rotation and subtalar joint pronation.

Although there is hip internal rotation during crossover cutting, the trunk and pelvis movements impose an external rotational torque on the femur. Because the limb is maintained in relative internal rotation and the femur is externally rotated over the tibia of the planted foot, the crossover cutting is described as the functional equivalent of a clinical pivot shift maneuver used to test the integrity of the anterior cruciate ligament (ACL) and for anterolateral rotary instability.[31] Thus, the crossover cutting, similar to sidestep, imposes a great demand on the knee joint. For example, torques on the knee joint can reach 140 Nm for an athlete with 75 kg of body mass.[38] Although the demands on the knee joint are similar in both cutting maneuvers, the foot loading characteristic is different in a crossover cutting as compared with sidestep cutting. In crossover cutting, the load acts mainly on the lateral aspect of the foot and the peak pressure occurs on the lateral portion of forefoot.[33] Another kinematic pattern

that is also observed only during crossover cutting is hip adduction in the support leg when the contralateral leg is crossing the body. This movement is accompanied by eccentric contraction of the gluteus medius, a muscle that has its fascial sheet fused with the deep surface of the tensor fascia lata.[41] Thus, the lateral structures of the hip, including the gluteus medius and tensor fascia lata, must have adequate strength and stiffness to control excessive hip adduction and to prevent the occurrence of injuries around the hip.

Cutting mechanisms vary substantially among sports and individuals. The variability observed in cutting biomechanics reports are possibly due to differences among subjects in terms of techniques, cutting angle, movement speed during the maneuver, or the type of movement performed immediately before the cutting maneuver (e.g., running or landing from a jump). For example, cutting movements performed with cutting angles at approximately 90° require greater values for the breaking and propelling forces.[32] The presence of a defensive opponent during the maneuvers can also alter the kinematic and kinetic parameters normally reported by biomechanical investigations on cutting mechanisms. Larger medial GRFs and larger hip abduction and knee valgus angles are observed during sidestep cutting when the presence of defensive opponent is simulated.[42] In addition, parameters such as cutting technique can influence the athlete's performance. Besier and colleagues,[38] demonstrated that athletes who perform the sidestep cutting with a knee joint varus moment maintained greater speeds and achieved greater cutting angles than those who performed the same task with a valgus moment on the knee. Thus, cutting technique may affect not only the player's performance but also the loads placed on the knee joint.

Biomechanics of Heading

Soccer is the only contact sport in which players frequently hit the ball with their head, called *heading the ball* or *heading*, during matches or training. Scoring a goal, defending, gaining control, or passing the ball with the head is an integral part of soccer. To accomplish these tasks, different types of headers are normally used in soccer.[43] In a clearing header, the player has to impact the ball to produce maximum force to drive the ball back in a safe direction. A passing header advances the ball over a small distance toward an open area or a teammate. Finally, a shooting header must drive the ball, with appropriate speed and direction, to reach the goal accurately (Table 12-5).[44] Heading in soccer may be performed in multiple ways, which depends on the aim of the action, the game situation (e.g., position of the ball and of the player during heading), and the technique used. Furthermore, players can head the ball while on the ground, when running, jumping vertically, and diving. For example, a shooting header can be performed with different strategies. In a game situation in which the player is positioned approximately perpendicular to the goal and the ball

Table 12-5

Types of Heading

Type of Heading	Definition
Clearing header	Header that projects the ball high into the air to drive the ball back in the direction from which it came
Shooting header	Header that generates sufficient ball speed and direction to elude the goal-keeper in an attempt to score a goal
Passing header	Header that drives the ball over a small distance towards a teammate or an open area

is moving above his or her head, the player may be required to jump and slightly rotate the head and neck laterally to intercept the ball and redirect it toward the goal. In a different situation, in which the ball has been rebounded by the goalkeeper and moves in the direction and at the height of the player's head, the player may be required to impact the ball forward using mostly upper body anterior displacement while standing on the ground. Therefore, heading is a complex, multimodal component of soccer that involves and imposes mechanical demands on the whole body.[43,44]

Despite the several heading strategies that may be required during a soccer game, the main header types share similar mechanical features such as stability demands for the cervical joints, the temporal characteristics and magnitude of the electromyographic activities of the cervical muscles, and the forces applied on the forehead and ball.[45] These similarities are due to the fact that the distinct headings have the same overall function: transferring mechanical energy from the body kinetic chain to the ball to redirect it toward a desired target. To describe the main mechanical demands imposed on the musculoskeletal system during headings, this section focuses on a heading action executed with the aim of propelling the ball forward, regardless of header type.

Heading can be temporally divided into three consecutive phases: preparation, impact, and follow-through (Figure 12-3).[43] During the preparation phase, hip and trunk extension may occur, with backward displacement of the trunk, neck, and head. Subsequently, these motions are reversed and there are hip and trunk flexion and forward displacement of the same segments.[43,44] These motions allow the player to accelerate the upper body forward prior to the impact moment, in an attempt to contact the ball with greater velocity and then transferring a larger amount of kinetic energy to the ball. During this phase, the musculoskeletal system must function as a spring.[8] The flexor muscles of the hips and trunk are the main structures responsible for this function, producing the required flexor net torques.

Initially, they stretch and contract eccentrically to absorb and store potential energy during the hip and trunk extension. During hip and trunk flexion, these muscle groups are shortened and return energy to the system.[12] They also contract concentrically to add energy to the kinetic chain. In the absence of initial extension of the hips and trunk, the concentric contractions are responsible for generating the energy of the forward displacement of the upper body. The upper limbs and trunk motions occur in an antiphase fashion. The upper limbs are displaced forward (with shoulder flexion) during the backward displacement of the trunk, and are displaced backward (with shoulder extension and elbow flexion) during the trunk forward displacement. The upper limbs have the role of providing inertial anchoring for the trunk, enhancing the power of the forward displacement of the upper body, with the involvement of the shoulder extensor and scapulae retractor muscles. The arms also improve balance, by compensating for the initial backward projection of the center of mass of the trunk-head unit.[44]

Clinical Relevance Summary - Heading

- Cervical stability and stiffness are required during heading to minimize cervical angular motion, causing the head-neck-trunk complex to move together as a unit, allowing effective transfer of mechanical energy from the kinetic chain to the ball.
- Combined actions of the muscles of the hip, knee, and ankle are necessary to produce an effective jump during heading, without overloading any of these joints.

The instant of ball contact with the player's head, with its resulting ball deformation, is called the *impact phase*. The duration of this phase of heading has been consistently reported as lasting from 10 ms to 23 ms. The magnitude of the head acceleration during the impact period is approximately 20 g (1 g = 9.8 m/s^2) for a ball traveling at 42 km/hr (26 mph).[46] However, during real game conditions, the ball reaches speeds from 120 to 130 km/hr (76 to 81 mph).[44] Therefore, the ball may convey an impact force of approximately 2000 N to the player's head,[47] imposing a large mechanical demand on the musculoskeletal system.

During the follow-through phase, the hip and trunk flexion continue to occur but decelerate.[43] The musculoskeletal system has a damping function, absorbing and dissipating the kinetic energy related to the upper body linear and angular motions. Extensor net torques must be produced at the hips and trunk. The stretching of myofascial structures and eccentric contractions of the extensor muscles of the hips and trunk are mainly responsible for this energy absorption and dissipation.[16]

The head has a small mass and the cervical muscles have small cross-sectional areas and short moment arms, which

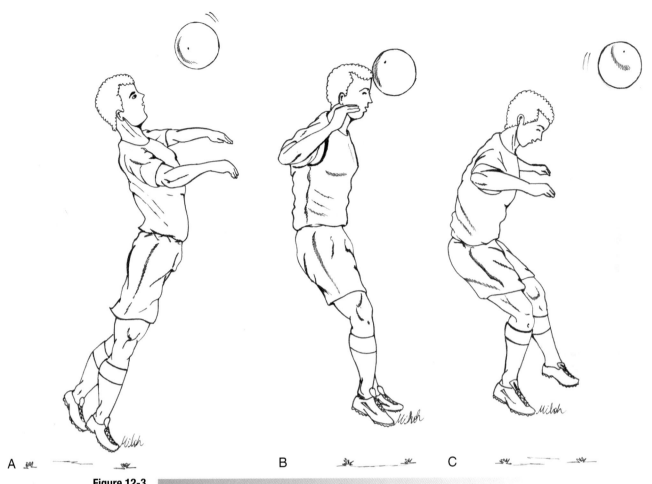

Figure 12-3
Heading phases. **A,** Preparation phase. **B,** Impact phase. **C,** Follow-through phase. See text for details.

limit the capacity of the head-neck complex to generate inertial and active torques and to deal with energy flows between the body and the ball. To meet such mechanical demands, the neuromusculoskeletal system exploits the greater masses and inertial properties of the other segments of the upper body. The cervical joints must have high stiffness and stability to transfer mechanical energy from the kinetic chain to the ball. Cervical stiffness is also needed to absorb and dissipate the energy transferred from the ball to the body originating from internal reactive forces.[10] Cervical stability is required during the whole heading action, during which there is minimal cervical angular motion (i.e., motion of the head in relation to the trunk), making the head-neck-trunk complex move together as one single unit.[43] Consequently, the linear and angular motions of the head (in a global coordinate system) accompany the trunk motion.

During the preparation phase, appropriate neck stiffness is necessary to make the motions of the head in phase with the trunk motion,[43] and thus to take advantage of the acceleration produced at the hips and trunk. The cervical flexor muscles, especially the sternocleidomastoid, are active during this phase[43,45] to create a flexor torque that offsets the extensor torques produced by the head weight and moment of inertia (about the cervical axes of rotation). During the impact phase, the cervical joints must have the greatest amount of stiffness. Such behavior produces a "sum of masses," which increases the kinetic energy of the head-neck-trunk unit, allowing an effective transfer of mechanical energy from the kinetic chain to the ball. Great trunk stiffness is also required for such function. High cervical stiffness during impact also permits the energy transferred from the ball to the head to flow through the upper body. Hence, the reaction forces imparted by the ball can be distributed and dissipated through the kinetic chain. This energy flow prevents high rotational cervical accelerations and excessive energy absorption by the cervical structures. Increased cervical stiffness during the impact moment is mostly generated by co-contraction of the cervical flexors and extensors, which begins a few milliseconds before and ends a few milliseconds after the impact.[43,45] Because of the very short duration of the ball-impact phase, the muscles do not have enough time to generate responsive contraction adjustments before the end of the phase.[43] Therefore, part of the increased cervical stiffness, especially the stiffness generated at ball impact, relies on the inherent and pre-existing passive and architectural properties of the cervical myofascial structures.[48] During the follow-through phase, cervical stability is also necessary to allow the kinetic energy of the anterior displacement of the head-neck-trunk to be dissipated by the stretching and by eccentric contractions[16] of the extensor muscles of the hips and trunk. The cervical extensor muscles, especially the trapezius, are active,[43,45] producing an extensor torque that offsets the flexor torques produced by the head weight and moment of inertia (about the cervical axes of rotation).

The minimal cervical angular motion suggests that the muscle contractions during heading are predominantly isometric.[43] However, some eccentric and concentric contractions probably occur in different internal compartments of these muscles (mainly during the perturbations created by the ball impact). Thus, energy-generating, energy-absorbing, and energy-dissipative capabilities of the cervical muscles are also required for proper heading performance. The impact force and the amount and timing of muscle activation depend on the type of heading. For example, when the objective is to perform a passing header, the player must apply less force and allow motion at the neck to refine the action and obtain more precision.[45] In this case, less coactivation of neck muscles will be observed, as well as an uncoupling between trunk and neck motions.

Heading is a skill that is frequently embedded in other body motions. Jumping is a task that often occurs associated with heading. For example, jumping as high as possible to reach the ball is a common requirement for effective heading in soccer. In fact, the height achieved during a vertical jump is a predictor of different performance levels among soccer players.[49,50] From the initial lower limb flexion to the take-off phase of vertical jumps, the lower limbs go into a flexed position and from there, they have to generate the necessary force to propel the entire body into the air. This mechanical function is similar to the vertical dynamics of a mass-spring model or a pogo stick.[8,51] During hip and knee flexion and ankle dorsiflexion, the lower limbs absorb and store potential energy. Subsequently, during extension of the hip and knee and plantar flexion of the ankle, this energy is returned and more energy is added to the system according to the desired height to be achieved by the head. There are bilateral hip and knee extensor net torques and ankle plantar flexion net torque during these motions. Eccentric contractions followed by concentric contractions and stretching followed by shortening of the hip and knee extensors and ankle plantar flexors are the main mechanisms of the mass-spring dynamics of jumping. The activity of the antagonists of these muscle groups has a crucial role in increasing the joints' stiffness (which

is positively correlated with jumping vertical height) by co-contraction.[52]

Inverse dynamic calculations have estimated that the percentage contribution of work done during jumping in soccer players was 43% for the hip, 29% for the knee, and 28% for the ankle. It has been shown that players who jump higher than their teammates (10 cm or more) produce greater power at the ankle joint.[53] Because the energy flow between anatomically close and remote segments and joints and that the kinetic parameters of each joint, estimated through inverse dynamics, do not provide sufficient information about the forces and energy sources that generate such parameters, it is not possible to affirm that the hip muscles are required more than the knee and ankle muscles.[9] For example, a three-dimensional model of the musculoskeletal system, which considers energy flows, indicates that the plantar flexors generate approximately twice the power produced by the gluteus maximus.[54] The energy produced at each joint flows through the kinetic chain, and thus the torques produced at each joint may be influenced by the forces produced in all of the joints involved in the jumping dynamics.[9] Therefore, the combined actions of the muscles of the hips, knees, and ankles are necessary to produce an effective jump, without overloading any of these joints.

There is a high variability of jump technique among soccer players. Some of them emphasize motion and force generation at the knee joint, whereas others generate more forces at the hip joint. In addition, high values for work production at the hip joint has been associated with low values at the knee joint.[53] The variability in jumping pattern indicates that soccer athletes exploit the strategy that is more compatible with their available force production capabilities.[10] Therefore, it is important to consider the contribution of three lower limb joints when planning jumping training and injury prevention programs for soccer players.

After jumping and heading the ball, the athletes land on the ground. Landing involves movements designed to dissipate the kinetic energy through muscle power and joint torques of the lower extremity.[55] On landing, the GRF must be attenuated by ankle dorsiflexion and knee and hip flexion. This lower limb flexion acts like a damping spring to decrease inertial torque of the landing player. In addition, hip and knee joint flexion-extension angular velocities at the initial foot contact with the ground significantly affect the peak GRF during landing. Thus, eccentric contractions of the hip and knee extensor muscles during landing are necessary to reduce knee joint resultant force.[15,56] During landing, there are external torques of hip adduction and knee abduction (valgus).[57] To land with an adequate lower limb alignment in the frontal and transverse planes of movement, an adequate amount of strength and proper activation timing of the muscles of the hip and knee is needed, especially the hip abductors and external rotators. Strength and adequate stiffness of the hip muscles are required to control the adduction and internal rotation of the hip. In addition to this proximal-to-distal effect observed during landing from a jump, distal-to-proximal effects may also happen. The vertically directed GRF normally generates foot pronation during landing;[58] however, it depends on the current foot position and on the anatomical alignment of the foot and tibia. Because the foot is the first body segment to receive the impact force during landing, alignment disorders of the foot and tibia may induce excessive subtalar joint pronation or supination. Excessive foot pronation may lead to excessive hip adduction and internal rotation and knee abduction. These abnormal joint actions may influence the alignment of the lower limbs and the patterns of force transmission along the kinetic chain.

Biomechanics of Soccer-Related Injuries

One of the basic objectives of studying soccer kinetic and kinematic characteristics and, more specifically, the interplay between the athlete's capability and demand during soccer is to provide information that may assist in reducing the player's susceptibility to injury and improving performance. In this view, injury prevention and performance depend on the capability of the musculoskeletal system to deal with the resulting stress caused by the flow of forces (energy) through the kinetic chain. Classic approaches involve the identification of intrinsic and extrinsic factors associated with injury production, but capability-demand reasoning recognizes that factors such as the player's anatomic characteristics, game versus practice situations, and the use of inadequate equipment or field conditions can produce increased demands on the body segments. On the other hand, adequate levels of strength, stiffness, and endurance define the capability of the player's musculoskeletal system. When the stress (energy) applied to a particular tissue exceeds a critical limit (i.e., above the player's capability), injury occurs. Therefore, the aim of any injury prevention program should be to achieve a balance between the player's capabilities and the demands imposed by the sport.

The most common injuries during soccer practice involve the lower extremity.[30] Upper extremity injuries are less common than lower extremity injuries and usually occur after a fall to the ground or collision with another player. In fact, upper extremity injuries are more common in goalkeepers than in any other soccer playing position.[30] The majority of injuries observed in soccer are traumatic. For example, a high proportion of ankle and foot injuries results from player-to-player contact in tackling events.[59] In general, tackling produces lateral or medial forces that create a great demand in eversion or inversion of the foot and ankle during weight-bearing.[59] However, during soccer activity many musculoskeletal injuries are also related to overuse mechanisms. Because of the great variability of situations in which injuries may occur, in this section, the stress demand and musculoskeletal injuries for each component of soccer (kicking, cutting, and heading) are discussed separately. Because many pathological conditions share common causal mechanisms, the approach taken in this section is to group some conditions into one description to avoid unnecessary repetition. However, some overlap among the soccer components may occur, as different mechanisms or movement patterns may produce similar pathological conditions.

Kicking-Related Injuries

The musculoskeletal system must have the capability of withstanding the mechanical demands inherent to the kicking action by exploiting the whole kinetic chain to execute the task with maximum performance and minimum injury risk. The biomechanical characteristics of the player and the interactions with the performed task and the environmental conditions may increase the demands imposed on the musculoskeletal system during kicking. Kicking-related pathological conditions occur when kicking demands overcome the system's capability and are often related to inappropriate energy flow between the upper body and the lower swinging limb. Impaired muscle function and altered passive stiffness of myofascial structures at the trunk, pelvis, and support limb leads to compensatory changes in the lower swing-limb mechanics to allow for an effective kick. These compensations constitute increased demands on lower limb structures. Although many acute, overuse, and contact injuries may be related to the mechanics of kicking, this section focuses on muscle strains, tendinopathies, painful hip and knee conditions, and lumbopelvic dysfunctions, which are some of the most common pathological conditions that affect soccer players.[2,60,61]

Clinical Relevance Summary – Kicking Injuries

- Kicking-related pathological conditions are often related to inappropriate energy flow between the upper body and the lower swinging limb, which requires excessive locally generated torques and imposes increased demands on lumbopelvic, hip, and knee structures.
- Injuries of the knee and hip joints of the lower swing limb and of the lumbopelvic complex may arise as a result of eccentric and concentric weaknesses of muscles such as the oblique abdominis, the nonkicking-side pectoralis major and hip internal rotators, during the backswing, leg-cocking, and leg-acceleration phases, respectively. Eccentric weakness of muscles such as the nonkicking-side latissimus dorsi and bilateral gluteus maximus may also overload lower swing-limb structures, during the follow-through phase.

Hip and Knee Injuries

Insufficient contribution of the upper body in the spring function of kicking creates excessive requirements of locally generated hip flexor and adductor torques and knee extensor torques. For instance, during the backswing phase of kicking, eccentric weakness and decreased passive stiffness of the oblique abdominis and hip internal rotators of the support limb may lead to excessive demands for eccentric activity of the hip flexors (especially during the instep kick) and adductors (especially during the sidestep kick) and knee extensors. As a result, injuries such as rectus femoris and adductor magnus strains and tendinopathies may occur.[61] Concentric weakness of the same muscles at the trunk and support limb may require, during leg cocking and leg acceleration phases, compensatory vigorous concentric contractions of the hip flexors and adductors and knee extensors of the swing limb to generate additional energy to the kinetic chain. This augmented muscle recruitment also increases the possibility of developing tendinopathies of the proximal or distal insertions of these muscles. In addition, knee extensors compensatory actions overload patellofemoral joint structures[62] such as the articular cartilage, subchondral bone, patellar retinaculi, and infrapatellar fat pad, which predisposes the development of anterior knee pain.

Hamstrings Strain

During the follow-through phase of kicking, impaired functions of the trunk, pelvis, and support limb muscles, which are involved in the kicking damping function, result in excessive locally generated torques of hip extension and knee flexion at the swing limb. Eccentric weakness and decreased passive stiffness of muscles such as the nonkicking-side latissimus dorsi, the kicking-side gluteus maximus, and external hip rotators of the support limb may require excessive eccentric activity of the swing-limb hamstrings to absorb and dissipate energy for limb deceleration. Such a mechanism often results in the occurrence of hamstrings strains.[2,61] In the presence of an associated hamstring eccentric weakness or previous strain, this injury is even more likely to occur.[63]

Pelvic Dysfunctions and Groin Pain

Deficient transverse plane rotational energy transfers from the upper trunk and support limb to the pelvis decrease the contribution of pelvic forward acceleration and deceleration (toward the nonkicking side) to the necessary swing limb acceleration and deceleration during kicking. This condition requires greater sagittal plane torques at the swing limb hip and at the pelvis, predisposing the athlete for pelvic dysfunctions. For example, the presence of femoral retroversion with increased internal rotation stiffness at the hip of the support limb hampers the necessary pelvic forward rotation. Compensatory locally generated torques by the hip flexors and adductors in the swing limb, during leg cocking and leg acceleration, may create excessive anteversion torques on the kicking side innominate bone. Weakness of the internal oblique abdominis at the kicking side also contributes for decreased torque of pelvic forward rotation. In addition, it may result in smaller upward-directed forces imposed upon the ipsilateral pubis in comparison with the downward-directed forces imparted by hip flexors and adductors. Furthermore, compensatory locally generated hip extension torques during the follow-through phase result in excessive retroversion torques imposed on the same innominate bone. Such compensations and imbalances may lead to instability and excessive torsional and shear stresses at the symphysis pubis and sacroiliac (SI) joints. Osteitis pubis and sacroiliitis are commonly resulting dysfunctions[64] of these altered movement patterns and force distribution. In addition, proximal tendinopathies of the hip adductors (groin pain) and distal tendinopathies of abdominal muscles are frequently associated conditions.[65]

Back Pain

Appropriate trunk transverse and sagittal planes stiffness, and the resulting spine stability, is crucial for energy dissipation and flow among the segments involved in the kicking kinetic chain. Decreased myofascial passive stiffness and weakness of the muscles that participate in the regulation of trunk stiffness may overload spine structures. Bilateral impaired eccentric functions of muscles such as the oblique and rectus abdomini, latissimus dorsi, and gluteus maximus produce poor mechanical energy dissipation capacity at the trunk. Weakness and low endurance of these muscles and of the transversus abdominis and multifidus may also lead to decreased trunk stiffness.[66,67] These factors, and the associated repetitive extension, flexion, and longitudinal rotations of the spine segments will probably result in high stresses on the intersegmental discs, facet joints, and spinal ligaments. Consequently, acute and overuse injuries and degenerative changes at the thoracolumbar spine may result in back pain.[60] It is also important to be aware that back symptoms may also occur as a result of referred pain originated from kicking-related injuries at the SI and hip joints.[64]

Cutting-Related Injuries

Cutting is frequently embedded in different playing actions during soccer matches and practices. Normally, decelerating and sprinting actions are followed by players' direction changes. The characteristics of fast deceleration and sudden direction changes observed exclusively during cutting impose specific demands on the individual's musculoskeletal system. These demands are closely related to development of different soccer-related injuries in the lower extremities. Musculoskeletal injuries such as ligament sprains, adductor muscle strains and patellofemoral pain occur frequently in noncontact situations as a result of cutting. In this section, the specific demands promoted by cutting and its potential to injury production are discussed in detail.

Knee Injuries

The combination of rotational forces and deceleration observed in cutting creates opportunities for ligament, tendon, and patellofemoral joint injuries.[30,68] Stresses produced by cutting may account for the majority of noncontact ACL injuries during soccer games. A typical noncontact ACL injury mechanism is a combination of knee valgus or varus at near full extension and rotation of the tibia with the foot planted on the ground.[69,70] Increased rotational forces on the knee joint occur during both cutting maneuvers. However, crossover cutting is considered one of the most dangerous noncontact situations for the ACL because of the combination of femur external rotation and relative tibia internal rotation of the support limb.[31] Adequate performance and injury prevention during cutting depend on, in addition to other factors, the player's correct biomechanical alignment, adequate muscle function, and proper muscle and joint stiffness. These factors are necessary to promote correct movement patterns and consequently reduce the stress demands on the kinetic chain. The rotational demand on the knee joint depends on the coordinated mechanics of the hip and ankle-foot joints. In sidestep cutting, for example, a reduced hip-joint stiffness can allow excessive internal rotation of the femur in the support limb during direction changes. Excessive femoral internal rotation has been associated with greater adduction (valgus) torque in the knee joint, which increases the load on the ACL.[71] Differences between genders in relation to the biomechanics of the lower limb during cutting are used to explain the greater rate of ACL injury in female soccer athletes. In general, females have greater abduction (genu valgum) angles and adduction torque at the knee joint, greater internal rotation of the femur, subtalar pronation, and smaller knee-flexion angles than male athletes. This combination of excessive femoral internal rotation along with subtalar joint pronation results in increased valgus loading at the knee joint, which could explain the increased risk of knee injuries in female soccer players. In addition, it has been argued that the association between valgus loading and proximal anterior tibial shear forces increases the stresses applied to the ACL.[70] The quadriceps muscles are the major contributor to the anterior shear force at the proximal end of the tibia through the patellar tendon. During cutting maneuvers, the deceleration that occurs prior to the change in direction is associated with strong quadriceps action at knee angles lower than 40°, increasing the loading on the ACL.[28,29,72] Thus, cutting imposes an increased demand on the musculoskeletal system, as this action simultaneously applies rotational and shear forces at the knee joint. This increased demand suggests that proximal hip-pelvis stabilization and adequate strength and stiffness of the hamstrings are necessary to control and resist the anterior shear force of the tibia, preventing an excessive loading on the ACL.[68,72,73]

The presence of structural lower limb alignment abnormalities, in addition to changes in hip joint stiffness, may also increase the stress demand on the knee joint. A rearfoot varus deformity, for example, can generate compensatory movements such as excessive subtalar pronation and internal rotation of the tibia and femur during a sidestep cut, which also increases the load on the ACL. Therefore, the high incidence of ACL injury in female soccer athletes during cutting can be explained by the presence of greater hip adduction, femur internal rotation, and subtalar pronation angles with the consequent increased knee abduction angle and valgus loading. In addition to the contribution of the altered amount of hip joint stiffness to ACL ruptures, stiffness changes can also alter the movement pattern efficiency and, consequently, the performance of the athlete during cutting. Decreased hip joint stiffness allows the dissipation of part of the energy generated by pelvic and trunk movements, decreasing the energy transfer through the kinetic chain. This altered force transmission mechanism can result in poor performance, such as reduced velocity during direction changes and inadequate cutting angles.

The excessive stress demands on the knee joint are also related to development of knee overuse injuries in athletes who perform repetitive cutting maneuvers.[30] The inappropriate movement patterns previously discussed also impose a great demand over patellofemoral joint and patellar tendon. During the direction change phase in both cutting maneuvers, the absence of sufficient proximal strength and stiffness produce excessive hip adduction and internal rotation of the femur. This altered movement pattern promotes excessive lateral patellar tracking and increases retropatellar contact forces.[74] Inappropriate proximal stiffness can also result in movement patterns that contribute to dynamic alteration of the patella and tendon alignment. As a result, increased longitudinal or shear stresses are applied to the patellar tendon, which contribute to the development of a tendinopathy.[75] Structural abnormalities, such as a rearfoot varus deformity, can also play a role in the development of patellofemoral pain or patellar tendinopathy.[74] Foot malalignment can promote excessive subtalar pronation with consequently excessive tibial internal rotation, resulting in abnormal stress demand on the patellofemoral joint and patellar tendon during the execution of cutting.

Ankle and Foot Injuries

Although foot and ankle injuries may occur mostly during contact with another player, as observed in tackling situations, the majority of noncontact ankle sprains are observed during rotational movements with the foot planted on the ground.[76] For example, during crossover cutting, there is an increased susceptibility to lateral ankle sprains caused by a greater demand of foot inversion in the support limb caused by the athlete's direction change. A similar demand can be observed during sidestep cutting, when the swing limb plants on the ground after rolling the ball. Although the peroneal muscles are thought to be the primary muscles responsible for preventing excessive foot inversion,[77] decreases in ankle eversion strength have been shown not to be a risk factor for lateral ankle sprain.[78] The demands on the foot and ankle joints during cutting also depend on the dynamics of the lower extremity. During direction changes on the support leg (crossover) or when the swing limb plants on the ground (sidestep), there is an increased adduction torque in the hip joint. As a result, in addition to the demand of activity of the ankle evertor muscles, there is the necessity of hip abductor muscles contraction to control this increased frontal plane motion in the hip joint. The inability of the hip abductor muscles to properly absorb the laterally directed energy applied to the hip joint, by eccentric contractions, increases kinetic chain stress demand, altering foot motions. The deceleration of the lateral body displacement during cutting is achieved by balanced energy absorption at the hip and ankle joints. In this view, adequate strength and hip stiffness are necessary to control stress demand both on the hip and ankle joints. In addition to acute injuries, overuse foot injuries can be observed during cutting resulting from altered foot-loading patterns. The previously discussed differences in loading patterns between cutting maneuvers, such as increase lateral or medial foot loading, can explain the occurrence of metatarsal stress fractures commonly observed in soccer players.[33]

Muscle Strains

Muscle strains occur when muscles are stretched during contraction (i.e., eccentric or isometric loading). Strains of the adductor muscles have been suggested as the main cause of groin pain in soccer players.[79] During sidestep cutting, there is an increased risk of adductor muscle strains because of the movements required for direction changes and body propulsion. In the plant-and-cut phase of cutting, the initial lateral displacement of the body requires the hip to have frontal-plane stability. To increase hip stiffness, there is a co-contraction of the hip abductors and adductors.[80] The hip abduction, which occurs during the cut phase, stretches the activated adductor muscles (eccentric contraction). The capability of these muscles to resist injury depends on the amount of energy they can absorb. However, energy flows within the kinetic chain depend on the status of other muscles that work synergistically with those that act to accelerate or decelerate the body. During a sidestep cut, the actions of the contralateral external oblique and ipsilateral internal oblique abdominal muscles are crucial to an efficient energy transfer from the trunk to the support limb. In this case, strength imbalances between abdominal and adductor muscles may increase the susceptibility of adductor muscles to injury. The inability of the adductor and oblique muscles to act as a force couple may result in adductor muscle strains and increase shear forces directed to the pubic symphysis, and result in the development of groin pain, which is a common pathological condition caused by kicking. In addition to poor eccentric strength and inadequate force coupling, muscle fatigue is another factor that may reduce the capacity of the musculoskeletal system to deal with the demands of cutting. In this case, repetitive cutting movements during a soccer match, which produces continuous dissipative demands, may lead to premature muscle fatigue. Adductor muscle fatigue may decrease their efficiency to act as a dissipative mechanism and increase the chance of muscle strain.[81,82]

Heading-Related Injuries

During a soccer game, it is estimated that the player heads the ball an average five to six times. At the end of his or her professional life (approximately 15 years), the player receives approximately 5250 head impacts.[83] This high demand on the musculoskeletal system may play an important role in the development of traumatic brain injuries and impose cumulative stresses on the structures of the neck and head. The applied stresses on the neck and head may cause brain concussions, degenerative cervical spine disorders, and cognitive deficits. In addition, heading frequently involves complex body motions, such as jumping and landing, which subject the lower limbs to increased demands. The embedding of heading in jumping and landing makes the lower limbs susceptible to acute and overuse injuries, such as tendinopathy and ACL rupture. In this section, the mechanisms on the contribution of heading to these injuries are discussed.

> **Clinical Relevance Summary – Heading and Jumping/Landing Injuries**
>
> - The applied stresses to the neck and head may cause brain concussions, degenerative cervical spine disorders, and cognitive deficits if excessive mechanical energy reaches the head as consequence of poor heading technique.
> - During soccer, the patellar tendon is cyclically stretched in an excessive manner, when jumping and landing loads are not dissipated or properly transferred by the hip and ankle muscles. The knee is an intermediate joint in the lower kinetic chain and it depends on the kinetics and kinematics of the hip and ankle joints to attenuate or adequately distribute the forces.

Head Injuries and Concussion

Head and neck injuries constitute from 4% to 22% from all soccer injuries. Most of these injuries affect the head and a minor part involve the neck.[47] This injury incidence includes all types of injury, such as face fractures, lacerations, concussions, and eye injuries. Concussions have an incidence of 3.3% to 2.8% of all injuries in men and women soccer players respectively.[47] This condition is defined as a head injury followed by any type of alteration in brain functioning, caused directly or indirectly by rotational forces transmitted to the head. Immediate concussion symptoms include brief loss of consciousness, dizziness, cognitive or memory dysfunction, vomiting, nausea, photophobia, and loss of balance. Delayed signs and symptoms may include fatigue, depression, sleep irregularity, and an inability to perform daily activities.[84]

The incidence of brain injury in soccer depends on the competitive level of the game.[85,86] It has been shown that 70% of the head injuries occur during matches and the most frequent injury mechanisms are head-to-head contact, followed by the contact of the head with another body part (elbow, arm, or hand). None of the concussion cases reported in soccer were due to the intentional contact of the player's head with the ball.[86] During heading, considering a ball velocity from 7 to 10 m/s (23 to 33 ft/s), the rotational acceleration of the head can reach 200 to 360 rad/s^2 (11,460 to 20,630 deg/s^2). According to biomechanical analyses, the safe acceleration threshold is 1800 rad/s^2 (103,131 deg/^{2}), which is more easily reached during rotational impacts in comparison with linear ones.[21] In addition, it has been shown that the head impact is increased when the head mass/ball mass ratio is reduced. Thus, although the rotational acceleration values are frequently below injury threshold, children and women may present greater risk of head injury resulting from lower head mass/ball ratio, a thinner cranium, and weaker neck muscles (which act to attenuate the forces applied to the head after ball contact).[85] In addition, children normally demonstrate poor heading techniques, which when properly performed (using the head, neck, and trunk as a unit) may reduce the amount of mechanical energy that reaches the brain. Another factor that must be considered is that the mass of the ball and, by its turn, the energy applied to the cranium, may increase up to 20% when it is wet, for example because of rain. However, one of the most important factors for head injury prevention is the proper execution of heading. In this case, the player must stabilize the head, neck, and trunk into a greater mass unit, which reduces the head acceleration to a given force and decreases the head/ball mass ratio.[44,84]

Chronic Brain Injury (Cognitive Dysfunction)

Soccer players, even retired ones, may have chronic brain injuries (characterized by anatomic and neurophysiological changes) that can be assessed by means of computed tomography, neurological tests, and electroencephalogram.[47] Cognitive changes and intelligence deficits are also found in soccer players and seem to be more common in players considered as typical headers. Chronic brain injuries are due to the repetitive neck and head movements produced during heading or due to the impacts on the head.[86] In both cases, the brain damage may develop from the linear acceleration of the brain, which causes compression and increasing of the internal brain pressure or from rotational acceleration, which produces shear forces between the brain and the cranium.[21]

Cervical Injuries

The constant use of the head to defend, score, and pass the ball during soccer matches and practices increase the demand on the musculoskeletal structures of the cervical spine. When the players stabilize the head by means of the co-contraction of the extensors and flexors of the neck, they reduce the rotational acceleration of the head in relation to the trunk.[45] This reduced acceleration decreases the risk of injuries to the brain and neck. Considering the high demand to the neck structures during soccer, it was found that the degenerative changes found in 40-year-old soccer players were similar to those found in nonathletes 50 years old or older.[87] These premature changes in the cervical spine structures seem to be caused by repetitive heading during years of soccer practice and could be minimized by an adequate conditioning of the cervical spine muscles.[87]

Cervical muscle strains or ligament sprains are the most common problem related to frequent heading of the ball. Repetitive stress or improper technique, which could apply forces inappropriately to the neck structures or fail to dissipate or transfer them to the trunk muscles, can be associated with these injuries in soccer. Insufficient energy dissipation or transference increases the demand to the cervical spine and possibly results in muscle strains caused by the cervical muscles' eccentric contraction, which may lead to tensile failure at their myotendinous junction.[88]

Patellar Tendinopathy

Injuries to the lower limbs occur during jumping and landing, which are an integral part of heading. To reach the ball with the head, the player frequently jumps during soccer matches. Jumping applies high loads to the joints, tendons, and muscles of the lower limbs. The knee is an intermediate joint in the lower kinetic chain, and, therefore, it depends on the kinetics and kinematics of the hip and ankle joints to attenuate or adequately distribute the forces reaching the musculoskeletal system. It has been demonstrated that, during landing from vertical jumps, the patellar tendon receives forces up to 8000 N.[89] If forces of such magnitude are not dissipated or properly transferred to other body structures, the patellar tendon will be cyclically stretched in an excessive manner during practices and games. Environmental conditions (e.g., inadequate training or game turf), lower extremity malalignments (e.g., tibia, forefoot, and rearfoot varus and knee valgus), pelvis and hip instabilities (e.g., weak hip external rotators and oblique abdominal muscles) and muscle fatigue may, in fact, alter force distribution and increase the demands imposed on the patellar tendon during soccer-related activities such as jumping, landing, and running. Because soccer practice demands long-lasting and regular loading of the musculoskeletal system, the patellar tendon structure may not have adequate time for appropriate repair. Continual imposition of loading may produce collagen cross-linking damage, cystic formation, and nonfunctional neovascularization. These changes are characteristic of tendinosis (chronic tendinopathy), which differ from other forms of tendinopathies such as traumatic or frictional paratenonitis.[75]

Anterior Cruciate Ligament Injury

In soccer, 25% of the ACL injuries are a consequence of landing from jumps. In addition, women soccer players have two to eight times more ACL injuries than men.[70,71] This greater incidence of ACL injuries has been related to some form of altered neuromuscular control that results in increased valgus knee angle (2.5 times greater), 20% increase in GRF, and more erect posture during landing.[57] It has been observed that female athletes adopt a stiffer landing mechanism to decrease their downward momentum.[90] They reach peak hip and knee flexion angles earlier, and land with smaller joint angles when compared with men. Thus, greater amounts of force are applied in a briefer period to the musculoskeletal system. This strategy results in greater impact forces with less work produced by the hip and knee extensors. In this case, the ankle is used to absorb most of the energy and the body remains more erect during landing, after heading. The reduced participation of the larger muscles of the hip and knee produces increased loading to the noncontractile structures, such as the ACL.[91] Compared with women, male soccer players have a lower risk of landing injuries, because they use the ankle strategy less frequently and rely more on energy absorption by the hip and knee joints, probably because of their greater muscle strength.[92]

In noncontact ACL injuries during landing, a fast deceleration occurs in the joints of the lower limbs, when the hip is in adduction and internal rotation, whereas the knee is in valgus with external rotation.[93] Some athletes, especially women, have a significant increase in frontal plane motions (hip adduction and knee valgus) during landing (Figure 12-4).[58,94,95] The increased knee valgus angle has been considered as a prediction factor for ACL injuries.[57] The so-called lack of neuromuscular control may be, in fact, due to an inadequate stabilizing function of the hip and pelvis muscles (weakness and low stiffness of the hip abductor and external rotators and abdominal oblique muscles). There is evidence that women with weaker hip abductor and external rotator muscles have greater knee valgus angles (approximately 4°).[96] In addition, foot

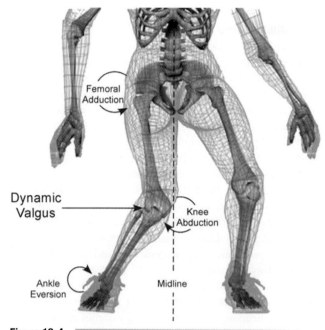

Figure 12-4

Kinematics of the lower limb during landing: Excessive hip adduction leading to excessive knee valgus. (From Hewett TE, Myer GD, Ford KR, et al: Biomechanical measures of neuromuscular control and valgus loading of the knee predict anterior cruciate ligament injury risk in female athletes: A prospective study, *Am J Sports Med* 33(4):492-501, 2005.)

malalignment may increase hip internal rotation forces, contributing to greater frontal plane motions. After foot alignment correction, the knee valgus angle has been shown to be significantly reduced during landing.[97] In addition, better hip and pelvic stabilization capabilities may increase the ability of the quadriceps and hamstring muscles to resist the forces imposed on the lower limbs during jumping and landing.[97] This contribution of different muscles of the kinetic chain to the heading components, such as jumping and landing, must be considered when evaluating the soccer athlete or planning rehabilitation and preventive programs for ACL injuries.

Implications for Rehabilitation

Soccer is a sport that requires the involvement of all body parts for the proper execution of its main components. However, most biomechanical analyses of soccer have concentrated on the demands imposed on specific joints or body segments. This approach is not only limited, but less fruitful, as it neglects to consider the complex interactions among these body segments. For example, the lack of strength and adequate stiffness of the oblique abdominals and pectoralis major muscles may require an increased force production by the hip flexors and adductors during kicking. Repetitive exigencies of the adductor muscles in kicking may result in muscle and tendon strains or in the development of pubic symphysis. Thus, the understanding of the causes and consequences of a local injury requires a global assessment of the player and the knowledge about the complex biomechanical interactions of the musculoskeletal system.

The previous sections of this chapter focused on outlining the demands imposed by soccer components and how they come about to produce pathological conditions. The other side of the story is the athlete. To play soccer properly and safely, the player must meet the demands that are frequently imposed by the execution of the soccer components. The presence of a weak link in the player's kinetic chain may result in reduced performance or increased risk of developing a given pathological condition. The ability of the player to generate and transfer the proper energy to the required movement, or distribute the excessive forces among all body parts to protect the musculoskeletal system defines the player capacity. It is in the understanding of the relationship between task demand and player's capacity that lies the main role of the rehabilitation professional. Reducing demands and increasing the player capacity are the foundations of an effective rehabilitation program directed toward reducing the risk of injuries or improving the player's performance.

Clinical Point - Rehabilitation

Reducing demands and increasing the player capacity are the foundations of an effective rehabilitation program directed toward reducing the risk of injuries or improving the player's performance.

Classical biomechanical analysis considers that most of the forces applied to or produced by the body are solely transmitted through joints.[9,14] Biomechanical models based on this assumption frequently find forces that easily exceed the capacity of any biological tissue to withstand them. Conversely, it has been suggested that the human body acts in synergistic manner, in which its continuing connective tissue network (i.e., muscles, tendons, ligaments, capsules, and fascia) acts to redistributes the forces among all body structures. Recent concepts derived from the works on tensegrity[98-100] and myofascial force transmission[101,102] seem to indicate that forces flow within the musculoskeletal system in an integral manner. This understanding shifts the focus on the analysis and treatment of separated body parts to the assessment and rehabilitation of the whole.

Rehabilitation of the soccer athlete entails a clinical reasoning approach by the sport rehabilitation professional. In essence, clinical reasoning requires the practitioner to think globally, act locally, and then act again globally. In clinical terms, it means that the rehabilitation team must understand the demands imposed by soccer; assess globally the athlete (looking for weak links in the kinetic chain); treat locally the areas that have inadequate strength, stiffness, endurance, or demonstrate improper alignment; and, finally, treat the

athlete functionally (training proper movement patterns) in the sport components that are related to the injury process. For example, a soccer player who has a complaint of groin pain may have the following mismatches between the sport demands and his or her musculoskeletal capacities:

1. A player frequently involved in running and cutting actions that have a reduced range of hip internal rotation (e.g., hip retroversion) will impose increased torsional stress on the SI joint. If this player, at the same time, has weak trunk or pelvic stabilizer muscles, resulting excessive motion of the SI joint will lead to increased stress to the pubic symphysis.

2. A constant running player (midfield or backside) who supinates the foot during heel strike because of inadequate lower limb alignment (e.g., rearfoot varus, with altered running line of progression) will have reduced shock absorption by the quadriceps muscles, as a result of insufficient knee flexion. If the player has weak gluteal, latissimus dorsi, abdominals, or other lumbothoracic fascia muscle stabilizers, the SI joint or lower back will be overstressed and pain may result.

3. A soccer kicker who has inefficient movement patterns caused by weakness of the oblique abdominals, pectoralis major, or upper limb muscles will excessively use the hip muscles to propel the ball during free kicks or long passes. In this case, increased action of the hip adductors is triggered by the lack of adequate force transmission through the kinetic chain, increasing the stress on the adductor muscles or pubic symphysis.

In all of the previous examples, local structures such as hip adductors or pubic symphysis are not the source of the problem, but only the location of the complaint. Initially, to treat such patients, it is necessary to assess the kinetic chain capability in relation to the sport demand (global thinking). Second, the rehabilitation team must work on weak structures that were ascertained to require improvement (local acting). Finally, the proper movement patterns or skills must be trained according to the demands normally applied functionally during soccer matches (global acting). This type of approach indicates that the athlete, not the pathologic condition, is the focus of the intervention.

The body is a continuous network of interconnected elements. In soccer, the presence of weak links in this kinetic chain is the main threat to the musculoskeletal system. However, the failure of the rehabilitation professional to recognize the global nature of the injury-producing factors is an even greater threat to the player. The understanding of the complex relations among the sport requirements and the musculoskeletal system's capability is the key factor for the proper treatment of the athlete. The demands of soccer are multiple, as many of the sport components overlap during games and practices. However, the understanding of how the musculoskeletal system is organized to deal with the forces arising from the interaction between the athlete and environment is a primary step toward planning an adequate intervention.

References

1. Fédération Internationale de Football Association: Big Count, *Fifa Magazine* 25(7):11–17, 2007.
2. Arnason A, Gudmundsson A, Dahl HA, et al: Soccer injuries in Iceland, *Scand J Med Sci Sports* 6(1):40–45, 1996.
3. Andersen TE, Floerenes TW, Arnason A, et al: Video analysis of the mechanisms for ankle injuries in football, *Am J Sports Med* 32(1 Suppl):69S–79S, 2004.
4. Dvorak J, Junge A: Football injuries and physical symptoms. A review of the literature, *Am J Sports Med* 28(5 Suppl):S3–9, 2000.
5. Nunome H, Asai T, Ikegami Y, et al: Three-dimensional kinetic analysis of side-foot and instep soccer kicks, *Med Sci Sports Exerc* 34(12):2028–2036, 2002.
6. Barfield WR: The biomechanics of kicking in soccer, *Clin Sports Med* 17(4):711–728, 1998.
7. Brophy RH, Backus SI, Pansy BS, et al: Lower extremity muscle activation and alignment during the soccer instep and side-foot kicks, *J Orthop Sports Phys Ther* 37(5):260–268, 2007.
8. Full RJ, Koditschek DE: Templates and anchors: Neuromechanical hypotheses of legged locomotion on land, *J Exp Biol* 202(Pt 23): 3325–3332, 1999.
9. Zajac FE, Neptune RR, Kautz SA: Biomechanics and muscle coordination of human walking. Part I: Introduction to concepts, power transfer, dynamics and simulations, *Gait Posture* 16(3):215–232, 2002.
10. Fonseca ST, Ocarino JM, Silva PLP, et al: Integration of stresses and their relationship to the kinetic chain. In Magee DJ, Zachazewski JE, Quillen WS, editors: *Scientific foundations and principles of practice in musculoskeletal rehabilitation*, St Louis, 2007, Saunders.
11. De Proft E, Clarys J, Bollens E, et al: Muscle activity in the soccer kick. In Reilly T, Lees A, Davids K, Murphy WJ, editors: *Science and football*, London, 1988, E & FN Spon.
12. Lindstedt SL, Reich TE, Keim P, et al: Do muscles function as adaptable locomotor springs? *J Exp Biol* 205(Pt 15):2211–2216, 2002.
13. Weiss PL, Hunter IW, Kearney RE: Human ankle joint stiffness over the full range of muscle activation levels, *J Biomech* 21(7): 539–544, 1988.
14. Robertson DG, Winter DA: Mechanical energy generation, absorption and transfer amongst segments during walking, *J Biomech* 13(10):845–854, 1980.
15. Seyfarth A, Blickhan R, Van Leeuwen JL: Optimum take-off techniques and muscle design for long jump, *J Exp Biol* 203 (Pt 4):741–750, 2000.
16. Lindstedt SL, LaStayo PC, Reich TE: When active muscles lengthen: Properties and consequences of eccentric contractions, *News Physiol Sci* 16:256–261, 2001.
17. Butler DL, Grood ES, Noyes FR, et al: Biomechanics of ligaments and tendons, *Exerc Sport Sci Rev* 6:125–181, 1978.
18. Sasaki K, Neptune RR: Muscle mechanical work and elastic energy utilization during walking and running near the preferred gait transition speed, *Gait Posture* 23(3):383–390, 2006.
19. Shan G, Westerhoff P: Full-body kinematic characteristics of the maximal instep soccer kick by male soccer players and parameters related to kick quality, *Sports Biomech* 4(1):59–72, 2005.
20. Isokawa M, Lees A: A biomechanical analysis of the instep kick motion in soccer. In Reilly T, Lees A, Davids K, Murphy WJ, editors: *Science and football*, London, 1988, E & FN Spon.
21. Lees A, Nolan L: The biomechanics of soccer: A review, *J Sports Sci* 16(3):211–234, 1998.
22. Bezodis N, Trewartha G, Wilson C, et al: Contributions of the non-kicking-side arm to rugby place-kicking technique, *Sports Biomech* 6(2):171–186, 2007.
23. Stecco A, Masiero S, Macchi V, et al: The pectoral fascia: Anatomical and histological study, *J Bodyw Mov Ther* 13(3): 255–261, 2009.
24. Plagenhof S: *Patterns of human motion: A cinematographic analysis*, Upper Saddle River, 1971, Prentice-Hall.
25. Cabri J, De Proft E, Dufour W, et al: The relation between muscular strength and kick performance. In Reilly T, Lees A, Davids K, Murphy WJ, editors: *Science and football*, London, 1988, E & FN Spon.
26. Vleeming A, Pool-Goudzwaard AL, Stoeckart R, et al: The posterior layer of the thoracolumbar fascia—its function in load transfer from spine to legs, *Spine* 20(7):753–758, 1995.
27. Bangsbo J, Peitersen B: *Soccer systems and strategies*, Champaign, IL, 2000, Human Kinetics.
28. Landry SC, McKean KA, Hubley-Kozey CL, et al: Neuromuscular and lower limb biomechanical differences exist between male and female elite adolescent soccer players during an unanticipated side-cut maneuver, *Am J Sports Med* 35(11):1888–1900, 2007.
29. Landry SC, McKean KA, Hubley-Kozey CL, et al: Neuromuscular and lower limb biomechanical differences exist between male and female elite adolescent soccer players during an unanticipated run and crosscut maneuver, *Am J Sports Med* 35(11):1901–1911, 2007.
30. Manning MR, Levy RS: Soccer, *Phys Med Rehabil Clin North Am* 17(3):677–695, 2006.
31. Nyland JA, Caborn DN, Shapiro R, et al: Crossover cutting during hamstring fatigue produces transverse plane knee control deficits, *J Athl Train* 34(2):137–143, 1999.
32. Schot P, Dart J, Schuh M: Biomechanical analysis of two change-of-direction maneuvers while running, *J Orthop Sports Phys Ther* 22(6):254–258, 1995.
33. Queen RM, Haynes BB, Hardaker WM, et al: Forefoot loading during 3 athletic tasks, *Am J Sports Med* 35(4):630–636, 2007.
34. Nyland JA, Shapiro R, Caborn DN, et al: The effect of quadriceps femoris, hamstring, and placebo eccentric fatigue on knee and ankle dynamics during crossover cutting, *J Orthop Sports Phys Ther* 25(3):171–184, 1997.
35. Farley CT, Blickhan R, Saito J, et al: Hopping frequency in humans: A test of how springs set stride frequency in bouncing gaits, *J Appl Physiol* 71(6):2127–2132, 1991.
36. Andrews JR, McLeod WD, Ward T, et al: The cutting mechanism, *Am J Sports Med* 5(3):111–121, 1977.
37. Smith N, Dyson R, Hale T, et al: Contributions of the inside and outside leg to maintenance of curvilinear motion on a natural turf surface, *Gait Posture* 24(4):453–458, 2006.
38. Besier TF, Lloyd DG, Cochrane JL, et al: External loading of the knee joint during running and cutting maneuvers, *Med Sci Sports Exerc* 33(7):1168–1175, 2001.
39. Gracovetsky S: Musculoskeletal function of the spine. In Winters JM, Woo SLY, editors: *Multiple muscle systems: Biomechanics and movement organization*, New York, 1990, Springer Verlag.
40. Sanders B, Nemeth WC: Hip and thigh injuries. In Zachazewski JE, Magee DJ, Quillen WS, editors: *Athletic injuries and rehabilitation*, Philadelphia, 1996, WB Saunders Company.
41. Grant JCB, Smith CG: The musculature. In Schaeffer JP, editor: *Morris human anatomy—A complete systematic treatise*, ed 11, New York, 1953, McGraw-Hill Book Company Inc.
42. McLean SG, Lipfert SW, van den Bogert AJ: Effect of gender and defensive opponent on the biomechanics of sidestep cutting, *Med Sci Sports Exerc* 36(6):1008–1016, 2004.
43. Shewchenko N, Withnall C, Keown M, et al: Heading in football. Part 1: Development of biomechanical methods to investigate head response, *Br J Sports Med* 39 Suppl 1:i10–25, 2005.
44. Mehnert MJ, Agesen T, Malanga GA: "Heading" and neck injuries in soccer: A review of biomechanics and potential long-term effects, *Pain Physician* 8(4):391–397, 2005.

45. Bauer JA, Thomas TS, Cauraugh JH, et al: Impact forces and neck muscle activity in heading by collegiate female soccer players, *J Sports Sci* 19(3):171–179, 2001.

46. Naunheim RS, Bayly PV, Standeven J, et al: Linear and angular head accelerations during heading of a soccer ball, *Med Sci Sports Exerc* 35(8):1406–1412, 2003.

47. Tysvaer AT: Head and neck injuries in soccer. Impact of minor trauma, *Sports Med* 14(3):200–213, 1992.

48. Brown IE, Loeb GE: A reductionist approach to creating and using neuromusculoskeletal models. In Winters J, Crago P, editors: *Biomechanics and neuro-control of posture and movement*, New York, 2000, Springer-Verlag.

49. Smith R, Ford KR, Myer GD, et al: Biomechanical and performance differences between female soccer athletes in National Collegiate Athletic Association Divisions I and III, *J Athl Train* 42(4):470–476, 2007.

50. Wisloff U, Castagna C, Helgerud J, et al: Strong correlation of maximal squat strength with sprint performance and vertical jump height in elite soccer players, *Br J Sports Med* 38(3):285–288, 2004.

51. Laffaye G, Bardy BG, Durey A: Leg stiffness and expertise in men jumping, *Med Sci Sports Exerc* 37(4):536–543, 2005.

52. Nagano A, Komura T, Yoshioka S, et al: Contribution of non-extensor muscles of the leg to maximal-effort countermovement jumping, *Biomed Eng Online* 4:52, 2005.

53. Vanezis A, Lees A: A biomechanical analysis of good and poor performers of the vertical jump, *Ergonomics* 48(11–14):1594–1603, 2005.

54. Nagano A, Komura T, Fukashiro S: Optimal coordination of maximal-effort horizontal and vertical jump motions—A computer simulation study, *Biomed Eng Online* 6:20, 2007.

55. Devita P, Skelly WA: Effect of landing stiffness on joint kinetics and energetics in the lower extremity, *Med Sci Sports Exerc* 24(1):108–115, 1992.

56. Yu B, Lin CF, Garrett WE: Lower extremity biomechanics during the landing of a stop-jump task, *Clin Biomech* (Bristol, Avon) 21(3):297–305, 2006.

57. Hewett TE, Myer GD, Ford KR, et al: Biomechanical measures of neuromuscular control and valgus loading of the knee predict anterior cruciate ligament injury risk in female athletes: A prospective study, *Am J Sports Med* 33(4):492–501, 2005.

58. Kernozek TW, Torry MR, H Van Hoof, et al: Gender differences in frontal and sagittal plane biomechanics during drop landings, *Med Sci Sports Exerc* 37(6):1003–1012; discussion 1013, 2005.

59. Giza E, Fuller C, Junge A, et al: Mechanisms of foot and ankle injuries in soccer, *Am J Sports Med* 31(4):550–554, 2003.

60. Lundin O, Hellstrom M, Nilsson I, et al: Back pain and radiological changes in the thoraco-lumbar spine of athletes. A long-term follow-up, *Scand J Med Sci Sports* 11(2):103–109, 2001.

61. Volpi P, Melegati G, Tornese D, et al: Muscle strains in soccer: A five-year survey of an Italian major league team, *Knee Surg Sports Traumatol Arthrosc* 12(5):482–485, 2004.

62. Kujala UM, Kettunen J, Paananen H, et al: Knee osteoarthritis in former runners, soccer players, weight lifters, and shooters, *Arthritis Rheum* 38(4):539–546, 1995.

63. Gabbe BJ, Bennell KL, Finch CF, et al: Predictors of hamstring injury at the elite level of Australian football, *Scand J Med Sci Sports* 16(1):7–13, 2006.

64. Major NM, Helms CA: Pelvic stress injuries: the relationship between osteitis pubis (symphysis pubis stress injury) and sacro-iliac abnormalities in athletes, *Skeletal Radiol* 26(12):711–717, 1997.

65. Jansen JA, Mens JM, Backx FJ, et al: Diagnostics in athletes with long-standing groin pain, *Scand J Med Sci Sports* 18(6):679–690, 2008.

66. Brown SH, McGill SM: How the inherent stiffness of the in vivo human trunk varies with changing magnitudes of muscular activation, *Clin Biomech* (Bristol, Avon) 23(1):15–22, 2008.

67. Howarth SJ, Beach TA, Callaghan JP: Abdominal muscles dominate contributions to vertebral joint stiffness during the push-up, *J Appl Biomech* 24(2):130–139, 2008.

68. Bonci CM: Assessment and evaluation of predisposing factors to anterior cruciate ligament injury, *J Athl Train* 34(2):155–164, 1999.

69. Olsen OE, Myklebust G, Engebretsen L, et al: Injury mechanisms for anterior cruciate ligament injuries in team handball: A systematic video analysis, *Am J Sports Med* 32(4):1002–1012, 2004.

70. Yu B, Garrett WE: Mechanisms of non-contact ACL injuries, *Br J Sports Med* 41 Suppl 1:i47–51, 2007.

71. Pollard CD, Sigward SM, Powers CM: Gender differences in hip joint kinematics and kinetics during side-step cutting maneuver, *Clin J Sport Med* 17(1):38–42, 2007.

72. Houck J, Yack HJ: Associations of knee angles, moments and function among subjects that are healthy and anterior cruciate ligament deficient (ACLD) during straight ahead and crossover cutting activities, *Gait Posture* 18(1):126–138, 2003.

73. Lloyd DG: Rationale for training programs to reduce anterior cruciate ligament injuries in Australian football, *J Orthop Sports Phys Ther* 31(11):645–654; discussion 661, 2001.

74. Ireland ML, Willson JD, Ballantyne BT, et al: Hip strength in females with and without patellofemoral pain, *J Orthop Sports Phys Ther* 33(11):671–676, 2003.

75. Cook JL, Khan KM: What is the most appropriate treatment for patellar tendinopathy? *Br J Sports Med* 35(5):291–294, 2001.

76. Junge A, Dvorak J: Soccer injuries: A review on incidence and prevention, *Sports Med* 34(13):929–938, 2004.

77. Ergen E, Ulkar B: Proprioception and ankle injuries in soccer, *Clin Sports Med* 27(1):195–217, 2008.

78. Barker HB, Beynnon BD, Renstrom PA: Ankle injury risk factors in sports, *Sports Med* 23(2):69–74, 1997.

79. Ibrahim A, Murrell GA, Knapman P: Adductor strain and hip range of movement in male professional soccer players, *J Orthop Surg* (Hong Kong) 15(1):46–49, 2007.

80. Neptune RR, Wright IC, van den Bogert AJ: Muscle coordination and function during cutting movements, *Med Sci Sports Exerc* 31(2):294–302, 1999.

81. Garrett WE, Jr.: Muscle strain injuries: Clinical and basic aspects, *Med Sci Sports Exerc* 22(4):436–443, 1990.

82. Mair SD, Seaber AV, Glisson RR, et al: The role of fatigue in susceptibility to acute muscle strain injury, *Am J Sports Med* 24(2):137–143, 1996.

83. Smodlaka VN: Medical aspects of heading the ball in soccer, *Phys Sportsmed* 12:127–131, 1984.

84. Aubry M, Cantu R, Dvorak J, et al: Summary and agreement statement of the 1st International Symposium on Concussion in Sport, Vienna 2001, *Clin J Sport Med* 12(1):6–11, 2002.

85. Delaney JS, Frankovich R: Head injuries and concussions in soccer, *Clin J Sport Med* 15(4):216–219; discussion 212–213, 2005.

86. Kirkendall DT, Jordan SE, Garrett WE: Heading and head injuries in soccer, *Sports Med* 31(5):369–386, 2001.

87. Kartal A, Yildiran I, Senkoylu A, et al: Soccer causes degenerative changes in the cervical spine, *Eur Spine J* 13(1):76–82, 2004.

88. Zmurko MG, Tannoury TY, Tannoury CA, et al: Cervical sprains, disc herniations, minor fractures, and other cervical injuries in the athlete, *Clin Sports Med* 22(3):513–521, 2003.

89. Alexander RM, Vernon A: The dimensions of knee and ankle muscles and the forces they exert, *J Hum Movement Stud* 1:115–123, 1975.

90. Zhang SN, Bates BT, Dufek JS: Contributions of lower extremity joints to energy dissipation during landings, *Med Sci Sports Exerc* 32(4):812–819, 2000.

91. Decker MJ, Torry MR, Wyland DJ, et al: Gender differences in lower extremity kinematics, kinetics and energy absorption during landing, *Clin Biomech* (Bristol, Avon) 18(7):662–669, 2003.

92. Fonseca ST, Vaz DV, Aquino CF, et al.: Muscular co-contraction during walking and landing from a jump: Comparison between genders and influence of activity level, *J Electromyogr Kinesiol* 16(3):273–280, 2006.

93. Ireland ML: Anterior cruciate ligament injury in female athletes: Epidemiology, *J Athl Train* 34(2):150–154, 1999.

94. Hewett TE, Paterno MV, Myer GD: Strategies for enhancing proprioception and neuromuscular control of the knee, *Clin Orthop Relat Res* (402):76–94, 2002.

95. Lephart SM, Ferris CM, Riemann BL, et al: Gender differences in strength and lower extremity kinematics during landing, *Clin Orthop Relat Res* (401):162–169, 2002.

96. Heinert BL, Kernozek TW, Greany JF, et al: Hip abductor weakness and lower extremity kinematics during running, *J Sport Rehabil* 17(3):243–256, 2008.

97. Joseph M, Tiberio D, Baird JL, et al: Knee valgus during drop jumps in National Collegiate Athletic Association Division I female athletes: The effect of a medial post, *Am J Sports Med* 36(2):285–289, 2008.

98. Ingber DE: Tensegrity I. Cell structure and hierarchical systems biology, *J Cell Sci* 116(Pt 7):1157–1173, 2003.

99. Ingber DE: Tensegrity II. How structural networks influence cellular information processing networks, *J Cell Sci* 116(Pt 8):1397–1408, 2003.

100. Levin SM: A different approach to the mechanics of the human pelvis: Tensegrity. In: Vleeming A, Mooney V, Dorman TA, et al, editors: *Movement, stability and low back pain*, New York, 1997, Churchill Livingstone.

101. Huijing PA: Muscular force transmission necessitates a multilevel integrative approach to the analysis of function of skeletal muscle, *Exerc Sport Sci Rev* 31(4):167–175, 2003.

102. Huijing PA, Jaspers RT: Adaptation of muscle size and myofascial force transmission: A review and some new experimental results, *Scand J Med Sci Sports* 15(6):349–380, 2005.

APPLIED BIOMECHANICS OF RUNNING

Scott T. Miller

Introduction

The evaluation and management of running injuries present a tremendous challenge to the health care provider. When evaluating the client with a running injury, the clinician must be aware of the numerous differences in anatomic alignment and mechanics that occur during running in comparison with walking. It is essential that the clinician look at both the proximal and distal ends of the kinetic chain. Furthermore, the activity of running causes an increase in ground reaction forces and pressures acting on the plantar surface of the foot. These variations in anatomic alignment, ground reaction force, and plantar pressures can significantly influence and possibly magnify abnormalities in lower extremity alignment resulting in overuse or repetitive trauma to body tissues. Successful treatment depends on the ability of the clinician to recognize and manage those biomechanical factors that can lead to excessive tissue stresses.

Numerous surveys have been conducted to determine the most common running injuries. One of the first epidemiological studies on running injuries was conducted by James and colleagues in 1978.[1] They reported that 30% of all injuries occurred in the knee, with another 13% of patients having shin splints, and an additional 7% diagnosed with plantar fasciitis. Lutter reported similar results in a survey of 171 runners, with 50% of all injuries occurring in the foot and 29% in the knee.[2] A subsequent survey of 540 runners conducted by Kerner and D'Amico in 1983 found that 28% had shin splints and 25% had knee pain.[3]

Further studies have looked at the causal factors and treatment of common overuse running injuries involving the pelvis, hip, and thigh.[4-9] Paluska identified muscle strains and tendinopathy as the most common cause of hip pain, which typically results from sudden acceleration and deceleration maneuvers, directional changes, or eccentric contraction.[4] Hamstring muscle strain injury is one of the most common injuries seen in running sports and strength deficits have been identified as the common cause, specifically the concentric action of the hip extensors and the eccentric contraction of the hamstrings.[5,6] Apophysitis and avulsion fractures may affect younger runners and produce localized pain at the muscle attachment sites, as well as disorders such as slipped capital femoral epiphysis and Legg-Perthes disease.[4,8] Iliotibial band syndrome (ITBS) was identified as a common cause of sharp or burning pain at either the lateral hip or knee. Bursitis was found to be prevalent, because of repetitive activity or acute trauma, at the trochanteric, ischial, or iliopectineal bursae. Paluska[4] also discusses less common running injuries such as snapping hip syndrome, acetabular labral tears, and sports hernias, and Clement and colleagues[9] looked at 71 athletes with exercise-induced stress injuries to the femur, in which 89.2% indicated running as the most common activity at the time of injury.

The results of these earlier epidemiological surveys and studies indicate that the most common problem affecting the runner is injury of the knee complex, followed by lower leg and foot injuries. In addition to the data published on the incidence of overuse injuries to the pelvis, hip, and thigh, it becomes obvious that the clinician must evaluate the entire lower extremity (proximal and distal) when treating the injured runner. To highlight those anatomical and mechanical factors that can result in overuse injuries during running, this chapter first describes the kinematic or movement patterns associated with the running cycle. Next, the electromyographic (EMG) activity of lower extremity

Note: This chapter includes content from previous contributions by Thomas G. McPoil, PhD, PT, ATC, and Mark W. Cornwall, PhD, PT, as it appeared in the predecessor of this book: Zachazewski JE, Magee DJ, Quillen WS, editors: *Athletic Injuries and Rehabilitation*, Philadelphia, 1996, WB Saunders.

musculature as well as the ground reaction force and plantar pressure patterns that occur during running are discussed. Finally, variations in lower extremity alignment that can cause abnormal movement patterns of the lower extremity during running and lead to overuse injuries are reviewed. In reviewing the pathomechanics of overuse injuries, the importance of orthosis (foot orthotic) intervention and footwear selection is discussed as a treatment option for the successful management of overuse running injuries. For more information on bone and soft tissue repetitive stress injuries, see Chapters 21 and 22 in *Pathology and Intervention in Musculoskeletal Rehabilitation*, the third volume in this series.

Biomechanics of Running

Running Kinematics

The Running Cycle

Running is basic to almost every athletic activity. The primary objective of running is to move the body rapidly over the ground toward a specific target or goal. This is accomplished by repeatedly propelling the body forward through the alternating movements of each lower extremity as the tibia advances over the foot.

The running cycle has been previously described by numerous authors,[10-14] who have broken the act of running into a series of strides or cycles. Each stride is further divided into a stance or *support phase* and a flight or *recovery phase*. Thus, a support and a flight phase for the same extremity constitutes one stride. The periods of support and flight have been further divided into six separate components, or subphases (Figure 13-1). The three components of the support phase are foot strike, midsupport, and takeoff. The three components of the recovery phase are follow-through, forward swing, and foot descent.

Running Cycle Phases and Subphases
• Support or stance phase
• Foot strike
• Midsupport
• Takeoff
• Recovery or flight phase
• Follow-through
• Forward swing
• Foot descent

The support phase begins with *foot strike*, which occurs when the foot initially contacts the ground and continues until the plantar surface of the foot is fully plantigrade to the support surface. Next, *midsupport* starts from the point at which the foot is in full contact with the ground and continues until the heel starts to leave the ground. Finally, *takeoff* begins when the heel starts to leave the ground and continues until the toes are completely free of the supporting surface. The primary purposes of the support phase are to (1) re-establish contact with the supporting surface; (2) provide a stable base of support for the advancing opposite limb in its flight phase; and (3) reverse the retarding influence of the early stance phase, as well as (4) accelerate the runner's mass forward to the next cycle.

The initial component of the flight or recovery phase is *follow-through*, which starts at the end of takeoff, when the trailing foot leaves the ground, and continues until that foot discontinues any further posterior or backward motion. Next is *forward swing*, which begins with the initiation of forward movement of the foot and stops when the foot reaches the most forward position. Finally, *foot descent* starts at the point of maximal hip flexion, with the foot at its most forward position. Foot descent continues until foot strike,

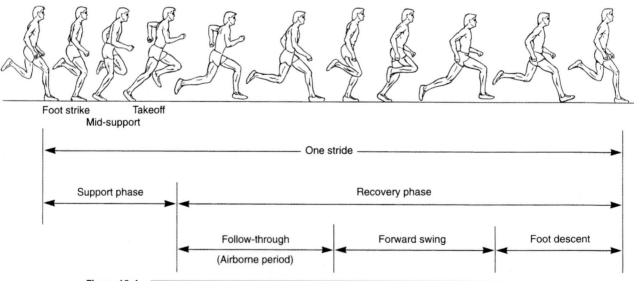

Figure 13-1
The running cycle and its various components.

at which time a new cycle is initiated. The primary purpose of the flight or recovery phase is to add momentum to the center of mass by means of the swinging limb.

During the flight or recovery phase, the airborne or non-support period occurs. This is the period in which neither foot is in contact with the ground, in contrast to walking where one foot is always in contact with the ground. Because there is a brief period where neither foot is in contact with the ground, when the swinging foot recontacts the ground at foot strike, the magnitude of ground reaction force is substantially increased in comparison with walking. Various studies have indicated that the ground reaction force during running may be as much as two to three times greater than seen when walking.[15,16] This increase in the magnitude of ground reaction force is an example of Newton's second law of motion, which states that force is equivalent to mass times acceleration. If an individual's mass remains constant and he or she accelerates his or her mass, then the ground reaction forces at foot strike will be increased. This is certainly the case when going from walking to running. Furthermore, a by-product of this change in ground reaction force is an increase in both the amplitude and the rate of foot pronation during the support phase of running. These factors, which are unique to running, can combine to result in an injury that would not necessarily occur during walking.

Joint Movements During Running

The amount of joint movement that occurs at the hip, knee, and ankle during the running cycle is different from that which occurs during the walking cycle. A summary of joint movements in the lower extremity during running is found in Table 13-1. As previously noted, overuse injuries to the knee region are commonly seen in runners. To illustrate one of the major differences between running and walking, the position of the knee joint when the foot makes contact with the ground is significantly different. During walking, the knee joint is either completely extended or flexed approximately 5° at the time of heel strike. In contrast, at the instant of foot strike while running, the knee joint is already in at least 20° of flexion. This flexed position of the knee is important to assist the runner in attenuating impact forces that are being applied through the lower extremity. Unfortunately, this greater degree of knee flexion also causes increased compressive forces between the patella and femur. This is an important factor, considering the extremely high incidence of knee injuries in runners, particularly to the patellofemoral joint. This flexed position of the knee joint at foot strike also implies that the flexibility of the soleus muscle is just as important as the flexibility of the gastrocnemius when assessing range of motion in runners. Furthermore, this supports the importance that the subtalar joint has on the rotatory component of the tibia and the subsequent alignment and tracking of the patella (e.g., foot pronation

Table 13-1

Typical Range-of-Motion Values for the Lower Extremities During Running

Running Phase	Joint	Motion
Foot strike* to midsupport†	Hip	45° to 20° flexion at midsupport
	Knee	20° to 40° flexion by midsupport
	Ankle	5° plantar flexion to 10° dorsiflexion
Midsupport to takeoff‡	Hip	20° flexion to 5° extension
	Knee	40° to 15° flexion
	Ankle	10° to 20° dorsiflexion
Follow-through§	Hip	5° to 20° hyperextension
	Knee	15° to 5° flexion
	Ankle	20° to 30° plantar flexion
Forward swing¶	Hip	5° to 20° hyperextension
	Knee	15° to 5° flexion
	Ankle	20° to 30° plantar flexion
Foot descent‖	Hip	65° to 40° flexion
	Knee	130° to 20° flexion
	Ankle	0° to 5° dorsiflexion to 5° plantar flexion

*Foot strike begins when the foot first touches the ground and continues until the foot is firmly fixed.
†Midsupport starts when the foot is fixed and continues until the heel leaves the ground.
‡Take-off begins when the heel starts to rise and continues until the toes leave the ground.
§Follow-through begins as the trailing foot leaves the ground and continues until the foot ceases rearward motion. It includes the airborne period.
¶Forward swing starts with forward motion of the foot and stops when the foot reaches its most forward position.
‖Foot descent starts after the recovering foot has reached its most forward position, reverses direction, and then terminates with foot strike.

influences tibial internal rotation and supination influences tibial external rotation).

To effectively manage overuse injuries associated with running, it is important to have an understanding of the changes in range of motion at the hip, knee, and ankle joints throughout the different phases of gait. From foot strike to midsupport, hip joint flexion decreases from 45° to 20°, whereas knee joint flexion increases from 20° to 40°. The position of the ankle (talocrural) joint at foot strike is 5° plantar flexed, with progression to 10° dorsiflexion by the midsupport phase.

From midsupport to takeoff, the hip joint moves from 20° of flexion to a 5° extended position, helping to propel the runner's mass forward in preparation for the next foot strike. The knee joint decreases the amount of its flexion by moving from a 40° to a 15° position. Finally, the talocrural joint moves from a 10° dorsiflexed position to a 20° dorsiflexed position.

During the flight or recovery phase, the swinging limb assists in increasing the forward momentum of the runner, thereby improving efficiency. During the follow-through phase of recovery, the hip joint, starting from a 5° position, moves into further hyperextension of 20° supporting the importance of proper gluteus maximus strength and neuromuscular recruitment. The knee joint starts in a 15° flexed position and moves to within 5° of full extension. The talocrural joint moves from a 20° plantar flexed position to approximately 30° of plantar flexion. As was previously mentioned, during forward swing, the hip joint moves into its most maximally flexed position. Thus, the hip joint moves a total of 85° from a 20° extended position into a 65° flexed position. At the same time, the knee joint undergoes 125° of motion, moving from a 5° flexed position to almost 130° of flexion. This amount of knee joint motion is significantly greater than that during walking, which is only 65° to 70°, and is related to the greater amount of momentum generated by the lower limbs during running. Finally, the talocrural joint will move from 30° of plantar flexion to a position of neutral (0°). Finally, during foot descent, the hip joint will move from a 65° flexed position to 40° of flexion, whereas the knee joint moves from 130° of flexion to 20° of flexion in preparation for foot strike. The talocrural joint will move from 0° to 5° of dorsiflexion to 5° of plantar flexion in preparation for foot strike.

Stride Length Characteristics

A major issue when evaluating a client's running cycle is the optimal stride length for that individual runner, as well as variations in stride length that can occur with different speeds of running. In general, stride length increases as the speed of the runner increases. However, there are variations depending on whether the person is running on level ground, uphill, downhill, or on a treadmill. Cavanagh[17] notes that when running uphill, stride length decreases, whereas during downhill running, stride length is typically increased. Landry and Zebas note that improved running performance is generally associated with increased stride rate, but not necessarily with increased stride length.[18] Cavanagh and Williams demonstrated that at a specific running speed, each individual has a stride length that appears to be optimal in terms of using the most efficient metabolic energy necessary for running.[19] Their study further showed that forcing an individual to lengthen or shorten his or her stride could possibly increase energy cost by 1% to 2%. This is an important point for clinicians to remember when they are considering advising runners to decrease or increase their stride length. In some cases, it might seem impractical to suggest that runners change their self-selected stride length because of the possibility of increasing energy costs, but certain injuries may dictate a recommendation to modify stride length. For example, the individual who is having heel pain might be advised to reduce or shorten

his or her stride length. By shortening his or her stride, the runner with a diagnosis of plantar fasciitis can enhance the possibility of contacting the ground with the midfoot rather than with the rearfoot, thereby decreasing impact stress to the heel tissues. This midfoot contact will also allow for a more efficient transition to the forefoot by not decelerating the body like runners who aggressively foot strike on their heels with every stride.

Stride Length

Each runner has an optimal stride length and stride length changes (increases) as the runner's speed increases and may vary if running surface is level, uphill, or downhill or on treadmill.

Finally, stride length can also vary depending on the comfort level of a runner on a treadmill. For example, if an individual is uncomfortable or inexperienced on a treadmill during a gait evaluation, that runner will often tend to shorten his or her stride length. In some cases, the runner will actually present as a forefoot striker versus the natural "outdoor running" stride. This forefoot strike position is inherently more rigid and provides increased stability for the runner. This is an important factor that the clinician needs to determine as it may influence any subsequent recommendations on footwear or the need for a foot orthosis.

Foot Placement During Running

Another factor that differs between walking and running is a variation in the base of gait, or the distance between the midpoints of the heels. Murray and colleagues reported that in walking, the typical base of gait for both men and women was approximately 2 to 4 inches (5 to 10 cm).[20,21] However, in running, this value approaches zero or can even fall on or cross over the line of progression (midline).[17] The reason for this decrease in base of gait during running is because of an increase in the functional limb varus of the entire support leg. *Functional limb varus* is defined as the angle between the bisection of the lower leg and the floor. An increase in functional limb varus results during the period of single-limb support when the pelvis is shifted laterally over the single supporting lower extremity. During running, the entire center of mass of the body must be placed over the single support foot. During walking, however, even though there is a period of single limb support, the movement of the body's center of mass is not usually displaced completely over the single support foot. Bogdan and colleagues were the first to report that there was an increase in functional limb varus during running.[22] In their report, Bogdan and colleagues noted that there was an approximate 10° increase in functional limb varus in running as compared with walking.

McPoil and Cornwall assessed five female and five male cross-country runners using two-dimensional videography to determine the change in functional limb varus during running in comparison with walking.[23] The average increase in functional limb varus when going from walking to running was approximately 5°. Figure 13-2 illustrates the increase in functional limb varus in a runner while walking and running.

Recognition of this increase in functional limb varus by the clinician is important when evaluating the runner, as a change in alignment can increase both valgus stress at the knee and pronation of the foot. The clinician should attempt to evaluate the change in the angle of the lower leg to the floor when evaluating runners with lower extremity injuries. This is accomplished by having the individual shift his or her weight laterally while standing with both feet in contact with the ground (Figure 13-3, *A*) and then assuming a position of single-limb support (see Figure 13-3, *B*). We have found that the average increase in single-limb varus when shifting from standing on both feet to standing on a single limb is approximately 5°.

The clinician must also consider the effect of functional limb varus on foot movement. If the amount of functional limb varus increases during running, a greater degree of foot pronation is required to allow the foot to remain plantigrade to the supporting surface. Thus, even if the runner does not excessively pronate during walking, the increase in functional limb varus during the running cycle will cause a greater degree of pronation during running. This increased amount of foot pronation may lead to excessive soft tissue stress in the lower extremity. The end result may lead to the development of any number of pathological conditions involving the foot, lower leg, knee, thigh, hip, or pelvis. Because of the greater amount of foot pronation required during running, clinicians should counsel their clients in the use of proper running footwear that matches their specific foot type and biomechanics. Generally speaking, that is a shoe that has adequate rearfoot stabilization. Running shoes with enhanced rearfoot stabilization features can assist in controlling excessive foot pronation, thereby reducing soft tissue stress while running. Further discussion on footwear recommendations and foot orthotic management may be found in a later section.

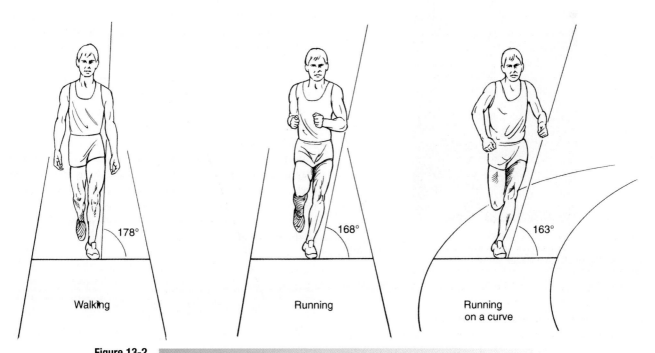

Figure 13-2
The effect of walking and running on functional limb varus.

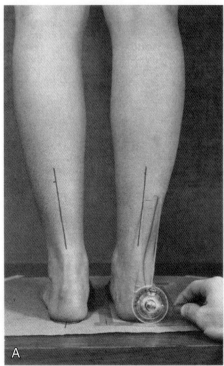

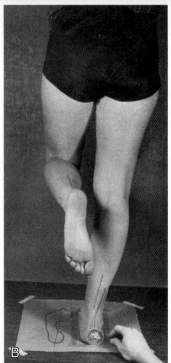

Figure 13-3

Static assessment of functional limb varus. Bilateral-limb stance assessment (**A**) and single-limb stance assessment (**B**).

in functional limb varus causes increased foot pronation to allow the plantar surface of the foot to fully contact the supporting surface. Several investigations have studied the pattern of rearfoot motion during the running cycle[24-26] and have reported that the period of pronation is longer during running than walking. Other studies have also shown that the magnitude of foot pronation is also greater during running than during walking. Another factor that affects rearfoot motion during running is the increase in ground reaction forces, which can cause greater acceleration of foot pronation.

Studies that have analyzed rearfoot motion have used both two- and three-dimensional analysis techniques.[25-33] In general, these studies have defined rearfoot motion as the movement of the calcaneus in relation to the lower one-third of the leg. Three-dimensional rearfoot analysis has been shown to be significantly different from two-dimensional analysis during running. These differences are caused primarily by projection errors onto the plane of a single camera placed behind the subject.[25,26] In 1990, Areblad and colleagues compared two-dimensional and three-dimensional measurement of rearfoot inversion and eversion during running and found that as the alignment angle between the foot and camera axis increased, so did the differences between the two measurement methods.[25] They advised the use of a three-dimensional model when studying motion between the foot and lower leg during running. Soutas-Little and colleagues also made a comparative study of two- and three-dimensional analysis of foot motion during running.[26] Although they found that projection errors did occur when measuring foot inversion and eversion with two-dimensional analysis techniques, the rearfoot motion determined from two-dimensional measurements approximated that determined from three-dimensional measurements during much of the running cycle support phase.

Although several authors have attempted to look not just at rearfoot and midfoot motion during walking, no studies to date have attempted to assess both rearfoot and midfoot motion during the running cycle. Based on published rearfoot motion studies, the clinician should expect the rate or speed of pronation, as well as the total magnitude of pronation, to increase during the running cycle. Thus, appropriate shoes and the use of foot orthoses must be considered if the clinician desires to control or modify the amount and speed of rearfoot pronation as part of the management program.

Rearfoot Motion During Running

Of major interest to the clinician treating a runner is the effect of the running cycle on the pattern of foot motion. The preceding section discussed the fact that the increase

Foot Pronation During Running

The rate or speed and amount of pronation increases during running.

Furthermore, the concept of resupination after the midsupport phase of the stance cycle is an important consideration in two-dimensional gait analysis. As previously stated, there are no published studies to date on this concept, but the assumption is that the delay in the derotation (or external rotation) of the tibia has the potential for increasing soft tissue stresses on proximal structures, including the ITB, patellofemoral joint, posterior tibialis, and plantar fascia. Clinically speaking, it appears that footwear changes alone are typically insufficient, and a foot orthosis with medial rearfoot to forefoot posting may be necessary.

Another foot evaluation concept to consider is the onset at which the majority of subtalar joint pronation occurs. Whether the majority of pronation occurs early in the stance phase (early pronation) or later in the stance phase (late pronation) may dictate the need for a footwear modification or the addition of a customized foot orthosis. *Early pronation* is the amount of movement measured between foot strike and midsupport of stance phase. *Late pronation* is the amount of movement measured after midsupport leading up to takeoff. One limitation in currently available running footwear is the ability to effectively control late pronation near takeoff. Sell and colleagues described a method of evaluating subtalar joint motion in a relaxed weight-bearing position using an inclinometer (Figure 13-4, *A*).[34] In this study, testers were able to determine the subtalar-joint-neutral position, the resting position, and the difference between these two measurements using an inclinometer for calcaneal position and navicular height. Intratester and intertester reliabilities (ICC 2, 1), standard errors of measurement, and 95% confidence intervals were determined. Intertester and intratester reliability for calcaneal position ranged from 0.68 to 0.91 for all measurements and navicular height ranged from 0.73 to 0.96 for all measurements. Thus, the testers concluded that these weight-bearing measurement techniques were reliable and acceptable for clinical and research purposes.[34] Although there are no studies to date to support evaluating pronation in a loaded (partial squat) position, this concept could potentially provide additional static weight-bearing information as it relates to the dynamic response of the subtalar joint in a more functional position during takeoff (Figure 13-4, *B, C*). To standardize the testing procedure for the measurement in the squatting position, the athlete is instructed to squat until 20° of ankle dorsiflexion is achieved. This amount of ankle joint dorsiflexion was selected based on the typical range of motion values for the ankle during take-off while running (see Table 13-1). Both evaluation techniques (resting and squatting position) can be used to compare the relative change in the degrees of pronation to determine whether the majority of total pronation is evident early (resting position) or late (squatting position). This will then assist in the clinical decision making process of whether a shoe change is sufficient or if the addition of a foot orthosis is recommended. A clinical example is illustrated in Table 13-2.

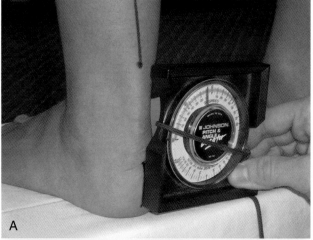

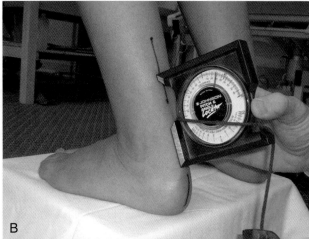

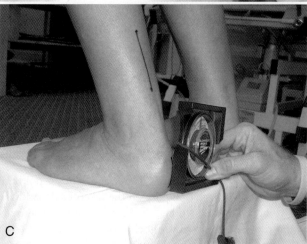

Figure 13-4

Static assessment of subtalar joint motion. Relaxed position described by Sell and colleagues[34] in a relaxed position (**A**) and modified technique in a partial squatting (20 degrees of ankle dorsiflexion) position (**B, C**). (Reprinted with permission from Agility Physical Therapy & Sports Performance, Portage, Michigan.)

Table 13-2

Clinical Example: Comparison of Early versus Late Pronation in Decision Making

Case Example	Subtalar Joint Motion		Clinical Observation	Clinical Recommendations
	*Relaxed Stance**	*Partial Squat†*		
"Early pronator"	10° of pronation	12° of pronation	Of the 12° measured, the majority of the motion was observed early in the static relaxed position consistent with the period between the foot-strike and midfoot support phase of running.	Try a footwear change to a stability shoe to control rearfoot motion.
"Late pronator"	5° of pronation	14° of pronation	Of the 14° measured, the majority of the motion was observed later in the static partial-squat position consistent with the period of take-off during running.	Consider the use of a foot orthosis with medial rear-foot to forefoot posting to assist with keeping the foot in a more neutral position, along with a stability or straight-last cushion shoe.

*Sell et al.[34] method for evaluating subtalar joint pronation using an inclinometer in a relaxed weight-bearing position.
†Modified technique using Sell et al.[34] method of evaluating subtalar joint using an inclinometer in a dorsiflexed (partial squatting) position of 20°.

Pronation During Stance Phase

- Early pronation—Pronation that takes place from heel strike to midsupport during stance phase
- Late pronation—Pronation that takes place from midsupport to take off during stance phase

---

Pelvic Drop During Running

The clinician should also consider the maximum amount of downward pelvic obliquity or pelvic drop (to the contralateral side) observed during the support phase of running using two- or three-dimensional videography (Figure 13-5). In the frontal plane, the pelvis reaches a point of maximum downward obliquity on the takeoff side, and the hip is in slight abduction.[35-37] Schache and colleagues[37] found the average downward pelvic obliquity to be 5.4° ± 2.6° at takeoff. There are several factors that can influence pelvic drop in runners. Research appears to indicate a relationship between hip abduction weakness and injury. Fredericson and colleagues studied 24 distance runners (14 females, 10 males) with ITBS to assess differences in hip abduction strength as compared with 30 controls (14 females, 16 males).[38] They found that runners with ITBS had weaker hip abductors on their injured side compared with the noninjured side and controls. Niemuth and colleagues also identified an association between hip

abductor muscle group strength imbalances and lower extremity overuse injuries in 30 recreational runners with a single-leg overuse injury.[7] Cichanowski and colleagues identified injured limb hip abductors to be significantly weaker ($p = 0.003$) than the noninjured side and the control group ($p = 0.010$) in 13 female collegiate athletes with unilateral patellofemoral pain syndrome.[39] Research indicates that deficits in hip abduction strength could, in theory, correspond to pelvic drop on the contralateral side. Therefore, the presence of pelvic drop or hip abduction weakness could be a significant evaluative finding. Gluteus medius activation pattern also needs to be considered in frontal plane pelvic drop. Previous research has identified changes in gluteus medius EMG latency and amplitude in subjects with chronic conditions.[40-43] Beckman and Buchaman reported a decreased latency of gluteus medius muscle recruitment in subjects with hypermobile ankles when compared with a healthy control group.[40] These findings indicate gluteus medius muscle dysfunction related to onset or amplitude, not necessarily strength. Thus, addressing gluteus medius strength alone may not be sufficient to return the runner to preinjury status. Finally, gluteus medius muscle fatigue could contribute to frontal plane pelvic drop. Research has shown that hip abduction peak torque and fatigability were not significantly correlated, suggesting that strength and fatigability should be evaluated separately.[44] Meanwhile, Eggen and colleagues[45] found that knee valgus movement increased following isometric hip abductor fatigue. Understanding that the stance phase of running is a closed kinetic chain

Figure 13-5

Two-dimensional rear view analysis of downward pelvic obliquity. **A,** Left stance leg measuring 3.5° of maximum downward pelvic obliquity. **B,** Right stance leg measuring 10.3° of maximum downward pelvic obliquity. (Reprinted with permission from Agility Physical Therapy & Sports Performance, Portage, Michigan.)

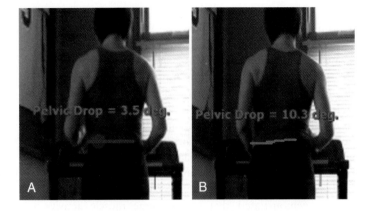

activity, the lower extremity might compensate for frontal plane pelvic drop via increased genu valgum. These studies point toward a relationship between frontal plane pelvic drop and gluteus medius muscle fatigue.

In summary, excessive pelvic drop can potentially increase the soft tissue stresses at the hip, knee, and foot through the functional limb varus angulations. This is commonly attributed to lack of functional strength, neuromuscular recruitment, or endurance of the gluteus medius on the stance leg.

Important Clinical Point

The stance phase of running is a closed kinetic chain activity, which requires proximal stability to control the absorption of contact forces. If proximal instability is present, the body may be put at a biomechanical disadvantage for absorbing contact forces, which, in turn, can place the runner at an increased risk for lower extremity injury. Hip abductor weakness, specifically gluteus medius, has been found to have an association with injury, and is therefore often addressed during the rehabilitation of runners.[7,38,46,47]

Muscle Activity During Running

In general, investigations of muscle action during running have demonstrated increased magnitudes of EMG activity in comparison with walking.[48] In addition, the duration of EMG activity has been found to be longer during the support phase of running in comparison with the stance phase of walking.[48] However, the reader should be aware that the majority of researchers have used surface electrodes, rather than indwelling or fine-wire electrodes, to study EMG activity because of the velocity and intensity of the motions required for running.

Hip Joint

Hip joint flexors have been shown to have a greater period of EMG activity during the forward swing of running than during the swing phase of walking. The rectus femoris muscle is active during the early support phase and then diminishes toward the end of the support phase.[49-51] The lack of appreciable activity during the late support and early swing phases shows that muscle contraction is not responsible for limiting hip extension. The hip joint extensors, specifically the gluteus maximus, demonstrate EMG activity early in the foot-descent period, and this activity continues through the first 40% of the support phase.[14] Whereas the hip joint abductors demonstrate similar EMG activity in both walking and running, the adductors show increased EMG activity throughout the entire support phase.

Knee Joint

At the time of foot strike, the quadriceps muscle is very active in preparation for the rapid loading that occurs at this time. The quadriceps muscle group reaches peak activity during the early support phase.[49-51] Quadriceps muscle activity during this period of the running cycle facilitates the shock attenuation process as the hip, knee, and ankle joints undergo flexion to create a shortening of the lower extremity. The hamstring muscles have been shown to be active from before foot strike until the hip joint completes its period of extension later in the support phase.[50,51] The activity reported before foot strike is responsible for slowing the rapidly extending knee in preparation for loading.[50-52] The later activity helps to propel the runner's body mass forward.

Ankle Joint

The tibialis anterior muscle is active at the instant of foot strike so as to provide a stable base of support by co-contracting with the triceps surae muscles.[50-52] The muscle's activity during the early portion of the support phase is much more variable than at other times in the running cycle. The tibialis anterior muscle has been shown to be both active as well as absent from foot strike until the foot is plantigrade to the ground.[50,51,53,54] The observed absence of tibialis anterior activity might be caused by the variation in foot placement at contact by different runners. A rearfoot striker may need the tibialis anterior muscle to contract eccentrically to allow smooth plantar flexion after foot strike. A midfoot striker, however, would already be in a plantigrade position and therefore would not need the muscular contraction for support.[55] Finally, during the swing phase of running, there is a small amount of activity to prevent the toes from contacting the ground.[50-52] As mentioned earlier, co-contraction of the triceps surae and tibialis anterior muscles has been reported at the instant of foot strike. Continued high activity during early support helps to control the eccentric dorsiflexion that is occurring at this time.[50,51,53,54] During the later portion of the support phase, activity in the triceps surae muscles continues and helps propel the runner's body into the air.[50,51] Mann and Hagy[53] demonstrated that triceps surae muscle activity ceased before toe-off when running at speeds of 2.7 m/s. If the running speed increased to 5.4 m/s, the muscle was found to be active all the way until toe-off.

In summary, the phasic activity of muscles during running is very similar to that during walking, except that the magnitude of activity is increased during running.[56] As the speed of running increases, so does the integrated EMG activity.[51,56-59] Ito and colleagues[60] showed that integrated EMG activity increased during the swing phase but remained constant during the contact phase as running speed increased from 3.7 to 9.3 m/s. To date, there has been very little research on what effect, if any, orthotic devices or footwear have on muscular activity in the foot and lower extremity during running.

Running Kinetics

Influence of Ground Reaction Forces

During walking, the vertical component of the ground reaction force acting through the lower extremity throughout the stance phase is approximately 125% of body weight. The vertical component of the ground reaction force is typically greater during the latter half of the walking cycle when the propulsion period is occurring. Several studies have shown that the vertical component of ground reaction force during distance running is usually 150% to 200% greater than during slow walking.[61,62] Cavanagh and LaFortune noted that the typical distance runner who runs approximately 130 km (80.8 miles) a week subjects each lower extremity to approximately 40,000 such impacts over a 7-day period.[61] Drez states that vertical force values of two to three times body weight can occur at foot strike during running and jogging.[63] He further notes that there are approximately 800 foot strikes on each foot in a 1-mile run.

Drez also notes that for this reason, adequate midsole cushioning in a running shoe is necessary to help the body attenuate or lessen the effect of these impact forces. Others are in agreement that a shock-absorbing orthoses (semiflexible) is generally indicated versus a rigid device in the management of lower extremity overuse injuries to assist in the attenuation of impact forces associated with running.[64-69]

To lessen or attenuate the increased ground reaction forces that occur during running, the body must provide a mechanism similar to the shock absorber used in a car. The shock absorber is designed to attenuate forces acting on the car by shortening to absorb energy. The shock absorber consists of two solid cylinders, one smaller in diameter than the other, and a spring that is positioned between the two cylinders. At rest, the spring is in its normal, or fully lengthened, position. When the car travels over a bump, the smaller cylinder moves within the larger diameter cylinder and the spring compresses, absorbing energy. Thus, the spring goes from a state of potential energy at rest to a state of kinetic energy when the car encounters a bump in the road (Figure 13-6, *A*).

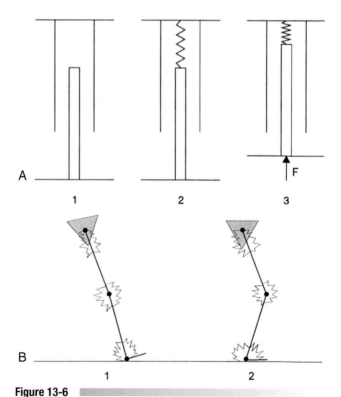

Figure 13-6

Shock attenuation model. **A,** Diagram *1* illustrates a simple plunger and cylinder system. Diagram *2* depicts the system with a shock attenuation spring added. Diagram *3* shows the system compressed under some compressive load *(F)*. **B,** Diagrams *1* and *2* illustrate the shock attenuation model applied to the lower extremities during walking. See text for further explanation.

To provide a system similar to the automobile shock absorber, the lower extremity must also permit shortening and absorption of energy. During the support phase of running, simultaneous movements of the hip, knee, and ankle joints cause a shortening of the lower extremity. To function as the spring in the automobile shock absorber, the muscles surrounding the hip, knee, and ankle articulations contract eccentrically during the early support phase.[70] Thus, shock attenuation during running is created by movements of the lower extremity articulations, which cause a shortening of the lower limb and energy absorption via contraction of the muscles surrounding the joints of the lower extremity (see Figure 13-6, *B*). Theoretically, the effectiveness of this anatomical shock absorber could be reduced by muscle fatigue or loss of flexibility, which may explain the occurrence of stress reactions or fractures in highly trained athletes during the middle or later part of their competitive season. It could also be hypothesized that a loss of shock absorption could occur if the runner has not undergone appropriate muscular endurance training for the distance he or she intends to run.

Another factor that affects the magnitude of the vertical force component of the ground reaction force is variation in running speed. The results of a study done by Hamill and colleagues indicate that although the events in ground reaction force curves occurred at the same relative time, an increase in magnitude of both vertical force and relative impulses at greater speeds was observed.[71] Relative impulse was defined as the amount of time the force was applied over the areas of the foot.

Cavanagh and LaFortune, in studying ground reaction forces that occurred during distance running, observed that runners could be classified by the first point of ground contact made by their foot.[61] Based on the part of the shoe contacting the ground at foot strike, those individuals who made contact with the posterior one-third of the shoe were classified as rearfoot strikers, whereas those runners whose initial contact with the ground was in the middle one-third of the shoe were classified as midfoot strikers. The plots of the center of pressure and three-dimensional wire diagrams illustrate the differences observed in the patterns of initial contact between rearfoot and midfoot strikers (Figures 13-7 and 13-8). Rearfoot strikers demonstrate a double-peak vertical force component of the ground reaction force, whereas midfoot strikers have a single-peak vertical force component (Figure 13-9). Nigg noted that the large initial spike in the vertical force component pattern of the rearfoot striker occurred just as the heel was making contact with the ground and referred to this as the *impact peak*.[72] Nigg also found that in most rearfoot runners, this peak occurred at approximately 20 ms after the initiation of ground contact. Cavanagh has stated that if any muscular activity is instituted to help reduce impact forces, it must be initiated before foot strike in rearfoot strikers, because the impact peak occurs very quickly.[17]

Runner Classification by Foot Strike

- Rearfoot strikers—posterior ⅓ of shoe strikes ground first
- Midfoot strikers—middle ⅓ of shoe strikes ground first
- Forefoot strikers—anterior ⅓ of shoe strikes ground first

Heil has reported that runners who make initial contact with the forefoot experienced a reduced ground reaction force when compared with rearfoot strikers.[73] Heil stated that this was because the calf muscles act as a shock-absorbing system to help reduce impact loads. However, forefoot contact also causes a significant increase in the tensile loading of the Achilles tendon. Becker has noted that midfoot strikers keep the knee and hip in a slight degree of flexion and thus absorb the shock

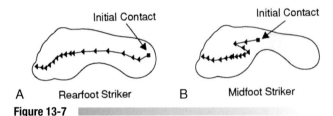

Figure 13-7
Center of pressure paths for a rearfoot and midfoot striker.

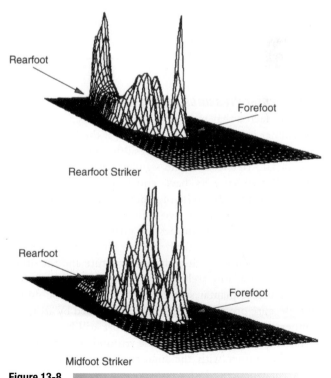

Figure 13-8
Plantar pressure plot for a rearfoot and midfoot striker.

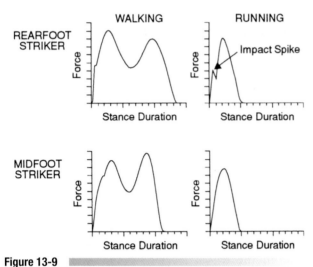

Figure 13-9

Typical vertical ground reaction force patterns for rearfoot and midfoot strikers during walking and running.

of contact in a more elastic fashion.[74] McMahon and colleagues reported that running with the knees bent reduced the magnitude of vertical ground reaction forces and diminished the transmission of mechanical shock through the lower extremity and foot.[75] They also reported, however, that this style of running produced an increased force in the muscles of the leg and could require as much as a 50% increase in the rate of oxygen consumption. They referred to this increased oxygen requirement as the "cost of cushioning." Becker has also reported that in both heel and forefoot strikers, impact forces were decreased by the degree of pronation, which he noted is principally controlled by the anterior and posterior tibial muscles.[74]

Foot Plantar Pressures During Running

Another factor that must be considered when evaluating the runner is how the plantar surface of the foot contacts the supporting surface and the resulting plantar pressures that occur. To illustrate the significance of plantar pressures, if two runners have equal body weight, equal height, and the same style of running, including identical stride length, then these two runners theoretically would generate similar magnitudes of ground reaction force when running at identical speeds. However, if one of these runners has a high-arch foot structure and the other runner has a low-arch foot structure, the pressures applied to the plantar surface of their feet will be different. Because pressure is equal to force divided by area, the runner with the low-arch foot structure will have greater surface area in contact with the ground in comparison with the runner with the high-arch foot structure and thus will experience lower pressures on the plantar surface of the foot.

Nachbauer and Nigg evaluated the effect of arch height of the foot on ground reaction forces in running.[76] They found that impact forces were not significantly different for low-arch and high-arch individuals, even though a link has been suggested between running injuries and type of foot arch. However, it is important to realize that even though ground reaction forces may not be significantly different, the pressures acting through the plantar surface of the foot may be different. The runner with a more mobile or pronatory foot type that allows increased plantar surface area of the foot to make contact with the ground will experience less overall pressure than the person with a less mobile, or supinatory, foot type, as he or she has decreased plantar surface area in contact with the ground. Figure 13-10 shows the area in contact with the ground for two different individuals, a person with a low arch and a person with a high arch. As can be seen in the runner with the high-arch foot structure, only the supporting surface of the heel and forefoot make contact. Unlike the person with the low-arch foot structure, there is no midfoot contact with the ground, and thus plantar surface area is reduced, causing increased plantar pressures under the foot.

This has important implications for the clinician when prescribing footwear. The individual with a pes cavus, or high-arch, foot structure may be using a running shoe that has good midsole cushioning properties, but he or she will still have reduced plantar surface area contacting the shoe. In the management of these individuals, some type of foot orthosis or accommodative arch support should be placed within the shoe to increase the total area of contact within the running shoe and reduce plantar pressures.

Summary

To effectively evaluate and treat the runner, not only must the pattern of joint motion during the running cycle be considered, but the effect of muscle activity, ground reaction forces, and plantar pressures acting on the lower extremity and foot must also be taken into account. These kinematic and kinetic factors, as well as their effect on the lower extremity during running, have been reviewed.

Clinical Point

If abnormalities exist in lower extremity alignment, the changes in the pattern of joint motion, muscle activity, ground reaction forces, and plantar pressures associated with running can exacerbate the already increased level of stress on soft tissues as well as dynamic muscle stabilizers and contribute to the development of overuse injuries.

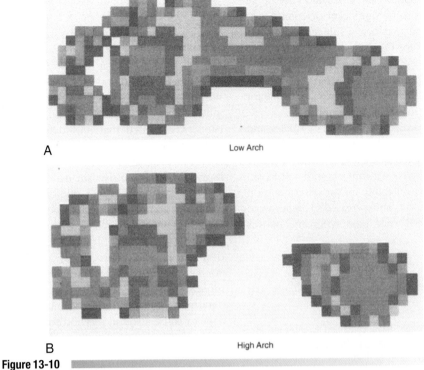

A   Low Arch

B   High Arch

Figure 13-10
Surface area in a high-arch and a low-arch individual.

Pathomechanics

Numerous abnormalities in the anatomical alignment of the lower extremity and foot, as well as limitations in soft tissue mobility, have been identified as causal factors in lower extremity overuse running injuries. These various abnormalities are discussed relative to lower extremity malalignment and foot pronation.

Lower Extremity Malalignment

Root and colleagues identified several structural abnormalities in the lower extremity as factors extrinsic to the foot that were compensated for by abnormal foot pronation.[77] These extrinsic factors included tibial varus, internal and external tibial or malleolar torsion, internal and external femoral torsion, as well as leg-length discrepancies. Root and colleagues also noted that limitations in the normal degree of flexibility of the calf, hamstring, and iliopsoas muscles could cause or accentuate abnormal lower extremity alignment during activity. Excessive pronation in the foot has also been identified as one of the factors that can cause excessive stress at the patellofemoral joint. Excessive pronation of the foot can cause the lower leg to be maintained in a prolonged period of internal rotation. This prolonged period of lower leg internal rotation can alter the normal patellar tracking pattern during both walking and running.

Structural Abnormalities Leading to Abnormal Foot Pronation[75]

- Coxa vara/valga
- Internal (medial) femoral torsion
- External (lateral) femoral torsion
- Tibial varum
- Internal (medial) tibial torsion
- External (lateral) tibial torsion
- Leg length discrepancies
- Muscle inflexibility (especially calf, hamstrings and iliopsoas)
- Rearfoot (calcaneal) varus
- Forefoot varus
- Forefoot valgus
- Morton toe

Numerous authors have reported a strong link between knee pain and excessive subtalar joint pronation.[73,78-80] Heil has indicated that various extrinsic factors, including genu varum, genu valgum, coxa vara, coxa valga, and abnormal internal and external rotations of the tibia and the femur, can lead to excessive pronation because of a change in the normal foot and lower extremity alignment.[81]

In a study that examined the causal factors associated with patellofemoral pain in runners, Messier and colleagues noted that the only significant discriminatory anthropometric variable that was identified from numerous measurements, including isokinetic assessments, was an increased

Q angle.[82] Arch index, leg length, and ankle and knee range of motion were not found to be significant discriminators. Moss and colleagues found that heavy subjects and those with a larger static quadriceps Q angle were more likely to have patellofemoral stress syndrome.[83] Because an activity such as running involves numerous repetitions of knee extension, Moss and colleagues[83] noted that it was possible for a small variation in the Q angle to cause symptoms.

A more recent study, however, conducted by Caylor and colleagues found no significant difference in the Q angle between 52 patients with anterior knee pain syndrome and a control group of 50 subjects without anterior knee pain syndrome.[84] The intratester reliability for the determination of the Q angle was quite good, but increased Q angles were not responsible for anterior knee pain syndrome in this group of patients.

Important Clinical Point: Managing Knee Pain in Runners

As running and multisport events have continued to increase in popularity, so has the incidence of knee pain. This common overuse injury manifests itself in various forms or diagnoses, including patellar tendinitis, patellofemoral pain syndrome, or iliotibial band (ITB) friction syndrome. The causal factors for these types of injuries have been discussed in the literature with a common consensus that there may be a problem proximally or a problem distally. However, it is astounding how many clinicians still continue to treat the symptoms at the knee. It is critical in the successful management of running athletes to address the hip and the ankle and foot, as well as the knee. Some key areas to evaluate:

Hip
- Gluteus medius and hip lateral rotator strength
- Recruitment pattern for both gluteus maximus and medius
- Flexibility of iliopsoas (can inhibit gluteus maximus function consistent with lower crossed syndrome described by Janda[85,86])
- Length flexibility and fascial mobility of the ITB

Ankle and Foot
- Talocrural (ankle) joint mobility, especially dorsal glide
- The ability to "lock out" the oblique midtarsal joint with supination
- Mobility assessment for subtalar joint, midtarsal joint and first ray
- Appropriate shoe recommendations consistent with the runner's foot type
- Foot orthosis recommendations considering both rearfoot and forefoot

There is sufficient research to support the need for the continued drive toward evidence-based practice. Furthermore, the research completed provides a foundation and a stimulus for further research to answer the "burning questions" that still exist. The chance of successfully managing a runner with ITB friction syndrome by simply performing ultrasound over the bursa, instructing him or her in seated isometric vastus medialis oblique (VMO) quadriceps sets, and recommending a motion-control shoe (without looking at the athlete's feet) as a treatment plan is not only unlikely, it is a sign of poor treatment. One should think "function" and look at the "big picture."

Foot Pronation

Abnormal foot pronation has been identified as a major cause of foot, lower leg, knee, thigh, and hip running injuries, including plantar fasciitis, ITB friction syndrome, patellofemoral pain and medial shin pain ("shin splints" or *medial tibial stress syndrome*). Schuster, in describing the influence of the environment on the foot of long distance runners, indicated that foot deformities, such as rearfoot (calcaneal) varus, tibial varus, and forefoot varus, were a common cause of extreme structural imbalance within the foot, causing excessive pronation.[87] Excessive pronation of both the rearfoot and midfoot during running causes increased stress on the soft tissues surrounding the various joints of the foot, including the capsule, ligaments, and plantar aponeurosis. More importantly, there can be an over-reliance on lower leg and foot musculature in an attempt to control excessive foot mobility and provide a more stable foot structure. Thus, a thorough evaluation to determine whether these various foot abnormalities exist appears to be a sound method to predict which individuals might develop lower quarter injuries.

In a study that attempted to determine the causal factors associated with selected running injuries, Messier and Pittala collected anthropometric and motion data on runners affected with ITB friction syndrome, shin splints, or plantar fasciitis.[88] The groups studied consisted of a control group of 19 healthy subjects, a shin splint group (17 subjects), a plantar fasciitis group (15 subjects), and an ITB group (13 subjects). All of the runners underwent an evaluation that included foot prints, determination of plantar flexion and dorsiflexion range of motion, hamstring and lower leg flexibility testing, and assessment of Q angle and leg length. The authors also determined total rearfoot motion and time from maximal pronation to maximal supination by analyzing film records. The results of their study indicated that the only significant discriminator between the plantar fasciitis group and the control group was that the fasciitis group had greater plantar flexion range of motion. No other significant differences could be validated statistically. They did note, however, that the ITB friction syndrome group had a significantly higher arch foot structure than the control group, and the shin splint and ITB friction groups had less ankle dorsiflexion range of motion than the control group. The results of this study seem to question the accepted theory that structural deformities in the foot cause a deviation in alignment leading to the development of foot problems.

Ross and Schuster conducted a similar study in which they attempted to predict injuries in distance runners.[89] They evaluated 63 runners, measuring inversion and eversion of the subtalar joint, the position of the subtalar joint (to determine whether a varus or valgus deformity of the hindfoot existed), forefoot varus or valgus, and the amount of available dorsiflexion at the ankle with the knee joint both flexed and extended. They also performed two weight-bearing measurements: resting calcaneal stance position and neutral calcaneal stance position. Based on their results and considering the cause of lower extremity injuries studied, the authors concluded that there was not one single "cause-and-effect" factor responsible for running injuries.

Warren and Jones attempted to determine those anatomic factors that could be used to predict plantar fasciitis in long distance runners.[90] Forty-two runners were classified as (1) having no history of plantar fasciitis, (2) currently having plantar fasciitis, or (3) having recovered from plantar fasciitis. Various measurements were taken on each subject, including leg length, degree of pronation from neutral, arch height of the foot, and dorsiflexion and plantar flexion of the ankle. The results of the study were interesting in that the control group who had never had a history of plantar fasciitis actually had a greater degree of pronation than both of the other two groups. These authors noted that perhaps plantar fasciitis was caused by excessive overuse stress rather than faulty biomechanics. Little has been written regarding the runner with a high-arch and hypomobile foot structure. Schuster noted that runners with high-arch foot structure had an extremely rigid foot, and their joint ranges of motion were usually less than average.[87] He further noted, as has been previously discussed, that they had a much smaller weight-bearing pattern and difficulty in attenuating impact forces. Thus, the runner with limited rearfoot motion could be classified as having decreased shock attenuation and increased plantar pressures, especially in the forefoot, secondary to limited midfoot loading.

Use of the Load-Deformation Curve to Explain Running Injuries

Although numerous factors have been outlined as possible causes of overuse injuries in the lower extremity and foot, it does not appear that any study to date has been able to accurately predict which individuals will develop lower extremity overuse injuries. Furthermore, the literature strongly suggests that it is extremely difficult to pinpoint the actual cause of an overuse injury. Often individuals who exhibit the most profound lower extremity and foot malalignments are asymptomatic, whereas those individuals with an "ideal" runner's alignment—including symmetric hip rotation, no evidence of external or internal malleolar torsion, and a "normal" foot structure with minimal pronation—can be highly susceptible to overuse injuries. Because of these problems, we believe that a tissue stress model that is based on the load-deformation curve can assist the clinician in understanding the effect of lower extremity and foot malalignments on the development of overuse injuries in runners.

Each individual runner has his or her own level of tolerance for the amount of tissue stress that can be withstood during the activity of running. The importance of this individual level of tissue stress tolerance can be illustrated using the load-deformation curve (Figure 13-11). The load-deformation curve consists of two regions or zones: an elastic region and a plastic region.[91] A load-deformation curve is commonly used by material engineers to explain the degree of deformation that occurs when a load is applied to an object. The region or area separating the elastic and plastic regions is termed the *microfailure zone*. Although deformation occurs when the load is applied, the object being tested can completely recover from the deformation, provided the deformation does not exceed the microfailure zone. If deformation of the object exceeds the microfailure zone and enters the plastic region, then permanent, nonrecoverable deformation will occur.

The deforming force may be from a single load or the summation of several loadings. To illustrate the effect of loads applied to soft tissue during running, using the

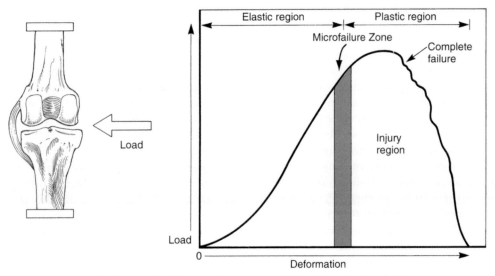

Figure 13-11
Schematic of the load-deformation principle of soft tissue.

load-deformation curve, the elastic region represents the normal "give and take" of soft tissues as the foot is loaded and unloaded during the running cycle. As long as the runner maintains the level of tissue stress within this elastic region, the amount of soft tissue stress will most likely be tolerated and an overuse injury will be avoided.

The various factors that contribute to excessive tissue stress include the amount of stress applied to the soft tissues, the amount of extrinsic and intrinsic muscle activity required to enhance foot stability, and the degree of abnormal lower extremity and foot alignment. If these factors can be balanced so that the tissues never go beyond the elastic range and enter the microfailure zone, then injury will be avoided. If runners increase their running speed or the training distance is accelerated too quickly, soft tissues may enter the microfailure zone, resulting in an overuse stress injury. If the runner does not rest the injured tissues when microtrauma is present, the stressed tissues can eventually be taken beyond the microfailure zone and into the plastic range, with the result being a breakdown of soft tissues, muscle guarding, and pain. The load-deformation curve also provides a model to explain the effectiveness of footwear and foot orthoses in precluding excessive tissue stress by restricting excessive motion and preventing soft tissues from entering the microfailure zone.

Footwear Considerations in the Management of Running Injuries

It is evident that the cause of overuse running injuries is a multifactorial problem and successful management often relies on sound decision-making by the clinician. One key factor is the consideration of matching the appropriate footwear to an individual's foot classification, including alignment, mobility and biomechanical factors related to running. Clinically, footwear recommendations are a necessary complement to the various treatment approaches for running injuries, including therapeutic exercise for lower quarter imbalances, foot orthosis intervention, or the judicious use of modalities.

To provide appropriate recommendations on running footwear, having a basic understanding of how the shoe is constructed is important. The key features of a running shoe include the outsole, midsole, and upper. The outsole is the bottom of the shoe and is generally made from carbon or blown rubber. The midsole is the shock-absorbing layer between the outsole and the "upper" part of the shoe. This midsole is the most important part of a running shoe, as the construction and materials used will impact the levels of both cushioning and stability in the shoe. The amount of cushioning in the shoe is generally proportionate to the shoe's heel height. The two types of cushioning generally found in running shoes are ethylene vinyl acetate (EVA) and polyurethane (PU). Increased stability in a shoe is accomplished through the incorporation of a heavier-density

EVA or PU in combination with the existing cushioning materials. This type of construction is referred to as a *dual density midsole*. Finally, the "upper" is the soft body of the shoe that encloses the foot and is usually made of a combination of materials, from lightweight, durable synthetic mesh to heavier materials such as leather. The materials and construction of the upper provide stability, comfort, and a snug fit. Features to consider in the upper include the *last* (the shape of the shoe), the *toe box* (the front of the shoe), the *heel counter* (the part holding the heel, which can vary in stiffness for increased stability), and the *Achilles notch* (a groove in the heel piece to protect the tendon from irritation). Running footwear can be divided into four primary categories related to their overall cushioning and stability properties (Box 13-1). The shoe categories are (1) light cushion, (2) straight last cushion, (3) stability, and (4) motion control.

A *light cushion* running shoe (Figure 13-12, *A*) is best for a true supinatory foot or for someone who is an underpronator. This foot type is generally fairly rigid in nature with pes cavus presentation, and thus does not absorb shock during the initial contact phase of running. A light cushion running shoe is not a very substantial shoe and is constructed of single-density material for the midsole with minimal arch support. This shoe is extremely flexible through the arch to allow the foot as much motion as possible. In general, a light cushion shoe will break down rather quickly (typically in less than 400 miles [643 km]).

A *straight last cushion* running shoe (see Figure 13-12, *B*) is a newer category shoe, described by one author as a hybrid shoe that is a transition shoe between a light cushion shoe and a stability shoe (described in the following paragraph). This type of shoe is best for someone who is an underpronator, but still presents with some forefoot or rearfoot alignment concerns (e.g., forefoot varus or calcaneal varus). This foot type is generally somewhat rigid, but more accurately does not have the necessary motion available at the subtalar joint to accommodate for the positional faults (e.g., uncompensated forefoot varus). This unique shoe still employs the single-density cushioning material for the midsole, while providing more inherent stability based on the geometry of the shoe (straight last construction) versus implementing a dual-density midsole or stability system commonly seen in the stability shoes. Clinically, this shoe provides a more stable platform for the foot and foot orthosis to function without the extrinsic influence of the shoe, which may or may not be desirable.

A *stability* running shoe (see Figure 13-12, *C*) is best for someone who is a mild to moderate overpronator. This type of shoe generally has enough mobility in the subtalar joint to assist in shock absorption during stance phase. This shoe encompasses some additional stability through the midsole with some type of added stability feature like a dual density material found in most brands or the Graphite Rollbar system found exclusively in the New Balance shoes. A stability

Box 13-1 Classifications and Characteristics of Running Shoe Types

Light Cushion Shoe
- Indication: Supinatory foot
- Traditional cushion shoe typically with more of a curved last shape
- Central or peripheral slip last construction
- Midsole materials (EVA or PU) depending on body weight, but usually lean to lighter-weight EVA
- Single-density midsole
- Very flexible through the midfoot
- Midsole cushioning units (rearfoot and forefoot)

Straight Last Cushion Shoe
- Indication: Neutral to supinatory foot that is unstable
- Newer *transition* shoe that bridges the gap between a traditional cushion and stability mostly by the geometry of the shoe
- Straight last shape
- Midsole materials (EVA or PU) depending on body weight, but usually lean to lighter-weight EVA
- Single-density midsole
- Midsole cushioning units (rearfoot and forefoot)
- May use stability pillars (e.g., Brooks Dyad series) with less flexibility noted through the midfoot as compared with a traditional cushion shoe
- Firmer heel counter

Stability Shoe
- Indications: Neutral to mild overpronator
- Semicurved last shape
- Combination or peripheral last construction
- Midsole materials (EVA or PU) depending on body weight
- Firmness of medial midsole or stabilization device depending of range on stability shoe. Lower end stability shoes may not have a stabilization device.
- Some flexibility through the midfoot and firm heel counter

Motion Control Shoe
- Indications: Moderate-to-severe overpronator
- Straighter last shape
- Board or combination last construction*
- Midsole materials (EVA or PU) depending on body weight
- Firmer medial midsole or stabilization device
- Reinforced and extended heel counter
- Will sometimes use higher medial side versus lateral side (wedge) for increased early motion control

Common Last Types

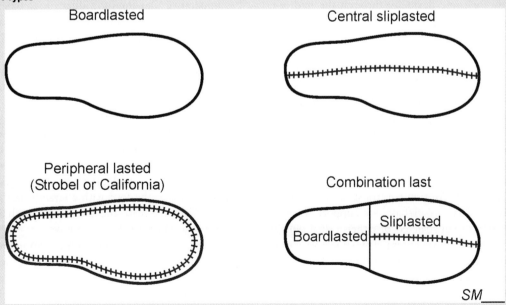

Boardlasted

Central sliplasted

Peripheral lasted
(Strobel or California)

Combination last

Boardlasted   Sliplasted

SM___

Data from Gazelle Sports, Grand Rapids, Michigan and Agility Physical Therapy and Sports Performance, Portage, Michigan.
EVA, Ethylene vinyl acetate; PU, polyurethane.
*Board last construction primarily used with older running shoes and basketball shoes. Combination last primarily used now in newer running shoes.

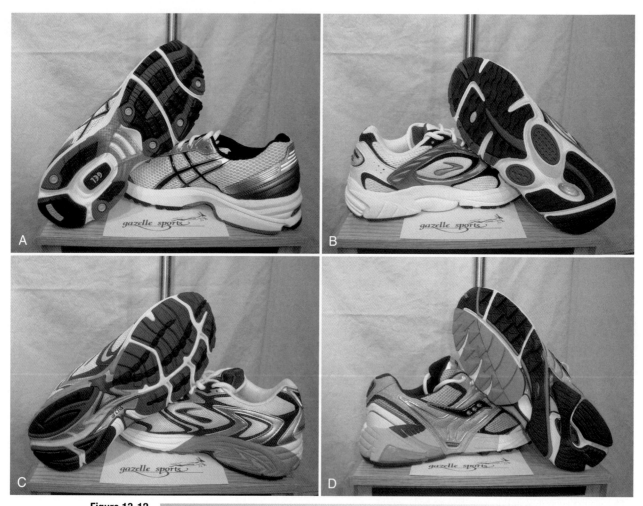

Figure 13-12
Running shoe categories. **A,** Light cushion. **B,** Straight last cushion. **C,** Stability. **D,** Motion control.
(Reprinted with permission from Gazelle Sports, Grand Rapids, Michigan.)

shoe does allow for some flexibility through the midfoot, but has enough rigidity to provide pronation control.

Finally, a *motion control* shoe (see Figure 13-12, *D*) is designed for the moderate-to-severe overpronator. This foot type generally has the same forefoot and rearfoot alignment concerns, but by stark contrast to the more rigid foot, has an excessive amount of subtalar or midtarsal joint motion available. A foot type that can compensate for a forefoot or calcaneal varus can present dynamically as an overpronator (at midsupport) or as a late pronator (at takeoff). This causes the foot to roll inward, placing excessive stress on soft tissue structures proximal to the foot, including lower leg, knee, hip, and back. Motion control shoes are straight-lasted and have a very broad base for support. Motion control shoes are also constructed of either a dual density midsole or a Graphite Rollbar system. This shoe is very rigid through the midsole, much more so than the stability shoe, to provide maximum pronation control.

When making footwear recommendations, there are several factors to consider that can influence the type of shoe that is ideal for each individual runner. Most important,

it is imperative that the individual's foot type matches the shoe by evaluating whether the runner has a flexible or rigid foot type. Next, consider whether the runner has an overall neutral, varus, or valgus alignment. In the case in which a runner has a forefoot varus combined with a rigid foot type, this is clinically a challenging foot type to manage. Furthermore, overstabilizing someone's foot can be just as detrimental to the soft tissue structures of the lower extremity as understabilizing the foot. Finally, consideration needs to be made with an individual who has significantly different foot types (e.g., left foot is supinatory foot; right foot is an overpronator). In this example, the best clinical decision may be to understabilize the foot with a straight-last cushion shoe and selectively increase the stability through a customized foot orthosis (Box 13-2).

Other factors to take into consideration are the type of foot striker (e.g., midfoot versus forefoot); the distance the runner is training for (e.g., 5 K versus marathon); body weight (e.g., heavier versus lighter runner); selecting a training shoe versus a racing shoe; the width of the runner's foot (e.g., selecting the shoe manufacturer that has a wider

Box 13-2 Clinically Important Point: Possible Footwear Recommendations Based on Foot Type

Case Example		Shoe Recommendation	Orthosis Recommendation
#1	Rigid foot type (underpronator)	Straight last cushion	Semiflexible
	Forefoot varus (uncompensated)		Full-length device
			Medial posting into the forefoot only leaving the rearfoot in neutral

Clinical Rationale: This individual does not have enough motion to compensate for the forefoot deformity, so overstabilization of the rearfoot (subtalar joint) is undesirable. By placing this individual in a straight last cushion shoe, a good stable foundation allows the orthosis to function. By only posting the forefoot, the alignment concern will be addressed with less influence on the rearfoot.

#2	Left foot = underpronator	Straight last cushion	Semiflexible
	Right foot = overpronator		Full-length device
	Forefoot varus bilaterally		L = Medial posting into the forefoot only
			R = Medial posting from the rearfoot to the forefoot

Clinical Rationale: This individual does not have enough motion to compensate for his or her forefoot deformity only on the left, but does have the necessary available range of motion on the right in the subtalar joint. Placing the individual in a straight last cushion shoe will allow a good stable foundation for the orthosis to function while not overstabilizing the left foot. The orthotic can then be individually adjusted to meet the needs of each foot.

toe box); whether or not an orthosis will be used in the shoe; and the runner's past history of running injuries.

Footwear Recommendations

- Make sure foot type (e.g., flexible, rigid) matches type of shoe.
- Determine whether athlete has a neutral, varus, or valgus foot.
- Remember both feet may not be the same.
- What type of foot striker is the runner (heel, micfoot, forefoot)?
- What distance does the runner run per week?
- What is the runner's weight?
- What type of shoe is needed?
- Is there a history of past injuries?
- Will the runner be wearing an orthotic in the shoe?

Orthosis Management for Running Injuries

Philosophy of Orthotic Therapy

The use of a foot orthosis (commonly referred to as an *orthotic*) to address lower extremity overuse running injuries by controlling foot abnormalities has been recommended by various health care professionals for years.[64-69,92-100] Despite the disagreement in the literature as to what type of foot orthosis has shown to be superior (e.g., rigid versus semiflexible; full-length), successful treatment using orthotics depends on careful evaluation of the runner and formulation of a properly fitted device. There are several advantages and disadvantages of each device that need to be factored into the decision-making process by the prescribing clinician (Table 13-3). The normal foot functions most efficiently when no deformities

are present that predispose it to injury or exacerbation of existing injuries. However, in many cases, when a lower limb overuse injury is present, there are lower extremity extrinsic or primary-foot abnormalities present. An orthosis can be used to control abnormal compensatory movements of the foot by "bringing the floor to the foot."[101] This will allow the foot to function more efficiently in a subtalar-joint-neutral position and provide the necessary support so that the foot does not have to move abnormally.

When making a clinic decision regarding the type of device to use, it is important to have an understanding of how the device is to function. There are two basic types of orthoses:

Clinical Point—Orthosis Goal

The goal of the orthosis is to create a biomechanically balanced kinetic chain by using a device capable of controlling motion-related pathological conditions in the foot and leg by maintaining the foot in or as close to a subtalar-joint-neutral position as possible.

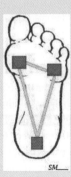

(Illustration reprinted with permission from Agility Physical Therapy & Sports Performance, Portage, Michigan.)

Table 13-3

Rigid versus Semiflexible Orthoses—Advantages and Disadvantages

Type	Advantage	Disadvantage
Rigid orthosis	Rearfoot—arch support High control acquired Several different available materials Intrinsic* corrections from a neutral mold Rigid materials less likely to break down Able to get into a low-profile shoe	No forefoot support or correction Sacrifices shock absorption More difficult to make adjustments Typically, not a comfortable with impact athletes
Semiflexible orthosis	Rearfoot–forefoot support Motion control acquired with shock absorption Several different available materials Extrinsic† posting on neutral module (shell) Adjustments are easy to accomplish Typically more comfortable for impact athletes Able to address several forefoot abnormalities	Semiflexible materials will eventually break down Less likely to achieve the high control More difficult to get into a lower profile shoe

Data from Biocorrect Custom Foot Orthotics Lab, Kentwood, Michigan.

*Intrinsic posting is a means of achieving the recommended corrections by modifying the shape of the rigid material from the original neutral mold.

†Extrinsic posting is a means of achieving the recommended corrections by adding different durometer (stiffness) materials to a neutral shell, which can be easily adjusted by using a grinder (to reduce) or by adding additional materials (to increase).

Biomechanical Orthosis

Biomechanical orthoses are either hard, semirigid or flexible devices that are used to help maintain the foot at or near subtalar joint neutral (Figure 13-13). These rigid, semirigid or flexible "shells" are used to correct forefoot and/or rearfoot deformities that are thought to be causing pathology. The rigid and semirigid shells are molded from a neutral cast. These shells use noncompressible postings (i.e., wedges of different angles to limit foot movement) on the medial or lateral side of the forefoot and/or rearfoot to correct the pathological deformities. The rigid-type shell can be made from carbon graphite, acrylic rohadur or (polyethylene) hard plastic. The hard plastic shell is used when control requirements are paramount to firmly restrain excessive foot motion. However their rigidity results in the loss of some shock absorption and are most commonly used to correct walking deformities. For the more active sports specific individuals, a semirigid shell may be used. These shells are made from thermoplastic, rubber or leather. A semi-rigid device can provide both shock absorption and motion control under increased loading while retaining its original shape. Flexible devices are made of felt or dense foam and offer more shock absorption and less control but have a disadvantage in that they do not maintain their rigidity and wear out faster. The flexible devices are often used as a temporary correction or to determine if the orthotic will correct the problem and, if so, then a semi-rigid device is made and used.[99,102-104]

Accommodative Orthosis

Accommodative orthoses are the flexible devices mentioned in the biomechanical orthoses section above that allow the foot to compensate but are not concerned about maintaining the foot in the subtalar neutral position. These devices are used in people with congenital malformations, restricted ROM, neurological and neuromuscular problems, or physiological old age. Flexible, soft materials are used to fabricate the shell (felt or dense foam) and are designed to yield to the forces applied to the foot on weight bearing rather than resist them.[102-104]

When specifically dealing with running athletes, it is one author's experience that a semiflexible, full-length device (i.e., full length at the foot) using extrinsic posting on a neutral module (see Figure 13-13, C) is recommended for several clinical reasons. First, the functions of the foot during the gait cycle are adaptation, shock absorption, rigid support for leverage, and torque conversion. More specifically, at foot strike, the foot acts as a shock absorber to the impact forces and then adapts to the uneven surfaces. If the prescribed device is rigid (e.g., carbon fiber), this rigidity creates the potential for decreased shock absorption by the device attenuated through the soft tissue structures and less ability for the foot to adapt to the surface. Furthermore, at take-off, the foot has to return to a rigid lever to transmit the explosive force from the lower extremity to the running surface. In cases in which the clinician has noted primary abnormalities of the foot related to the forefoot (e.g., forefoot varus), consideration needs to be given to addressing this alignment issue with a full-length device to assist in the transition back to a rigid foot from a supple foot. Finally, most researchers concur that the use of orthotic therapy is both a "science and an art." There are advantages to using extrinsically posted, neutral-module devices (versus intrinsically designed modules) such as ease of modifications or adjustments. With extrinsically posted

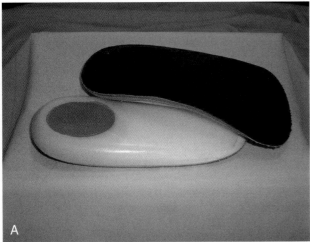

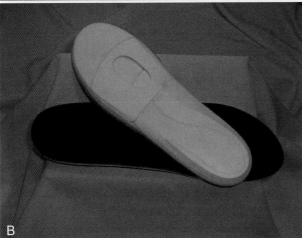

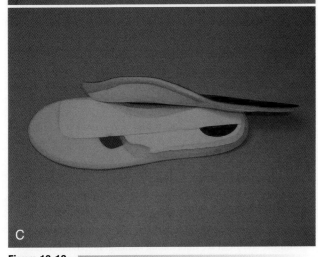

Figure 13-13

Biomechanical orthosis. **A,** Rigid, sulcus-length device. **B,** Semiflexible, full-length device. **C,** Semiflexible, full-length device with rearfoot to forefoot medial posting. (Reprinted with permission from Biocorrect Custom Foot Orthotics Lab, Kentwood, Michigan.)

devices, different types and density of materials can be selected for support and posting. For example, the use of felt, cork, and EVA are common supportive or posting materials used for this type of orthosis. There is also variability in the stiffness (durometer) rating of such materials as EVA depending on the desired function of the material or the weight of the patient.

Regardless of the clinician's philosophy regarding orthotic therapy or the type of orthosis that is used, the goal is to create biomechanical balance at the foot that will subsequently influence the proximal kinetic chain that the patient will wear. A device that is uncomfortable or painful is undesirable and will be detrimental to the overall rehabilitation process.

Conclusion

Clearly, research to date indicates that the cause of running injuries is a multifactorial problem. Although clinicians often emphasize abnormal anatomic alignment as a primary cause of running injuries, anatomic malalignment can be considered only one of numerous factors leading to injury. Because running injuries are often the result of repetitive stress over an extended duration, management of the individual with a running injury requires the clinician to have a thorough understanding of joint kinematics, ground reaction forces, muscle activity, and plantar pressures affecting the body while running. To effectively treat the runner with an overuse injury of the lower extremity and foot, the clinician must understand normal running mechanics so that he or she can determine the causes of repetitive trauma and inflammation secondary to tissue stress. Furthermore, considerations of both the proximal and distal ends of the kinetic chain are essential. Only then will the runner be provided with optimal treatment and a rehabilitation program that will lead to a return to full activity.

References

1. James SL, Bates BT, Osternig LR: Injuries to runners, *Am J Sports Med* 6:40–50, 1978.
2. Lutter LD: Injuries in the runner and jogger, *J Am Podiatr Med Assoc* 70:45–50, 1980.
3. Kerner JA, D'Amico JC: A statistical analysis of a group of runners, *J Am Podiatr Med Assoc* 73:160–164, 1983.
4. Paluska SA: An overview of hip injuries in running, *Sports Med* 35:991–1014, 2005.
5. Yu B, Queen RM, Abbey AN, et al: Hamstring muscle kinematics and activation during overground sprinting, *J Biomech* 41: 3121–3126, 2008.
6. Sugiura Y, Saito T, Sakuraba K, et al: Strength deficits identified with concentric action of the hip extensors and eccentric action of the hamstrings predispose to hamstring injury in elite sprinters, *J Orthop Sports Phys Ther* 38:457–464, 2008.
7. Niemuth PE, Johnson RJ, Myers MJ, Thieman TJ: Hip muscle weakness and overuse injuries in recreational runners, *Clin J Sports Med* 15:14–21, 2005.

8. Kocher MS, Tucker R: Pediatric athlete hip disorders, *Clin Sports Med* 25:241–253, 2006.
9. Clement DB, Ammann W, Taunton JE, et al: Exercise-induced stress injuries to the femur, *Int J Sports Med* 14:347–352, 1993.
10. Slocum DB, James SL: Biomechanics of running, *JAMA* 205:97–100, 1968.
11. James SL, Brubaker CE: Biomechanics of running, *Orthop Clin North Am* 4:605–611, 1973.
12. Adrian MJ, Kreighbaum E: Mechanics of distance-running during competition. In Jokl E, editor: *Biomechanics III*, Baltimore, 1973, University Park Press.
13. Deshon DE, Nelson RC: A cinematographical analysis of sprint running, *Res Q* 35:451–455, 1964.
14. Mann RA, Hagy J: Biomechanics of walking, running and sprinting, *Am J Sports Med* 8:345–350, 1980.
15. Roy B: Caracteristiques biomecaniques de la course d'endurance, *Can J Appl Sports Sci* 7:104–116, 1982.
16. Sprague P, Mann RV: The effects of muscular fatigue on the kinetics of sprint running, *Res Q Exerc Sport* 54:60–66, 1983.
17. Cavanagh PR: The biomechanics of lower extremity action in distance running, *Foot Ankle* 7:197–217, 1987.
18. Landry M, Zebas CJ: Biomechanical principles in common running injuries, *J Am Podiatr Med Assoc* 75:48–52, 1985.
19. Cavanagh PR, Williams KW: The effect of stride length variation on oxygen uptake during distance running, *Med Sci Sports Exerc* 14:30–34, 1982.
20. Murray MP, Drought AB, Kory RC: Walking patterns of normal men, *J Bone Joint Surg Am* 46:335–360, 1964.
21. Murray MP, Kory RC, Sepic BS: Walking patterns of normal women, *Arch Phys Med Rehabil* 51:637–650, 1970.
22. Bogdan RJ, Jenkins D, Hyland T: The runner's knee syndrome. In Rinaldi RR, Sabia M, editors: *Sports medicine*, Mount Kisco, NY, 1978, Futura Publishing.
23. McPoil TG, Cornwall MW: *Influence of running on functional limb varus*, Unpublished data, 1992.
24. Bates BT, Osternig LR, Mason BR, et al: Functional variability of the lower extremity during the support phase of running, *Med Sci Sports Exerc* 11:328–331, 1979.
25. Areblad M, Nigg BM, Ekstrand J, et al: Three-dimensional measurement of rearfoot motion during running, *J Biomech* 23:933–940, 1990.
26. Soutas-Little RW, Beavis GC, Verstraete MC, et al: Analysis of foot motion during running using a joint co-ordinate system, *Med Sci Sports Exerc* 19:285–293, 1987.
27. Engsberg JR, Andrews JG: Kinematic analysis of the talocalcaneal/talocrural joint during running support, *Med Sci Sports Exerc* 19:275–284, 1987.
28. Rodgers MM, LeVeau BF: Effectiveness of foot orthotic devices used to modify pronation in runners, *J Orthop Sports Phys Ther* 4:86–90, 1982.
29. Nigg BM, Herzog W, Read LJ: Effect of viscoelastic shoe insoles on vertical impact forces in heel-toe running, *Am J Sports Med* 16:70–76, 1988.
30. Nigg BM, Morlock M: The influence of lateral heel flare of running shoes on pronation and impact forces, *Med Sci Sports Exerc* 19:294–301, 1987.
31. Stacoff A, Reinschmidt C, Stussi E: The movement of the heel within a running shoe, *Med Sci Sports Exerc* 24:695–701, 1992.
32. Clarke TE, Frederick EC, Hamill CL: The effects of shoe design parameters on rearfoot control in running, *Med Sci Sports Exerc* 15:376–381, 1983.
33. Reinschmidt C, Stacoff A, Stussi E: Heel movement within a court shoe, *Med Sci Sports Exerc* 24:1390–1395, 1992.
34. Sell KE, Verity TM, Worrell TW, et al: Two measurement techniques for assessing subtalar joint position: a reliability study, *J Orthop Sports Phys Ther* 19:162–167, 1994.
35. Novacheck TF: The biomechanics of running, *Gait Posture* 7:77–95, 1998.
36. Schache AG, Bennell KL, Blanch PD, Wrigley TV: The coordinated movement of the lumbo-pelvic-hip complex during running: a literature review, *Gait Posture* 10:30–47, 1999.
37. Schache AG, Blanch PD, Rath D, et al: Three-dimensional angular kinematics of the lumbar spine and pelvis during running, *Human Mov Sci* 21:273–293, 2002.
38. Fredericson M, Cookingham CL, Chaudhari AM, et al: Hip abductor weakness in distance runners with iliotibial band syndrome, *Clin J Sports Med* 10:169–175, 2000.
39. Cichanowski HR, Schmitt JS, Johnson RJ, Niemuth PE: Hip strength in collegiate female athletes with patellofemoral pain, *Med Sci Sports Exerc* 39:1227–1232, 2007.
40. Beckman SM, Buchanan TS: Ankle inversion injury and hypermobility: Effect on hip and ankle muscle electromyography onset latency, *Arch Phys Med Rehabil* 76:1138–1143, 1995.
41. Sims KJ, Richardson CA, Brauer SG: Investigation of hip abductor activation in subjects with clinical unilateral hip osteoarthritis, *Ann Rheum Dis* 61:687–692, 2002.
42. Long WT, Dorr LD, Healy B, Perry J: Functional recovery of noncemented total hip arthroplasty, *Clin Orthop Relat Res* 288:73–77, 1993.
43. Watanabe H, Shimada Y, Sato K, et al: Gait analysis before or after varus osteotomy of the femur for hip osteoarthritis, *Biomed Mater Eng* 8:177–186, 1998.
44. Jacobs C, Uhl TL, Seeley M, et al: Strength and fatigability of the dominant and nondominant hip abductors, *J Athl Train* 40:203–206, 2005.
45. Eggen JM, Carcia CR, Gansneder BM, Shultz SJ: Hip abductor fatigue affects knee motion during the landing phase of a drop jump, *J Athl Train* 38(2, Suppl):S22, 2003.
46. Ireland ML, Willson JD, Ballantyne BT, Davis IM: Hip strength in females with and without patellofemoral pain, *J Orthop Sports Phys Ther* 33(11):671–676, 2003.
47. Leetun DT, Ireland ML, Wilson JD, et al: Core stability measures as risks for lower extremity injury in athletes, *Med Sci Sports Exerc* 36(6):926–934, 2004.
48. Boden F, Volkert R, Menke W, et al: Computer-assisted electromyographic running studies of athletic shoes with various sole configurations. In Segesser B, Pforringer W, editors: *The shoe in sport*, Chicago, 1989, Year Book Medical.
49. Brandell BR: An analysis of muscle coordination in walking and running gaits. In Jokl E, editor: *Biomechanics III*, Baltimore, 1973, University Park Press.
50. Elliott BC, Blanksby BA: A biomechanical analysis of the male jogging action, *J Hum Mov Stud* 5:42–51 1979.
51. Elliott BC, Blanksby BA: The synchronization of muscle activity and body segment movements during a running cycle, *Med Sci Sports Exerc* 11:322–327, 1979.
52. Frigo C, Pedotti A, Santambrogio G: A correlation between muscle and ECG activities during running. In Terauds J, Dale G, editors: *Science in athletics*, Del Mar, CA, 1979, Academic Press.
53. Mann RA, Hagy JL: The function of the toes in walking, jogging, and running, *Clin Orthop Relat Res* 142:24–29, 1994.
54. Dietz V, Schmidtbleicher D, Noth J: Neuronal mechanisms of human locomotion, *J Neurophysiol* 42:1212–1222, 1979.
55. Williams KR: Biomechanics of running, *Exerc Sports Sci Rev* 13:389–441, 1985.
56. Miyashita M, Matsui M, Miura M: The relation between electrical activity in muscle and speed of walking and running.

In Vredenbregt J, Wartenweiler JW, editors: *Biomechanics II*, Baltimore, 1971, University Park Press.

57. Hoshikawa T, Matsui H, Miyashita M: Analysis of running pattern in relation to speed. In Jokl E, editor: *Biomechanics III*, Baltimore, 1973, University Park Press.
58. Komi PV: Biomechanical features of running with special emphasis on load characteristics and mechanical efficiency. In Nigg B, Kerr B, editors: *Biomechanical aspects of sport shoes and playing surfaces*, Calgary, 1983, University of Calgary, 1983.
59. Knuttgen HG: Oxygen uptake and pulse rate while running with undetermined and determined stride lengths at different speeds, *Acta Physiol Scand* 52:366–371, 1961.
60. Ito A, Fuchimoto T, Kaneko M: Quantitative analysis of EMG during various speeds of running. In Winter DA, Normal RW, Wells RP, et al, editors: *Biomechanics IX*, Champaign, IL, 1985, Human Kinetics Publishers.
61. Cavanagh PR, LaFortune MA: Ground reaction forces in distance running, *J Biomech* 13:397–406, 1980.
62. Dickinson JA, Cook SD, Leinhardt TM: The measurement of shock waves following heel strike while running, *J Biomech* 18:415–422, 1985.
63. Drez D: Running footwear: Examination of the training shoe, the foot, and functional orthotic devices, *Am J Sports Med* 8:140–141, 1980.
64. Michaud TC, Nawoczenski DA: The influence of two different types of foot orthoses on first metatarsophalangeal joint kinematics during gait in a single subject, *J Manipulative Physiol Ther* 29:60–65, 2006.
65. Saxena A, Haddad J: The effect of foot orthoses on patellofemoral pain syndrome, *J Am Podiatr Med Assoc* 93:264–271, 2003.
66. MacLean CL, Davis IS, Hamill J: Short- and long-term influences of a custom foot orthotic intervention on lower extremity dynamics, *Clin J Sport Med* 18:338–343, 2008.
67. McNicol K, Taunton JE, Clement DB: Iliotibial tract friction syndrome in athletes, *Can J Appl Sport Sci* 6:76–80, 1981.
68. Gross ML, Napoli RC: Treatment of lower extremity injuries with orthotic shoe inserts. An overview, *Sports Med* 15:66–70, 1993.
69. Gross ML, Davlin LB, Evanski PM: Effectiveness of orthotic shoe inserts in the long-distance runner, *Am J Sports Med* 19:409–412, 1991.
70. Dillman CJ: A kinetic analysis of the recovery leg during sprint running. In Cooper J, editor: *Biomechanics*, Chicago, 1971, Athletic Institute.
71. Hamill J, Bates BT, Knutzen KM, et al: Variations in ground reaction force parameters at different running speeds, *Hum Movement Sci* 2:47–56, 1983.
72. Nigg BM: *Biomechanics of running shoes*, Champaign, IL, 1986, Human Kinetics Publishers.
73. Heil B: Lower limb biomechanics related to running injuries, *Physiotherapy* 78:400–406, 1992.
74. Becker N-L: Specific running injuries and complaints related to excessive loads: Medical criteria of the running shoe. In Segesser B, Pforringer W, editors: *The shoe in sport*, Chicago, 1987, Year Book Medical.
75. McMahon TA, Valiant G, Frederick EC: Groucho running, *J Appl Physiol* 62:2326–2337, 1987.
76. Nachbauer W, Nigg BM: Effects of arch height of the foot on ground reaction forces in running, *Med Sci Sports Exerc* 24:1264–1269, 1992.
77. Root ML, Orien WP, Weed JH: *Clinical biomechanics, Vol 2: Normal and abnormal function of the foot*, Los Angeles, 1977, Clinical Biomechanics Corporation.
78. McConnell J: The management of chondromalacia patellae: A long term solution, *Aust J Physiother* 32:215–223, 1986.

79. James SL: Chondromalacia of the patella in the adolescent. In Kennedy JC, editor: *The injured adolescent knee*, Baltimore, 1979, Williams & Wilkins.
80. Buchbinder MR, Napora NJ, Biggs EW: The relationship of abnormal pronation to chondromalacia of the patella in distance runners, *J Am Podiatr Med Assoc* 69:159–162, 1979.
81. Heil B: Running shoe design and selection related to lower limb biomechanics, *Physiotherapy* 78:406–412, 1992.
82. Messier SP, Davis SE, Curl WW, et al: Etiologic factors associated with patellofemoral pain in runners, *Med Sci Sports Exerc* 23:1008–1015, 1991.
83. Moss RI, DeVita P, Dawson ML: A biomechanical analysis of patellofemoral stress syndrome, *J Athl Training* 27:64–69, 1992.
84. Caylor D, Fites R, Worrell TW: The relationship between quadriceps angle and anterior knee pain syndrome, *J Orthop Sports Phys Ther* 17:11–16, 1993.
85. Janda V, editor: *Movement patterns in the pelvic and hip region with special reference to pathogenesis of vertebrogenic disturbances*, Prague, Czechoslovakia, 1964, Charles University.
86. Jull GA, Janda V: Muscles and motor control in low back pain: assessment and management. In Twomey LT, Taylor JR, editors: Physical therapy of the low back, New York, 1987, Churchill-Livingstone.
87. Schuster RO: Foot types and the influence of environment on the foot of the long distance runner, *Ann NY Acad Sci* 301:881–887, 1977.
88. Messier SP, Pittala KA: Etiologic factors associated with selected running injuries, *Med Sci Sports Exerc* 20:501–505, 1988.
89. Ross CF, Schuster RO: A preliminary report on predicting injuries in distance runners, *J Am Podiatr Med Assoc* 73:275–277, 1983.
90. Warren BL, Jones CJ: Predicting plantar fasciitis in runners, *Med Sci Sports Exerc* 19:71–73, 1986.
91. Cornwall MW: Biomechanics of noncontractile tissue: A review, *Phys Ther* 64:1869–1873, 1984.
92. Bates BT, Osternig L, Mason B: Foot orthotic devices to modify selected aspects of lower extremity mechanics, *Am J Sports Med* 7:338–342, 1979.
93. Cavanaugh PR: *An evaluation of the effects of orthotics force distribution and rearfoot movement during running*. Paper presented at meeting of American Orthopedic Society for Sports Medicine, Lake Placid, 1978.
94. Collona P: Fabrication of a custom molded orthotic using an intrinsic posting technique for a forefoot varus deformity, *Phys Ther Forum* 8:3, 1989.
95. Gill E: Orthotics, *Runner's World*, Feb:55–57, 1985
96. Itay S: Clinical and functional status following lateral ankle sprains: Follow-up of 90 young adults treated conservatively, *Orthop Rev* 11:73–76, 1982.
97. Rogers MM, LeVeau BF: Effectiveness of foot orthotic devices used to modify pronation in runners, *J Orthop Sports Phys Ther* 4:86–90, 1982.
98. Subotnick SI: The flat foot, *Phys Sports Med* 9:85–91, 1981.
99. Subotnick SI, Newell SG: *Podiatric sports medicine*, Mt Kisko, NY, 1975, Futura.
100. Williams JGP: The foot and chondromalacia—a case of biomechanical uncertainty, *J Orthop Sports Phys Ther* 2:50–51, 1980.
101. Hunter S, Dolan M, Davis M: *Foot orthotics in therapy and sports*, Champaign, IL, 1996, Human Kinetics Publishers.
102. American Physical Rehabilitation Network: *When the feet hit the ground...everything changes*. Program outline and prepared notes—a basic manual, Sylvania, OH, 2000.
103. American Physical Rehabilitation Network: *When the feet hit the ground...take the next step*. Program outline and prepared notes—an advanced manual, Sylvania, OH, 1994.
104. Voight M, Hoogenboom B, Prentice W: *Musculoskeletal interventions: techniques for therapeutic exercise*, New York, McGraw-Hill, 2006.

Additional Suggested Readings

Bates BT, Osternig, LR, Mason B, et al: Lower extremity function during the support phase of running. In Asmussen E, Jorgensen K, editors: *Biomechanics VI-B*, Baltimore, 1978, University Park Press.

Blair SN, Kohl HW, Goodyear NN: Rates and risks for running injuries: Studies in three populations, *Res Q* 58:221–228, 1987.

Brubaker CE, James SL: Injuries to runners, *J Sports Med* 2:189–198, 1974.

Clancy WG: Runners' injuries: Part I, *Am J Sports Med* 8:137–138, 1980.

Clancy WG: Runners' injuries: Part II, Evaluation and treatment of specific injuries, *Am J Sports Med* 8:287–289, 1980.

Claremont AD, Hall SJ: Effects of extremity loading upon energy expenditure and running mechanics, *Med Sci Sports Exerc* 20: 167–172, 1988.

Clement DB, Taunton JE, Smart GW, et al: A survey of overuse running injuries, *Phys Sports Med* 9:47–58, 1981.

Cureton TK: Mechanics of track running: Review of the research that has been done to determine factors in running efficiency, *Scholastic Coach* 4:7, 1935.

Dal Monte A, Fucci S, Manoni A: The treadmill used as a training and a simulator instrument in middle- and long-distance running. In Cerquiglini S, Vernarando A, Wartenweiler J, editors: *Biomechanics III*, Basel, Switzerland, 1973, Karger.

D'Amico JC, Rubin M: The influence of foot orthoses on quadriceps angle, *J Am Podiatr Med Assoc* 76:337–340, 1986.

Dillman CJ: Kinematic analyses of running. In Wilmore JH, Keogh JF, editors: *Exercise and sport sciences reviews*, New York, 1975, Academic Press.

Dyson GHG: *The mechanics of athletics*, New York, 1977, Holmes & Meirer.

Elliott BC, Blanksby BA: A cinematographic analysis of overground and treadmill running by males and females, *Med Sci Sports Exerc* 8:84–87, 1976.

Elliott BC, Blanksby BA: Optimal stride length considerations for male and female recreational runners, *Br J Sports Med* 13:15–18, 1979.

Hamill J, Bates BT: A kinetic evaluation of the effects of in vivo loading on running shoes, *J Orthop Sports Phys Ther* 10:47–53, 1988.

Hamill J, Freedson PS, Boda W, et al: Effects of shoe type on cardio-respiratory responses and rearfoot motion during treadmill running, *Med Sci Sports Exerc* 20:515–521, 1988.

Hoffman K: The relationship between the length and frequency of stride, stature and leg length, *Sport VIII* 3:11, 1965.

Ikai M: Biomechanics of sprint running with respect to the speed curve. In Jokl E, editor: *Biomechanics I*, Basel, Switzerland, 1968, Karger.

Jones RE: A kinematic interpretation of running and its relationship to hamstring injury, *J Health Phys Ed Rec* 41:83, 1970.

Lilletvedt J, Kreighbaum E, Phillips RL: Analysis of selected alignment of the lower extremity related to the shin splint syndrome, *J Am Podiatr Med Assoc* 69:211–217, 1979.

Luhtanen P, Komi PV: Mechanical factors influencing running speed. In Asmussen E, Jorgensen K, editors: *Biomechanics VI-B*, Baltimore, 1978, University Park Press.

Mann RA, Baxter DE, Lutter LD: Running symposium, *Foot Ankle* 1:190–224, 1981.

Mero A, Komi PV: Force-, EMG-, and elasticity-velocity relationships at submaximal, maximal and supramaximal running speeds in sprinters, *Eur J Appl Physiol* 55:553–561, 1986.

Miller S, Hunter S, Prentice W: Rehabilitation of the ankle and foot. In Voight ML, Hoogenboom BJ, Prentice WE, editors: *Musculoskeletal interventions: techniques for therapeutic exercise*, New York, 2007, McGraw Hill.

Miura M, Kobayashi K, Miyashita M, et al: Experimental studies on biomechanics in long distance running. In Matsui H, editor: *Review of our researches*, Nagoya, Japan, 1973, Department of Physical Education, University of Nagoya.

Montgomery L, Nelson F, Norton J, et al: Orthopedic history and examination in the etiology of overuse injuries, *Med Sci Sports Exerc* 21:237–243, 1989.

Nelson RC, Brooks CM, Pike NL: Biomechanical comparison of male and female distance runners, *Ann NY Acad Sci* 301:793–807, 1977.

Nelson RC, Gregor RJ: Biomechanics of distance running: A longitudinal study, *Res Q* 47:417–424, 1976.

Nilsson J, Thorstensson A, Halbertsma J: Changes in leg movements and muscle activity with speeds of locomotion and mode of progression in humans, *Acta Physiol Scand* 123:457–475, 1985.

Noble CA: Iliotibial band friction syndrome in runners, *Am J Sports Med* 8:232–234, 1980.

Payne AH: A comparison of the ground forces in race walking with those in normal walking and running. In Asmussen E, Jorgensen K, editors: *Biomechanics VI-A*, Baltimore, 1978, University Park Press.

Robbins SE, Gouw GJ, Hanna AM: Running-related injury prevention through innate impact-moderating behavior, *Med Sci Sports Exerc* 21:130–139, 1989.

Robbins SE, Hanna AM, Gouw GJ: Overload protection: avoidance response to heavy plantar surface loading, *Med Sci Sports Exerc* 20:85–92, 1988.

Rubin BD, Collins HR: Runner's knee, *Phys Sports Med* 8:49–58, 1980.

Sinning WE, Forsyth HL: Lower-limb actions while running at different velocities, *Med Sci Sports Exerc* 2:28–34, 1970.

Slocum DB, Bowerman W: The biomechanics of running, *Clin Orthop* 23:39–45, 1962.

Smart G, Taunton J, Clement D: Achilles tendon disorders in runners—a review, *Med Sci Sports Exerc* 4:231–243, 1980.

Smith WB: Environmental factors in running. *Am J Sports Med* 8:138–140, 1980.

Stanton P, Purdam C: Hamstring injuries in sprinting—the role of eccentric exercise, *J Orthop Sports Phys Ther* 10:343–349, 1989.

Warren B: Anatomical factors associated with predicting plantar fasciitis in long-distance runners, *Med Sci Sports Exerc* 16:60–63, 1984.

CHAPTER

14

APPLIED BIOMECHANICS OF SWIMMING

Marilyn M. Pink, George T. Edelman, Russell Mark, and Scott A. Rodeo

Introduction

When clinicians think "overhead athlete," swimming is one of the sports that come to mind. Some of the other sports include throwing and pitching, volleyball, and tennis. In the past, the mechanics of the "overhead athlete" were sometimes viewed collectively. Most of the "overhead" sports are mechanically at risk during humeral abduction and elevation with external rotation. That is not the case with the swimmer. It is now clear that the requirements of each sport are distinct, and the precise requirements are able to be defined. Thus, this chapter provides an opportunity to describe the specific biomechanics of swimming as they relate to the clinician.

One unique aspect of swimming mechanics is that the power comes from the muscles of the shoulder girdle. In most sports, there is a ground reaction force and power is transmitted from the legs through the trunk and scapula and out the arms. In swimming, however, the body is being pulled over the arms. Thus the arms are the propulsive mechanism, and the shoulders are quite vulnerable, especially if the scapula cannot act as a stable base for the glenohumeral control muscles. Therefore, one of the primary foci of this chapter is the shoulder.

Because the shoulder is the focus, the most visually apparent pathomechanical clue to impending injury is that of axial rotation and humerus position. The visually apparent pathomechanics are discussed, as are the pathomechanics that are harder to see. These pathomechanics are related to their effect on shoulder injury. In addition, shoulder

muscle firing patterns in the normal and the painful shoulder are discussed.

The emphasis of this chapter is identifying injury early and taking steps to minimize anatomic damage. To identify the subtle signs of impending injury, a bridge between the coach and on-deck personnel and the medical team must be built. Hence, this chapter presents such a framework and offers the clinician a problem-solving approach to minimize anatomic damage in the swimmer's shoulder.

Swimmer Characteristics

Unfortunately, approximately half of competitive swimmers develop shoulder pain severe enough to cause them to alter their training schedule at some point during their swimming career.[1] In a survey of 532 collegiate swimmers and 395 master swimmers, not only did approximately half the swimmers have a history of 3 or more weeks of shoulder pain that forced them to alter their training, but more than half of the injured swimmers also had a recurrence. These data point to the need for long-term intervention in the competitive swimmer.

In a separate unpublished survey of 233 competitive swimmers on 17 collegiate teams, the location of pain was queried, as were the positions during the stroke of the most intense pain.[2] The anterior-superior region of the shoulder was identified in 44% of the swimmers as the area of pain. Diffuse pain was identified in 26% of the swimmers, with lesser frequencies reported for the anterior-inferior region of the shoulder (14% of the swimmers), posterior-superior region (10% of the swimmers), and posterior-inferior region (4% of the swimmers). It is likely that swimmers who identified diffuse pain had not acknowledged the pain when it was more localized, and the inciting symptoms were masked by inflammation or more severe damage.

This chapter includes content from previous contributions by Marilyn M. Pink, PhD, PT, and Frank W. Jobe, MD, as it appeared in the predecessor of this book, Zachazewski JE, Magee DJ, Quillen WS, editor: *Athletic Injuries and Rehabilitation*, Philadelphia, 1996, WB Saunders.

During the freestyle stroke, 70% of the "most pain" occurred during the first half of pull-through.[2] Another vulnerable point of the stroke appeared during the first half of recovery (18% of the symptoms were elicited during this phase) (Figure 14-1). During the first half of the pull-through, the arm is unilaterally pulling the body over the arm as the arm generates the propulsive force. The humerus has a common tendency to be hyperextended relative to the trunk rotation toward the submerged side (Figure 14-2, *A*). In this position, the humeral head is pushing anteriorly. Any anterior impingement, labral damage, or inflammation would be aggravated in this position.

Toward midrecovery, the humerus is swinging the forearm forward. When the elbow is too high and close to the body, the humerus is in hyperextension, which is most likely causing the pain. It has been suggested that the humerus is moving into maximal external rotation, and this has been equated to the late cocking phase of the baseball pitch. Although it is true that at this point the humerus is as far into external rotation as it goes during the freestyle stroke, it is nowhere near the degree of maximal external rotation required during the baseball pitch. During the midrecovery phase of the freestyle stroke, the humerus is closer to neutral rotation than it is to "maximal" external rotation. This singular fact underscores the issue that the mechanics of injury in the swimmer are unique for that sport; indeed, they are unique for each stroke within swimming. A grouping of all overhead athletes does injustice to the understanding of specific injury mechanics.

Based on the knowledge of where the shoulder hurt during swimming and which phase of the stroke provoked the injury, an anatomical study was designed to determine the proximity of soft tissues with skeletal tissue. Nine cadaver shoulders were placed in the positions during the first half of pull-through, and cross-sections were taken. Five of the specimens exhibited bursal and intraarticular contact with the rotator cuff. This is now called a *double squeeze* (of the rotator cuff). Three of these specimens also revealed the biceps tendon in contact with the coracoacromial arch. Two other specimens demonstrated intra-articular contact only,

and two demonstrated bursal contact only.[2] Two of the specimens with intra-articular cuff contact demonstrated greater tuberosity contact with the acromion. The site of intra-articular contact was the most common in the anterior-superior labrum (five specimens). Cadaver specimens greatly simplify the issue of shoulder problems in swimmers because they cannot account for the inflammation that would accompany the microtrauma of injury. The inflammation could cause more, or different, areas of contact. The cadavers cannot account for any pathological instability or muscular fatigue or substitution mechanics that may occur. Although simplified, this cadaver model allows a clinician to understand the multiplicity of anatomical contact areas (bursal and intra-articular areas) during the most painful phase of the freestyle stroke.

The Strokes

The shoulder is the primary area of interest to clinicians working with swimmers because of its vulnerability to injury. The visually apparent mechanics related to potential shoulder injury in the freestyle, backstroke, and butterfly strokes is that of humeral position relative to the axis of the body. Figures 14-2, these three strokes and demonstrates the problem of humeral hyperextension relative to body axis. For the purposes of this chapter, *humeral hyperextension* is defined as a combination of humeral abduction and extension (i.e., the humerus is behind the long-axis of the body while the arm is abducted). This position places stress on the anterior joint structures. Too much or too little body rotation changes the position of the humerus relative to the body axis, and thus is related to humeral hyperextension. Whether these faulty mechanics cause the pathological muscle firing patterns or whether weak or fatigued muscles cause these faulty mechanics is a bit like the issue of the chicken and the egg. The changes in muscle firing patterns are not as visually apparent as is the body rotation; however, knowledge of the faulty muscle firing patterns defines the underlying issues and allows the clinician to effectively and efficiently diagnose and treat the problem.

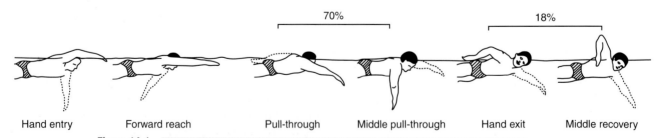

Figure 14-1

Painful phases of the freestyle stroke. Seventy percent of painful symptoms are identified during the first half of pull-through. Eighteen percent of symptoms are identified during the first half of recovery. (From Pink MM, Tibone JE: The painful shoulder in the swimming athlete, *Orthop Clin North Am* 31[2]:248, 2000.)

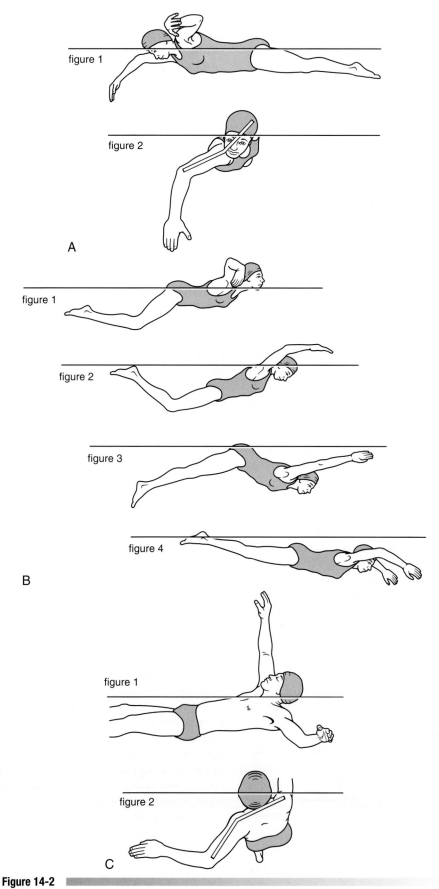

Figure 14-2

Humeral hyperextension. **A,** During the freestyle stroke. Hand exit *(left)* and hand entry *(right)*.
B, During the butterfly stroke. **C,** During the backstroke.

The following is intended to be a synopsis of the key factors in each of the four competitive strokes. There are multiple excellent books and articles on swimming mechanics for those with an interest in more detail. Some of the articles are referenced herein. Two books on basic swim mechanics are those by Ernest Maglischo[3] and Cecil M. Colwin.[4]

Freestyle Stroke

Mechanics

The basic arm mechanics—with the arm position marking different phases of the freestyle stroke—are as follows (Figure 14-3):

1. The arm enters the water and extends forward in front of the shoulder. The underwater pull-through starts with the *early pull-through* phase, which is marked by the initiation of the backward arm movement. The palm and forearm should face the backward direction with the fingertips pointing down for *as long as possible.*
2. The point at which the humerus is perpendicular to the body is called the *mid pull-through.*
3. Subsequent to mid pull-through is the *late pull-through.* The hand continues back and passes next to the hip until it exits the water, leading with the elbow.
4. After the arm exits the water, the *recovery phase* begins, when the arm is swung above the water to bring the arm into position to pull once again.

The arm motion is accompanied by axial rotation of the body. Many swimmers are taught to rotate, yet some degree of rotation will naturally occur toward the side of arm entry. As the arm is entering and the elbow is extending, the shoulder and side of the body rotate below the surface of the water. During the recovery, that same shoulder and side of the body begin to counter-rotate above the surface of the water (while the opposite shoulder is rotated down).

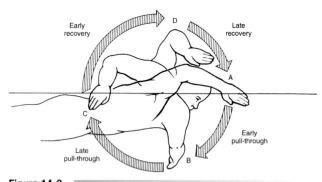

Figure 14-3

Phases of the swimming stroke. (From Pink M, Perry J, Browne A, et al: The normal shoulder during freestyle swimming, *Am J Sports Med* 19:569–576, 1991.)

As previously mentioned, it has been noted that shoulder pain occurs most frequently in two phases of the stroke: (1) the early pull-through to mid pull-through and (2) hand exit to mid-recovery.[2] There is potential in both of these phases for humeral hyperextension that could likely cause pain (see Figure 14-2, *A*). When adjusting to mitigate the pain, the swimmer will most likely seek a path of least resistance and decrease efficiency of the arm stroke while shortening the pull-through phase. One of the easiest ways to see this is during an increase in stroke count.

Swimmers with painful shoulders may begin to use a wider hand-entry and a wider pull-through to diminish the pinching of an inflamed supraspinatus. A wide hand-entry and wide pull-through, combined with the body rotation, can increase the likelihood of humeral hyperextension.

It is important to take notice of the shoulder complex in relation to trunk rotation when a swimmer takes a breath. Observations of elite swimmers from an underwater front view shows a maximum trunk rotation of approximately 30° to 40° down from the surface of the water on each side. The purpose of the rotation should be to aid in the forward progression, not to rotate the body onto its side. It is common for a swimmer to rotate excessively during a breathing cycle, sometimes rotating as much as 90°. In other words, if a swimmer breathes to the right side, there will be a tendency to rotate onto the left side too much. A situation of over-rotating like this is a no-win situation. If the swimmer maintains the optimal pull-through mechanics, the excessive trunk rotation may lead to humeral hyperextension. If the swimmer avoids the humeral hyperextension by keeping the arm in front of the body, it is a major mechanical flaw that will not maximize propulsion.

Another way that the injured swimmer may reduce humeral hyperextension is to adjust the timing of the arm strokes to a "catch-up" timing as opposed to being symmetrically opposite each other. "Catch-up" timing is when the arm phases overlap slightly, so that the recovery arm is on the late recovery while the underwater arm is still in the early pull-through. This reduces body rotation during the early to mid pull-through, thus decreasing the chances for humeral hyperextension.

During the hand exit to mid-recovery, humeral hyperextension can be reduced by swinging the arm wider and decreasing elbow flexion. The elbow does not have to be very high or close to the body (i.e., the emphasis should not be on a high elbow recovery). The recovery should be relaxed and controlled, and it is acceptable to swing the hand around to the side.

The recovery phase should be led by the elbow. Some swimmers try to lead with the hand. They overemphasize the finish motion of the pull-through and actively flick the wrist out of the water upon exit. When they flick the wrist, they are also typically increasing the humeral hyperextension, which increases the vulnerability of the shoulder. Also, it typically changes the initiation of recovery by increasing humeral internal rotation.

Muscle Activity

Clinically, the key to potential pathological conditions in the shoulder during the freestyle stroke may be related to the serratus anterior. In swimmers with normal shoulders, the serratus anterior continually fires above 20% of its maximum.[5] This muscle appears to be stabilizing the scapula in a protracted position as the arm pulls the body over itself. When a muscle continually fires above 20%, it is susceptible to fatigue.[6] With the distances required during swim training, the serratus anterior is certainly vulnerable to fatigue. Indeed, in swimmers with painful shoulders, the serratus anterior demonstrates significantly less muscle action during a large portion of pull-through (Figure 14-4, A). Although the serratus anterior diminishes its action during pull-through, the rhomboids increase their activity (Figure 14-4, B). It may be that, in an attempt to stabilize the scapula during the absence of the serratus anterior, the primary muscles available are the rhomboids. Yet the action of the rhomboids (retraction and downward rotation of the scapula) is the exact opposite of the serratus anterior (protraction and upward rotation). This may well be positioning the acromion to impinge on the rotator cuff.

Another muscle to consider when studying muscle activity during the freestyle stroke is the subscapularis. In swimmers with normal shoulders, this muscle also continually fires above 20% of its maximum.[5] And, in swimmers with painful shoulders, there is significantly less activity during pull-through (Figure 14-4, C).[7]

Of interest, the primary "power" muscles of the shoulder during swimming (the latissimus dorsi and the pectoralis major) demonstrate no significant differences when comparing normal versus painful shoulders. So it appears that these muscles may not be integral in the prevention of injury (Figures 14-4, D and 14-4, E).[7] Also of note, neither the supraspinatus, teres minor, nor posterior deltoid exhibit any significant differences in muscle activity between painful and nonpainful or normal shoulders (Figures 14-4, F–H).[7]

As a clinician, one application of this research information is to ensure there is both a strengthening and endurance component for the serratus anterior and the subscapularis in a swimmer's conditioning program. Another application is to watch for the initial signs of fatigue in these muscles, as that may be the start of a chain of injury.

Butterfly
Mechanics

The butterfly stroke is a bilateral activity, as opposed to a reciprocal, unilateral pattern in the freestyle and backstroke. The pull pattern and body motion are also different, with the butterfly stroke typically consisting more of an S-shaped pulling pattern (Figure 14-5) and the upper body pivoting up and down about the hips, instead of rotating about the central axis as in freestyle and backstroke.

The hands enter the water with the arms extended forward and in front of the shoulder. The upper body presses down at the same time the arms enter the water to generate a more dynamic motion on entry and support the swimmer's forward motion. The hands and arms should remain extended forward during the upper body press, as opposed to aiming downward. This being the case, the magnitude of the upper body press has a great influence on the subsequent motion of the early pull-through and on susceptibility to shoulder pain. Swimmers who press the chest down such that the hands and arms are above the torso are generally in a more risky shoulder position in the early pull-through because this leads to the humeral hyperextension (the humerus is behind the axis of the body). The pulling pattern for a swimmer with a deep upper body press tends to go wide and well outside the shoulder on the early pull-through. If a swimmer is experiencing shoulder pain in the early pull-through, a possible corrective measure for the mechanics is a change in the depth of the upper body press and focusing on keeping the arms in line or in front of the body.

During late pull-through and the beginning of the recovery phase, there is also a chance for the shoulder to be at risk. At the beginning of the late pull-through, the arms are bent and the hands are underneath the hips. The arms then extend, with the hands sweeping outward and the arms lifting upward to exit the water and transition into the recovery phase. There is potential for the humerus to be internally rotated during the arm exit and early recovery phase. A swimmer should not overemphasize the end of late pull-through and lift the hands out of the water too high; instead, he or she should keep his or her hands as close to the surface of the water as possible in the early recovery phase.

With the undulating body motion in the butterfly, the swimmer takes a breath by lifting the upper body upward throughout the underwater pull-through. The swimmer should use the forces generated by the pull-through to lift the upper body just enough for the shoulders and head to clear the surface, but it is common for swimmers to forcefully arch the back and throw the head upward to do this. This action, followed by lunging forward on arm entry, can stress the spine and lower back.

Muscle Activity

As with the freestyle stroke, the pattern of disruptive muscle firing patterns during the butterfly are primarily seen in the muscles attaching to the scapula. The two muscles with clinically relevant muscle firing changes in the painful shoulder during the butterfly are the serratus anterior and the teres minor.[8] In swimmers with painful shoulders,

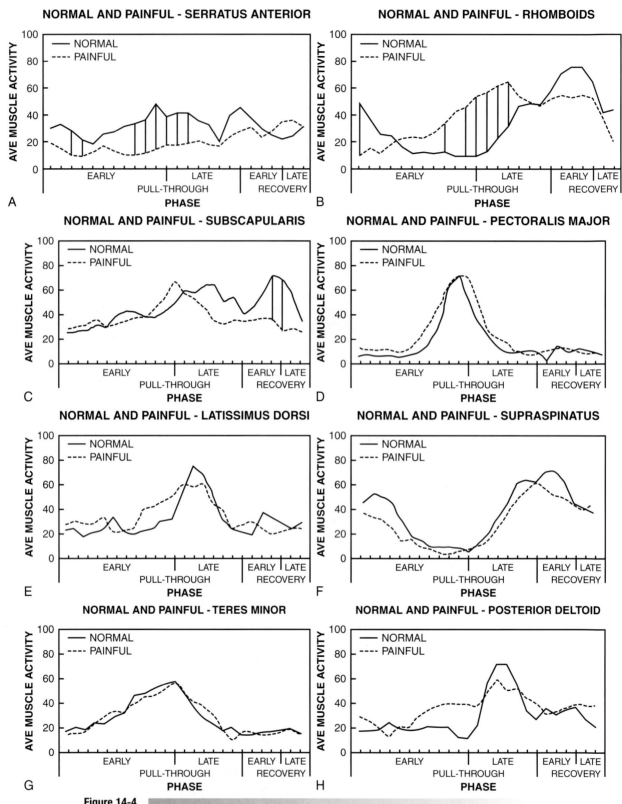

Figure 14-4

Normal and painful shoulders muscle firing during the freestyle. **A,** Serratus anterior. **B,** Rhomboids. **C,** Subscapularis. **D,** Pectoralis major. **E,** Latissimus dorsi. **F,** Supraspinatus. **G,** Teres minor. **H,** Posterior deltoid. (From Scovazzo ML, Browne A, Pink M, et al: The painful shoulder during freestyle swimming: An electromyographic cinematographic analysis of twelve muscles, *Am J Sports Med* 19[6]:579-581, 1991.)

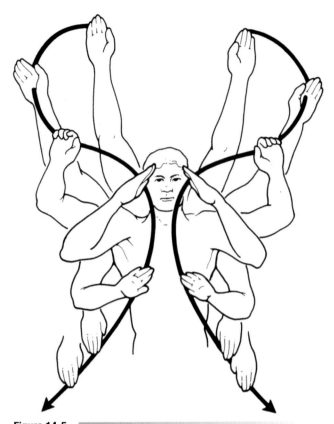

Figure 14-5
S-shaped pull of the freestyle swimming stroke. (From Pink M, Perry J, Browne A, et al: The normal shoulder during freestyle swimming, *Am J Sports Med* 19:569–576, 1991.)

the hand entry is wider than that of the swimmers with normal shoulders. This is also one of the two common points at which swimmers experience shoulder pain during the butterfly stroke.[2] With the wider hand entry, the scapula does not need as much upward rotation or protraction, as evidenced by the decreased activity in the serratus anterior. The teres minor also reveals significantly less action, most likely caused by the altered scapular and humeral position.

During the powerful pulling in the butterfly stroke, the swimmers with painful shoulders continue to demonstrate

less action in the serratus anterior. This muscle is not firing enough to stabilize the scapula or to assist with the pulling of the body over the arm. The decreased firing may be attributable to fatigue. In the normal shoulders, the serratus anterior constantly fires above 20% (which, as previously discussed, leaves it susceptible to fatigue). In the painful population, the serratus anterior may have become fatigued, hence the markedly depressed muscle activity and the resultant unstable scapula.

With an unstable or "floating" scapula, the teres minor is unable to control the humeral rotation caused by the powerful pectoralis major. Therefore, these two muscles (the serratus anterior and the teres minor), which are attached to the scapula, lack the synergistic interplay to assist with propulsion and balance the rotatory humeral motion (Figure 14-6).

At the end of the recovery phase, the teres minor also exhibits decreased muscle activity in the swimmer with a painful shoulder. This is most likely because the muscle is preparing for the wider hand entry, and thus does not require as much action.

The butterfly is not a stroke in which the swimmer puts in the same yardage as the freestyle stroke without a rest period between sets. Therefore, the concern is not as great for fatigue in the butterfly as it is for the freestyle. Yet the fact that the swimmers who perform the butterfly actually train largely with the freestyle stroke cannot be overlooked and fatigue must be considered.

Backstroke
Mechanics
The backstroke is similar to the freestyle stroke in that the arms stroke reciprocally and are supported by a trunk rotation and a leg kick. Obviously, the major difference between the backstroke and the freestyle is that the backstroke is performed supine. In the backstroke, the shoulder is vulnerable to injury similarly to the freestyle, and the relationship between the arm and the body orientation is important to note.

The phases are the same for the two strokes. The beginning of the pull-through is marked by the hand entry of the

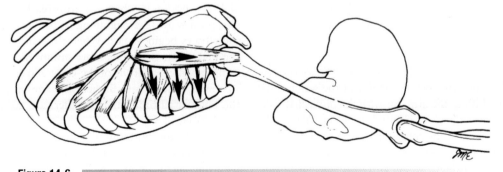

Figure 14-6
With a floating scapula during the butterfly stroke there is no stable base and the teres minor and serratus anterior cannot function adequately.

swimmer with the arm extended above the head. The arm becomes submerged and the hand and arm press toward the feet. The mid pull-through phase begins when the humerus is perpendicular to the body. The arm continues to move toward the feet, and at the end of the late pull-through, the elbow straightens out with a slight downward press before lifting out of the water to start the recovery phase. The elbow is fully extended throughout the recovery phase and travels straight over the top of the water and overhead to the point of hand entry.

The timing of the body rotation as it relates to the arm entry and early pull-through is important. To maximize performance and minimize shoulder vulnerability, the body should be rotating in synchrony with the arm. In other words, if the humerus is oriented 30° below the surface, the torso should be rotated a similar amount below the surface at that time. However, oftentimes this is not the case, because it is typical for the timing of the body rotation to lag behind the arm mechanics. Common symptoms of a late body rotation are a hand entry that crosses inside the shoulder width and a hand entry with the back of the hand. In this situation, in which the arm stroke leads the body rotation, the humerus is hyperextended. For the body rotation and arm motion to be in sync, it is important that the body rotation is initiated at the mid-recovery phase so that at hand entry, the shoulders are horizontal in the water. The body rotation continues as the arm is submerged and the early pull-through is started. The swimmer should rely on the leg kick and the late pull-through to properly execute the body rotation.

Variations across swimmers in the mechanics of the early pull-through phase can also affect the degree of shoulder vulnerability. After the hand enters the water, the early pull-through can vary in depth, palm orientation, and direction of the initial motions. Although observations of today's elite backstrokers show that their palms rotate toward the feet very shortly after hand entry and their arms stay to the side of the body, many swimmers have been taught to press downward immediately after entry to have a deep pull. A deep, early pull-through can lead to a humeral hyperextension because the body is not rotated enough—or soon enough. If a swimmer is experiencing shoulder pain in the early pull-through phase of backstroke and the swimmer is observed to have a straight arm and deep initial pull, then some stress on the shoulder may be relieved with a suggestion to keep the pull more shallow and the arm closer to the body.

At the end of the late pull-through, when the hand exits the water, it is important that the hand exit the water with the thumb first. Lifting the arm out with the pinky first will result in excessive humeral internal rotation. This will increase the pinching of the supraspinatus on the undersurface of the acromion. The hand then rotates during mid-recovery so that the hand can enter the water with the pinky first and the palm rotated out.

Muscle Activity

The muscle action during the backstroke, by mere virtue of the swimmer being on his or her back, is widely different from that of the other strokes. The muscles most active during the powerful pull-through are the teres minor and the subscapularis[9]; and obviously, these two muscles were not designed for power. Even during the peak moments of pulling, the latissimus dorsi reveals 30% less action than does the teres minor and the subscapularis in swimmers with normal shoulders. So, not only is the backstroke swimmer at risk because of the aforementioned humeral hyperextension and levering of the humeral head anteriorly, but these athletes require the small rotator cuff muscles to perform as power muscles.

In addition, during pull-through, the teres minor and subscapularis are constantly active at approximately 30% maximum voluntary contraction. Thus it appears that these two rotator cuff muscles are functioning as power drivers as well as endurance muscles.

At the same time as the depressed activity in the teres minor in the backstrokers with painful shoulders, the rhomboids also exhibit less action.[10] Apparently, the scapula is not retracted properly in early recovery and hence there may be less clearance for the humeral head under the acromion.

A third rotator cuff muscle, the supraspinatus, demonstrates suppressed activity toward mid pull-through in the swimmers with painful shoulders.[10] Given the decreased action in three of the four rotator cuff muscles, one can reasonably conclude that there could be difficulty in depressing the humeral head for adequate clearance of the acromion during pull-through.

Breaststroke
Mechanics

The breaststroke is the oldest of all competitive swim strokes, and it is unique in that the arms do not exit the water. In this stroke, the legs are more of the propeller or power drivers than are the arms. It appears that the least number of complaints of shoulder pain appear to occur with the breaststroke. And, the issue of body rotation along with humeral hyperextension is minimal. This stroke uses a bilateral arm motion in which the arms reach forward and then sweep outward (the beginning of the pull-through), while the elbows begin to flex. When the hands are in line with the mid-chest, the hands move inward in a circular pattern until they meet in front of the chest and are thrust forward (recovery) once again. Because the arms remain in front of the body at all times, the shoulders are not at high risk in the breaststroke.

Just like the butterfly, the body motion in the breaststroke is centered around the hips. The swimmer breathes by lifting the head up as well, but because the breaststroke arm motion leads to a much more natural lifting of the upper body, the spine and lower back are not as susceptible to pain as in the butterfly stroke.

The kicking motion most frequently used in competition is the whip kick, a symmetric, bilateral action (Figure 14-7).

The kick motion starts with the legs fully extended horizontally. The knees bend and move forward as the heels are brought as close to the buttocks as possible. When the heels reach their highest point, the feet rotate outward so that the toes point to the side, and will also move wide of the knees. The knees and feet push backward and inward from that position until reaching full extension with the legs together again. Forward propulsion is generated primarily by the force of the inside of the feet and lower leg pushing directly against the water. The

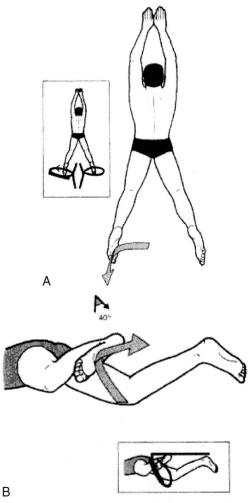

Figure 14-7

Whip kick. **A,** Propulsion generated during the inward portion of the insweep of the breaststroke kick. **B,** Propulsion is produced during the downward portion of the insweep of the breaststroke kick. The illustration shows how water can be displaced backward by the combination of direction and angle of attack during the first downward portion. (From Costill DL, Maglischo EW, Richardson AB, International Olympic Committee: *Swimming,* An IOC Medical Commission Publication, pp 102-103, Oxford, 1992, Wiley-Blackwell.)

feet and knee orientation during the propulsive portion of the kick can create issues with the knee, and the forceful inward motion can lead to a pulled groin muscle. A swimmer can reduce the risk of injury in these cases with proper warm-up and conditioning.

Muscle Activity

During pull-through, breaststroke swimmers with painful shoulders demonstrate an increase in activity in the subscapularis and the latissimus dorsi.[11] The increased subscapularis activity, along with a decrease in the action of the teres minor, leads to a relative increase in internal rotation. The increased internal rotation places the arm in a position that is vulnerable to impingement. The increase in latissimus dorsi action may assist with humeral head depression to relieve the impingement.

Subtle Signs of Injury
Pain versus Soreness

Soreness versus pain: One is expected in the competitive athlete and the other is a signal of potential anatomical damage. Thus, it is appropriate to spend a moment discussing the difference between "pain" and "soreness." The perception of pain may be influenced by the society in which the person lives. Some cultures are more reticent to admit to pain than others. For example, baseball players in Japan in the late 1800s were not allowed to admit to pain, but rather would say "Kayui" or "it itches." Groups of athletes can be their own societies. In our training rooms today, we might see the opposite of the Japanese ball players from the 1800s: Upon inquiry and examination, we may find that a good portion of the pain that was initially reported by athletes in the training room may end up being soreness. When societies shift their perception of pain, the relative nature of the pain scale interpretation must shift also. Therefore, it is worth asking an athlete if the feeling is really one of pain or one of soreness. Soreness can be expected. It is natural for intense workouts to cause soreness.

The feeling of "soreness" is loosely herein defined as a generalized feeling in the muscles, whereas the feeling of "pain" is loosely defined as a deeper, and sometimes sharper, more localized feeling. True pain infers the potential for anatomical damage. This damage means it is probably time to see a physician—and perhaps time to cease training until the issue is resolved. The words to communicate pain versus soreness may offer a challenge. Yet every athlete knows what true pain is.

Pain scales are common in medicine. When a nonathlete patient is recovering from surgery, he or she may be encouraged to take his or her pain medications when the pain hits a "3" or "4." The relative shift in the pain scale is very different for competitive athletes. Coaches and strength and conditioning professionals want to break the athletes down with high-level training to ultimately make them stronger. In the case of the swimmer, this is usually mid-season.

Pain exists on a continuum—and yet with our interpretation and discussion of pain, we are trying to fit it into categories. Although the categorization of pain is easiest for discussion purposes, it is not entirely accurate. So, when combining the categorical discussion along with societal influence, interpretation of a pain scale can be difficult in this population. The true accuracy comes from an integration of the pain scale with observations of the athlete, the on-deck personnel, and the medical professionals.

Athlete's Pain Scale

An athlete's pain scale is suggested in Figure 14-8. This scale is currently under investigative study, and hence the reliability and validity are unknown. The authors choose to present it, however, to make the point of differentiating pain from soreness, as well as the point that an athlete's perception of pain may well require a different interpretation from that of a nonathlete.

The standard 10-cm horizontal line is used for this pain scale, which has a mark at every centimeter, with the 0 and the 10 numerically identified (see Figure 14-8). The different zones of white to red are used for the purpose of communicating with the health care professional. The color codes are not necessarily presented to the athlete.

White Zone (0-3). Symptoms in the white zone indicate fatigue and soreness from training rather than true pain. This zone is a normal part of the intensity of training in a competitive athlete. The athlete can continue to train and continue with his or her exercise conditioning program when pain is reported in this zone. As the athlete increases

the intensity of pain on the scale, the athlete may progress to "shampoo arm syndrome" (i.e., it is hard for the athlete to lift his or her arm to shampoo his or her hair in the shower after workout) and faulty mechanics by the end of the workout. As the athlete reaches a level 3 pain, ice is recommended, and the athlete needs to make certain he or she is performing his or her conditioning program appropriately. At this point, mechanics are normal at the beginning of the workout, and may have adapted by the end of the workout because of fatigue. Within this zone, the athlete is still able to complete a full workout but may need to minimize certain strokes to avoid pain. Pain may last 2 to 4 hours after practice, but is resolved upon waking the next day.

Yellow Zone (4-5). The yellow zone is the "heads-up" zone, signaling caution, yet basically managed by the athlete and the coach. Almost all competitive athletes reach this zone at some point in the season. The coach is trying to break down the athlete so that he or she can then progress to the next level of performance. If the athlete's pain increases throughout this zone, his or her mechanics may become faulty, stroke disciplines modified, and workout distances decreased. Minor performance inconsistencies develop early in this zone, yet the athlete can still compete well enough to win. As this zone progresses, the performance diminishes. Pain may be experienced with forceful arm movements during swimming. Pain may last 4 to 8 hours following a workout, and could be experienced on waking the next day. Management strategies for this zone include a longer-than-normal warmup with slow swimming. It is recommended that sprint sets and hand paddles be eliminated from practice. Fins can be used during

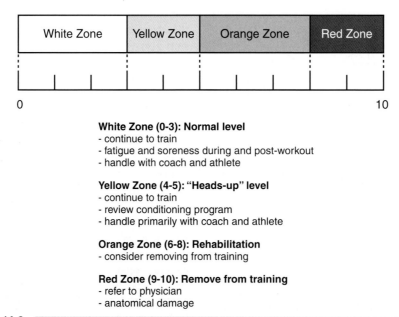

Figure 14-8
Athlete's pain scale.

practice to unweigh the shoulders. To maintain a feel of the water, the athlete can kick in a side-lying or vertical position, but with the involved arm down by the side. The conditioning program should be reviewed with the athlete before and after a workout with a level 4 pain. Once again, adaptations in the program performed after the workouts are probably secondary to fatigue (and simple planar motions may exhibit scapular asymmetry), whereas substitution patterns in the program before a workout need attention. The true pain is probably localized (the soreness and fatigue are generalized). Ice is recommended after practice and before bedtime. If the athlete cannot return to pain-free swimming within 7 to 10 days of modifying the stroke, workout, and conditioning program, referral to sports medicine staff may be appropriate.

Orange Zone (6-8). The orange zone is the rehabilitation zone. Once the pain duration consistently spills into the next day (level 6), the swimmer should be referred to sports medicine staff. This could be the start of potential anatomical damage. The power portion of the upper-extremity conditioning program should be considered and probably discontinued by the time the swimmer's pain is in this zone. Early in this zone (level 6), the coach may want to consider a 3-day rest from workouts. If the swimmer does not improve with a 3-day rest, then a referral to a physician is appropriate.

Red Zone (9-10). This zone represents anatomical damage. The athlete is unable to perform at a competitive level, must stop swimming altogether for an undetermined period, and needs to be under the care of a physician, physical therapist, or athletic trainer.

Mechanical Changes

Mechanical changes in the body go hand-in-hand with fatigue, soreness, and pain. Swimmers will modify their stroke because of these factors before they decrease workouts. The mechanical changes caused by fatigue are identified prior to the pain modifications. These alterations obviously show up toward the end of the workout as fatigue increases. When the fatigue-induced mechanical changes show up early in the workout, then the swimmer may need a recovery workout or a day of rest. The butterfly is likely the first stroke to demonstrate mechanical changes, followed by the freestyle and the backstroke. The breaststroke is likely the most mechanically enduring stroke related to fatigue, soreness, and pain.

Mechanical flaws and adaptations are easiest to see from the underwater vantage point. Ideally, all pools would have underwater windows, both laterally and under the pool. A more practical solution is the use of underwater video, which has become an affordable and valuable analysis tool. The most subtle changes in mechanics will be very difficult for a relatively naïve eye to catch, and the use of digital video analysis software can aid a coach and clinician to diagnose mechanics.

Because the medical personnel are not typically on-deck with the swimmers and coaches, it behooves sports clinicians to be a bridge between the clinics and the deck. Thus, it is important that sports clinicians converse with the coaches and on-deck personnel about the subtle mechanical changes that may lead to anatomical damage.

Because the freestyle is the most used stroke, the mechanical changes caused by fatigue, soreness, and pain are noted herein for that stroke. Table 14-1 presents some of the more common potential mechanical changes in the freestyle stroke.

Clinical Implications

Repetitive overuse appears to be a major contributor to shoulder pain in swimmers. In addition to the aforementioned mechanics, which can lend to impingement, other contributing factors for swimmer's shoulder include (1) overuse and subsequent fatigue of the muscles around the shoulder, scapula, and upper back; and (2) glenohumeral laxity. These factors are all related, because impingement may be caused by altered glenohumeral kinematics resulting from muscle fatigue or glenohumeral laxity. Other associated findings include muscle imbalances and inflexibility, such as tightness of the pectoral muscles, and sometimes inflexibility of the posterior capsule and posterior rotator cuff.

Muscle Fatigue and Dysfunction

Because the shoulder is an inherently unstable joint, muscle forces are critical for maintaining stability, proper motion, and painless function. As previously discussed, performance of the swimming stroke requires a highly coordinated pattern of muscles firing at precisely the right time to provide the most efficient and powerful stroke. If one muscle fatigues, it is as if one cog in a machine is malfunctioning. When that one muscle fatigues, it affects the function of other muscles in the kinetic chain.

Muscle dysfunction increases impingement by loss of the humeral head depressor function of the rotator cuff and loss of upward rotation and elevation of the scapula. Loss of the stabilizing effect of muscles may be especially problematic in swimmers with associated shoulder laxity (discussed in the following section). Fatigue of the abdominal and pelvic muscles may also contribute by affecting scapular kinematics and body position in the water.

Laxity

Many competitive swimmers have an element of shoulder laxity.[12,13] A certain degree of laxity may be advantageous by allowing a swimmer to achieve both a body position that

Table 14-1

Common Freestyle Mechanical Changes Caused by Fatigue, Soreness, and Pain

Mechanical Change	Effect on Stroke
Wider hand entry and lateral underwater hand motion	Hand starts wide and "slides" under the belly Less force on the shoulder Flatter hand entry Avoids Neer and Hawkins impingement positions
Shorten underwater reach after hand entry	Hand does not extend as far forward under water after hand entry Avoids positions that mimic Neer and Hawkins impingement positions
Leading with elbow rather than hand during catch and early pull-through	Attempts to decrease amount of force on hand and forearm
Early hand exit	Minimizes humeral internal rotation Looks similar to hand exit with butterfly stroke
Decreased trunk rotation	Related to shorter underwater reach and early hand exit Attempts maintain stroke rate
Premature rotation and lifting of head prior to breathing	Attempts to get arm out of water earlier and with less force in final position of stroke
"Dropped" elbow on recovery	Decreased elbow flexion and height More lateral swing Attempts to avoid painful internal rotation of humerus

reduces drag and a longer sweep during the pull-through phase. It is well-established that there is a narrow distinction between physiological laxity (normal) and pathological instability (abnormal). Normal laxity may increase over time because of repetitive overuse and eventually become a pathological condition. Shoulder stability is controlled by static (i.e., glenohumeral ligaments and capsule) and dynamic (rotator cuff muscles) factors. Loss of the static component (i.e., glenohumeral capsular laxity) requires a greater contribution from the rotator cuff, which can result in muscle overload and eventual muscle fatigue, as described previously. The challenge for the clinician is to distinguish between normal laxity and abnormal instability.

Previous studies have documented the presence of increased joint laxity and glenohumeral instability in swimmers. Bak and Faunø reported that 37 out of 49 competitive swimmers had increased humeral head translation with associated apprehension.[14] Furthermore, McMaster and colleagues found a significant correlation between shoulder laxity and shoulder pain in a group of 40 elite-level swimmers.[15] The presence of underlying generalized joint hypermobility was reported by Zemek and Magee.[13] These authors reported both increased glenohumeral laxity and increased generalized joint hypermobility in elite swimmers. These studies suggest that a combination of acquired and inherent factors contribute to shoulder laxity in swimmers.

The most common pattern of instability is anteroinferior, but there is often a component of multidirectional instability. Subluxation can occur during the backstroke as the hand enters the water with the swimmer on his or her back with the arm in full flexion and external rotation. Posterior instability symptoms, although less common, may be exacerbated because of the position of the arm in flexion, adduction, and internal rotation.

Impingement

Swimmers usually have a nonoutlet type of impingement, in which altered kinematics rather than subacromial pathological changes (i.e., acromial osteophyte or coracoacromial ligament abnormalities) results in abnormal contact. Such impingement may be subacromial (the bursal surface of the rotator cuff against the anteroinferior acromion) or intra-articular (the articular surface of the rotator cuff or biceps tendon impinges on the anterosuperior glenoid and labrum). The position of the shoulder during the recovery phase of the stroke (forward flexion and internal rotation) is a classic position for subacromial impingement. At the end of the pull-through phase of the stroke, the arm goes into hyperextension, which pushes the humeral head anteriorly, which also exacerbates impingement. Use of a video analysis system to document impingement during the freestyle stroke found that impingement occurred when the hand entered the water and in the middle of the recovery phase.[16] The mean duration of impingement was nearly 25% of the total stroke time. This study demonstrated that impingement was most likely in swimmers who have excessive internal rotation during the pulling phase, delayed initiation of external rotation of the arm during the recovery phase, and decreased upward scapular rotation.[17] Hydrodynamic forces exerted by the water may also exacerbate impingement. At the point at which the hand enters the water, the hydrodynamic force exerted on the hand generates a large moment about the shoulder joint caused by the long moment arm in this position. This moment will forcibly elevate the arm, possibly increasing impingement.[16]

Alternatively, intra-articular impingement may occur during the swimming stroke as the articular surface of the rotator cuff can impinge against the anterosuperior labrum adjacent to the biceps attachment as the arm is placed into forward flexion and internal rotation. Such a mechanism could account for the frequent localization of pain around the biceps tendon in swimmers. The position of forward elevation, adduction, and internal rotation may also result in impingement of the coracoid process on the lesser tuberosity and subscapularis tendon.

Muscle fatigue caused by overuse may also contribute to impingement. The normal rotator cuff functions to stabilize the glenohumeral joint and acts as a humeral head depressor, preventing subacromial impingement. It is known that loss of the humeral head depressor function of the rotator cuff results in superior migration of the humeral head and increases the risk of impingement.[18]

Conditioning, Prevention, and Rehabilitation

Stretching

Given the discussion on laxity as well as underwater videography indicating that no extraordinary shoulder joint motion is necessary for a fast, efficient stroke, there is little reason to consider an excessive stretching program for swimmers. As a matter of fact, the stretching performed by many swimmers may actually be harmful to the capsuloligamentous structures. Thus, it is probably more important for swimmers to stop traditional stretching practices than it is to begin proper stretching based on individual physiology. The four stretches demonstrated in Figure 14-9 should no longer be considered in a dry-land program for swimmers.

Stretching is athlete-specific. A simple shoulder screen (Figure 14-10) for coaches and on-deck personnel has been developed to review the flexibility of all members of the team effectively and efficiently. There are three positions for each athlete to review:

Suggested Flexibility Screen for Swimmers

- Tight streamline position (see Figure 14-10)
- 90/90 position (see Figure 14-10)
- 45° position (see Figure 14-10)

---

1. **Tight Streamline Position—½ Sit Against the Wall.** This position is a sport-specific, functional position that assesses mobility in the scapulothoracic and glenohumeral joints as well as the length of the latissimus dorsi. The swimmer should be able to complete this desired motion without difficulty with the lumbar

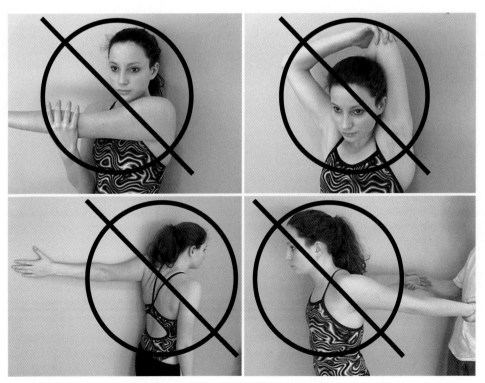

Figure 14-9
Stretches that swimmers should NOT do.

Tight Streamline –$\frac{1}{2}$ Sit Against Wall: Assume the following tight streamline position.
(In order to 'pass' this position, all of the 5 questions in this section must be answered with a 'Yes'.)

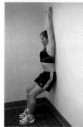

Are the elbows in full extension?	YES	NO
Are the arms by the ears?	YES	NO
Are the hands clasped?	YES	NO
Are the hands in contact with the wall?	YES	NO
Is the low back in contact with the wall?	YES	NO

90/90 Position: Lie supine with knees bent and feet on surface. Assume 90° of shoulder abduction in the coronal plane and 90° of glenohumeral external rotation.
(In order to 'pass' this position, all 4 of the questions in this section must be answered with a 'Yes'.)

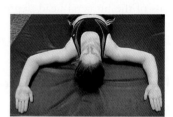

Are the shoulders flat on the floor?	YES	NO
Do the forearms and elbows rest comfortably on the floor?	YES	NO
When the swimmer is asked to press his/her wrists into the surface, are the wrists flat on the surface?	YES	NO
Is the back flat the surface?	YES	NO

45 Position: In standing with the humerus in full adduction (arm by your side), bend your elbows to 90° and externally rotate to 45° or beyond.
(In order to 'pass' this position, both of the questions in this section must be answered with a 'Yes'.)

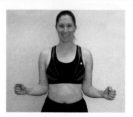

Do the shoulders rotate to 45° or beyond?	YES	NO
Do the elbows maintain contact with the trunk?	YES	NO

If a swimmer is able to achieve at least two of the positions above, then he/she is well served with the stretching program herein. If the swimmer fails in 2 or all of the positions, then a customized stretching routine from a health care professional is recommended.

Figure 14-10
Shoulder range of motion screen for swimmers.

spine flat against the wall, full elbow extension, and clasped hands against the wall.

2. **90/90 Position.** This position is completed in supine position. It assesses mobility of the inferior and anterior glenohumeral joint capsule as well as the blended anterior band of the inferior glenohumeral and the middle glenohumeral ligaments.[19] Shortening of the pectoralis group is also identified with this position. The swimmer should be able to rest his or her forearm, wrist, and elbow comfortably on the floor in this position while maintaining 90° of elbow flexion and 90° of glenohumeral abduction. The posterior shoulder joint muscles should be in contact with the floor or table.

3. **45° Position.** This position specifically assesses the length of the subscapularis. A competitive swimmer needs to be able to achieve this position with 45° of external rotation while keeping the humerus in an adducted position.

If the swimmer is able to achieve at least two of these positions, then the athlete is well served with the stretching program described in Figure 14-11. If the swimmer is unable to achieve two or more of the positions in the shoulder screen, then consultation with a sports medicine professional is encouraged to help identify the origin of the restriction and develop a customized stretching program for that individual.

Based on the physical demands of swimming, understanding the biomechanics of the stroke and respecting the capsuloligamentous structures, the focus of the recommended stretches is to target the at-risk connective tissue while avoiding insult to the static stabilizers. Observationally, it appears that only three muscle groups of the glenohumeral joint may be at risk of shortening in the swimmer. Those three groups are the (1) pectoralis muscles, (2) latissimus dorsi, and (3) subscapularis. If these muscles have been tight for a prolonged period, there is also a risk of tightness in the capsuloligamentous complex.

However, swimmers tend to have more tightness in the low back than in the shoulder. Although the back is not necessarily at risk during the swim stroke, the "common" posture of the swimmer with forward shoulders, lordotic back, and genu recurvatum indicates that the soft tissue structures in the lumbar spine may shorten. In the long run, this is known to be a potential cause of back problems.

Although there is little, if any, research literature on the musculoskeletal requirements and common limitations of the lower extremity, a swimmer ideally has good range of motion (ROM) at the hip and at the ankle. If there are tight hip flexors, they could contribute to a low back problem. And if there is a limitation in ankle plantar flexion ROM, kicking efficiency could be decreased.

Based on these observations and if the swimmer "passes" the shoulder screen in Figure 14-10, an appropriate dry-land stretching routine can be found in Figure 14-11.

It is recommended that swimmers stretch at a time unrelated to working out or racing (at least several hours prior to getting in the water). Pre-exercise stretching has been found to compromise muscle performance for up to 1 hour.[20-25] Postexercise stretching is not encouraged. Stretching fatigued muscles tends to facilitate muscle spindle and inhibit Golgi tendon organ firing.[26,27] General guidelines for stretching include completing a specific static stretch that targets muscle tissue one to three times for 15 to 30 seconds each, approximately 5 days a week is appropriate.[28-31] Instead of pre-exercise stretching, a longer warmup in the water with increasing intensity is recommended.

Conditioning the Uninjured Swimmer

Given the muscle functions described previously, the following is an offered infrastructure intended to assist the health care professional in designing a conditioning program for the uninjured swimmer that is specific not only to swimming, but also specific for the individual's competitive strokes. Numerous studies identify optimal exercises for the different muscles.[32-41] The suggested optimal exercises are simply that: a suggestion for a starting point in considering the conditioning program.

A program for competitive butterfly, backstroke, and breaststroke swimming will, most likely, include the exercises for the freestyle stroke because most swimmers (regardless of competitive strokes) put in large distances with the freestyle. Coaches are encouraged to implement the strength and endurance program after practice or several hours before practice (Table 14-2). Exercising the muscles of the shoulder complex directly before practice may lead to fatigue and subsequent faulty stroke mechanics.[7]

Rehabilitation

Given the currently known specificity of muscle requirements in the competitive swimmer, the work of the rehabilitation professional can be much more focused than ever before. The intent of these few paragraphs is to give the professional the scaffolding on which to build the nonsurgical rehabilitation program.

A swimmer's inflamed shoulder is treated the same as the inflamed shoulder of any individual. Rest from offending activities, ice, and anti-inflammatory medication may be necessary as well as potential application of modalities such as iontophoresis, ultrasound, or high-voltage galvanic stimulation. Once the inflammatory process is halted, gentle stretches such as those described in the conditioning program are suggested. Consideration needs to be given to safe arcs of motion for the stretches. Identification of the weak

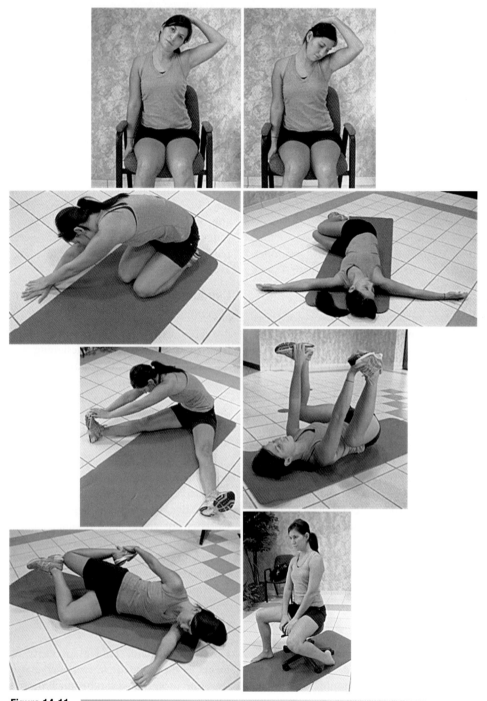

Figure 14-11
Dry-land stretching recommendations for swimmers.

muscles begins at this stage. As reinforcement to the afore-mentioned material, each swimming stroke carries different muscle injury risk requiring varying levels of strength and endurance.

Once the weak components for the glenohumeral muscles are identified, the specific exercise program can be developed. The optimal exercise program takes into consid-eration not only those exercises that optimally recruit the specific muscles within a safe and efficient range, but they also use the most effective type of contraction (i.e., isomet-ric or concentric). For example, if the rhomboids were muscles needing strengthening, the optimal exercise is an isometric contraction while the muscles are in the maxi-mally shortened state. Although it is beyond the scope of

Table 14-2

Muscles at Risk During the Swim Stroke and Suggested Exercises

Stroke	Muscles at Risk	Strength or Endurance	Suggested Optimal Exercises
Freestyle	Serratus anterior	Strength	Push-up plus
			Military press
		Endurance	Scaption moving from medial rotation → lateral rotation with low load—use time as a measure rather than repetitions
			Upper-body exercises, boxing, or fencing maneuver
	Subscapularis	Strength and endurance	Medial rotation—low load, high number of reps
Butterfly	Serratus anterior	Strength and endurance	Suggestions as with freestyle
	Teres minor	Strength and endurance	Lateral rotation with humeral elevation—low loads—fairly quick motions—high number of repetitions
			Lateral rotation with humerus ≈30° off the trunk—can be higher load and slower than lateral rotation with humeral elevation
Backstroke	Teres minor	Strength and endurance	Suggestions as with butterfly
	Subscapularis	Strength and endurance	Suggestions as with freestyle
	Rhomboids	Strength	Retraction with an isometric hold
	Supraspinatus	Strength	Flexion—challenging load to complete 15 repetitions
Breaststroke	Supraspinatus	Strength	Suggestions as with backstroke
	Upper trapezius	Strength	Shoulder shrugs

Table 14-3

Return to Swimming Benchmarks

Criteria to Allow Swimming	Swimming Activity Allowed
Benchmark 1	
Reach above shoulder height pain free	Swim 1000-2000 yards slowly and comfortably while
Pain-free resisted movements 0° to 90°	avoiding antagonizing swim strokes and sprint sets
Benchmark 2	
Pain free with resisted shoulder motions	Add 500 yards every three workouts
Pain free with most activities of daily living	Avoid double workouts at this time
Pain free with swimming 2000 yards	
Benchmark 3	
Pain free swimming 4000 to 5000 yards	Short sprint sets
	Incorporate all swim strokes

this chapter to discuss the specific muscle physiology for each muscle, health care practitioners have such information available to them.

Any individual with shoulder problems benefits from cardiovascular and muscle endurance rehabilitation. Walking, rowing, stationary bicycling, and use of the elliptical are all ways to maintain aerobic conditioning. Muscle endurance training is another integral part of the rehabilitation program for swimmers. Endurance training can be addressed with low-resistance and high-repetition activities.

Plyometric training has also been found to improve endurance. Swanik and colleagues[42] studied the effect of plyometric training on shoulder proprioception, kinesthe-

sia, and selected muscle performance in a group of Division I female swimmers. After a 6-week period of a plyometric training program that focused on the internal rotators of the shoulder complex, both proprioception and kinesthesia significantly improved. The Swanik study confirmed that plyometric exercises for the competitive swimmer helps to promote endurance, glenohumeral joint stability, and neuromuscular efficiency.

Return to Swimming Program

Maintaining a feel for the water is critical during the rehabilitation process and, as a result, coordinating a timely return to the pool is essential. There are specific benchmarks in the swimmer's return to a pool program (Table 14-3) based on their progress. Adherence to a slow, progressive program ensures a healthy return to the sport they love.

Conclusion

The mechanics of swimming are different from that of the "overhead" athlete. Indeed each of the four swim strokes need to be considered independently. With the high rate of injury and reinjury, it is important for clinicians to understand the mechanics and the cause of injury and reinjury for each stroke. Such an understanding will not only allow the clinician and on-deck personnel to catch the subtle signs of injury, but it will also minimize the risk of potential injury and maximize the rehabilitative outcomes.

References

1. Stocker D, Pink MM, Jobe FW: Comparison of shoulder injury in collegiate and masters level swimmers, *Clin J Sports Med* 5:4–8, 1995.
2. Pink MM, Tibone JE: The painful shoulder in the swimming athlete, *Orthop Clin North Am* 31(2):247–261, 2000.
3. Maglischo EW: *Swimming fastest*, Champaign, IL, 2003, Human Kinetics.
4. Colwin CM: *Breakthrough swimming: stroke mechanics, training methods, racing techniques*, Champaign, IL, 2002, Human Kinetics.
5. Pink M, Perry J, Browne A, et al: The normal shoulder during freestyle swimming, *Am J Sports Med* 19:569–576, 1991.
6. Monad H: Contractility of muscle during prolonged static and static dynamic activity, *Ergonomics* 28:81, 1985.
7. Scovazzo ML, Browne A, Pink M, et al: The painful shoulder during freestyle swimming: an electromyographic and cinematographic analysis of twelve muscles, *Am J Sports Med* 19:577–582, 1991.
8. Pink M, Jobe, FW, Perry J, et al: The painful shoulder during the butterfly stroke: an electromyographic and cinematographic analysis of twelve muscles, *Clin Orthop Relat Res* 288:60–72, 1993.
9. Pink M, Jobe FW, Perry J, et al: The normal shoulder during the backstroke: an EMG and cinematographic analysis of twelve muscles, *Clin J Sports Med* 2:6–12, 1992.
10. Perry J, Pink M, Jobe FW, et al: The painful shoulder during the backstroke: an EMG and cinematographic analysis of twelve muscles, *Clin J Sports Med* 2:13–20, 1992.
11. Ruwe PA, Pink M, Jobe FW, et al: The normal and painful shoulder during the breaststroke: an EMG and cinematographic analysis of twelve muscles, *Am J Sports Med* 6:709–796, 1993.
12. Rupp S, Berninger K, Hopf T: Shoulder problems in high level swimmers—impingement, anterior instability, muscular imbalance? *Int J Sports Med* 16(8):557–562, 1995.
13. Zemek MJ, Magee DJ: Comparison of glenohumeral joint laxity in elite and recreational swimmers, *Clin J Sport Med* 6(1):40–47, 1996.
14. Bak K, Faunø P: Clinical findings in competitive swimmers with shoulder pain, *Am J Sports Med* 25(2):254–260, 1997.
15. McMaster WC, Roberts A, Stoddard T: A correlation between shoulder laxity and interfering pain in competitive swimmers, *Am J Sports Med* 26(1):83–86, 1998.
16. Yanai T, Hay JG, Miller GF: Shoulder impingement in front-crawl swimming: I. A method to identify impingement, *Med Sci Sports Exerc* 32(1):21–29, 2000.
17. Yanai T, Hay JG: Shoulder impingement in front-crawl swimming: II. Analysis of stroking technique, *Med Sci Sports Exerc* 32(1):30–40, 2000.
18. Paletta GA Jr., Warner JJ, Warren RF, et al: Shoulder kinematics with two-plane x-ray evaluation in patients with anterior instability or rotator cuff tearing, *J Shoulder Elbow Surg* 6(6):516–527, 1997.
19. Turkel SJ, Panio MW, Marshall JL, Girgis FG: Stabilizing mechanisms preventing anterior dislocation of the glenohumeral joint, *J Bone Joint Surg* 63: 1208–1217, 1981.
20. Knudson DV, Magnusson P, McHugh M: Current issues in flexibility fitness, *Pres Council Phys Fitness Sports* 3:1–6, 2000.
21. Kokkonen JA, Nelson AG, Cornwell A: Acute muscle stretching inhibits maximal strength performance, *Res Q Exerc Sport* 69:411–415, 1998.
22. Fowles JR, Sale DG, MacDougall JD: Reduced strength after passive stretch of the human plantar flexors, *J Appl Physiol* 89:1179–1188, 2000.
23. Cornwell AG, Nelson A, Heise G, Sidaway B: Acute effects of passive muscle stretching on vertical jump performance, *J Hum Mov Stud* 40:307–324, 2001.
24. Knudson D, Bennett K, Corn R, et al: Acute effects of stretching are not evident in the kinematics of the vertical jump, *J Strength Cond Res* 15(1):98–101, 2001.
25. Cramer JT, Housh TJ, Johnson GO, et al: Acute effects of static stretching on peak torque in women, *J Strength Cond Res* 18(2):236–241, 2004.
26. Nelson HL, Hutton RS: Dynamic and static stretch responses in muscle spindle receptors in fatigued muscle, *Med Sci Sports Exerc* 17:445–450, 1985.
27. Hutton RS, Nelson DL: Stretch sensitivity of Golgi tendon organ in fatigued gastrocsoleus muscle, *Med Sci Sports Exerc* 18:69–74, 1986.
28. Decoster LC, Scanlon RL, Horn KD, Cleland J: Standing and supine hamstring stretching are equally effective, *J Athl Train* 39(4):330–334, 2004.
29. Bandy WD, Irion JM, Briggler M: The effect of time and frequency of static stretching on flexibility of the hamstring muscles, *Phys Ther* 77:1090–1096, 1997.
30. Bandy WD, Irion JM: The effect of time on static stretch on the flexibility of the hamstring muscles, *Phys Ther* 74:845–852, 1994.
31. Bandy WD, Irion JM, Briggler M: The effect of static stretch and dynamic range of motion training on the flexibility of the ham string muscles, *J Orthop Sports Phys Ther* 27:295–300, 1998.
32. Blackburn TA, McLeod WD, White B, Wofford L: EMG analysis of posterior rotator cuff exercises, *J Athl Train* 25:40–45, 1990.
33. Moseley JB, Jobe FW, Pink M, et al: EMG analysis of the scapular muscles during a shoulder rehabilitation program, *Am J Sports Med* 20(2):128–134, 1992.
34. Wilk KE, Arrigo C: Current concepts in the rehabilitation of the athletic shoulder, *J Orthop Sports Phys Ther* 18:365–378, 1993.
35. Lear LJ, Gross MT: An electromyographical analysis of the scapular stabilizing synergists during a push-up progression, *J Orthop Sports Phys Ther* 28(3):146–157, 1998.
36. Kibler WB: Shoulder rehabilitation: principles and practice, *Med Sci Sports Exerc* 30:540–550, 1998.
37. Decker MJ, Hintermeister RA, Faber KJ, Hawkins RJ:. Serratus anterior muscle activity during selected rehabilitation exercises, *Am J Sports Med* 27(6):784–791, 1999.
38. Blackburn TA, Guido TA: Rehabilitation after ligamentous and labral surgery of the shoulder: guiding concepts, *J Athl Train* 35(3):373–381, 2000.

39. Voight ML, Thomson BC: The role of the scapula in the rehabilitation of shoulder injuries, *J Athl Train* 35(3):364–372, 2000.

40. Ekstrom R, Donatelli R, Soderberg G: Surface electromyographic analysis of exercises for the trapezius and serratus anterior muscles, *J Orthop Sports Phys Ther* 33:247–258, 2003.

41. Reinold M, Wilk KE, Fleisig GS, et al: Electromyographic analysis of the rotator cuff and deltoid musculature during common shoulder external rotation exercises, *J Orthop Sports Phys Ther* 34:385–394, 2004.

42. Swanik KA, Lephart SM, Swanik CB, et al: The effects of shoulder plyometric training on proprioception and selected muscle performance characteristics, *J Shoulder Elbow Surg* 11(6):579–586, 2002.

APPLIED BIOMECHANICS OF BASEBALL PITCHING

Glenn S. Fleisig, Rafael F. Escamilla, and James R. Andrews

Introduction

Baseball pitching is one of the fastest and most stressful throwing motions in all of sport. The prevalence of overuse injury due to pitching is well documented.[1-4] Because of the popularity of baseball and the risk of injury from repetition, a number of papers have been published on pitching biomechanics.[5-18] An understanding of pitching biomechanics includes knowledge of kinematics, kinetics, and electromyography (EMG). *Kinematics* describes how something is moving without stating the cause—quantifying linear and angular displacement, velocity, and acceleration. *Kinetics* explains why an object moves the way it does, quantifying the forces and torques that cause the motion. *EMG* measures muscle activity during the motion. The experimental set-up used in quantifying pitching biomechanics is shown in Figure 15-1. Pitching kinematic measurements are defined in Figure 15-2 and Figure 15-3, pitching kinetic measurements are defined in Figure 15-4, and pitching EMG for each muscle are presented as a percent of a maximum voluntary isometric contraction (MVIC). In this chapter, the following topics relative to baseball pitching are presented:

1. Adult baseball pitching kinematics, kinetics (and associated pathological conditions), and EMG findings while throwing the fastball pitch
2. Kinematic and kinetic comparisons among fastball, curveball, slider, and change-up baseball pitches
3. Kinematic and kinetic comparisons among youth, high school, college, and professional levels
4. Kinematic and kinetic comparisons between adult male and female baseball pitchers
5. A kinematic and kinetic comparison between baseball pitching and football passing
6. Common shoulder and elbow injuries in pitching
7. Implications for rehabilitation

Adult Baseball Pitching Kinematics, Kinetics (and Associated Pathological Conditions), and Electromyography During Pitching Phases

Previously defined pitching phases are shown in Figure 15-5.[5,10,19] It is important to understanding that although the entire body is used during each pitching phase, pitching kinematics, kinetics, and EMG findings are different in each phase. To maximize performance and minimize stress on the body throughout the pitching phases, an athlete's body should function as a *kinetic chain*. The kinetic chain mechanism involves neuromuscular coordination (i.e., sequential movements of body segments) in such a manner as to transfer energy up the body from the ground to the legs, hips, trunk, upper arm, forearm, hand, and finally to the ball.[20,21] The better the body works together to build force, the greater the potential velocity will be at the distal end where the object is released, and less stress will be manifested on any single body segment.

Pitching Phases[5,10,19]

- Windup
- Stride
- Arm cocking
- Arm acceleration
- Arm deceleration
- Follow-through

During overhead pitching, movements are initiated from the larger base segments, and terminate with the smaller distal segments. There are primarily seven segments that

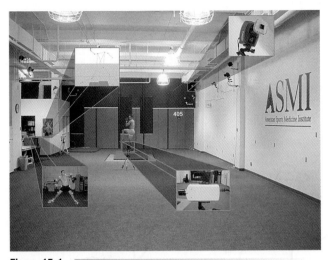

Figure 15-1

Experimental set-up for quantifying pitching biomechanics.

have both angular and linear movements during the throw: (1) lower extremity, (2) pelvis, (3) trunk, (4) shoulder girdle, (5) upper arm, (6) forearm, and (7) wrist and hand. These segments rotate about axes through the ankle, knee, hip, intervertebral, sternoclavicular, shoulder, elbow, radioulnar, wrist, and finger joints.

To rotate and accelerate a body segment, an athlete applies a torque (or "twisting force") at a given joint. In pitching, the lower extremity, pelvis, and trunk are the larger base segments that produce the muscular torques needed to accelerate the smaller distal upper extremity segments. These larger base segments have greater rotational inertia (i.e., resistance to rotation, which is a function of mass and mass distribution); thus they generate smaller angular velocities as they rotate. However, the smaller distal segments have less rotational inertia; therefore, the torque applied to these segments results in greater angular velocities.

Elastic properties of muscle and connective tissue can also affect joint torques, as they enhance recoil tendencies after a segment has been placed on stretch. As proximal segments are accelerated forward, distal segments 'lag

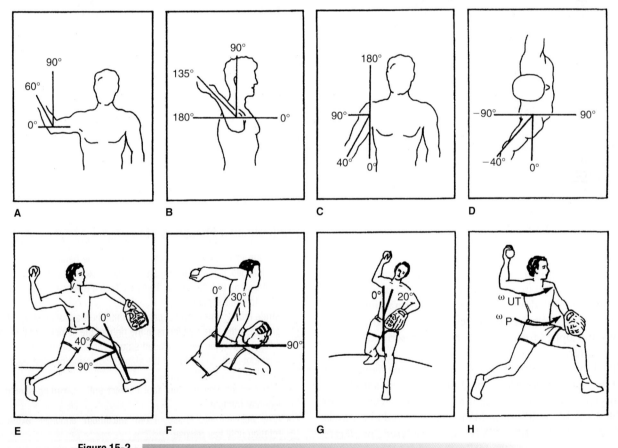

Figure 15-2

Definition of kinematic parameters. **A,** Elbow flexion. **B,** Shoulder external and internal rotation. **C,** Shoulder abduction. **D,** Shoulder horizontal adduction (positive values) and horizontal abduction (negative values). **E,** Lead knee flexion. **F,** Forward trunk tilt. **G,** Lateral trunk tilt. **H,** Pelvis angular velocity (ω_P) and upper torso angular velocity (ω_{UT}). (From Escamilla RF, Fleisig GS, Barrentine SW, et al: Kinematic comparison of throwing different types of baseball pitches, *J Appl Biomech* 14:1-23, 1998.)

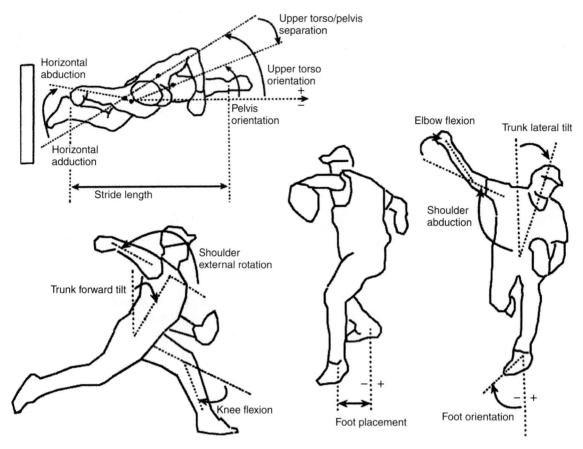

Figure 15-3

Definition of kinematic parameters (continued): Stride length, horizontal abduction and adduction, upper torso orientation, pelvis orientation, foot placement, foot orientation. (From Chu Y, Fleisig GS, Simpson KJ, et al: Biomechanical comparison between elite female and male baseball pitchers, *J Appl Biomech* 25:22-31, 2009.)

back' and are placed on stretch. An evoked stretch reflex and stored elastic energy from series and parallel elastic components—such as connective tissue, tendons, and muscles—can further enhance voluntary muscle force throughout sequential movements. This elastic energy may be lost or diminished when abnormal mechanics occur during the pitching phases, such as opening up the pelvis and upper torso prematurely, as described later in this chapter.

Pitching kinematics, kinetics, and EMG are summarized in Table 15-1, Table 15-2, and Table 15-3, respectively. To help generalize phase comparisons in muscle activity from Table 15-3, 0% to 20% of an MVIC is considered low muscle activity, 21% to 40% MVIC is considered moderate muscle activity, 41% to 60% MVIC is considered high muscle activity, and greater than 60% MVIC is considered very high muscle activity.[19] Baseball pitching kinematics, kinetics (and associated pathological conditions), and EMG findings are discussed for each pitching phase.

Definitions—Phases of Throwing

- Windup Phase: From first movement until the hands separate. As the lead leg lifts up, causing the hip and knee to flex, all the weight is placed on the stance leg. This results in a balanced position just prior to hand separation.
- Stride Phase: From hand separation until the lead foot contacts the ground. If the lead foot lands to the right of the stance foot (left for a left-handed pitcher), a closed stance results. Conversely, if the lead foot lands to the left of the stance foot (right for a left-handed pitcher), an open stance results.
- Arm Cocking Phase: From foot contact until maximum shoulder external rotation.
- Arm Acceleration Phase: From maximum shoulder external rotation until ball release.
- Arm Deceleration Phase: From ball release until maximum shoulder internal rotation (approximately zero degrees of rotation).
- Follow-Through Phase: From maximum shoulder internal rotation until a balanced position is achieved.

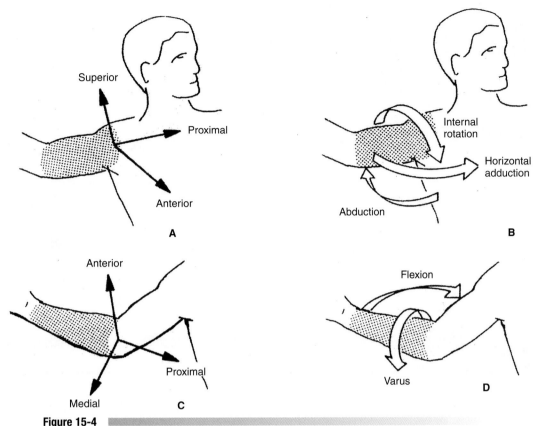

Figure 15-4

Definition of kinetic parameters. **A,** Forces applied by the trunk to the upper arm at the shoulder. **B,** Torques applied by the trunk to the upper arm about the shoulder. **C,** Forces applied by the upper arm to the forearm at the elbow. **D,** Torques applied by the upper arm to the forearm about the elbow. (From Fleisig GS, Andrews JR, Dillman CJ, Escamilla RF: Kinetics of baseball pitching with implications about injury mechanisms, *Am J Sports Med* 23:233-239, 1995.)

Windup

The objective of the windup phase is to put the thrower in a good starting position. The windup begins when the athlete initiates the first motion and ends with maximum knee lift of the stride leg. The time from when the stance foot pivots to when the knee has achieved a maximum height and the pitcher is in a balanced position is typically between 0.5 and 1.0 seconds (Figure 15-6).[5,12] During the windup, no lateral movement toward home plate should occur.

The athlete typically begins with the weight evenly distributed on both feet. The stance foot then pivots to a position parallel with the rubber (see Figure 15-5 B). The lead leg is lifted by concentric action of the hip flexors, and the lead side (left side for a right handed thrower) faces the target. The stance leg bends slightly controlled by eccentric action from the quadriceps muscle, and remains in a fairly fixed position because of isometric action of the quadriceps until a balanced position is achieved (see Figure 15-5 C). Isometric action from the hip abductors

of the stance leg prevent a downward tilting of the opposite side pelvis, while the hip extensors and flexors of the stance leg help control and stabilize the hip. The shoulders are partially flexed and abducted, and held in this position by the shoulder flexors and abductors.[22,23] In addition, elbow flexion is maintained by the elbow flexors.[24]

Table 15-3 demonstrates that the greatest activity during this phase is from the upper trapezius, serratus anterior, and anterior deltoids.[19] Concentric muscle action occurs in these muscles to upwardly rotate and elevate the scapula and abduct the shoulder as the arm is initially brought overhead, and then eccentric muscle action occurs to control downward scapular rotation and shoulder adduction as the hands are lowered to approximately chest level. The rotator cuff muscles, which have a duel function as glenohumeral joint compressors and rotators, have their lowest activity during this phase. Because upper extremity muscle activity is low,[19] shoulder and elbow forces and torques generated are also low.[5,10] Consequently, very few, if any, shoulder and elbow injuries occur during this phase.

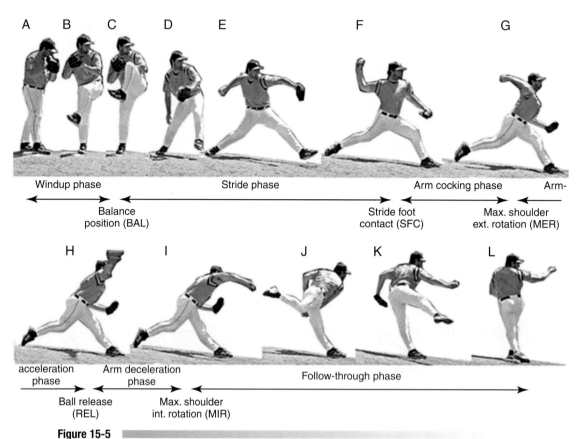

Figure 15-5

Pitching phases and key events. (From Chu Y, Fleisig GS, Simpson KJ, et al: Biomechanical comparison between elite female and male baseball pitchers, *J Appl Biomech* 25:22-31, 2009.)

Stride

The stride phase begins at the end of the windup, when the lead leg begins to fall and move toward the target and the two arms separate from each other (see Figure 15-5 D). During the stride, both arms should smoothly break down, swing apart, and then up. This phase, which ends when the lead foot first contacts the ground (see Figure 15-5 F), lasts between 0.50 and 0.75 seconds (see Figure 15-6).[7,12] There are many muscles activated, and to a higher degree, during the stride compared with the windup. Low to moderate forces, torques, and muscle activity typically occur during this phase.[10,19]

As the phase begins, the lead leg strides toward the target as the stance leg remains in contact with the ground. Eccentric action of the hip flexors controls the lowering of the lead leg. It is still unclear how much of the stride is pushing off the rubber, and how much is simply "falling" off the rubber. In either case, the forward movement is probably initiated to some degree by hip abduction, followed by knee and hip extension from the stance leg. As the lead leg falls downward and forward, the lead hip begins to externally rotate, initiated by concentric action of the hip external rotators, while the stance hip begins to internally rotate, initiated by concentric action of the hip internal rotators.

The stride length at lead foot contact is approximately 70% to 80% of the pitcher's height when measured from ankle to ankle (Figure 15-7; see Table 15-1),[24] and approximately 80% to 90% of the pitcher's height when measured from the rubber to the lead ankle (see Table 15-1 and Figure 15-7).[5,12] At foot contact, the lead foot orientation (foot angle) should be approximately 5° to 20° inward in a closed position, as shown in Figure 15-7.[25] Moreover, the lead foot placement should be approximately 0 to 25 cm closed (note that Figure 15-7 shows an open foot placement position).[25] For a right-handed pitcher, a closed-foot placement position is positioning the lead foot slightly to the right of a line from the rubber to home plate.

The placement and position of the lead foot is very important in pitching, as is lead knee flexion. The lead knee should be flexed approximately 35° to 55° at lead foot contact (see Table 15-1).[5,12] Appropriate lead knee flexion and foot placement and orientation at lead foot contact help the lead leg act as a stable brace over which the upper body can rotate during the arm-cocking and arm-acceleration phases. If the lead foot is positioned excessively closed, pelvis rotation can be impeded and the athlete ends up "throwing across the body," which may minimize the contribution of the lower body in later phases of the pitch. Conversely if the

Table 15-1

Kinematic and Temporal Measurements (Mean ± SD) During American Professional Baseball Pitching

	Kinematic Parameter ($n = 11$)	Temporal Parameter ($n = 11$)
Lead Foot Contact		
Stride length (% height)	91 ± 8	NA
Shoulder abduction (°)	88 ± 8	NA
Shoulder horizontal adduction (°)	−27 ± 10	NA
Shoulder external rotation (°)	45 ± 19	NA
Lead knee flexion (°)	49 ± 4	NA
Elbow flexion (°)	89 ± 12	NA
Arm-Cocking Phase		
Maximum pelvis angular velocity (°/s)	673 ± 48	34 ± 17% of pitch
Maximum upper torso angular velocity (°/s)	1248 ± 73	52 ± 7% of pitch
Maximum elbow flexion (°)	104 ± 12	57 ± 15% of pitch
Maximum shoulder horizontal adduction (°)	16 ± 7	NA
Maximum shoulder external rotation (°)	181 ± 8	80 ± 7% of pitch
Arm-Acceleration Phase		
Maximum elbow extension angular velocity (°/s)	2565 ± 280	90 ± 7% of pitch
Maximum shoulder internal rotation angular velocity (°/s)	7844 ± 954	100 ± 8% of pitch
Average shoulder abduction (°)	98 ± 5	NA
Instance of Ball Release		
Lead knee flexion (°)	32 ± 9	NA
Forward trunk tilt (°)	36 ± 7	NA
Lateral trunk tilt (°)	22 ± 12	NA
Elbow flexion (°)	21 ± 5	NA
Shoulder horizontal adduction (°)	8 ± 8	NA
Ball velocity (m/s)	38.0 ± 1.3	NA

From Escamilla RF, Fleisig GS, Barrentine SW, et al: Kinematic and kinetic comparisons between American and Korean professional baseball pitchers, *Sports Biomech* 1:213-228, 2002.

NA, Not applicable; *SD*, standard deviation.

Note: Temporal parameters were defined as a percentage of the pitch completed, measured from lead foot contact to the kinematic parameter shown, in which 0% corresponded to lead foot contact and 100% corresponded to the instant of ball release.

foot is positioned excessively open, pelvis rotation may occur too early. This results in improper timing, causing energy from pelvis rotation to be applied to the upper trunk prematurely.[26] Consequently, the pitcher may throw with too much "arm," because the energy generated from the pelvis rotation may be dissipated instead of being applied up the kinetic chain to the throwing arm.

Improper *foot placement* and orientation at lead foot contact can also result in increased shoulder forces during the arm-cocking phase. Fleisig[9] demonstrated that shoulder anterior force increased 3 N during the arm-cocking phase for every centimeter (approximately 0.5 inch) that foot placement was in the *open position* at lead foot contact (from Figure 15-7, the foot is positioned in an open placement position, which is to the left of a line drawn from the rubber

to home plate for a right-handed pitcher). For example, a 20-cm (8-inch) open foot placement would result in an estimated 60-N increase in shoulder anterior force. Because the mean shoulder anterior force in adult pitching is approximately 380 N during the arm cocking phase (see Table 15-2), a 60-N increase results in approximately a 15% increase in shoulder anterior force.

An *open foot orientation* (i.e., foot points out [externally rotated], which is the opposite of the illustration shown in Figure 15-7) can also result in increased shoulder anterior force. Fleisig[9] demonstrated that shoulder anterior force increased 2 N during the arm-cocking phase for every degree that the foot orientation is externally rotated at lead foot contact. For example, a 45° open foot orientation would result in an estimated 90-N increase in shoulder

Table 15-2

Kinetic Measurements (Mean ± SD) During American Professional and Collegiate Baseball Pitching

Parameter	Fleisig et al.[10] (n = 26)	Werner et al.[35] (n = 7)	Feltner and Dapena[36] (n = 8)
Arm-Cocking Phase			
Shoulder Kinetics			
Maximum anterior shear force (N)	380 ± 90		
Maximum proximal force (N)	660 ± 110		
Maximum horizontal adduction torque (Nm)	100 ± 20		110 ± 20
Maximum internal rotation torque (Nm)	67 ± 11		90 ± 20
Elbow Kinetics			
Maximum medial shear force (N)	300 ± 60		
Maximum varus torque (Nm)	64 ± 12	120	100 ± 20
Maximum elbow extension torque (Nm)		40	20 ± 10
Arm-Acceleration Phase			
Elbow Kinetics			
Maximum anterior shear force (N)	360 ± 60		320 ± 60
Maximum flexor torque (Nm)	61 ± 11	55	
Arm-Deceleration Phase			
Shoulder Kinetics			
Maximum posterior shear force (N)	400 ± 90		390 ± 240
Maximum inferior shear force (N)	310 ± 80		
Maximum proximal force (N)	1090 ± 110		860 ± 120
Maximum adduction torque (Nm)	83 ± 26		
Maximum horizontal adduction torque (Nm)	97 ± 25		
Elbow Kinetics			
Maximum anterior shear force (N)	260 ± 70		
Maximum proximal force (N)	900 ± 100	780	830 ± 80

Data from Fleisig GS, Andrews JR, Dillman CJ, Escamilla RF: Kinetics of baseball pitching with implications about injury mechanisms, *Am J Sports Med* 23:233-239, 1995; Werner SL, Fleisig GS, Dillman CJ, Andrews JR: Biomechanics of the elbow during baseball pitching, *J Orthop Sports Phys Ther* 17(6):274-278, 1993; Feltner M, Dapena J: Dynamics of the shoulder and elbow joints of the throwing arm during a baseball pitch, *Int J Sports Biomech* 2:235-259, 1986.
SD, Standard deviation.

anterior force, which is approximately a 25% increase in shoulder anterior force.

During the stride, both shoulders abduct, externally rotate, and horizontally abduct as a result of the concentric muscle action of several muscles, including the deltoids, supraspinatus, infraspinatus, teres major, serratus anterior, and upper trapezius (see Table 15-3). The supraspinatus has its highest activity during the stride phase as it works to not only abduct the shoulder but also to help compress and stabilize the glenohumeral joint.[19] The deltoids exhibit high activity during this phase to initiate and maintain the shoulder in an abducted position.[19] Moreover, the trapezius and

serratus anterior have moderate to high activity as they assist in stabilizing, upward rotating, and elevating the scapula. At lead foot contact, shoulder abduction is approximately 80° to 100° (Figure 15-8; see Table 15-1).[5,12] The shoulder abductors are responsible for abducting and holding the arm in this position, while the rotator cuff muscles help maintain proper humeral head position within the glenoid fossa.[19]

At lead foot contact, the throwing arm is positioned slightly behind the trunk in approximately 10° to 35° of horizontal abduction (see Table 15-1, Figure 15-3, and Figure 15-8).[5,25] The posterior deltoid, latissimus dorsi,

Table 15-3

Muscle Activity (Mean ± SD) During the Phases of Baseball Pitching, Expressed as % MVIC

Muscles	N	Windup	Stride	Arm-Cocking Phase	Arm-Acceleration Phase	Arm-Deceleration Phase	Follow-Through Phase
Scapular							
Upper trapezius	11	18 ± 16	64 ± 53	37 ± 29	69 ± 31	53 ± 22	14 ± 12
Middle trapezius	11	7 ± 5	43 ± 22	51 ± 24	71 ± 32	35 ± 17	15 ± 14
Lower trapezius	13	13 ± 12	39 ± 30	38 ± 29	76 ± 55	78 ± 33	25 ± 15
Serratus anterior (sixth rib)	11	14 ± 13	44 ± 35	69 ± 32	60 ± 53	51 ± 30	32 ± 18
Serratus anterior (fourth rib)	10	20 ± 20	40 ± 22	106 ± 56	50 ± 46	34 ± 7	41 ± 24
Rhomboids	11	7 ± 8	35 ± 24	41 ± 26	71 ± 35	45 ± 28	14 ± 20
Levator scapulae	11	6 ± 5	35 ± 14	72 ± 54	76 ± 28	33 ± 16	14 ± 13
Glenohumeral							
Anterior deltoid	16	15 ± 12	40 ± 20	28 ± 30	27 ± 19	47 ± 34	21 ± 16
Middle deltoid	14	9 ± 8	44 ± 19	12 ± 17	36 ± 22	59 ± 19	16 ± 13
Posterior deltoid	18	6 ± 5	42 ± 26	28 ± 27	68 ± 66	60 ± 28	13 ± 11
Supraspinatus	16	13 ± 12	60 ± 31	49 ± 29	51 ± 46	39 ± 43	10 ± 9
Infraspinatus	16	11 ± 9	30 ± 18	74 ± 34	31 ± 28	37 ± 20	20 ± 16
Teres minor	12	5 ± 6	23 ± 15	71 ± 42	54 ± 50	84 ± 52	25 ± 21
Subscapularis (lower third)	11	7 ± 9	26 ± 22	62 ± 19	56 ± 31	41 ± 23	25 ± 18
Subscapularis (upper third)	11	7 ± 8	37 ± 26	99 ± 55	115 ± 82	60 ± 36	16 ± 15
Pectoralis major	14	6 ± 6	11 ± 13	56 ± 27	54 ± 24	29 ± 18	31 ± 21
Latissimus dorsi	13	12 ± 10	33 ± 33	50 ± 37	88 ± 53	59 ± 35	24 ± 18
Elbow and Forearm							
Triceps brachii	13	4 ± 6	17 ± 17	37 ± 32	89 ± 40	54 ± 23	22 ± 18
Biceps brachii	18	8 ± 9	22 ± 14	26 ± 20	20 ± 16	44 ± 32	16 ± 14
Brachialis	13	8 ± 5	17 ± 13	18 ± 26	20 ± 22	49 ± 29	13 ± 17
Brachioradialis	13	5 ± 5	35 ± 20	31 ± 24	16 ± 12	46 ± 24	22 ± 29
Pronator teres	14	14 ± 16	18 ± 15	39 ± 28	85 ± 39	51 ± 21	21 ± 21
Supinator	13	9 ± 7	38 ± 30	54 ± 38	55 ± 31	59 ± 31	22 ± 19
Wrist and Fingers							
Extensor carpi radialis longus	13	11 ± 8	53 ± 24	72 ± 37	30 ± 20	43 ± 24	22 ± 14
Extensor carpi radialis brevis	15	17 ± 17	47 ± 26	75 ± 41	55 ± 35	43 ± 28	24 ± 19
Extensor digitorum communis	14	21 ± 17	37 ± 25	59 ± 27	35 ± 35	47 ± 25	24 ± 18
Flexor carpi radialis	12	13 ± 9	24 ± 35	47 ± 33	120 ± 66	79 ± 36	35 ± 16
Flexor digitorum superficialis	11	16 ± 6	20 ± 23	47 ± 52	80 ± 66	71 ± 32	21 ± 11
Flexor carpi ulnaris	10	8 ± 5	27 ± 18	41 ± 25	112 ± 60	77 ± 42	24 ± 18

Modified from Fleisig GS, Escamilla RF, Andrews JR: Biomechanics of throwing. In Zachazewski JE, Magee DJ, Quillen WS, editors: *Athletic injuries and rehabilitation*, p 338, Philadelphia, 1996, WB Saunders. Adapted from DiGiovine NM, Jobe FW, Pink M et al: An electromyographic analysis of the upper extremity in pitching, *J Shoulder Elbow Surg* 1:15-25, 1992.

SD, standard deviation.

Windup, From initial movement to maximum knee lift of stride leg; *stride*, from maximum knee lift of stride leg to when lead foot of stride leg initially contacts the ground; *arm-cocking phase*, from when lead foot of stride leg initially contacts the ground to maximum shoulder external rotation; *arm-acceleration phase*, from maximum shoulder external rotation to ball release; *arm-deceleration phase*, from ball release to maximum shoulder internal rotation; *follow-through phase*, from maximum shoulder internal rotation to maximum shoulder horizontal adduction.

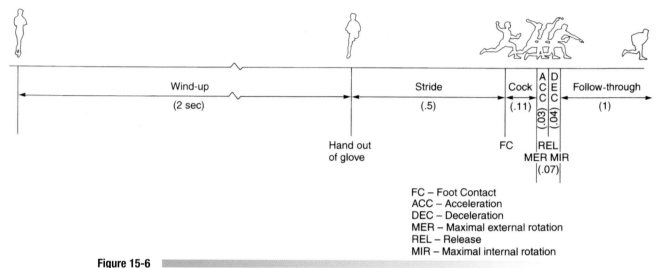

Figure 15-6

Approximate time lengths for pitching phases: wind-up, stride, arm cocking *(COCK)*, arm acceleration *(ACC)*, arm deceleration *(DEC)*, and follow-through. Events shown separating phases: hand out of glove, foot contact *(FC)*, maximum shoulder external rotation *(MER)*, ball release *(REL)*, and maximum internal rotation *(MIR)*.

teres major, and posterior rotator cuff (i.e., infraspinatus and teres minor) are responsible for horizontally abducting the shoulder, while the rhomboids and middle trapezius retract the scapula (see Table 15-3).[19] At lead foot contact, the pelvis orientation is in an open position (positive values, as shown in Figure 15-3) of approximately 20° to 30°,[25,26] and the upper torso orientation is in a closed position of approximately 10° to 20° (negative values, as shown in Figure 15-3).[25,26] The closed upper torso orientation places the trunk musculature, such as the abdominals, obliques, and paraspinal muscles, on stretch. Moreover, the horizontally abducted shoulder places the horizontal shoulder adductors on stretch. Therefore, the elastic energy stored in these muscles and associated connective tissue caused by being stretched can be transferred up the kinetic chain during the arm-cocking phase. The stretch reflex may also be evoked as these muscles are quickly stretched, summating the energy that can be transferred up the kinetic chain during the arm-cocking phase. This elastic energy may not be generated and transferred appropriately in a pitcher who does not exhibit a normal sequence of pelvis, upper torso, and shoulder spatial orientations.

A shoulder external rotation of approximately 45° to 70° at lead foot contact (Figure 15-9; see Table 15-1) causes the forearm to rotate up toward a vertical position.[5,12] If the arm is late in rotating upward, shoulder proximal (i.e., the force that resists shoulder distraction) force may increase. Fleisig[9] demonstrated for every degree the arm is late rotating up at lead foot contact, shoulder proximal force increased 1.5 N during the arm-cocking phase. For example, given a mean shoulder external rotation of 45° at lead foot contact (see Table 15-1), a shoulder external rotation

of 0° (i.e., forearm parallel with ground) at lead foot contact would result in an increase in shoulder proximal force of 70 N during arm cocking. Given a mean shoulder proximal force of 660 N during arm cocking (see Table 15-2),[10] a 70-N increase results in a 10% increase in shoulder proximal force.

Elbow flexion of the throwing arm at foot contact is approximately 80° to 100° (see Table 15-1).[5,12] Eccentric and isometric actions from the elbow extensors of the throwing arm help control elbow flexion, while the pronator muscles pronate the forearm as the shoulder abducts and externally rotates (see Table 15-3).[19] EMG has shown that the wrist and finger extensors have very high activity during the stride, causing the wrist to move from a position of slight flexion to a position of hyperextension (see Table 15-3).[19] These muscles act concentrically as they work against gravity, with the throwing palm and ball initially facing downward as the shoulder abducts.

Arm Cocking

Arm cocking begins at lead foot contact and ends at maximum shoulder external rotation, as the upper body is rotated to face the target (see Figure 15-5 F, G). This phase lasts between 0.10 to 0.15 seconds (see Figure 15-6).[7,12] High to very high forces, torques, and muscle activity typically occur during this phase.[10,19]

The quadriceps of the lead leg initially exhibit an eccentric action to decelerate knee flexion after lead foot contact, and then an isometric action to stabilize the lead leg. High activity from the gluteus maximus also occurs to help stabilize the hip.[27] This emphasizes the importance of lower

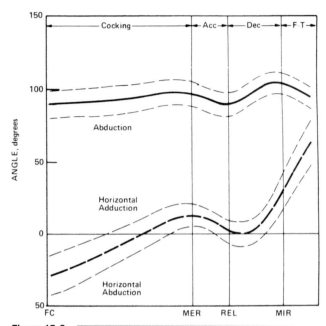

Figure 15-8
Shoulder abduction and horizontal adduction. *Acc,* Arm acceleration; *Cocking,* arm cocking; *Dec,* arm deceleration; *FC,* time of foot contact; *F-T,* follow-through; *MER,* maximum shoulder external rotation; *MIR,* maximum internal rotation; *REL,* ball release. (From Dillman CJ, Fleisig GS, Andrews JR: Biomechanics of pitching with emphasis upon shoulder kinematics, *J Orthop Sports Phys Ther* 18:402-408, 1993.)

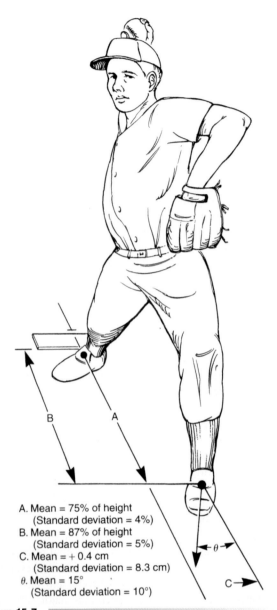

A. Mean = 75% of height
   (Standard deviation = 4%)
B. Mean = 87% of height
   (Standard deviation = 5%)
C. Mean = + 0.4 cm
   (Standard deviation = 8.3 cm)
θ. Mean = 15°
   (Standard deviation = 10°)

Figure 15-7
Stride length, foot placement, and foot orientation measurements during baseball pitching. (Modified from Dillman CJ, Fleisig GS, Andrews JR: Biomechanics of pitching with emphasis upon shoulder kinematics, *J Orthop Sports Phys Ther* 18:402-408, 1993.)

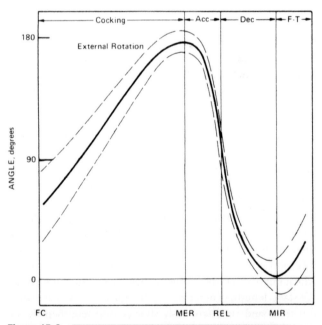

Figure 15-9
External/internal rotation. *Acc,* Arm acceleration; *Cocking,* arm cocking; *Dec,* arm deceleration; *FC,* time of foot contact; *F-T,* follow-through; *MER,* maximum shoulder external rotation; *MIR,* maximum internal rotation; *REL,* ball release. (From Dillman CJ, Fleisig GS, Andrews JR: Biomechanics of pitching with emphasis upon shoulder kinematics, *J Orthop Sports Phys Ther* 18:402-408, 1993.)

extremity strength in overhead pitching.[28] At this time, the thrower's body should be stretched out in the direction of the target. The kinetic energy that is generated from the larger lower extremity and trunk (i.e., pelvis and upper torso) segments is transferred up the body to the smaller upper extremity segments.[7,11,29] The pitching arm lags behind as the trunk rapidly rotates forward to face the hitter as both hips internally rotate. The pelvis achieves a maximum rotation of approximately 400 deg/sec to 700 deg/sec (see Table 15-3).[7,12] Maximal pelvis rotation occurs approximately 0.03 to 0.05 seconds after foot contact, which is approximately 35% of the time from lead foot contact to ball release (see Table 15-1).[12,26] As the hips rotate to face the target, the trunk rotators are placed on stretch, which will produce a recoil effect for the subsequent shoulder rotation. Shortly after the pelvis begins its rotation, the upper torso begins transverse rotation about the spinal column (see Table 15-1).[12,26] Maximum upper torso angular velocity of approximately 900 deg/sec to 1300 deg/sec (approximately twice as large as pelvis angular velocity) is achieved.[7,12] This action occurs 0.05 to 0.07 seconds after lead foot contact, which is approximately 50% of the time from lead foot contact to ball release (see Table 15-1).[12,26] The sequence of attaining maximal pelvis rotation prior to maximal upper torso rotation is important in establishing proper timing and coordination for subsequent portions of the throw, and can also affect ball velocity.[26] Moreover, pitchers who delay upper torso rotation as late as possible (typically higher-skilled professional pitchers) minimize shoulder internal rotation torque.[30] When maximum shoulder external rotation occurs, both the pelvis and the upper torso are rotated approximately 90° and now face the hitter.[26] The abdominal and oblique musculature are also placed on stretch because of the hyperextension of the lumbar trunk that occurs as the upper torso rotates. High activity from the abdominals, obliques, and lumbar paraspinal muscles have been reported during the arm-cocking phase, which emphasizes the importance of strong trunk musculature in overhead pitching.[27]

As the trunk rotates to face the target, the throwing shoulder horizontally adducts, moving from a position of 20° to 30° of horizontal abduction at lead foot contact to a position of 15° to 20° of horizontal adduction at the time of maximum shoulder external rotation (see Table 15-1 and Figure 15-8).[7,12] During this time, a maximum shoulder horizontal adduction velocity (relative to the trunk) of approximately 500 deg/sec to 650 deg/sec is obtained.[7] Consequently, high to very high shoulder muscle activity is needed to keep the arm moving with the rapidly rotating trunk (see Table 15-3),[19] as well as control the resulting shoulder external rotation, which peaks near 180° (see Figure 15-9).[7]

The multiple functions of muscles are clearly illustrated during arm cocking. For example, the pectoralis major, anterior deltoid, and subscapularis act concentrically to horizontally adduct the shoulder and act eccentrically to control shoulder external rotation. The dual function of these muscles helps maintain an appropriate length-tension relationship by simultaneously shortening and lengthening, which implies that these muscles may be maintaining a near-constant length. Therefore, some muscles that have duel functions and simultaneously shorten and lengthen as the shoulder performs dual actions at the same time may in effect be acting isometrically. Muscle actions during pitching have important implications in training and rehabilitation.

The shoulder girdle muscles (i.e., levator scapulae, serratus anterior, trapezius, rhomboids, and pectoralis minor) show high to very high activity during the arm cocking phase (see Table 15-3).[19] High activity from these muscles is needed to stabilize the scapula and properly position the scapula in relation to the horizontally adducting and rotating shoulder.[19] The scapular protractors are especially important during this phase to resist scapular retraction by eccentric and isometric action during the early part of this phase, and cause scapular protraction by concentric action during the latter part of this phase. The serratus anterior is the most active, as it provides both stabilization and protraction to the scapula (see Table 15-3).[19] During late arm cocking, the serratus anterior is important in providing upward rotation and protraction of the scapula, allowing the scapula to move with the horizontally adducting humerus. The middle trapezius, rhomboids, and levator scapulae, which oppose the scapular motion created by the serratus anterior, have also been shown to be quite active (see Table 15-3).[19] Dysfunction of the scapula muscles may adversely affect normal function of the glenohumeral muscles. Moreover, scapular muscle imbalances may lead to abnormal scapular movement and position relative to the humerus, increasing injury risk to the shoulder.

Gowan and colleagues[31] demonstrated that subscapularis activity is nearly twice as great in professional pitchers as in amateur pitchers during this phase. In contrast, muscle activity from the pectoralis major, supraspinatus, serratus anterior, and biceps brachii was approximately 50% greater in amateur pitchers than in professional pitchers. From these data, professional pitchers may exhibit better pitching efficiency, requiring less muscular activity compared with amateurs.

Glousman and colleagues[32] compared shoulder muscle activity between healthy pitchers with no pathologic, conditions of the shoulder to pitchers with chronic anterior shoulder instability caused by anterior glenoid labral tears. Pitchers diagnosed with chronic anterior instability exhibited greater muscle activity in the biceps brachii and supraspinatus and less muscle activity in the pectoralis major, subscapularis, and serratus anterior. Chronic anterior instability results in excessive stretch of the anterior capsule, which may stimulate mechanoreceptors within the capsule, resulting in excitation of the biceps brachii and supraspinatus and inhibition of the pectoralis major, subscapularis, and serratus anterior.[32] Increased activity in the biceps brachii and supraspinatus help compensate for anterior shoulder instability as these muscles enhance glenohumeral stability. Rodosky and colleagues[33] reported that as the humerus abducts and maximally externally rotates, the long head of the bicep helps enhance anterior stability of the glenohumeral joint and decreases stress placed on the inferior glenohumeral ligament. Decreased activity from the pectoralis major and subscapularis, which act eccentrically to decelerate the externally rotating shoulder, may accentuate shoulder external rotation and increase the stress on the anterior capsule.[32] Decreased activity in the serratus anterior may cause the scapula to be abnormally positioned relative to the externally rotating and horizontally adducting humerus, and a deficiency in scapular upward rotation may decrease the subacromial space and increase the risk of impingement and pathological conditions of the rotator cuff.[34]

Interestingly, infraspinatus activity was less in pitchers with chronic anterior shoulder instability than in healthy pitchers.[32] The infraspinatus helps externally rotate and compress the glenohumeral joint. It is unclear whether chronic rotator cuff insufficiency results in shoulder instability, or whether chronic shoulder instability results in rotator cuff insufficiency caused by excessive activity.

Because both the triceps brachii (long head) and biceps brachii (both heads) cross the shoulder, they both show moderate activity during this phase to enhance shoulder stabilization (see Table 15-3).[19] In contrast to the moderate triceps activity reported by DiGiovine and colleagues,[19] Werner and colleagues[35] reported that triceps activity was highest during arm cocking. Because elbow extensor torque peaks during this phase,[35,36] high eccentric contractions by the triceps brachii is needed to help control the rate of elbow flexion that occurs throughout the initial 80% to 90% of this phase.[7] High triceps activity is also needed to initiate and accelerate elbow extension, which occurs during the final 10% to 20% of this phase as the shoulder continues externally rotating.[7] Therefore, during arm cocking, the triceps initially acts eccentrically to control elbow flexion, and then acts concentrically to initiate elbow extension during the latter portion of arm cocking.

Throughout the arm-cocking phase, the shoulder remains abducted approximately 80° to 100° (see Figure 15-8). The forearm and hand segments lag behind the rapidly rotating trunk and shoulder, with the shoulder achieving a maximum external rotation of approximately 165° to 180° (see Table 15-1 and Figure 15-9). The forearm now lies in a horizontal position approximately 90° backward from its vertical position obtained at or just after lead foot contact (see Figure 15-5). Shoulder external rotation magnitude is very important in pitching, as it influences the range of motion that ensues during the rapid acceleration phase, as well as ball velocity.[28] EMG has shown that as the shoulder externally rotates, the wrist and finger extensors have very high activity, placing the wrist in a hyperextended position (see Table 15-3).[19]

High shoulder joint forces and torques are generated during the arm cocking phase (Figure 15-10, Figure 15-11, and Figure 15-12; see Table 15-2). A peak force in the proximal direction of approximately 550 to 770 N (approximately 80% body weight) occurs near maximum shoulder external rotation (see Table 15-2 and Figure 15-10), and is needed to resist distraction caused by rapid pelvis and upper torso rotation.[10] This force in the proximal direction is generated dynamically by high activity from the rotator cuff muscles (see Table 15-3), which help keep the humeral head properly centered within the glenoid fossa. The posterior cuff muscles and latissimus dorsi generate a

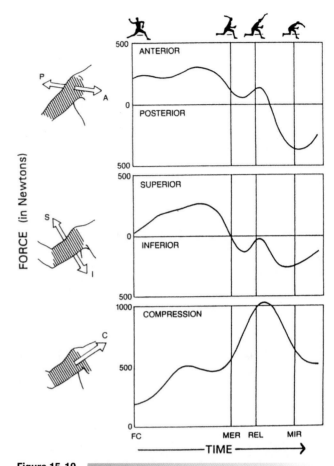

Figure 15-10

Forces applied to a pitcher's arm at the shoulder in anterior-posterior *(AP)*, superior-inferior *(SI)*, and compression (or "proximal") *(C)* directions. The instants of foot contact *(FC)*, maximum shoulder external rotation *(MER)*, ball release *(REL)*, and maximum internal rotation *(MIR)* torque are shown. (From Fleisig GS, Andrews JR, Dillman CJ, Escamilla RF: Kinetics of baseball pitching with implications about injury mechanisms, *Am J Sports Med* 23:233-239, 1995.)

posterior force to the humeral head which helps resist anterior humeral head translation, which may help unload the anterior capsule and anterior band of the inferior glenohumeral ligament.[10,23,32] The posterior cuff muscles also contribute to the extreme range of shoulder external rotation that occurs during this phase.

A peak shoulder internal rotation torque of 65 to 70 Nm is generated just before maximum shoulder external rotation (see Table 15-2, Figure 15-11, and Figure 15-12),[5,10] which implies that shoulder external rotation is progressively slowing down as maximum shoulder external rotation is approached. High to very high activity is generated by the shoulder internal rotators (see Table 15-3),[19] which act eccentrically during this phase to control the rate of shoulder external rotation. In addition, a maximum shoulder anterior force of approximately 290 to 470 N (see Table 15-2, Figure 15-10, and Figure 15-12) and a shoulder horizontal adduction torque of approximately

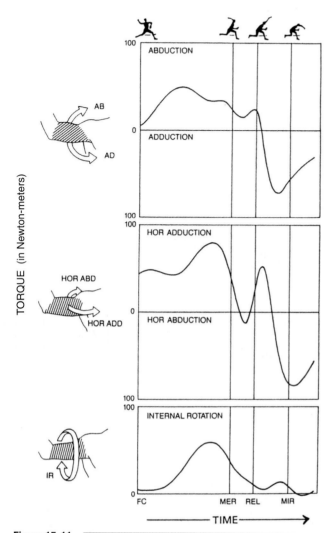

Figure 15-11

Torques applied to a pitcher's arm at the shoulder in abduction-adduction *(AB-AD)*, horizontal adduction-abduction *(HOR ABD, HOR ADD)*, and internal rotation *(IR)* directions. The instants of foot contact, maximum shoulder external rotation, ball release, and maximum internal rotation torque are shown. (From Fleisig GS, Andrews JR, Dillman CJ, Escamilla RF: Kinetics of baseball pitching with implications about injury mechanisms, *Am J Sports Med* 23: 233-239, 1995.)

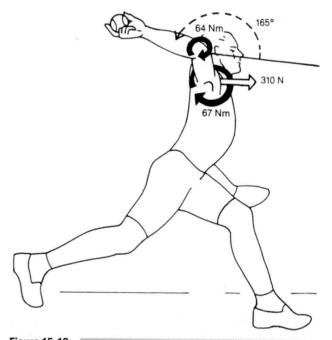

Figure 15-12

Shortly before maximum external rotation is achieved, a critical instant occurs; at this instant, a pitcher's shoulder is externally rotated 165°, and the elbow is flexed 95°. Among the loads generated at this time are 67 Nm of internal rotation torque, 310 N of anterior force at the shoulder, and 64 Nm of varus torque at the elbow. (From Fleisig GS, Andrews JR, Dillman CJ, Escamilla RF: Kinetics of baseball pitching with implications about injury mechanisms, *Am J Sports Med* 23:233-239, 1995.)

80 to 120 Nm (see Table 15-2 and Figure 15-11) is produced to resist posterior translation at the shoulder and keep the arm moving with the trunk.[10]

High elbow joint forces and torques are also generated throughout the arm-cocking phase (Figure 15-13; see Table 15-2 and Figure 15-12). Maximum elbow extensor torques of approximately 20 to 40 Nm have been reported during the arm-cocking phase (see Table 15-2 and Figure 15-13).[10,35,36] Consequently, the elbow flexors show some activity, but primarily during the middle third of the arm-cocking phase (see Table 15-3 and Figure 5-13).[19,24,35] A large valgus torque is produced at the elbow, caused in part by the large amount of shoulder external rotation (see

Figure 15-13). To resist this valgus torque, a maximum varus torque of approximately 50 to 75 Nm is generated shortly before maximum shoulder external rotation (see Figure 15-13 and Table 15-2).[10] The flexor and pronator muscle mass of the forearm display moderate to high activity which contribute to the varus torque (see Table 15-3).[19] Because these muscles originate at the medial epicondyle, they contract to help stabilize the elbow. Large tensile forces on the medial aspect of the elbow result from the valgus torque placed on the arm. Repetitive valgus loading may eventually lead to injury to the ulnar collateral ligament (UCL).[35,37] Furthermore, inflammation to the medial epicondyle or adjacent tissues may also occur, such as medial epicondylitis.[35,37]

An *in vitro* study by Morrey and An[38] demonstrated that the UCL contributed approximately 54% of the resistance to valgus stress. Assuming that the UCL produces 54% of a 64 Nm varus torque generated by elite adult pitchers,[10] the UCL would then provide 35 Nm of the varus torque. This is a similar magnitude to the 32 Nm failure load of the UCL reported by Dillman and colleagues.[39] Therefore, it initially appears that, during baseball pitching, the UCL is loaded near its maximum capacity.[10] However, in cadaveric research, the UCL ultimate strength may be considerably different compared with the *in vivo* strength of the UCL in

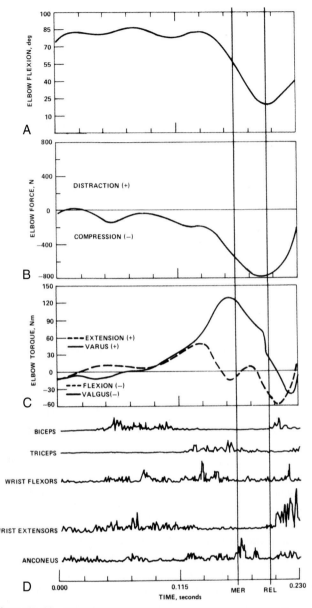

Figure 15-13 Time-matched measurements during the baseball pitch. **A,** elbow flexion, **B,** force applied at the elbow, **C,** torque applied at the elbow, and **D,** electromyographic muscle activity. (From Werner SL, Andrews JR, Fleisig GS, et al: Biomechanics of the elbow during baseball pitching, *J Orthop Sports Phys Ther* 17:274-278, 1993.)

a well-conditioned baseball pitcher, and cadaveric research does not account for muscle contributions (such as the flexor-pronator muscle mass of the forearm), which have been shown to unload strain on the UCL.[40] Muscle contraction during this phase may reduce the strain on the UCL by compressing the joint and enhancing joint stability.[35,40] For example, Buchanan and colleagues[40] reported that the muscles crossing the elbow, in particular the flexor/pronator muscle mass, may provide up to 34 Nm of varus torque with maximum muscle contractions. The

pronator teres has been found to be the largest contributor to varus torque, followed by the flexor carpi radialis and flexor carpi ulnaris.[40]

During arm cocking, a maximum elbow proximal force (i.e., a force that resists elbow distraction) of approximately 400 to 500 N is applied by the upper arm to the forearm to resist distraction of the forearm at the elbow (see Figure 15-13).[35] Valgus torque can also cause high compressive force on the lateral elbow, which can lead to lateral elbow compression injury at the radiocapitellar joint.[10] Specifically, a valgus torque can cause compression between the radial head and humeral capitellum.[35] According to the *in vitro* study by Morrey and An,[38] 33% of the varus torque needed to resist valgus torque applied by the forearm is supplied by the joint articulation. Thirty-three percent of the 64 Nm maximum varus torque generated during pitching is 21 Nm. Assuming that the distance from the axis of valgus rotation to the compression point between the radial head and the humeral capitellum is approximately 4 cm (1.6 inches), then the compressive force generated between the radius and humerus to produce 21 Nm of varus torque is approximately 500 N.[10] Muscle weakness or fatigue in the flexor-pronator muscle mass, or a loss of joint integrity on the medial side of the elbow (such as a sprained or torn UCL) can cause this compressive force to increase at the radiocapitellar joint.[35] Excessive or repetitive compressive force can result in avascular necrosis, osteochondritis dissecans, or osteochondral chip fractures.[35]

The elbow achieves a maximum flexion of approximately 80° to 90° approximately 30 ms before maximum shoulder external rotation (see Figure 15-13).[10,35] Maximum elbow flexion appears to be controlled by the triceps brachii, which shows moderate activity during the last third of the arm-cocking phase (see Table 15-3 and Figure 15-13).[19,35] This hypothesis is supported by data from Roberts,[41] who demonstrated that if the triceps brachii was paralyzed by a radial nerve block, the elbow "collapses" and continues flexing near its limit at approximately 145°.[41] This collapse is caused by an elbow flexion torque created by the rapidly rotating upper torso and arm. The triceps brachii appears to act eccentrically and then isometrically in resisting the "centripetal" elbow flexor torque that occurs during late arm cocking. Approximately 30 ms prior to maximum shoulder external rotation, the triceps brachii act concentrically to initiate elbow extension (see Figure 15-13).[10,35] The interactions between muscle activity, elbow joint force, elbow joint torque, and elbow range of motion are shown in Figure 15-13.

Arm Acceleration

Arm acceleration begins at maximum shoulder external rotation and ends at ball release (see Figure 15-5). The acceleration phase is very rapid, lasting approximately 0.03 to 0.04 seconds (see Figure 15-6).[5,12]

Moderate to high muscle activity occurs during this phase as the arm accelerates forward both linearly and angularly (see Table 15-3).[19,22,23]

Just prior to maximum shoulder external rotation, elbow extension begins (see Figure 15-13).[7] This movement is followed immediately by the onset of shoulder internal rotation.[7] The initiation of elbow extension before shoulder internal rotation allows the thrower to reduce the rotational inertia around the arm's longitudinal axis, resulting in greater internal rotation velocity. The shoulder internal rotators act concentrically to help produce an extremely high maximal internal rotation velocity of approximately 7000 deg/sec to 8000 deg/sec (see Table 15-1),[5,12] which is one of the fastest known movements in sports. Maximal shoulder internal rotation angular velocity occurs at approximately ball release.[5,12] EMG data show that the subscapularis is the most active shoulder internal rotator, followed by the latissimus dorsi and pectoralis major (see Table 15-3).[19,31,42]

As the elbow extends and the shoulder internally rotates, the trunk flexes forward from its hyperextended position to a neutral position at ball release.[5,12] High muscle activity from the trunk flexors (i.e., rectus abdominals and obliques) has been demonstrated during the acceleration phase, as well as from the lumbar paraspinal muscles and gluteus maximus.[27] Forward trunk tilt achieves a maximal angular velocity of approximately 300 deg/sec to 450 deg/sec.[5] Forward flexing of the trunk is enhanced by lead knee extension, providing a stable base around which the trunk rotates.[5] The lead knee extends approximately 15° to 20° from lead foot contact to ball release (see Table 15-1).[5] Forward trunk tilt may decrease (i.e., be more erect) if the lead knee continues flexing and moving forward, and in such cases ball velocity also is diminished.[28] This again illustrates the importance of lower extremity strength in the overhead thrower. At ball release, the trunk of a baseball pitcher is normally flexed forward from a vertical position approximately 30° to 40° (see Table 15-1).[5]

The throwing shoulder remains abducted approximately 80° to 100° throughout the acceleration phase, which implies that this is a strong position for the shoulder (see Table 15-1 and Figure 15-8).[7] This is true regardless of the type of pitching delivery (i.e., sidearm, three-quarters, or overhand) that occurs.[39] It is lateral trunk tilt, not shoulder abduction, that changes with varying types of pitching deliveries, with an overhand thrower tilting the trunk to the contralateral side (i.e., away from the throwing arm) more than a sidearm or three quarters thrower. In overhead pitching, trunk tilt normally deviates from a vertical position 20° to 30° away from the throwing arm (see Table 15-1).[7]

The rotator cuff muscles, trapezius, serratus anterior, rhomboids, and levator scapula have all demonstrated high levels of activity during the acceleration phase (see Table 15-3).[19] This implies that humeral head control and scapula stabilization are crucial during this phase. However, Gowan[31] has demonstrated that rotator cuff activity is significantly different between professional and amateur pitchers. Muscle activity in infraspinatus, teres minor, supraspinatus, and biceps were two to three times higher in amateur pitchers. In contrast, the muscle activity of the subscapularis, serratus anterior, and latissimus dorsi were greater in professional pitchers. These findings may imply that professional pitchers better coordinate the movements of their body segments to increase pitching efficiency. This improved efficiency may minimize glenohumeral instability during the arm cocking and acceleration phases, thus less rotator cuff muscle activity is needed. These findings also appear to support the results of previous EMG studies.[22,23]

Maximum elbow angular velocity during pitching occurs approximately half way through the acceleration phase, and reaches a peak of approximately 2100 deg/sec to 2400 deg/sec (see Table 15-1).[5,35] This rapid elbow extension may primarily be due to "centrifugal" force acting at the elbow as the trunk and arm rotate, for it is unlikely that the elbow extensors can shorten fast enough to generate the high angular velocity measured at the elbow.

Several studies have examined the role of the triceps brachii in extending the elbow during the acceleration phase of pitching. Roberts[41] reported that a pitcher with a paralyzed triceps caused by a differential nerve block was able to throw a ball more than 80% of the speed attained prior to the paralysis of the triceps brachii. This seems to support the concept that concentric action of the triceps brachii does not generate all of the elbow extension angular velocity, and that "centrifugal" force may be a major factor. EMG has shown high triceps brachii and anconeus activity during the arm-acceleration phase, suggesting that the triceps brachii probably initiate or contribute to the angular velocity generated during this phase.[19,22,24,35] However, these muscles may function more as arm stabilizers than as accelerators.[36]

Toyoshima and colleagues[29] compared "normal throwing" (i.e., using the entire body) to throwing using only the forearm to extend the elbow. The latter "forearm throw" involved a maximum voluntary effort to extend the elbow with the upper arm immobilized. If it is assumed that the triceps brachii shortened as fast as voluntarily possible during the "forearm throw," the resulting elbow angular velocity would be the maximum possible given a maximum triceps brachii contraction. Their results demonstrated that "normal throwing" generated approximately twice the elbow extension angular velocity as could be achieved during the "forearm throw." It was concluded that the elbow was swung open like a whip when the entire body was involved in the throw, and that the elbow extension angular velocity that occurred during "normal throwing" was due more to the rotary actions of other parts of the body, such as the hips, trunk, and shoulder, rather than by the elbow-extending capabilities of the triceps brachii. It was further stated that in "normal throwing" the elbow contributed less than 43% to ball velocity, and that a larger contribution percentage to ball velocity resulted from "body" rotations.

Ahn[43] used computer simulations and optimization techniques to compare theoretical data with experimental data during baseball pitching. His data demonstrated that hand velocity at ball release was approximately 80% of the experimental result when the resultant elbow joint torque was set to zero, approximately 95% of the experimental value when the resultant wrist joint torque was set to zero, and approximately 75% of the experimental value when both the resultant elbow and wrist joint torques were set to zero. He concluded that ball velocity at ball release was generated primarily by body segments other than the upper extremity, such as the legs, hips, and trunk.

At ball release, the elbow is almost fully extended, and positioned slightly anterior to the trunk. At release, the elbow is slightly flexed approximately 20°, and shoulder horizontal adduction is approximately 5° to 10° (see Table 15-1).

Shoulder internal rotation torque and elbow varus torque decrease during the arm acceleration phase as the arm begins rotating forward and generating speed (see Figures 15-11 and 15-13).[10] However, because the valgus stress at the elbow is near maximum at the beginning of the arm-acceleration phases when the elbow is extending, a wedging of the olecranon against the medial aspect of the trochlear groove and the olecranon fossa can occur. This impingement leads to osteophyte production at the posterior and posteromedial aspect of the olecranon tip and can cause chondromalacia and loose body formation.[4] Figure 15-13 demonstrated substantial varus torque being generated throughout the arm-cocking and arm-acceleration phases to resist this valgus stress. During arm cocking and acceleration, the elbow extends from approximately 85° to 20° of elbow flexion (see Figure 15-13).[10] This combination of elbow extension and resistance to valgus stress supports the "valgus extension overload" mechanism described by Wilson and colleagues.[4] In addition, Campbell and colleagues[44] found greater valgus torque (normalized by body weight × height) in 10-year-old pitchers than in professional pitchers at the instant of ball release, which they felt may be related to "little league" elbow syndrome in young pitchers.

A maximum elbow proximal force of approximately 800 to 900 N is produced at the elbow to prevent distraction of the forearm resulting from the "centrifugal" force acting on the forearm (see Table 15-2 and Figure 15-10).[10] In addition, a maximum elbow flexor torque of approximately 50 to 60 Nm (see Table 15-2 and Figure 15-13)[10,35] is generated by low to moderate activity from the elbow flexors.[19,24] Contraction of the elbow flexors in this phase resists elbow distraction, enhancing elbow joint stability, and also controls the rate of elbow extension. The final segment to impart force to the ball is the hand, which moves from a hyperextended wrist position at maximum shoulder external rotation to a neutral wrist position at ball release.[45] The wrist flexors (i.e., flexor carpi radialis, flexor carpi ulnaris, and flexor digitorum) have been shown to be active during this phase of pitching (see Table 15-3).[19] Their activity may initially be eccentric to slow down the hyperextending wrist at the beginning of the acceleration phase.[45] However, as they continue to fire, they concentrically contract and flex the wrist as ball release is approached.[45] In addition, the pronator teres is also active during this phase to pronate the forearm (see Table 15-3).[19] Mean ball velocity for college and professional pitchers average approximately 75 to 85 mph (see Table 15-1).[5,12]

Arm Deceleration

This arm-deceleration phase, which lasts between 0.03 to 0.05 seconds (see Figure 15-6), goes from ball release to maximum shoulder internal rotation (see Figure 15-5I). The trunk and hips continue to flex and the lead knee and throwing elbow continue to extend until almost full extension is reached. Moderate to high activity has been reported in the lumbar paraspinals, abdominal and oblique muscles, and gluteus maximus.[27] The stance leg now starts moving upward in reaction to the flexing trunk and hips. The moving of the arm forward, down, and across the body may be a natural occurrence in pitching to minimize injury potential at the elbow and shoulder.[46]

Shoulder internal rotation continues until approximately 0° (i.e., neutral position). Pronation occurs at the radioulnar joint,[45] with the pronator teres exhibiting moderate activity (see Table 15-3).[19] The biceps brachii and supinator muscles act eccentrically to decelerate the rapidly pronating forearm (see Table 15-3).[19] The biceps brachii also act eccentrically to decelerate elbow extension, as does the brachialis.

The posterior muscles of the shoulder have been identified as having a paramount role in resisting shoulder distraction and anterior subluxation forces.[5,10,22,23] These muscles include the infraspinatus, supraspinatus, teres major and minor, latissimus dorsi, and posterior deltoid. Contraction of the teres major, latissimus dorsi, and posterior deltoid also helps to decelerate the shoulder abduction that occurs during this phase. The lower trapezius, rhomboids, and serratus anterior have all been shown to be quite active, thus providing stability to the scapula (see Table 15-3).[19] The teres minor, which is often an isolated source of rotator cuff pain, has demonstrated the highest activity of all the glenohumeral muscles during this phase (see Table 15-3), providing a posterior restraint that may limit humeral head anterior translation, horizontal adduction, and shoulder internal rotation.[19,23]

Comparing professional and amateur pitchers, Gowan and colleagues[31] reported that amateur pitchers had more than twice as much muscle activity in the biceps and posterior deltoid. This may imply that amateur pitchers incur greater posterior shoulder stress compared with professional pitchers because of a less efficient throwing pattern.

The wrist and finger flexors also had very high muscle activity during this phase (see Table 15-3).[19] These muscles continue contracting and flexing the wrist. In addition, the wrist and finger extensor muscles demonstrate low to moderate activity (see Table 15-3),[19] perhaps acting eccentrically to decelerate the flexing wrist and fingers.

Large shoulder and elbow forces and torques are needed during arm deceleration to slow the rapidly moving arm (see Table 15-2).[5,10] Maximum proximal forces of approximate body weight are needed at both the elbow (800 to 1000 N) and shoulder (1000 to 1200 N) to prevent distraction at these joints (see Table 15-2, Figure 15-10, and Figure 15-13).[10,35] These shoulder and elbow proximal forces are two to three times greater than other shoulder and elbow forces generated during pitching (see Table 15-2).[10,35]

A maximum shoulder posterior force of approximately 310 to 490 N and a maximum shoulder horizontal abduction torque of approximately 75 to 125 Nm are applied to the arm to resist shoulder horizontal adduction and anterior humeral head translation (see Table 15-2 and Figure 15-11).[5,10] In addition, a maximum shoulder inferior force of approximately 230 to 390 N and a maximum shoulder adduction torque of approximately 60 to 110 Nm are produced to resist shoulder abduction and superior humeral head translation (see Table 15-2, Figure 15-10, and Figure 15-11).[5,10]

Follow-Through

The follow-through phase begins at the time of maximum shoulder internal rotation and ends when the arm completes its movement across the body and a balanced position is obtained (see Figure 15-5). This phase typically lasts approximately 1 second (see Figure 15-6). Energy in the throwing arm continues to be dissipated back through the kinetic chain. A long arc of deceleration from the throwing arm, as well as sufficient forward tilting of the trunk, allows energy to be absorbed by the large musculature of the trunk and legs. This absorption helps reduce the stress placed on the throwing arm. All the body's weight is now borne by a straight or almost-straight lead leg. The trunk and hips continue flexing and the stance leg continues moving upward (see Figure 15-5).

As in the deceleration phase, the posterior shoulder muscles continue to act eccentrically, continuing to decelerate the horizontally adducting shoulder. Shoulder joint forces and torques generated during the follow-through are generally lower than joint forces and torques generated during the deceleration phase (see Figures 15-10, 15-11).[10]

The serratus anterior has demonstrated the highest activity of all scapular rotators in this phase (see Table 15-3),[19] acting concentrically or isometrically. However, the middle trapezius and rhomboids act eccentrically to decelerate scapular protraction (see Table 15-3).[19] As in the deceleration phase, EMG has shown that the wrist and finger extensor muscles had low to moderate activity during the follow-through, implying that they act eccentrically to decelerate the flexing wrist (see Table 15-3).[19]

Kinematic and Kinetic Comparisons Among Fastball, Curveball, Slider, and Change-Up Baseball Pitches

Kinematic (Table 15-4), temporal (Table 15-5), and kinetic (Table 15-6) differences among fastball, curveball, slider, and change-up pitches in adult pitchers have been reported by Escamilla and colleagues,[7] Barrentine and colleagues,[45] and Fleisig and colleagues.[17] Fleisig and colleagues reported that 10 of 15 kinematic variables measured demonstrated significant differences among the four pitch variations (see Table 15-4). Most significant differences among pitches were at the instant of ball release. Elbow flexion, shoulder horizontal adduction, and knee flexion were greater in the change-up than in the other pitches. The curveball demonstrated greater forward and lateral trunk tilt compared with the fastball and change-up. Similarly, Escamilla and colleagues[7] also reported that approximately two thirds (18 of 26) of the kinematic variables measured demonstrated significant differences among the four pitch variations. The greatest number of kinematic differences (14 of 26) occurred between the fastball and change-up groups, which implies that disguising the change-up to look like the fastball may be challenging, but it is important for the fastball and change-up to look similar to fool the hitter. The fewest kinematic differences (2 of 26) occurred between the fastball and slider groups. The change-up group had the smallest knee and elbow flexion at lead foot contact and the greatest knee and elbow flexion at ball release. During the arm-cocking and arm-acceleration phases, peak shoulder, elbow, and trunk angular velocities were generally greatest in the fastball and slider groups and smallest in the change-up group. At ball release, the change-up group had the most upright trunk and the greatest horizontal shoulder adduction, whereas the curveball group had the most lateral trunk tilt. Understanding kinematic differences can help a pitcher select and learn different pitches, and help a batter learn how to identify different pitches.

Forearm, wrist, and hand kinematics have also been reported during different pitch types.[45,47] The forearm is supinated more during the arm-cocking phase for a curveball (approximately 40°) compared with a fastball

Table 15-4

Kinematic Comparisons (Mean ± SD) Among Fastball, Curveball, Change-Up, and Slider Baseball Pitches in Collegiate Baseball Pitchers

	Fastball ($n = 21$)	Curveball ($n = 20$)	Change-Up ($n = 19$)	Slider ($n = 6$)	Comparison*
Lead Foot Contact					
Elbow flexion (°)	86 ± 16	89 ± 13	84 ± 16	80 ± 10	*(f)
Shoulder external rotation (°)	46 ± 25	45 ± 29	45 ± 26	41 ± 27	
Lead knee flexion (°)	38 ± 9	37 ± 9	35 ± 9	34 ± 11	*(b,e)
Stride length between ankles (% height)	70 ± 4	70 ± 4	70 ± 4	71 ± 2	
Foot position (m)	−0.19 ± 0.14	−0.23 ± 0.13	−0.20 ± 0.14	−0.18 ± 0.14	*(a,f)
Foot orientation (°)	19 ± 11	19 ± 11	18 ± 9	7 ± 8	
Arm-Cocking Phase					
Maximum elbow flexion (°)	99 ± 11	101 ± 10	98 ± 12	96 ± 6	
Maximum shoulder horizontal adduction (°)	18 ± 6	19 ± 6	21 ± 6	16 ± 6	*(b,e)
Maximum shoulder external rotation (°)	178 ± 7	180 ± 6	177 ± 8	183 ± 10	
Ball Release					
Elbow flexion (°)	29 ± 6	29 ± 6	33 ± 6	26 ± 4	*(b,e,f)
Shoulder abduction (°)	96 ± 9	98 ± 10	99 ± 10	94 ± 9	*(b,d,e)
Shoulder horizontal adduction (°)	12 ± 8	14 ± 7	16 ± 7	11 ± 10	*(b,e,f)
Forward trunk tilt (°)	33 ± 7	37 ± 8	33 ± 8	36 ± 9	*(a,f)
Lateral trunk tilt (°)	23 ± 9	26 ± 10	19 ± 8	22 ± 9	*(a,d,f)
Lead knee flexion (°)	29 ± 12	32 ± 11	39 ± 12	27 ± 10	*(b,e,f)

From Fleisig GS, Kingsley DS, Loftice JW et al: Kinetic comparison among the fastball, curveball, change-up, and slider in collegiate baseball pitchers, *Am J Sports Med* 34:423-430, 2006.

SD, Standard deviation.

*Significant difference (*p* < 0.01) among fastball, curveball, and change-up. *Post-hoc* pair-wise significant difference (p < 0.05): *a,* fast versus curve; *b,* fast versus change; *c,* fast versus slider; *d,* slider versus curve; *e,* slider versus change; *f,* change versus curve

(approximately 20°), which may also may be related to the risk of injury.[47] The wrist was extended more in the fastball (approximately 40°) compared with the curveball (approximately 30°) during late cocking and acceleration phases.[47] Moreover, Barrentine and colleagues[45] and Sakurai and colleagues[47] reported that during arm cocking, peak wrist extension for the fastball and change-up was greater than for the curveball, whereas forearm supination was greater in the curveball compared with the fastball and change-up. At ball release, the forearm was in a supinated position for the curveball, but a fairly neutral position for the fastball and change-up.

Angular velocity kinematic and temporal measurements among pitch type variations are shown in Table 15-5. Ball velocity decreased significantly from fastball to slider to change-up to curveball. Although the curveball had the lowest ball velocity, it was the change-up that generated significantly less angular velocities in the upper trunk, elbow, and shoulder than the three other pitch types. There were no significant differences in any of the temporal parameters.

Kinetic measurements among pitch type variations are shown in Table 15-6. There was only one significant kinetic difference between the fastball and curveball and between the fastball and the slider. Shoulder and elbow kinetics were significantly less for the change-up compared with the fastball, curveball, and slider. This implies that the change-up may have a lower injury risk potential to the shoulder and elbow compared with the other three pitches, and the fastball and curveball may have similar injury risk potential because of the similar joint loads they produce.

Perhaps nowhere is the topic of pitch types as important as it is with youth baseball. Even though previous

Table 15-5

Magnitude and Timing of Maximum Velocity Comparisons (Mean ± SD) Among Fastball, Curveball, Change-Up, and Slider Baseball Pitches in Collegiate Baseball Pitchers

	Fastball (n = 21)	Curveball (n = 20)	Change-Up (n = 19)	Slider (n = 6)	Comparison*
Arm-Cocking Phase					
Maximum pelvis angular velocity (°/s)	596 ± 112	562 ± 91	536 ± 89	546 ± 42	*(a,b)
Maximum pelvis angular velocity (% of pitch)	30 ± 17	34 ± 17	29 ± 15	38 ± 18	
Maximum upper trunk angular velocity (°/s)	1120 ± 95	1071 ± 85	1025 ± 65	1107 ± 60	*(a,b,e,f)
Maximum upper trunk angular velocity (% of pitch)	50 ± 9	51 ± 6	49 ± 10	52 ± 9	
Arm-Acceleration Phase					
Maximum elbow extension angular velocity (°/s)	2206 ± 263	2160 ± 234	1971 ± 215	2264 ± 158	*(b,e,f)
Maximum elbow extension angular velocity (% of pitch)	93 ± 3	93 ± 3	94 ± 2	93 ± 3	
Ball velocity (m/s)	77 ± 3	64 ± 3	67 ± 3	70 ± 4	*(a,b,c,d,f)
Arm-Deceleration Phase					
Maximum shoulder internal rotation velocity (°/s)	6518 ± 946	6484 ± 857	5799 ± 778	6356 ± 721	*(b,e,f)
Maximum internal rotation velocity (% of pitch)	104 ± 2	104 ± 2	105 ± 2	102 ± 2	

From Fleisig GS, Kingsley DS, Loftice JW et al: Kinetic comparison among the fastball, curveball, change-up, and slider in collegiate baseball pitchers, *Am J Sports Med* 34:423-430, 2006.

SD, Standard deviation.

*Significant difference ($p < 0.01$) among fastball, curveball, and change-up. *Post-hoc* pair-wise significant difference (p < 0.05): *a*, fast versus curve; *b*, fast versus change; *c*, fast versus slider; *d*, slider versus curve; *e*, slider versus change; *f*, change versus curve.

Note: Timing parameters expressed on a normalized time scale as a percent of pitch, in which 0% was the time of lead foot contact and 100% was the time of ball release.

studies showed no significant increases in elbow and shoulder kinetics with breaking pitches, many people believe that curveballs are more stressful than fastballs in younger, less experienced pitchers. Dun and colleagues[48] repeated the biomechanical comparison among pitch types with adults,[7,17] but this time, youth pitchers (10 to 15 years old) were employed. Once again, elbow and shoulder forces and torques were less in the change-up than in the fastball and curveball (Table 15-7).[48] Furthermore, forces and torques for youth pitchers were significantly less during the curveball than during the fastball. These results suggest that the curveball is not a primary contributor to elbow injuries in youth pitchers. Avoiding overuse (such as high pitch counts, year-round baseball, and multiple teams) and poor mechanics are most likely more important for minimizing the risk of youth pitching injuries.[6,12,49,50]

Baseball Pitching Kinematic and Kinetic Comparisons Among Youth, High School, College, and Professional Levels

Kinematic (Table 15-8), temporal (Table 15-9), and kinetic (Table 15-10) differences among youth, high school, college, and professional pitchers have been reported by Fleisig and colleagues.[12] Of the 16 position and velocity parameters tested, six had significant differences among competition levels (see Table 15-8). Five of the six parameters that exhibited significant differences were velocity parameters, which were generally significantly greater in college and professional pitchers compared with youth and high school pitchers. No significant differences were observed in temporal measurements (see Table 15-9).

All eight kinetic parameters were significantly different among youth, high school, college, and professional

Table 15-6

Joint Kinetic Comparisons (Mean ± SD) Among Fastball, Curveball, Change-Up, and Slider Baseball Pitches in Collegiate Baseball Pitchers

	Fastball ($n = 21$)	Curveball ($n = 20$)	Change-Up ($n = 19$)	Slider ($n = 6$)	Comparison*
Arm-Cocking Phase					
Elbow varus torque (Nm)	82 ± 13	79 ± 14	71 ± 12	81 ± 5	*(b,f)
Shoulder internal rotation torque (Nm)	84 ± 13	81 ± 14	73 ± 13	84 ± 6	*(b,e,f)
Arm-Acceleration Phase					
Wrist flexion (Nm)	0.4 ± 0.3	0.5 ± 0.3	0.4 ± 0.3	0.5 ± 0.2	
Elbow flexion torque (Nm)	40 ± 9	41 ± 16	32 ± 9	37 ± 14	*(f)
Elbow proximal force (N)	988 ± 110	934 ± 103	857 ± 138	1040 ± 53	*(a,b,e,f)
Shoulder horizontal adduction torque (Nm)	111 ± 29	109 ± 20	98 ± 20	130 ± 35	*(b,c,d,e,f)
Shoulder proximal force (N)	1056 ± 157	998 ± 155	910 ± 169	1145 ± 113	*(b,d,e,f)
Arm-Deceleration Phase					
Shoulder adduction torque (Nm)	110 ± 27	116 ± 34	100 ± 23	127 ± 33	*(b,e,f)

From Fleisig GS, Kingsley DS, Loftice JW et al: Kinetic comparison among the fastball, curveball, change-up, and slider in collegiate baseball pitchers, *Am J Sports Med* 34:423-430, 2006.

SD, Standard deviation.

*Significant difference ($p < 0.01$) among fastball, curveball, and change-up. *Post-hoc* pair-wise significant difference (p < 0.05): *a*, fastball versus curveball; *b*, fastball versus change-up; *c*, fastball versus slider; *d*, slider versus curveball; *e*, slider versus change-up; *f*, change-up versus curveball.

Table 15-7

Joint Kinetic Comparisons (Mean ± SD) Among Fastball, Curveball, and Change-Up Baseball Pitches in Youth (10 to 15 Years Old) Baseball Pitchers

	Fastball ($N = 29$)	Curveball ($N = 29$)	Change-Up ($N = 29$)	Comparison* ($N = 29$)
Arm-Cocking Phase				
Elbow varus torque (Nm)	34.8 ± 15.4	31.6 ± 15.2	29.0 ± 14.8	a, b, c
Shoulder internal rotation torque (Nm)	35.2 ± 15.6	31.9 ± 15.3	29.5 ± 15	a, b, c
Arm-Acceleration Phase				
Wrist flexion torque (Nm)	1.5 ± 1.3	2.3 ± 1.9	1.1 ± 1.1	a, b, c
Forearm supination torque (Nm)	0.9 ± 0.7	1.2 ± 0.9	0.7 ± 0.6	a, b, c
Elbow flexion torque (Nm)	16.4 ± 7.2	14.4 ± 7.5	12.9 ± 6.8	a, b
Elbow proximal force (N)	461.9 ± 163.2	428.2 ± 164.3	377.9 ± 164.9	a, b, c
Shoulder horizontal adduction torque (Nm)	39.1 ± 18.7	38.2 ± 18.9	32.9 ± 17.6	b, c
Shoulder proximal force (N)	465.6 ± 169.9	433.3 ± 170.7	384.2 ± 165.4	a, b, c
Arm-Deceleration Phase				
Shoulder adduction torque (Nm)	43.1 ± 21.1	44 ± 21.2	34.7 ± 17.5	b, c

From Dun S, Loftice J, Fleisig GS et al: A biomechanical comparison of youth baseball pitches: Is the curveball potentially harmful? *Am J Sports Med* 36(4):686-692, 2008.

SD, Standard deviation.

*Significant difference ($P < 0.01$) among pitch types. *Post-hoc* pair-wise significant difference (p < 0.05): *a*, fastball versus curveball; *b*, fastball versus change-up; *c*, curveball versus change-up.

Table 15-8

Kinematic Differences (Mean ± SD) Among Youth, High School, College, and Professional Baseball Pitchers

	Youth (n = 23)	High School (n = 33)	College (n = 115)	Professional (n = 60)	Significant Differences
Lead Foot Contact					
Stride length from rubber to lead ankle (% height)	85 ± 8	85 ± 9	85 ± 6	86 ± 5	
Shoulder external rotation (°)	67 ± 28	64 ± 25	55 ± 29	58 ± 26	
Elbow flexion (°)	74 ± 17	82 ± 17	85 ± 18	87 ± 15	*b, c
Lead knee flexion (°)	43 ± 12	50 ± 9	48 ± 12	46 ± 8	
Arm-Cocking Phase					
Maximum pelvis velocity (°/s)	650 ± 110	640 ± 90	670 ± 90	620 ± 80	†f
Maximum upper torso velocity (°/s)	1180 ± 110	1130 ± 110	1190 ± 100	1200 ± 80	†a, d, e
Maximum elbow flexion (°)	95 ± 12	100 ± 14	99 ± 15	98 ± 15	
Maximum shoulder horizontal adduction (°)	21 ± 8	20 ± 9	20 ± 8	17 ± 9	
Maximum shoulder external rotation (°)	177 ± 12	174 ± 9	173 ± 10	175 ± 11	
Arm-Acceleration Phase					
Maximum elbow extension angular velocity (°/s)	2230 ± 300	2180 ± 340	2380 ± 300	2320 ± 300	†b, d, e
Maximum shoulder internal rotation angular velocity (°/s)	6900 ± 1050	6820 ± 1380	7430 ± 1270	7240 ± 1090	*d
Ball Release					
Elbow flexion (°)	24 ± 7	23 ± 7	23 ± 6	23 ± 5	
Shoulder horizontal adduction (°)	11 ± 9	10 ± 8	9 ± 9	9 ± 10	
Forward trunk tilt (°)	32 ± 9	31 ± 9	33 ± 10	33 ± 9	
Lead knee flexion (°)	36 ± 11	43 ± 13	39 ± 13	38 ± 13	
Ball speed (m/s)	28 ± 1	33 ± 2	35 ± 2	37 ± 2	†a, b, c, d, e, f

From Fleisig GS, Barrentine SW, Zheng N et al: Kinematic and kinetic comparison of baseball pitching among various levels of development, *J Biomech* 32:1371–1375, 1999.

SD, Standard deviation.

*Significant differences ($p < 0.05$) among four levels.

†Significant differences ($p < 0.01$) among four levels.

Post-hoc pair-wise significant difference ($p < 0.05$) between a, youth and high school; b, youth and college; c, youth and professional; d, high school and college; e, high school and professional; and f, college and professional.

pitchers (see Table 15-10).[12] Joint forces and torques increased with each level of competition, which may be due to greater muscle strength at each higher level. The greater shoulder and elbow angular velocities produced by higher-level pitchers were most likely caused by the greater joint forces and torques generated during the arm-cocking and arm-acceleration phases. Because joint kinetics increased with the level of competition, a higher-level pitcher may be more susceptible to arm injury. However, such relationships can only be discussed in theory, as joint kinetic values represent the combination of forces in muscles, tendons, ligaments, and bone that connect adjacent body segments. Furthermore, the magnitude of force needed to produce injury most likely varies among levels of competition, because of differences in muscle mass and tissue strength.

Although increased kinetics cannot be proven to increase the risk of injury, interpretation of the data with knowledge of functional anatomy can be insightful. For example, elbow varus torque is produced by tension in the UCL, tension in the flexor-pronator muscle mass, and compression in the radiocapitellar joint.[10,36] Thus, greater varus torque generated by college and professional pitchers (see Table 15-10) may imply that they are at higher risk for UCL tear, muscle strain,

Table 15-9

Temporal Differences (Mean ± SD) Among Youth, High School, College, and Professional Baseball Pitchers

	Youth (n = 23)	High School (n = 33)	College (n = 115)	Professional (n = 60)
Arm-Cocking Phase				
Maximum pelvis angular velocity (% of pitch)	37 ± 16	39 ± 20	34 ± 18	34 ± 14
Maximum upper torso angular velocity (% of pitch)	49 ± 11	50 ± 11	51 ± 11	52 ± 7
Maximum shoulder external rotation (% of pitch)	80 ± 6	81 ± 5	81 ± 5	81 ± 5
Arm-Acceleration Phase				
Maximum elbow angular velocity (% of pitch)	92 ± 3	91 ± 3	91 ± 5	91 ± 4
Ball release (sec)	0.150 ± 0.025	0.150 ± 0.020	0.145 ± 0.020	0.145 ± 0.015
Arm-Deceleration Phase				
Maximum shoulder internal rotation angular velocity (% of pitch)	103 ± 2	102 ± 3	102 ± 5	102 ± 4

From Fleisig GS, Barrentine SW, Zheng N et al: Kinematic and kinetic comparison of baseball pitching among various levels of development, *J Biomech* 32:1371-1375, 1999.
SD, Standard deviation.
Note: No significant differences ($p < 0.05$) found.
Note: Timing parameters expressed on a normalized time scale as a percent of pitch, in which 0% was the time of lead foot contact and 100% was the time of ball release.

Table 15-10

Kinetic Differences (Mean ± SD) Among Youth, High School, College, and Professional Baseball Pitchers

	Youth (n = 23)	High School (n = 33)	College (n = 115)	Professional (n = 60)	Significant Differences
Arm Cocking Phase					
Elbow varus torque (Nm)	28 ± 7	48 ± 13	55 ± 12	64 ± 15	†a, b, c, d, e
Shoulder internal rotation torque (Nm)	30 ± 7	51 ± 13	58 ± 12	68 ± 15	†a, b, c, d, e
Shoulder anterior force (N)	210 ± 60	290 ± 70	350 ± 70	390 ± 90	†a, b, c, d, e
Arm-Acceleration Phase					
Elbow flexion torque (Nm)	28 ± 7	45 ± 9	52 ± 11	58 ± 13	†a, b, c, d, e
Arm-Deceleration Phase					
Elbow proximal force (N)	400 ± 100	630 ± 140	770 ± 120	910 ± 140	†a, b, c, d, e
Shoulder proximal force (N)	480 ± 100	750 ± 170	910 ± 130	1070 ± 190	†a, b, c, d, e
Shoulder posterior force (N)	160 ± 70	280 ± 100	350 ± 160	390 ± 240	†a, b, c, d, e
Shoulder horizontal abduction torque (Nm)	4014	6925	8949	10985	†b, c, e, f

From Fleisig GS, Barrentine SW, Zheng N et al: Kinematic and kinetic comparison of baseball pitching among various levels of development, *J Biomech* 32:1371-1375, 1999.
SD, Standard deviation.
†Significant differences ($p < 0.01$) among four levels.
Post-hoc pair-wise significant differences ($p < 0.05$) between *a*, youth and high school; *b*, youth and college; *c*, youth and professional; *d*, high school and college; *e*, high school and professional; and *f*, college and professional.

avascular necrosis, osteochondritis dissecans, or osteochondral chip fractures.[51-54] Furthermore, the combination of varus torque and elbow extension may lead to osteophyte production at the posterior and posteromedial aspect of the olecranon tip, which can cause chondromalacia and loose body formation.[51-54] These common elbow injuries will be discussed subsequently in the "Common Elbow Injuries in Throwing" section of this chapter.

Because kinetics are different between youth and adult pitching, and because both levels throw the same size and weight ball, Fleisig and colleagues[18] investigated kinematics and kinetics of youth baseball pitching using standard and lightweight baseballs. Pitching the lightweight ball produced no difference in arm position, but greater shoulder, elbow, and ball velocities. With the lightweight ball, pitchers produced decreased kinetics, such as significant decreases in elbow varus torque and shoulder internal rotation torque. These data suggest that playing with lightweight baseballs may reduce the risk of overuse injury in the youth pitcher and also help develop arm speed. However, before introducing lightweight baseballs into the youth game, the effect of lighter, faster-pitched balls for the batters and fielders should also be considered.

Fleisig and colleagues[13] reported a trend of decreased variability in kinematics with development level. Most of the significant improvements in kinematic consistency occurred from the youth to high school level. To help increase consistency in the younger pitcher, coaches may focus on a more consistent and stable windup and stride. Particular attention can be given to the positioning of the front leg as it lands on the front of the mound. In general, increased consistency with higher levels (college and professional) is most likely a natural process acquired from experience and physical development. Furthermore, young pitchers who do not achieve consistent mechanics may not perform well enough to advance to higher levels.

Stodden and colleagues[55,56] investigated kinematic constraints associated with the acquisition of overarm throwing in boys and girls approximately 10 years of age. These authors reported that step, trunk, humerus, and forearm kinematics progress through developmental levels. The differences in kinematics between levels reflect increased energy that is generated and transferred within the system. Taking a contralateral step and increasing stride length promote increased linear and angular rotation velocities of the trunk, which provide increased energy that can be transferred to the upper extremity. To optimize the use of this increased energy, it is vital to have the humerus and forearm in proper position at stride foot contact. Higher-skilled throwers exploit certain mechanical and neuromuscular principles such as segmental inertial characteristics and the stretch-reflex mechanism, which promote increased energy generation and transfer to the ball. Increased energy trans-fer results in high distal segment angular velocities and ultimately high ball velocities.

Dun and colleagues[57] investigated the effects of age on the pitching kinematics among younger (20 years of age or younger) and older (27 years of age or older) professional baseball pitchers. Six position variables were found to be significantly different between the two groups. At the instant of lead foot contact, the older group had a shorter stride, a more closed pelvis orientation, and a more closed upper trunk orientation. The older group also produced less shoulder external rotation during the arm-cocking phase, more lead knee flexion at ball release, and less forward-trunk tilt at ball release. Ball velocity and body segment velocity variables showed no significant differences between the two groups. Thus, differences in specific pitching kinematic variables among professional baseball pitchers of different age groups were not associated with significant differences in ball velocities between groups. The current results suggest that both biological changes and technique adaptations occur during the career of a professional baseball pitcher.

Kinematic and Kinetic Comparisons Between Adult Male and Female Pitchers

Chu and colleagues[25] performed a biomechanical comparison between elite female and male baseball pitchers, reporting kinematic (Table 15-11), temporal (Table 15-12), and kinetic (Table 15-13) differences. Results demonstrated that females had general similarities to males in pitching kinematics, but there were some differences. At lead foot contact, the female pitcher had a shorter and more open stride and less separation between pelvis and upper torso orientations (see Table 15-11). The female athlete had lower peak angular velocities for throwing elbow extension and lead knee extension (see Table 15-11). At the instant of ball release, the female had greater lead knee flexion and less ball velocity (see Table 15-11). The time from lead foot contact to ball release took longer in females, and females achieved peak knee extension angular velocity later compared with males (see Table 15-12). Peak shoulder and elbow forces and torques were considerably less in females compared with males (see Table 15-13). However, it is unclear whether these lower kinetics in females equate to a lower risk of injury to the shoulder and elbow.

Kinematic and Kinetic Comparisons Between Baseball Pitching and Football Passing

Fleisig and colleagues[15] compared pitching kinematics and kinetics between 26 baseball pitchers and 26 football quarterbacks at high school and college levels. Of 21 kinematic parameters, 20 were significantly different between baseball pitchers and football passers (Table 15-14). At lead

Table 15-11

Kinematic Comparisons (Mean ± SD) Between Male and Female Adult Baseball Pitchers

Variable	Female	Male	P value
Balance Position (Windup)			
Stride knee max height (% body height)	50 ± 9	N/A	N/A
Stride knee max height (cm above stride hip)	3.2 ± 13.9	N/A	N/A
Upper torso orientation (°)	−24 ± 13	N/A	N/A
Pelvis orientation (°)	−18 ± 9	N/A	N/A
Lead Foot Contact			
Lead knee flexion (°)	50 ± 14	55 ± 16	0.464
Foot placement (m)	−0.01 ± 0.14	−0.14 ± 0.10	0.018*
Stride length (% body height)	70.3 ± 8.4	78.4 ± 6.7	0.021*
Foot orientation (°)	−5 ± 19	−5 ± 13	0.965
Upper torso orientation (°)	−5 ± 21	−17 ± 14	0.144
Upper torso/pelvis separation (°)	40 ± 15	56 ± 15	0.018*
Shoulder abduction (°)	99 ± 13	91 ± 7	0.082
Shoulder horizontal abduction (°)	19 ± 18	22 ± 15	0.666
Shoulder external rotation (°)	59 ± 35	54 ± 24	0.679
Elbow flexion (°)	98 ± 25	97 ± 26	0.897
Arm-Cocking Phase			
Maximum upper torso angular velocity (°/s)	1190 ± 240	1250 ± 20	0.519
Maximum shoulder external rotation (°)	180 ± 10	171 ± 8	0.095
Arm-Acceleration Phase			
Maximum shoulder internal rotation angular velocity (°/s)	5630 ± 1590	5850 ± 2400	0.807
Maximum shoulder horizontal adduction angular velocity (°/s)	660 ± 250	750 ± 240	0.384
Maximum elbow extension angular velocity (°/s)	2060 ± 370	2980 ± 740	0.001*
Ball Release			
Lead knee flexion (°)	62 ± 14	41 ± 19	0.008*
Lead knee extension angular velocity (°/s)	80 ± 190	320 ± 180	0.007*
Forward trunk tilt (°)	28 ± 7	33 ± 13	0.252
Lateral trunk tilt (°)	16 ± 11	25 ± 10	0.061
Overall upper torso rotation (°)	118 ± 25	121 ± 19	0.648
Shoulder abduction (°)	89 ± 6	90 ± 10	0.750
Shoulder horizontal adduction (°)	9 ± 8	7 ± 15	0.688
Shoulder external rotation (°)	136 ± 14	122 ± 29	0.139
Elbow flexion (°)	31 ± 10	27 ± 7	0.247
Ball velocity (m/s)	26.8 ± 1.5	36.3 ± 1.8	<0.001*

From Chu Y, Fleisig GS, Simpson KJ et al: Biomechanical comparison between elite female and male baseball pitchers, *J Appl Biomech* 25:22-31, 2009.

N/A, Not available; *SD,* standard deviation.

*Female and male groups significantly different ($p < 0.05$).

Table 15-12

Temporal Comparisons (Mean ± SD) Between Male and Female Adult Baseball Pitchers

Variables	Female	Male	p value
Time from lead foot contact to ball release (seconds)	0.163 ± 0.026	0.141 ± 0.021	0.048*
Arm-Cocking Phase			
Maximum pelvis angular velocity (% of pitch)	33 ± 26	33 ± 32	0.997
Maximum elbow flexion (% of pitch)	39 ± 18	30 ± 22	0.274
Maximum upper torso angular velocity (% of pitch)	56 ± 17	42 ± 19	0.075
Maximum shoulder external rotation (% of pitch)	76 ± 10	81 ± 5	0.169
Arm-Acceleration Phase			
Maximum elbow extension angular velocity (% of pitch)	95 ± 5	93 ± 4	0.478
Maximum forward trunk angular velocity (% of pitch)	104 ± 27	89 ± 12	0.111
Maximum shoulder internal rotation angular velocity (% of pitch)	107 ± 4	105 ± 7	0.309
Arm-Deceleration Phase			
Maximum knee extension angular velocity (% of pitch)	120 ± 24	98 ± 26	0.050*

From Chu Y, Fleisig GS, Simpson KJ et al: Biomechanical comparison between elite female and male baseball pitchers, *J Appl Biomech* 25:22-31, 2009.
SD, Standard deviation.
*Female and male groups significantly different ($p < 0.05$).
Note: Timing parameters expressed on a normalized time scale as a percent of pitch, in which 0% was the time of lead foot contact and 100% was the time of ball release.

Table 15-13

Kinetic Comparisons (Mean ± SD) Between Female Adult Baseball Pitchers and Previously Reported Values for Male Adult Baseball Pitchers

Variables	Female	Fleisig et al.[10a]	Fleisig et al.[12b]	Escamilla et al.[5c]
Arm-Cocking Phase				
Maximum elbow varus torque (Nm)	46 ± 9	64 ± 12	55 ± 12	
Maximum elbow varus torque (% body weight × body height)	4 ± 1			3.9 ± 0.7
Maximum shoulder internal rotation torque (Nm)	48 ± 11	67 ± 11	58 ± 12	
Maximum shoulder internal rotation torque (% body weight × body height)	4 ± 1			4.1 ± 0.7
Arm-Deceleration Phase				
Maximum elbow proximal force (N)	453 ± 60	900 ± 100		
Maximum elbow proximal force (% body weight)	64 ± 10			
Maximum shoulder proximal force (N)	510 ± 108	1090 ± 110	910 ± 130	
Maximum shoulder proximal force (% body weight)	73 ± 25			134.5 ± 17.2

From Chu Y, Fleisig GS, Simpson KJ et al: Biomechanical comparison between elite female and male baseball pitchers, *J Appl Biomech* 25:22-31, 2009.
SD, Standard deviation.
[a]26 professional and college participants.
[b]115 college participants.
[c]11 professional participants.

Table 15-14

Kinematic Differences (Mean ± SD) Between Baseball Pitching and Football Passing

Parameter	Pitching (n = 26)	Passing (n = 26)
Lead Foot Contact		
Stride length between ankles (% height)[†]	74 ± 5	61 ± 8
Shoulder abduction (°)	93 ± 12	96 ± 13
Shoulder horizontal adduction (°)[†]	−17 ± 12	7 ± 15
Shoulder external rotation (°)*	67 ± 24	90 ± 33
Elbow flexion (°)[†]	98 ± 18	77 ± 12
Lead knee flexion (°)[†]	51 ± 11	39 ± 11
Arm-Cocking Phase		
Maximum pelvis angular velocity (°/s)[†]	660 ± 80	500 ± 110
Maximum shoulder horizontal adduction (°)[†]	18 ± 8	32 ± 9
Maximum upper torso angular velocity (°/s)[†]	1170 ± 100	950 ± 130
Maximum elbow flexion (°)[†]	100 ± 13	113 ± 10
Maximum shoulder external rotation (°)*	173 ± 10	164 ± 12
Arm-Acceleration Phase		
Maximum elbow extension angular velocity (°/s)[†]	2340 ± 300	1760 ± 210
Average shoulder abduction (°)[†]	93 ± 9	108 ± 8
Ball Release		
Ball velocity (m/s)[†]	35 ± 3	21 ± 2
Shoulder horizontal adduction (°)[†]	7 ± 7	26 ± 9
Elbow flexion (°)[†]	22 ± 6	36 ± 8
Forward trunk tilt (°)*	32 ± 10	25 ± 8
Lateral trunk tilt (°)[†]	124 ± 9	116 ± 5
Lead knee flexion (°)[†]	40 ± 12	28 ± 9
Arm-Deceleration Phase		
Maximum shoulder internal rotation angular velocity (°/s)[†]	7550 ± 1360	4950 ± 1080
Minimum elbow flexion (°)[†]	18 ± 5	24 ± 5

From Fleisig GS, Escamilla RF, Andrews JR et al: Kinematic and kinetic comparison between baseball pitching and football passing, *J Appl Biomech* 12: 207-224, 1996.
SD, Standard deviation.
*$p < 0.01$.
[†]$p < 0.001$.

foot contact, baseball pitchers had a greater stride length, shoulder horizontal abduction, elbow flexion, and lead knee flexion, and less shoulder external rotation, compared with football passers. These data imply that, compared with baseball pitchers, football passers rotate their arms up quicker, lead with the elbow, and flex the lead knee and elbow less.

During the arm-cocking phase, baseball pitchers rotated their pelvis and upper torso with greater angular velocity and had greater shoulder external rotation, whereas football passers had greater shoulder horizontal adduction and elbow flexion (see Table 15-14).[15] Moreover, compared with passers, maximum pelvis and upper torso angular velocities in pitchers occurred earlier in arm cocking and maximum shoulder external rotation occurred later in arm cocking (Table 15-15). During the arm-acceleration phase, baseball pitchers had greater elbow extension angular velocity and less shoulder abduction compared with football passers (see Table 15-14). Compared with passers, maximum elbow extension angular velocity in pitchers occurred earlier in the arm acceleration phase (see Table 15-15). At ball release, baseball

Table 15-15

Temporal Comparisons (Mean ± SD) Between Baseball Pitching and Football Passing

Variables	Pitching ($n = 26$)	Passing ($n = 26$)
Time from lead foot contact to ball release (seconds)*	0.145 ± 0.022	0.207 ± 0.037
Arm-Cocking Phase		
Maximum pelvis angular velocity (% of pitch)*	35 ± 19	56 ± 12
Maximum shoulder horizontal adduction (% of pitch)	49 ± 17	55 ± 21
Maximum upper torso angular velocity (% of pitch)*	50 ± 8	62 ± 10
Maximum elbow flexion (% of pitch)	53 ± 14	53 ± 11
Maximum shoulder external rotation (% of pitch)†	81 ± 4	71 ± 14
Arm-Acceleration Phase		
Maximum elbow extension angular velocity (% of pitch)*	92 ± 3	95 ± 2
Maximum forward trunk angular velocity (% of pitch)*	99 ± 16	76 ± 14
Arm-Deceleration Phase		
Maximum shoulder internal rotation angular velocity (% of pitch)*	103 ± 2	106 ± 2
Minimum elbow flexion (% of pitch)*	103 ± 2	107 ± 3

From Fleisig GS, Escamilla RF, Andrews JR et al: Kinematic and kinetic comparison between baseball pitching and football passing, *J Appl Biomech* 12:207–224, 1996.

SD, Standard deviation.

*$p < 0.001$.

†$p < 0.01$.

Note: Timing parameters expressed on a normalized time scale as a percent of pitch, where 0% was the time of lead foot contact and 100% was the time of ball release.

pitchers had greater ball velocity, lateral trunk tilt, forward trunk tilt, and lead knee flexion, whereas football passers had greater shoulder horizontal adduction and elbow flexion (see Table 15-14). Just after ball release, during arm deceleration, baseball pitchers had greater shoulder internal rotation angular velocity and less elbow flexion. Maximum shoulder internal rotation angular velocity and minimum elbow flexion occurred earlier in pitchers compared with passers.

Of 11 kinetic variables, only three demonstrated significant differences (Table 15-16).[15] The lower incidence of rotator cuff injury in passers compared with pitchers may be related to less shoulder proximal force in passers (660 ± 120 N) compared with pitchers (850 ± 140 N). The risk of subacromial impingement may also be less in football passers compared with pitchers because they do not externally rotate their shoulders as much during the arm-cocking stage (see Table 15-14). The lower incidence of elbow injury in passers compared with pitchers may be related to less elbow proximal force in passers (620 ± 110 N) compared with pitchers (710 ± 110 N).

The kinetic data (see Table 15-16) show that football passing did not produce higher forces or torques compared with baseball pitching.[15] One explanation for why the incidence of shoulder and elbow injuries is lower for quarterbacks than pitchers is that passers exhibit less motion in their legs, pelvis, and upper torso compared with pitchers. Another justification for the lower incidence of injury in passers is that quarterbacks throw much less than pitchers, play in fewer games, and have a greater rest period between games.

Common Shoulder Injuries in Pitching

Pathological conditions in the thrower's shoulder are often complex and multifaceted, involving the rotator cuff, the labrum-biceps complex, and the capsule. Both static (capsulolabral complex) and dynamic stabilizers (rotator cuff and scapular rotators) control the movement and stability of the humeral head within the glenoid cavity. A summary of pathomechanics associated with increased shoulder kinetics and decreased ball velocity is shown in Table 15-17.

Internal impingement, in which the supraspinatus or infraspinatus tendons impinge on the posterosuperior labrum, is one of the most common soft tissue injuries seen in throwers.[58,59] With a capsular injury, internal impingement may result secondary to excessive anterior humeral head translation. Contributing factors to internal impingement include

Table 15-16

Kinetic Differences (Mean ± SD) Between Baseball Pitching and Football Passing

Parameter	Pitching ($n = 26$)	Passing ($n = 26$)
Arm-Cocking Phase		
Maximum shoulder anterior force (N)	310 ± 50	350 ± 80
Maximum shoulder horizontal adduction torque (Nm)	82 ± 13	78 ± 19
Maximum shoulder internal rotation torque (Nm)	54 ± 10	54 ± 13
Maximum elbow medial force (N)	260 ± 50	280 ± 60
Maximum elbow varus torque (Nm)	51 ± 10	54 ± 13
Arm-Acceleration Phase		
Maximum elbow flexion torque (Nm)	47 ± 9	41 ± 8
Arm-Deceleration Phase		
Maximum shoulder proximal force (N)*	850 ± 140	660 ± 120
Maximum elbow proximal force (N)†	710 ± 110	620 ± 110
Maximum shoulder adduction torque (Nm)*	79 ± 23	58 ± 34
Follow-Through Phase		
Maximum shoulder posterior force (N)	310 ± 110	240 ± 120
Maximum shoulder horizontal abduction torque (Nm)	85 ± 51	80 ± 34

From Fleisig GS, Escamilla RF, Andrews JR et al: Kinematic and kinetic comparison between baseball pitching and football passing, *J Appl Biomech* 12:207-224, 1996.

SD, Standard deviation.

*$p < 0.01$.

†$p < 0.001$.

excessive shoulder external rotation, internal rotation deficit caused by posterior cuff or capsule tightness, anterior capsule-labrum injuries, excessive shoulder horizontal abduction, muscle imbalances, and scapular dyskinesis.[58,60,61] A protective factor in helping to prevent internal impingement is humeral head and glenoid retroversion, which is believed to occur by throwing in childhood.[62,63]

Shoulder Injuries in Pitchers

- Posterior internal impingement
- Anterior instability
- Strain of posterior shoulder muscles
- Superior labrum anterior-posterior (SLAP) tears
- Stress fracture of proximal humeral physis
- Spiral humeral fractures
- Suprascapular nerve entrapment
- Quadrilateral space syndrome
- Snapping scapula

External (subacromial) impingement, in which the bursal surface of the supraspinatus tendon, the subacromial bursa, and the long biceps tendon impinge on the undersurface of the acromion, is a common soft tissue injury seen in older throwers, but typically not common in younger throwers.[10,34,64] The rotator cuff muscles generate shear and compressive forces to depress, rotate, and center the humeral head within the glenoid fossa. Consequently, they help prevent superior translation of the humeral head caused largely by deltoid activity. When these muscles function abnormally, such as when a partial or complete rotator cuff thickness tear occurs, superior translation of the humeral head may occur as the result of muscle fatigue and weakness, causing the bursal surface of the supraspinatus, the subacromial bursa, and the long biceps tendon to abrade against the undersurface of the acromion.

Anterior shoulder instability is also common in throwers, especially baseball pitchers. During shoulder external rotation, the anterior capsule and anterior band of the inferior glenohumeral ligament are stretched and help resist humeral head anterior translation. Repeated stretching of the anterior capsule can further stress the joint, leading to chronic inflammation and damage to the anterior capsular structures and anterior labrum. Laxity within the joint can exacerbate this problem, resulting in further anterior shoulder instability. Muscle imbalances, such as overpowering anterior shoulder muscles and weak posterior shoulder

Table 15-17

Summary of Pathomechanics Associated With Increased Kinetics and Decreased Ball Velocity

Phase/Event	Proper Mechanics	Pathomechanics → Consequences
Windup	Lift front leg	
Maximum knee height	Pitcher is balanced	
Stride	Front leg goes down and forward Arms separate, swing down, and up	↓ Push off rubber, ↓ ball velocity
Lead foot contact	Front foot is planted slightly to third-base side (for a right-handed pitcher) Front foot is pointed slightly inward Shoulder is abducted approximately 90°, with approximately 60° of external rotation	↓ Stride length, ↓ ball velocity Front foot open (position or angle) ↑ Shoulder and elbow force Improper shoulder external rotation ↑ Shoulder and elbow kinetics Excessive shoulder external rotation ↓ ball velocity ↓ Shoulder horizontal abduction ↓ ball velocity
Arm-cocking phase	Pelvis rotation, followed by upper trunk rotation Shoulder externally rotates, and trunk arches	Early pelvis rotation ↓ ball velocity Late pelvis rotation ↑ shoulder and elbow kinetics ↓ Pelvis rotation velocity ↓ ball velocity Poor timing between pelvis rotation and upper trunk rotation ↓ ball velocityPoor timing between pelvis rotation and upper trunk rotation ↑ shoulder internal rotation torque
Maximum shoulder external rotation	Shoulder external rotation is approximately 180° Elbow flexion is approximately 90°	↓ Shoulder external rotation ↑ ball velocity Excessive shoulder horizontal adduction and elbow flexion ↑ shoulder kinetics

Table 15-17

Summary of Pathomechanics Associated With Increased Kinetics and Decreased Ball Velocity—cont'd

Phase/Event	Proper Mechanics	Pathomechanics → Consequences
Arm-acceleration phase	Elbow extends, followed by shoulder internal rotation Front knee extends	
Ball release 	The throwing shoulder is abducted approximately 90°	↑ Knee extension velocity ↑ ball velocity Improper shoulder abduction ↓ ball velocity Improper shoulder abduction ↑ elbow varus torque ↓ Forward trunk tilt ↓ ball velocity
Arm-deceleration phase	Shoulder internal rotation and front knee extension continue Trunk tilts forward	
Maximum internal rotation 	Shoulder external rotation is approximately 0°	
Follow-through phase	Arm crosses in front of body Trunk flexes forward	

From Fortenbaugh D, Fleisig GS, Andrews JR: Baseball pitching biomechanics in relation to injury risk and performance, *Sports Health: A Multidisciplinary Approach* 1:314-320, 2009.
↓ Decreased; ↑ increased.

muscles, can also contribute to the humeral head being pulled forward within the glenoid.

Because of the large eccentric loads on the posterior shoulder muscles during the deceleration and follow-through phases, these muscles are frequently injured during pitching. Most rotator cuff injuries in pitching are partial-thickness undersurface tears, which do not heal well.[10] If the rotator cuff muscles and other posterior shoulder muscles are weak, fatigued, or injured, the humeral head will distract and anteriorly translate out of the glenoid fossa.

This action can place abnormal stress on the posterior capsule and lead to "posterior capsule syndrome."[3] Repeated abrasions of the posteroinferior capsule structures has been described as creating an exostosis of the posteroinferior glenoid.[58]

Although the biceps has been considered to function primarily at the elbow, the biceps also contributes to shoulder abduction and flexion, especially when the shoulder is externally rotated and the forearm is supinated. Biceps activity, especially the long head, has been shown to be a significant contributor to shoulder abduction and flexion in a compromised shoulder, such as a torn rotator cuff.[32] Because the biceps long head originates at the anterosuperior glenoid labrum, its contraction could abnormally stress this portion of the labrum. This is especially true in pitching, because the biceps has been shown to eccentrically contract in decelerating the rapidly extending elbow. Andrews and colleagues[2,65] arthroscopically observed 73 throwing athletes who had labrum tears in their throwing shoulders. The long head of the biceps tendon appeared to have pulled the anterosuperior portion of the labrum off the glenoid, resulting in a superior labrum tear that is anterior to posterior in direction. This observation was verified arthroscopically by electrically stimulating the biceps muscle. When stimulated, the tendinous portion became taut near its attachment to the labrum, and actually lifted the labrum off the glenoid.[2,65]

Several other injuries may occur during overhead pitching. In youth, a common overuse injury is "little league shoulder,"[66] which involves a stress fracture of the proximal humeral physis. This can be caused by large rotational forces (torques) applied to humerus during shoulder external and internal rotation, resulting in humeral torsion. Excessive pitching during a game or a season, poor pitching mechanics, or throwing high-stress pitches (e.g., a curveball or slider) can exacerbate or cause little league shoulder.

Spiral fractures of the humeral shaft occasionally occurs in overhead pitching.[67] These injuries occur because of large rotational torques applied to the humerus.[5,68] They are more common in adults than children, and more common with excessive pitching and overuse. Spiral fractures are more common in throwing maximum-effort fastball, curveball, and slider pitches because of the greater shoulder internal rotation torques generated by these pitches.[17] The fracture occurs during the arm-cocking or arm-acceleration phases, and is associated with improper warmup and deconditioned pitchers. Moreover, they are common in older (> 30) recreational pitchers who pitch infrequently, and seldom occur in younger, well-conditioned pitchers.

Suprascapular nerve entrapment can occur in pitchers as the suprascapular nerve becomes entrapped in the suprascapular or spinoglenoid notches, resulting in atrophy and weakness in supraspinatus or infraspinatus muscles, and possible posterolateral shoulder pain if the entrapment occurs in the suprascapular notch.[69] If the entrapment occurs at the spinoglenoid notch, isolated atrophy occurs in the infraspinatus. It is believed to occur in approximately 5% of major league starting pitchers at the end of the season.[69] When pitching, the suprascapular nerve is susceptible to compressive and tensile loads because of its relatively fixed position under the rotator cuff and ligaments. Because the spinoglenoid ligament inserts into the posterior glenohumeral capsule, it tightens with horizontal adduction and internal rotation, thus compressing the nerve. Stretching of the nerve may be exacerbated by rapid scapular protraction combined with infraspinatus and supraspinatus contractions, which pull the nerve medially as it is tethered laterally.

Quadrilateral space syndrome can occur when the axillary nerve and posterior humeral circumflex artery are entrapped in the quadrilateral space between the teres minor above, teres major below, long triceps brachii head medially, and humerus laterally.[70] This entrapment can result in atrophy of the teres minor and deltoid with concomitant loss of shoulder abduction and external rotation strength, as well as diminished sensation over lateral deltoid. Tenderness and pain in quadrilateral space, especially during late arm cocking, may also occur.

A "snapping scapula" can also occur from repetitive pitching, especially during the deceleration and follow-through phases.[71,72] This pathological condition, which can be quite painful, is the result of an inflamed bursa located beneath the medial border of the scapula. This bursa provides lubrication as the scapula moves in relation to the thorax. During repeated and overuse conditions, bursitis can develop, resulting in both pain and a "snapping" sound as the swollen tissue impinges upon the thorax. A good follow-through can help minimize injury potential of the shoulder. A long arm arc of deceleration and sufficient forward trunk tilt (trunk approximately in a horizontal position) may help minimize stress on the shoulder complex.

Common Elbow Injuries in Pitching

Musculotendinous, joint, and neural injuries are the most common problems that occur in the throwing elbow.[51-54] A summary of pathomechanics associated with increased elbow kinetics and decreased ball velocity is shown in Table 15-17.[73] Pathological conditions of the elbow caused by pitching can be categorized into four areas.

Medial Compartment

Medial musculotendinous injuries are quite common, especially involving the muscles that originate at the medial epicondyle (medial epicondylitis).[51-54] These muscles, which are collectively referred to as the *flexor/pronator mass*, are composed primarily of the pronator teres, flexor carpi radialis, flexor digitorum superficialis, and flexor carpi ulnaris. During pitching, pain and tenderness can occur in the medial epicondyle region.[51-54] The flexor-pronator mass is loaded as a result of tensile force during the late arm-cocking and early acceleration phases of pitching. These dynamic contractile structures must apply a varus torque to the forearm to resist the valgus stress created by the throwing motion.

Elbow Injuries in Pitchers

- Medial epicondylitis
- Ulnar collateral ligament
- Ulnar neuritis
- Lateral epicondylitis
- Osteochondrosis of radiocapitellar joint
- Stress fracture of olecranon
- Hypertrophy of olecranon
- Loose bodies
- Bicipital tendinitis
- Radical nerve entrapment
- Pronator teres (median nerve) entrapment

Capsular and ligamentous tensile stress on the ulna and humerus may lead to osteophyte formation.[51-54] These osteophytes usually form distally at the ulnar attachment. Because the ulnar nerve lies near the medial capsule and UCL, these osteophytes may compress the nerve.[51-54] Furthermore, the repetitive valgus stress of the medial elbow during pitching can excessively stretch the ulnar nerve, contributing to ulnar neuritis.[51-54] The UCL, which also originates at the medial epicondyle, helps reinforce the medial elbow capsule, but may tear if excessively loaded.[51-54] The UCL is most susceptible to injury when the flexor-pronator muscle mass weakens and fatigues, or when repetitive pitching and overuse occurs. Moreover, Matsuo and Fleisig[74] reported that excessive or not enough shoulder abduction or lateral trunk tilt can increase elbow varus torque, increasing the risk of UCL injuries.

Lateral Compartment

Lateral musculotendinous injuries involve the wrist and finger extension musculature (supinator-extension muscle mass). These muscles, which originate at or near the lateral epicondyle, can cause lateral epicondylitis when abnormally stressed. These muscles are rapidly stretched and eccentrically loaded during the deceleration and follow-through phases in pitching.

Whereas the medial elbow is subject to high tensile stresses, the radiocapitellar joint is subject to high compressive forces.[51-54] These compressive forces occur between the radial head and the humeral capitellum. Degenerative changes in the articular cartilage of these structures can result from the repetitive compressive at the radiocapitellar joint. Consequently, loose body formations can occur as the articular cartilage fragments break off into the joint. Osteochondrosis of the radiocapitellar joint may also occur in preadolescent athletes before physeal closure.[51-54]

Posterior Compartment

The posterior region of the elbow is injured more than the anterior region, but less than the medial and lateral regions.[51-54] Because of repetitive extension of the elbow during pitching, the olecranon is continually and forcefully driven into the olecranon fossa.[51-54] Consequently, a stress fracture of the olecranon or a hypertrophic olecranon may develop.[51-54] Valgus stress that occurs during late arm cocking and early acceleration may exacerbate the problem by forcing the olecranon against the medial olecranon fossa (i.e., valgus extension overload).[4] Because of the repetitive trauma of the olecranon against the olecranon fossa, osteophytes may form and migrate anteriorly.[51-54] Loose bodies can also arise as the result of a shearing off of osteocartilaginous fragments. The triceps tendon can also be injured (triceps tendinitis) at its insertion on the olecranon. Furthermore, it may partially avulse off the olecranon.

Anterior Compartment

The anterior elbow is the least commonly injured region; however, anterior capsular sprains, flexor-pronator strains, bicipital tendinitis, and intra-articular loose bodies are problems that may occur in the anterior elbow.[51-54] In the throwing athlete, these pathological conditions can lead to incomplete elbow extension, especially during the acceleration phase of the throw.

Anterior pain can also result from neural injuries, such as radial nerve entrapment. Repetitive supination and pronation movements, such as those occurring during the throwing motion, can lead to entrapment.[51-54] For example, anterior pain can occur when the median nerve is entrapped between the two heads of the pronator teres. This is referred to as *pronator teres syndrome,* and occurs because of repetitive forearm pronation, which is seen during pitching.[51-54]

Implications for Rehabilitation

Because of the involvement of the full body in the pitching motion, it is important to condition the musculature of both the upper and lower body to maximize performance and minimize the risk of injury. The principle of the kinetic chain implies that weakness in any segment may result in a deficiency in performance. When an athlete with a deficiency in one section of the kinetic chain tries to compensate by altering mechanics, increased demands on other segments can result in injury.

It is especially important to evaluate a thrower's mechanics after rehabilitation from an injury. Improper mechanics may be related to either the cause of the initial injury or modifications resulting from the initial injury. In either case, improper mechanics should be corrected to prevent reinjury.

Clinical Essentials in Rehabilitation Pitchers

- Joint flexibility
- Pitching—specific high speed controlled motion
- Eccentric loading
- Throwing program

Joint flexibility and pitching-specific, high-speed, controlled motion are essential, and should be emphasized in a rehabilitation program for pitchers. Constrained exercises that include limited ranges of motion and joint speeds are useful early in rehabilitation, but have certain limitations. Another important concept in the design and selection of a rehabilitation program for the throwing athlete is that joint loads in pitching are largely eccentric. These eccentric loads occur primarily in the arm-cocking, arm-acceleration, and arm-deceleration phases. Exercises emphasizing eccentric contractions should therefore be performed with range of motions and speeds of movement specific to pitching. The best exercise for pitching rehabilitation is throwing. Under the guidance of a sport physical therapist or athletic trainer, a pitcher should include throwing in rehabilitation as soon as possible. An interval throwing program or other moderate throwing program may be appropriate. Joint loads do not reach maximal values when their velocity is maximal, but rather during the arm cocking and deceleration phases of the throw. In accordance with Newton's second law of motion, it is the *acceleration* of a segment, not the velocity, that is proportional to the net force acting on that segment. An analogy of a skater can be used. A skater who wishes to quickly skate a short distance needs to generate significant force to start the motion, minimal force to move at a fast speed, and significant force to stop the motion.

Conclusion

Pitching is a highly dynamic activity in which body segments move through large ranges of motion and high speeds of movement; consequently, large joint forces and torques are generated, especially at the elbow and shoulder. Biomechanical research has quantified these large loads, and proposed associated injury mechanisms. Differences have been shown among various types of baseball pitchers and among various types of pitches. A proper understanding of the pitching mechanism is helpful to physicians, therapists, trainers, and coaches in recommending appropriate conditioning and injury treatment.

References

1. Andrews JR: Bony injuries about the elbow in the throwing athlete, *Instr Course Lect* 34:323–331, 1985.
2. Andrews JR, Carson WG Jr, McLeod WD: Glenoid labrum tears related to the long head of the biceps, *Am J Sports Med* 13(5):337–341, 1985.
3. Jobe FW, Kvitne RS, Giangarra CE: Shoulder pain in the overhand or throwing athlete. The relationship of anterior instability and rotator cuff impingement, *Orthop Rev* 18(9):963–975, 1989.
4. Wilson FD, Andrews JR, Blackburn TA, McCluskey G: Valgus extension overload in the pitching elbow, *Am J Sports Med* 11(2):83–88, 1983.
5. Escamilla R, Fleisig G, Barrentine S, et al: Kinematic and kinetic comparisons between American and Korean professional baseball pitchers, *Sports Biomech* 1(2):213–228, 2002.
6. Escamilla RF, Barrentine SW, Fleisig GS, et al: Pitching biomechanics as a pitcher approaches muscular fatigue during a simulated baseball game, *Am J Sports Med*, 35(1):23–33, 2007.
7. Escamilla RF, Fleisig GS, Barrentine SW, et al: Kinematic comparisons of throwing different types of baseball pitches, *J Appl Biomech* 14(1):1–23, 1998.
8. Escamilla RF, Fleisig GS, Zheng N, et al: Kinematic comparisons of 1996 Olympic baseball pitchers, *J Sports Sci* 19(9):665–676, 2001.
9. Fleisig GS: The biomechanics of baseball pitching, (Dissertation), Birmingham, 1994, University of Alabama.
10. Fleisig GS, Andrews JR, Dillman CJ, Escamilla RF: Kinetics of baseball pitching with implications about injury mechanisms, *Am J Sports Med* 23(2):233–239, 1995.
11. Fleisig GS, Barrentine SW, Escamilla RF, Andrews JR: Biomechanics of overhand throwing with implications for injuries, *Sports Med* 21(6):421–437, 1996.
12. Fleisig GS, Barrentine SW, Zheng N, et al: Kinematic and kinetic comparison of baseball pitching among various levels of development, *J Biomech* 32:1371–1375, 1999.
13. Fleisig GS, Chu Y, Weber A, Andrews JR: Variability in baseball pitching biomechanics among various levels of competition, *Sports Biomech* 8(1):10–21, 2009.
14. Fleisig GS, Escamilla RF, Andrews JR: Biomechanics of throwing. In Zachazewski JE, Magee DJ, Quillen WS, editors: *Athletic injuries and rehabilitation*, Philadelphia, 1996, WB Saunders.
15. Fleisig GS, Escamilla RF, Andrews JR, et al: Kinematic and kinetic comparison between baseball pitching and football passing, *J Appl Biomech* 12:207–224, 1996.
16. Fleisig GS, Escamilla RF: Biomechanics of the elbow in the throwing athlete, *Oper Tech Sports Med* 4(2):62–68, 1996.
17. Fleisig GS, Kingsley DS, Loftice JW, et al: Kinetic comparison among the fastball, curveball, change-up, and slider in collegiate baseball pitchers, *Am J Sports Med* 34(3):423–430, 2006.
18. Fleisig GS, Phillips R, Shatley A, et al: Kinematics and kinetics of youth baseball pitching with standard and lightweight balls, *Sports Engin* 9:155–163, 2006.
19. DiGiovine NM, Jobe FW, Pink M, Perry J: Electromyography of upper extremity in pitching, *J Shoulder Elbow Surg* 1:15–25, 1992.
20. Feltner ME: Three-dimensional interactions in a two-segment kinetic chain. Part II: Application to the throwing arm in baseball pitching, *Int J Sport Biomech* 5:420–450, 1989.
21. Feltner ME, Dapena J: Three-dimensional interactions in a two-segment kinetic chain. Part I: General model, *Int J Sport Biomech* 5(4):403–419, 1989.
22. Jobe FW, Moynes DR, Tibone JE, Perry J: An EMG analysis of the shoulder in pitching. A second report, *Am J Sports Med* 12(3):218–220, 1984.

23. Jobe FW, Tibone JE, Perry J, Moynes D: An EMG analysis of the shoulder in throwing and pitching. A preliminary report, *Am J Sports Med* 11(1):3–5, 1983.

24. Sisto DJ, Jobe FW, Moynes DR, Antonelli DJ: An electromyographic analysis of the elbow in pitching, *Am J Sports Med* 15(3):260–263, 1987.

25. Chu Y, Fleisig GS, Simpson KJ, Andrews JR: Biomechanical comparison between elite female and male baseball pitchers, *J Appl Biomech* 25:22–31, 2009.

26. Stodden DF, Fleisig GS, McLean SP, et al: Relationship of pelvis and upper torso kinematics to pitched baseball velocity, *J Appl Biomech* 21:164–172, 2005.

27. Watkins RG, Dennis S, Dillin WH, et al: Dynamic EMG analysis of torque transfer in professional baseball pitchers, *Spine* 14(4):404–408, 1989.

28. Matsuo T, Escamilla RF, Fleisig GS, et al: Comparison of kinematic and temporal parameters between different pitch velocity groups, *J Appl Biomech* 17:1–13, 2001.

29. Toyoshima S, Hoshikawa T, Miyashita M, Oguri T: Contribution of the body parts to throwing performance. In Nelson RC, Morehouse CA, editors: *Biomechanics IV*, Baltimore, 1974, University Part Press.

30. Aguinaldo AL, Buttermore J, Chambers H: Effects of upper trunk rotation on shoulder joint torque among baseball pitchers of various levels, *J Appl Biomech* 23(1):42–51, 2007.

31. Gowan ID, Jobe FW, Tibone JE, et al: A comparative electromyographic analysis of the shoulder during pitching. Professional versus amateur pitchers, *Am J Sports Med* 15(6):586–590, 1987.

32. Glousman R, Jobe F, Tibone J, et al: Dynamic electromyographic analysis of the throwing shoulder with glenohumeral instability, *J Bone Joint Surg Am* 70(2):220–226, 1988.

33. Rodosky MW, Harner CD, Fu FH: The role of the long head of the biceps muscle and superior glenoid labrum in anterior stability of the shoulder, *Am J Sports Med* 22(1):121–130, 1994.

34. De Wilde L, Plasschaert F, Berghs B, et al: Quantified measurement of subacromial impingement, *J Shoulder Elbow Surg* 12(4):346–349, 2003.

35. Werner SL, Fleisig GS, Dillman CJ, Andrews JR: Biomechanics of the elbow during baseball pitching, *J Orthop Sports Phys Ther* 17(6):274–278, 1993.

36. Feltner ME, Dapena J: Dynamics of the shoulder and elbow joints of the throwing arm during a baseball pitch, *Int J Sport Biomech* 2:235–259, 1986.

37. Werner SL, Murray TA, Hawkins RJ, Gill TJ: Relationship between throwing mechanics and elbow valgus in professional baseball pitchers, *J Shoulder Elbow Surg* 11(2):151–155, 2002.

38. Morrey BF, An KN: Articular and ligamentous contributions to the stability of the elbow joint, *Am J Sports Med* 11(5):315–319, 1983.

39. Dillman CJ, Smutz C, Werner S: Valgus extension overload in baseball pitching, *Med Sci Sports Exerc* 23(suppl 4):S135, 1991.

40. Buchanan TS, Delp SL, Solbeck JA: Muscular resistance to varus and valgus loads at the elbow, *J Biomech Eng* 120(5):634–639, 1998.

41. Roberts EM: Cinematography in biomechanical investigation, In *Proceedings of the CIC Symposium on Biomechanics*, Chicago, 1971, The Athletic Institute.

42. Moynes DR, Perry J, Antonelli DJ, Jobe FW: Electromyography and motion analysis of the upper extremity in sports, *Phys Ther* 66(12):1905–1911, 1986.

43. Ahn BH: *A model of the human upper extremity and its application to a baseball pitching motion*, East Lansing, 1991, Michigan State University.

44. Campbell KR, Hagood SS, Takagi Y: Kinetic analysis of the elbow and shoulder in professional and little league pitchers, *Med Sci Sports Exerc* 26:S175, 1994.

45. Barrentine SW, Matsuo T, Escamilla RF, et al: Kinematic analysis of the wrist and forearm during baseball pitching, *J Appl Biomech* 14(1):24–39, 1998.

46. Dillman CJ, Fleisig GS, Andrews JR: Biomechanics of pitching with emphasis upon shoulder kinematics, *J Orthop Sports Phys Ther* 18(2):402–408, 1993.

47. Sakurai S, Ikegami Y, Okamoto A, et al: A three-dimensional cinematographic analysis of upper limb movement during fastball and curveball baseball pitches, *J Appl Biomech* 9:47–65, 1993.

48. Dun S, Loftice J, Fleisig GS, et al: A biomechanical comparison of youth baseball pitches: Is the curveball potentially harmful? *Am J Sports Med* 36(4):686–692, 2008.

49. Lyman S, Fleisig GS, Andrews JR, Osinski ED: Effect of pitch type, pitch count, and pitching mechanics on risk of elbow and shoulder pain in youth baseball pitchers, *Am J Sports Med* 30(4):463–468, 2002.

50. Petty DH, Andrews JR, Fleisig GS, Cain EL: Ulnar collateral ligament reconstruction in high school baseball players: Clinical results and injury risk factors, *Am J Sports Med* 32(5):1158–1164, 2004.

51. Andrews JR, Whiteside JA: Common elbow problems in the athlete, *J Orthop Sports Phys Ther* 17(6):289–295, 1993.

52. Azar FM, Andrews JR, Wilk KE, Groh D: Operative treatment of ulnar collateral ligament injuries of the elbow in athletes, *Am J Sports Med* 28(1):16–23, 2000.

53. Cain EL Jr., Dugas JR, Wolf RS, Andrews JR: Elbow injuries in throwing athletes: A current concepts review, *Am J Sports Med* 31(4):621–635, 2003.

54. Jobe FW, Nuber G: Throwing injuries of the elbow, *Clin Sports Med* 5(4):621–636, 1986.

55. Stodden DF, Langendorfer SJ, Fleisig GS, Andrews JR: Kinematic constraints associated with the acquisition of overarm throwing part I: Step and trunk actions, *Res Q Exerc Sport* 77(4):417–427, 2006.

56. Stodden DF, Langendorfer SJ, Fleisig GS, Andrews JR: Kinematic constraints associated with the acquisition of overarm throwing part II: Upper extremity actions, *Res Q Exerc Sport* 77(4):428–436, 2006.

57. Dun S, Fleisig GS, Loftice J, et al: The relationship between age and baseball pitching kinematics in professional baseball pitchers, *J Biomech* 40(2):265–270, 2007.

58. Meister K, Andrews JR, Batts J, et al: Symptomatic thrower's exostosis. Arthroscopic evaluation and treatment, *Am J Sports Med* 27(2):133–136, 1999.

59. Paley KJ, Jobe FW, Pink MM, et al: Arthroscopic findings in the overhand throwing athlete: Evidence for posterior internal impingement of the rotator cuff, *Arthroscopy* 16(1):35–40, 2000.

60. Meister K: Injuries to the shoulder in the throwing athlete. Part one: Biomechanics/pathophysiology/classification of injury, *Am J Sports Med* 28(2):265–275, 2000.

61. Meister K: Injuries to the shoulder in the throwing athlete. Part two: Evaluation/treatment, *Am J Sports Med* 28(4):587–601, 2000.

62. Crockett HC, Gross LB, Wilk KE, et al: Osseous adaptation and range of motion at the glenohumeral joint in professional baseball pitchers, *Am J Sports Med* 30(1):20–26, 2002.

63. Osbahr DC, Cannon DL, Speer KP: Retroversion of the humerus in the throwing shoulder of college baseball pitchers, *Am J Sports Med* 30(3):347–353, 2002.

64. Park SS, Loebenberg ML, Rokito AS, Zuckerman JD: The shoulder in baseball pitching: Biomechanics and related injuries—Part 1, *Bull Hosp Jt Dis* 61(1–2):68–79, 2002.

65. Andrews JR, Broussard TS, Carson WG: Arthroscopy of the shoulder in the management of partial tears of the rotator cuff: A preliminary report, *Arthroscopy* 1(2):117–122, 1985.

66. Carson WG Jr., Gasser SI: Little Leaguer's shoulder. A report of 23 cases, *Am J Sports Med* 26(4):575–580, 1998.

67. Ogawa K, Yoshida A: Throwing fracture of the humeral shaft. An analysis of 90 patients, *Am J Sports Med* 26(2):242–246, 1998.

68. Sabick MB, Torry MR, Kim YK, Hawkins RJ: Humeral torque in professional baseball pitchers, *Am J Sports Med* 32(4):892–898, 2004.

69. Cummins CA, Messer TM, Schafer MF: Infraspinatus muscle atrophy in professional baseball players, *Am J Sports Med* 32(1):116–120, 2004.

70. Redler MR, Ruland LJ, McCue FC: Quadrilateral space syndrome in a throwing athlete, *Am J Sports Med* 14(6):511–513, 1986.

71. Milch H: Snapping scapula, *Clin Orthop* 20:139–150, 1961.

72. Sisto DJ, Jobe FW: The operative treatment of scapulothoracic bursitis in professional pitchers, *Am J Sports Med* 14(3):192–194, 1986.

73. Fortenbaugh D, Fleisig GS, Andrews JR: Baseball pitching biomechanics in relation to injury risk and performance, *Sports Health: A Multidisciplinary Approach* 1:314–320, 2009.

74. Matsuo T, Fleisig GS: Influence of shoulder abduction and lateral trunk tilt on peak elbow varus torque for college baseball pitchers during simulated pitching, *J Appl Biomech* 22(2):93–102, 2006

APPLIED BIOMECHANICS OF COMMON WEIGHT TRAINING EXERCISES

Michael P. Reiman, Rafael F. Escamilla, and Loren Z. F. Chiu

Introduction

It has been suggested that the term *weightlifting* be reserved for the Olympic lifts, the snatch and clean and jerk. Therefore, we have chosen to entitle this chapter "Applied Biomechanics of Common Weight Training Exercises," which is all-encompassing, not only including the two weightlifting exercises, but also other commonly used weight training exercises. Because it is beyond the scope of this chapter to include every weight training exercise and joint in the body, the authors have chosen to focus on the spine, the lower extremities, and Olympic lifts as they relate to applied biomechanics. Therefore, this chapter has been divided into three primary sections: biomechanics of weight training exercises and the spine, biomechanics of weight training exercises and the lower extremities, and biomechanics of Olympic weightlifting exercises. Each section presents unique aspects as the amount and detail of the research for each relationship differs.

Biomechanics of Weightlifting Exercises and the Spine

Although it is beyond the scope of this chapter to describe every particular exercise as it relates to the spine, some of the more common specific exercise examples are described with respect to muscle electromyographic (EMG) activity, kinetics, and kinematics when available as reported. Research in this area is currently limited. This is especially the case when compared with the other two sections of this chapter: lower-extremity exercises and Olympic weightlifting exercises.

Functional Anatomy of the Spine
Functional Muscle Anatomy

The importance of trunk muscles in providing stability to the lumbar spine has been well documented and supported.[1-6] When the spine is loaded, trunk muscles need proper recruitment to provide optimal stability. Deficiency in a timely muscle activation in responses to sudden trunk loading has been documented among patients with low back pain,[7-10] leading to loss of spinal stability and recurrent injuries to the lumbar spine.[4,11] The isolated thoracolumbar spine was found to buckle under compressive loads exceeding 20 N[12] and the lumbar spine buckles under approximately 90 N.[13] The fact that level walking imparts up to 140 N on the lumbar spine[14] and holding an 80-pound (36.3-kg) object in front of the body with a neutral spine loads up to 2000 N.[15] This fact underlies the importance of muscle activation to maintain stability in realistic conditions. The various muscle groups must be recruited to stiffen and stabilize the spine.[1]

Muscle Activity During Weightlifting Exercises

Trunk stability is afforded by three interdependent subsystems (passive spinal osseoligamentous, active muscular, and motor control).[11] The active muscular subsystem has been further divided into local and global muscle groups.[1] The local muscular system, or inner muscle unit, consists of muscles predominantly involved in joint support or stabilization. These muscles are not movement-specific, but rather provide stability of the lumbar spine to allow movement of a peripheral joint.[1,16] These muscles either originate or insert (or both) into the lumbar spine[1] and include the transverse abdominis, lumbar multifidus (LM), internal oblique, diaphragm, and the muscles of the pelvic floor.[1,16,17]

Local Stabilizer Muscles

- Transverse abdominus
- Lumbar multifidus
- Internal oblique
- Diaphragm
- Pelvic floor muscles

Clinical Point

Local stabilizer muscles provide stability to the lumbar spine while allowing movement of peripheral joints.

The global muscle system, or outer muscle unit, is predominantly responsible for movement and consists of more superficial musculature that attaches from the pelvis to the rib cage or lower extremities. Major muscles in this group include the rectus abdominis, external oblique, erector spinae (ES), hamstrings, gluteus maximus, latissimus dorsi, hip adductors, and quadriceps.[1,16,17] These muscles transfer and absorb forces from the upper and lower extremities to the pelvis.[1]

Global Stabilizer Muscles

- Rectus abdominus
- External oblique
- Erector spinae
- Hamstrings
- Gluteus maximus
- Latissimus dorsi
- Hip adductors
- Quadriceps

Clinical Point

Global stabilizers transfer and absorb forces from the upper and lower extremities to the pelvis.

Trunk muscles often perform several functions simultaneously, depending on instantaneous demands. It should also be recognized that the most important muscles for trunk stability have been shown to rotate among the many muscles.[18,19] Whereas ES muscle activation occurs primarily to maintain appropriate lumbar spine posture, other muscles function primarily to generate torque.[20-22] Because it has been determined that no one or two muscles were consistently active across all of the various tasks required of human function[19,23] and in deference to the proposal that the exercises themselves are the most important component of spinal stability,[24] we delineate the specific spinal stabilization exercises as they have been reported.

Specific Exercise Examples Including Kinetics, Kinematics, and Pathomechanics

Squat Exercise

The squat exercise has been advocated as an important method for hip, knee, and back muscle training.[25-28] Weight-lifters and powerlifters use squatting as one of the most important parts of their training programs, and for the powerlifters, squatting is directly included during their competition performance.[29-31] Most research regarding kinetics, kinematics, and muscle EMG activity for the squat exercise has been devoted to the lower extremities, and therefore greater detail is devoted to this particular exercise in that section of this chapter.

It has been a long-held belief that, during the lifting task, the ES muscles provide the extensor force necessary to resist the weight of the upper body and any external loads in the hands.[32,33] ES muscle activity was found to be reduced in kyphotic postures during the squat type of lifting.[34-36] Kyphotic postures during a squat movement were found to demonstrate peak EMG activity of the ES muscle in the middle of the lift, whereas a lordotic posture demonstrated peak ES muscle EMG activity early in the lift.[36] As an individual continues deeper into his or her squat posture, the ES muscles undergo a "silent phase" of EMG activity known as *flexor relaxation*.[37,38] It has since been discovered that the extensor function of the lumbar part of the ES muscles is then taken over by the thoracic part of the ES,[39] although the EMG activity of the entire ES muscle group decreases as the spine flexes (Figure 16-1).

It is generally accepted that the closer the load is placed to the body, the more significantly diminished are the resultant compressive forces to the lumbar spine (Figure 16-2). This is a strategy that is employed more effectively in the semi–squat lift (load between the feet and knees) than with the stoop or squat lift (Figure 16-3). This posture has traditionally been accepted as the norm for these reasons.

Conflicting findings regarding the specific type of lift posture with static lifting tasks have been discovered. Although lumbar flexion was much greater in lifts from the kyphotic initial position, the torques required around L3 were similar between the two different postures (kyphotic and lordotic), although somewhat larger initially in lifts from a kyphotic posture.[36] The largest torques were

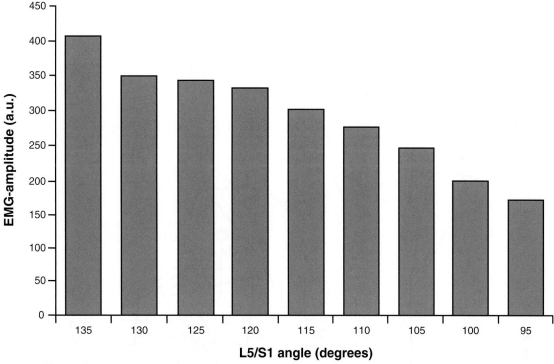

Figure 16-1

Example of maximal electromyographic values expressed in arbitrary units determined during standard isometric contractions at the L3 level for a range of L5/Sl joint angles (95" indicates maximal flexion). (From Toussaint HM, de Winter AF, de Haas Y, et al: Flexion relaxation during lifting: Implication for torque production by muscle activity and tissue strain at the lumbo-sacral joint, *J Biomech* 28[2]: 199-210, 1995.)

sustained by flexed lumbar spines during periods of little or no ES muscle activity.[36] More recent results[40] suggest that the tensile strain on tissues in the lower lumbar spine was not affected by lift style. Squat lifting over stoop lifting (Figure 16-4) as the technique of choice resulted in reduced net moments, muscle forces, and internal spinal loads,[41-43] although a freestyle lifting mechanism has also been advocated.[44] Most recently, in a comparison study between the squat and stoop lift, it was concluded that although the range of motion (ROM) at the waist, hip, knee, and ankle was different between squat and stoop lifts, the maximum lumbar joint movement was not significantly different between the two lifting methods when lifting three different box loads (5, 10, and 15 kg [11, 22, and 33 lb]) (Figure 16-5, also see Figure 16-4).[45]

Trunk muscle coactivation is thought to increase trunk stiffness and potentially reduce risk of injury, even in flexed or kyphotic postures. Increasing torso muscle coactivation leads to a linear-type increase in trunk stiffness throughout trunk extension ROM.[41] Stiffness in trunk flexion and lateral flexion, however, only increased with muscle coactivation until approximately 40% and 60% of ROM respectively.[46] A "yielding" phenomenon similar to the "flexor relaxation" phenomenon previously described was seen after these points in each respective ROM.[41]

Adding to the potential for injury is the fact that the compressive loads sustained during squatting can be extremely high. Half-squats performed with barbell loads of 0.8 to 1.6 times body weight (BW) demonstrated compressive loads between 6 to 10 times BW.[47] Even higher compressive loads were found in powerlifters.[48] Cholewicki and colleagues[48] estimated compressive loads on L4 and L5 of powerlifters to be up to 17,192 N. Because the spine is inherently unstable, as previously described in this chapter, how the spine can withstand such forces might be questioned. Motor control of trunk flexion posture, advanced technique with such lifts, and systematic training of the spinal musculature over years has been postulated to account for high-level athletes' ability to successfully perform such lifts without injury.[24] Adams and colleagues[49] suggested that a fully flexed spine is weaker than one that is moderately flexed. In a strictly biomechanical model analysis, Gunning and colleagues[50] used a porcine spine model to demonstrate that a fully flexed spine is 20% to 40% weaker than if it were in a neutral posture. A more neutral spine posture is also more effective at reducing total joint shear, compared with a flexed spine posture straining the interspinous ligament complex and therefore imposing an anterior shear force on the superior vertebra (Figure 16-6).[51]

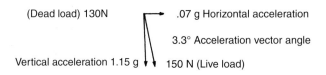

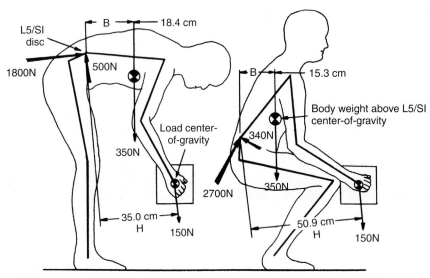

Figure 16-2
An approximate 50% variance in lumbar movements at the L5/S1 segments when comparing squat and stoop lifts. (From Chaffin DB, Andersson GB: *Occupational biomechanics,* ed 2, New York, 1991, John Wiley & Sons.)

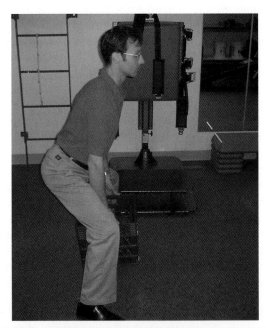

Figure 16-3
A semi-squat lift. (From Jacobs K: *Ergonomics for therapists,* ed 3, St Louis, 2007, Mosby.)

Clinically Relevant Points Regarding Squatting

- Squatting is important for training the back, hip, and knee musculature
- Electromyographic activity of erector spinae muscles decreases as the spine flexion angle increases
- Conflicting findings exist regarding torques, tensile loads, and compressive loads on the lumbar spine with respect to the type of lift posture
- Posture types include:
  - Semi-squat lift with load between the lower extremities (see Figure 16-3)
  - Stoop lift (see Figures 16-2 and 16-4)
  - Squat lift (see Figures 16-2 and 16-4)
- Spinal compressive loads during squatting can be extremely high

Pushing and Pulling Exercises

It has been suggested that on average, 9% to 20% of low-back injuries may be associated with either a pushing or pulling task.[52-55] Lett and McGill[56] determined the main contributing factors to the forces produced on the low back were the quantity of the load being pushed or pulled, the handle height from which the load is pushed or pulled, and

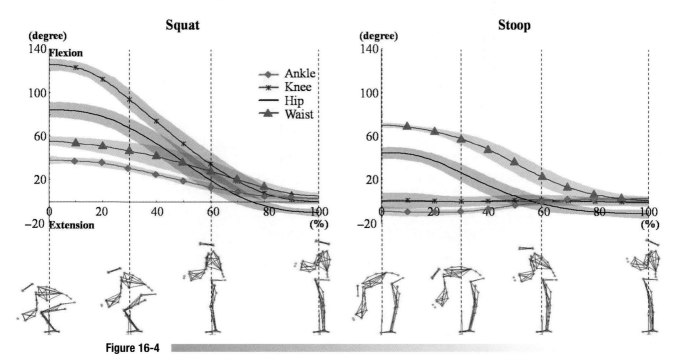

Figure 16-4
Joint angles in sagittal plane during squat and stoop lifting. (From Hwang S, Kim Y, Kim Y: Lower extremity joint kinetics and lumbar curvature during squat and stoop lifting, *BMC Musculoskel Dis* 10:15, 2009.)

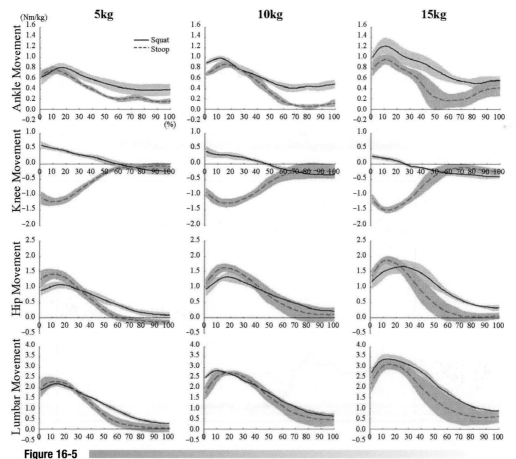

Figure 16-5
Joint moments during squat and stoop lifting at various loads. (From Hwang S, Kim Y, Kim Y: Lower extremity joint kinetics and lumbar curvature during squat and stoop lifting, *BMC Musculoskel Dis* 10:15, 2009.)

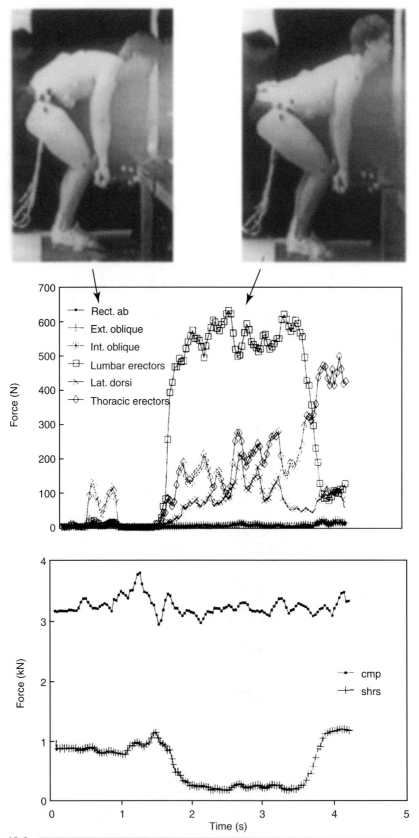

Figure 16-6

Comparison of a fully flexed spine versus a more neutral posture associated with myoelectric silence in the back extensors, loaded posterior passive tissues, and shearing forces on the lumbar spine. (From McGill SM: Biomechanics of low back injury: Implications on current practice and the clinic, *J Biomech* 30[5]:465-475, 1997.)

the experience level and technique of the participant. Technique especially was found to influence the amount of loading of the spine.[53] Novice lifters were particularly vulnerable to increased compressive loads with a push-and-pull exercise when compared with more experienced individuals.[53]

Rowing is another exercise that involves trunk flexion and therefore the potential of the flexor relaxation phenomenon. The potential for this phenomenon is actually much greater because of repeated trunk flexion of extreme ROM. Lumbar flexion has been shown to increase significantly during a rowing trial, as was the magnitude of EMG activity of the LM and other ES musculature.[54,55] Findings showed that young adult rowers attained relatively high levels of lumbar flexion during the rowing stroke, and these levels continued to increase during the course of the rowing trial.[55]

Spinal compressive forces are also a significant issue with rowing, even though the individual is not in an upright posture. Peak spinal compressive forces as high as 6066 N for men and 5031 for women have been measured in rowers.[54] The combination of increased hip flexion, increased EMG activity of the lumbar ES and LM, and particularly the exceedingly high compressive forces encountered during this activity should caution the clinician as the application of such an exercise in a rehabilitation continuum.

Spinal loading during many forms of the push-up is substantial. Plyometric forms of the push-up require much higher levels of muscle activity and therefore result in higher spine loading.[24] Compression loads have been measured in various forms of the push-up: 1838 N with a traditional push-up, 2840 N with both hands on a ball-type of push-up, 4699 N with a clapping push-up, and as high as 5848 N of compression force on the spine with a one-arm push-up.[57] Performing push-ups on labile surfaces only moderately increased spinal compressive loads.[57] EMG activity of the contralateral rectus abdominis was higher than the ipsilateral rectus abdominis in a staggered-hand-placement push-up (i.e., right hand more cranial than left and vice versa).[57] Moderate activation levels in the trunk flexors and lower activation in the trunk extensors has been suggested to challenge the musculature surrounding the lumbar spine with a standard push-up, provided that a neutral spine posture is maintained.[57] For lumbar spine vertebral joint rotational stiffness, the abdominal muscles contributed $64.32 \pm 8.5\%$, $86.55 \pm 1.13\%$, and $83.84 \pm 1.95\%$ on average around the sagittal, frontal, and transverse axes respectively.[58] The muscles primarily involved were the rectus abdominis and external and internal obliques, with minimal contribution from the transverse abdominis, LM, and ES.[58]

A vertically oriented Bodyblade with large-amplitude oscillation resulted in the greatest activation levels of the internal oblique and external oblique muscles (48% and 46% of maximum voluntary isometric contraction [MVIC] respectively). This particular technique was also associated with L4-L5 compressive forces as high as 4328 N.[59] The rectus abdominis and external and internal oblique muscles exhibited a continuous activation pattern, independent of the oscillation plane, whereas the LM and ES changed from continuous activation in the horizontal plane to phasic patterns in the vertical plane with the oscillating pole.[60] Compressive loads were not measured with the oscillating pole.

Clinically Relevant Points Regarding Push-Pull Activities

- 9% to 20% of low back injuries may be associated with push-pull activities
- Spinal compressive loads are also significant with push-pull activities
- Spinal compressive loads and spine musculature activation varies with the type of push-up exercise performed

---

Trunk Flexion Exercises

Bent-knee sit-ups have been recommended to decrease psoas muscle activity and decrease its resultant compressive force on the lumbar spine caused by length-tension relationships. Juker and colleagues[61] found psoas muscle activation levels to be higher during bent-knee sit-ups than with straight-knee sit-ups. It is postulated that the shortened psoas muscle must contract to higher levels of activation given its compromised length with the bent-knee situp.[61] This bent-knee position for sit-ups also imposes approximately 3300 N of compression force on the spine.[62] A bent-knee sit-up in which the client first isometrically contracts the hamstrings was originally thought to inhibit the psoas muscle, but actually was found to produce some of the highest levels of psoas muscle activation of any sit-up exercise as a result of the psoas requirement to overcome the trunk extensor movement created by the hamstring contraction.[62] Abdominal curls or "crunches," although going through a much smaller amplitude of motion, still demonstrated large compressive forces on the L4-L5 in at least one study,[19] with values ranging from 2615 N to 3422 N. The EMG MVIC values ranged from 30% to 32% for the rectus abdominis to 30% for left internal oblique and 44% for right internal oblique with the same exercise.[19] Higher MVIC values for upper rectus abdominis (62%), lower rectus abdominis (55%), and external oblique (52%) have been reported with the curl-up exercise in another study.[63]

Trunk Extension Exercises

Recent EMG comparison analysis with various exercises has supported an interaction between various muscle groups in affording stability to the lumbar spine. Using EMG during three bridging exercises, Stevens and colleagues found that the relative muscle activity and the ratio of the abdominal obliques seemed to alter depending on the task and the presumable need for stability.[64] These authors concluded that their findings supported the assumption that during these bridging exercises, all back muscles contribute in a similar way to control spine positions and movements in a healthy population.[64] Mean EMG amplitudes of the longissimus thoracis (LT) and LM MVIC values during various bridging exercises has been investigated by multiple authors.[65-67] Performing a bridging movement varied slightly depending on how it was performed (Table 16-1). Compressive loads on the spine were not measured in any of these studies. Average compression loads on L4-L5 have been measured with supine bridging to neutral with bilateral shoulders on ground and lifting pelvis with either one or both legs.[19] Values ranged from 2387 N to 3231 N for bridging with bilateral legs and from 2707 N to 3656 N for bridging with one leg on the ground and the other extended.[19]

The "dying bug" or "dead bug" exercise in which the contralateral upper and lower extremity is lifted from the supine position has been advocated as an integral part of a properly designed stabilization program. EMG analysis established that the rectus abdominis and oblique muscles were equally active with three different progression levels of this exercise.[68] The same authors also assessed three different progression levels of exercises in the quadruped position. They concluded that the ES and gluteus maximus both demonstrated significant activation above resting, especially with elevation of ipsilateral lower extremity, although neither muscle exceeded 41% of MVIC. The authors speculated that these relatively low levels of activation would most likely not be sufficient to produce strengthening in healthy subjects.[68]

The "Superman" exercise (prone lying, arms above head) exerts more than 6000 N or more than 1300 pounds of compressive force on the lumbar spine. The "bird dog" or quadruped exercise, in which contralateral upper and lower extremity are lifted to horizontal from the quadruped position, has been advocated as an alternative to the prone "Superman" exercise in which bilateral upper and lower extremities are lifted simultaneosly.[24] The "bird dog" exercise decreased the load to 3000 N while still producing a maximum voluntary contraction range of 30% to 40% in the primary muscles involved.[19] Other MVIC percentage values of various trunk muscles are listed in Table 16-2.

Unstable Surface Exercises

The use of changing unstable surfaces is also an increasing trend in stabilization training programs. EMG analysis comparing a curl-up exercise found increased abdominal activity when the exercise was performed on the unstable surfaces. It was concluded that much higher demands were placed on the motor control system when on unstable surfaces and therefore these exercises were more likely appropriate for later stages of rehabilitation.[72] In addition, performing stabilization exercises on exercise balls has also been a popular method of stabilization training. No change in the internal oblique/rectus abdominis ratio between stabilization exercises performed on or off a ball was found. Significant increase in activation of the rectus abdominis with performance of a single–leg hold and at the top of a hook-lying press-up on the ball was identified.[73] Although trunk strengthening demonstrated improvement on unstable surfaces in normals[73,74] and nonspecific chronic low back pain patients were reported to have trunk muscle activation levels similar to normals,[75] the assumption that the use of an exercise ball will always create a greater challenge for the musculoskeletal system is not universally supported.[69]

Table 16-1

Mean MVIC Values (%) of Longissimus Thoracis and Lumbar Multifidus Muscles During Various Bridging Exercises

Exercise	Muscle %MVIC
Bridge while lying supine on the floor to neutral pelvis position (shoulders on ground)	LT = 37 ± 12[65] LT = 39 ± 15[66] LT = 12.8 ± 9.9 to 13.9 ± 8.5 for men; 33.8 ± 23.7 to 37.1 ± 25.8 for women[67] LM = 39 ± 13[65]
Bridge while lying supine on the floor to neutral pelvis position with bilateral shoulders on gymnastics ball	LT = 35 ± 13[65] LM = 38 ± 14[65]
Bridging to neutral pelvis position with bilateral knees extended and feet on gymnastics ball (shoulders on ground)	LT = 42 ± 13[65] LM = 44 ± 12[65]
Unilateral bridge to neutral pelvis position with one leg extended and NWB (shoulders on ground)	LT = 40 ± 16[66] LT = 13.0 ± 8.6 on NWB leg to 26.7 ± 12.3 on WB for men; 25.5 ± 16.2 on NWB leg to 71.4 ± 52.2 on the WB leg for women[67] LM = 44 ± 18[66]

LM, Lumbar multifidus; *LT,* longissimus thoracis; *MVIC,* maximum voluntary isometric contraction; *NWB,* nonweight bearing; *WB,* weightbearing.

Table 16-2

Mean MVIC Values (%) of Various Muscles During Various Quadruped Exercises

Exercise	Muscle %MVIC
Ipsilateral leg raise only	LM = 23.3 $\pm$ 17.4[69] and 22[70]
Contralateral leg raise only	LM = 15.8 $\pm$ 9.2[69] and 14[70]
Ipsilateral arm and leg extension ("bird dog")	LM = 28 for ipsilateral and 22 for contralateral[70] LM = 48.1 $\pm$ 6.2 for men and 56.6 $\pm$ 30.2 for women[71] EO = 30 $\pm$ 18[66], 10.4 $\pm$ 5.3 to 21.3 $\pm$ 6.7[69] RA = 8 $\pm$ 7[66], 5.1 $\pm$ 2.4 to 5.9 $\pm$ 4[69]
Contralateral arm and leg extension	LM = 22.8 $\pm$ 14.1 to 23.1 $\pm$ 13.0[69]
"Superman" exercise	LT = 36 $\pm$ 18[66]

EO, External oblique; *LM,* lumbar multifidus; *LT,* longissimus thoracis; *MVIC,* maximum voluntary isometric contraction; *RA,* rectus abdominus.

Commercial Devices

There are multiple commercial devices advocating improved core strengthening. Limited research is available for support of such claims. The Power Wheel and hanging knee-up with straps recruited greater abdominal muscle activity than a traditional crunch, bent-knee sit-up, or reverse crunch in a study comparing various devices with traditional exercises.[76] In another study with similar comparisons, the Ab Slide and Torso Track activated trunk abdominal musculature to a greater degree than the crunch or bent-knee sit-up while minimizing low back and hip flexion activity.[77] The authors concluded that the Power Wheel, reverse crunch, and bent-knee sit-up may be problematic for some individuals with low back pain because of the relatively high rectus femoris muscle activity.[76]

Recommendations and Alternative Exercise Options

As it is readily apparent, research is lacking in relationship to the spine and applied biomechanical analysis. Continued research will assist in determining the kinetics, kinematics, and muscle activity with the various exercises currently employed by the clinician. Although no single exercise has been confirmed with quantitative data to challenge all of the trunk musculature while sparing the back from excessive compressive loads,[62] three exercises have been advocated: curl-ups for rectus abdominis; progressions of the "bird dog" for the back extensors; and several variations of the side bridge for the obliques, transversus abdominus, latissimus dorsi, and quadratus lumborum.[24] Systematic progression of these exercises with an emphasis on trunk muscle endurance, as well as emphasis on lumbar spine neutral posture and trunk movement coming specifically from bilateral hip joints should be the mainstay of all lifting programs.[19] Therefore, stability should be the emphasis for the spine, whereas the mobility during the specific lifts comes from the bilateral hip joints. Continued research will determine the best "spine saving" exercises.

> **Clinically Relevant Points Regarding Stabilization Exercises for the Spine**
>
> - Involve various movements (flexion and extension primarily discussed in the literature)
> - MVIC values of various muscles vary amongst different forms of the same type of exercise
> - MVIC values of various muscles also vary amongst different exercises
> - Can be performed on unstable surfaces
> - Can be performed with various commercial devices
>
> *MVIC,* Maximum voluntary isometric contraction.

Biomechanics of Lower Extremity Exercises

This section discusses lower-extremity biomechanics while performing select squat, deadlift, and lunge exercises. Lower-extremity muscle activity is presented regarding a variety of squat, lunge, and deadlift exercises performed with technique variations, involving muscle activity from the rectus femoris, vastus lateralis (VL) and vastus medialis (VM), medial and lateral hamstrings, gastrocnemius, gluteus maximus, and hip adductors. Knee kinetics and pathomechanics are presented regarding squat and lunge exercises. Specifically, the section discusses patellofemoral joint compressive force and stress and tibiofemoral force (compressive and shear, including cruciate ligament tensile force).

The following exercises are discussed in this section:

- Barbell squat, a one- and two-leg squat both on a flat surface and on a stability ball,
- Wall squat, which is divided into *wall squat long* (with the feet placed so that at 90° knee flexion, the knees are over the ankles and the tibia is vertical) and *wall*

squat short (with the feet positioned half the distance from the wall compared with the wall squat long so that at 90° knee flexion, the knees are positioned approximately 8 to 10 cm [approximately 3 to 4 inches] beyond the toes)

- Ball squat long and ball squat short, which are performed in a similar fashion as the wall squat long and wall squat short except the client rolls up and down the wall using a Swiss ball positioned between the back and the wall, instead of sliding up and down the wall
- Forward lunge long (a long stride is used so when the lead knee is flexed 90°, the lead tibia is in a vertical position) and forward lunge short (a forward lunge with a stride length half the distance of the forward lunge long) so that at 90° lead knee flexion, the lead knee is positioned approximately 8 to 10 cm (approximately 3 to 4 inches) beyond the toes of the same leg
- Side lunge
- Barbell deadlift (both sumo and conventional styles)

Lower-Limb Weightlifting Exercises

- Barbell squat (flat surface)
- Barbell squat (on balance ball)
- Wall squat long
- Wall squat short
- Ball squat long
- Ball squat short
- Forward lunge long
- Forward lunge short
- Side lunge
- Barbell deadlift (Sumo and conventional)

Muscle Activity During Squat, Deadlift, and Lunge Exercises

Mean muscle activity, quantified by EMG and normalized by MVIC, are shown in Table 16-3 and Table 16-4 for a variety of squat,[78] deadlift,[79] and lunge[78] exercises. As previously defined, EMG between 0% to 20% of an MVIC represents low muscle activity, 21% to 40% of an MVIC represents moderate muscle activity, 41% to 60% of an MVIC represents high muscle activity, and 61% to 100% of an MVIC represents very high muscle activity.[80] Table 16-3 displays muscle activity using BW only as external resistance, and Table 16-4 displays muscle activity using a 12-repetition maximum (12 RM) as external resistance.

Not surprisingly, muscle activity was greater when the 12 RM was employed as resistance compared with BW.

Compared with using BW as resistance, using the 12 RM as resistance resulted in 70% to 100% greater quadriceps activity, 60% to 70% greater hamstrings and thigh adductor activity, and 150% to 200% greater gastrocnemius and gluteus maximus activity.

Quadriceps and hamstrings activity was greatest in the one-leg squat and side-lunge exercises, which produced high quadriceps activity and moderate hamstrings activity (see Table 16-3). The remaining exercises in Table 16-3 produced moderate quadriceps activity and low to moderate hamstrings activity. Moreover, gluteus maximus activity was greatest in the one-leg squat, producing moderate muscle activity, whereas thigh adductor activity was greatest in the forward lunge with a long stride, producing moderate muscle activity. Gastrocnemius activity was low in all exercises.

Quadriceps and gluteus maximus activity was greatest in the forward lunge long and forward lunge short, which produced very high quadriceps activity, whereas hamstrings activity was greatest in the convention and sumo style deadlifts, which produced moderate to high hamstrings activity (see Table 16-4). The remaining exercises in Table 16-4 produced moderate to high quadriceps activity and low to moderate hamstrings activity. Moreover, hip adductor activity was greatest in the side lunge, producing moderate to high muscle activity, whereas gastrocnemius activity was greatest in the conventional style deadlift, producing moderate muscle activity. Data from Table 16-4 demonstrates that squat, lunge, and deadlift exercises collectively are very effective in recruiting the quadriceps musculature, and moderately effective in recruiting the hamstrings, gluteus maximus, hip adductors, and gastrocnemius.

In addition to the squat data provided in Tables 16-3 and 16-4, several other papers have reported lower-extremity muscle activity during squat exercises.[81-96] Escamilla and colleagues[83] and Wilk and colleagues[93] quantified quadriceps, hamstring, and gastrocnemius activity using a 12-RM load during the barbell squat. Quadriceps activity progressively increased as the knee flexed and decreased as the knees extended, with peak activity occurring at approximately 80° to 90° of knee flexion. Similar results were observed in several other studies.[84,86,89,91,92,95] Quadriceps activity remained fairly constant beyond 80° to 90° knee flexion, which has also been observed in other studies.[92,95,96] Hence, descending beyond 90° knee flexion, which is near the parallel squat position, may not enhance quadriceps development.

Escamilla and colleagues[83] reported that the two vasti muscles produce 40% to 50% more activity than the rectus femoris, which is in agreement with squat data from Escamilla and colleagues,[84] Wretenberg and colleagues,[94] Wright and colleagues,[96] and Isear and colleagues.[86] The lower activity observed in the rectus femoris compared with the vasti muscles may be due to its biarticular function as both a hip flexor and knee extensor. Increased activity from

Table 16-3

Lower Extremity Mean (SD) EMG Activity Expressed as a Percent of a Maximum Isometric Voluntary Contraction During the Knee Extending (90° to 0°) Ascent Phase of Squat and Lunge Exercises Using Bodyweight Only as Resistance

	Rectus Femoris	Vastus Medialis	Vastus Lateralis	Lateral Hamstrings	Medial Hamstrings	Gastrocnemius	Gluteus Maximus	Adductors
One-leg squat on ground	33(23)	51(34)	47(29)	19(16)	17(14)	11(9)	20(15)	24(16)
One-leg squat on balance ball	37(26)	57(38)	50(33)	20(17)	19(15)	12(12)	24(20)	21(17)
Two-leg squat on ground	20(15)	29(21)	23(17)	11(11)	8(6)	5(6)	9(7)	9(7)
Two-leg squat on balance ball	23(19)	29(21)	21(15)	15(16)	14(14)	8(8)	10(10)	11(8)
Wall squat short	26(21)	35(28)	33(26)	10(9)	8(9)	7(7)	9(9)	13(11)
Wall squat long	20(15)	33(25)	28(20)	10(9)	11(12)	6(7)	11(11)	10(8)
Ball squat short	22(15)	30(22)	26(18)	9(8)	6(6)	6(5)	7(8)	9(6)
Ball squat long	21(16)	30(22)	26(17)	8(9)	6(6)	5(5)	7(7)	9(7)
Forward lunge short with stride	26(22)	41(30)	38(29)	12(10)	11(8)	8(8)	17(17)	17(12)
Forward lunge long with stride	28(28)	44(39)	38(30)	16(13)	15(12)	9(8)	18(19)	25(19)
Forward lunge short with stride up to 4" bench	29(23)	37(31)	31(26)	12(11)	11(9)	7(7)	17(18)	17(14)
Forward lunge long with stride up to 4" bench	26(21)	46(38)	32(28)	16(12)	15(12)	8(7)	19(19)	26(20)
Side lunge with stride	36(28)	49(37)	47(38)	17(15)	14(12)	9(8)	18(17)	18(14)
Side lunge with stride up to 4" bench	37(30)	50(41)	41(29)	17(15)	17(15)	9(9)	18(17)	16(13)

EMG, Electromyographic; *SD,* standard deviation.

the rectus femoris would increase hip flexor torque, with a concomitant increase in the amount of hip extensor torque needed from the hamstrings, gluteus maximus, and adductor magnus (ischial fibers) to extend the hip. The rectus femoris is probably more effective as a knee extensor during the squat when the trunk is more upright, because it is in a lengthened position compared with when the trunk is tilted forward in hip flexion. Compared to each other, the VM and VL produced approximately the same amount of activity, which is in agreement with data from other studies.[84,88,91,93]

Hamstring activities from Escamilla and colleagues[83,84] and Wilk and colleagues[93] were highest during the squat ascent, with the lateral hamstrings showing greater overall activity than the medial hamstrings. Peak hamstring activity between approximately 30% to 80% of a MVIC, occurs near 50° to 70° knee flexion. In contrast, peak hamstring activity was approximately 12% MVIC, 15% MVIC, and 20% MVIC, respectively, with peak values occurring between 10° and 60° knee flexion based on data from Isear and

colleagues,[86] Ninos and colleagues,[89] and Stuart and colleagues.[92] The lower hamstring activities in these latter studies are probably due to subjects squatting with a lower relative external load, and perhaps squatting with a more erect trunk. Subjects in the Isear and colleagues[86] study used no external lifting load, whereas subjects in the Ninos and colleagues[89] and the Stuart and colleagues[92] studies used lifting loads of 25% BW and 28% BW, respectively, while subjects in Escamilla and colleagues[83,84] studies lifted loads equal to 140% to 160% BW. Because many of the subjects in the Escamilla and colleagues studies[83,84] were powerlifters and used the power squat position with the trunk tilted forward 30° to 45° from vertical, greater hamstring activity was generated. Greater hamstring activity with greater forward trunk tilt during the squat has also been reported by Ohkoshi and colleagues.[97]

Several studies have reported gastrocnemius activity and force during the squat.[82-84,86] Escamilla and colleagues[83] observed moderate gastrocnemius activity during the squat, which progressively increased as the knees flexed and

Table 16-4

Lower Extremity Mean (SD) EMG Activity Expressed as a Percent of a Maximum Isometric Voluntary Contraction During the Knee Extending (90° to 0°) Ascent Phase of Squat, Lunge, and Deadlift Exercises Using Each Subject's 12-Repetition Maximum as Resistance

	Rectus Femoris	Vastus Medialis	Vastus Lateralis	Lateral Hamstrings	Medial Hamstrings	Gastrocnemius	Gluteus Maximus	Adductors
One-leg squat on ground	47(15)	79(20)	78(22)	29(12)	25(14)	25(9)	57(24)	26(11)
Wall squat short	51(17)	71(24)	70(17)	12(9)	7(5)	16(8)	24(12)	17(10)
Wall squat long	48(15)	69(19)	67(16)	12(7)	10(5)	8(6)	28(12)	20(12)
Ball squat short	47(29)	58(37)	48(33)	16(13)	11(9)	7(6)	21(20)	17(11)
Ball squat long	39(26)	53(35)	45(34)	13(11)	10(8)	6(6)	17(13)	16(10)
Forward lunge short without stride	50(20)	75(23)	76(23)	16(8)	14(7)	19(9)	53(31)	22(15)
Forward lunge short with stride	67(32)	88(31)	84(29)	16(11)	16(12)	21(11)	64(32)	28(15)
Forward lunge long without stride	32(11)	63(20)	62(19)	23(11)	21(10)	20(11)	50(29)	28(14)
Forward lunge long with stride	67(30)	104(36)	102(30)	31(17)	27(17)	29(16)	62(29)	37(18)
Side lunge without stride	43(16)	77(18)	72(15)	22(13)	18(11)	19(9)	41(23)	30(13)
Side lunge with stride	55(25)	87(22)	92(27)	31(12)	23(16)	25(12)	52(21)	42(22)
Sumo-style deadlift	24(14)	63(21)	59(27)	41(16)	40(23)	31(18)	38(26)	26(19)
Conventional-style deadlift	26(18)	56(19)	54(27)	41(15)	37(24)	39(24)	32(22)	21(19)

EMG, Electromyographic; *SD*, standard deviation.

decreased as the knees extended. Escamilla and colleagues[83] and Isear and colleagues[86] reported peak gastrocnemius activity between 60° to 90° knee flexion. Because the ankle dorsiflexes during the descent and plantar flexes during the ascent, it is a common belief that the gastrocnemius contracts eccentrically during the descent to help control the rate of ankle dorsiflexion, and concentrically during the ascent to aid in ankle plantar flexion.

Several studies have investigated the effects of varying foot positions on quadriceps, hamstrings, and gastrocnemius activity.[84,85,89,90] Escamilla and colleagues[84] reported no significant differences in quadriceps, hamstrings, or gastrocnemius activity between two foot positions (feet pointing straight ahead and feet turned outward 30°). Signorile and colleagues[90] reported no significant differences in VM, VL, and rectus femoris activity among three foot positions (feet pointing straight ahead, toes pointed outward as far as possible, and toes pointed inward approximately 30°). Ninos and colleagues[89] reported no significant differences in quadriceps or hamstrings activity between two foot positions (self-selected neutral position

and foot turned outward 30°). Hung and Gross[85] examined the effects of foot wedges on VM oblique (VMO) and VL activity. Their study varied foot angle by changing forefoot inversion and eversion (by using 10° medial and lateral wedges) rather than changing forefoot adduction and abduction. These authors reported no significant EMG differences in VMO/VL ratios among the foot positions. EMG data from the aforementioned studies demonstrate that varying foot positions do not appear to affect quadriceps, hamstrings, or gastrocnemius activity during the squat.

Several studies have investigated the effects of stance width (narrow stance and wide stance) on knee muscle activity during the squat.[84,87,98,99] Escamilla and colleagues[84] found that gastrocnemius activity was 21% greater in the narrow-stance barbell squat compared with the wide-stance barbell squat. In addition, there was no significant differences in quadriceps or hamstrings activity between narrow- and wide-stance squats, which is in agreement with EMG data from McCaw and Melrose,[87] which also employed similar narrow and wide stances. Tesch,[99] using magnetic resonance imaging immediately after performing the squat, also showed no differences in quadriceps or hamstrings activity between narrow- and wide-stance squats. Anderson and colleagues[98] found no significant differences in VMO/VL ratios between narrow and wide stances during the BW squat, but did report significantly greater VMO/VL ratios with increasing knee flexion angles (0° to 30°, 0° to 60°, 0° to 90°). These results imply that increasing knee flexion angles during the BW squat elicited greater activity of the VMO relative to the VL. One additional study[81] investigated the effects of moving the feet forward while performing a machine squat exercise. This author reported that a more forward foot position during a machine squat increased quadriceps and hamstrings activity.

In addition to the lunge data provided in Tables 16-3 and 16-4, a few other studies have reported lower-extremity muscle activity during lunge exercises.[92,100,101] Farrokhi and colleagues[100] reported that performing the forward lunge with the trunk tilted forward significantly increased gluteus maximus and biceps femoris EMG compared with performing the forward lunge with the trunk erect. These lunge EMG data are similar to squat EMG data reported by Ohkoshi and colleagues.[97] Both Hefzy and colleagues[101] and Stuart and colleagues[92] reported co-contraction of the quadriceps and hamstrings during the lunge, although Stuart and colleagues[92] reported increased quadriceps activity with decreased hamstrings activity. Because trunk position was not reported by Stuart and colleagues,[92] the decreased hamstrings activity may have resulted from maintaining an erect trunk position during the lunge.

Kinetics and Pathomechanics During Squat Exercises

Tibiofemoral Forces

Several studies have quantified tibiofemoral shear (anterior cruciate ligament [ACL] and posterior cruciate ligament [PCL] loading) or compressive forces during squat exercises.[82-84,92,93,102-107] These studies reported low to moderate posterior shear forces and PCL loading during the squat, with PCL loading increasing as knee flexion increased. A few of these studies also showed low ACL loading during the squat,[104-107] but only at knee flexion angles between 0° to 60°. When tibiofemoral forces were normalized as a percent of BW plus load lifted, the normalized peak posterior shear forces (PCL loading) ranged from 29% to 99%, normalized peak anterior forces (ACL loading) ranged from 4% to 14%, and normalized compressive force ranged from 54% to 367%. It can be concluded from these data that squat exercises moderately compress the tibiofemoral joint (primarily at higher knee angles), moderately load the PCL (primarily at higher knee angles), and minimally load the ACL (primarily at lower knee angles).

The relatively low ACL forces observed during the squat may in part be due to moderate hamstring activity, because several studies have demonstrated that the hamstrings help

unload the ACL by producing a posterior-directed force to the leg throughout the knee movement.[97,108-112] Quadriceps activity also affects the strain on the cruciate ligaments. Quadriceps force, via the patella tendon, exerts an anterior directed force on the leg (ACL loading) when the knee is flexed between 0° to 50°, and a posterior directed force on the leg (PCL loading) when the knee is flexed greater than 50° to 60°.[113,114]

Escamilla and colleagues[83,84] reported cruciate ligament loading during the barbell squat with a 12-RM intensity. During the squat ascent, a mean peak PCL tensile force of 1868 ± 878 N occurred at 63° knee flexion, whereas a mean peak compressive force of 3134 ± 1040 N occurred at 53° knee flexion. During the descent, a mean peak PCL tensile force of 1635 ± 369 N occurred at 95° knee flexion, whereas a mean peak compressive force of 2192 ± 930 N occurred at 81° knee flexion. There were no significant differences in compressive forces and PCL tensile forces between two foot angle conditions (feet straight and turned out 30°), and no significant differences in PCL tensile forces between two stance conditions (narrow stance and wide stance). However, the wide stance generated 15% to 16% significantly greater tibiofemoral compressive forces than the narrow stance. It is currently unknown at what magnitude tibiofemoral compressive force becomes injurious to knee structures, such as menisci and articular cartilage. Excessive loading of the menisci and articular cartilage can lead to degenerative changes. However, compressive forces have been demonstrated to be an important factor in knee stabilization by resisting shear forces and minimizing tibia translation relative to the femur.[115-118]

Escamilla and colleagues[119] reported cruciate ligament loading during the wall squat and one-leg squat with a 12-RM intensity (Table 16-5). During the squat-ascent phase, mean PCL forces were significantly greater during the wall squat long compared with the wall squat short between 70° and 0° knee angles, significantly greater in the wall squat long compared with the one-leg squat between 90° and 60° and 20° and 0° knee angles, and significantly greater in the wall squat short compared with the one-leg squat between 90° and 70° and 0° knee angles. For all three squat exercises, mean peak PCL force magnitudes occurred between 80° and 90° knee angles during the squat ascent, and were 723 ± 127 N for the wall squat long, 786 ± 197 N for the wall squat short, and 414 ± 133 N for the one leg squat. ACL forces, which were generated only during the one leg squat (31 to 59 N range), occurred between 0° and 40° knee angles. The mean peak ACL force magnitude during the one leg squat was 59 ± 52 N and occurred at 30° knee angle.

The mean peak PCL forces of approximately 400 N during the one-leg squat and approximately 750 N during the wall squat exercises may be problematic early after PCL reconstruction when the graft site is still healing. Moreover, during PCL reconstruction, at any given exercise intensity, it may be appropriate to employ the one-leg squat prior to

Table 16-5

Mean (±SD) Cruciate Ligament Forces (N) Among the Three Squat Types, Wall Squat Long, Wall Squat Short, and One-Leg Squat, and Between the Two Squat Phases (Squat Descent and Squat Ascent) as a Function of Knee Angle

Knee Angles for Descent Phase	Wall Squat Long	Wall Squat Short	One-Leg Squat	Significant Differences ($P < 0.05$) Between Squat Types
0°	482 ± 209	297 ± 152	−31 ± 52	WSL > WSS ($p = 0.002$); WSL > OLS ($p < 0.001$); WSS > OLS ($p < 0.001$)
10°	423 ± 205	243 ± 140	−36 ± 54	WSL > WSS ($p = 0.011$); WSL > OLS ($p < 0.001$); WSS > OLS ($p < 0.001$)
20°	316 ± 135	143 ± 131	−51 ± 77*	WSL > WSS ($p = 0.049$); WSL > OLS ($p < 0.001$); WSS > OLS ($p < 0.004$)
30°	261 ± 124	100 ± 100	−59 ± 52*	WSL > WSS ($p = 0.023$); WSL > OLS ($p < 0.001$)
40°	259 ± 121	109 ± 77	−22 ± 66*	WSL > WSS ($p = 0.014$); WSL > OLS ($p = 0.002$)
50°	295 ± 122	157 ± 70	64 ± 93*	WSL > WSS ($p = 0.005$); WSL > OLS ($p < 0.001$)
60°	348 ± 133*	231 ± 81	160 ± 97*	WSL > WSS ($p = 0.034$); WSL > OLS ($p < 0.001$)
70°	445 ± 136*	324 ± 101*	227 ± 81*	WSL > WSS ($p = 0.022$); WSL > OLS ($p < 0.001$)
80°	573 ± 149*	439 ± 129*	326 ± 118	WSL > WSS ($p = 0.017$); WSL > OLS ($p < 0.001$)
90°	659 ± 150	578 ± 158*	386 ± 121	WSL > OLS ($p < 0.001$); WSS > OLS ($p = 0.003$)

Knee Angles for Ascent Phase	Wall Squat Long	Wall Squat Short	One-Leg Squat	Significant Differences ($p < 0.05$) Between Squat Types
90°	723 ± 127	786 ± 197*	414 ± 133	WSL > OLS ($P < 0.001$); WSS > OLS ($P < 0.001$)
80°	757 ± 185*	702 ± 200*	391 ± 169	WSL > OLS ($P < 0.001$); WSS > OLS ($P < 0.001$)
70°	714 ± 181*	529 ± 177*	368 ± 157*	WSL > WSS ($P < 0.001$); WSL > OLS ($P < 0.001$); WSS > OLS ($P = 0.035$)
60°	542 ± 144*	366 ± 146	374 ± 178*	WSL > WSS ($P < 0.001$); WSL > OLS ($P = 0.002$)
50°	408 ± 137	267 ± 141	329 ± 172*	WSL > WSS ($P < 0.001$)
40°	355 ± 120	223 ± 174	266 ± 159*	WSL > WSS ($P = 0.020$)
30°	363 ± 141	206 ± 158	231 ± 132*	WSL > WSS ($P = 0.007$)
20°	436 ± 180	222 ± 139	209 ± 142*	WSL > WSS ($P < 0.001$); WSL > OLS ($P = 0.005$)
10°	539 ± 223	253 ± 155	88 ± 130	WSL > WSS ($P < 0.001$); WSL > OLS ($P < 0.001$)
0°	529 ± 249	274 ± 178	−37 ± 146	WSL > WSS ($P = 0.003$); WSL > OLS ($P < 0.001$); WSS > OLS ($P < 0.001$)

N, Ligament forces; *OLS*, one-leg squat; *WSL*, wall squat long; *WSS*, wall squat short.
Note: Anterior cruciate ligament forces are listed as negative values and posterior cruciate ligament forces are listed as positive values. An asterisk (*) indicates that there is a significant difference ($p < 0.05$) in cruciate ligament force at the specified knee angle between the squat descent and the squat ascent phases of a squat exercise.

wall squat exercises because there is less PCL loading during the one leg squat. In addition, it may be prudent to employ smaller knee angles (e.g., 0° to 50°) before progressing to larger knee angles (e.g., 50° to 100°) because PCL forces generally increase as knee angle increases. In contrast, wall squat exercises may be a better choice compared with the one-leg squat early after ACL reconstruction because of ACL forces generated during the one-leg squat. However, because peak ACL force during the one-leg squat were only approximately 60 N, it is not likely that the one-leg squat will produce forces that would be injurious to the healing ACL graft, and mild strain to the graft may enhance the healing process.[120] Nevertheless, after ACL reconstruction it may be safer to start with wall squat exercises and progress to the one-leg squat, and employ larger knee angles (e.g., 50° to 100°) before progressing to smaller knee angles (e.g., 0° to 50°) because ACL forces may be generated at smaller knee angles less than 50°.

During the one leg sit-to-stand, which is similar to the ascent phase of the one leg squat, Heijne and colleagues[121] reported a peak 2.8% ACL strain (calibrated to approximately 100 N) at 30° knee angle. Moreover, Kvist and Gillquist[122] reported a peak anterior shear ACL force of less than 90 N at 30° knee angle during the one leg BW squat, which is similar to the results in the Heijne and colleagues study.[121] Moreover, ACL forces as a function of knee angle in Escamilla and colleagues[119] are similar to ACL forces and knee angles reported by other authors.[104,106,107,121]

The ACL and PCL forces that are generated while performing squat exercises depend on which exercise technique is employed and whether external resistance was used. For example, in Beynnon and colleagues,[104] the subjects may have squatted using a more upright trunk position with relatively little forward trunk tilt, which suggests that these subjects may have used their quadriceps to a greater extent than their hamstrings.[97] This is important because hamstrings force has been shown to unload the ACL and load the PCL during the weight bearing squat exercise.[83,97,109] Ohkoshi and colleagues[97] reported no ACL strain at all knee angles tested (15°, 30°, 60°, and 90°) while maintaining a squat position with the trunk tilted forward, with 30° or more forward-trunk tilt being optimal for eliminating or minimizing ACL strain throughout the knee ROM, and recruiting relatively high hamstrings activity. In Escamilla and colleagues' study,[83,84] in which subjects also performed the squat with the trunk tilted forward approximately 30°, they also reported no ACL strain and relatively high hamstrings activity during the squat.

Squat exercises that involved anterior knee movement beyond the toes, such as the one-leg squat (10 ± 2 cm) and wall squat short (9 ± 2 cm),[119] tend to generate the greatest ACL forces and least PCL forces compared with squat exercises such as the wall squat long, in which the knee does not translate beyond the toes and which generated higher PCL forces and lower ACL forces.[119] Therefore, the one-leg squat and wall squat short may be preferable to the wall squat long during PCL rehabilitation. Anterior knee movement beyond the toes can influence quadriceps activity and patellar tendon force, which can influence cruciate ligament loading, especially at low knee angles. Zernicke and colleagues[123] estimated the force in the patellar tendon at approximately 17 times BW (at a relatively low knee angle) in a subject who used a considerable external load during a squat descent with an erect trunk and excessive anterior knee movement beyond the toes.

Patellofemoral Forces

Patellofemoral compressive forces produce stress (i.e., compressive force divided by contact area) on the articular cartilage of the patella and patellar surface of the femur. Excessive compressive force and stress, or repetitive occurrences of lower-magnitude force and stress, may contribute to patellofemoral degeneration and pathological conditions, such as chondromalacia patella and osteoarthritis.

There are several studies that have quantified patellofemoral compressive forces during squat exercises[82-84,94,106,124,125] Escamilla and colleagues,[83] employing a 12-RM intensity during the barbell squat, reported that patellofemoral compressive forces increased as the knees flexed, decreased as the knees extended, and were slightly greater during the descent compared with the ascent. During the descent, a peak compressive force of 4548 ± 1395 N occurred at 85° knee flexion, whereas during the ascent, a peak compressive force of

---

Clinically Relevant Points Regarding Lower Extremity Muscle Activity During Squat Exercises (One-Leg and Two-Leg Squat on Ground and on Balance Ball, Wall Squat, and Ball Squat)

Squatting Without Resistance (Bodyweight Only)
- Moderate quadriceps activity occurs regardless of technique employed
- Approximately twice as much quadriceps activity occurs in one-leg squat compared with two-leg squat
- Hamstrings, gluteus maximus, and hip adductor activities showed low to moderate activity during the one-leg squat, and low during the wall squat and ball squat
- Squatting on balance ball produced slightly greater hamstrings activity compared with squatting on flat surface
- Low gastrocnemius activity occurs during all squat exercises

Squatting With Resistance (12-Repetition Maximum Intensity)
- High quadriceps activity occurs in all squatting techniques, except during the ball squat in which only moderate quadriceps activity occurs
- Wall and ball squat short produced slightly more quadriceps activity compared with wall and ball squat long
- Hamstrings activity was high when the trunk was inclined forward at least 30°, such as during the barbell squat, and low when the trunk was more erect, such as during the wall squat and ball squat
- Moderate hamstrings activity occurred during the one-leg squat
- Gluteus maximus activity was moderate to high in the one-leg squat and moderate in the wall squat and ball squat
- Hip adductor and gastrocnemius activities were moderate in the one-leg squat and low in the wall squat and ball squat

---

4042 ± 955 N occurred at 95° knee flexion. These results are similar to those reported by several other authors.[82,94,125,126] Because peak compressive forces generally occur near maximum knee flexion and increase with lifting load,[83] individuals with patellofemoral disorders should avoid performing higher-intensity squats at high knee-flexion angles.

Escamilla and colleagues[84] reported no significant differences in compressive forces between squatting with the feet pointing straight ahead and squatting with the feet turned outward 30°. In addition, they reported a 15% increase in compressive forces with a wide stance squat compared with the narrow stance squat, but only during the squat descent.

Patellofemoral compressive forces generated during the barbell squat are four to seven times BW when squatting with moderate loads (65% to 75% of 1 RM).[82-84,94,106,124,125] Escamilla and colleagues[83] estimated patellofemoral joint stress at 20°, 30°, 60°, and 90° knee flexion to be approximately 1.15 MPa, 2.42 MPa, 7.69 MPa, and 11.6 MPa, respectively. Consequently, patellofemoral compressive force and stress both increase as the knees flex, reaching peak values near 80° to 90°° of knee flexion. Patellofemoral force and stress have been shown to remain relatively constant between 75° and 110° knee flexion.[83,124,127] Therefore, injury risk to the patellofemoral joint may not increase with knee angles between

75° and 110° because of similar magnitudes of patellofemoral stress during these knee angles, with the benefit of increased quadriceps, hamstrings, and gastrocnemius activity when training at higher knee angles (75° to 110°) compared with training at lower knee angles (0° to 70°).[83]

Escamilla and colleagues[124] compared patellofemoral force and stress among wall squat (wall squat long and short) and one-leg squat exercises using dumbbell weights, and these results are shown in Figure 16-7 and Figure 16-8. Like the barbell squat, patellofemoral force and stress generally increased with greater knee angles and decreased with smaller knee angles. For example, during the squat-ascent phase of the wall squat short, patellofemoral force ranged from approximately 75 to 1400 N between 0° and 50° knee angle and from approximately 2100 to 3650 N between 60° and 90° knee angles, and patellofemoral stress ranged from approximately 0.5 to 4.4 MPa between 0° and 50° knee angles and from approximately 5.9 to 8.9 MPa between 60° and 90° knee angles. Therefore, performing the squat in the functional range between 0° and 50° of knee flexion may be more appropriate for patellofemoral patients, because only low to moderate patellofemoral compressive forces were generated in this range.

Patellofemoral force and stress were significantly greater at 90° knee angle during the wall squat short compared with wall squat long and one-leg squat, significantly greater at 70° and 80° knee angles in the wall squat short and long compared with the one-leg squat, and significantly greater at 60° knee angle in the wall squat long compared with the wall squat short and one-leg squat.[124] The primary cause of the greater patellofemoral force and stress between 90° and 70° knee angles in the wall squat short compared with the one-leg squat was 30% to 40% greater estimated quadriceps force and 60% to 70% less estimated hamstrings force during the wall squat short compared with the one-leg squat.[124] One reason for greater quadriceps force and less hamstrings force in the wall squat short compared with the one-leg squat is because the trunk is erect in the wall squat short (more conducive to greater quadriceps activity and less hamstrings activity) and tilted forward 30° to 40° in the one-leg squat (more conducive to greater hamstrings activity and less quadriceps activity).

Unfortunately, it is currently unknown how much patellofemoral compressive force and stress is detrimental to the patellofemoral joint. There are many factors that may contribute to patellofemoral pathological conditions, such as overuse or trauma, dysfunctional extensor mechanism, weakness in the quadriceps or hip external rotators, tight quadriceps, hamstrings, or iliotibial band, lower-extremity malalignment, and excessive rear-foot pronation. Nevertheless, clinicians can use information regarding patellofemoral joint force and stress magnitudes among different weight-bearing exercises, technique variations, and functional

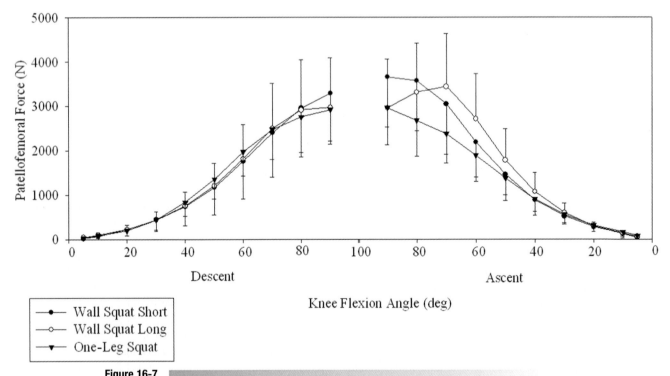

Figure 16-7

Mean (standard deviation) patellofemoral compressive force during the one leg squat and the wall squat. (From Escamilla RF, Zheng N, Imamura R, et al: Patellofemoral compressive force and stress during the one leg squat and wall squat, *Med Sci Sports Exerc* 41[4],879-888, 2009.)

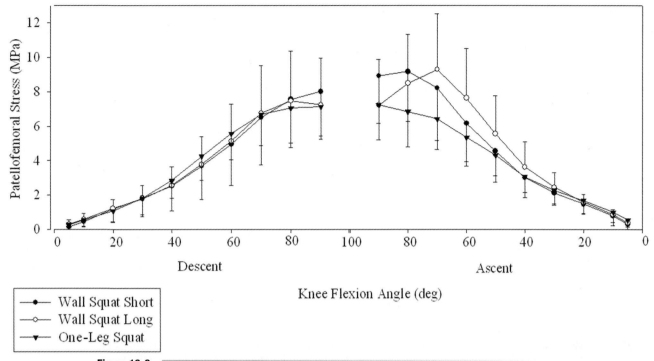

Figure 16-8
Mean (standard deviation) patellofemoral stress during the one-leg squat and the wall squat. (From Escamilla RF, Zheng N, Imamura R, et al: Patellofemoral compressive force and stress during the one leg squat and wall squat, *Med Sci Sports Exerc* 41[4],879-888, 2009.)

activities to be able to make informed decisions regarding which exercise they choose to employ during patellofemoral rehabilitation.

Clinically Relevant Points Regarding Compressive Loads at the Patellofemoral Joint During Squat Exercises

- Except at 60° to 90° knee angles, patellofemoral compressive force and stress were similar between the wall squat short and wall squat long
- Between 60° to 90° knee angles, wall squat exercises generally produced greater patellofemoral compressive force and stress compared with the one-leg squat
- When the goal is to minimize patellofemoral compressive force and stress, it may be prudent to employ a smaller knee angle range between 0° and 50° compared with a larger knee angle range between 60° to 90°
- During squatting, anterior knee translation beyond the toes should be discouraged because of higher patellofemoral force and stress generated compared with when knees are maintained over feet
- Peak patellofemoral force and stress during lunging are 40% to 50% less compared with the barbell squat, leg press, and seated leg extension exercises at the same relative intensity
- Patellofemoral force and stress are greater in the barbell squat compared with the leg press (same relative intensity) between 40° to 90° knee angle

Kinetics and Pathomechanics During Lunge Exercises

Tibiofemoral Forces

There have only been a few studies that have examined tibiofemoral forces during lunge exercises.[92,121,128,129] Escamilla and colleagues[128] examined forward lunging using a short step (forward lunge short) and a long step (forward lunge long) both with a stride (striding forward from the upright position and then returning back to the upright position) and without a stride (lunging with both feet remaining stationary). Mean cruciate ligament force values between forward lunge step length variations and between forward lunge stride variations are shown in Table 16-6. Mean PCL forces ranged between 69 and 765 N and were significantly greater in the forward lunge long compared with the forward lunge short between 0° to 80° knee angles. The PCL force generally increased progressively as knee angle increased and decreased progressively as knee angle decreased. Moreover, for a given knee angle, cruciate ligament forces were greater during the ascent phase compared with the descent phase.

The forward lunge short, which resulted in the lead knee translating forward beyond the toes of the same leg 8 ± 3 cm (3 ± 1 inches) at maximum knee flexion, generated greater ACL forces and smaller PCL forces compared with the forward lunge long, which maintained the lead knee over the foot throughout the knee ROM.[128] These results support the beliefs of some clinicians that cruciate ligament

Table 16-6

Mean (± SD) Cruciate Ligament Force (N) Values Between Forward Lunge Step Length Variations and Between Forward Lunge Stride Variations

Knee Angles for Descent Phase	Step Length Variations			Stride Variations		
	Long Step	Short Step	p Value	With Stride	Without Stride	p Value
0°	349 ± 202	69 ± 169	< 0.001*	86 ± 202	352 ± 177	< 0.001*
10°	396 ± 177	125 ± 157	< 0.001*	140 ± 208	362 ± 157	< 0.001*
20°	420 ± 205	136 ± 142	< 0.001*	192 ± 224	341 ± 203	< 0.001*
30°	387 ± 207	124 ± 97	< 0.001*	224 ± 219	285 ± 193	0.254
40°	383 ± 195	139 ± 71	< 0.001*	258 ± 210	264 ± 172	0.961
50°	422 ± 155	174 ± 73	< 0.001*	314 ± 187	282 ± 159	0.282
60°	474 ± 141	240 ± 70	< 0.001*	368 ± 155	344 ± 170	0.327
70°	521 ± 173	316 ± 85	< 0.001*	421 ± 141	413 ± 197	0.969
80°	570 ± 205	418 ± 101	< 0.001*	479 ± 142	508 ± 209	0.340
90°	591 ± 218	505 ± 127	0.030	524 ± 136	571 ± 219	0.184

Knee Angles for Ascent Phase	Step Length Variations			Stride Variations		
	Long Step	Short Step	p Value	With Stride	Without Stride	p Value
90°	682 ± 275	612 ± 157	0.326	602 ± 174	691 ± 262	0.046
80°	740 ± 247	610 ± 196	0.020	663 ± 224	686 ± 241	0.539
70°	765 ± 220	549 ± 195	< 0.001*	681 ± 248	632 ± 218	0.301
60°	744 ± 233	485 ± 194	< 0.001*	669 ± 266	560 ± 223	0.056
50°	706 ± 264	452 ± 219	< 0.001*	642 ± 281	514 ± 251	0.005
40°	676 ± 279	390 ± 184	< 0.001*	563 ± 285	509 ± 269	0.224
30°	657 ± 259	375 ± 201	< 0.001*	515 ± 285	522 ± 261	0.675
20°	580 ± 268	340 ± 163	< 0.001*	418 ± 263	502 ± 239	0.355
10°	488 ± 212	279 ± 142	< 0.001*	305 ± 168	448 ± 216	0.015
0°	412 ± 185	219 ± 150	< 0.001*	266 ± 183	360 ± 193	0.126

N, Ligament forces

*Significant difference ($p < 0.0025$) between step length variations or stride variations.

Note: Anterior cruciate ligament forces represent negative values and posterior cruciate ligament forces represent positive values.

Note: The mean values given for the two step length variations (long step and short step) were collapsed across the two stride variations (with stride and without stride), and the mean values given for the two stride variations were collapsed across the two step length variations.

loading is different between the forward lunge short and the forward lunge long.

When the goal is to minimize ACL loading, such as after ACL reconstruction, the forward lunge long may be a more appropriate and safer choice compared with the forward lunge short, especially the forward lunge short with stride, which was the only lunge variation that generated ACL loading.[128] Moreover, performing the lunge throughout a higher knee angle range may be preferred compared with a lower knee angle range, because ACL forces were only generated at smaller knee angles.[128]

When the goal is to minimize PCL loading, such as after PCL reconstruction, all lunge variations should be used cautiously, especially the forward lunge long at higher knee angles between 60° and 90°, where mean PCL forces ranged between 475 to 775 N.[128] Mean PCL forces ranged between 250 and 600 N for the forward lunge short.[128] Stuart and colleagues[92] also reported tibial posterior shear loads (i.e., PCL loading) throughout the knee ROM while

performing a forward lunge exercise using a 50 N barbell, which support the results of Escamilla and colleagues.[128]

During a BW lunge with a stride (step length was not measured), Heijne and colleagues[121] reported a mean ACL strain of approximately 1% or less (approximately 40 N or less) at knee angles less than 60° (i.e., no ACL strain at knee flexion angles greater than 60°), and a peak ACL strain of 1.8% (approximately 75 N) between 0° and 30° knee flexion. By comparison, the peak ACL force found by Escamilla and colleagues[128] was approximately 50 N in the forward lunge short with stride between 0° and 10° knee flexion angles. This demonstrates a remarkable similarity between the ACL lunge data between Escamilla and colleagues,[128] who calculated ACL loading by knee biomechanical modeling techniques, and the ACL strain lunge data by Heijne and colleagues,[121] who calculated ACL loading by direct measurement using force sensors within the ACL. The subjects in Heijne and colleagues' study[121] were patients who had force sensors implanted within the anteromedial bundle of a healthy ACL during arthroscopic surgery to repair damaged knee structures (partial meniscectomies, capsule and patellofemoral joint debridement). Immediately after surgery, these patients were asked to perform a variety of exercises, including the lunge, and the strain within the anteromedial bundle of the ACL was measured and referenced to an instrumented Lachman test. Unfortunately, Heijne and colleagues[121] did not measure PCL strain, so PCL loads cannot be compared among studies.

Estimated hamstring forces calculated by Escamilla and colleagues[128] during the forward lunge were 50% to 60% greater in the forward lunge long compared with the forward lunge short, which helps explain the greater PCL forces generated in the forward lunge long. Because the same trunk position was used during the forward lunge long and short, the greater hamstrings force during the forward lunge long appears to be related to a longer step length during the lunge. Trunk position may also affect cruciate ligament loading during the lunge. Farrokhi and colleagues[100] demonstrated that, compared with performing a forward lunge with a relatively erect trunk, performing the lunge with the trunk tilted forward approximately 30° to 45° resulted in significantly greater hip extensor impulse and significantly greater hamstrings activity. This greater hamstrings activity would likely result in an increase in hamstrings force compared with performing the lunge with a more erect trunk, which may result in greater PCL loading and less ACL loading.

Comparing with and without stride techniques, PCL forces were significantly greater without a stride between 0° and 20° knee angles.[128] Conversely, ACL forces were significantly greater with a stride compared to without a stride, but only between 0° and 10° knee-flexion angles during the forward lunge short with stride, in which ACL forces were between 0° and 50 N. One possible explanation for greater ACL forces with a stride and greater PCL forces without a stride is that with a stride produced 15% to 30% greater quadriceps forces between 0° and 20° knee flexion angles,[128] and higher quadriceps force at these lower knee angles has been shown to result in greater ACL loading.[114] Just after lead foot contact during the descent, when the knee was flexed 0° to 20°, peak ground reaction forces acting on the lead foot were 15% to 20% greater with a stride, because the body had more forward and downward acceleration compared to without a stride. Therefore, with a stride the lead foot had to push harder into the ground to slow down and control the rate of lead knee flexion, causing greater quadriceps activity. Therefore, when the goal is to minimize ACL loading, lunging without a stride may be a safer choice compared with lunging with a stride, because the ACL is less likely to be loaded without a stride compared to with a stride.[128]

Like the reconstructed ACL, it is unknown how much loading can safely occur in the reconstructed PCL, and graft type must also be considered. Because the ultimate strength

of the healthy PCL is approximately 4000 N,[130] all four lunge variations appear appropriate for healthy individuals. However, although the reconstructed PCL typically has equal or greater ultimate strength compared with the healthy PCL, it is unclear how much PCL loading may become injurious to the healing graft site during PCL rehabilitation.

Escamilla and colleagues[129] compared cruciate ligament loading between the forward lunge and side lunge both with and without a stride. Mean PCL forces ranged from 205 to 765 N, and were significantly greater in the forward lunge compared with the side lunge between 40° and 80° knee flexion angles. When the goal is to minimize PCL loading, the side lunge may be a better choice than the forward lunge.

Clinically Relevant Points Regarding Lower-Extremity Muscle Activity During Lunge Exercises

Lunging without Resistance (Bodyweight Only)
- Moderate quadriceps activity occurs regardless of technique employed
- Hamstrings, gluteus maximus, and hip adductor activities were low during the forward lunge and side lunge
- Hamstrings and hip adductor activities were slightly greater in the forward lunge long than the forward lunge short
- Low gastrocnemius activity occurs during all lunging techniques

Lunging with Resistance (12-Repetition Maximum Intensity)
- High quadriceps activity occurs in all lunging techniques employed
- Quadriceps activity was greater in the forward and side lunge with a stride compared to without a stride
- Quadriceps activity was greater in the forward lunge long with stride compared with the forward lunge short with stride, but quadriceps activity was less in the forward lunge long without stride compared with the forward lunge short without stride
- Quadriceps activity was greater in the forward lunge long with stride compared with the side lunge with stride, but quadriceps activity was less in the forward lunge long without stride compared with the side lunge short without stride
- Moderate hamstrings activity occurs during the forward and side lunge
- Hamstrings activity is greater in forward lunge long compared with the forward lunge short
- Hamstrings activity is similar between the forward lunge and side lunge
- High gluteus maximus activity occurs in the forward lunge, whereas moderate gluteus maximus activity occurs in the side lunge
- Gluteus maximus activity is greater in the forward lunge long compared than the side lunge
- Moderate hip adductor activity occurs in the forward lunge and side lunge
- Low to moderate gastrocnemius activity occurs during all lunging techniques

Patellofemoral Forces

Only two known studies have reported patellofemoral force and stress during lunging.[131,132] Escamilla and colleagues[132] reported patellofemoral force and stress between a short step lunge (forward lunge short) and long step lunge (forward lunge long) with and without a stride (Figure 16-9 and Figure 16-10). Patellofemoral joint force and stress curves were similar in shape to each other because of near proportional increases in patellofemoral joint forces and patellar contact areas with increased knee flexion. Patellofemoral joint force and stress increased progressively as knee flexion increased and decreased progressively as knee flexion decreased. One exception was at higher knee angles between 70° and 90°, in which patellofemoral joint force and stress began to plateau or decrease. This occurred because although patellar contact area increased nearly linearly between 70° and 90°, patellofemoral joint force did not increase proportionally, but instead began to plateau. These findings are consistent with patellofemoral joint force and stress data during the barbell squat studies of Escamilla and colleagues[83] and Salem and Powers.[127] Escamilla and colleagues[83] reported that patellofemoral joint forces increases until 75° or 80° knee flexion, and then began to plateau or slightly decrease. Salem and Powers[127] reported no significant differences in patellofemoral joint force or stress at 75°, 100°, and 110° knee flexion. Therefore, injury risk to the patellofemoral joint may not increase with knee angles between 75° and 110° because of similar magnitudes in patellofemoral joint stress during these knee angles, with the benefit of increased quadriceps, hamstrings, and gastrocnemius activity when training at higher knee angles (75° to 110°) compared with lower knee angles (0° to 70°).[6]

Between 70° and 90° of knee flexion, patellofemoral joint force and stress were significantly greater during the forward lunge short compared with the forward lunge long. Between 10° and 40° of knee flexion, patellofemoral joint force and stress were significantly greater when performing a forward lunge with a stride compared to without a stride. Therefore, when the goal is to minimize patellofemoral joint force and stress during the lunge, the forward lunge long may be preferred to the forward lunge short, and lunging without stride may be preferred to lunging with a stride. Moreover, a more functional knee flexion range between 0° and 50° may be appropriate during the early phases of patellofemoral rehabilitation because of lower patellofemoral joint force and stress. Higher knee angles between 60° and 90° may be more appropriate later in the rehabilitation process because of higher patellofemoral joint force and stress.

During the forward lunge short, the lead knee first begins translating beyond the distal toes at approximately 60° to 70° knee flexion angles, which is approximately

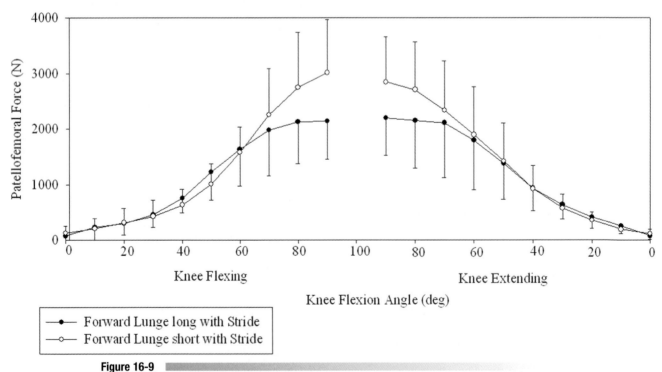

Figure 16-9

Mean (standard deviation) patellofemoral compressive force during the forward lunge long and short with a stride. (From Escamilla RF, Zheng N, Macleod TD, et al: Patellofemoral joint force and stress between a short- and long-step forward lunge, *J Orthop Sports Phys Ther* 38[11]:681-690, 2008.)

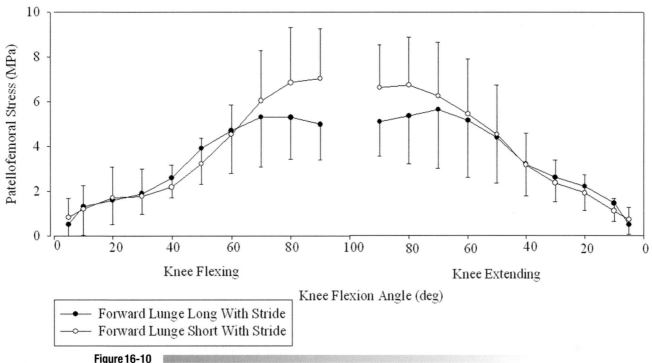

Figure 16-10

Mean (standard deviation) patellofemoral stress during the forward lung long and short with a stride. (From Escamilla RF, Zheng N, Macleod TD, et al: Patellofemoral joint force and stress between a short- and long-step forward lunge, *J Orthop Sports Phys Ther* 38[11]:681-690, 2008.)

when patellofemoral joint force and stress are initially greater in the forward lunge short compared with the forward lunge long.[132] The lead knee continues translating beyond the toes as the lead knee continues flexing, translating 8 ± 3 cm (3 ± 1 inches) beyond the distal toes at maximum lead knee flexion.[132] These results support the belief of many clinicians and trainers that anterior lead knee translation beyond the toes during the forward lunge may be harmful to the patellofemoral joint, and should be avoided. In contrast, the lead knee did not translate beyond the toes throughout the knee ROM during the forward lunge long.[132] Because significantly greater patellofemoral joint force and stress occur between 70° to 90° knee angles during the forward lunge short compared with the forward lunge long, there appears to be a relationship between anterior knee translation and increased patellofemoral joint force and stress.

The greater patellofemoral force and stress in the forward lunge short compared with the forward lunge long, and with a stride compared to without a stride, is primarily the result of approximately 20% to 30% greater quadriceps forces in the forward lunge short compared with the forward lunge long, and approximately 40% greater quadriceps force with a stride compared to without a stride.[132] Quadriceps forces are greater with a stride because peak ground reaction forces acting on the lead foot, which generates a knee flexor torque throughout the lunge that is opposed by

the knee extensors, are approximately 15% to 20% greater with a stride compared to without a stride between 10° and 40° knee angles.[132] This occurs because with a stride the subjects have to forcefully push off the force platform to accelerate the body backward and upward and return the body back to the upright starting position. Because lunging without a stride results in both feet remaining stationary throughout the lunging motion, acceleration is minimal.

Escamilla and colleagues[131] reported patellofemoral force and stress magnitudes between a forward and side lunge with and without a stride. They reported that patellofemoral force and stress were greater in the side lunge compared with the forward lunge between 80° and 90° knee angles, and greater with a stride compared to without a stride between 10° and 50° knee flexion angles. From these data, it can be concluded that loading the patellofemoral joint is similar between forward and side lunges except at higher knee angles, in which patellofemoral loading is greater in the side lunge. Performing forward and side lunges without a stride within a smaller knee angle range (e.g., 0° to 50°) may be easier and safer to start with earlier during patellofemoral rehabilitation when the goal is to minimize patellofemoral compressive force and stress, whereas performing forward and side lunges with a stride may be more appropriate later during patellofemoral rehabilitation because of greater patellofemoral compressive force and stress compared to without a stride.

Biomechanics of Competitive Weightlifting

The sport of *weightlifting* refers to competition in two disciplines—the snatch and the clean and jerk. It is important to distinguish the sport of weightlifting from weight lifting, weight training, powerlifting, and bodybuilding because of the distinct objectives of the sport and the characteristics of the competitive and training lifts.[133-136] As a sport, weightlifting evolved from a series of barbell and dumbbell lifts from the 19th century to the format introduced in the 1924 Olympic Games. In 1924, athletes competed in the one-hand snatch, one-hand clean and jerk, two-hands clean and press, two-hands snatch, and two-hands clean and jerk. After the 1924 Olympic Games, the one-hand lifts were dropped and only the two-hands press, snatch, and clean and jerk were performed until 1972, when the press was eliminated.

The *snatch* involves lifting a barbell from the floor to an overhead position in a single motion. The *clean and jerk* involves lifting a barbell first from the floor to the shoulders (i.e., the clean) and secondly from the shoulders to overhead (i.e., the jerk). In strength and conditioning, variations of these lifts such as the "power clean," "power snatch," "hang clean," and "hang snatch" are commonly used.[136] *Clean and snatch* is generally accepted as referring to a lift in which the barbell is lifted from the floor and caught either on the shoulders or overhead, respectively, in a full squat. The term *power* denotes a clean or snatch in which the barbell is caught in a partial squat. *Hang* denotes a clean or snatch in which the barbell is held in the hands in

the starting position rather than resting on the floor. The term *split* may also be used, referring to a clean or snatch in which the bar is caught with the legs split fore and aft.

The technique, and therefore biomechanics, of competitive weightlifting exercises has evolved during the last century. Early on, the snatch, clean, and jerk lifts were performed using the "splot style," an awkward shuffling of the feet to the sides and slightly fore and aft. The splot style evolved into the split style, which involved splitting the feet in a fore-aft manner, similar to a lunge. In the early 1950s, the squat style became more popular in the snatch and clean, as the performance of a deep knee bend did not require the lifter to pull the barbell as high to complete the lift. The split jerk is still preferred, although the push jerk (partial squat) and squat jerk (full squat) have been used successfully in competition. Another change in technique resulted from a change in the technical rules in 1964, which allowed nonviolent contact of the barbell against the thighs and pelvis. Both of these technical evolutions resulted in a shift to greater use of the knee extensor muscles—the squat technique during the recovery phase[137] and thigh contact during the pulling phase.[138,139] The final major evolution in technique occurred after elimination of the press in 1972, which shifted the emphasis of weightlifting from being a strength-oriented sport to a speed- and strength-oriented sport.[140]

Because of the evolution of weightlifting as a sport and as a training methodology, this section of the chapter discusses the biomechanics of modern weightlifting movements (i.e., squat snatch and clean, split jerk). Furthermore, the analyses of these lifts focus on technical styles used and data collected after 1972. The majority of data presented is collected from elite-level lifters, such as world and Olympic champions, under the assumption that they have optimized both their physiological capabilities and technical execution of these lifts.[31] Finally, the biomechanics of women weightlifters is discussed. Because women's weightlifting became an international sport in 1987, it is still relatively novel and comparison between men's and women's weightlifting provides relevant information regarding the human neuromuscular system.[141,142]

Segment Mechanics of the Snatch and Clean

The snatch and clean differ in terms of the grip width, the final position of the barbell, and the amount of weight that can be lifted; however, both movements involve the same sequence of movements and muscle activation of primary movers. Since 1972, two styles of performing the snatch and clean have been observed—the double knee bend and frog-style pulls.[139,143,144] The double knee bend–style pull is performed using an approximate shoulder width stance and has a sequence of knee extension, knee flexion, and knee extension, with continuous hip extension.[139,143-145] The frog-style pull is performed with the heels touching and rotated laterally in the transverse plane. Because of the orientation of the lower extremity, the sequence of this pull involves predominantly knee extension followed by hip extension.[138,139,143,144] A majority of elite lifters use the double knee bend pull, and empirical evidence from recent major international events (world championships and Olympic Games) has found no lifters using the frog-style pull. Therefore, this discussion of the snatch and clean focuses on the double knee bend technique.

Both the snatch (Figure 16-11) and clean (Figure 16-12) can be broken into seven distinct phases based on segment kinematics and kinetics and muscle activation.[146-148] These phases are (1) pre-lift, (2) first pull (FP), (3) second knee bend (SKB), (4) second pull (SP), (5) pull under the barbell, (6) amortization phase, and (7) recovery. The FP, SKB, and SP are collectively referred to as the *pulling phase*,[145] and the majority of research in weightlifting has analyzed the pulling phase. The duration of phases two through six are detailed in Table 16-7.

When performed properly, the barbell follows a characteristic trajectory during the pulling phase. Vorobyev[149] categorized pulling trajectories based on the initial direction of the barbell and the number of horizontal crossings of the barbell relative to an imaginary vertical line projected from the initial barbell position (Figure 16-13). Although there is considerable dissent over which trajectory is optimal,[150-152]

type A and B trajectories appear to be most common in world champions.[31,144,153,154] Type A and B trajectories are fairly similar, in that both are an S-shaped curve with the barbell pulled toward the lifter during the FP, followed by a forward trajectory during the end of the SKB and start of the SP, after which it arcs back toward the lifter during the pull-under phase. In the type A trajectory, the forward trajectory during the SKB and SP pushes the barbell forward of the vertical reference line, whereas the barbell always remains behind the vertical reference line in a type B trajectory. Type B trajectories are typically accompanied by the feet jumping backward.[152,155] Type C trajectories are generally considered improper because the amount of horizontal motion increases the work performed in lifting the barbell.[144,156]

To initiate the lift, the lifter assumes a partial squat position, in which the knee and shoulder are over or forward of the barbell. The shanks (tibia) are rotated forward approximately 25°, the angle of the knees is 70° to 75° in the snatch and 80° to 85° in the clean, and the angle of the hips 45° to 50° (note that *joint angles* refers to the angle between two adjacent segments). Gourgoulis et al.[157] observed that elite Greek women weightlifters had an initial knee angle of 60°. Center of pressure is located toward the forefoot, 30% to 50% behind the front of the feet.[158,159] In lifting the barbell from the ground, a static or dynamic start

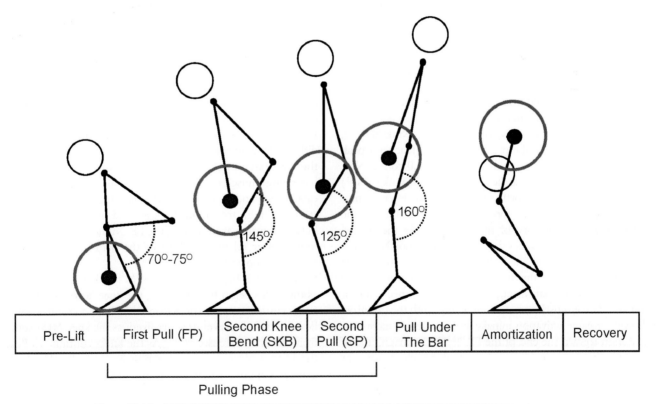

Figure 16-11
The seven phases of the snatch using the double knee bend pull.

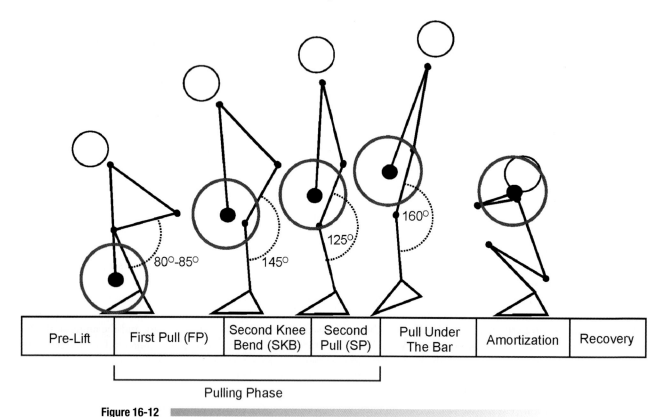

| Pre-Lift | First Pull (FP) | Second Knee Bend (SKB) | Second Pull (SP) | Pull Under The Bar | Amortization | Recovery |

Pulling Phase

Figure 16-12
The seven phases of the clean using the double knee bend pull.

may be employed. The static start involves pulling from the aforementioned positions, whereas a dynamic start may involve starting in a deeper squat and rising to these positions or performing a countermovement. There does not appear to be a clear advantage or disadvantage for any of these starting methods.[160]

As the barbell is lifted from the ground, the hips and knees extend and the ankles plantar flex. The hip extensors have the largest net joint moment (NJM) (3.5 to 5.5 NmkgBM^{-1}), which increases during the pre-lift phase and reaches a peak during the FP.[138,153,161] The knee extensor (1.0 to 2.2 NmkgBM^{-1}) and ankle plantar flexor (1.4 to 2.5 NmkgBM^{-1}) NJM also reach a peak shortly after lift-off. The lifter's center of pressure shifts from the fore to rear foot, resulting in the initial posterior trajectory of the barbell.[158] As the barbell passes mid-shank, the knees shift from an extensor NJM to a flexor NJM.[161-163] The knees, however, continue to extend; thus, the knee flexor musculature is acting eccentrically. It is important to note that throughout the FP, the knee extensor and knee flexor muscles are co-contracting, with the extensors showing greater activation initially and the flexors increasing activation toward the end of the FP.[162,164] The magnitude of co-contraction suggests that the actual muscle movement generated by the knee extensors is considerably larger than the NJM indicates.[138,162,163] In addition, the biarticular hamstring muscles are likely also contributing to hip extension during the FP.

Peak knee flexor NJM (−0.5 to −1.5 NmkgBM^{-1}) occurs before the end of the FP.[138] The FP is completed when the knees reach their first maximum extension. Elite weightlifters extend their knees to an angle of approximately 145° at the completion of the FP[154,157,165-167]; however, it has been noted that lower-caliber men lifters only reach 135° and elite women 130°.[157,165] The angle of the trunk relative to the ground remains relatively constant throughout the FP; therefore, as the knees extend, it becomes increasingly difficult to continue elevating the bar relying primarily on the hip extensors,[138,139,145] which include the biarticular hamstring muscles. Therefore, it is likely that in lower-caliber men and elite women, the hamstring muscles are not strong enough to extend the knee and hip joints, resulting in less extension at the end of the FP. Numerous studies have found lower relative strength of the hamstring muscles in women compared with men.[168,169]

As the SKB begins, the knee NJM is still flexor-dominant as the knees begin to flex. Thus, the knee flexors shift from an eccentric to concentric action.[161-163] This concentric knee flexor action, however, is short-lived, as the knee NJM shifts from flexor to extensor.[161-163] As the knees continue to flex, the knee extensors are now acting eccentrically. The SKB generates approximately 20° flexion of the knee, resulting in a knee angle of approximately 125°.[147,148,153,154,157,166,167] It is interesting to note that elite male lifters during the early 1970s flexed their knees up to 30° during the SKB.[165] The

Table 16-7

Duration of Phases 2 Through 6 in the Snatch and Clean, Observed in Laboratory and Competition Investigations

Weightlifters	Lift—Conditions	Duration				
		First Pull (s)	Second Knee Bend (s)	Second Pull (s)	Pull Under the Bar (s)	Amortization (s)
Greek National Men's Team[167]	Snatch—Laboratory	0.48 ± 0.07	0.14 ± 0.01	0.15 ± 0.01	0.24 ± 0.03	–
Greek Junior National Men's Team[167]	Snatch—Laboratory	0.51 ± 0.10	0.13 ± 0.02	0.26 ± 0.23	0.46 ± 0.05	–
Y. Zakharevich (USSR)—World Record[166]	Snatch—World record in competition	0.37	0.08	0.17	0.20	0.33
Finnish National Men's Team[148]	Snatch—Laboratory	0.54 ± 0.23	0.13 ± 0.04	0.20 ± 0.03	0.17 ± 0.02	–
Finnish Non-Elite[148]	Snatch—Laboratory	0.57 ± 0.09	0.14 ± 0.03	0.17 ± 0.03	0.18 ± 0.04	–
Finnish National Men's Team[148]	Clean—Laboratory	0.64 ± 0.18	0.13 ± 0.03	0.19 ± 0.04	0.17 ± 0.03	–
Finnish Non-Elite[148]	Clean—Laboratory	0.78 ± 0.18	0.14 ± 0.04	0.17 ± 0.03	0.16 ± 0.02	–
Greek National Men's Team[157]	Snatch—Laboratory	0.45 ± 0.04	0.15 ± 0.01	0.16 ± 0.01	0.23 ± 0.01	–
Greek National Women's Team[157]	Snatch—Laboratory	0.45 ± 0.04	0.14 ± 0.02	0.18 ± 0.02	0.26 ± 0.02	–
Greek National Men's Team[154]	Snatch—Competition	0.47 ± 0.06	0.16 ± 0.01	0.15 ± 0.01	0.23 ± 0.02	–
European Junior Men—56 kg & 62 kg[175]	Snatch—European junior championships	0.48 ± 0.04	0.14 ± 0.02	0.16 ± 0.03	0.36 ± 0.02	0.14 ± 0.06
European Junior Men—85 kg & 105 kg[175]	Snatch—European junior championships	0.54 ± 0.03	0.12 ± 0.02	0.16 ± 0.03	0.37 ± 0.02	0.15 ± 0.06

Note: Some investigations did not report data for all phases.

rationale for the greater knee flexion is unknown, but would be expected to increase the loading on the hip, knee, and ankle musculature. This style of lifting may be a residual effect of the press era when greater emphasis was placed on strength than speed strength.[140] Lower caliber men and elite women flex their knees 10° to 15° during the SKB, resulting in a similar knee angle to elite men at the end of the SKB and start of the SP.[157,165]

In addition to knee flexion, the SKB is characterized by a repositioning of the body.[145] As the knees flex, the ankles dorsiflex and the center of pressure shifts from the rear to mid-foot.[158,159] The trunk repositions from an inclined to vertical position. These events increase the ankle plantar flexion and knee extensor NJM and decrease the hip extensor and lumbar spine NJM.[138,145,153,161,163] The dorsiflexion at the ankles results in anterior translation of the tibia, thigh, and pelvis, and it is during this phase that the barbell makes contact with the upper thighs or pelvis. It is important to consider that at this point, the barbell has reached its maximum posterior horizontal displacement. Therefore, as the barbell continues to travel vertically, it brushes against the forward-moving thighs and pelvis, as opposed to the barbell being purposely pulled rearward and violently colliding with the thighs or pelvis.

The change in segment orientations during the SKB repositions the body into a mechanically advantageous position to impart vertical momentum to the barbell during the SP.[139,145] The knees shift from an eccentric action during the SKB to a concentric action during the SP, similar to the stretch-shortening cycle phenomenon observed during a countermovement jump.[162,163,170,171] In the SP, the hips and knees extend, and the ankles plantar flex in a rapid manner to increase the vertical velocity of the barbell. A second peak in the knee extensor (1.5 to 2.5 NmkgBM^{-1}) and ankle plantar flexor (0.6 to 2 NmkgBM^{-1}) NJM occurs.[138,153,161-163] In a longitudinal analysis of national and international caliber lifters, Garhammer[133,156] observed that the knee extensor NJM was particularly reflective of changes in performance (whether positive or negative). As load increases, knee extensor joint angular power during the SP also increases, but not ankle plantar-flexor or hip extensor joint angular power.[163] Knee extensor joint angular power (NJM × joint angular velocity) is also less variable than either hip extensor or ankle plantar flexor joint angular power.[172]

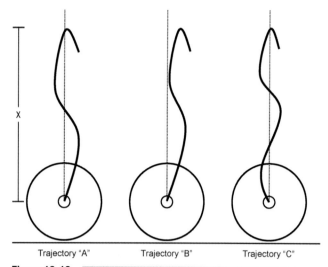

Trajectory "A" Trajectory "B" Trajectory "C"

Figure 16-13

Three trajectories of the weightlifting pull. X—the optimal height for raising the center of the barbell in the snatch (60% of lifter's height) and clean (50% of lifter's height).

These data highlight the importance of the knee extensors for generating propulsion during the SP.

The SP is completed when the barbell reaches maximum vertical velocity. Contrary to popular belief, the knees do not fully extend at the end of the SP.[153,154,157,166,167] For elite men lifters, the angle of the knees at the end of the SP is approximately 160°, whereas lower caliber men lifters reach a knee angle of 145° to 150° and elite women approximately 165°. Simultaneous to knee extension, the hips fully extend (reaching 180° ± 10°) and the ankles reach 20° to 30° of plantar flexion, with the heels raising off the ground.[153,154,157,165-167] At the end of the SP, the knee NJM shifts from extensor to flexor.[162] The knee flexor NJM likely prevents hyperextension of the knee and prepares the lifter for the pulling-under-the-bar phase.

Although the vertical momentum generated during the SP results in additional gain in barbell height, the lifter must rapidly reposition the body under the barbell to receive it overhead or on the shoulders. The acceleration of the lifter's center of mass during the pull under phase approaches 15 ms^{-2}, indicating that he or she is not in free fall, but is actively interacting with the barbell.[173] As with any object in free fall, the center of mass of the system obeys the principles of projectile motion; however, the lifter is able to reposition his or her body relative to the barbell by actively pulling on the barbell. The negative acceleration of the barbell is offset by the active interaction between the lifter with the barbell. This motion is aided by the hamstring, tibialis anterior, trapezius, and biceps brachii muscles.[147,164,174]

When performed properly, the lifter receives the barbell in the overhead or front squat position and transitions from the pull-under to the amortization phase when the barbell

is at its apex.[149,166] The squat positions achieved are similar to those occurring during the squatting exercise.[157,166] The barbell should not be received in the deepest squat position, however, as the falling barbell will push the lifter into a deeper squat. Elite junior weightlifters receive the bar at a knee angle of approximately 45° and reach a peak knee angle of approximately 38° during the amortization phase.[175] To maintain balance in the deep squat, the tibias are rotated anteriorly 30° to 40° and the torso maintains an upright position.[137,166] The stretch-shortening cycle phenomenon also occurs during the amortization phase as the hip and knee extensor and ankle plantar flexor muscles are active during the eccentric motion and transition to concentric motion. In addition, recent evidence indicates that the knee extensor NJM required to maintain static equilibrium decreases with contact between the soft tissues of the posterior thigh and shank.[176] The decreased requirement for static equilibrium allows the knee extensor NJM to be used for vertical propulsion during the recovery phase, which is often observed as a rapid rise from the deep squat position.

System Mechanics of the Snatch and Clean

The systematic activation of muscles during the first five phases of the snatch and clean result in a coordinated movement designed to displace a barbell of maximum weight in the vertical and horizontal directions such that the lifter can receive the barbell overhead or on the shoulders.[146,149,166] In the snatch, the barbell must be raised vertically to approximately 60% of the lifter's height, whereas for the clean, the barbell must be raised to approximately 50% of the lifter's height.[153,177] Mechanically, the work performed to raise the barbell these distances is a combination of a change in potential and kinetic energies.[177,178] The change in potential energy of the barbell is calculated from the displacement of the barbell from the floor to the height attained at the end of the SP and the change in kinetic energy is calculated from the peak vertical velocity minus the initial velocity of the barbell.[30,178,179] As the lifter's body rises, there is a change in potential energy to elevate the lifter's center of mass.[30,178] Work performed and changes in energy can also be calculated for a specific phase of the snatch or clean, such as the SP.[30,157,178,179]

The majority of the work performed during the pulling phase is to elevate the barbell, followed by work performed to raise the lifter's center of mass and finally work performed to achieve the peak vertical velocity of the barbell.[178] A small amount of work is also performed to move the barbell in the anterior-posterior directions; however, with type A and B trajectories, this work should be minimal. From analysis of elite weightlifters at the national and international level, greater than 95% of the total work done in the snatch and clean should be performed in the vertical direction.[144,156] Greater horizontal work is performed when a lifter uses the type C trajectory as well as deviations of the typical type A and B trajectories, as did Zaitsev, of the Soviet Union, in the 1978 World Weightlifting Championships. While winning the 110-kg class in 1978, Zaitsev employed an uncharacteristic type-A trajectory, with the barbell being caught forward of the vertical reference line.[144] It should be noted that in the same year, Rigert, also of the Soviet Union, cleaned a then–world record 223 kg weighing 94.4 kg with a 97% efficiency compared with Zaitsev, who cleaned 220 kg weighing 109 kg with 90% efficiency.[144] Rigert's lift was performed with a type-B trajectory.

An additional source of inefficient energy expenditure arises from elevating the barbell higher than is required to receive it in either the overhead or front squat position. This can occur either by extending the knees beyond 160° while generating propulsion during the SP or by reaching an excessive peak vertical barbell velocity. The former has been observed in elite Greek women compared with elite Greek men,[157] and college versus international[165] weightlifters. The latter is often observed in women[157,173,180] as well as during submaximal attempts.[147,181] In both laboratory investigations and studies of lifters in competition, peak vertical barbell velocity is lower for maximum attempts than submaximum attempts.[147,182] The lower barbell velocity also corresponds to changes in vertical ground reaction forces, which decrease with increasing load.[147,182] In addition, the shape of the force-time curve appears as a "U" shape as opposed to a "V" shape for maximum lifts, indicating that rather than higher peak forces, heavier lifts are characterized by near-maximal force applied for a longer period (Figure 16-14).[171] Elevating the barbell to a greater height by an increase in either or both potential or kinetic energies requires greater work to be performed. This greater amount of work, however, could be performed on a heavier barbell, lifting it to the minimum height required to pull under and receive the barbell. A peak vertical barbell velocity of 1.6 to 2 ms^{-1} in the snatch and 1.4 to 1.8 ms^{-1} in the clean appears to be sufficient, with taller lifters requiring greater barbell velocity than shorter lifters.[31,144,153,154,157,167]

Women tend to achieve greater peak vertical velocities when compared with men, despite being slightly shorter than men.[157] This translates to a greater relative peak barbell height, resulting in the barbell falling a greater distance to the lowest position in the amortization phase. Based on elite men weightlifters, an acceptable drop distance in either the snatch or clean is 10 to 15 cm (3.9 to 5.9 inches),[153,154,157,167,175] whereas elite women are observed to have a drop distance ranging from 19 to 47 cm (7.5 to 18.5 inches).[157,173,180] This suggests that women should be capable of lifting heavier weights; however, the technical differences discussed previously (i.e., less knee extension during the FP) may be a limiting factor in pulling heavier weights during the FP and into the SP position.

A consideration of power output during the pulling phase provides useful information about differences between men and women. Power is calculated from the mechanical work performed divided by the time required to perform work.[30,179] Typically, power has been calculated for the entire pulling phase (i.e., from lift-off to peak vertical barbell velocity) and during the SP only (Table 16-8).[30,31,144,178] For ease of analysis, work performed and power generated on the barbell rather than the lifter-barbell system can also be determined.[142,157,178,179,183] It should be noted that this calculation results in the average power during the given phase, and not the peak power generated. For elite men weightlifters, power output during the snatch and clean is similar for the same individual, whether evaluating the entire pulling phase or the SP alone.[30,144] This suggests that at the elite level, technical abilities have been optimized and that the limiting factor in the snatch and clean is the ability for muscles to perform work. For lower caliber lifters, differences in power generated during maximum snatch and clean attempts may be indicative of technical errors; therefore, assessing power generating capability can be used as a pedagogical tool.[30,178]

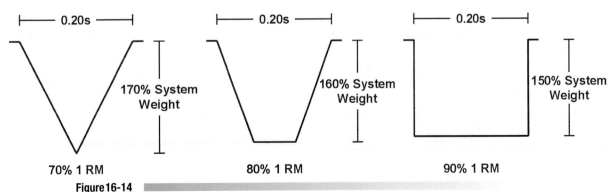

Figure 16-14

Theoretical shift from V- to U-shaped force-time curve. (Adapted from Garhammer J, Gregor R: Propulsion forces as a function of intensity for weightlifting and vertical jumping, *J Appl Sport Sci Res* 6[3]:131, 1992, using data from Häkkinen, et al, *Scand J Sports Sci* 6[2]:57-66, 1984.)

Table 16-8

Average Barbell Power for World and Olympic Champions During the Snatch, Clean, and Jerk

Competition	Lift	Average Power Output (W)									
		52 kg	56 kg	60 kg	67.5 kg	75 kg	82.5 kg	90 kg	100 kg	110 kg	110+ kg
1978 World Championships[144]	Snatch—pull	1619	2018	—	2460	2675	3057	3139	3216	3542	4021
	Snatch—Second pull	2784	3187	—	3239	3892	4765	4976	5243	5212	6088
	Clean—pull	1453	2200	—	2149	2803	2858	2837	3246	3877	—
	Clean—Second pull	2470	3364	—	2762	4846	4630	4700	5291	4387	—
	Jerk	2515	3451	—	2948	5060	4495	5072	—	5080	—
1984 Olympic Games[31]	Snatch—pull	—	1770	—	—	2533	2423	—	2920	—	3671
	Snatch—Second pull	—	3190	—	—	4052	3689	—	4714	—	5442
	Clean—pull	—	1677	—	—	2600	2268	—	2772	—	3360
	Clean—Second pull	—	3142	—	—	3877	3543	—	4983	—	6120
	Jerk	—	2825	—	—	3804	3548	—	4170	—	4321

Note: Data were not available for each lift for every athlete.

In elite men weightlifters, 31 to 37 WkgBM^{-1} power is generated during the entire pulling phase and 45 to 60 WkgBM^{-1} during the SP.[144] Power output for elite men weightlifters has remained relatively constant since the late 1970s, which parallels the small increases in the world records to the present day.[150] In the inaugural women's world championships in 1987, power output averaged 62% for the entire pulling phase and 73% for the SP relative to power generated by men (Table 16-9).[141] At the same time, the women's world records in the long jump and high jump were 85% of the records for men.[141] Given that the BW of elite women jumpers at the time was 85% that of men, it can be estimated that women generated approximately 72% (85% jump × 85% BW) as much power as men in performing world record jump attempts.[141] Thus, the power output generated during the SP is appropriate given physiological differences between men and women. However, the power generated during the FP and entire pulling phase is lower than would be expected.

Analysis of more recent lifts by women indicate that power generated during the SP approaches 80% of power generated by men[158,183]; however, power generated during the FP and entire pulling phase has not increased, despite a considerable increase in the women's world records for the snatch and the clean and jerk. Thus, while women are capable of generating large muscular forces during the mechanically advantageous SP, they are limited by their ability to generate muscular forces during the mechanically disadvantageous FP. In particular, the strength of the hamstring muscles should be considered because of its role in eccentrically extending the knee and concentrically extending the hip at the end of the FP.[161-163]

Clinically Relevant Points Regarding the Snatch and Clean

- Consist of seven distinct phases
- The pulling phases (first pull, second knee bend, second pull) require muscle forces to elevate the lifter and barbell (i.e., propulsion)
- The pull under and amortization phases require muscle forces to absorb impulse (i.e., braking)
- Requires a coordinated sequence of muscle actions to lift the barbell through an appropriate trajectory
- Excessive elevation of the barbell is energetically inefficient
- The hip extensor and ankle plantar-flexor muscles are primarily used to maintain proper body posture during the pulling phase
- The quadriceps and hamstrings are primarily used to generate propulsion during the pulling phase
- In receiving the barbell, a lifter actively repositions the body from an upright to a squatting position

Segment Mechanics of the Split Jerk

Considerably less research exists for the jerk than the snatch or clean. A major difference between the jerk versus the snatch and clean is that the lifter begins the jerk movement in an upright posture, which reduces the importance of the hip and back extensor musculature that are essential for the

FP and SKB. The jerk has been broken into seven distinct phases: (1) preliminary half squat, (2) active half squat, (3) braking, (4) thrust, (5) push under the bar, (6) support, and (7) recovery (Figure 16-15).[184,185] Weightlifting coaches often refer to the jerk as a *dip and drive and split*. The dip consists of phases 1 and 2, the drive phases 3 and 4, and the split phases 5, 6, and 7.

The preliminary half squat consists of the lifter flexing the knees and dorsiflexing the ankles, ending when the barbell begins to move downward. This initiates the active half squat, which ends when the falling barbell reaches maximum velocity. The peak downward velocity of the barbell ranges from 0.9 to 1 ms^{-1} and the knees reach an angle of approximately 130°.[148,185] Elite lifters have been observed performing these phases faster than lower-caliber lifters, achieving a higher downward barbell velocity and displaying a shorter time to peak velocity.[185,186] During the preliminary half-squat phase of the jerk, and the mechanically similar push press, a knee flexor NJM is observed.[137,187,188] No segment kinetic analyses of the hip and ankle exist for the jerk; however, an analysis of the push press, which involves a similar dip and drive motion found minimal (< 0.5 NmkgBM^{-1})

Table 16-9

Comparison of Relative Power Output for Men and Women World Champions in the Snatch and Clean

	Average Power Output (WkgBM^{-1})			
	Snatch—Pull	Snatch—Second Pull	Clean—Pull	Clean—Second Pull
Men—1978 World Champions	34.4 ± 2.5	52.7 ± 4.5	34.2 ± 3.6	52.5 ± 8.9
Women—1987 World Champions	22.5 ± 1.7	40.1 ± 5.0	21.0 ± 1.8	38.2 ± 3.3
% (Women/men)	65.4	76.1	61.4	72.8

Data from Garhammer J: A comparison of maximal power outputs between elite male and female weightlifters in competition, *Int J Sport Biomech* 7:3–11, 1991.

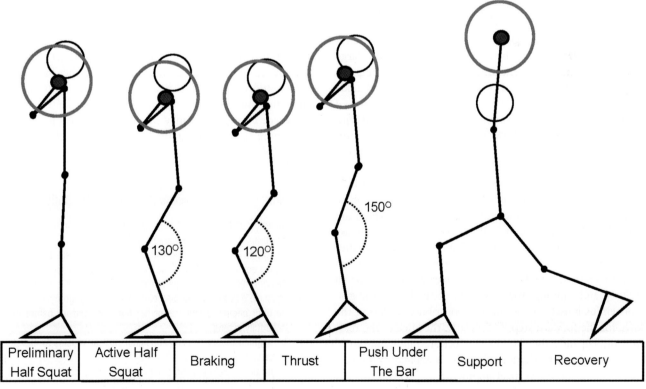

| Preliminary Half Squat | Active Half Squat | Braking | Thrust | Push Under The Bar | Support | Recovery |

Figure 16-15
The seven phases of the split jerk.

hip extensor and ankle plantar flexor NJM during the initial dip motion.[137] The knee flexor NJM likely increases the rate of performing the half squat, whereas the low hip and ankle NJM minimize resistance to movement.

As the barbell attains maximum downward velocity, the braking phase begins, ending when the knees reach maximum flexion. An additional 10° knee flexion occurs during the braking phase, with the knee extensors actively resist further flexion.[159] A rapid rise in the knee extensor NJM has been observed during this phase of the jerk and push press, as well as a large increase in vertical ground reaction force during the jerk.[137,147,148,187,188] The rapid rise in ground reaction force during the braking phase is similar to what is observed during the SKB phase of the snatch and clean, as well as during the squat in a countermovement jump.[145,147,148,171] The combined knee flexion with a rapidly increasing knee extensor NJM is indicative of a stretch-shortening cycle movement. Shortly after maximum knee flexion is attained, there is elastic deformation of the ends of the barbell, resulting in the ends of the barbell dropping lower than the center, increasing the load on the knee extensors.[188]

As the ends of the barbell reach their minimum height, the knees begin to extend, initiating the thrust phase. Similar to the SP in the snatch and clean, the end of the jerk thrust phase occurs when the barbell has reached maximum velocity.[30] The peak vertical velocity of the barbell should exceed 1.6 ms^{-1}, with taller lifters requiring a greater velocity than shorter lifters.[144,185,186] It has been observed that the ratio between the peak upward velocity to the peak downward velocity increases with the caliber of athlete.[186] As peak downward velocity is also higher for better lifters,[185,186] it highlights the importance of applying a large impulse to impart momentum to the barbell. This impulse is predominantly generated by the knee extensor and ankle plantar flexor muscles.[137,187,188] The large co-contraction of the quadriceps and hamstring muscles[147,148] combined with the high knee extensor NJM $(>4 \text{ NmkgBM}^{-1})$[187,188] indicate that the muscular force generated by the quadriceps during the jerk is considerably high.

As with the snatch and clean SP, the knees do not fully extend during the jerk thrust. At the end of the thrust phase and start of the push-under-the-bar phase, the knees are extended to approximately 150° to 160°.[185,186] An increase in the ankle plantar flexor NJM[137] indicates that the lifter raises onto his or her toes; however, this may not be occurring to increase the height of the barbell. Rather, as in walking and running, the activation of the biarticular gastrocnemius muscle at toe-off may contribute to flexing the knee for the forward step.[189] Similarly, the knee of the rear-moving leg must also flex. As the feet are rapidly removed from the platform, additional impulse is applied to the barbell, increasing its vertical momentum.[190] Prior to the barbell leaving the shoulders, the lifter aggressively pushes under the barbell, accelerating his or her body downward at -14 ms^{-2}, which imparts additional vertical impulse to the barbell.[173] If performed properly, the barbell should be received overhead at the instant it reaches its apex.

System Mechanics of the Split Jerk

During the "dip and drive" in the jerk, the optimal downward displacement of the lifter's center of mass ranges from 10% to 12% of the lifter's height.[186,190] A larger downward displacement indicates that the half squat was not performed rapidly enough or insufficient muscular force was generated during the braking phase. The larger downward displacement results in longer thrust duration.[185] Interestingly, longer thrust duration is associated with higher peak vertical barbell velocity and a higher peak height of the barbell; however, these are characteristic of low caliber rather than elite weightlifters.[185] These data are indicative of the importance of the push-under-the-bar phase, which, when performed properly, imparts sufficient vertical momentum to the barbell that the athlete is able to reposition into the split position and receive the barbell overhead.[190]

The longer-duration thrust phase may be an indicator of inefficient energy expenditure.[178] The greater change in potential energy during the thrust phase, and higher peak vertical barbell velocity at the end of the thrust phase increase the mechanical work that must be performed; however, power output is lower. As with the snatch and clean, it is preferable to perform the same amount of work to lift a heavier barbell, rather than to lift a lighter barbell to a greater height. A long duration of the thrust phase will also reduce power output during the jerk. Typically, in elite lifters, the average power during the jerk is comparable to the power generated during the SP of the snatch and clean.[30,144] However, some elite lifters generate considerably less power during the jerk than either the snatch or clean, which may suggest a technical fault, such as dipping too low or extending the duration of the thrust phase.[30,178]

Clinically Relevant Points Regarding the Split Jerk

- The jerk requires the rapid reversal of knee flexion to knee extension to apply vertical impulse to the barbell
- During this knee flexion and extension, the quadriceps are active, first eccentrically then concentrically, to generate propulsion
- The contribution of the arms to elevating the barbell is minimal
- Excessive elevation of the barbell is energetically inefficient
- The lifter begins to split his or her legs fore and aft before the knees fully extend
- The splitting motion applies additional vertical impulse to elevate the barbell
- The arms are used to push the lifter under the barbell

Injuries in Weightlifting

There is considerable discussion of the potential for injuries when performing weightlifting movements and their variations.[191-199] In considering the incidence of injuries, it is important to distinguish weightlifting, either as a sport or as training exercises, from other forms of resistance exercise because the muscles and joints stressed as well as the nature of the stresses are often different. Long-term assessments of weightlifters of varying abilities indicate that the incidence of injuries ranges from 2.4 to 3.3 per one thousand participation hours.[191,196] The incidence of injuries in youth and adolescents is considerably lower.[199,200] Injuries in weightlifting appear to be influenced by the weight of the barbell, and acute and long-term fatigue.[191,198] The most common injuries involve the low back and knee followed by the shoulder, wrist, and hand.[191,196,198,201] The majority of these injuries are acute (60%) rather than chronic (30%) or recurring (10%).[61] Most injuries to the low back (87%), knee (95%), and shoulder (92%) required less than one day to resolve and rarely more than one week.[191] Typically, these injuries were classified as a muscle strain or tendinitis.[191] More serious, although rare, injuries have been reported in competition, which include dislocation of the lunate,[202,203] wrist fractures,[204,205] dislocation of the elbow,[195] and rupture of the patellar ligament.[188]

Injuries in Weightlifting

Chronic
- Tendinosis—quadriceps tendon, patellar ligament
- Spondylolysis (Note: the incidence of spondylolysis in weightlifting has rarely been reported since the elimination of the clean and press from competition in 1972)

Acute
- Tendinitis—quadriceps tendon, patellar ligament, shoulder rotator cuff tendons and biceps tendon
- Muscle strains—quadriceps, shoulder muscles especially biceps and rotator cuff, lumbar spine muscles
- Fractures/dislocations—carpal bones, elbow (Note: these injuries are not common and are typically associated with maximum lifts in competition)

A potential concern in the low back is spondylolysis (fracture of the pars interarticularis), which was reported to have a high incidence in the 1970s and 1980s.[197,206-209] The mechanism of injury for pars interarticularis fracture is spinal hyperextension, which is augmented by heavy loading.[210] It should be noted, however, that a majority of weightlifters examined in these investigations participated in the sport prior to 1972, when the press was used in competition. During the decade preceding its removal from competition, the press had evolved from a strict upright pressing motion to one that involved an initial hyperextended trunk that preceded a rapid hip flexion–hip extension motion sequence. It was speculated that the hyperextension under load would injure the low back.[191] In 1978, Rossi[197] reported 21 of 58 weightlifters with low back pain had spondylolysis; however, in a follow-up paper in 1990,[209] an additional 39 weightlifters presented with low back pain, but only one had spondylolysis. This provides support for the notion that the press contributed to the incidence of spondylolysis, and not the snatch, clean, or jerk movements. In today's weightlifter, the majority of injuries appear to be muscle strains as a result of the high training volumes typically used.[191]

Similarly, the majority of knee injuries appear to be strains to the quadriceps tendon or patellar ligament.[191] It is commonly believed that the "bouncing" nature of the amortization phase of the clean, snatch, and jerk will result in injury to the knee joint, particularly the patellar ligament.[211] Zernicke and colleagues[188] reported a patellar ligament rupture during the braking phase of an attempted jerk of 175 kg by an 82.5-kg lifter in competition, in which the knee extensor NJM was 550 to 560 Nm and the tension in the ligament was estimated to be 14.5 KN. Prior to the moment of rupture, the knee extensor NJM peaked at 400 Nm and began to decrease as the barbell oscillated, first downward, then upward. However, a second downward oscillation of the barbell led to a rapid increase in the knee extensor NJM, resulting in rupture of the patellar ligament 0.06 seconds later. An analysis of a 165-kg jerk by a 104-kg lifter in a laboratory setting reported a peak knee extensor NJM of 350 Nm.[187] Knee extensor NJM during the amortization phase of the clean preceding the 165-kg jerk peaked at 400 Nm.[187] Normally, the braking phase of the jerk and amortization phase of the snatch and clean is reportedly at least 2.5 times longer than that found during the ligament rupture, which would result in a substantially lower loading rate and less peak demand on the quadriceps tendon and patellar ligament.[159,175,185,186] Thus, the second oscillation of the barbell may have been abnormal, and its high loading rate ultimately led to the patellar ligament rupture.[188]

When evaluating the potential for knee injuries during weightlifting, two factors must be considered when assessing the supposed stress due to "bouncing." First, the ultimate tensile strength of viscoelastic tissues, such as the patellar ligament, increases with strain rate.[188,212,213] While the loading rate reported by Zernicke and colleagues[188] was high, it appears to be considerably higher than that observed during normal performance of the jerk, as well for the snatch and clean.[137,153,163-165,187] Thus, a controlled "bounce" may actually afford greater protection for the quadriceps tendon and patellar ligament than a slower descent. In addition, slower squats are more likely to avulse the bony attachment than rupture the tendon and ligament midsubstance because of the different viscoelastic properties of tendon and ligament compared with bone.[212,214] With advances in modeling technology, future research should investigate the stresses imposed on these and other soft tissues during rapid dynamic movements such as those occurring in weightlifting.

The second factor to consider is the soft tissue reaction forces that occur in a deep squat. Zelle and colleagues[176] found that in an unloaded deep squat, thigh-calf contact resulted in reaction forces of 34% of BW, acting approximately 15 cm (5.9 inches) from the knee axis of rotation. This would result in a moment extending the knee of approximately 0.5 $NmkgBM^{-1}$, whereas the NJM flexing the knee in an unloaded squat with thigh contact is approximately 1 $NmkgBM^{-1}$.[215] Although it is unknown what the effect of soft tissue contact is on knee extensor NJM during the snatch and clean, this factor may considerably reduce the stress imposed on the quadriceps tendon and patellar ligament during these movements. Clearly, more research is required on this topic to assess the practical implications of soft tissue contact during human movement.

A recent case study has cast doubt on whether chronic pain and morphological changes to the patellar ligament result in weakening of the tissue.[216] Patellar tendinosis was diagnosed in an international caliber weightlifter from ultrasound evidence of local widening of the ligament with focal hypoechoic areas, irregular fiber structure, and neovascularization. Treatment of the neovascularization with a sclerosing agent (polidocanol) resulted in a decrease in pain and return to training in 2 weeks (including performing deep squats with 240 kg). Ligament morphology was unchanged at 2- and 4-month follow-ups, except a reduction of neovascularization. Similar results were reported in a larger study of various athletes who returned to physical activity after sclerosing treatment without ligament morphological changes.[217]

The incidence of shoulder instability has been reported to be high in weightlifters.[196] However, most of these reports have generally presented cases of recreational weight trainers and not competitive weightlifters.[218-220] Cahill[218] reported 19 cases of osteolysis of the distal clavicle requiring surgery, of which all performed weight training, and four were identified as "competitive weightlifters." However, the bench press and parallel bar dip exercises were implicated as contributing to most of these injuries. As these exercises are rarely performed by competitive weightlifters,[134,140,190] it is possible that some or all of these four cases were powerlifters. Furthermore, three of the four were followed up for 10 to 11 years prior to the article date (1982); thus, if they were competitive weightlifters, they would have competed in the press. Because of the similarity in motion for the press and bench press, it is reasonable to expect that similar injuries may occur for both exercises. However, the propulsive forces during the jerk are generated primarily by the lower extremities[163,187,188] and the weight of the barbell is only supported by the shoulders in the extended position, as opposed to when flexed as occurs during pressing exercises.

Retrospective assessments of active and retired weightlifters supports the notion that weightlifting exercises are not inherently dangerous, nor do injuries during weightlifting result in long-term disability.[192,193,221] The incidence of low back, hip, knee and shoulder osteoarthritis is no greater and in some cases less than the general population.[193] The use of free weight training alone is associated with a low relative risk for lumbar and cervical disc herniation.[221] Kujala et al.[194] has reported a higher incidence of tibiofemoral joint osteoarthritis in weightlifters than in runners and shooters, and patellofemoral joint osteoarthritis than runners, shooters, and soccer players. However, the 29 weightlifters selected for this investigation were a subsample of 40 weightlifters who had responded to an initial survey, which may skew the actual incidence of these degenerative conditions. The results are further confounded by the number of years the weightlifters participated in occupations involving kneeling and squatting and heavy labor compared with the other athlete groups. Finally, as the technique and mechanics of weightlifting have evolved since 1972, it is important to continue to assess the long-term effect of training and competition on joint health.

Conclusion

The biomechanics of weight training is complex because of the various kinetics, kinematics, muscle activity, and pathological conditions of each respective body part. Significant muscle activity is relevant to specific tasks and movements, as is the coordination of muscles activated. Compressive, tensile, and shear forces can be high with various forms of specific exercises, which may be significant for individuals with pre-existing pathological conditions. It is recommended the clinician use the included information in this chapter to prescribe the most efficacious exercise program for their clients. In particular, clinicians should consider how the mechanics of an exercise load the body, as well as how modifications of these mechanics may increase effectiveness and reduce risk of injury. This is especially relevant for those clients with a pathologic conditions of a particular body part that may respond less favorably to excessive forces.

References

1. Bergmark A: Stability of the lumbar spine. A study in mechanical engineering, *Acta Orthop Scand* [Suppl] (230):1–54, 1989.
2. Crisco JJ 3rd, Panjabi MM: The intersegmental and multisegmental muscles of the lumbar spine, A biomechanical model comparing lateral stabilizing potential, *Spine* 16:793–799, 1991.
3. Gardner-Morse M, Stokes IA, Laible JP: Role of muscles in lumbar spine stability in maximum extension efforts, *J Orthop Res* 13:802–808, 1995.
4. Cholewicki J, McGill SM: Mechanical stability of the in vivo lumbar spine: Implications for injury and chronic low back pain, *Clin Biomech* 11:1–15, 1996
5. Cholewicki J, Panjabi MM, Khachatryan A: Stabilizing function of trunk flexor-extensor muscles around a neutral spine posture, *Spine* 22:2207–2212, 1997.
6. Granata KP, Marras WS: Cost-benefit of muscle cocontraction in protecting against spinal instability, *Spine* 25:1398–1404, 2000.
7. Magnusson ML, Aleksiev A, Wilder DG, et al: Unexpected load and asymmetric posture as etiologic factors in low back pain, *Eur Spine J* 5:23–35, 1996.
8. Hodges PW, Richardson CA: Delayed postural contraction of transversus abdominis in low back pain associated with movement of the lower limb, *J Spinal Disor* 11:46–56, 1998.
9. Hodges PW, Richardson CA: Altered trunk muscle recruitment in people with low back pain with upper limb movement at different speeds, *Arch Phys Med Rehabil* 80:1005–1012, 1999.
10. Radebold A, Cholewicki J, Panjabi MM, Patel TC: Muscle response pattern to sudden trunk loading in healthy individuals and in patients with chronic low back pain, *Spine* 25:947–954, 2000.
11. Panjabi MM: The stabilizing system of the spine. Part I. Function dysfunction, adaptation, and enhancement, *J Spinal Disord* 5:383–389, 1992.
12. Lucas DB, Bresler B: *Stability of the ligamentous spine*, Report no. 40 from the Biomechanics Laboratory, University of California, San Francisco, Berkeley, 1961.
13. Crisco JJ, Panjabi MM, Yamamoto I, et al: Euler stability of the human ligamentous lumbar spine: Part II experiment, *Clin Biomech* 7:27–32, 1992.
14. Cromwell R, Schultz AB, Beck R, et al: Loads on the lumbar trunk during level walking, *J Orthop Res* 7:371–377, 2005.
15. El-Rich M, Shirazi-Adl A, Arjmand N: Muscle activity, internal loads, and stability of the human spine in standing postures: Combined model and in vivo studies, *Spine* 29:2633–2642, 2004.
16. Gibbons SGT, Comerford MJ: Strength versus stability. Part 1: Concept and terms, *Orthop Division Rev* March/April:21–27, 2001.
17. Solomonow M, Zhou B-H, Bratta RV, et al: Biomechanics and electromyography of a cumulative lumbar disorder: Response to static stretching, *Clin Biomech* 18:890–898, 2003.
18. Lavender SA, Tsuang YH, Andersson GB, et al: Trunk muscle cocontraction: The effects of moment direction and moment magnitude, *J Orthop Res* 10:691–700, 1992.
19. Kavcic N, Grenier S, McGill SM: Determining the stabilizing role of individual torso muscles during rehabilitation exercises, *Spine* 29:1254–1265, 2004.
20. Pope MH, Andersson GB, Broman H, et al: Electromyographic studies of the lumbar trunk musculature during the development of axial torques, *J Ortho Res* 4:288–297, 1986.
21. Aspden RM: The spine is an arch. A new mathematical model, *Spine* 14:266–274, 1989.
22. McGill SM: Electromyographic activity of the abdominal and low back musculature during the generation of isometric and dynamic axial trunk torque: Implications for lumbar mechanics, *J Orthop Res*, 9:91–103, 1991.
23. Cholewicki J, Van Velt JJ: Relative contribution of trunk muscles to the stability of the lumbar spine during isometric exertions, *Clin Biomech* 17:99–105, 2002.
24. McGill SM. *Ultimate back fitness and performance*, Waterloo, Ontario, Canada, 2004.Wabuno.
25. Chandler TJ, Stone MH: The squat exercise in athletic conditioning: A review of the literature, *Natl Strength Condit Assoc J* 13:52–58, 1991.
26. Hattin HC, Pierrynowski MR, Ball KA: Effect of load, cadence, and fatigue on tibio-femoral joint force during a half squat, *Med Sci Sports Exerc* 5:613–618, 1989.
27. McLaughlin TM, Dillman CJ, Lardner TJ: A kinematic model of performance in the parallel squat by champion powerlifters, *Med Sci Sports* 2:128–133, 1977.
28. McLaughlin TM, Lardner TJ, Dillman CJ: Kinetics of the parallel squat, *Res Q* 2:175–189, 1978.
29. Coaches' Roundtable. The squat and its application to athletic performance, *Natl Strength Condit Assoc J* 6:10–22, 1984.
30. Garhammer J: Power production by Olympic weightlifters, *Med Sci Sports Exerc* 1:54–60, 1980.
31. Garhammer J: Biomechanical profiles of Olympic weightlifters, *Int J Sports Biomech* 1:122–130, 1985.
32. Hutton WC, Adams MA: Can the lumbar spine be crushed in heavy lifting? *Spine* 7:586–590, 1982.
33. Schultz AB, Andersson GBJ: Analysis of loads on the lumbar spine, *Spine* 6:76–82, 1981.
34. Delitto RS, Rose SJ, Apts DW, Electromyographic analysis of two techniques for squat lifting, *Phys Ther* 67:1329–1334, 1987.
35. Hart DL, Stobbe TJ, Jaraiedi M: Effect of posture on lifting, *Spine* 12:138–145, 1987.
36. Holmes JA, Damaser MS, Lehman SL: Erector spinae activation and movement dynamics about the lumbar spine in lordotic and kyphotic squat-lifting, *Spine* 17(3):327–334, 1992.
37. Floyd WF, Silvers PHS: The function of the erector spinae muscles in certain movements and postures in man, *J Physiol* 129:184–203, 1955.
38. Floyd WF, Silvers PHS: Function of erector spinae in flexion of the trunk, *Lancet* 1:133–134, 1951.
39. Toussaint HM, de Winter AF, de Haas Y, et al: Flexion relaxation during lifting: Implication for torque production by muscle activity and tissue strain at the lumbo-sacral joint, *J Biomechanics* 28(2):199–210, 1995.
40. Gill KP, Bennett SJ, Savelsbergh GJP, et al: Regional changes in spine posture at lift onset with changes in lift distance and lift style, *Spine* 32(15):1599–1604, 2007.
41. Shirazi-Adl A, El-Rich M, Pop DG, Parninpour M: Spinal muscle forces, internal loads and stability in standing under various postures and loads-application of kinematics-based algorithm, *Eur Spine J* 14(4):381–392, 2005.
42. Bazrgari B, Shirazi-Adl A, Arjmand N: Analysis of squat and stoop dynamic liftings: Muscle forces and internal spinal loads, *Eur Spine J* 16(5):687–699, 2007.
43. Bazrgari B. Shirazi-Adl A: Spinal stability and role of passive stiffness in dynamic squat and stoop lifts, *Comput Methods Biomech Biomed Engin* 10(5):351–360, 2007.
44. Arjmand N, Shirazi-Adl A: Biomechanics of changes in lumbar posture in static lifting, *Spine* 30(23):2637–2648, 2005.
45. Hwang S, Kim Y, Kim Y: Lower extremity joint kinetics and lumbar curvature during squat and stoop lifting, *BMC Musculoskel Dis* 10:15, 2009.

46. Brown SHM, McGill SM: How the inherent stiffness of the in vivo human trunk varies with changing magnitudes of muscular activation, *Clin Biomech* 23:15–22, 2008.

47. Cappozzo A, Felici F, Figura F, et al: Lumbar spine loading during half-squat exercises, *Med Sci Sports Exerc* 17:613–620, 1985.

48. Cholewicki J, McGill SM, Norman RW: Lumbar spine loads during the lifting of extremely heavy weights, *Med Sci Sports Exerc* 23:1179–1186, 1991.

49. Adams MA, McNally DS, Chinn H, et al: Posture and the compressive strength of the lumbar spine, *Clin Biomech* 9:5–14, 1994.

50. Gunning JL, Callaghan JP, McGill SM: The role of prior loading history and spinal posture on the compressive tolerance and type of failure in the spine using a porcine trauma model, *Clin Biomech* 16(6):471–480, 2001.

51. McGill SM: Biomechanics of low back injury: Implications on current practice and the clinic, *J Biomech* 30(5):465–475, 1997.

52. Kumar S: Upper body push-pull strength of normal young adults in sagittal plane at three heights, *Ind Ergon* 15:427–436, 1995.

53. Caldwell JS, McNair PJ, Williams M: The effects of repetitive motion on lumbar flexion and erector spinae muscle activity in rowers, *Clin Biomech* 18(8):704–711, 2003.

54. Anderson K, Behm DG: Maintenance of EMG activity and loss of force output with instability, *J Strength Cond Res* 18:637–640, 2004.

55. Schibye B, Sogaaro K, Martinsen D, et al: Mechanical load on the low back and shoulders during pushing and pulling of two wheeled waste containers compared with lifting and carrying of bags and bins, *Clin Biomech* 16:549–559, 2001.

56. Lett KK, McGill SM: Pushing and pulling: Personal mechanics influence spine loads, *Ergonomics* 49(9):895–908, 2006.

57. Freeman S. Karpowicz A, Gray J, et al: Quantifying muscle patterns and spine load during various forms of the pushup, *Med Sci Sports Exerc* 38(3):570–577, 2006.

58. Howarth SJ, Beach TAC, Callaghan JP: Abdominal muscles dominate contributions to vertebral joint stiffness during the push-up, *J Appl Biomech* 24:130–139, 2008.

59. Moreside JM, Vera-Garcia FJ, McGill SM: Trunk muscle activation patterns, lumbar compressive forces, and spine stability when using the Bodyblade, *Phys Ther* 87(2):153–163, 2007.

60. Anders C, Wenzel B, Scholle HC: Activation characteristics of trunk muscles during cyclic upper-body perturbations caused by an oscillating pole, *Arch Phys Med Rehabil* 89:1314–1322, 2008.

61. Juker D, McGill SM, Kropf P, et al: Quantitative intramuscular myoelectric activity of lumbar portions of psoas and the abdominal wall during a wide variety of tasks, *Med Sci Sports Exerc* 30(2):301–310, 1998.

62. Axler C, McGill SM: Low back loads over a variety of abdominal exercises: Searching for the safest abdominal challenge, *Med Sci Sports Exerc* 29(6):804–811, 1997.

63. Willett GM, Hyde JE, Uhrlaub MB, et al: Relative activity of abdominal muscles during commonly prescribed strengthening exercises, *J Strength Cond Res* 15(4):480–485, 2001.

64. Stevens VK, Bouche KG, Mahieu NN, et al: Trunk muscle activity in healthy subjects during bridging stabilization exercises, *BMC Musculoskelet Disord* 20:75, 2006.

65. Ekstrom RA, Osborn RW, Hauer PL: Surface electromyographic analysis of the low back muscles during rehabilitation exercises, *J Orthop Sports Phys Ther* 38(12):736–745, 2008.

66. Ekstrom RA, Donatelli RA, Carp KC: Electromyographic analysis of core trunk, hip, and thigh muscles during 9 rehabilitation exercises, *J Orthop Sports Phys Ther* 37(12):754–762, 2007.

67. Arokoski JP, Valta T, Airaksinen O, et al: Back and abdominal muscle function during stabilization exercises, *Arch Phys Med Rehabil* 82:1089–1098, 2001.

68. Souza GM, Baker LL, Powers CM: Electromyographic activity of selected trunk muscles during dynamic spine stabilization exercises, *Arch Phys Med Rehabil* 82:1551–1557, 2001.

69. Drake JDM, Fischer SL, Brown SHM, et al: Do exercise balls provide a training advantage for trunk extensor exercises? A biomechanical evaluation, *J Manipulative Physiol Ther* 29:354–362, 2006.

70. Stevens VK, Vleeming A, Bouche KG, et al: Electromyographic activity of trunk and hip muscles during stabilization exercises in four-point kneeling in healthy volunteers, *Eur Spine J* 16:711–718, 2007.

71. Arokoski JPA, Kankaanpää M, Valta T, et al: Back and hip extensor muscle function during therapeutic exercises, *Arch Phys Med Rehabil* 80:842–850, 1999.

72. Vera-Garcia FJ, Grenier SG, McGill SM: Abdominal muscle response during curl-ups on both stable and labile surfaces, *Phys Ther* 80:564–569, 2000.

73. Marshall PW, Murphy BA: Core stability exercises on and off a Swiss ball, *Arch Phys Med Rehabil* 86:242–249, 2005.

74. Behm DG, Leonard AM, Young WB, et al: Trunk muscle electromyographic activity with unstable and unilateral exercises, *J Strength Cond Res* 19(1):193–201, 2005.

75. Arokoski JPA, Valta T, Kankaanpää M, et al: Activation of lumbar paraspinal and abdominal muscles during therapeutic exercises in chronic low back pain patients, *Arch Phys Med Rehabil* 85:823–832, 2004.

76. Escamilla RF, Babb E, DeWitt R, et al: Electromyographic analysis of traditional and nontraditional abdominal exercises: Implications for rehabilitation and training, *Phys Ther* 86(5):656–671, 2006.

77. Escamilla RF, McTaggart MSC, Fricklas EJ, et al: An electromyographic analysis of commercial and common abdominal exercises: Implications for rehabilitation and training, *J Orthop Sports Phys Ther* 36(2):45–57, 2006.

78. Escamilla RF, Bonacci L, Burnham T, et al: A biomechanical analysis of squatting and lunging type exercises, *Med Sci Sports Exerc* 38(5):S97, 2006.

79. Escamilla RF, Francisco AC, Fleisig GS, et al: A three-dimensional biomechanical analysis of sumo and conventional style deadlifts, *Med Sci Sports Exerc* 32(7):1265–1275, 2000.

80. DiGiovine NM, Jobe FW, Pink M, Perry J: Electromyography of upper extremity in pitching, *J Shoulder Elbow Surg* 1:15–25, 1992.

81. Blanpied PR: Changes in muscle activation during wall slides and squat-machine exercise, *J Sport Rehabil* 8(2):123–134, 1999.

82. Dahlkvist NJ, Mayo P, Seedhom BB: Forces during squatting and rising from a deep squat, *Eng Med* 11(2):69–76, 1982.

83. Escamilla RF, Fleisig GS, Zheng N, et al: Biomechanics of the knee during closed kinetic chain and open kinetic chain exercises, *Med Sci Sports Exerc* 30(4):556–569, 1998.

84. Escamilla RF, Fleisig GS, Zheng N, et al: Effects of technique variations on knee biomechanics during the squat and leg press, *Med Sci Sports Exerc* 33(9):1552–1566, 2001.

85. Hung YJ, Gross MT: Effect of foot position on electromyographic activity of the vastus medialis oblique and vastus lateralis during lower-extremity weight-bearing activities, *J Orthop Sports Phys Ther* 29(2):93–105, 1999.

86. Isear JA Jr., Erickson JC, Worrell TW: EMG analysis of lower extremity muscle recruitment patterns during an unloaded squat, *Med Sci Sports Exerc* 29(4):532–539, 1997.

87. McCaw ST, Melrose DR: Stance width and bar load effects on leg muscle activity during the parallel squat, *Med Sci Sports Exerc* 31(3):428–436, 1999.

88. Mirzabeigi E, Jordan C, Gronley JK, et al: Isolation of the vastus medialis oblique muscle during exercise, *Am J Sports Med* 27(1):50–53, 1999.

89. Ninos JC, Irrgang JJ, Burdett R, Weiss JR: Electromyographic analysis of the squat performed in self-selected lower extremity neutral rotation and 30 degrees of lower extremity turn- out from the self-selected neutral position, *J Orthop Sports Phys Ther* 25(5):307–315, 1997.

90. Signorile JF, Kwiatkowski K, Caruso JF, Robertson B: Effect of foot position on the electromyographical activity of the superficial quadriceps muscles during the parallel squat and knee extension, *J Strength Cond Res* 9(3):182–187, 1995.

91. Signorile JF, Weber B, Roll B, et al: An electromyographical comparison of the squat and knee extension exercises, *J Strength Cond Res* 8(3):178–183, 1994.

92. Stuart MJ, Meglan DA, Lutz GE, et al: Comparison of intersegmental tibiofemoral joint forces and muscle activity during various closed kinetic chain exercises, *Am J Sports Med* 24(6): 792–799, 1996.

93. Wilk KE, Escamilla RF, Fleisig GS, et al: A comparison of tibio-femoral joint forces and electromyographic activity during open and closed kinetic chain exercises, *Am J Sports Med* 24(4): 518–527, 1996.

94. Wretenberg P, Feng Y, Arborelius UP: High-and low-bar squatting techniques during weight-training, *Med Sci Sports Exerc* 28(2):218–224, 1996.

95. Wretenberg P, Feng Y, Lindberg F, Arborelius UP: Joint moments of force and quadriceps activity during squatting exercise, *Scand J Med Sci Sports* 3:244–250, 1993.

96. Wright GA, Delong TH, Gehlsen G: Electromyographic activity of the hamstrings during performance of the leg curl, stiff-leg deadlift, and back squat movements, *J Strength Cond R* 13(2):168–174, 1999.

97. Ohkoshi Y, Yasuda K, Kaneda K, et al: Biomechanical analysis of rehabilitation in the standing position, *Am J Sports Med* 19(6):605–611, 1991.

98. Anderson R, Courtney C, Carmeli E: EMG analysis of the vastus medialis/vastus lateralis muscles utilizing the unloaded narrow-and wide-stance squats, *J Sport Rehabil* 7(4):236–247, 1998.

99. Tesch PA: Muscle meets magnet, Stockholm, 1993, PA Tesch AB.

100. Farrokhi S, Pollard CD, Souza RB, et al: Trunk position influences the kinematics, kinetics, and muscle activity of the lead lower extremity during the forward lunge exercise, *J Orthop Sports Phys Ther* 38(7):403–409, 2008.

101. Hefzy MS, al Khazim M, Harrison L: Co-activation of the hamstrings and quadriceps during the lunge exercise, *Biomed Sci Instrum* 33:360–365, 1997.

102. Andrews JG, Hay JG, Vaughan CL: Knee shear forces during a squat exercise using a barbell and a weight machine. In Matsui H, Kobayashi K, editors: *Biomechanics VIII-B*, Champaign, 1983, Human Kinetics.

103. Ariel BG: Biomechanical analysis of the knee joint during deep knee bends with heavy loads. In Nelson R, Morehouse C, editors: *Biomechanics IV*, Baltimore, 1974, University Park Press.

104. Beynnon BD, Johnson RJ, Fleming BC, et al: The strain behavior of the anterior cruciate ligament during squatting and active flexion-extension. A comparison of an open and a closed kinetic chain exercise, *Am J Sports Med* 25(6):823–829, 1997.

105. Hattin HC, Pierrynowski MR, Ball KA: Effect of load, cadence, and fatigue on tibio-femoral joint force during a half squat, *Med Sci Sports Exerc* 21(5):613–618, 1989.

106. Nisell R, Ekholm J: Joint load during the parallel squat in powerlifting and force analysis of in vivo bilateral quadriceps tendon rupture, *Scand J Sports Sci* 8(2):63–70, 1986.

107. Toutoungi DE, Lu TW, Leardini A, et al: Cruciate ligament forces in the human knee during rehabilitation exercises, *Clin Biomech* 15(3):176–187, 2000.

108. Aune AK, Ekeland A, Nordsletten L: Effect of quadriceps or hamstring contraction on the anterior shear force to anterior cruciate ligament failure. An in vivo study in the rat, *Acta Orthop Scand* 66(3):261–265, 1995.

109. More RC, Karras BT, Neiman R, et al: Hamstrings—An anterior cruciate ligament protagonist. An in vitro study, *Am J Sports Med* 21(2):231–237, 1993.

110. Ortiz GJ, Schmotzer H, Bernbeck J, et al: Isometry of the posterior cruciate ligament. Effects of functional load and muscle force application, *Am J Sports Med* 26(5):663–668, 1998.

111. Yasuda K, Sasaki T: Muscle exercise after anterior cruciate ligament reconstruction. Biomechanics of the simultaneous isometric contraction method of the quadriceps and the hamstrings, *Clin Orthop* (220):266–274, 1987.

112. Yasuda K, Sasaki T: Exercise after anterior cruciate ligament reconstruction. The force exerted on the tibia by the separate isometric contractions of the quadriceps or the hamstrings, *Clin Orthop* (220):275–283, 1987.

113. Castle TH Jr., Noyes FR, Grood ES: Posterior tibial subluxation of the posterior cruciate-deficient knee, *Clin Orthop* (284): 193–202, 1992.

114. Herzog W, Read LJ: Lines of action and moment arms of the major force-carrying structures crossing the human knee joint, *J Anat* 182:213–230, 1993.

115. Hsieh HH, Walker PS: Stabilizing mechanisms of the loaded and unloaded knee joint, *J Bone Joint Surg Am* 58(1):87–93, 1976.

116. Shoemaker SC, Markolf KL: Effects of joint load on the stiffness and laxity of ligament-deficient knees. An in vitro study of the anterior cruciate and medial collateral ligaments, *J Bone Joint Surg Am* 67(1):136–146, 1985.

117. Markolf KL, Bargar WL, Shoemaker SC, Amstutz HC: The role of joint load in knee stability, *J Bone Joint Surg Am* 63(4):570–585, 1981.

118. Yack HJ, Washco LA, Whieldon T: Compressive forces as a limiting factor of anterior tibial translation in the ACL-deficient knee, *Clin J Sports Med* 4:233–239, 1994.

119. Escamilla RF, Zheng N, Imamura R, et al: Cruciate ligament force during the wall squat and one leg squat, *Med Sci Sports Exerc* 41(2):408–417, 2009.

120. Fitzgerald GK: Open versus closed kinetic chain exercise: Issues in rehabilitation after anterior cruciate ligament reconstructive surgery, *Phys Ther* 77(12):1747–1754, 1997.

121. Heijne A, Fleming BC, Renstrom PA, et al: Strain on the anterior cruciate ligament during closed kinetic chain exercises, *Med Sci Sports Exerc* 36(6):935–941, 2004.

122. Kvist J, Gillquist J: Sagittal plane knee translation and electromyographic activity during closed and open kinetic chain exercises in anterior cruciate ligament-deficient patients and control subjects, *Am J Sports Med* 29(1):72–82, 2001.

123. Zernicke RF, Garhammer J, Jobe FW: Human patellar-tendon rupture: A kinetic analysis, *J Bone Joint Surg Am* 59(2):179–183, 1977.

124. Escamilla RF, Zheng N, Imamura R, et al: Patellofemoral compressive force and stress during the one leg squat and wall squat, *Med Sci Sports Exerc* 41(4):879–888, 2009.

125. Reilly DT, Martens M: Experimental analysis of the quadriceps muscle force and patello-femoral joint reaction force for various activities, *Acta Orthop Scand* 43(2):126–137, 1972.

126. Nisell R, Ekholm J: Patellar forces during knee extension, *Scand J Rehabil Med* 17(2):63–74, 1985.

127. Salem GJ, Powers CM: Patellofemoral joint kinetics during squatting in collegiate women athletes, *Clin Biomech* (Bristol, Avon) 16(5):424–430, 2001.

128. Escamilla RF, Zheng N, Hreljac A, et al: Cruciate ligament force between the forward lunge long and short with and without a stride, In *Annual Meeting of the American Society of Biomechanics*, Palo Alto, CA, 2007.

129. Escamilla RF, Zheng N, Macleod TD, et al: Cruciate ligament tensile forces during lunging with varying techniques, *Med Sci Sports Exerc* 41(5):S81, 2009.

130. Race A, Amis AA: The mechanical properties of the two bundles of the human posterior cruciate ligament, *J Biomech* 27(1): 13–24, 1994.

131. Escamilla RF, Zheng N, MacLeod TD, et al: Patellofemoral compressive force and stress during the forward and side lunges with and without a stride, *Clin Biomech* (Bristol, Avon) 23(8):1026–1037, 2008.

132. Escamilla RF, Zheng N, Macleod TD, et al: Patellofemoral joint force and stress between a short- and long-step forward lunge, *J Orthop Sports Phys Ther* 38(11):681–690, 2008.

133. Garhammer J: Weight lifting and training. In Vaughan CL, Editor: *Biomechanics of sport*, Boca Raton, 1989, CRC Press.

134. Garhammer J, Takano B: Training for weightlifting, In Komi PV, Editor: *Strength and power in sport*, Oxford, 2003, Blackwell Scientific.

135. Newton H: Weightlifting? Weight Lifting? Olympic Lifting? Olympic Weightlifting? *Strength Cond J* 21(3):15–16, 1999.

136. Chiu LZF, Schilling BK: A primer on weightlifting: From sport to sports training, *Strength Cond J* 27(1):42–48, 2005.

137. Chiu LZF, Salem GJ: Comparison of joint kinetics during free weight and flywheel resistance exercise, *J Strength Cond Res* 20(3):555–562, 2006.

138. Garhammer J: *Biomechanical analysis of selected snatch lifts at the U.S. Senior National Weightlifting Championships*, In Proceedings of the International Congress of Physical Activity, Quebec City, QC, 1976, Symposia Specialists Inc.

139. Garhammer J: Energy flow during Olympic weight lifting, *Med Sci Sports Exerc* 14(5):353–360, 1982.

140. Laputin NP, Oleshko VG: *Managing the training of weightlifters* [Russian]. Kiev, 1982, Zdorov'ya Publishers. Translated by A. Charniga Jr.

141. Garhammer J: A comparison of maximal power outputs between elite male and female weightlifters in competition, *Int J Sport Biomech* 7:3–11, 1991.

142. Garhammer J, Kauhanen H, Häkkinen K: *A comparison of performances by women at the 1987 and 1998 World Weightlifting Championships*, In Proceedings of the Science for Success Congress, Jyväskylä, Finland, 2002.

143. Garhammer J: Longitudinal analysis of highly skilled Olympic weightlifters. In Terauds J, Editor: *Science in weightlifting*, Del Mar, CA, 1979.

144. Garhammer J: Biomechanical characteristics of the 1978 world weightlifting champions, In *Biomechanics VII-B*, Baltimore, 1981, University Park Press.

145. Enoka RM: The pull in Olympic weightlifting, *Med Sci Sports* 11(2):131–137, 1979.

146. Frolov VI, Lelikov SI, Efimov NM, et al: Snatch technique of top-class weightlifters [Russian], *Teoriya i Praktika Fizicheskoi Kultury* 6:59–61, 1977. Translated by M. Yessis.

147. Häkkinen K, Kauhanen H, Komi PV: Biomechanical changes in the Olympic weightlifting technique of the snatch and clean and jerk from submaximal to maximal loads, *Scand J Sports Sci* 6(2):57–66, 1984.

148. Kauhanen H, Häkkinen K, Komi PV: A biomechanical analysis of the snatch and clean & jerk techniques of Finnish elite and district level weightlifters, *Scand J Sports Sci* 6(2):47–56, 1984.

149. Vorobyev AN: *A textbook on weightlifting*, Budapest, 1978, International Weightlifting Federation. Translated by WJ Brice.

150. Garhammer J: *Weightlifting performance and techniques of men and women*, In Proceedings of the International Conference on Weightlifting and Strength Training, Lahti, Finland, 1998, Gummerus Printing.

151. Newton H: *Explosive lifting for sports*, Champaign, IL, 2002, Human Kinetics.

152. Stone MH, O'Bryant HS, Williams FE, et al: Analysis of bar paths during the snatch in elite male weightlifters, *Strength Cond* 20(4):30–38, 1998.

153. Baumann W, Gross V, Quade K, et al: The snatch technique of world class weightlifters at the 1985 World Championships, *Int J Sport Biomech* 4:68–89, 1988.

154. Gourgoulis V, Aggeloussis N, Mavromatis G, et al: Three-dimensional kinematic analysis of the snatch of elite Greek weightlifters, *J Sport Sci* 18:643–652, 2000.

155. Schilling BK, Stone MH, O'Bryant HS, et al: Snatch technique of collegiate national level weightlifters, *J Strength Cond Res* 16(4):551–555, 2002.

156. Garhammer J: Performance evaluation of Olympic weightlifters, *Med Sci Sports* 11(3): 284–287, 1979.

157. Gourgoulis V, Aggeloussis N, Antoniou P, et al: Comparative 3-dimensional kinematic analysis of the snatch technique in elite male and female Greek weightlifters, *J Strength Cond Res* 16(3):359–366, 2002.

158. Garhammer J, Taylor L: *Center of pressure movements during weightlifting*, In Proceedings of the 2nd International Symposium on Biomechanics in Sports, Colorado Springs, CO, 1984.

159. Breniére Y, Do MC, Gatti L, et al: A dynamic analysis of the squat snatch, In *Biomechanics VII-B*, Baltimore, MD, 1981, University Park Press.

160. Lee Y-H, Huwang C-Y, Tsuang Y-H: Biomechanical characteristics of preactivation and pulling phases of snatch lift, *J Appl Biomech* 11:288–298, 1995.

161. Chiu LZF: *Acute Physiologic and Neuromuscular Responses to High-Power Resistance Exercise*, Unpublished Doctoral Dissertation, Division of Biokinesiology and Physical Therapy, University of Southern California, Los Angeles, 2008.

162. Enoka RM: Muscular control of a learned movement: The speed control system hypothesis, *Exper Brain Res* 51:135–145, 1983.

163. Enoka RM: Load- and skill-related changes in segmental contributions to a weightlifting movement, *Med Sci Sports Exerc* 20(2):178–187, 1988.

164. Connan A, Moreaux A, Van Hoecke J: Biomechanical analysis of the two-hand snatch, In *Biomechanics VII-B*, Baltimore, MD, 1981, University Park Press.

165. Burdett RG: Biomechanics of the snatch technique of highly skilled and skilled weightlifters, *Res Q Exerc Sport* 53(3): 193–197, 1982.

166. Roman RA, Treskov VV: Snatch technique of world record holder Yuri Zakharevich [Russian], *Tyazhelaya Atletika* 1:10–16, 1983. Translated by M. Yessis.

167. Gourgoulis V, Aggeloussis N, Kalivas V, et al: Snatch lift kinematics and bar energetics in male adolescent and adult weightlifters, *J Sports Med Phys Fit* 44:126–131, 2004.

168. Lephart SM, Ferris CM, Riemann BL, et al: Gender differences in strength and lower extremity kinematics during landing, *Clin Orthop Rel Res* 401:162–169, 2002.

169. Pincivero DM, Campy RM, Coelho AJ: Knee flexor torque and perceived exertion: A gender and reliability analysis, *Med Sci Sports Exerc* 35(10):1720–1726, 2003.

170. Bosco C, Komi PV: Potentiation of the mechanical behavior of the human skeletal muscle through prestretching, *Acta Physiol Scand* 106(4):467–472, 1979.

171. Garhammer J, Gregor R: Propulsion forces as a function of intensity for weightlifting and vertical jumping, *J Appl Sport Sci Res* 6(3):129–134, 1992.

172. Kipp K, Harris C, Sabick M, et al: Lower extremity joint power production during Olympic weightlifting exercise [abstract], *Med Sci Sports Exerc* 38(5):S296, 2006.

173. Deming L, Kangwei A, Yunde W: *Three dimensional analysis of the clean and jerk techniques for female elite Chinese weightlifters*, In Proceedings of the 11th International Symposium on Biomechanics in Sports, Amherst, MA, 1993.

174. Lehr RP, Poppen R: An electromyographic analysis of Olympic power and squat clean, In Terauds J, Editor: *Science in weightlifting*, Del Mar, CA, 1979, Academic Publishers.

175. Campos J, Poletaev P, Cuesta A, et al: Kinematical analysis of the snatch in elite male junior weightlifters of different weight categories, *J Strength Cond Res* 20(4):843–850, 2006.

176. Zelle J, Barink M, Loeffen R, et al: Thigh-calf contact force measurements in deep knee flexion, *Clin Biomech* 22:821–826, 2007.

177. Nelson RC, Burdett RG: *Biomechanical analysis of Olympic weightlifting*, In Proceedings of the International Congress of Physical Activity, Quebec City, QC, 1976.

178. Garhammer J: A review of power output studies of Olympic and powerlifting: Methodology, performance prediction, and evaluation tests, *J Strength Cond Res* 7(2):76–89, 1993.

179. Chiu LZF, Schilling BK, Fry AC, et al: The influence of deformation on barbell mechanics during the clean pull, *Sports Biomech* 7(2):260–273, 2008.

180. Hoover DL, Carlson KM, Christensen BK, et al: Biomechanical analysis of women weightlifters during the snatch, *J Strength Cond Res* 20(3):627–633, 2006.

181. Campbell DE, Pond JW, Trenbeath WG: Cinematographic analysis of varying loads of the power clean, In Terauds J, Editor: *Science in weightlifting*, Del Mar, CA, 1979, Academic Publishers.

182. Campillo P, Chollet D, Micallef JP: Localisation de points critiques lors du tirage à l'arraché en haltérophilie, *Sci Sports* 13:90–92, 1998.

183. Garhammer J: Barbell trajectory, velocity and power changes: Six attempts and four world records, *Weightlifting USA* 19(3):27–30, 2001.

184. Frolov VI, Levshunov NP: The phasic structure of the jerk from the chest [Russian], *Tyazhelaya Atletika* 11:25–28, 1982. Translated by A Charniga Jr.

185. Grabe SA, Widule CJ: Comparative biomechanics of the jerk in Olympic weightlifting, *Res Q Exerc Sport* 59(1):1–8, 1988.

186. Roman RA, Shakirzyanov MS: *The snatch, the clean & jerk* [Russian]. Moscow, 1978, Fizkultura I Sport. Translated by A Charniga Jr.

187. Whittle MW, Sargeant AJ, Johns L: Computerised analysis of knee moments during weightlifting, In de Groot G, Hollander AP, Huijing PA, et al, Editors: *Biomechanics XI-B*, Amsterdam, 1988, Free University Press

188. Zernicke RF, Garhammer J, Jobe FW: Human patellar-tendon rupture, *J Bone Joint Surg Am* 59(2):179–183, 1977.

189. Neptune RR, Kautz SA, Zajac FE: Contributions of the individual ankle plantar flexors to support, forward progression and swing initiation during walking, *J Biomech* 34:1387–1398, 2001.

190. Roman RA: *The training of the weightlifter* [Russian]. Moscow, 1986, Fizkultura I Sport. Translated by A Charniga Jr.

191. Calhoon G, Fry AC: Injury rates and profiles of elite competitive weightlifters, *J Athl Tr* 34(3):232–238, 1999.

192. Fitzgerald B, McLatchie GR: Degenerative joint disease in weight-lifters: Fact or fiction? *Br J Sports Med* 14(2–3):97–101, 1980.

193. Granhed H, Morelli B: Low back pain among retired wrestlers and heavyweight lifters, *Am J Sports Med* 16(5):530–533, 1988.

194. Kujala UM, Kettunen J, Paananen H, et al: Knee osteoarthritis in former runners, soccer players, weight lifters, and shooters, *Arthritis Rheum* 38(4):539–546, 1995.

195. Kuland DN, Dewey JB, Brubaker CE, et al: Olympic weight-lifting injuries, *Phys Sports Med* 6(11):111–119, 1978.

196. Raske Å, Norlin R: Injury incidence and prevalence among elite weight and power lifters, *Am J Sports Med* 30(2):248–256, 2002.

197. Rossi F: Spondylolysis, spondylolisthesis and sports, *J Sports Med Phys Fitness* 18(4):317–340, 1978.

198. Stone MH, Fry AC, Ritchie M, et al: Injury potential and safety aspects of weightlifting movements, *Strength Cond* 16(3):15–21, 1994.

199. Hamill BP: Relative safety of weightlifting and weight training, *J Strength Cond Res* 8(1):53–57, 1994.

200. Byrd R, Pierce K, Rielly L, et al: Young weightlifter's performance across time, *Sports Biomech* 2(1):133–140, 2003.

201. Mölsä J, Kauhanen H, Häkkinen K: *Sports injuries among junior weightlifters*, In Proceedings of the International Conference on Weightlifting and Strength Training, Lahti, Finland, 1998.

202. Miller SJ, Smith PA: Volar dislocation of the lunate in a weight lifter, *Orthopedics* 19(1):61–63, 1996.

203. Wooten JR, Jones DH: An unusual weightlifting injury, *Injury* 19:446–454, 1988.

204. Gumbs VL, Segal D, Halligan JB, et al: Bilateral distal radius and ulnar fractures in adolescent weight lifters, *Am J Sports Med* 10(6):375–379, 1982.

205. Lewis DC, Johnson SR: Spontaneous dislocation of the lunate in a weightlifter, *Injury* 21(4):252–254, 1990.

206. Aggrawal ND, Kaur R, Kumar S, et al: A study of changes in the spine in weight lifters and other athletes, *Br J Sports Med* 13:58–61, 1979.

207. Dangles CJ, Spencer DL: Spondylolysis in competitive weight lifters [abstract], *Am J Sports Med* 15(6):624–625, 1987.

208. Kotani PT, Ichikawa N, Wakabayashi W, et al: Studies of spondylolysis found among weight lifters, *Br J Sports Med* 6(1):4–8, 1971.

209. Rossi F, Dragoni S: Lumbar spondylolysis: Occurrence in competitive athletes, *J Sports Med Phys Fitness* 30:450–452, 1990.

210. Alexander MJL: Biomechanical aspects of lumbar spine injuries in athletes: A review, *Can J Appl Sport Sci* 10(1):1–20, 1985.

211. Ariel BG: Biomechanical analysis of the knee joint during deep knee bends with heavy loads. In Nelson RC, Morehouse C, Editors, *Biomechanics IV*, Baltimore, MD, 1974, University Park Press.

212. Whiting WC, Zernicke RF: *Biomechanics of musculoskeletal injury*, ed 2, Champaign, IL, 2008, Human Kinetics.

213. Yamamoto N, Hayashi K: Mechanical properties of rabbit patellar tendon at high strain rate, *Biomed Mater Eng* 8(2):89–90, 1998.

214. Grenier R, Guimont A: Simultaneous bilateral rupture of the quadriceps tendon and leg fractures in a weightlifter: A case report, *Am J Sports Med* 11(6):451–453, 1983.

215. Fry AC, Smith JC, Schilling BK: Effect of knee position on hip and knee torques during the barbell squat, *J Strength Cond Res* 17(4):629–633, 2003.

216. Gisslén K, Öhberg L, Alfredson H: Is the chronic painful tendinosis tendon a strong tendon? *Knee Surg Sports Traumatol Arthrosc* 14:897–902, 2006.

217. Alfredson H, Öhberg L: Neovascularisation in chronic painful patellar tendinosis—Promising results after sclerosing neovessels outside the tendon challenge the need for surgery, *Knee Surg Sports Traumatol Arthrosc* 13(2):74–80, 2005.

218. Cahill BR: Osteolysis of the distal part of the clavicle in male athletes, *J Bone Joint Surg Am* 64(7):1053–1058, 1982.

219. Fees M, Decker T, Snyder-Mackler L, et al.: Upper extremity weight-training modifications for the injured athlete: A clinical perspective, *Am J Sports Med* 26(5):732–742, 1998.

220. Neviaser TJ: Weight lifting. Risk and injuries to the shoulder, *Clin Sports Med* 10(3):615–620, 1991.

221. Mundt DJ, Kelsey JL, Golden AL, et al: An epidemiologic study of sports and weight lifting as possible risk factors for herniated lumbar and cervical discs, *Am J Sports Med* 21(6):854–860, 1993.

CHAPTER

17

DELAYED-ONSET MUSCLE SORENESS

William T. Stauber and Corrie A. Mancinelli

Introduction

The pain or discomfort in skeletal muscles following unaccustomed exercise, particularly exercise involving eccentric muscle actions or lengthening contractions, is commonly called *delayed onset muscle soreness (DOMS)*. Unlike pain resulting from direct injury to a muscle such as a laceration, strain, or muscle contusion, DOMS does not begin until hours after the cessation of the injurious activity (Table 17-1).[1] The soreness continues for several days regardless of whether there is further activity. However, further exercise training will not exacerbate the soreness,[2] but actually diminishes the response, particularly to a subsequent, repeated bout of the same exercise.[3]

Soreness is a curious type of muscle pain. The intensity of the soreness changes with movement or pressure. Active contraction, passive stretching, and manual palpation of the exercised muscle increases the discomfort. In fact, one of the accepted methods for documenting this type of pain is to apply manual pressure to the muscle and note whether pain is experienced by the subject.[4] The experience of pain on palpation is called *tenderness*.

Differentiation between DOMS and muscle pain should be made. A wide variety of conditions, including exercise, can produce muscle pain (Table 17-2). The common "burning" experience from exercise is thought to be a result of local disturbances following alterations in pH and ion homeostasis that stimulate free nerve endings. In healthy individuals, the burning pain subsides within a couple of minutes of cessation of activity. This reduction in pain experience is due to the removal of acids, the return of high-energy phosphate stores, and the restoration of ionic gradients.

Another type of pain, closely related to burning results from muscle cramps. The reason for the similarity in experience stems from physiological outcome of a muscle cramp. A muscle cramp is the result of uncontrolled, muscle activation caused by high stimulation frequencies in muscles working often in shortened positions. Stretching the muscle relieves a cramp but actually exacerbates DOMS.

A muscle cramp is similar to a voluntary isometric muscle action held at the same tension level for the same amount of time. During any high-tension isometric muscle action, blood flow to active muscles decreases because of the high compressive forces generated by the muscle. However, because only parts of the muscle are contracted during a cramp, a shearing force on the connective tissue between active and inactive portions probably also contributes to the nociceptor activation.[5] Thus, is useful to generalize and say that the causes of muscle pain are different than the causes of DOMS—the subject of this discussion.

Causes of Muscle Pain

- Trauma (strain)
- Local muscle soreness immediately after exercise
- Muscle cramping
- Delayed onset muscle soreness

Pain and Tenderness

Normally, active contractions, muscle stretch, or weak pressure on muscle tissue do not elicit pain or soreness. This lack of responsiveness of muscle nociceptors to everyday experiences is due to the high threshold for activation of these receptors.[6] However, severe pressure to a skeletal muscle can usually produce a nociceptic response and, under certain conditions, even referred pain. The muscle receptors responsible for pressure-mediated pain are called high-threshold mechanosensitive (HTM) muscle receptors.[6]

423

Table 17-1

Muscle Strain Continuum

Damage	Failure	Disruption
Subcellular	Sarcomere, sarcolemma, cytoskeleton, extracellular matrix	Disruption in structures smaller than myofiber
Cellular	Myofiber	Rupture and retraction of one or more muscle cells
Organ	Muscle	Rupture of a fascicle or the entire muscle, involving myofiber fascia, and blood vessels (e.g., hamstring tears)

Table 17-2

Muscle Pain Experience

Finding	Presence (+) or Absence (−) of Pain
Degeneration/regeneration	−
Ischemia at rest	−
Inflammation	+ or −
Ischemic exercise	+
Defective energy metabolism	+
Acute fiber necrosis	+
Connective tissue damage	+
Eccentric muscle action (delayed onset)	+
Intramuscular injection (delayed onset)	+

Clinical Point

The muscle receptors responsible for pressure-mediated pain are called *high-threshold mechanosensitive (HTM) muscle receptors*.[6]

The HTM receptors in skeletal muscles have no direct contact with the myofibers but are commonly associated with blood vessels and to a lesser degree with connective tissue.[6] This anatomical arrangement may help explain why muscle pain is normally minimal in myopathies such as Duchenne muscular dystrophy even though there is marked degeneration of muscle and myofiber necrosis. In contrast, inflammatory conditions such as myositis[7] and vasculitis[8] can be quite painful because inflammatory mediators increase the responsiveness of nociceptors.

For example, the responsiveness of HTM receptors to pressure or movement can be increased by administration of bradykinin,[9] serotonin,[10] and high concentrations of potassium ions[11] (Figure 17-1). In vivo, these sensitizing agents are commonly produced in response to tissue damage and inflammation. However, the sensitization of muscle nociceptors by tissue damage is not a nonspecific process. Thus, purinergic receptors can be activated by adenosine triphosphate (ATP) released by disruption of cell membranes. Similarly, vanilloid receptors are activated by protons resulting from a decrease in pH caused by ischemia (swelling) and inflammation. Bradykinin is produced as part of the inflammatory process by proteases released from neutrophils, macrophages, and mast cells (Figure 17-2) that act on tissue kininogens. Bradykinin binds to the B_2 receptor on the nociceptor ending (see Figure 17-1) resulting in the activation of a cascade of intracellular reactions, leading to an increase in responsiveness of bradykinin binding to the B_1 receptor and the sensitivity of sodium channels to depolarizing stimuli.[6] Thus, many algesic compounds can be produced locally from tissue damage and inflammation that act on directly muscle nociceptors.

The sensitization of muscle nociceptors (see Figure 17-1) in response to damaged muscle and inflammation is, at present, the preferred explanation for the subjective experience of DOMS.[6] In humans, soreness, as determined by a reduction in the pressure-pain threshold, was documented in response to intramuscular injections of either serotonin or bradykinin; combinations of serotonin and bradykinin induced muscle hyperalgesia and tenderness.[12] In addition, bradykinin and serotonin, among other compounds with the potential for peripheral sensitization of muscle nociceptors, were elevated in the painful upper trapezius muscle of volunteers with active trigger points.[13] In contrast, decreased sensitization of HTM receptors resulted from intramuscular injection of the serotonin antagonist, granisetron, into the masseter muscle in human volunteers and patients with craniofacial myalgia.[14] Thus, if warranted, pharmacological intervention to reduce DOMS may, in the future, be possible.

Location of the Soreness

Because DOMS is a common experience following activities that contain lengthening contractions,[15] not all sports or occupational activities would be expected to result in muscle soreness. For example, muscle-shortening contractions such as level cycling and swimming rarely result in soreness. In contrast, even walking downhill for a couple of miles can result in DOMS of the dorsiflexor muscles, but not the knee extensor muscles. Thus, the location of DOMS is activity-dependent and often muscle specific.

Because the location of soreness can be grossly quantified using pressure algometers[16-18] and sophisticated computer-controlled methods are now available, it will soon be possible to identify regional differences in muscle soreness. The idea that the area of the myotendon

High-Threshold Mechnosensitive Receptor

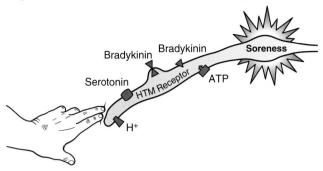

Figure 17-1

Mechanosensitive receptors become sensitive to pressure (tenderness) in response to many substances.

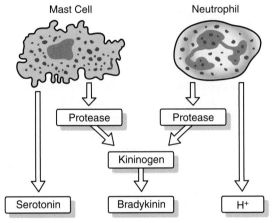

Figure 17-2

Resident mast cells and infiltrating neutrophils can produce substances that are hyperalgesic such as bradykinin and serotonin.

junction would be more prone to damage caused by a concentration of forces at that region has gained favor as the distal portion of some muscles appeared to be more sensitive to DOMS.[19] However, alterations in pressure-pain threshold can be measured in other areas, including the more central region of the biceps brachii muscles.[20] Attempts have been made to map the soreness as a function of the surface area of quadriceps muscles using a standardized grid placed on the leg and a threshold force of 50 N. These studies revealed regional differences do exist.[21] For example, the location of the soreness was found in the distal portion of the vastus medialis and the proximal part of the vastus lateralis, whereas the rectus femoris was absent of muscle soreness.[22] Regional differences were also noted in the quadriceps muscles before and after a bout of downhill running—proximal and distal regions were more sensitive.[23] For practical reasons, most investigators choose a point that is easily located and reproduced in repeated trials, but may be problematic if regional differences do exist or change with time.

Time Course of DOMS

It is widely recognized that DOMS does not appear immediately after an exercise protocol,[1] even though a performance deficit can be measured in the volunteers and stiffness documented.[24,25] Most studies revealed that soreness was present at 24 hours and peaked at approximately 48 hours.[26] A gradual decline occurred over several days and generally the pain was resolved by approximately 5 to 7 days.[27] However, there have been a few examples of pain lasting longer and of greater magnitude[28] perhaps as a result of the compression of tissues (e.g., compartment syndrome)[29,30] or differences in lymphatic return (e.g., lymphedema). Nevertheless, DOMS can be generally considered a temporary condition that will resolve itself with time over several days and without intervention.

> **Clinical Point**
>
> Delayed onset muscle soreness can be generally considered a temporary subjective condition that will resolve itself over several days and without intervention.

Models to Study Muscle Soreness

To produce DOMS in humans, activated or contracted muscles are stretched (lengthening contractions) using a variety of methods ranging from free weights[31] to dynamometers.[32] Generally, many repetitions with short rest times between contractions are used with single-joint movements (e.g., lengthening of active knee extensor or elbow flexor muscles) or complex limb movements such as downhill walking or running.

Because DOMS is subjectively experienced by humans, researchers rely on reports of resting pain via visual analog scales (VASs) or pain evoked by pressure (pressure-pain threshold) or movement. Two types of protocols are commonly used in humans to produce DOMS: (1) voluntary or electrically activated skeletal muscles exposed to repeated lengthening contractions[33] (Figure 17-3) using typically the elbow flexor, knee extensor, or ankle dorsiflexor muscles; and (2) downhill running, stepping, or walking. Because these activities recruit different muscle fibers within different anatomical muscles with diverse architecture and fascial compartments, outcome measures would be expected to have large variability. For example, it is quite easy to produce extreme soreness in the elbow flexor muscles of untrained individuals with only 30 repetitions.[33] However, to produce DOMS in the knee extensor muscle, used more frequently in activities of daily living, hundreds of repetitions were used[34,35] and downhill running required 15 bouts of 10 floor descents.[36] Surprisingly, even repeated isometric muscle actions at long muscle

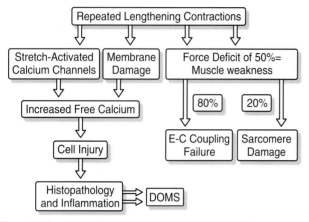

Figure 17-3
Repeated lengthening contractions can lead to delayed onset muscle soreness and muscle weakness by different mechanisms.

lengths of the elbow flexor muscles can produce damage and soreness.[37] Other models for inducing muscle soreness include injections of noxious materials into human muscles[14,38] and are beyond the scope of this discussion.

Relationship Between Load, Repetition Number, Velocity of Movement and Muscle Length

It is common experience that low loads, small numbers of repetitions and slow velocities of movement do not always result in DOMS. However, only a few studies have evaluated the effects of submaximal protocols;[32,39-41] a systematic study of load and repetition number on DOMS has not been undertaken. From the studies available, it appears that the minimum number of maximal lengthening contractions of the elbow flexor muscles required to produce DOMS was two repetitions[41] and a load of only 10% of maximum if the number of repetitions was large.[32]

Load

Factors That Can Lead to DOMS

- Load
- Number of repetitions
- Velocity of movement
- Length of muscle

The magnitude of the load or level of muscle contraction (percent of maximum voluntary contraction [MVC]) as a determinant for DOMS has been studied. Differences in pain during straightening of the injured elbow flexor muscles, but not during palpation (although a trend was clearly evident), were reported following 36 lengthening contractions using

loads of 84% and 112% of MVC.[39] Also, using two different protocols, another study found that using 10% of isometric elbow flexor strength with 600 repetitions was no different in producing DOMS than using 30 repetitions at 100%.[32]

Repetition Number

DOMS increases as a function of the number of times the muscle experiences lengthening contractions. Increasing the number of repetitions from 2 to 6 to 24 demonstrated a dose-response effect, but the magnitude of the increase in soreness was not linear. Increasing the number of repetitions further from 24 to 70 resulted in increased soreness.[42] This study did provide evidence that the early contractions were more important in producing DOMS.

Velocity of Movement

Unlike studies on animals, the effect of velocity of movement with maximally activated muscles has not been performed in humans without additional confounding variables. Using relatively low angular velocities of elbow movement, faster velocities produced greater DOMS than lower velocities.[43] Similar findings were reported for differences between 30° and 210° per second using an isokinetic dynamometer and human elbow flexor muscles.[44] Unfortunately, the study standardized the total time under contraction by using different numbers of repetitions for the two groups. Thus, repetition number alone could have resulted in the same outcome.

Muscle Length

Early studies on the role of mechanical factors in the development of DOMS revealed that there was a length-dependent component.[45] Exercises at longer muscle lengths produced more soreness.[37] Partial range-of-motion (ROM) exercises have been used for knee extension (150° to 80°)[46] and elbow flexion (120° to 180°)[32] to produce soreness. Most studies use large ROM exercises for the elbow flexor muscles.

Thus, load and repetition number are important factors in magnitude of the DOMS reported, but large variability between subjects prevents conclusive statements. Large variability is not the result of total work performed or peak torque.[47]

Performance Deficit

In 1902, Hough[48] first hypothesized that the muscle damage that occurred following unaccustomed exercise was the result of mechanical stress to the muscles (see Figure 17-3). Working with simple equipment and using himself as a subject, Hough described his experience and functional outcome of this type of exercise-induced muscle damage and hypothesized the mechanism of injury. Hough observed that the reduction in muscle force immediately after exercise preceded the onset of muscle soreness, which began the day after the exercise session. It is remarkable that continued exercise with sore, weakened elbow flexor muscles did not exacerbate the injury or alter the repair process.[49,50]

The decrease in muscle performance or loss of function, usually measured as a decreased maximal isometric force (weakness), is due to a reduction in the muscles intrinsic ability to produce force (see Figure 17-3).[51] The majority of the force decrement occurs early in a series of repeated lengthening contractions in both voluntary and electrically active muscles in humans[33] and in electrically active muscles in animals.[52-55]

More detailed studies on animals have revealed that force-generating[56] and transmitting components[57] of skeletal muscles are compromised with repeated lengthening contractions. Both the force generator (sarcomere) and activating system (excitation-contraction [E-C] coupling) have been observed to be disrupted following repeated lengthening contractions (see Figure 17-3).[58] Of these two, E-C coupling damage perhaps is responsible for 75% of the force decline.[59] During the early contractions, it is probable that unstable sarcomeres become overstretched (sarcomere popping),[58] which, in turn, causes the transverse (T) tubule, structurally associated with the sarcomere, to shear,[60] disconnecting it from the sarcolemma. Thus, the T tubule and associated sarcoplasmic reticulum, called a *triad,* would become functionally detached from the sarcolemma and unable to respond to subsequent action potentials. The reduction in release-activator calcium from disconnected triads would result in a decline in force output or weakness. Although these cellular disruptions would alter the force-producing capability of muscle, they would not necessarily lead to plasma membrane rupture unless the overstretched sarcomeres are attached to the plasma membrane via costameres.[61] Some type of membrane damage is presumed to be a precursor for myofiber necrosis and subsequent inflammation (see Figure 17-3).

It has been shown in rats that increasing the rest interval between successive lengthening contractions prevented histopathological changes in spite of a 50% decrease in muscle force.[52] Thus, muscle weakness occurred without evidence of cellular pathology. What appears to be lacking in human studies has been efforts to define the threshold for muscle soreness. Although tissue damage may be a prerequisite for DOMS, the factors involved in muscle weakness can occur independently from those that produce soreness (see Figure 17-3).

Histopathological Changes

Although the magnitude of the force deficit (weakness) diminishes with increasing repetition number in humans[62] and animals,[52] the amount of cellular pathology continues to increase,[54] providing indirect support for two distinct

processes occurring over time: contraction failure and histopathological changes (see Figure 17-3). Contraction failure results primarily from mechanical events occurring more prominently during the early repetitions while the events, eventually leading to histopathological changes, increase in magnitude throughout the course of repeated lengthening contractions. Thus, it is not surprising that the magnitude of the force deficit does not correlate with soreness or markers of muscle damage such as creatine kinase (CK).[63] In addition, in animal studies, weakness could be produced from 30 lengthening contractions with or without histopathological changes.[52] Perhaps the soreness would correlate best with the degree of histopathologic changes that, in turn, varies with the loss of cellular integrity. Loss of cellular integrity may increase with repetition number.

Following lengthening contractions, the membrane-associated protein, dystrophin, is lost[64-66] indicating a loss of cell membrane integrity (Figure 17-4). Such membrane disruptions can lead to cell death caused by calcium overload[67] as high concentrations of extracellular calcium enter the cell (see Figure 17-4) and overcome the cellular buffering capacity leading to cell death.[68] Dead cells become necrotic and require phagocytic cell action to remove the cellular debris. Necrotic myofibers can be easily observed in rat muscles 48 hours after a single bout of repeated lengthening contractions[52,66,69] and after long-distance running in humans.[70] Some of these necrotic myofibers are infiltrated by phagocytic cells (neutrophils and macrophages) but still contain some detectable myosin.[52] Thus, histopathological changes appear to result from loss of myofiber integrity.

Evidence for loss of myofiber integrity following a bout of repeated lengthening contractions is provided by observations of extracellular dyes,[71] technetium pyrophosphate,[70] and proteins such as albumin[72] and fibronectin[70] inside myofibers. These perturbations of the cell membrane also allow intracellular, muscle-specific proteins to exit. Many studies have provided evidence for myofiber injury as muscle specific proteins such as creatine kinase (CK) (see Figure 17-4), myoglobin and myosin fragments could be measured in the blood following different protocols known to contain exercises that produce muscle injury.[73] Myoglobin appears early

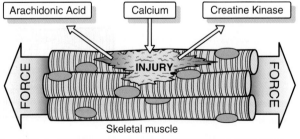

Figure 17-4

Skeletal muscle injury can result in plasma membrane injury and the production of arachidonic acid, increased influx of extracellular calcium, and release of intracellular proteins such as creatine kinase.

in the blood and could be a direct indicator of myofiber injury as it can pass easily the capillary wall.[74] With a similar time course, fatty acid–binding protein appears in the blood with a peak between 2 to 4 hours.[73] CK appears later,[73] perhaps requiring lymphatic clearance[75] to arrive in the circulation. Lastly, the time course of myosin fragments[73] might support a role in neutrophil action as the proteases released from neutrophils during removal of cellular debris would be capable of fragmenting but not completely degrading contractile proteins. The protein fragments could then pass directly into the blood.

Inflammation

Because the weakness observed as a function of lengthening contractions would not produce DOMS, developing inflammation following associated tissue damage is a likely candidate (see Figure 17-3). Inflammation is a complex cellular and chemical reaction in blood vessels and adjacent tissues to an injury. Typically, acute inflammation is characterized by hyperemia, edema, and diapedesis of neutrophils and macrophages. Inflammation is commonly accompanied by pain. Although others have presented arguments to the contrary,[76] the arrival of inflammatory cells into the injured muscle especially around blood vessels, may be the prerequisite for pain.

Evidence of an inflammation state in injured muscles has been long appreciated (see review[77]); both vascular and cellular responses have been identified. Unlike studies on the location of muscle pain, inflammation was distributed throughout the muscle.[34] When technetium-99m–labeled white blood cells (WBCs) were given to subjects prior to 300 repeated lengthening contractions of the knee extensor muscles, the entire muscle contained WBCs at 24 hours later together with an increase in DOMS.[34] In a subsequent study, labeled neutrophils were used to provide evidence that DOMS is associated with inflammation but not with muscle damage.[78]

Because neutrophils and macrophages can be identified in injured muscles,[52,78,79] chemoattractants such as leukotriene B4 released by injured cells may play a role in their recruitment[80] (Figure 17-5). Unfortunately, no attempts at measuring leukotrienes in injured skeletal muscles in vivo have been reported and inhibition of lipoxygenase (LIPOX) has only been reported for isolated rat muscles.[81] Thus, the role of LIPOX must be inferred from the presence of neutrophils in injured human muscle. However, activation of LIPOX initially depends on the production of arachidonic acid.

The production of arachidonic acid (see Figure 17-5) and the generation of inflammation results from the activation of the enzyme, phospholipase A2. In turn, arachidonic acid results in the activation of 5-LIPOX and cyclo-oxygenase (COX). The activation of COX leads to the production of prostaglandins, which could contribute to pain, edema, and vasodilation—typical of inflamed tissue.

Mast Cells

One additional candidate for the production of sensitizing agents is mast cell degranulation. Human mast cells contain proteolytic enzymes that could activate kininogens leading to bradykinin production[82] and have been shown

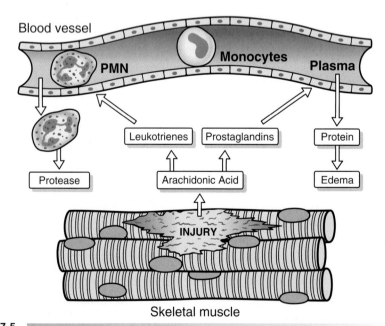

Figure 17-5

Membrane injury can lead to the release of arachidonic acid from muscle resulting in cellular infiltration mediated by leukotriene signaling and protein extravasation by prostaglandin interaction with vascular endothelial cells. The infiltrating neutrophils and macrophages can release enzymes such as proteases.

to release stored serotonin[83] (see Figure 17-2). Thus, mast cell degranulation could provide the necessary chemical mediators for sensitization even in the absence of loss of myofiber integrity.

Some evidence exists for mast cell degranulation following repeated lengthening contractions in both animal[84] and human[57] skeletal muscles. Because mast cells are generally found near neurovascular elements, blood vessels, and the connective tissue interstitium,[85] they are ideally situated to influence nearby nociceptors. Overstretched connective tissue from myofiber rupture[86] or disruption of the supporting extracellular matrix (ECM)[57] could provide a nonphysiological stretch to some mast cells, causing a leakage of granules and release of noxious agents. Mechanical manipulation of certain tissues can produce mast cell degranulation[87] and mast cell degranulation can itself be injurious to muscle.[88]

Connective Tissue

In contrast to direct damage to myofibers, tissue swelling[89] and disruption of the ECM[57] following muscle injury may be important in the cause of muscle soreness. It is well recognized that extreme passive stretching can produce pain because HTM receptors located in the connective tissues around muscles are activated by excessive deformation. In addition, myofibers appear swollen.[30,90] Therefore, swelling of cells and degradation of ECM could potentially result in soreness if the expansion of the muscle (swelling) exceeded the threshold for mechanical activation of the receptors. A disrupted and partially degraded matrix would serve as an excellent oncotic material promoting tissue water accumulation. Evidence for ECM breakdown was observed 2 days after exercise by the presence of collagen breakdown products in the urine.[91] Expanded ECM can also be observed around injured human myofibers.[57] Thus the environment around injured myofibers would favor the accumulation of water resulting in a swollen muscle.

Evidence for muscle swelling following repeated lengthening contractions has been reported using ultrasound imaging[26] and magnetic resonance imaging.[46,92] However, swelling alone is not sufficient to produce soreness unless the additional water was held in a closed compartment.[30] The soreness increases as the limb is moved or the muscles are palpated as if the tissue pressure within the muscle must exceed some threshold for activation of the HTM receptors. Therefore, sensitization of the receptors by chemical mediators released in response to muscle injury would still appear critical for DOMS.

The connective tissue, in addition to containing HTM receptors, also contains resident neutrophils and T cells.[93] After downhill running to produce muscle damage, more T cells and neutrophils were found in the epimysium from those subjects who experienced DOMS compared with those who exercised but did not experience DOMS.[93] The

activation of resident cells in the matrix may be necessary for DOMS.[93] Thus, the connective tissue surrounding the myofibers could play a major role in DOMS and may also help explain why markers of myofiber injury do not correlate with the magnitude of DOMS.

Prevention and Attenuation of DOMS

To our knowledge, no treatment or manipulation can fully protect an untrained muscle from developing DOMS in elbow flexor muscles following a series of repeated lengthening contractions even as little as two maximal lengthening contractions.[41] However, attenuation of DOMS to a second bout of lengthening contractions produced by an initial bout of exercises has been referred to as the *repeated bout effect*[50] and may last as long as 6 months.[94] This repeated bout effect was first observed as a stepwise marked reduction in DOMS for elbow flexor muscles when high-force lengthening contractions were repeated 2 weeks and 4 weeks following an initial bout.[95] In contrast, force deficits were only slightly reduced with each successive bout, indicating that the force-generating system was repeatedly disrupted. Remarkably, no increase in plasma CK was measured following the second and third bout. This study supports the hypothesis that DOMS does not require myofiber disruption of sufficient magnitude to allow the exit of intracellular proteins.

Subsequently, many studies have verified this observation that prior exposure to lengthening contractions attenuates the soreness following repeated exercise trials.[96] For example, only 24 contractions were necessary to dramatically attenuate soreness produced 2 weeks later by 70 maximal lengthening contractions.[42] In contrast, some exercises may actually exacerbate the problem[97] perhaps by producing shorter muscles.[98]

Treatment of DOMS

Just as the exact mechanisms leading to DOMS are not completely understood, its treatment and the effects of those treatments on the condition are at present questionable (Figure 17-6).

Pharmacological Management of DOMS

If the inflammatory response is a major contributor to DOMS, then anti-inflammatory agents should be useful in the management of DOMS. However, anti-inflammatory drugs have shown mixed results for treating DOMS. The administration of 400 mg of ibuprofen given 4 hours before or 1200 mg given 24 hours after exercise was somewhat effective in decreasing perceived soreness and enhancing recovery of muscle force at 24 to 48 hours after exercise-induced injury.[21] In contrast, no significant effect of ibuprofen or other nonsteroidal anti-inflammatory drugs (NSAIDs)

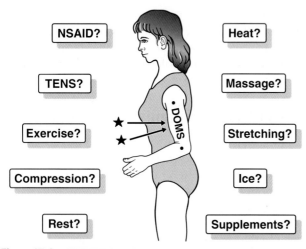

Figure 17-6
Schematic representation interventions commonly used for delayed onset muscle soreness.

on DOMS has also been reported.[99-103] Regardless of the type of NSAID, dosage, or time of delivery (e.g., before or after exercise), NSAIDs produced little reduction in DOMS. For example, no improvements in DOMS, muscle strength or endurance time were reported for 16 subjects receiving 2400 mg of ibuprofen twice (24 hours before and 72 hours after) compared with placebo controls using a single bout of downhill running to produce muscle injury.[100] Interestingly, CK activity was actually higher in the ibuprofen group.[100] However, using repeated lengthening contractions of the elbow flexor muscles, a reduction in CK activity was observed in individuals treated with 2400 mg of ibuprofen for 5 days before and 10 days after exercise[104]—no measurements of DOMS were conducted.

Because diclofenac inhibits both the COX and LIPOX pathways of arachidonic acid metabolism,[105,106] it might be more effective in treating DOMS. Indeed, decreased muscle soreness and CK activity following elbow exercise has been reported for diclofenac.[106] In addition, another NSAID that alters both the COX and LIPOX pathways, ketoprofen, has also been shown to decrease muscle soreness when 100 mg was given 36 hours after the exercise.[107]

Because prostaglandin E (PGE_2) plays an important role in healing, inhibition of COX by NSAIDs could impair muscle healing by reducing PGE_2 synthesis. Impaired recovery of muscle function after lengthening contractions of the elbow flexor muscles resulted in NSAID-treated subjects.[108] Fifteen subjects were given either 300 mg of flurbiprofen or a placebo 24 hours before and for 14 days after exercise protocol.[108] Flurbiprofen did not reduce DOMS, swelling, or stiffness but did adversely lower the maximal force, suggesting that additional weakness resulted from NSAID administration. Furthermore, studies with animals have demonstrated that NSAIDs can have adverse effects on skeletal muscle healing following injury.[109]

In summary, the use of NSAIDs for the prevention and treatment of DOMS is equivocal. Reported discrepancies may exist because of the mode of exercise used and whether or not soreness truly developed. In addition, the type of drug, the dosage, and the timing of administration were different in these studies, and all used small sample sizes. Furthermore, repeated lengthening contractions may not produce a classic inflammatory response.[108,110] Finally, because the literature does not provide strong support for using NSAIDs to treat or prevent DOMS and these drugs are not benign, routine use of NSAIDs for DOMS cannot be recommended.

Physical Modalities for DOMS
Cryotherapy
Experimental evidence has been reported that cryotherapy reduced the signs and symptoms of acute soft tissue injury.[111] The decrease in tissue temperature associated with cryotherapy is thought to limit the degree of injury by stimulating cutaneous receptors to cause sympathetic vasoconstriction and by slowing the extravasation of blood proteins to decrease swelling. In addition, a decrease in tissue temperature would decrease cellular metabolism and reduce the production of metabolites.[112] Cold also dulls or diminishes the sensation of pain.[112] Taken together, cryotherapy would be expected to reduce DOMS. Despite its widely accepted use among athletes, little or no benefit has been reported using cryotherapy to treat DOMS.[113-116]

Immersion in Cold. Subjects performed a total of 40 maximal lengthening contractions of the elbow flexor muscles to produce injury and the injured arm was immersed in cold water (15°C [59°F]) for 15 minutes immediately after the exercise bout and every 12 hours for a total of seven sessions.[113] Although the relaxed elbow angle and CK activity were significantly lower for the cryotherapy group, there was no effect on tenderness or loss of strength.[113] A similar study, using 64 lengthening contractions, employed five repeated immersions of the injured arm using colder water (5°C [41°F]) for 20 minutes each.[114] Each immersion was separated by 60 minutes. Again, no beneficial reduction in DOMS was reported.[114]

Lower-extremity muscles have also been subjected to lengthening contractions and followed with immersion in cold (5°C [41°F]) or tepid water (24°C [75°F]).[117] In addition to measurement of perceived soreness, thigh circumference, serum CK, and isometric strength, tests of lower-extremity function were included, such as a hop test for distance and a sit-to-stand test. Surprisingly, the cold-immersion treatment resulted in increased soreness during the sit-to-stand test 24 hours after exercise.[117]

In addition to treatments of the injured areas, whole-body ice immersion has been recommended, but its effectiveness to reduce DOMS remains unknown (see "Contrast

Baths" section). In addition, the discomfort of prolonged whole-body immersion in ice water and the risk of hypothermia precludes its use.

Ice Massage. The effects of ice massage on DOMS in the elbow flexor muscles was studied with 15- to 20-minute applications immediately, 24, or 48 hours following damaging exercise.[115] No differences in ROM or soreness were observed between treated and untreated arms. In fact, an increase in soreness was reported in subjects following the 24-hour treatment.[115] Similarly, when used immediately after exercise or 24 or 48 hours after exercise, ice massage was found to be ineffective in the treatment of DOMS.[118]

Ice massage was used in combination with exercise to assess its role in the prevention and treatment of DOMS by comparing the intervention to ice massage and exercise alone.[116] Prior to an exercise protocol to induce DOMS, ROM, strength, perceived soreness, and serum CK levels were measured and again at 2, 4, 6, 24, 48, 72, 96, and 120 hours after exercise. None of the treatments was able to significantly reduce DOMS. In fact, it appeared that the use of ice in the treatment of DOMS may actually be contraindicated[116] as the ice massage group had the highest peak soreness at rest, highest serum CK levels, and the lowest peak total ROM of all the groups tested.

In summary, it is possible that increasing the duration of the application of cold or the number of cold applications may prove beneficial in reducing DOMS. However, because prolonged cryotherapy (greater than 20 minutes in duration) may actually cause nerve injury,[119] prolonged applications are not recommended. In contrast to its effectiveness with acute soft tissue injury, cryotherapy (ice massage or ice water immersion, single or multiple applications, before or after exercise) appears to have little or no effect on minimizing DOMS. This observation may result from the differences in physiological processes that result in DOMS and perhaps also the inability of cryotherapy to markedly reduce intramuscular temperatures.[120]

Thermotherapy

Thermotherapy has been shown to increase tissue temperature, local blood flow, muscle elasticity and metabolite production[121]—potentially important factors for reducing DOMS if intramuscular temperature can actually be elevated by thermotherapy. Typical hot water immersion (hydrotherapy) has been reported to have no effect on reducing DOMS in leg extensor muscles.[122] However, using a unique injury protocol to the back extensor muscles and a commercially available heat wrap, the positive effects of continuous low-level heat versus cold pack therapy were reported.[123] Approximately 8 hours of low-level heat (40°C [104°F]) was provided and the device allowed the subject to continue to be active while wearing the wrap. The heat wrap group used the device for 8 hours on two

occasions, first starting at 18 hours after exercise and then again at 32 hours after exercise. The cold pack intervention used a gel pack for 15 to 20 minutes every 4 hours between 18 and 42 hours after exercise while lying prone or supine. Using self-reporting as a measure of function and pain, the heat wrap served as a preventive measure, starting 4 hours before the exercise bout, resulting in a substantial decrease in low back pain and smaller deficits in function. Furthermore, when subjects were tested 24 hours after exercise, the heat wrap again provided superior pain relief compared with the cold pack.[123] Although the findings are interesting, no objective measures of soreness and function were used. The results may also be unique to the muscles tested.

Contrast Baths

Alternating heat and cold-water immersions have been purported to assist with recovery after exercise.[124] Based on anecdotal experience by athletes, warm spas with cold plunges or contrast hot-cold baths have been recommended. Contrast baths are commonly used by physical therapists and athletic trainers for a variety of conditions, but little is known about the effectiveness of using such a modality for the prevention and treatment of DOMS. It has been speculated that contrast baths create a pumping action through alternating vasodilation and vasoconstriction.[124] Typical protocols consist of a warm to cold duration ratio of 3:1 or 4:1, with temperatures of 38°C to 44°C (100°F to 111°F) for warm water and 10°C to 18°C (50°F to 64°F) for cold water. Treatment starts with 10 minutes of warm-water submersion followed by 1 minute of cold water and then 4 minutes of warm water. The cycle continues for 30 minutes, ending with warm water.[125] However, for the injured athlete, the cycle should end with cold water to promote vasoconstriction.[124] As expected, many different protocols exist with differing warm/cold ratios, temperatures, cycle times, and frequency of use.

Using whole-body immersion and 1 minute of cold water (15°C [59°F]) immersion followed by 1 minute of warm water (38°C [100°F]) for a total of 14 minutes following lengthening contractions of the legs in a bilateral leg-press exercise, contrast baths resulted in reduction of perception of pain at 24, 48, and 72 hours after the exercise protocol compared with 14 minutes of continuous cold- or hot-water immersion.[122] However, immersion of only the lower extremity to the pelvis for contrast baths of 1 minute of cold water (8°C to 10°C [46°F to 50°F]) immersion followed by 2 minutes of warm water (40°C to 42°C [104°F to 108°F]) for a total of 15 minutes did not reduce soreness compared with rest.[126] If indeed valid, a pumping action stimulated by alternating vasodilation and vasoconstriction of blood vessels[122] should have resulted from both protocols.[122,126] No adequate explanation was provided to account for the different outcomes to contrast baths involving the whole body or injured limb.

Ultrasound and Phonophoresis

Ultrasound has been commonly used to decrease pain and edema and to increase the rate of healing in musculoskeletal conditions. Ultrasound uses high-frequency sound waves to transmit energy into tissues and the absorption of ultrasonic waves is believed to produce both thermal and nonthermal physiological effects. The thermal effects include increased blood flow, increased extensibility of tissues, and a proinflammatory response. Nonthermal effects include cavitation or pressure-induced increases in fluid flow and acoustic microstreaming or the unidirectional movement of fluids along cell membranes. In vitro studies have revealed that cavitation and microstreaming can stimulate fibroblasts[127] during repair and tissue regeneration. By extension, ultrasound has been found useful for promoting wound healing[128,129] and scar tissue dissolution[130] as well as enhancing angiogenesis.[131]

Continuous ultrasound has a greater thermal effect than pulsed ultrasound. However, either continuous ultrasound or ultrasound pulsed at low intensity will have nonthermal effects. Most ultrasound is delivered at a frequency of 1 MHz or 3 MHz, with the lower frequency providing a greater depth of penetration up to 5 cm (2 inches). Absorption is higher in tissues rich in protein like skeletal muscle.[132]

Using pulsed ultrasound (1 MHz, 0.8 W/cm^2), a reduction in pain and tenderness of the knee extensor muscles and an acceleration in muscle performance following injury has been reported.[133] However, others found no effect.[134,135] For example, using similar pulsed ultrasound (1 MHz, 0.8 W/cm^2) for the treatment of DOMS at both low (172.8 J) and high (345.6 J) doses, no significant differences for pain ratings or pain thresholds were observed for either ultrasound group, a "sham" ultrasound group, or a control group.[134] In another study, also using injured elbow flexor muscles, pulsed ultrasound (1 MHz, 1.5 W/cm^2) was administered twice per day for 3 days following the exercise bout with no reduction in perceived soreness.[135] There appears to be no convincing evidence to support the sole use of pulsed ultrasound for the treatment of DOMS.

Warmup, prior to exercise, has been proposed as a possible intervention for DOMS.[136] Because ultrasound can be used as a form of passive warmup prior to intense exercise, continuous ultrasound was applied to the elbow flexors for 10 minutes at 1 MHz, 1.5 W/cm^2 prior to repeated lengthening contractions.[137] Muscle tissue temperature did increase by approximately 1°C to 2°C in the ultrasound-treated group, but no effects of continuous ultrasound were found on perceived soreness. In contrast, continuous ultrasound (1 MHz, 1.5 W/cm^2) to the elbow flexor muscles actually worsened DOMS.[138] However, DOMS was attenuated when the ultrasound was combined with an anti-inflammatory agent, trolamine salicylate, for phonophoresis.[138]

The range of ultrasound treatments possible for effectively treating or preventing DOMS as well as influencing repair processes has yet to be fully considered in skeletal muscles injured by repeated lengthening contractions. Perhaps future studies will reveal areas of usefulness, but it appears, from the data available, that the use of ultrasound therapy will be of little benefit. In fact, definitive evidence for a clinical effect of ultrasound in the treatment of other soft tissue injuries is lacking.[132]

Iontophoresis

The transdermal delivery of anti-inflammatory drugs by means of low-voltage direct current to move charged compounds across the skin is called *iontophoresis*. Because transdermal administration of trolamine salicylate by phonophoresis did attenuate DOMS,[138] other methods of transdermal delivery such as iontophoresis would be expected to be beneficial. Using a stepping exercise to induce muscle damage in female volunteers, the effects of dexamethasone administered by iontophoresis 24 hours after the exercise on DOMS was tested.[22] Dexamethasone (2 mL) and lidocaine (1 mL) were combined and delivered by iontophoresis at 2 mA for 5 minutes, 3 mA for 5 minutes, and 4 mA for 10 minutes. A placebo group underwent the exact procedure using 3 mL of lidocaine and a control group underwent no intervention. The investigators mapped out the soreness and calculated an intensity of soreness by using a probe that measured the force of pressure needed to induce discomfort. The delivery site of the iontophoresis was also selected from the two areas identified with the most intense muscle soreness in all subjects (vastus medialis and lateralis). A single treatment of dexamethasone iontophoresis was effective in decreasing muscle soreness 48 hours after exercise.[22] Given the depth of penetration of drugs delivered by iontophoresis, it would be surprising to find marked analgesic action. Still, more studies are needed to determine whether multiple treatments or earlier treatments closer to the time of insult would be more effective and whether men respond differently than women.

Electrophysical Agents for Pain

Electrophysical agents, particularly transcutaneous electrical nerve stimulation (TENS), has been reported to be effective in modulation of pain.[139] However, using electrophysical agents for the treatment of DOMS has proven to be equivocal. For example, a decrease in soreness was reported when TENS was applied 48 hours after three maximal lengthening contractions using the elbow flexor muscles.[140] For this application, electrodes were placed over the musculotendinous junction and the site reported as the location of greatest soreness (most often the belly of the brachialis). TENS was delivered continuously at a pulse rate of 90 pulses per second (pps) and phase duration of 20 microseconds with the amplitude sufficient to provide tingling without any muscle activation (i.e., sensory-level stimulation). In contrast, using exhausting exercise, no analgesic effects were reported using either low- or high-frequency TENS.[141] Another study also using both high- and low-frequency TENS provided by an interferential current generator also failed to find reduction in DOMS in volunteers subjected to exhausting exercise.[142] Using sensory-level electrical stimulation (TENS) and a high-voltage unit set at a frequency of 120 pps, soreness perception was reduced during the treatment but did not last long afterward.[143] Similar findings of lack of prolonged effect were reported for repeated treatments over several days[144] using high voltage to produce TENS.[144] Thus, it was possible for traditional TENS to be an effective treatment when the degree of muscle injury was small (e.g., three repetitions) and the attenuation was planned to be temporary (e.g., during the treatment only). However, when the damage was large, such as is produced by exhaustive exercise, TENS was ineffective.

Microcurrent electrical neuromuscular stimulation (MENS) is a subsensory stimulation using electrical current amplitudes (< 1000 μA) below the level necessary for sensory nerve activation. None of the studies available using MENS reported any reduction in DOMS. Both continuous stimulation for 48 hours[145] and intermittent treatments[146-148] were conducted for varying times after muscle injury without effect. At present, MENS has no role in treating DOMS.

Compression

If exercise-induced muscle tissue injury leads to an influx of fluid (edema) that results in an elevation of intramuscular pressure and this swelling contributes to the activation of HTM receptors, then modalities that promote movement of fluid away from the muscle would be expected to result in less soreness and improved physical performance. Compression has been studied and results have been mixed depending on the type and duration of compression used. Intermittent compression can briefly reduce swelling and stiffness[149] and would be expected to temporarily reduce the activation of HTM receptors in injured muscles. In contrast, if fluids could actually be squeezed out by external limb compression, constant compression would be expected to have a more profound effect. Constant compression using a compressive sleeve did reduce the perception of soreness and swelling following elbow flexor contractions.[150] The compression garments used were made of raschel fabric with 25% elastic fabric and provided a 10-mm Hg compressive force. The compression was provided for 24 hours per day for 5 days after exercise. In addition to the decrease in soreness, recovery of muscle force output and power were also hastened in this study. Although this study shows promising results for the treatment of DOMS, use of compression sleeves for all extremities may not be practical during an athlete's training.

Massage

Massage, like compression, may also help move fluid away from involved muscles. Massage has been touted as a modality that facilitates recovery after intense exercise and can be used to enhance physical performance. A wide variety of techniques are commonly used for massage. For classic western massage or Swedish massage, the most common form of massage used for athletes, five basic techniques are used: effleurage, pétrissage, tapotement, friction, and vibration.[151,152] The progression of the massage advances from distal to proximal and usually lasts between 10 and 30 minutes.[152,153] A typical treatment begins and ends with light gliding strokes with the palm of the hand, known as *effleurage*. The initial effleurage strokes then progress to deeper stroking known as *pétrissage*. Pétrissage involves a kneading motion or lifting, pressing, or rolling of the tissues. Tapotement, friction, and vibration can be added before the final effleurage strokes. Tapotement involves stimulating the tissues either with repetitive percussion strokes or tapping and is commonly used before and during competition.[152] Friction techniques that involve circular movements with the palm or fingertips purportedly can be added for the specific purpose of reducing muscle spasm following injury.[152] Vibration or shaking is purportedly used for reduction in muscle tone.[151]

Massage is considered to have a number of physiological and psychological benefits that may contribute to pain modulation and tissue repair aided in part by increased circulation and lymphatic flow.[154] However, using exercise-induced muscle damage to the quadriceps muscles, massage did not alter blood flow to muscles, but did reduce soreness to some degree.[155] In contrast, light exercise alone improved blood flow and temporarily reduced soreness.[155] Although exercise might be expected to increase lymphatic return in active muscles, massage was unable to increase lymphatic flow or to reduce edema in humans.[151] Despite these findings, a significant reduction in soreness was reported following a 30-minute massage using a distal (hand) to proximal (shoulder) sequence with combinations of effleurage, pétrissage, and cross-fiber massage together with shaking.[156]

The effectiveness of a single massage technique, pétrissage, on the subjective reporting of soreness has been tested for its effectiveness on reducing DOMS.[157] Pétrissage administered immediately following eccentric exercise did not alleviate DOMS examined 24 and 48 hours later. In contrast, soreness was reduced in 48 hours by the combined effects of effleurage, tapotement, and pétrissage given 2 hours after repeated lengthening contractions of the knee flexor muscles.[158] Standardized techniques of effleurage, pétrissage, and vibration composed the massage treatment for a group of collegiate women volleyball and basketball players who were subjected to unaccustomed, intense training.[159] Two days later, both reports of perceived soreness and measurements of the pressure-pain threshold (algometry) revealed that DOMS was reduced immediately after the 17-minute massage as well as providing some improvement in physical performance (shuttle run and vertical jump).[159]

In summary, some evidence is available to support the use of massage to treat DOMS. Unfortunately, the attenuation of soreness is not profound and the mechanism of action is unknown. Because a wide variety of factors are probably involved,[156] additional well-controlled studies are needed to provide a scientific basis for its action and further insight into the best application.

Stretching

Stretching prior to and after activity is thought to protect an individual from injury and soreness.[160] However, a systematic review using pooled data from five studies revealed that static stretching used before and after exercise produced small but insignificant reductions in muscle soreness.[160] Stretching reduced soreness on average of less than 2 mm on a 100-mm VAS.[160] However, no objective recordings of soreness were used. Using an algometer in addition to soreness ratings (VAS), the effect of static stretching prior to exercise was tested using hamstring muscle injury to produce DOMS.[161] Four 20-second static stretches prior to 100 repetitions of resisted lengthening contractions of the knee flexor muscles produced no preventive effect on DOMS measured with either method in 10 female volunteers.[161] Using knee extensor muscles, passive static stretching (three times for 30 seconds) was performed before and immediately after intensive eccentric exercise and three times daily for the following 7 days; passive stretching did not reduce muscle soreness at any point examined.[162] However, both static and ballistic stretching can independently produce muscle soreness, with the greatest soreness ratings resulting from static stretching.[163] Because stretching might actually increase soreness, a control group using only the stretching protocols should be required in future studies such as daily stretching (training) prior to exercise. If chronic stretching can actually result in longer muscles as limb distraction does,[164] longer muscles would be less susceptible to injury from lengthening contractions[165] and thus DOMS might be prevented by prior training with stretching.

Warmup

An active warmup of 100 shortening contractions performed just before a damaging exercise bout was successful at decreasing soreness and ROM associated with DOMS.[166] However, using a similar warmup exercise did not result in change.[136] Furthermore, using an exhausting stepping exercise, no effect of warmup on soreness was reported.[167] Because the magnitude of the force during lengthening is a major factor in producing muscle injury,[168] fatiguing exercise could result in lower forces and thus lower injury potential during certain activities but not others. However, fatigue did not offer any protection in preventing muscle injury by repeated lengthening contractions under controlled conditions.[169] Thus, warmup exercises consisting of active contractions of muscles before a damaging bout of lengthening contractions would not confer much protection if any.

Exercise Immediately After DOMS-Producing Protocols

Mixed results have been obtained for exercises performed immediately following protocols designed to produce DOMS. For example, upper-arm ergometry was performed for 8 minutes immediately following the injury protocol and again 24 hours later.[146] The arm exercise did not improve soreness measured at 24, 48, and 72 hours after the initial exercise bout.[146] Repeating the same activity but using submaximal contractions (25) also did not reduce the soreness on the day following DOMS-inducing exercise.[170] In contrast, when light exercise (i.e., elbow flexion with a 5-pound dumbbell for two bouts of 25 repetitions) was repeated daily following a bout of lengthening contractions, improvements in soreness ratings were reported.[171] Decreased soreness was also measured following high-velocity (300°/sec) isokinetic exercise using concentric muscle actions performed on the day following the injury protocol.[172] Using maximal voluntary efforts and reciprocal knee flexion and extension movements, six bouts of 20 repetitions with a rest of 3 minutes between bouts were performed as a successful therapeutic intervention. It is difficult to resolve these conflicting findings without knowledge of changes in intramuscular tissue pressure, inflammatory cell infiltrates and algesic mediators.

Alternative Therapies and Nutritional Supplements

Hyperbaric Oxygen Therapy

Hyperbaric oxygen therapy (HBOT) has been used by elite athletes as a means of hastening recovery following injury. Using 100% oxygen at a pressure of 2.5 atm, daily exposures for 60 minutes each were ineffective at reducing soreness ratings for injured elbow flexor muscles.[173,174] In contrast, increased soreness has been reported to result from HBOT at 48 and 72 hours following the exercise bout.[175]

Acupuncture

Acupuncture has been recognized as an effective modality for pain management,[176,177] yet little is known about the effects of acupuncture on DOMS. However, following repeated lengthening contractions of the elbow flexor muscles to produce DOMS, needling at traditional acupuncture points or at points identified as most tender by palpation did not reduce pain (VAS) or soreness (algometry).[178]

Homeopathy

The homeopathic approach has been advocated by some using *Arnica*, which is thought to have analgesic[179] and anti-inflammatory properties.[180] However, no benefit was found for *Arnica* in the treatment of DOMS whether used as a sublingual pellet[181] or as a topical cream.[182]

Nutritional Supplements

Nutritional supplements have also been used to treat or prevent DOMS. In a study using only six subjects, L-carnitine (3 g/day for 3 weeks prior to exercise) decreased pain (VAS) and soreness (pain threshold) following knee extensor exercise.[183]

Although coenzyme Q10 (120 mg/day) reduced angina pectoris following myocardial infarction,[184] it may actually be detrimental to skeletal muscle.[185] Prior administration of coenzyme Q10 resulted in an increase in markers of muscle damage following cycle ergometry that was not seen in placebo controls.[185]

Other antioxidants such as vitamins C and E have been used without definitive results. The treatment of DOMS using vitamin C[186] or E[187] alone did not result in any measurable benefit, whereas an antioxidant mixture did reduce

DOMS.[188] Perhaps antioxidant therapy might decrease DOMS if secondary free radical damage produced by inflammatory cells arriving in injured muscles were reduced.

Conclusion

This review has focused on many factors resulting from strain injury to skeletal muscles most likely to produce DOMS and some that coexist with muscle injury (Figure 17-7) as well as a wide variety of approaches for the prevention and treatment of DOMS. No attempt was made to evaluate factors involved in perception of soreness including anticipatory fear of pain, anxiety, and catastrophizing.[189] From the studies reviewed, only limited success in reducing DOMS has been reported, providing evidence that local algesic factors, once produced by injured muscle (see Figure 17-7), will continue to sensitize HTM receptors to encode pressure or movement as pain or tenderness until they are removed by the cessation

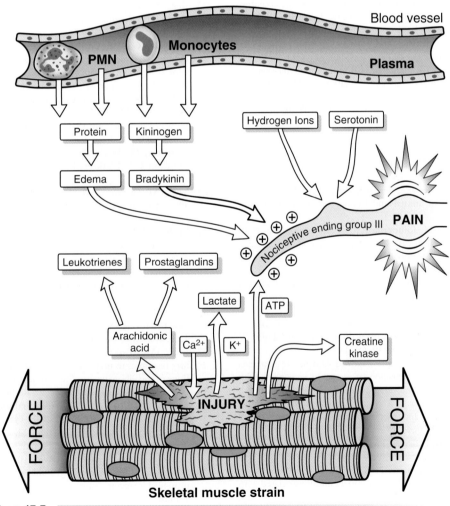

Figure 17-7
Muscle injury and delayed onset muscle soreness.

of the inflammatory response. However, some limited success in reduction of DOMS was obtained by compression, massage, and mild exercise perhaps by reducing tissue pressure and hence the stimulus for HTM receptor activation. Further advances may be forthcoming once standardization of protocols and muscle groups such as using the elbow flexor muscles subjected to 50 lengthening contractions are tested between research groups for consistency. In addition, objective measurements of tenderness such as determination of a pressure-pain threshold are required before interventions can be compared across studies. To date, DOMS appears to be an inevitable part of life for active individuals and, although continual training will prevent subsequent soreness during repeated exercises, vigorous unaccustomed activities will produce DOMS even in trained individuals. Because DOMS is transient, it will always resolve within a few days even without intervention.

References

1. Clarkson PM, Byrnes WC, McCormick KM, et al: Muscle soreness and serum creatine kinase activity following isometric, eccentric, and concentric exercise, *Int J Sports Med* 7(3):152–155, 1986.
2. Nosaka K, Newton M: Repeated eccentric exercise bouts do not exacerbate muscle damage and repair, *J Strength Cond Res* 16(1):117–122, 2002.
3. Clarkson PM, Nosaka K, Braun B: Muscle function after exercise-induced muscle damage and rapid adaptation, *Med Sci Sports Exerc* 24(5):512–520, 1992.
4. Nosaka K, Chapman D, Newton M, Sacco P: Is isometric strength loss immediately after eccentric exercise related to changes in indirect markers of muscle damage? *Appl Physiol Nutr Metab* 31(3):313–319, 2006.
5. Simons DG, Mense S: Understanding and measurement of muscle tone as related to clinical muscle pain, *Pain* 75(1):1–17, 1998.
6. Graven-Nielsen T, Mense S: The peripheral apparatus of muscle pain: Evidence from animal and human studies, *Clin J Pain* 17(1):2–10, 2001.
7. Philen RM, Eidson M, Kilbourne EM, et al: Eosinophilia-myalgia syndrome. A clinical case series of 21 patients. New Mexico Eosinophilia-Myalgia Syndrome Study Group, *Arch Intern Med* 151(3):533–537, 1991.
8. Ali Z, Ranganathan P, Perry A, Gelbart M: Localized striated muscle vasculitis in rheumatoid arthritis, *J Clin Rheumatol* 13(1):35–37, 2007.
9. Mense S, Meyer H: Bradykinin-induced modulation of the response behaviour of different types of feline group III and IV muscle receptors, *J Physiol* 398:49–63, 1988.
10. Ernberg M, Lundeberg T, Kopp S: Pain and allodynia/hyperalgesia induced by intramuscular injection of serotonin in patients with fibromyalgia and healthy individuals, *Pain* 85(1–2):31–39, 2000.
11. Kumazawa T, Mizumura K: Thin-fibre receptors responding to mechanical, chemical, and thermal stimulation in the skeletal muscle of the dog, *J Physiol* 273(1):179–194, 1977.
12. Jensen K, Tuxen C, Pedersen-Bjergaard U, et al: Pain and tenderness in human temporal muscle induced by bradykinin and 5-hydroxytryptamine, *Peptides* 11(6):1127–1132, 1990.
13. Shah JP, Danoff JV, Desai MJ, et al: Biochemicals associated with pain and inflammation are elevated in sites near to and remote from active myofascial trigger points, *Arch Phys Med Rehabil* 89(1):16–23, 2008.
14. Christidis N, Nilsson A, Kopp S, Ernberg M: Intramuscular injection of granisetron into the masseter muscle increases the pressure pain threshold in healthy participants and patients with localized myalgia, *Clin J Pain* 23(6):467–472, 2007.
15. Clarkson PM, Hubal MJ: Exercise-induced muscle damage in humans, *Am J Phys Med Rehabil* 81(11 Suppl):S52–S69, 2002.
16. Fischer AA: Reliability of the pressure algometer as a measure of myofascial trigger point sensitivity, *Pain* 28(3):411–414, 1987.
17. Reeves JL, Jaeger B, Graff-Radford SB: Reliability of the pressure algometer as a measure of myofascial trigger point sensitivity, *Pain* 24(3):313–321, 1986.
18. Jaeger B, Reeves JL: Quantification of changes in myofascial trigger point sensitivity with the pressure algometer following passive stretch, *Pain* 27(2):203–210, 1986.
19. Newham DJ, Mills KR, Quigley BM, Edwards RH: Pain and fatigue after concentric and eccentric muscle contractions, *Clin Sci (Lond)* 64(1):55–62, 1983.
20. Nussbaum EL, Gabison S: Rebox effect on exercise-induced acute inflammation in human muscle, *Arch Phys Med Rehabil* 79(10):1258–1263, 1998.
21. Hasson SM, Daniels JC, Divine JG, et al: Effect of ibuprofen use on muscle soreness, damage, and performance: A preliminary investigation, *Med Sci Sports Exerc* 25(1):9–17, 1993.
22. Hasson SM, Wible CL, Reich M, et al: Dexamethasone iontophoresis: Effect on delayed muscle soreness and muscle function, *Can J Sport Sci* 17(1):8–13, 1992.
23. Baker SJ, Kelly NM, Eston RG: Pressure pain tolerance at different sites on the quadriceps femoris prior to and following eccentric exercise, *Eur J Pain* 1(3):229–233, 1996.
24. Chleboun GS, Howell JN, Conatser RR, Giesey JJ: Relationship between muscle swelling and stiffness after eccentric exercise, *Med Sci Sports Exerc* 30(4):529–535, 1998.
25. Jones DA, Newham DJ, Clarkson PM: Skeletal muscle stiffness and pain following eccentric exercise of the elbow flexors, *Pain* 30(2):233–242, 1987.
26. Howell JN, Chleboun G, Conatser R: Muscle stiffness, strength loss, swelling and soreness following exercise-induced injury in humans, *J Physiol* 464:183–196, 1993.
27. Ebbeling CB, Clarkson PM: Exercise-induced muscle damage and adaptation, *Sports Med* 7(4):207–234, 1989.
28. Sayers SP, Clarkson PM, Rouzier PA, Kamen G: Adverse events associated with eccentric exercise protocols: Six case studies, *Med Sci Sports Exerc* 31(12):1697–1702, 1999.
29. Birtles DB, Rayson MP, Jones DA, et al: Effect of eccentric exercise on patients with chronic exertional compartment syndrome, *Eur J Appl Physiol* 88(6):565–571, 2003.
30. Friden J, Sfakianos PN, Hargens AR: Muscle soreness and intramuscular fluid pressure: Comparison between eccentric and concentric load, *J Appl Physiol* 61(6):2175–2179, 1986.
31. Gibala MJ, MacDougall JD, Tarnopolsky MA, et al: Changes in human skeletal muscle ultrastructure and force production after acute resistance exercise, *J Appl Physiol* 78(2):702–708, 1995.
32. Peake JM, Nosaka K, Muthalib M, Suzuki K: Systemic inflammatory responses to maximal versus submaximal lengthening contractions of the elbow flexors, *Exerc Immunol Rev* 12:72–85, 2006.
33. Nosaka K, Newton M, Sacco P: Responses of human elbow flexor muscles to electrically stimulated forced lengthening exercise, *Acta Physiol Scand* 174(2):137–145, 2002.
34. MacIntyre DL, Reid WD, Lyster DM, et al: Presence of WBC, decreased strength, and delayed soreness in muscle after eccentric exercise, *J Appl Physiol* 80(3):1006–1013, 1996.
35. Beaton LJ, Tarnopolsky MA, Phillips SM: Contraction-induced muscle damage in humans following calcium channel blocker administration, *J Physiol* 544(Pt 3):849–859, 2002.
36. Yu JG, Thornell LE: Desmin and actin alterations in human muscles affected by delayed onset muscle soreness: A high resolu-

tion immunocytochemical study, *Histochem Cell Biol* 118(2): 171–179, 2002.

37. Jones DA, Newham DJ, Torgan C: Mechanical influences on long-lasting human muscle fatigue and delayed-onset pain, *J Physiol* 412:415–427, 1989.

38. Nosaka K: Changes in serum enzyme activities after injection of bupivacaine into rat tibialis anterior, *J Appl Physiol* 81(2): 876–884, 1996.

39. Evans GF, Haller RG, Wyrick PS, et al: Submaximal delayed-onset muscle soreness: Correlations between MR imaging findings and clinical measures, *Radiology* 208(3):815–820, 1998.

40. Nosaka K, Newton M: Difference in the magnitude of muscle damage between maximal and submaximal eccentric loading, *J Strength Cond Res* 16(2):202–208, 2002.

41. Nosaka K, Sakamoto K, Newton M, Sacco P: The repeated bout effect of reduced-load eccentric exercise on elbow flexor muscle damage, *Eur J Appl Physiol* 85(1–2):34–40, 2001.

42. Clarkson PM, Tremblay I: Exercise-induced muscle damage, repair, and adaptation in humans, *J Appl Physiol* 65(1):1–6, 1988.

43. Kulig K, Powers CM, Shellock FG, Terk M: The effects of eccentric velocity on activation of elbow flexors: Evaluation by magnetic resonance imaging, *Med Sci Sports Exerc* 33(2): 196–200, 2001.

44. Chapman D, Newton M, Sacco P, Nosaka K: Greater muscle damage induced by fast versus slow velocity eccentric exercise, *Int J Sports Med* 27(8):591–598, 2006.

45. Newham DJ, Jones DA, Ghosh G, Aurora P: Muscle fatigue and pain after eccentric contractions at long and short length, *Clin Sci (Lond)* 74(5):553–557, 1988.

46. Mair J, Koller A, Artner-Dworzak E, et al: Effects of exercise on plasma myosin heavy chain fragments and MRI of skeletal muscle, *J Appl Physiol* 72(2):656–663, 1992.

47. Chapman DW, Newton MJ, Zainuddin Z, et al: Work and peak torque during eccentric exercise do not predict changes in markers of muscle damage, *Br J Sports Med* 242:585–591, 2008.

48. Hough T: Ergographic studies in muscular soreness, *Am J Physiol* 7:76–92, 1902.

49. Ebbeling CB, Clarkson PM: Muscle adaptation prior to recovery following eccentric exercise, *Eur J Appl Physiol Occup Physiol* 60(1):26–31, 1990.

50. Nosaka K, Clarkson PM: Muscle damage following repeated bouts of high force eccentric exercise, *Med Sci Sports Exerc* 27(9):1263–1269, 1995.

51. Warren GL, Ingalls CP, Lowe DA, Armstrong RB: What mechanisms contribute to the strength loss that occurs during and in the recovery from skeletal muscle injury? *J Orthop Sports Phys Ther* 32(2):58–64, 2002.

52. Stauber WT, Willems ME: Prevention of histopathologic changes from 30 repeated stretches of active rat skeletal muscles by long inter-stretch rest times, *Eur J Appl Physiol* 88(1–2):94–99, 2002.

53. Warren GL, Ingalls CP, Shah SJ, Armstrong RB: Uncoupling of in vivo torque production from EMG in mouse muscles injured by eccentric contractions, *J Physiol* 515 (Pt 2):609–619, 1999.

54. Hesselink MK, Kuipers H, Geurten P, Van Straaten H: Structural muscle damage and muscle strength after incremental number of isometric and forced lengthening contractions, *J Muscle Res Cell Motil* 17(3):335–341, 1996.

55. Lieber RL, Friden J: Muscle damage is not a function of muscle force but active muscle strain, *J Appl Physiol* 74(2):520–526, 1993.

56. Friden J, Sjostrom M, Ekblom B: Myofibrillar damage following intense eccentric exercise in man, *Int J Sports Med* 4(3):170–176, 1983.

57. Stauber WT, Clarkson PM, Fritz VK, Evans WJ: Extracellular matrix disruption and pain after eccentric muscle action, *J Appl Physiol* 69(3):868–874, 1990.

58. Morgan DL, Allen DG: Early events in stretch-induced muscle damage, *J Appl Physiol* 87(6):2007–2015, 1999.

59. Warren GL, Ingalls CP, Lowe DA, Armstrong RB: Excitation-contraction uncoupling: Major role in contraction-induced muscle injury, *Exerc Sport Sci Rev* 29(2):82–87, 2001.

60. Yeung EW, Balnave CD, Ballard HJ, et al: Development of T-tubular vacuoles in eccentrically damaged mouse muscle fibres, *J Physiol* 540(Pt 2):581–592, 2002.

61. Capetanaki Y, Bloch RJ, Kouloumenta A, et al: Muscle intermediate filaments and their links to membranes and membranous organelles, *Exp Cell Res* 313(10):2063–2076, 2007.

62. Nosaka K, Muthalib M, Lavender A, Laursen PB: Attenuation of muscle damage by preconditioning with muscle hyperthermia 1-day prior to eccentric exercise, *Eur J Appl Physiol* 99(2): 183–192, 2007.

63. Warren GL, Lowe DA, Armstrong RB: Measurement tools used in the study of eccentric contraction-induced injury, *Sports Med* 27(1):43–59, 1999.

64. Biral D, Jakubiec-Puka A, Ciechomska I, et al: Loss of dystrophin and some dystrophin-associated proteins with concomitant signs of apoptosis in rat leg muscle overworked in extension, *Acta Neuropathol* 100(6):618–626, 2000.

65. Stauber WT, Miller GR, Gibala MJ, MacDougall JD: Use of double labeling and photo CD for morphometric analysis of injured skeletal muscle, *J Histochem Cytochem* 43(11):1179–1184, 1995.

66. Komulainen J, Takala TE, Kuipers H, Hesselink MK: The disruption of myofibre structures in rat skeletal muscle after forced lengthening contractions, *Pflugers Arch* 436(5):735–741, 1998.

67. Wrogemann K, Pena SDJ: Mitochondrial calcium overload: A general mechanism for cell-necrosis in muscle diseases, *Lancet* 1:672–674, 1976.

68. Trump BF, Berezesky IK: Calcium-mediated cell injury and cell death, *FASEB J* 9(2):219–228, 1995.

69. Lowe DA, Warren GL, Ingalls CP, et al: Muscle function and protein metabolism after initiation of eccentric contraction-induced injury, *J Appl Physiol* 79(4):1260–1270, 1995.

70. Crenshaw AG, Friden J, Hargens AR, et al: Increased technetium uptake is not equivalent to muscle necrosis: Scintigraphic, morphological and intramuscular pressure analyses of sore muscles after exercise, *Acta Physiol Scand* 148(2):187–198, 1993.

71. Petrof BJ, Shrager JB, Stedman HH, et al: Dystrophin protects the sarcolemma from stresses developed during muscle contraction, *Proc Natl Acad Sci USA* 90(8):3710–3714, 1993.

72. McNeil PL, Khakee R: Disruptions of muscle fiber plasma membranes. Role in exercise-induced damage, *Am J Pathol* 140(5):1097–1109, 1992.

73. Sorichter S, Puschendorf B, Mair J: Skeletal muscle injury induced by eccentric muscle action: Muscle proteins as markers of muscle fiber injury, *Exerc Immunol Rev* 5:5–21, 1999.

74. Simionescu N, Simionescu M, Palade GE: Permeability of muscle capillaries to exogenous myoglobin, *J Cell Biol* 57(2):424–452, 1973.

75. Feola M, Glick G: Cardiac lymph flow and composition in acute myocardial ischemia in dogs, *Am J Physiol* 229(1):44–48, 1975.

76. Malm C, Nyberg P, Engstrom M, et al: Immunological changes in human skeletal muscle and blood after eccentric exercise and multiple biopsies, *J Physiol* 529(Pt 1):243–62, 2000.

77. Smith LL: Acute inflammation: The underlying mechanism in delayed onset muscle soreness? *Med Sci Sports Exerc* 23(5): 542–551, 1991.

78. MacIntyre DL, Sorichter S, Mair J, et al: Markers of inflammation and myofibrillar proteins following eccentric exercise in humans, *Eur J Appl Physiol* 84(3):180–186, 2001.

79. Tidball JG, Berchenko E, Frenette J: Macrophage invasion does not contribute to muscle membrane injury during inflammation, *J Leukoc Biol* 65(4):492–498, 1999.

80. Armstrong RB: Initial events in exercise-induced muscular injury, *Med Sci Sports Exerc* 22(4):429–435, 1990.

81. Duncan CJ, Jackson MJ: Different mechanisms mediate structural changes and intracellular enzyme efflux following damage to skeletal muscle, *J Cell Sci* 87(Pt 1):183–188, 1987.

82. Kozik A, Moore RB, Potempa J, et al: A novel mechanism for bradykinin production at inflammatory sites. Diverse effects of a mixture of neutrophil elastase and mast cell tryptase versus tissue and plasma kallikreins on native and oxidized kininogens, *J Biol Chem* 273(50):33224–33229, 1998.

83. Kushnir-Sukhov NM, Brown JM, Wu Y, et al: Human mast cells are capable of serotonin synthesis and release, *J Allergy Clin Immunol* 119(2):498–499, 2007.

84. Stauber WT, Fritz VK, Vogelbach DW, Dahlmann B: Characterization of muscles injured by forced lengthening. I. Cellular infiltrates, *Med Sci Sports Exerc* 20(4):345–353, 1988.

85. Nahirney PC, Dow PR, Ovalle WK: Quantitative morphology of mast cells in skeletal muscle of normal and genetically dystrophic mice, *Anat Rec* 247(3):341–349, 1997.

86. Ogilvie RW, Armstrong RB, Baird KE, Bottoms CL: Lesions in the rat soleus muscle following eccentrically biased exercise, *Am J Anat* 182(4):335–346, 1988.

87. The FO, Bennink RJ, Ankum WM, et al: Intestinal handling-induced mast cell activation and inflammation in human postoperative ileus, *Gut* 57(1):33–40, 2008.

88. Lazarus B, Messina A, Barker JE, et al: The role of mast cells in ischaemia-reperfusion injury in murine skeletal muscle, *J Pathol* 191(4):443–448, 2000.

89. Chleboun GS, Howell JN, Conatser RR, Giesey JJ: The relationship between elbow flexor volume and angular stiffness at the elbow, *Clin Biomech* 12(6):383–392, 1997.

90. Friden J, Sfakianos PN, Hargens AR, Akeson WH: Residual muscular swelling after repetitive eccentric contractions, *J Orthop Res* 6(4):493–498, 1988.

91. Brown SJ, Child RB, Day SH, Donnelly AE: Indices of skeletal muscle damage and connective tissue breakdown following eccentric muscle contractions, *Eur J Appl Physiol Occup Physiol* 75(4):369–374, 1997.

92. Foley JM, Jayaraman RC, Prior BM, et al: MR measurements of muscle damage and adaptation after eccentric exercise, *J Appl Physiol* 87(6):2311–2318, 1999.

93. Malm C, Sjodin TL, Sjoberg B, et al: Leukocytes, cytokines, growth factors and hormones in human skeletal muscle and blood after uphill or downhill running, *J Physiol* 556(Pt 3):983–1000, 2004.

94. Nosaka K, Sakamoto K, Newton M, Sacco P: How long does the protective effect on eccentric exercise-induced muscle damage last? *Med Sci Sports Exerc* 33(9):1490–1495, 2001.

95. Newham DJ, Jones DA, Clarkson PM: Repeated high-force eccentric exercise: Effects on muscle pain and damage, *J Appl Physiol* 63(4):1381–1386, 1987.

96. Nosaka K, Newton MJ, Sacco P: Attenuation of protective effect against eccentric exercise-induced muscle damage, *Can J Appl Physiol* 30(5):529–542, 2005.

97. Whitehead NP, Allen TJ, Morgan DL, Proske U: Damage to human muscle from eccentric exercise after training with concentric exercise, *J Physiol* 512(Pt 2):615–620, 1998.

98. Butterfield TA, Leonard TR, Herzog W: Differential serial sarcomere number adaptations in knee extensor muscles of rats is contraction type dependent, *J Appl Physiol* 99(4):1352–1358, 2005.

99. Kuipers H, Keizer HA, Verstappen FT, Costill DL: Influence of a prostaglandin-inhibiting drug on muscle soreness after eccentric work, *Int J Sports Med* 6(6):336–339, 1985.

100. Donnelly AE, Maughan RJ, Whiting PH: Effects of ibuprofen on exercise-induced muscle soreness and indices of muscle damage, *Br J Sports Med* 24(3):191–195, 1990.

101. Grossman JM, Arnold BL, Perrin DH, Kahler DM: Effect of ibuprofen on delayed onset muscle soreness of the elbow flexors, *J Sport Rehabil* 4:253–263, 1995.

102. Barlas P, Craig JA, Robinson J, et al: Managing delayed-onset muscle soreness: Lack of effect of selected oral systemic analgesics, *Arch Phys Med Rehabil* 81(7):966–972, 2000.

103. Bourgeois J, MacDougall D, MacDonald J, Tarnopolsky M: Naproxen does not alter indices of muscle damage in resistance-exercise trained men, *Med Sci Sports Exerc* 31(1):4–9, 1999.

104. Pizza FX, Cavender D, Stockard A, et al: Anti-inflammatory doses of ibuprofen: Effect on neutrophils and exercise-induced muscle injury, *Int J Sports Med* 20(2):98–102, 1999.

105. Brooks PM, Day RO: Nonsteroidal antiinflammatory drugs—Differences and similarities, *N Engl J Med* 324(24):1716–1725, 1991.

106. Donnelly AE, McCormick K, Maughan RJ, et al: Effects of a non-steroidal anti-inflammatory drug on delayed onset muscle soreness and indices of damage, *Br J Sports Med* 22(1):35–38, 1988.

107. Sayers SP, Knight CA, Clarkson PM, et al: Effect of ketoprofen on muscle function and sEMG activity after eccentric exercise, *Med Sci Sports Exerc* 33(5):702–710, 2001.

108. Howell JN, Conaster RR, Chleboun GS, et al: The effect of nonsteroidal anti-inflammatory drugs on recovery from exercise-induced muscle injury. 2. Ibuprofen, *J Musculoskeletal Pain* 6:69–83, 1998.

109. Almekinders LC, Gilbert JA: Healing of experimental muscle strains and the effects of nonsteroidal antiinflammatory medication, *Am J Sports Med* 14(4):303–308, 1986.

110. Nosaka K, Clarkson PM: Changes in indicators of inflammation after eccentric exercise of the elbow flexors, *Med Sci Sports Exerc* 28(8):953–961, 1996.

111. Michlovitz S: Cold therapy modalities: Frozen peas and more. In Michlovitz S, Nolan T, editors: *Modalities for therapeutic intervention*, ed 4, Philadelphia, 2005, FA Davis Company.

112. Enwemeka CS, Allen C, Avila P, et al: Soft tissue thermodynamics before, during, and after cold pack therapy, *Med Sci Sports Exerc* 34(1):45–50, 2002.

113. Eston R, Peters D: Effects of cold water immersion on the symptoms of exercise-induced muscle damage, *J Sports Sci* 17(3):231–238, 1999.

114. Paddon-Jones DJ, Quigley BM: Effect of cryotherapy on muscle soreness and strength following eccentric exercise, *Int J Sports Med* 18(8):588–593, 1997.

115. Yackzan L, Adams C, Francis KT: The effects of ice massage on delayed muscle soreness, *Am J Sports Med* 12(2):159–165, 1984.

116. Isabell WK, Durrant E, Myrer W, Anderson S: The effects of ice massage, ice massage with exercise, and exercise on the prevention and treatment of delayed onset muscle soreness, *J Athl Train* 27(3):208–217, 1992.

117. Sellwood KL, Brukner P, Williams D, et al: Ice-water immersion and delayed-onset muscle soreness: A randomised controlled trial, *Br J Sports Med* 41(6):392–397, 2007.

118. Howatson G, Gaze D, van Someren KA: The efficacy of ice massage in the treatment of exercise-induced muscle damage, *Scand J Med Sci Sports* 15(6):416–422, 2005.

119. Meeusen R, Lievens P: The use of cryotherapy in sports injuries, *Sports Med* 3(6):398–414, 1986.

120. Myrer JW, Measom G, Fellingham GW: Temperature changes in the human leg during and after two methods of cryotherapy, *J Athl Train* 33(1):25–29, 1998.

121. Michlovitz S, Rennie S: Heat therapy modalities: Beyond fake and bake. In Michlovitz S, Nolan T, editors: *Modalities for therapeutic intervention*, ed 4, Philadephia, 2005, FA Davis Company.

122. Vaile J, Halson S, Gill N, Dawson B: Effect of hydrotherapy on the signs and symptoms of delayed onset muscle soreness, *Eur J Appl Physiol* 102(4):447–455, 2008.

123. Mayer JM, Mooney V, Matheson LN, et al: Continuous low-level heat wrap therapy for the prevention and early phase treatment of delayed-onset muscle soreness of the low back: A randomized controlled trial, *Arch Phys Med Rehabil* 87(10):1310–1317, 2006.

124. Cochrane DJ: Alternating hot and cold water immersion for athlete recovery: A review, *Phys Ther Sport* 5(1):26–32, 2004.

125. Bukowski EL, Nolan TP. Hydrotherapy: The use of water as a therapeutic agent. In Michlovitz S, Nolan T, editors: *Modalities for therapeutic intervention*, ed 4, Philadelphia, 2005, FA Davis Company.

126. Vaile JM, Gill ND, Blazevich AJ: The effect of contrast water therapy on symptoms of delayed onset muscle soreness, *J Strength Cond Res* 21(3):697–702, 2007.

127. Webster DF, Harvey W, Dyson M, Pond JB: The role of ultrasound-induced cavitation in the "in vitro" stimulation of collagen synthesis in human fibroblasts, *Ultrasonics* 18(1):33–37, 1980.

128. Byl NN, McKenzie AL, West JM, et al: Low-dose ultrasound effects on wound healing: A controlled study with Yucatan pigs, *Arch Phys Med Rehabil* 73(7):656–664, 1992.

129. Young SR, Dyson M: Effect of therapeutic ultrasound on the healing of full-thickness excised skin lesions, *Ultrasonics* 28(3):175–180, 1990.

130. Francis CW, Onundarson PT, Carstensen EL, et al: Enhancement of fibrinolysis in vitro by ultrasound, *J Clin Invest* 90(5):2063–2068, 1992.

131. Young SR, Dyson M: The effect of therapeutic ultrasound on angiogenesis, *Ultrasound Med Biol* 16(3):261–269, 1990.

132. Speed CA: Therapeutic ultrasound in soft tissue lesions, *Rheumatology* (Oxford), 40(12):1331–1336, 2001.

133. Hasson S, Mundorf R, Barnes W, et al: Effect of pulsed ultrasound versus placebo on muscle soreness perception and muscular performance, *Scand J Rehabil Med* 22(4):199–205, 1990.

134. Craig JA, Bradley J, Walsh DM, et al: Delayed onset muscle soreness: Lack of effect of therapeutic ultrasound in humans, *Arch Phys Med Rehabil* 80(3):318–323, 1999.

135. Stay JC, Richard MD, Draper DO, et al: Pulsed ultrasound fails to diminish delayed-onset muscle soreness symptoms, *J Athl Train* 33(4):341–346, 1998.

136. Evans RK, Knight KL, Draper DO, Parcell AC: Effects of warm-up before eccentric exercise on indirect markers of muscle damage, *Med Sci Sports Exerc* 34(12):1892–1899, 2002.

137. Symons TB, Clasey JL, Gater DR, Yates JW: Effects of deep heat as a preventative mechanism on delayed onset muscle soreness, *J Strength Cond Res* 18(1):155–161, 2004.

138. Ciccone CD, Leggin BG, Callamaro JJ: Effects of ultrasound and trolamine salicylate phonophoresis on delayed-onset muscle soreness, *Phys Ther* 71(9):666–675, 1991.

139. Rao VR, Wolf SL, Gersh MR: Examination of electrode placements and stimulating parameters in treating chronic pain with conventional transcutaneous electrical nerve stimulation (TENS), *Pain* 11(1):37–47, 1981.

140. Denegar CR, Perrin DH: Effect of transcutaneous electrical nerve stimulation, cold, and a combination treatment on pain, decreased range of motion, and strength loss associated with delayed onset muscle soreness, *J Athl Train* 27(3):200–206, 1992.

141. Craig JA, Cunningham MB, Walsh DM, et al: Lack of effect of transcutaneous electrical nerve stimulation upon experimentally induced delayed onset muscle soreness in humans, *Pain* 67 (2–3):285–289, 1996.

142. Minder PM, Noble JG, ves-Guerreiro J, et al: Interferential therapy: Lack of effect upon experimentally induced delayed onset muscle soreness, *Clin Physiol Funct Imaging* 22(5):339–347, 2002.

143. Butterfield DL, Draper DO, Ricard MD, et al: The effects of high-volt pulsed current electrical stimulation on delayed-onset muscle soreness, *J Athl Train* 32(1):15–20, 1997.

144. Tourville TW, Connolly DA, Reed BV: Effects of sensory-level high-volt pulsed electrical current on delayed-onset muscle soreness, *J Sports Sci* 24(9):941–949, 2006.

145. Lambert MI, Marcus P, Burgess T, Noakes TD: Electro-membrane microcurrent therapy reduces signs and symptoms of muscle damage, *Med Sci Sports Exerc* 34(4):602–607, 2002.

146. Weber MD, Servedio FJ, Woodall WR: The effects of three modalities on delayed onset muscle soreness, *J Orthop Sports Phys Ther* 20(5):236–242, 1994.

147. Allen JD, Mattacola CG, Perrin DH: Effect of microcurrent stimulation on delayed-onset muscle soreness: A double-blind comparison, *J Athl Train* 34(4):334–337, 1999.

148. Denegar CR, Yoho AP, Borowicz AJ, Bifulco N: The effects of low-volt, microamperage stimulation on delayed onset muscle soreness, *J Sport Rehabil* 1(2):95–102, 1992.

149. Chleboun GS, Howell JN, Baker HL, et al: Intermittent pneumatic compression effect on eccentric exercise-induced swelling, stiffness, and strength loss, *Arch Phys Med Rehabil* 76(8):744–749, 1995.

150. Kraemer WJ, Bush JA, Wickham RB, et al: Influence of compression therapy on symptoms following soft tissue injury from maximal eccentric exercise, *J Orthop Sports Phys Ther* 31(6):282–290, 2001.

151. Callaghan MJ: The role of massage in the management of the athlete: A review, *Br J Sports Med* 27(1):28–33, 1993.

152. Weerapong P, Hume PA, Kolt GS: The mechanisms of massage and effects on performance, muscle recovery and injury prevention, *Sports Med* 35(3):235–256, 2005.

153. Cafarelli E, Flint F: The role of massage in preparation for and recovery from exercise, An overview, *Sports Med* 14(1):1–9, 1992.

154. Wright A, Sluka KA: Nonpharmacological treatments for musculoskeletal pain, *Clin J Pain* 17(1):33–46, 2001.

155. Tiidus PM, Shoemaker JK: Effleurage massage, muscle blood flow and long-term post-exercise strength recovery, *Int J Sports Med* 16(7):478–483, 1995.

156. Smith LL, Keating MN, Holbert D, et al: The effects of athletic massage on delayed onset muscle soreness, creatine kinase, and neutrophil count: A preliminary report, *J Orthop Sports Phys Ther* 19(2):93–99, 1994.

157. Lightfoot JT, Char D, McDermott J, Goya C: Immediate postexercise massage does not attenuate delayed onset muscle soreness, *J Strength Cond Res* 11:119–124, 1997.

158. Hilbert JE, Sforzo GA, Swensen T: The effects of massage on delayed onset muscle soreness, *Br J Sports Med* 37(1):72–75, 2003.

159. Mancinelli CA, Davis DS, Aboulhosn L, et al: The effects of massage on delayed onset muscle soreness and physical performance in female collegiate athletes, *Phys Ther Sport* 7:5–13, 2006.

160. Herbert RD, Gabriel M: Effects of stretching before and after exercising on muscle soreness and risk of injury: Systematic review, *BMJ* 325(7362):468, 2002.

161. Johansson PH, Lindstrom L, Sundelin G, Lindstrom B: The effects of preexercise stretching on muscular soreness, tenderness and force loss following heavy eccentric exercise, *Scand J Med Sci Sports* 9(4):219–225, 1999.

162. Lund H, Vestergaard-Poulsen P, Kanstrup IL, Sejrsen P: The effect of passive stretching on delayed onset muscle soreness, and other detrimental effects following eccentric exercise, *Scand J Med Sci Sports* 8(4):216–221, 1998.

163. Smith LL, Brunetz MH, Chenier TC, et al: The effects of static and ballistic stretching on delayed onset muscle soreness and creatine kinase, *Res Q Exerc Sport* 64(1):103–107, 1993.

164. Caiozzo VJ, Utkan A, Chou R, et al: Effects of distraction on muscle length: Mechanisms involved in sarcomerogenesis, *Clin Orthop Relat Res* 403:S133–S145, 2002.

165. Brockett CL, Morgan DL, Proske U: Human hamstring muscles adapt to eccentric exercise by changing optimum length, *Med Sci Sports Exerc* 33(5):783–790, 2001.

166. Nosaka K, Clarkson PM: Influence of previous concentric exercise on eccentric exercise-induced muscle damage, *J Sports Sci* 15(5):477–483, 1997.

167. High DM, Howley ET, Franks BD: The effects of static stretching and warm-up on prevention of delayed-onset muscle soreness, *Res Q Exerc Sport* 60(4):357–361, 1989.

168. Warren GL, Hayes DA, Lowe DA, Armstrong RB: Mechanical factors in the initiation of eccentric contraction-induced injury in rat soleus muscle, *J Physiol* 464:457–475, 1993.

169. Morgan DL, Gregory JE, Proske U: The influence of fatigue on damage from eccentric contractions in the gastrocnemius muscle of the cat, *J Physiol* 561(Pt 3):841–850, 2004.

170. Donnelly AE, Clarkson PM, Maughan RJ: Exercise-induced muscle damage: Effects of light exercise on damaged muscle, *Eur J Appl Physiol Occup Physiol* 64(4):350–353, 1992.

171. Sayers SP, Clarkson PM, Lee J: Activity and immobilization after eccentric exercise: I. Recovery of muscle function, *Med Sci Sports Exerc* 32(9):1587–1592, 2000.

172. Hasson S, Barnes W, Hunter M, Williams J: Therapeutic effect of high speed voluntary muscle contractions on muscle soreness and muscle performance, *J Orthop Sports Phys Ther* 10:499–507, 1989.

173. Mekjavic IB, Exner JA, Tesch PA, Eiken O: Hyperbaric oxygen therapy does not affect recovery from delayed onset muscle soreness, *Med Sci Sports Exerc* 32(3):558–563, 2000.

174. Harrison BC, Robinson D, Davison BJ, et al: Treatment of exercise-induced muscle injury via hyperbaric oxygen therapy, *Med Sci Sports Exerc* 33(1):36–42, 2001.

175. Bennett M, Best TM, Babul S, et al: Hyperbaric oxygen therapy for delayed onset muscle soreness and closed soft tissue injury, *Cochrane Database Syst Rev* (4):CD004713, 2005.

176. Berman BM, Lao L, Langenberg P, et al: Effectiveness of acupuncture as adjunctive therapy in osteoarthritis of the knee: A randomized, controlled trial, *Ann Intern Med* 141(12): 901–910, 2004.

177. Pomeranz B: Scientific research into acupuncture for the relief of pain, *J Altern Complement Med* 2(1):53–60, 1996.

178. Barlas P, Robinson J, Allen J, Baxter GD: Lack of effect of acupuncture upon signs and symptoms of delayed onset muscle soreness, *Clin Physiol* 20(6):449–456, 2000.

179. Robertson A, Suryanarayanan R, Banerjee A: Homeopathic Arnica montana for post-tonsillectomy analgesia: A randomised placebo control trial, *Homeopathy* 96(1):17–21, 2007.

180. Cheung K, Hume P, Maxwell L: Delayed onset muscle soreness: Treatment strategies and performance factors, *Sports Med* 33(2):145–164, 2003.

181. Vickers AJ, Fisher P, Smith C, et al: Homoeopathy for delayed onset muscle soreness: A randomised double blind placebo controlled trial, *Br J Sports Med* 31(4):304–307, 1997.

182. Gulick DT, Kimura IF, Sitler M, et al: Various treatment techniques on signs and symptoms of delayed onset muscle soreness, *J Athl Train* 31(2):145–152, 1996.

183. Giamberardino MA, Dragani L, Valente R, et al: Effects of prolonged L-carnitine administration on delayed muscle pain and CK release after eccentric effort, *Int J Sports Med* 17(5): 320–324, 1996.

184. Singh RB, Wander GS, Rastogi A, et al: Randomized, double-blind placebo-controlled trial of coenzyme Q10 in patients with acute myocardial infarction, *Cardiovasc Drugs Ther* 12(4): 347–353, 1998.

185. Malm C, Svensson M, Sjoberg B, et al: Supplementation with ubiquinone-10 causes cellular damage during intense exercise, *Acta Physiol Scand* 157(4):511–512, 1996.

186. Connolly DA, Lauzon C, Agnew J, et al: The effects of vitamin C supplementation on symptoms of delayed onset muscle soreness, *J Sports Med Phys Fitness* 46(3):462–467, 2006.

187. Avery NG, Kaiser JL, Sharman MJ, et al: Effects of vitamin E supplementation on recovery from repeated bouts of resistance exercise, *J Strength Cond Res* 17(4):801–809, 2003.

188. Bloomer RJ, Goldfarb AH, McKenzie MJ, et al: Effects of antioxidant therapy in women exposed to eccentric exercise, *Int J Sport Nutr Exerc Metab* 14(4):377–388, 2004.

189. George SZ, Dover GC, Fillingim RB: Fear of pain influences outcomes after exercise-induced delayed onset muscle soreness at the shoulder, *Clin J Pain* 23(1):76–84, 2007.

MEDICAL CONDITIONS IN SPORT

Dhiren J. Naidu

Introduction

Traditionally, sport medicine injuries are believed to be primarily of the musculoskeletal system. In fact, a sport medicine practitioner will commonly see injuries and illnesses outside the musculoskeletal system. A study from the University of Arizona showed that management of medical problems accounted for the highest incidence of visits to the team physician at the collegiate level.[1] This chapter focuses on some common and difficult medical conditions of which sport medicine providers should be aware.

Cardiovascular System

The prevalence of cardiovascular disease and the risk of sudden cardiac death in athletes is low.[2,3] In the United States, the number of athletes who die from cardiovascular causes is approximately 300 of the 10 to 15 million athletes participating in organized sport per year. Because of the high profile of professional athletes and perhaps their perceived invincibility, sudden death, although a relatively rare occurrence, seems to have an enormous impact on both the public and health care providers.

At the 36th Bethesda Conference, the generally accepted tenant was that young trained athletes with underlying cardiovascular abnormalities had an increased relative risk of 2.5 for sudden cardiac death in comparison with nonathletes.[2,4-6] This is thought to be due to the unique physiological and psychological stresses of intense training and competition. Because of the increased physiological stresses, deaths usually occur during athletic competition.

Note: This chapter includes content from previous contributions by James C. Puffer, MD, as it appeared in the predecessor of this book—Zachazewski JE, Magee DJ, Quillen WS, editors: *Athletic Injuries and rehabilitation*, Philadelphia, 1996, WB Saunders.

In young athletes, the most common fatal condition is hypertrophic cardiomyopathy (HCM) followed by congenital anomalies of the coronary arteries. Atherosclerotic heart disease is the most common fatal condition in older athletes.

The American Heart Association recommends further screening if an athlete presents with specific history or physical examination findings. Risk factors include exertional chest pain, a heart murmur, easy fatigability, syncope, shortness of breath, or a history of high blood pressure. Physical examination findings may include a heart murmur, abnormal blood pressure, irregular heart rate, or any stigmata of Marfan' syndrome.[7] Obtaining information about family history is also important. If there is a history of premature sudden death or heart disease in a relative younger than 50 years of age, further screening is necessary.

Risk Factors for Sudden Cardiac Death

- Exertional chest pain
- Heart murmur
- Easy fatigability
- Syncope
- Shortness of breath
- Hypertension
- Family history of premature sudden death
- Heart disease in a relative younger than 50 years of age
- Irregular heart rate or palpitations

Hypertrophic Cardiomyopathy (HCM)

HCM is the most common form of sudden unexpected cardiac death in both young people and competitive athletes.[8] In most cases, sudden death occurs in people younger than 30.[2] The most common pathological finding is in the cardiac muscle. The cardiac muscle is asymmetrically hypertrophied and an associated nondilated left ventricle is present. The septal thickness is at least 15 mm thick and the left ventricular (LV) cavity is less than 45 mm in cases of HCM.[9] Currently, echocardiography is the gold standard for the detection of HCM. HCM is rare in the setting of a normal electrocardiogram (ECG). ECG findings are relatively nonspecific, but include LV hypertrophy and ST segment and T wave abnormalities.

Currently, a diagnosis of HCM excludes participation in competitive and noncompetitive sports, with the exception of low-intensity sports.

Athletic Heart Syndrome

In athletes, there is a well-accepted condition described as *athlete's heart syndrome*. This may be confused with HCM as both conditions are characterized by an enlarged heart. Isometric or endurance training trigger physiological adaptations and structural cardiac remodeling, including increased left ventricle wall thickness, enlarged ventricular and atrial cavity dimensions, and increased cardiac mass.[10] The athlete's heart has a septal thickness of less than 15 mm and the LV cavity is larger than 55 mm (Table 18-1).[9]

Hypertension

Athletes and physically active people are thought to be free of high blood pressure (hypertension) because of their high level of fitness. In athletes, the overall presence of hypertension is approximately 50% less than the general population.[11]

Certain populations of athletes are at increased risk of hypertension. These include black athletes, elderly athletes, obese athletes, diabetic athletes, those with renal disease, or athletes with family history of hypertension.

Hypertension may occur in early adulthood. As people age, the prevalence of hypertension increases. For example, 5% to 10% of adults aged 20 to 30 are affected and 20% to 25% of adults aged 30 to 60 are affected.[12]

Interestingly, 80% of athletes who have blood pressure higher than 142/92 at a preparticipation medical examination eventually develop chronic elevated blood pressure.[13]

Table 18-1

Heart Differences in Athletic Heart Syndrome and Hypertrophic Cardiomyopathy

	Athletic Heart Syndrome	Hypertrophic Cardiomyopathy
Septal thickness	< 15 mm	> 15 mm
Left ventricular cavity size	> 55 mm	< 45 mm

Blood pressure, in the hemodynamic sense, can be conceptualized as a product of both cardiac output and peripheral vascular resistance.[14] In young athletes, hypertensive changes in blood pressure are most commonly the result of a significant increase in cardiac output, with minimal changes in peripheral vascular resistance. Heart rate, renal blood flow, plasma renin activity, and catecholamines are all elevated in the young hypertensive athlete, and cardiac output is increased 10% to 20% more than that seen in normal subjects. The hypertension of young athletes, therefore, has been characterized as a *hyperadrenergic* or *hyperdynamic hypertension*. On the other hand, in middle-aged or older athletes, hypertensive blood pressure change is most likely a reflection of significant increases in peripheral vascular resistance with no change or a decrease in cardiac output.

When clinically evaluating an athlete with hypertension, the history should focus on behaviors that may affect blood pressure. These include a high intake of sodium and saturated fats (e.g., in processed and "fast" foods) and the use of alcohol, drugs (specifically stimulants taken before competitions or cocaine), tobacco, or anabolic steroids.[15] Many over-the-counter medications, including nonsteroidal anti-inflammatory drugs, caffeine, diet pills, and decongestants, can also cause blood pressure to rise. In women, the estrogen in oral contraceptive pills can also lead to hypertension.

Patients should also be questioned about the use of herbs and dietary supplements, with special attention given to substances purported to increase energy or control weight. These supplements often contain "natural" substances such as guarana, ma huang, and ephedra, which are stimulants.

Risk Factors for Hypertension

- High sodium intake
- Excessive alcohol consumption
- Illicit drug use (e.g., cocaine)
- Anabolic steroid use
- Stimulant use
- High stress
- Male gender
- Black race
- Family history of hypertension
- Diabetes mellitus
- Smoking
- Obesity

The physical examination should include proper measurement of blood pressure, which may include serial measurements. Laboratory tests that exclude other medical causes of hypertension may include an ECG; a complete blood count; urinalysis; and measurements of sodium, potassium, blood urea nitrogen, creatinine, fasting glucose, total low-density lipoprotein, and high-density lipoprotein cholesterol levels.

Treatment includes both nonpharmacological and pharmacological therapy. Nonpharmacological therapy includes dietary changes aimed at restricting sodium intake. Intake of potatoes, bananas, and other foods high in potassium may provide some protection against high blood pressure.[16] A weight loss of 10 pounds can reduce blood pressure.[17] Changes of lifestyle to include limiting alcohol intake to less than two beers per day.[15] Regular aerobic exercise (moderate level of exercise), muscle relaxation, meditation, and other stress management techniques can also be helpful.[18]

From a pharmacological perspective, the ideal antihypertensive agent for use in competitive athletes should be free of any depressant effect on the myocardium, have no arrhythmogenic potential, preserve the redistribution of blood flow to exercising muscle, and not interfere with efficient substrate use for energy demands.[19] In the young athlete, the agents that meet all these criteria are the angiotensin-converting enzyme (ACE) inhibitors. The use of beta blockers should be discouraged because of their known ability to impair LV function, their unfavorable effect on serum lipids, and their negative influence on the mobilization of lipids during prolonged submaximal exercise. Likewise, diuretics are unsuitable first-line agents for the athlete because of their unfavorable effect on serum lipids, their potential to cause hypokalemia and hypomagnesemia, and their negative influence on volume status. For the older patient, appropriate first-line agents include the calcium-channel blockers and the ACE inhibitors. A combination of both these agents may be beneficial in treating the older athlete whose blood pressure is resistant to treatment with either agent used singly. The hypertensive black athlete deserves special mention because of the volume-dependent nature of the hypertension. The patient may respond to very small doses of diuretic such as 12.5 mg of hydrochlorothiazide daily. Other options for this population include antiadrenergic agents as well as the calcium-channel blockers. For the athlete participating in events at which drug testing will be done, special consideration must be given to the choice of therapeutic agents, because beta blockers (in some events) and diuretics are banned by both the International Olympic Committee and the World Anti-Doping Agency.

Recommendations from the 26th Bethesda conference for exercise in athletes with hypertension include no restrictions if an athlete has high normal blood pressure or controlled mild to moderate hypertension (< 140/90 mm Hg). If hypertension is uncontrolled (> 140/90 mm Hg) or there is any end organ damage present, then low-intensity dynamic exercise is recommended.

Marfan Syndrome

Marfan syndrome is a genetic (autosomal dominant) disorder of connective tissue with an estimated prevalence of 1:5000 to 1:10,000 in the general population.[20-23]

Clinical characteristics include abnormalities of the ocular, skeletal, and cardiovascular systems (Table 18-2).[22-24] The diagnosis is made if major criteria are present in two organ systems and a third is involved, or when there is a family history of Marfan syndrome.[22,23] The skeletal abnormalities include arm span/height ratio of greater than 1.05, tall stature, arachnodactyly (long, spiderlike fingers and toes), long and thin limbs, hyperextensibility, scoliosis, and chest wall deformities. Lens dislocations make up the ocular abnormality. Cardiovascular abnormalities include progressive dilatation of the aortic or descending root, which is the ultimate cause of death. Mitral valve prolapse with mitral regurgitation and lateral ventricle systolic dysfunction may also predispose to life threatening arrhythmias. Clinically, symptoms are relatively nonspecific and may include fatigue, shortness of breath, syncope, or presyncopal-type episodes. Aortic rupture usually results in sudden death. It is generally recommended that athletes with Marfan syndrome have regular cardiac evaluations and not compete in high-intensity or contact sports. In certain situations, they may compete in low-intensity and low-dynamic sports.

Coronary Artery Abnormalities

Congenital coronary artery abnormalities are the second most common cause of exercise-associated death in young patients. The most commonly reported coronary abnormality in the young athlete at autopsy is anomalous left coronary artery that originates from the right sinus of Valsalva and then makes an abrupt turn to travel between the pulmonary artery and aorta.[8] Anomalous right coronary arteries and single coronary arteries have been reported as well. It is next to impossible to screen for abnormalities for this condition on physical examination. An athlete who presents with syncope, syncopal-type episodes, or chest pain requires investigation and consultation by a cardiologist.

Table 18-2
Marfan Syndrome Abnormalities

Skeletal	Ocular	Cardiovascular
Arm span:height ratio of > 1.05	Lens dislocations	Progressive dilatation of aortic root
Tall stature		Progressive dilatation of descending root
Arachnodactyly		Mitral valve prolapse
Long, thin limbs		Mitral regurgitation
Hyperextensibility		Left ventricle systolic dysfunction
Scoliosis		
Chest wall deformities		

Coronary Artery Disease

In older athletes, arthrosclerotic coronary artery disease is the most common cause of sudden death. The incidence of sudden death for recreational joggers between the ages of 30 and 64 years was found to be approximately one sudden death per year for every 7620 joggers.[25] The absolute number of jogging deaths was low; however, there was an approximate seven times greater chance of dying suddenly while exercising versus being sedentary. In the middle-aged athlete, especially those who are starting a new exercise regime, it is important to assess cardiac risk factors. Modifiable risk factors such as smoking, high cholesterol, hypertension, obesity, and proper blood sugar levels should be controlled if abnormalities are present.[26]

Cardiac Risk Factors

- Smoking
- High cholesterol
- Hypertension
- Physical inactivity
- Obesity
- Diabetes mellitus
- Increasing age
- Male gender
- Black race

Commotio Cordis

Commotio cordis is a cause of sudden and unexpected death in young athletes resulting from a precordial blow to the chest.[8] It is more common in youth baseball, softball, ice hockey, football, and lacrosse. Death is usually caused by the projectiles used in these sports. Blows are typically of low energy (30 to 40 mph [48 to 66 km/hr]); however, high-velocity blows can occur from lacrosse balls or hockey pucks (90 mph [145 km/hr]). Collapse of the athlete can be instantaneous or preceded by brief periods of consciousness. Even in a case of a structurally normal heart, there is only a 15% survival rate; however, survival rates seem to be increasing with the use of prompt cardiopulmonary resuscitation and defibrillation protocols.[27] Strategies for prevention include equipment changes such as softer-than-normal safety balls and better chest equipment.[28] Also, the importance of immediate access to resuscitative equipment such as automated external defibrillators will help decrease mortality rates.[29,30]

Pulmonary System

Exercise-Induced Bronchospasm

Exercise-induced bronchospasm (EIB) is an obstruction of transient airflow that usually occurs 5 to 15 minutes after physical exertion. The National Asthma Education and Prevention Program in the United States describes EIB as the presence of symptoms in relation to athletic performance or a significant decrease in forced expiratory volume at 1 second in relation to exercise.

The symptoms of EIB include shortness of breath, wheezing, decreased exercise endurance, chest pain or tightness with exercise, cough, upset stomach, and a sore throat. The symptoms must occur during or following approximately 5 minutes of exercise. Most athletes with EIB have a normal physical examination. A pulmonary function test is the most objective way to diagnose EIB. Between 80% and 90% of patients with asthma also have EIB.[31] It is thought that unrecognized EIB occurs in 29% of athletes presenting for athletic preparticipation examinations.[32]

Treatment includes a variety of nonpharmacological and pharmacological treatments. The goal is to prevent or reduce the symptoms of EIB for the exercise to take place at varying intensity levels. Nonpharmacological measures include increasing physical conditioning; warming up for at least 10 minutes before exercise; covering mouth and nose with a scarf or mask during cold weather; and exercising in a warm, humidified environment. Other important measures include avoiding aeroallergens and pollutants, cooling down, gradually lowering the intensity of the exercise before stopping, and exercising at least 2 hours after a meal.[33] These measures can decrease both the frequency and intensity of bronchospasm.

Pharmacological therapy is usually started with an inhaled beta-agonist medication (e.g., betamethasone or albuterol [Ventolin]) that acts as a bronchodilator and opens up the airways for easier ventilation. Prophylactically, medication should be used 15 minutes prior to exercise. The use of a beta agonist may be repeated as necessary. Long-acting beta agonists have been shown to protect against EIB for 12 hours; however, continuous use leads to significant side effects, such as tachyphylaxis.[34]

Cromolyn and nedocromil are anti-inflammatory agents that work in cooperation with beta agonists. They can help by inhibiting both the early bronchospastic and late inflammatory stage of EIB.[35] Inhaled corticosteroids (e.g., fluticasone [Advair]) are also found to be effective in the treatment of EIB. They usually need to be used for 4 weeks to obtain maximal effectiveness. This medication should be reserved if it is thought that inflammation is a primary component of EIB. In the setting of Olympic, collegiate, and most professional sports, the use of an inhaled corticosteroid requires the use of a therapeutic use exemption form.

Upper Respiratory Tract Infection

Upper respiratory tract infections are the most common infections in the athletic population. They are usually viral and self-limiting (5 to 10 days). Treatment focuses on decreasing symptoms and athletes can usually continue to be physically active. If an athlete is febrile with myalgias (diffuse muscle pain), they should refrain from exercising because of a theoretical risk of developing viral myocarditis.[36] If an athlete has developed influenza, it usually occurs in winter or early spring and is associated with a rapidly rising fever, headache, and cough. Before treating with antiviral medication (e.g., zanamivir, amantadine), a rapid enzyme immunoassay should take place.

Pharyngitis (inflammation of the pharynx) is commonly viral and presents with a sore throat. In a minority of cases, pharyngitis is due to a bacterial infection, specifically beta-hemolytic streptococci. Typically, a fever of more than 38°C (100.4°F) is present, along with tender enlarged cervical lymph nodes, swelling of the tonsils, erythema, and exudate in the setting of little or no cough or upper respiratory symptoms. Before treating with antibiotics (e.g., penicillin [Pen V], amoxicillin [Amoxil]), a rapid enzyme immunoassay should be done.

Asthma

Asthma is a chronic inflammatory disorder of the airways. The inflammation causes airflow obstruction, which, in the presence of certain triggers, may cause acute bronchoconstriction that may be life threatening if not treated. Clinical features usually include wheezing; shortness of breath; chest tightness; and a dry, nonproductive cough.

Common Triggers for Asthma and Airway Bronchospasm

- Cigarette smoke
- Exercise
- Molds
- Dust
- Anxiety
- Stress
- Cold weather
- Weather changes
- General pollution

Treatment of asthma includes the use of a medication, such as an inhaled steroid, to work against the inflammation component of the disease. A bronchodilator is used for the relief of symptoms caused by the triggers. If symptoms worsen over time, pulmonary function tests should be considered along with further medications to act against the inflammatory component of the condition.

Altitude Sickness

Many activities, such as backpacking, mountain climbing, and downhill skiing involve traveling to extreme heights. If activities include traveling to heights above 10,000 feet (3048 m), the athlete may be at risk for altitude-related illness. There are three main types of high-altitude illness. They include acute mountain sickness, high-altitude pulmonary edema (HAPE) and high-altitude cerebral edema (HACE). Both HAPE and HACE are life-threatening manifestations of altitude illness and fortunately only occur in 0.1% to 4.0% of athletes traveling to high altitude.[37]

Upper Symptoms of Altitude Sickness

- Headache
- Lightheadedness
- Confusion
- Weakness
- Insomnia
- Gastrointestinal upset
- Shortness of breath at rest
- Coughing
- Balance difficulties

Symptoms of high-altitude illness include headache, lightheadedness, weakness, insomnia, and gastrointestinal upset. More severe symptoms include shortness of breath at rest, coughing, confusion, and balance difficulties.

The best treatment for high-altitude illness is to descend to a lower altitude. If symptoms are mild, athletes may be able to stay at that altitude to allow their bodies to acclimatize. If symptoms are more severe, immediate descent of 1500 to 2000 feet (457 to 610 m) should occur. There may be a need for further descent until the symptoms completely resolve.

Pharmacological treatment for prevention and treatment of severe high-altitude illness include acetazolamide, nifedipine, and dexamethasone.

High-altitude illness may be prevented by decreasing the rate of ascent. Ascending slowly allows for gradual acclimatization and leads to a lower likelihood of developing acute mountain sickness.[37] Guidelines for graded ascent include climbing from 1000 to 2000 feet per night (300 to 600 m) when above 10,000 feet (3048 m).[38,39] It is also recommended to descend to a lower altitude to sleep. For example, if skiing at an elevation of 10,000 feet (3048 m) during the day, an athlete should sleep the night before and the night after below an elevation of 8500 feet (2591 m).

For more information on altitude disorders and other environmental conditions, see Chapter 5.

Gastrointestinal System

Gastrointestinal problems can be part of a normal response to intense exercise. In some surveys, up to 80% of runners had gastrointestinal complaints.[40] Lower gastrointestinal tract problems seem to be more common; however, upper gastrointestinal complaints do occur. Common upper gastrointestinal complaints include heartburn, reflux, nausea, vomiting, bloating, and epigastric pain. Lower gastrointestinal tract complaints include cramping, urge to defecate, diarrhea, rectal bleeding, and flatulence.[41]

Upper Gastrointestinal Symptoms

- Heartburn
- Epigastric pain
- Chest pain
- Nausea
- Vomiting
- Bloating
- Hematemesis (vomiting bright red blood)

Gastrointestinal Reflux Disease

Gastrointestinal reflux is a common complaint in athletes.[42] It is thought to occur when exercise is performed within 3 hours of a meal and is due to lower esophageal sphincter relaxation. It is important to rule out other medical conditions such as an abdominal ulcer, hiatus hernia, or even cardiac disease if epigastric or chest pain is a presenting complaint. Abdominal ulcers and hiatus hernias can be investigated by endoscopic gastroscopy and cardiac disease by blood testing for cardiac enzymes and obtaining an ECG.

Treatment of reflux includes ensuring an empty stomach prior to exercise and avoiding large, solid meals prior to intense exercise. From a medication perspective, antacid medications are a good starting point. These usually help for exercise less than 1 hour in duration. If further medication is needed, treatment with H2 antagonists (e.g., ranitidine [Zantac]) or proton pump inhibitors (e.g., omeprazole [Losec] or pantoprazole [Pantoloc]) should be considered. If reflux is ignored, it could lead to further complications such as gastric ulceration, gastritis, and ultimately an upper gastrointestinal bleed.

Runner's Diarrhea

Runner's diarrhea or "runner's trots" is a common complaint in long-distance running.[43] Priebe studied runners and, in 30% of the cases, this exercise-induced phenomenon occurred.[44] Symptoms included the passing of watery stools, lower abdominal pain, and urgency of defecation, with some patients passing blood in the stool. The exact mechanism is not entirely understood; however, anxiety, increased intestinal motility, and possible hormonal influences may be a few causes. A treating physician should take a good history of supplements, including the use of caffeine, stimulants, and electrolyte supplementation, which may contribute to the condition.

The treatment should include proper dietary intake prior to exercise, the use of low-fiber and low-fat foods, as well as ensuring an empty stomach prior to exercise. Occasionally, medication such as loperamide may need to be used before competition. An antibiotic such as ciprofloxacin may be needed if there is an infectious cause for the diarrhea.

Acute Gastroenteritis

Acute gastroenteritis is the second most common viral infection in adolescents and young adults.[41] The symptoms include nausea, vomiting, abdominal cramping, diarrhea, myalgias, and fever. The symptoms are usually debilitating for a short period and stop the athlete from competing.

The infection is usually self-limited and lasts only 2 to 3 days. Treatment includes the use of clear, electrolyte-rich fluids such as sport drinks. Before return to sporting activity, no signs of dehydration (i.e., low blood pressure, low body weight) should be present. Antimotility agents and antidiarrheal agents (e.g., loperamide) may be useful to help treat the symptoms in the acute period. If the athlete is traveling and an infectious cause is suspected, then the diarrhea component should be considered a "traveler's diarrhea." In this case, antibiotic treatment (e.g., trimethoprim and sulfamethoxazole [Bactrim] or ciprofloxacin) should be considered.

Lower Gastrointestinal Bleeding

Lower gastrointestinal bleeding may occur after strenuous exercise. It is thought that relative ischemia is a mechanism for this.[45] Hypoperfusion caused by shunting of blood flow from the intestinal tract to the muscle and skin is thought to occur. Also, in a relatively dehydrated state, the trauma of running causes excessive movement of the cecum (cecal slap syndrome) and resultant hemorrhagic lesions can occur. In an intense performance setting, it is possible to see gross bloody diarrhea with a large amount of darker, clotted blood. In this case, a full evaluation is needed to rule out medical problems such as hemorrhoids or even malignancy. A full gastrointestinal work up may include a colonoscopy for evaluation of the lower gastrointestinal tract.

Lower Gastrointestinal Symptoms

- Abdominal cramping
- Urge to defecate
- Diarrhea
- Rectal bleeding
- Flatulence

Hematology

Anemia

Athletes may suffer from iron deficiency leading to symptoms of fatigue and ultimately decreased performance. True anemia should not be confused with "sports anemia." Sports anemia is truly a dilutional pseudoanemia that is associated with exercise.[45] In endurance athletes, reduction in both red blood cell mass and hemoglobin concentrations have been shown after a 20-day course of training.[46] In addition, increased plasma volume has been found in these athletes. The increased plasma volume combined with reduced red blood cell mass leads to the dilutional or pseudoanemia.

Causes of Iron Deficiency Anemia

- Inadequate intake
- Decreased absorption
- Increased loss

"True" iron deficiency anemia occurs from inadequate intake, decreased absorption, and increased loss of iron. Dietary intake varies for different populations. For example, the recommended daily intake for men is half of what is required for premenopausal women.[41] When increasing activity, dietary requirements may increase further.

Inadequate absorption of iron may also contribute to anemia. Iron from sources such as meat have different rates of absorption than iron from vegetables. In some cases, as with endurance athletes, reduced blood flow to the intestine may also decrease absorption rates.

Athletes have many possible sites of blood loss. The gastrointestinal tract is the most likely location of loss, usually occurring through the lower tract. Running may also cause mechanical and subsequently ischemic damage to the bowel. Blood loss from the urinary tract may stem from bladder wall damage secondary to mechanical trauma from running. Finally, red blood cell destruction in the foot and lower extremity muscles may also occur. Clinically, loss through the lower gastrointestinal tract could present with dark stools, hematuria may present as frank blood in the urine and bruising may be present in the lower extremities if mechanical damage is the cause of red blood cell destruction.

Evaluation of the athlete who is anemic should include a review of dietary intake as well as a complete blood cell count and a peripheral blood smear. Also, a serum ferritin level, as well as folate and vitamin B_{12} levels should be part of a laboratory work up as these are all potential causes for anemia.

Because iron deficiency may cause poor performance, athletes should receive appropriate supplementation. This should be guided by the sport medicine team, which may include a nutritionist. See Chapter 4, "Nutrition Counseling and Athletes," for additional information.

Sickle Cell Trait

Sickle cell trait is a genetic abnormality carried by up to 10% of the black population in the United States. People with sickle cell trait have one copy of the sickle cell gene. If two copies of the sickle cell gene are present, then abnormal red blood cells are produced, which can lead to a sickling crisis and can possibly be fatal. The incidence of sickle cell trait in the National Football League has been found to be 6.7%.[47] Because of the remote chance of death resulting from a sickling crisis, there is no policy or restrictions on athletes competing. Early symptoms of a sickling crisis may include bone, abdominal, and joint pain. Dehydration and high altitude are two factors that may precipitate a sickling crisis. Medical attention should be sought if an athlete experiences these symptoms.

Infections

Infectious Mononucleosis

Infectious mononucleosis is commonly referred to as *mono*. It is caused by the Epstein-Barr virus. It occurs in up to 3% of college-age students.[48] Athletes usually present with fever, sore throat, fatigue, malaise, and enlarged lymph nodes. Physical examination findings include a fever of 39°C to 40°C (102°F to 104°F), lymphadenopathy (swelling of the lymph nodes), an enlarged spleen, enlarged tonsils, and an erythematous palate. Laboratory abnormalities include an elevated white blood cell count with an increase in neutrophils, increased liver function tests, and positive serological findings. Complications occur in less than 1% of patients, and may include splenic rupture, encephalitis (swelling of the brain), meningitis, and hemolytic anemia.[48]

Clinical Findings in Mononucleosis

- Fever
- Sore throat
- Fatigue
- Malaise
- Enlarged lymph nodes
- Enlarged spleen
- Enlarged tonsils
- Erythematous oropharynx (inflamed oropharynx)

Treatment of mononucleosis includes symptomatic treatment to reduce fever and the pain of a sore throat. Isolation is not necessary because the condition is not highly contagious; it is usually spread through saliva contact between individuals. Athletes should rest from sporting activities until all acute symptoms have resolved, they are afebrile, laboratory tests normalize, and when the spleen has returned to normal size. Premature return risks the possibility of a ruptured spleen, which can occur even while at rest with and without contact. Despite the use of ultrasound, it is often difficult to assess whether a spleen is enlarged because of variability in spleen size. However, the majority of splenic ruptures occur within 21 days of the onset of symptoms; therefore, most asymptomatic athletes can return to play after 4 weeks.

HIV/AIDS and Hepatitis

Human immunodeficiency virus (HIV) is the cause of acquired immunodeficiency syndrome (AIDS). HIV infects and seriously damages the body's immune system. Without the protection of the immune system, people with AIDS suffer from fatal infections and cancers. People can be infected with HIV for many years before becoming symptomatic. Other serious viral infections include hepatitis B (HBV) and hepatitis C (HCV). The hepatitis viruses infect the liver, causing serious illness, and may even be fatal.

Transmission of HIV occurs through sexual activity with the exchange of semen or vaginal and cervical secretions. Also, needle-stick injuries, blood transfusions, and blood into an open wound can result in HIV transmission. HBV and HCV are also transmitted in similar ways to HIV.

The risk of transmission of HIV in sport is exceedingly low. Only 3 in 1000 health care workers have become infected after being stuck with a needle contaminated with HIV-infected blood.[47] Using known prevalence and exposure rates combined with conversion rates similar to those of health care workers, the risk of being infected by HIV in the National Football League was much less than 1 in 1,000,000 game exposures.[49]

Sport-specific prevention includes using protective equipment designed to prevent bloody injuries, dealing with bloody wounds immediately, and removing players from participation if blood is visible. Stressing the importance of universal precautions for all athletes, coaches, and training and medical staff is essential.

A position statement from the Canadian Academy of Sport Medicine states that an HIV-positive individual should not be excluded from participating in sport exclusively on the basis of his or her HIV infection.[50]

Staphylococcus Infections

Staphylococcus aureus is a bacteria that can cause bothersome, contagious skin infections. Two common infections are impetigo and folliculitis.[51]

Impetigo is a skin infection that is easily spread with close contact with skin. It is commonly spread in wrestling. The lesions can be either larger, fluid-filled vesicles or smaller vesicles.

Active lesions preclude an athlete from participating in organized wrestling. Diagnosis is made clinically and may be confirmed with bacterial cultures. Treatment includes washing areas to keep the skin clean. When the lesions become more widespread, antibiotic treatment should be initiated.

Folliculitis refers to an infected hair follicle. Lesions are somewhat tender and are pustular in nature. If a deeper infection occurs, the lesions usually contain a large amount of pus and are referred to as *furunculosis*. The lesions usually occur on the buttock area, along the belt line, and in the groin and axillary area. When the lesions become widespread, antibiotic treatment should be initiated.

Methicillin-Resistant *Staphylococcus Aureus*

Community-acquired methicillin-resistant *Staphylococcus aureus* (MRSA) is a variant of hospital-acquired MRSA, which was first reported in 1963. MRSA infections are becoming more common in athletes and active individuals. The first reported cases were in a high school wrestling team in 1993 and a British rugby club in 1998. Because of their resistance to standard beta-lactam antibiotics, these conditions are concerning to athletes as well as the public.[52]

Most MRSA infections initially manifest as folliculitis or other skin findings such as pimples, pustules, or boils. Typically, the athlete may describe his or her presentation as an "infected pimple" or "insect bite." Some MRSA infections may progress to abscess formation. In other cases, the infection may manifest as a life-threatening illness, such as a rapidly progressing sepsis or pneumonia.

The initial clinical examination usually reveals limited area of redness, warmth, and swelling, with and without pus drainage. Occasionally, the patient may have swelling and pain in a joint. In more advanced cases, moderate to severe pain at the site of the infection may be reported; the pain may be due to soft tissue necrosis.

In severe cases of MRSA infection, endocarditis, septicemia, necrotizing fasciitis, osteomyelitis, multisystem organ failure, or death may occur. Severe cases may progress extremely fast from the initial skin infection.

The most common route of transmission of MRSA is through an open wound, such as a superficial abrasion or from contact with an MRSA carrier. Other methods of transmission include poor hand washing, poor personal hygiene (i.e., not showering after workouts), sharing personal items (e.g., razors, towels, clothing), or a failure to properly clean and disinfect exercise and training equipment.

Methicillin-Resistant *Staphylococcus aureus* Prevention and Management Strategies

- Practice routine hand washing using soap and warm water or using an alcohol-based hand sanitizer
- Immediately shower following activity
- Patients with open wounds, scrapes, or scratches should avoid whirlpools
- Avoid sharing towels, razors, and daily athletic gear
- Properly wash athletic gear and towels after each use
- Maintain clean facilities and equipment
- Refer to physician for active skin lesions that do not respond to initial therapy
- Use bacterial cultures to establish proper diagnosis
- Care for and cover skin lesions appropriately before participation

Because of the potentially serious effects of an MRSA infection, measures should be taken to prevent skin infections in athletes. First, all wounds should be covered. If a wound cannot be adequately covered, removal of an athlete from practice or game should be considered. Second, good hygiene should be encouraged, including showering and washing with soap after all practices and competitions. Third, discourage sharing of towels and personal items such as razors, clothing, and equipment. If equipment must be shared, then a thorough cleaning routine must be established. Athletes must be encouraged to report skin lesions to training staff. In turn, training staff must be educated in the first aid of wounds and in the recognition of potentially infected wounds.[53]

Other Medical Conditions

Diabetes Mellitus

Diabetes mellitus is a metabolic disorder characterized by the presence of hyperglycemia (high sugar levels in blood) resulting from defective insulin secretion, defective insulin action, or both. The chronic hyperglycemia of diabetes is associated with significant long-term sequelae, including dysfunction of kidneys, eyes, nerves, heart, and blood vessels.[54]

Importantly, with proper blood glucose control, athletes can perform at top level; athletes with diabetes have competed in professional sports such as hockey and football and won gold medals at Olympic games.

There are two main types of diabetes. Type 1 diabetes (insulin-dependent) is a result of pancreatic beta-cell destruction, which leads to absence of insulin production. Type 2 diabetes (non–insulin dependent) usually occurs in adulthood. It is characterized by reduced sensitivity to the action of insulin, impairment of pancreatic beta-cell insulin secretion, and excessive glucose production from the liver.

A definitive diagnosis of diabetes is usually made by testing the blood. A fasting plasma glucose level greater than 7.0 mmol/L is diagnostic.[54]

A well-controlled diabetic must be extra cautious during exercise. In types 1 and 2 diabetes, excessive insulin availability results in increased muscle glucose uptake and decreased glucose production in the liver. This produces a drop in blood glucose levels. A diabetic must ingest carbohydrates before exercise, avoid exercise during peak insulin action (depends on medication used), and avoid injecting into large active muscle groups.

Hypoglycemia and hyperglycemia are two emergent medical conditions that may occur in diabetics. Symptoms of hypoglycemia include the sudden onset of weakness, lethargy, and headaches, as well as cool, moist skin. Quick administration of carbohydrate will rapidly eliminate these symptoms. Hyperglycemic symptoms may include irritability; labored breathing; abdominal pain; acidic or fruity breath odor; hypotension; and a rapid, weak pulse. These people should be immediately transported to an emergency facility.

Symptoms of Hypoglycemia

- Sudden onset of weakness
- Lethargy
- Headaches
- Cool, moist skin

Clinical Note

Hypoglycemia is treated by quick administration of carbohydrates.

Symptoms of Hyperglycemia

- Irritability
- Labored breathing
- Abdominal pain
- Acidic odor to breath
- Hypotension
- Rapid, weak pulse

Pharmacological therapy is the cornerstone of treatment for diabetics, with proper glucose control being the goal. Usually athletes use a rapid-acting insulin (onset within 5 to 15 minutes) approximately three times per day with meals. Also, either an intermediate-acting (onset within 1 to 2 hours) or long-acting insulin (onset after 2 hours) is used at nighttime. Another treatment option includes the administration of continuous insulin through a subcutaneous pump, which avoids peaks of insulin at times of injection. However, the pump may not be durable enough to withstand the physical forces from sport. Along with other benefits, regular exercise decreases glucose instability.[55] If hypoglycemia is a regular occurrence, then the insulin dose should be adjusted accordingly. Fluid replacement is also important to avoid dehydration, which occurs secondarily to increased glucose levels.

From a musculoskeletal perspective, diabetics have an increased prevalence of certain conditions that include adhesive capsulitis of the shoulder, carpal tunnel syndrome, and flexor tenosynovitis.[56]

Proteinuria

Proteinuria refers to protein being present in urine. This is not visible to the human eye and is a microscopic diagnosis. This occurs in many sports and can be present in up to 70% of athletes after exertion.[57]

Proteinuria is usually caused by alteration in renal blood flow. It usually occurs with 30 minutes of exercise and clears in 24 to 48 hours. The amount of protein in the urine directly correlates with the intensity of exercise.

Benign orthostatic proteinuria may occur in younger athletes. Protein collects in the urine when standing. When the child is sleeping or lying flat, there is no protein collected in the urine. Therefore, urine samples are positive before bed and negative for protein in the morning. If the morning samples contain protein, then a more formal work up for renal disease should take place.[57]

Hematuria

Hematuria refers to blood in the urine. Up to 13% of the population has hematuria with no symptoms.[58] Sports hematuria is a benign and transient condition that usually resolves in 24 to 72 hours.

Hematuria can originate in the kidney or from the bladder. In athletes, renal hematuria can be traumatic or nontraumatic. Nontraumatic renal hematuria is due to decreased renal blood flow leading to ischemia at the cellular level in the nephron and subsequent passage of red blood cells. Traumatic renal hematuria occurs from obvious direct contact to the kidney. This may also occur indirectly from repetitive running, jumping, and jarring that occurs during sport.

Hematuria originating from the kidney may be gross hematuria (i.e., visible to the eye). Urological cystoscopic examination reveals contusions of the bladder wall. The contusions are caused by repetitive contact of the posterior bladder wall against the bladder base. This may be prevented by maintaining proper hydration to keep the bladder partially full.

If hematuria persists for more than 48 to 72 hours, further investigations should take place to rule out renal disease or cancer. To prevent exercise-induced hematuria, the athlete is encouraged to maintain adequate hydration before, during, and after exercise.

Conjunctivitis

Conjunctivitis is commonly referred to as "pink eye." The main causes include chemical irritation or infection by bacteria or viruses. The use of antibiotic solutions or ointments is indicated only when bacterial infection is likely. Infection with the herpes virus can be particularly worrisome, and these patients should be referred to an ophthalmologist for definitive care. Conjunctival infection and eye pain can also present as a result of eye trauma (usually a finger or other object injuring the eye) and subsequent corneal abrasion. The use of fluorescein dye instilled in the eye and examination by an ophthalmoscope's cobalt blue light will reveal the characteristic fluorescent stain on the cornea that confirms an abrasion. The eye should then be patched and treated with antibiotic drops. The athlete should be followed by the physician until the abrasion heals.

Otitis Externa

Otitis externa refers to an inflammatory condition to the external auditory canal. This is commonly referred to as "swimmer's ear." It is usually caused by chemical irritation, allergies, or infections. Essentially, water washes out cerumen (ear wax), which is protective, water-repellent, and has some antibacterial properties.

Athletes usually complain of ear fullness, discomfort, and possibly hearing loss. Otoscopic examination usually reveals erythema, swelling, absence of cerumen, and occasionally discharge. Treatment usually is by otic topical drops, which usually contain an antibiotic and an anti-inflammatory such as hydrocortisone.

Prevention includes drying the ear after swimming by tilting the head and jumping and drying the ear with a towel. Athletes may also use silicone ear plugs, avoid touching the ear, or use a drying agent in the ear after each swim.[59]

Overtraining

Overtraining syndrome has been referred to as "staleness," "overreaching," and "chronic fatigue."[60] It manifests with both physiological and psychological symptoms that can adversely affect an athlete's performance. Simply, it is the point at which an athlete exceeds her or his capacity for exercise.

Common Findings in Overtrained Athletes

- Increased morning heart rate
- Unexplained weight loss
- Prolonged excessive thirst
- Alteration in sleep habits
- Psychological malaise

The most common changes in overtrained athletes include an increase in morning heart rate, unexplained weight loss, prolonged excessive thirst, alteration in sleep habits, and psychological malaise.[61] Other common physiological indicators include changes in blood pressure, delayed return to resting heart rate, and elevated basal metabolic rate and body temperature. Also labored breathing, aching, and bowel complaints occur.[61] Psychological symptoms include sleep dysfunction, poor self-confidence, drowsiness, lack of motivation, irritability, emotional lability, fatigue, depression, anxiety, and anorexia.

It is thought that the causes of overtraining are associated with physical training and competition. The length of competitive season, monotony of training, lack of positive reinforcement, feelings of helplessness, abusiveness from fellow athletes or coaches, and high pressure levels may all be contributors.[61]

The first step to treating overtraining is to recognize it. After recognition, the physical symptoms should first be treated. This usually involves decreasing or discontinuing training for a time. An athlete logbook for self-analysis is an important tool. The logbook should include training details, comments on training (i.e., likes and dislikes), well-being rating, causes of stress or dissatisfaction, and any injuries or illness that may occur.[41] Addressing the psychological symptoms of overtraining is more difficult. In mild cases, changes in workout and training regimens may be helpful.[62] However, in more severe cases, completely discontinuing training and professional psychological and psychiatric treatment may be needed.

Myositis Ossificans

There are two types of myositis ossificans: *myositis ossificans traumatica* and *myositis ossificans progressiva*. Myositis ossificans progressiva, which is also called *fibrous dysplasia ossificans progressiva,* is a rare progressive congenital condition in which multiple muscles ossify. The condition can be lethal.[63] The more common type of myositis ossificans is myositis ossificans traumatica, which is discussed in this section.

Myositis ossificans traumatica is a complication of a contusion combined with the formation of an intramuscular hematoma. This development of heterotopic (ectopic) bone in soft tissue adjacent to bone is commonly associated with trauma, surgery, or a disease such as heterotopic ossification. Most commonly, it is seen in the quadriceps, brachialis, anterior hip muscles, and the soleus muscles.[64-66] The importance of this condition rests in the fact that contusions are usually viewed as minor injuries by coaches and athletes and thus are not treated with much concern, although appropriate, carefully controlled management of the initial injury can prevent or lessen the possible development of myositis ossificans.

The most common cause of myositis ossificans traumatica is trauma and occurs primarily in contact sports such as football, rugby, ice hockey, and lacrosse.[64-69] The signs and symptoms of developing myositis ossificans include a palpable, often immobile mass that is increasingly tender or painful and progressive loss of joint motion. Other possible indicators of the development of myositis ossificans include increase in pain or decrease in range of motion following one or two treatment sessions, the persistent palpable warmth at the injury site, or the palpation of increased indurations in the hematoma. In some cases, the symptoms and findings may be confused with a femoral stress fracture or, more seriously, malignant bone tumors that are similar both clinically and histopathologically to heterotopic bone. Therefore, an extremely accurate history is essential. Early diagnosis of myositis ossificans is extremely difficult, and, as a precaution, hematomas that occur in the muscles listed previously or ones that are very painful should be treated as myositis ossificans until proven otherwise. This may prolong the treatment initially, but in the long term is more likely to lead to an earlier resolution of the problem.

Provided the hematoma that forms in the muscle is given sufficient time to be reabsorbed and provided additional stresses are not applied to the injured tissue, normal recovery with reabsorption of the hematoma and no development of the myositis occurs. However, if the injury is treated too vigorously or the injury site is continually traumatized, mesenchymal cells derived from the fascial planes and muscle sheaths that are part of the reparative granulation tissue may invade the hematoma site and mature into osteoblasts and proliferate to form immature or heterotopic bone. Over time (6 weeks to 6 months), the amount of bone formed maximizes, but can take up to 2 years to fully mature, with the immature bone being replaced by trabecular bone. Because of the strong possibility of developing myositis ossificans in the muscles mentioned previously, any hematoma to these muscles must be treated with extreme care for at least 2 weeks, by which time a normal hematoma should begin to resolve.

Roentgenographic signs of injury are present in the fifth or sixth weeks following injury. The initial appearance on x-ray examination is that of a fluffy calcification with indistinct margins lying in the soft tissue anterior to the bone (Figure 18-1). As the lesion matures, it may enlarge, and margins become more distinct. It may coalesce with the actual bone itself, at which stage the mass may become smaller. Radionuclide bone scans may be used to assess the maturity of the lesion (they would be negative if the bone is mature). However, bone scans can be confusing if done prior to the typical radiographic changes becoming evident.

Following the formation of a hematoma, risk factors that should be avoided include continuing to play after injury, early massage, forceful passive stretching of the injured area, the application of heat to the area, too-rapid progression of rehabilitation, premature return to activity, reinjury to the same area, and innate predisposition to the ectopic bone formation.

Early treatment of myositis ossificans consists primarily of relative rest and gentle range-of-motion exercises.[68-71] The athlete should follow a regimen of protected weight-bearing with crutches for lower-limb injuries and avoid any heavy lifting in upper-limb injuries. Rest and immobilization should continue until pain and inflammation subside. Following the acute period (1 to 6 weeks), there may be considerable loss of motion resulting from restricted muscle function. Early rehabilitation should be conservative and consists of careful active range-of-motion and strengthening (pain-free and nonresisted) exercises. Forceful passive stretching should be avoided for at least 4 months. Until there is a definitive decision that myositis ossificans is not occurring, any rehabilitation programs should not involve intense exercise. Any strengthening or range-of-motion

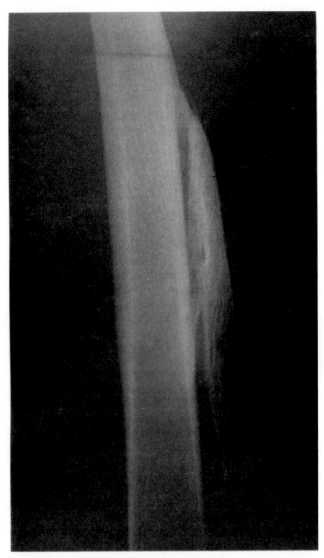

Figure 18-1

X-ray film of myositis ossificans.

bone scan shows quiescence of activity. This is generally 9 to 12 months following injury, but could take up to 2 years. O'Donoghue[72] states that early surgery usually results in recurrence and that an adequate incision should be made to fully visualize the entire mass. When surgery is performed, care must be taken in determining the pathological diagnosis because osteogenic sarcoma and myositis ossificans look very similar under microscopic examination, but treatment is radically different.[73] An accurate medical history is often the only way to distinguish between the two.

Prevention of myositis is the best treatment by padding and protecting the muscles. Coaches, trainers, clinicians, and athletes could understand the potential seriousness of this injury and recognized the need for a careful progressive rehabilitation program.

Conclusion

This chapter attempts to dispel the common belief that sports medicine injuries are solely caused by insults to the musculoskeletal system. Although most athletes are healthy and an active lifestyle should be encouraged, medical conditions that preclude competition in sport should not be ignored. It is very important for all health care practitioners involved with sport to err on the side of caution and not simply assume that symptoms are due to exercise. The importance of referring these cases to physicians cannot be overstated.

exercises must be pain free. Anti-inflammatory agents such as indomethacin may be given, and all activities are reduced. The athlete should be re-evaluated frequently. If there is no progression of the condition, once pain subsides, gentle range-of-motion and strengthening exercises can be initiated; however, exercise progression should be slow and cautious.

If there is no improvement of a hematoma injury after 10 days, prednisone or a course of diphosphonates should be administered. Return to activity can be considered when the bone mass show signs of stabilizing or maturing (which may take several months). In some cases, full range of motion may not be possible and the criteria may need to be modified. However, even large ossific masses are compatible with full range of motion and good function.

Surgery is indicated only to reduce the mass effect of the ectopic bone and should never be done until the

References

1. Hirsh FJ: The generalist as a team physician, *Phys Sports Med* 7:89–95, 1979.
2. Maron BJ, Shirani J, Poliac LC, et al: Sudden death in young competitive athletes: Clinical, demographic, and pathological profiles, *JAMA* 276:199–204, 1996.
3. Corrado D, Basso C, Schiavon M, Thiene G: Screening for hypertrophic cardiomyopathy in young athletes, *N Engl J Med* 339: 364–369, 1998.
4. Basso C, Maron BJ, Corrado D, Thiene G: Clinical profile of congenital coronary artery anomalies with origin from the wrong aortic sinus leading to sudden death in young competitive athletes, *J Am Coll Cardiol* 35:1493–1501, 2000.
5. Glover DW, Maron BJ: Profile of preparticipation cardiovascular screening for high school athletes, *JAMA* 279:1817–1819, 1998.
6. Maron BJ, Araújo CG, Thompson PD, et al: Recommendations for preparticipation screening and the assessment of cardiovascular disease in masters athletes: An advisory for healthcare professionals from the working groups of the World Heart Federation, the International Federation of Sports Medicine, and the American Heart Association Committee on Exercise, Cardiac Rehabilitation, and Prevention, *Circulation* 103(2):327–334, 2001.
7. Maron BJ, Thompson PD, Puffer JC, et al: Cardiovascular preparticipation screening of competitive athletes: A statement for health professionals from the Sudden Death Committee (clinical cardiology) and Congenital Cardiac Defects Committee (cardiovascular disease in the young), American Heart Association, *Circulation* 94:850–856, 1996.
8. Maron BJ: Sudden death in young athletes, *N Engl J Med* 349:1064–1075, 2003.

9. Huston TP, Puffer JC, Rodney WM: The athletic heart syndrome, *N Engl J Med* 313:24–32, 1985.

10. Pluim BM, Zwingerman AH, van der Laarsed A, van der Wall EE: The athlete's heart: A meta-analysis of cardiac structure and function, *Circulation* 101:336–344, 2000.

11. Lehmann M, Durr H, Merkelbach H, Schmid A: Hypertension and sports activities: Institutional experience. *Clin Cardiol* 13:197–208, 1990.

12. Gifford RW Jr, Kirkendall W, O'Connor DT, Weidman W: Office evaluation of hypertension. A statement for health professionals by a writing group of the Council for High Blood Pressure Research, American Heart Association, *Circulation* 79:721–731, 1989.

13. Tanji JL: Tracking of elevated blood pressure values in adolescent athletes at 1-year follow-up, *Am J Dis Child* 145:665–667, 1991.

14. Messerli FH, Garavaglia GE: Cardiodynamics of hypertension: A guide to selection of therapy, *J Clin Hypertens* 3:100S–108S, 1986.

15. The sixth report of the Joint National Committee on Prevention, Detection, Evaluation, and Treatment of High Blood Pressure, *Arch Intern Med* 157:241–346, 1997.

16. Whelton PK, He J, Cutler JA, et al: Effects of oral potassium on blood pressure. Meta-analysis of randomized controlled clinical trials, *JAMA* 277:1624–1632, 1997.

17. The Trials of Hypertension Prevention Collaborative Research Group: Effects of weight loss and sodium reduction intervention on blood pressure and hypertension incidence in overweight people with high-normal blood pressure, *Arch Intern Med* 157:657–667, 1997.

18. Petrella RJ: How effective is exercise training for the treatment of hypertension? *Clin J Sport Med* 8:224–231, 1998.

19. Chick TW, Halperin AK, Gacek EM: The effect of antihypertensive medications on exercise performance: A review, *Med Sci Sports Exerc* 20(5):447–454, 1988.

20. Dietz HC, Cutting GR, Pyeritz RE, et al: Marfan syndrome caused by a recurrent de novo missense mutation in the fibrillin gene, *Nature* 352:337–339, 1991.

21. Robinson PN, Godfrey M: The molecular genetics of Marfan syndrome and related microfibrillopathies, *J Med Genet* 37:9–25, 2000.

22. Pyeritz RE: Marfan syndrome and other disorders of fibrillin. In Rimoin DL, Connor JM, Pyeritz RE, Korf B, editors: *Principles and practice of medical genetics*, ed 4, Edinburgh, 2002, Churchill Livingstone.

23. Dr Paepe A, Devereux RB, Dietz HC, et al: Revised diagnostic criteria for the Marfan syndrome, *Am J Med Genet* 62:417–426, 1996.

24. Januzzi JL, Isselbacher EM, Fattori R, et al: Characterizing the young patient with aortic dissection: Results from the International Registry of Aortic Dissection (IRAD), *J Am Coll Cardiol* 43:665–669, 2004.

25. Thompson DD, Funk EJ, Carleton RA, Sturner WQ: Incidence of death during jogging in Rhode Island from 1975 through 1980, *JAMA* 247:2535–2538, 1982.

26. American Heart Association website. Accessed 2008 from www.americanheart.org.

27. Maron BJ, Gohman TE, Kyle SB, et al: Clinical profile and spectrum of commotio cordis, *Am J Cardiol* 89:210–213, 2002.

28. Weinstock J, Maron BJ, Song C, et al: Commercially available chest wall protectors fail to prevent ventricular fibrillation induced by chest wall impact (commotio cordis), *Heart Rhythm* 1:692, 2004.

29. Strasburger JF, Maron BJ: Images in clinical medicine: commotio cordis, *N Engl J Med* 347:1248, 2002.

30. Link MS, Maron BJ, Stickney RE, et al: Automated external defibrillator arrhythmia detection in a model of cardiac arrest due to commotio cordis, *J Cardiovasc Electrophysiol* 14:83–87, 2003.

31. Kawabori I, Pierson WE, Conquest LL, Bierman CW: Incidence of exercise-induced asthma in children, *J Allergy Clin Immunol* 58:447–455, 1976.

32. Rupp NT, Guill MF, Brudno DS: Unrecognized exercise-induced bronchospasm in adolescent athletes, *Am J Dis Child* 146:941–944, 1992.

33. Tan RA, Spector SL: Exercise-induced asthma, *Sports Med* 25:1–6, 1998.

34. Bisgaard H: Long-acting beta(2)-agonists in management of childhood asthma: A critical review of the literature, *Pediatr Pulmonol* 29:221–234, 2000.

35. Cavallo A, Cassaniti C, Glogger A, Magrini H: Action of nedocromil sodium in exercise-induced asthma in adolescents, *J Investig Allergol Clin Immunol* 5:286–288, 1995.

36. Ilback NG, Fohlman J, Friman G: Exercise in coxsackie B3 myocarditis: Effects on heart lymphocyte subpopulations and the inflammatory reaction, *Am Heart J* 117(6):1298–1302, 1989.

37. Schneider M, Bernasch D, Weymann J, et al: Acute mountain sickness: Influences of susceptibility, preexposure, and ascent rate, *Med Sci Sports Exerc* 34(12):1886–1891, 2002.

38. Murdoch D: How fast is too fast? Attempts to define a recommended ascent rate to prevent acute mountain sickness, *Int Soc Mountain Med Newsletter* 9(1):3–6, 1999.

39. Hackett P, Roach R: High-altitude medicine. In Auerbach P, editor: *Wilderness medicine: Management of wilderness and environmental emergencies*, ed 4, St Louis, 2001, Mosby.

40. Mellion MB, Walsh WM, Madden C, et al: *Team physician's handbook*, ed 3, Philadelphia, 2002, Hanley & Belfus.

41. Brukner P, Khan K: *Clinical sports medicine*, ed 3, Sydney, Australia, 2006, McGraw-Hill.

42. Shawdon A: Gastro-oesophageal reflux and exercise. Important pathology to consider in the athletic population, *Sports Med* 20(2):109–116, 1995.

43. Rao SS, Beaty J, Chamberlain M, et al: Effects of acute graded exercise on human colonic motility, *Am J Physiol* 276(5 Pt 1):G1221–1226, 1999.

44. Priebe M, Priebe J: Runners diarrhea—Prevalence and clinical symptomatology, *Am J Gastroenterol* 73:872–878, 1984.

45. Fields KB: The athlete with anemia. In Fields KB, Fricker PA, editors: *Medical problems in athletes*, Malden, MA, 1997, Blackwell Scientific.

46. Dressendorfer RH, Wade CE, Amsterdam EA: Development of pseudo-anemia in marathon runners during a 20-day road race. *JAMA* 246:1215–1218, 1981.

47. Murphy JR: Sickle cell hemoglobin (Hb AS) in black football players, *JAMA* 225:981–982, 1973.

48. Ryan AJ, Evans AS Hoogland RJ, Seifert M: Infectious mononucleosis in athletes, *Phys Sports Med* 6:41–56, 1978.

49. Henderson DK, Feahey B, Wily M, et al: Risk of occupational transmission of human immunodeficiency virus type 1 (HIV-1) associated with clinical exposures, *Ann Intern Med* 113:740–746, 1990.

50. Brown LS, Drotman P: What is the risk of HIV infection in athletic competition? 9th International Conference on AIDS, *Berlin*, June 1993.

51. Robinson J: Canadian *Academy of Sport Medicine: Position statement: HIV as it relates to sport*. Updated 2007. Available at http://www.casm-acms.org/pg_Statements.php.

52. Centers for Disease Control and Prevention: *Community Associated-MRSA Information for the Public*. Available at http://www.cdc.gov/ncidod/dhqp/ar_mrsa_ca_public.html.

53. National Athletic Trainers' Association: *Official statement from the National Athletic Trainers' Association on Community-Acquired MRSA Infections (CA-MRSA)*, March 2005. Available at http://www.nata.org/statements/official/MRSA_Statement.pdf.

54. Canadian Diabetes Association: Canadian Diabetes Association 2008 Clinical Practice Guidelines. Available at http://www.diabetes.ca/for-professionals/resources/2008-cpg/.

55. Landry GL, Allen DB: Diabetes Mellitus and exercise, *Clin Sports Med* 11(2):403–418, 1992.

56. Smith LL, Burnet SP, McNeil JD: Musculoskeletal manifestations of diabetes mellitus, *Br J Sports Med* 37(1):30–35, 2003.

57. Carroll MF, Tenite JL: Proteinuria in adults: A diagnostic approach. *Am Fam Physician* 62:1333–1340, 2000

58. Abarbanel J, Benet AE, Lask D, Kimche D: Sports hematuria, *J Urol* 143:887–890. 1990.

59. Micheli L, Smith A, Bachl N, et al, editors: *FIMS team physician manual*, ed 1, Hong Kong, 2001, Lippincott Williams & Wilkins Asia Ltd.

60. Ryan AJ, Burke ER, Falsetti HL, et al: Overtraining of athletes (round table). *Phys Sportsmed* 11:92–110, 1983.

61. Johnson MB, Thiese SM: A review of overtaining syndrome—Recognizing the signs and symptoms, *J Athl Train* 27(4):352–354, 1992.

62. Henschen KP: Prevention and treatment of athletic staleness and burnout, *Sci Period Res Technol Sport* 10:1–8, 1990.

63. Dixon TF, Mulligam L, Nassium R, Stevenson FH: Myositis ossificans progressiva, *J Bone Joint Surg Br* 36:445–449, 1954.

64. Finerman GA, Shaporo MS: Sports-induced soft-tissue calcification. In Leadbetter WB, Buckwalter JA, Gordon SL, editors: *Sports induced inflammation*, Park Ridge, IL, 1989, American Academy of Orthopedic Surgeons.

65. Huss CD, Fuhl JJ: Myositis ossification of the upper arm, *Am J Sports Med* 8:419–424, 1980.

66. Jackson DW, Feazin JA: Quadriceps contusions in young athletes. *J Bone Joint Surg Am* 55:95–105, 1973.

67. Beiner J, Jokl P: Muscle contusion and myositis ossificans traumatica, *Clin Orthop Relat Res* 403:S110–S119, 2002.

68. Aronen JG, Garrick JG, Chronister RD, McDeritt ER: Quadriceps contusions: Clinical results of immediate immobilization in 120 degrees of knee flexion, *Clin J Sports Med* 16:383–387, 2006.

69. Wieder DL: Treatment of traumatic myositis ossificans with acetic acid iontophoresis. *Phys Ther* 72:133–137, 1992.

70. Jackson DW: Managing myositis ossificans in the young athlete, *Phys Sportsmed* 3:56–61, 1975.

71. Lipscomb AB, Thomas ED, Johnson RK: Treatment of myositis ossificans traumatica, *Am J Sports Med* 4:111–120, 1976.

72. O'Donoghue DH, editor: *Treatment of injuries to athletes*, ed 4, Philadelphia, 1984, WB Saunders.

73. La Roux DA: Chondrosarcoma and myositis ossificans, *J Manipulative Physiol Ther* 21:640–648, 1998.

DERMATOLOGICAL CONSIDERATIONS IN ATHLETICS

Donald W. Groot and Patricia A. Johnston

The Skin

The skin is not simply a sack in which the organs, bones, and muscles of the body are housed. It is in itself a vital organ that teams with nerves, blood vessels, pigment cells, and glands. The skin is the largest organ of the body and is highly visible and vulnerable. In its protective role, the skin is often the first and only part of the body to be injured in athletic activity.

The skin protects the body from harmful external factors such as trauma, ionizing radiation, ultraviolet light, and toxic fumes and chemicals. Through dilation or contraction of blood vessels and excretion from the sweat glands the skin monitors and manages temperature fluctuations that could disrupt the functioning of the internal organs. It also signals many internal diseases, providing early warning signs for such conditions as hormonal imbalance, internal cancer, diabetes, and the acquired immunodeficiency syndrome virus.

Although the skin is unique, varying from individual to individual and from race to race as well as from one area of the body to the next, its basic structure is the same in all individuals. The skin is divided into three layers: the epidermis, the dermis, and fat (Figure 19-1).

The epidermis is the top layer of the skin. It extends along the surface, dipping into the dermis to surround hair follicles and oil glands. At a molecular level the epidermis is very effective at blocking the entry of foreign materials to the deeper layers of the skin and the internal organs.

The epidermis is made up of two types of cells: keratinocytes and dendritic cells. The clear appearance of the dendritic cells differentiates them from the keratinocyte cells, which contain cytoplasm and are connected by intracellular bridges. The keratinocytes are arranged in layers, whereas the dendritic cells are distributed throughout the epidermis. The basal cell layer of the keratinocytes is a single layer of elongated cells that borders the dermis. The many-sided squamous cells form the next layer. The thickness varies from 5 to 10 cells laid down in a meshlike fashion. At its interface with the next layer of granular cells, the squamous cells flatten. The granular cell layer varies in thickness with the horny layer. Where the horny layer is thin, such as the skin of the back, the granular layer is only one to three cells deep. Where the horny layer is thick, such as on the palm of the hand or sole of the foot, the granular layer may be 10 cells thick. The granular cells are characterized by their diamond shape. Their cytoplasm contains keratohyaline granules, which contain tonofibrils that keep the skin flexible. This is in contrast to the keratin granules of the nails and hair, which are hard because they are devoid of tonofibrils. The fourth horny layer of the epidermis is highly keratinized. As new skin cells, produced in the deeper layers of the epidermis, push upward, the dead cells of the superficial horny layer, known as the *stratum corneum,* are sloughed. This turnover takes 3 weeks on average.[1]

The mucosa of the mouth differs from other skin surfaces in that the epidermis does not contain a granular or horny layer except on the hard palate and dorsum of the tongue.[1]

Three types of dendritic cells are present in the epidermis: melanocytes, Langerhans cells, and indeterminate dendritic cells. Indeterminate dendritic cells are thought to be related to the Langerhans cells, which are part of the immunological system. These epidermal Langerhans cells provide a first-response reaction to foreign antigens that come in contact with the skin. The melanocytes produce melanin, which is transferred to and stored in the basal-cell layer of the epidermis, providing the skin with its color.[1]

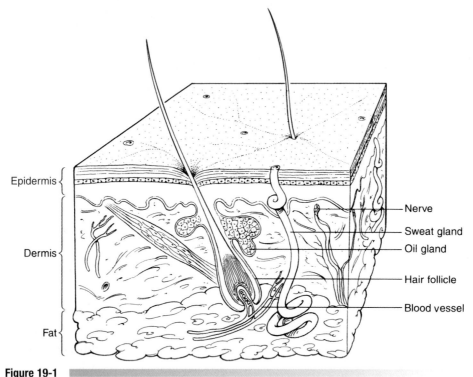

Figure 19-1

Elements of the skin.

The nails of the fingers and toes originate from the epidermis of the nail matrix, which is the moon-shaped structure at the proximal end of the nail (Figure 19-2). The cells of the nail plate are not vital and consist of keratinized cells.[1]

The dermis is the second layer of the skin. Divided into two layers, the papillary dermis and the reticular dermis, it contains the building blocks of the skin. Collagen, a fibrous protein, is the most abundant fibroblast of the dermal connective tissue. Collagen provides strength and structure to the skin; it is most abundant in the deeper reticular layer of the dermis but is also found in the papillary dermis. Elastins, also a major component of the reticular dermis, are elastic proteins that give the skin tone and suppleness, so that it will snap back into place when stretched. The breakdown of fibrous and elastic proteins is responsible for many of the signs of aging, such as sagging skin and wrinkles.

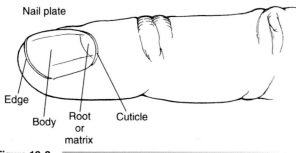

Figure 19-2

Elements of the nail.

The papillary dermis contains blood vessels that deliver essential nutrients to and remove wastes from the skin. The complex system of nerves in the papillary dermis makes the skin one of the most sensitive organs of the body.

The glands of the skin are found in the papillary dermis, although they extend into the basal layer of the epidermis. Sebaceous glands secrete lipids to lubricate the skin; eccrine glands release sweat to regulate fluctuations of body temperature; and apocrine gland secretions are responsible for body odor. These glands vary in their location, size, and distribution. For example, eccrine glands are most abundant in the palms of the hands and soles of the feet and are nonexistent along the vermilion borders of the lips.

Although the hair follicle is an appendage of the epidermis, it extends into the papillary dermis, where it receives its blood supply and surrounding network of nerves (Figure 19-3). The hair follicle is alive and grows at an average rate of ½ to 1 inch (1.3 to 2.5 cm) per month. The shaft or visible portion of the hair consists of dead, keratinized cells.[2]

A layer of fat underlies the dermis. It plays an important role in providing a protective pad between the skin and the underlying skeletal and muscular structures. Subcutaneous fat is also responsible for giving the skin a full, healthy look.[2]

In its role as an interface between the body and an often hostile environment, the skin is subject to frequent and often damaging abuse. This is particularly the case with athletes. In mild cases, sports-related skin injuries may simply be annoying, yet in severe cases may impede an athlete's ability to perform.

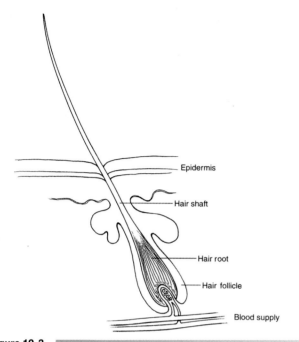

Figure 19-3
A single strand of hair.

Skin Conditions Caused by Trauma

- Lacerations and abrasions
- Purpura (bruising) and hematomas
- Dirt tattoos
- Piezogenic papules
- Leg veins
- Herpes zoster
- Aphthous ulcer (canker sore)
- Pyogenic granuloma
- Surfer's nodules

Frequently, a direct causal relationship can be established between the athletic activity and a skin condition. Blisters are an obvious example. In other circumstances, a pre-existing skin condition is aggravated by the athletic activity. Acne under protective padding, known as *acne mechanica,* is an example.

Age also affects the way in which the skin responds to trauma. As time passes, the skin breaks down with repetitive trauma. Blisters and bruises are more likely to occur, and the skin does not heal as well, increasing the likelihood of unacceptable scarring. The passage of time also affects the efficiency with which the sebaceous glands produce the natural lubricating oils of the skin, creating dry skin problems, especially with exposure to environmental factors such as wind and chlorine in pools.

The most common dermatological problems in athletes are caused by trauma, equipment, heat and sweat, communal contact, and environmental exposure.[3]

Conditions Caused by Trauma

It is difficult to participate in any sport without experiencing some form of trauma to the skin. Lacerations and bruising are typical, but other traumatically induced skin problems may result in irritating discomfort.

Lacerations and Abrasions

Lacerations are categorized according to the depth of the wound. A superficial laceration or abrasion involves the epidermis and possibly a small superficial portion of the dermis.

A partial-thickness wound extends into the dermis but does not sever it entirely, whereas a full-thickness wound involves the entire dermis.

Superficial and partial-thickness wounds generally re-epithelialize without direct intervention. The wound should be cleansed with water and any dirt gently removed. A medicated (antibiotic) dressing, such as mupirocin (Bactroban) or sodium fusidate (Fucidin) ointment under a semiocclusive (e.g., Mepore) bandage, may be applied to stanch any bleeding and to protect the wound from infection. After an initial 24-hour period when re-epithelialization has begun, the dressing is changed.

Full-thickness wounds, which sever the dermis, take longer to heal. If the skin is cut so that two opposing edges can be brought together, suturing is the treatment of choice. Absorbable sutures are used to repair the deep dermal and subcutaneous layers. This is important to strengthen the closure. The epidermal layers are generally brought together with nonabsorbable sutures that are removed after an average of 5 to 14 days, depending on the location of the wound. Care must be taken to avoid tension at the epidermal margins, as this contributes to tissue necrosis and the subsequent formation of weak scar tissue. If there is poor blood supply to the wound or infection, the healing process will be compromised.

Adhesive materials, such as n-Butyl-2 cyanoacrylate (Histoacryl), are becoming popular alternatives to superficial sutures for joining the epidermal borders of wounds. They eliminate the risk of cross-hatch scarring when excess tension is placed on the sutures; also, there are no sutures to be removed.

Steri-strip and butterfly bandages are effective in cases of superficial and partial-thickness lacerations in which the two opposing epidermal edges can be brought together easily and held in place by the tape.

If a piece of the skin has been removed, suturing may not be possible. A major loss of skin may require direct intervention with grafting. However, in many instances, the wound can be left to heal on its own after it has been thoroughly cleansed.

The removal of dirt and debris from a wound is important for proper healing. If debris is left behind, permanent discoloration in the form of a "dirt tattoo" may result. Running water through the wound may be adequate; however, if the wound is dirty, a more aggressive approach is required. Under local anesthetic, the wound is scrubbed with a disposable, sterile, surgical brush that contains an antiseptic cleansing solution. Any foreign material, such as glass or gravel, is carefully removed and necrosis of the tissue debrided.

Once the wound is properly prepared, healing can take place. Some areas of the body heal faster and better than others depending largely on the blood supply to the region. For example the face heals faster than the legs. The body lays down a base of granulation tissue with a circular pattern of collagen fibers to fill in the missing dermis. This process causes the wound to contract, drawing the epidermal edges closer together. The skin loses its ability to retain water in the damaged area, contributing to the formation of a scab from the inflammatory deposits. Although the scab plays an important role in the control of infection, it can also slow the healing process. To encourage more rapid epithelialization it is best to keep a wound moist with an appropriate dressing. A topical antibiotic, such as sodium fusidate or mupirocin ointment under a semiocclusive (e.g., Mepore) dressing, will reduce the risk of infection and will promote healing.

Scarring is inevitable with full-thickness wounds. The cosmetic result may vary according to intrinsic and extrinsic factors. Intrinsic factors include a hereditary predisposition for scar formation or poor nutrition; extrinsic factors include poor surgical technique, infection, compromised blood supply, use of topical or systemic steroids, and foreign materials in the wound. Scars may be categorized as *normal, hypertrophic, keloid,* or *atrophic.* A normal scar, although never regaining the strength of tissue that has not been traumatized, is flat and similar in color to the surrounding skin. Hypertrophic and keloid scars are both overgrown, the difference lying in the mass of scar tissue deposited and the tendency for recurrence. Keloid scars tend to be extensively overgrown and have a high rate of recurrence despite numerous interventional therapies. Atrophic scars are deficient in collagen and tend to be weak and depressed.

Types of Scars

- Normal
- Hypertrophic
- Keloid
- Atrophic

Purpura (Bruising) and Hematomas

Purpura, the medical term for bruising, is derived from the Greek name for a mollusk, *porphyra,* from which a deep purple dye can be obtained. Bruising occurs when blood escapes into the skin or the mucous membranes; it is characterized by a purplish-red discoloration of the skin resulting from red cell extravasation.[3]

Although the cause of red cell extravasation varies, in sports, bruising is largely the result of blunt trauma. The two types of bruises most commonly seen in athletes are petechiae and ecchymoses. Petechiae are purpuric lesions, which are less than 3 mm in diameter, and often occur in groups.[4] An example of petechiae may be seen in a hockey player who has been checked into the boards. His garment may leave a pattern of tiny vascular eruptions that match the weave of the cloth.[3] This is known as "jersey bruise" or *patterned petechiae* (Figure 19-4). *Ecchymosis* is a bruise larger than 3 mm in diameter.

Types of Bruising

- Petechiae
- Ecchymosis
- Hematoma

An ice pack applied with pressure immediately after the trauma will help stop the bleeding and control swelling. With time, the macrophage cells of the body will clear away the blood cell particles, and the bruise will gradually fade from a deep purple or red discoloration to a green or yellow tone and finally disappear.

A unique type of petechiae bruising found only in athletes, adolescents in particular, is referred to as "black heel" or "black palm." It is characterized by a grouping of bluish black specks on the back of the heel or the padded portion of the palm. It is due to the rupturing of the papillary capillaries in the skin. Athletes who participate in high-impact sports that involve jumping, twisting, and sudden

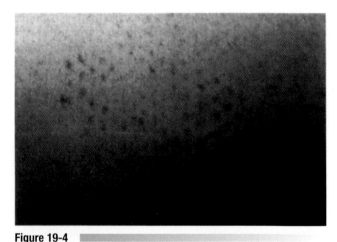

Figure 19-4

Patterned petechiae ("boarded" hockey player).

shearing movements or stops, such as basketball, football, lacrosse, tennis, and squash, are candidates for a black heel. Black palm has been reported in athletes participating in sports involving friction and pressure to the palm of the hand, such as weight lifting, tennis, mountain climbing, and golf.[5,6] No intervention is required for this condition, as there is no associated pain or functional disruption of the foot or hand. Reassurance that these black skin lesions do not represent mole cancer is often sought by the athlete. Once the sport is stopped for the season, the condition spontaneously disappears.

Another type of ecchymotic condition unique to athletes is known as "runner's rump." Postecchymotic hyperpigmentation occurs in the cleft of the buttocks owing to the constant repetitive contact between the cheeks of the buttocks. The condition is asymptomatic and subsides with a decrease in running.[6]

Hematomas may occur when the blood does not seep into the skin or mucous membranes but becomes trapped and pools in a confined space, such as under the fingernail or toenail (subungual hematoma). They may have to be drained, especially in circumstances in which the pressure from the trapped blood is very painful, as is the case with subungual hematomas. A needle into the collection of blood may aspirate enough blood to relieve the pressure. Massage assists absorption of the loculated serous blood components of clear hematomas (seromas) that may be trapped in skeletal soft tissue.

Dirt Tattoos

"Dirt tattoos" occur when dirt or other debris is embedded in the skin from a traumatic injury, such as a fall on an asphalt surface while cycling or running. This is sometimes referred to as "road rash" (Figure 19-5).

If a wound is properly cleansed after an injury, dirt tattoos are usually prevented. In instances in which the

debris has been incorporated into the skin during the healing process, no amount of cleansing will remove the resulting discoloration.

The advent of laser technology has made it possible to remove dirt tattoos with a minimal risk of scarring. The type of laser selected for the surgery is important. Lasers that target the pigment in the skin, leaving the remaining tissue relatively untouched, ensure the best results. Several lasers have the color-specific selectivity to remove blue, black, and brown discolorations in the skin, including the Q-switched Alexandrite and the single- or double-frequency Nd:YAG lasers.

The selective affinity of the laser light for certain discolorations allows the laser surgeon to remove pigment from the skin with minimal disruption to the surrounding tissue. The energy emitted by the laser light when it hits the targeted pigment causes a microscopic fragmentation of the pigment particles. The macrophage cells of the immune system then carry the minuscule waste particles away.[2]

The methods of tattoo removal used in the past generally left unsightly scars. Resurfacing techniques such as salabrasion (salt scraping), dermabrasion (mechanical scraping), lasabrasion (laser vaporization), and chemical peels as well as surgical techniques such as skin grafting were the only available options for the removal of tattoos. The new target-specific lasers have driven these techniques into obsolescence.

Decorative tattoos are popular among some athletes. The trend is to tattoo a team logo or insignia into the skin. These tattoos may be removed in a similar fashion to dirt tattoos, although red and yellow pigments are more resistant to laser therapy.[7]

Piezogenic Papules

Piezogenic papules have been reported in athletes participating in prolonged endurance events such as marathons and triathlons (Figure 19-6).[6] These skin-colored bumps

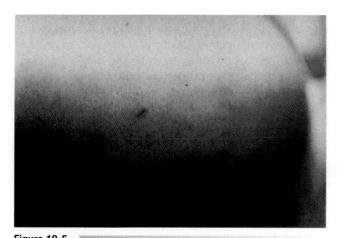

Figure 19-5
Dirt tattoo (cyclist fall on asphalt).

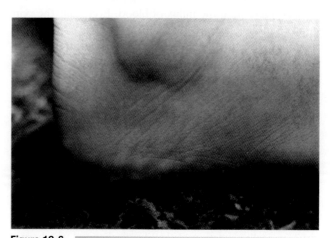

Figure 19-6
Piezogenic papules (squash player).

most commonly occur on the medial and lateral aspects of the heel and are due to a herniation of the subcutaneous fat into the dermis.[4]

The athlete may experience pain only when the foot is weight-bearing. However, the pain can be such that it will prevent the athlete from continuing with the sport. These papules have been reported, with no associated pain, in the general population. Therefore, there is some speculation as to why some individuals with this condition are prone to pain. Such factors as faulty weight bearing, bony spurs, and secondary inflammatory changes to the deep dermis have been discussed.[5]

Intralesional injections of the cortisone triamcinolone acetonide (Kenalog) will shrink the fat, providing relief to the individual who suffers pain. If there is no associated pain, intervention is not indicated except for cosmetic reasons.[8] Orthotic support to the heel has been of benefit to some.[6]

Leg Veins

Repetitious, high-impact sports, such as running and aerobic dancing, can dilate and weaken the walls of the small superficial veins of the legs, leaving spiderlike venous patterns on the skin. This condition is four times more common in women than in men.[9] Although harmless, many individuals find this condition cosmetically disturbing.

If the veins are blushlike and indistinct, treatment with a vascular laser, such as the flash lamp pulse dye laser, will suffice. The light from this laser passes harmlessly through the epidermis and is selectively absorbed by the targeted vessels. Upon contact, a microscopic fragmentation of the blood vessels occurs, resulting in a localized bruise. The macrophage cells remove the debris, leaving normal intact skin behind.[2]

Sclerotherapy is still the treatment of choice for well-defined superficial vessels. An irritating solution, such as salt, sugar, and alcohol in various concentrations, is injected into the small spiderlike veins using a fine needle. The solution inflames the walls of the vein, causing them to adhere to one another, preventing the influx of blood. Eventually the vein shrinks and disappears. Deeper reticular vessels respond well to a long-pulse 1064 Nd:YAG laser. Larger varicose veins are sometimes treated with foam sclerosants; however, veins that are too large need to be surgically ligated.

Herpes Zoster

Herpes zoster is a virus that lies dormant in the nervous system. A traumatic blow to the spine or exhaustion can stimulate the virus to run down a nerve root with a linear distribution on the surface of the skin, resulting in the condition commonly known as "shingles." It is believed that herpes zoster results when a latent form of the chickenpox virus (varicella) is activated. Unlike chickenpox, the herpes zoster rash is not generally contagious and is localized to an area innervated by a single nerve. It occurs on only one side of the body.[10]

The rash is characterized initially by painful red bumps (papules) that fill with a clear fluid, giving a blisterlike appearance (vesicles). The vesicles then become infected (pustules). As the pustules dry up, a crust is formed that falls off in the final stages of healing.[11] Scars may result. The initial stages of the virus may be accompanied by a high fever, headache, and general malaise. The entire cycle may take 3 to 4 weeks.

When the initial signs of the virus are noted, oral acyclovir (Zovirax) or valacyclovir (Valtrex) has been found to be the most effective agent for aborting the disease cycle. It should be administered immediately. Once the virus has taken hold, the medication loses its effect. Because the drug is of little value once the rash reaches the vesicular stage, early diagnosis is crucial.

Aphthous Ulcer (Canker Sore)

Aphthous ulcers, superficial erosions of the mucous membrane lining of the mouth, are sometimes caused by blunt trauma to the face. The ulcers can be very painful and may interfere with eating. Bacterial infections may exacerbate the discomfort and contribute to further deterioration of the tissue. Tantum Oral Rinse, a mild topical analgesic, may be used to control inflammation and alleviate the discomfort. In more severe cases, cortisone injections have provided some relief. Vaporization of the ulcer with the carbon dioxide (CO_2) laser has been helpful in promoting the healing process.[12]

Mouth guards protect the teeth from fractures in contact sports, and the smooth outer surface may also help prevent ulcers from resulting when the mucosal lining is forced against the teeth from a blow to the face.

Pyogenic Granuloma

Pyogenic granulomas are benign vascular tumors that may occur after traumatic injury. Their color range is bright red to reddish-brown. The size, shape, and texture of these lesions tend to vary. They frequently form crusts and ulcerate, although some show a transition from vascular tissue to vascular and fibrous tissue, forming a hemangioma. Continuous trauma to the same area contributes to ongoing necrosis and bleeding of the tumor. Surgical excision or laser vaporization is generally the treatment of choice.

Surfer's Nodules

Surfer's nodules are small, benign, fibrotic growths that occur in the dermis and subcutaneous tissue of the skin on the top of the feet of dedicated surfers. They result from continuous localized trauma and hemorrhaging. Over time the lesion may calcify, contributing to bone deformities in the area. However, in most cases the condition is not symptomatic.

Surfers rarely seek treatment, as the nodules tend to have symbolic meaning for them.[6]

Conditions Caused by Equipment

Equipment-related skin problems are more common in some sports, such as hockey and football, than in others. Occlusive material, chemicals in cloth, and friction or pressure from the garments contribute to a wide variety of skin conditions. Prevention plays an important role in the management of equipment-related skin problems.

Skin Conditions Caused by Equipment

- Acne mechanica
- Folliculitis
- Alopecia
- Subungual hemorrhages
- Ingrown toenails
- Blisters
- Calluses and corns
- Lichen simplex chronicus
- Chafing
- Pseudobursitis
- Dermatitis

Acne Mechanica

A combination of friction, pressure, and heat from occlusive clothing and equipment may cause swelling of the pore openings of an athlete's skin, preventing the oil glands from draining properly. The trapped oil ferments, causing the gland to become irritated, inflamed, and in some cases infected, resulting in acne (Figure 19-7). The problem is common in the regions of the back, neck, shoulders, and face because of the high concentration of oil glands in these areas. It is particularly troublesome in sports that require heavy padding and protective equipment, such as hockey

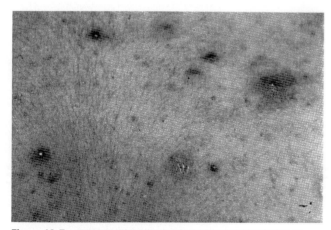

Figure 19-7
Acne mechanica (football shoulder pad).

and football, and in which taut, occlusive garments are worn. Other sports in which there appears to be a relatively high incidence of acne mechanica include cross-country skiing, speed skating, competitive cycling, and aerobic dancing. Golfers, hikers, and mountain climbers may experience acne mechanica along the strap lines of the equipment that they carry on their back and over their shoulders. Weight lifters may notice that the problem is particularly troublesome on their back because of contact with plastic-covered weight benches.[6]

Undergarments made of absorbent material specially designed to wick moisture away from the skin, such as Coolmax, Supplex, and Drylette, will help keep the skin dry and control the irritating friction caused by garments that do not absorb moisture and breathe, such as nylon. A thin cotton lining between the skin and the garment is also helpful. Proper cleansing of the skin immediately after an activity is important. Using a mild soap, the involved areas should be gently scrubbed with lukewarm water and a rough washcloth. Aggressive cleansing, particularly with abrasive soaps, may cause further swelling of the pore openings, compounding the problem.

Generally, over-the-counter preparations for the treatment of acne mechanica have little effect, although preparations containing benzoyl peroxide may be helpful in drying up some lesions.

Application of a sulfur mixture, such as Sulfacet lotion, may help open the pores to encourage better drainage of the oil from the glands and decrease inflammation from bacterial overgrowth. Sulfur lotions may be very drying, so they should be used sparingly. To further control inflammation, 1% hydrocortisone powder may be added to the lotion.

Medications for acne are categorized as *topical* or *systemic*. Tretinoin, a member of the retinoid (vitamin A) family, is a topical antibacterial and pore-opening agent that has proved effective in controlling milder forms of acne mechanica. Unfortunately, the antibacterial drugs that are taken systemically for other forms of acne, such as tetracycline, erythromycin, and minocycline, are not as effective for acne mechanica. However, they may help prevent a milder form of acne from becoming infected and cystic. Isotretinoin (Accutane), which is the best medication currently available for pustulocystic acne, controls the secretions of the sebaceous glands, preventing the build-up of thick oils in the pores. Unfortunately, it can wreak havoc with athletes, as the side effects may interfere with their performance. Aching muscles and joints, lack of energy, general lethargy, and dehydration are among the expected side effects when isotretinoin is prescribed.

Folliculitis

Folliculitis, inflammation and infection of the hair follicles, is a problem for some athletes, particularly on the scalp, when helmets are required to protect the head from injury. It may also occur in padded areas of athletes who are particularly hairy, such as on the thighs or back and shoulders. Contributing factors are occlusion, heat, pressure, and friction. Folliculitis is characterized by raised red bumps around the hair follicles. When scar tissue forms, it is referred to as *folliculitis keloidalis*. This condition is more common in black athletes because the pressure from the athletic equipment pushes the ends of the tightly curled hair back into the skin, which reacts to the embedded keratin of the hair shaft. *Keloid* refers to a dense overgrowth of fibrous tissue forming a large, raised scar. These scars tend to be cosmetically unacceptable, especially when they occur on the forehead and cheeks. Prevention in some individuals may be as simple avoiding short haircuts.

Medical intervention is generally not required with folliculitis unless bacterial infection is involved. Then a topical antibacterial agent, such as clindamycin, may be recommended; some cases require a systemic antibiotic, such as minocycline. The formation of keloid scars may require injections of cortisone, which flatten the scar. Resurfacing with a vaporization laser smoothes out the lumpy fibrous tissue and blends the edges to the normal surrounding tissue. This approach often helps to cosmetically improve the appearance of the scar. Excision is generally not recommended, because the scar tissue will usually recur.

Alopecia

Alopecia refers to loss of hair, which can occur in athletes as a result of friction from equipment causing the hair shaft to fracture (Figure 19-8). A snug-fitting helmet may help prevent this problem. Hair styling to camouflage the problem will improve the appearance of a bald patch. Once the offending equipment is no longer required, the hair usually grows back. If permanent damage to the hair follicle occurs, replacement surgery may be required. In this case, a patch of normal hair from another area of the head is used to replace the bald spot, using grafting techniques.

Subungual Hemorrhages

Chronic, repetitive contact of the edge of the toenail plate with athletic footwear will cause hemorrhaging under the nails. The condition is characterized by a blue-black discoloration under the nails that is tender on palpation. Subungual hemorrhaging of the toes has been referred to as "skier's toe,"[13] "tennis toe,"[14] and "jogger's toe" (Figure 19-9).[15] The condition can occur in any sport in which the toenail and the athletic footwear are in repetitive, abrupt contact. In some cases the nail matrix is damaged, impeding the growth of the nail and resulting in a permanently disfigured nail plate.

If the hemorrhaging is significant, the blood may need to be drained to relieve the pain caused by the built-up pressure under the nail. The finger or toe is frozen with a ring block, which numbs the nerves of the digit. Using an extremely hot paper clip, nail drill, or twirling scalpel, a small hole is created in the nail plate through which the blood can drain. Electrocautery or a vaporization laser (CO_2) will serve the same purpose but obviously requires more sophisticated equipment. Relief from pain is immediate once the digit regains normal sensation as the local anesthetic wears off.

Properly fitting footwear is essential to prevent chronic hemorrhaging. One should avoid footwear that is too short or does not allow adequate room for unrestricted vertical movement of the toes. Keeping the toenails trimmed to the margin where the skin and nail come in contact will also help to control the problem.

Ingrown Toenails

Another condition of the toenail that can be particularly troublesome to the athlete is referred to as *ingrown nails*. Rather than the nail plate growing in an anterior direction, it tends to grow peripherally, cutting deep into the skin. When this occurs, the spicules of nail need to be removed to prevent acute pain and infection. Alternatively, the edge of the nail may be elevated with a piece of tape, paper, or

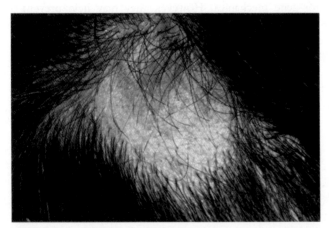

Figure 19-8
Traction alopecia (hockey helmet–induced).

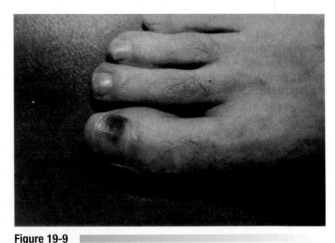

Figure 19-9
Jogger's toe (marathoner).

pledget of cotton wool to encourage the nail to grow above and beyond the inflamed skin.

The first step in prevention is to ensure properly fitting footwear that has adequate anterior and vertical movement in the toe box. Trimming the nails straight across with V-shaped grooves notched into the nail edge will encourage anterior, inward growth of the nail. Rubbing a glass slide across the middle of the nail will also stimulate the nail to grow toward the center rather than peripherally into the soft tissue of the skin.[3]

Persistent problems with ingrown toe nails may require removal of a portion of the nail matrix to prevent growth of the problematic portion of the nail.

Blisters

Repetitive friction will cause a separation within the epidermis or between the epidermis and the dermis. The resulting gap fills with fluid exudates and, in some cases, blood, resulting in what is commonly referred to as a *blister*.

Footwear that fits properly is the first step in preventing blisters. Absorbent socks are also important, as the tropical environment of athletic footwear also contributes to the formation of blisters. Foot powders such as Zeasorb cellulose powder are helpful in keeping the feet dry. Talcum is not recommended because it is essentially a powdered rock that, contrary to general belief, is not effective in absorbing moisture and can be abrasive. In areas particularly prone to blister formation, a protective dressing such as Spenco 2nd Skin may be applied prophylactically or, once the blister has formed, to protect the area from further trauma and to relieve discomfort. In those sports in which blisters may occur on the hands, such as cycling and gymnastics, protective gloves should be worn.

The management of blisters is fairly straightforward. Under sterile conditions, the blister should be drained; otherwise, pressure in the area can cause further peripheral separation and a more extensive blister. Draining will also help relieve the pain. The epidermal covering should be left intact until underlying healing takes place, at which time the covering will dry up and slough on its own. This helps prevent infection and promote rapid re-epithelialization. To drain the blister, a sterile needle should be used to puncture the epidermal covering. The excess fluid is aspirated or allowed to drain into a dressing. This procedure is repeated several times over a 24-hour period, if necessary, to release fluid build-up. A protective dressing is applied to discourage further friction to the involved area.[3]

Calluses and Corns

Calluses and corns are medically referred to as *conditions of hyperkeratosis,* which is an excessive overgrowth of the superficial layer of keratin on the surface of the epidermis. Hyperkeratosis occurs in areas of chronic friction. The friction may be mild in areas of structural abnormality or bony prominence, or it may be excessive in areas where the underlying structure is normal but the tissue is subjected to repeated stress (e.g., hands of a gymnast, heels of a runner). Architectural imbalance of the foot, poor walking or running habits, and poorly fitting footwear may all contribute to the formation of calluses and corns.[16]

Calluses commonly occur on the feet but may appear on any part of the body that is subject to repeated external pressure and friction, as may be the case with athletic equipment or padding. For example, calluses commonly occur on the hands of cyclists, oarsmen, gymnasts, golfers, and individuals who play racket sports.[6]

Padded, well-ventilated gloves help prevent calluses of the hands, and properly fitting footwear is the first step to the management of calluses on the feet. Further intervention may or may not be indicated. Some individuals view their calluses as a natural protection from blisters. Others find that calluses tend to contribute to the formation of blisters or eventually interfere functionally with performance. Soaking the feet in warm water will soften the callus such that it is easy to pare down with an abrasive material such as pumice stone or a scalpel in cases of very thick keratin. Regular applications of salicylic acid plasters, which gradually eat away at the keratin, have also proved effective. Generally, once the offending source of friction has been removed, the skin will return to normal without intervention.[6]

Corns are distinguished from calluses by a deep central core of keratin. They tend to be exclusive to the feet and occur over the bony prominence of the toes and lateral edge of the metatarsals. *Keratoma* is a medical term commonly used for cornlike formations on the bottom of the feet. Because of the tenderness of corns they are particularly annoying to athletes.

Warts (verrucae) underlying calluses may sometimes be misdiagnosed as corns. A simple test helps distinguish the two. A corn is more painful under direct pressure than a wart, whereas a wart is more painful when pinched.[5]

Correction of poorly fitting footwear and orthotics for architectural imbalances that contribute to the formation of hyperkeratosis are important to the prevention of repetitive formation of corns after treatment. To remove the core, cantharidin (an extract from the blister beetle) is applied to the lesion and kept under a salicylic acid plaster for three days. A blister forms under the keratosis, separating it from the underlying dermis. The resulting blister may be quite tender. It does, however, make the removal of the core and the surrounding keratosis easier. Recurrence is common.[6]

Lichen Simplex Chronicus

Thickening of the skin caused by chronic rubbing or scratching is referred to as *lichen simplex chronicus.* Individuals who develop lichen simplex chronicus in areas where the buttocks are continually rubbing against the metal seat of a rowing machine are said to have "rower's rump."[6] The condition is relatively asymptomatic and will self-resolve with cessation of the activity.

Chafing

Chafing occurs in areas of prolonged friction and usually involves coarse, sweaty garments. Erosion of the skin of the areolae and nipples is particularly troublesome to male long-distance runners wearing loose-fitting T-shirts. The nipple may bleed and is very tender because of the chafing. A popular solution is the application of petroleum jelly to the nipple. Although helpful, it is not always effective. To avoid the problem, several options are available: snug, non-occlusive, absorbent undergarments; no shirt at all; or a piece of circular adhesive tape applied over each of the nipples.[6,17] Women are less prone to the problem because of the soft exercise brassieres that are now available. Chafing between the upper thighs is characterized by inflamed, tender skin, sometimes accompanied by a burning sensation. To prevent the problem, long, close-fitting shorts or tights made of nonocclusive, absorbent material should be worn. Loose-fitting shorts and pants should be avoided.

A mild cortisone cream, such as HydroVal cream, applied two to three times a day to chafed nipples or skin will provide rapid relief and encourage healing in the area.

Pseudobursitis

Pseudobursitis is characterized by swelling, inflammation, and tenderness in an area of chronic friction, causing a subcutaneous pocket to form in which serous fluid gathers. Hence the names *pseudobursitis* or "false bursitis" are used because the fluid does not gather in an established bursa but in a friction-induced sac.

This condition is common to hockey defensemen because the extra padding at the front of the skate rubs under the pressure of the laces (Figure 19-10). Pseudobursitis among hockey players is often referred to as "skate bite," reflecting the painful nature of the condition.

At one time, surgical removal of the lesion was the treatment of choice. Today, however, potent topical cortisone salves, such as Dermovate or Temovate ointment, applied regularly to the area, controls the inflammation and decreases the discomfort. Once the offending equipment is no longer worn or proper protection is provided, the condition resolves on its own, and the cortisone treatments are no longer necessary.

Dermatitis

Dermatitis and *eczema* are terms used synonymously to describe conditions in which the skin is inflamed. The causes are many and varied, but characteristically the skin

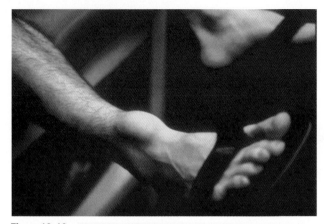

Figure 19-10
Skate or lace bite. Swelling over extensor tendons. (From Magee DJ: *Orthopedic physical assessment,* ed 5, St Louis, 2008, Saunders, p 850.)

is red, itchy, and scaly, and accompanied by vesicular papules. Laymen's terms abound for this condition and generally are sport-specific. For example, hockey players refer to dermatitis as "gunk," a term not found in any medical dictionary.

A common cause of dermatitis and allergic reactions in athletes is the chemicals in garments. Formaldehyde, which is used in fabric to prevent mildew and wrinkling and to preserve color, is very irritating to the skin when leached out with sweat (Figure 19-11).

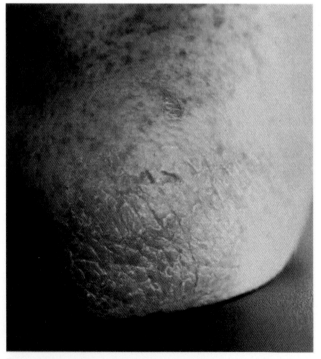

Figure 19-11
Contact dermatitis (elbow pad formaldehyde eczema).

Some individuals are hereditarily predisposed to irritable skin, a condition referred to as *atopic dermatitis.* Athletes with this condition are particularly susceptible to equipment-related irritation of the skin as well as environmental factors such as chemicals in swimming pools.

Cortisone salves such as HydroVal applied frequently may be used to relieve the dermatitis, once present. However, prevention is important in controlling the condition. Careful washing of clothing will help prevent contact dermatitis. Detergent should be used sparingly in the wash, as detergents and softeners are a source of skin irritation in themselves. Bleach should be avoided, as it may activate rubber elastic, making it more allergenic. A cup of powdered milk added to the second rinse cycle will remove the formaldehyde in new clothing. The formaldehyde molecules bind with milk caseins and are flushed away with the rinse cycle (Table 19-1).[8]

Conditions Caused By Heat and Sweat

The skin of the athlete is often immersed in a tropical-type environment because of the rise in body temperature through exertion and the body's natural cooling mechanism, sweating. Infectious organisms such as bacteria, viruses, and fungi thrive in this type of environment, and skin problems may result.

The stratum corneum, or superficial layer of the epidermis, plays an important role in preventing the invasion of infective micro-organisms. To serve this purpose well, the stratum corneum must be dry and intact. The macerating

Table 19-1
Prophylactic Measures for Skin Conditions

Measure	Rationale
Wear full or partial underclothing of soft, 100% cotton	Prevents dermatitis caused by sweat gland leaching of chemicals and dyes. Draws moisture away from the skin, preventing maceration of the stratum corneum and avoiding the development of a breeding ground for bacterial and fungal infections
Use a minimal amount of detergent (¼ cup) when washing clothing. Avoid bleach. Add powdered milk to the second rinse cycle to wash away formaldehyde in new garments	Detergents, bleach, and softeners are sources of irritation. Bleach can activate rubber and elastic, making them more allergenic. Formaldehyde in new clothing will bind to caseins in the powdered milk. These will be flushed away with the rinse water
Use protective dressings such as Spenco 2nd Skin on skin surfaces exposed to trauma or friction	Provides a buffer against trauma and friction and protects blisters from further injury
Use a moisturizer immediately after showering	Controls dryness and reduces the likelihood of asteatotic eczema. This is particularly important in cool, dry climates. Scaly, cracked skin is more susceptible to contact dermatitis and infections
Use a protective wrap such as Pro-Wrap Foam underadhesive tape	Adhesive tape can irritate the skin when next to the skin or when being removed
Wear properly fitting equipment, especially footwear	Reduces friction. For example, individually casted skates and water molding of skate boots will immobilize the foot, reducing friction
Wear protective clothing	Layer clothing in various ambient temperatures to allow for adjustment to changes in body heat. Wet/dry suits, underwater boots and gloves, and bathing caps provide protection in the water. Wide-brim hats, tightly woven cloth, and sunglasses protect against the sun's rays
Wear protective creams	A broad-spectrum sunscreen with an SPF of 15 or more will protect against UVA and UVB wavelengths of light. Apply when the skin is cool and dry. Oil-based ointments, such as petroleum jelly, should be used on the lips and around the nostrils to protect them from dehydration caused by cold and wind conditions
Postpone shaving and washing exposed skin surfaces when participating in sports in cold temperatures	The natural oils of the skin provide insulation from the wind and cold

Adapted from Groot DW, Johnston PJ: A review of sports-related skin problems, *Can J CME* 2:19-27, 1990.
SPF, Sun protectant factor; *UVA,* ultraviolet A; *UVB,* ultraviolet B.

effect of heat and moisture on the skin lowers its defenses, making it vulnerable to infection.

Conditions Caused by Heat and Sweat
• Intertrigo • Miliaria • Acrochordons • Pitted keratolysis

Intertrigo

Intertrigo is a condition in which the skin becomes inflamed because of moisture and constant friction in skin folds. It differs from chafing in that chafing is caused by friction between two skin surfaces or the skin and a garment, whereas intertrigo is caused by the maceration of the stratum corneum in areas where moisture has difficulty escaping, such as skin folds. In athletes, this commonly occurs in the groin or axillary regions. The symptoms include burning, itching, and redness of the skin. Secondary bacterial (candidiasis) or fungal (tinea) infections may accompany intertrigo. In severe cases, the skin becomes eroded and weeping. Blockage of the sweat pores in these areas causes small sweat gland cysts known as *miliaria*. Loose, absorbent, cotton underclothing is the first step in drawing moisture away from the skin. The area should be cleansed frequently, and, when thoroughly dry, a fine, absorbent dusting powder such as Zeasorb cellulose powder should be applied. Talcum powders should be avoided, as they can be abrasive and do not absorb moisture well. Underarm deodorants and antiperspirants can be irritating to the skin and should be avoided as long as the condition persists. Emollients, such as silicone-based creams (e.g., Prevex), may help reduce friction in more severe cases. If antibacterial, antifungal, and mild cortisone preparations are prescribed, the emollient should be applied on top of these to maximize the absorption of the active therapeutic agent into the skin. In cases in which the skin is actually eroded, wet medicated compresses, such as Buro Sol, may help in the healing process.

Miliaria

Miliaria refers to damage to the sweat gland, and, depending on the extent of damage, it may be classified as *crystallina*, *rubra*, or *profunda*.

Miliaria crystallina refers to a superficial obstruction of the sweat duct. It is found in individuals who sweat profusely and is characterized by multiple groupings of thin, clear-walled vesicles.[18]

Miliaria rubra, sometimes referred to as "prickly heat rash," is caused by increased body temperature with associated profuse sweating (Figure 19-12). It is commonly seen

Figure 19-12
Miliaria rubra (prickly heat rash).

in individuals who wear occlusive exercise garments or who exercise in hot, humid environments. Crops of erythematous papules cause a very uncomfortable prickly sensation in the skin. Because the sweat cannot escape through the blocked pores, it leaks into the epidermis, resulting in a crop of irritated, itchy papules and vesicles.[18]

Miliaria profunda is the result of chronic miliaria rubra and involves more extensive damage to the sweat duct. This condition is relatively uncommon except in the tropics; it is characterized by asymptomatic, pale, hard papules under the surface of the skin and may cause discomfort.[18]

Generally speaking, there is no effective treatment for miliaria. It is best managed by avoiding those circumstances that promote the condition by causing an increase in body temperature and profuse sweating. Unfortunately, for the athlete this is more easily said than done. Occlusive clothing that does not breathe, or excessive clothing in the case of outdoor sports, should be avoided. Frequent changes to clean absorbent cotton or silk clothing that draws moisture away from the skin are important. Molecularly fine dusting powder, such as Zeasorb cellulose powder, may be helpful. Cool showers or baths will offer some relief, followed by an application of calamine lotion. Because calamine lotion can be drying to the skin, a moisturizer applied over it may be required. However, moisturizers in themselves can create problems by plugging the sweat pores and aggravating the condition. As a last resort, acetaminophen (e.g., Tylenol or Tempra) taken to lower the body temperature may be helpful.

Acrochordons

Acrochordons are frequently referred to as "skin tags." They are small, benign polyps that are characteristically soft, pedunculated, and pigmented. Acrochordons generally appear in regions of chronic friction, such as the neck, the armpits, the groin creases, and under the breasts. Skin, like muscle and bone, tends to grow in the direction of physical stress and friction. In these areas the skin is confused with the multiplicity of movements and simply grows outward. Combined with sweat and heat, these lesions may become irritated and itchy.

Although acrochordons are benign, most individuals seek treatment for cosmetic purposes. Several effective techniques are used to remove these lesions. Small lesions may be clipped with surgical scissors, and cryotherapy, electrocauterization, tying off with stitches, and laser vaporization are effective techniques for removal of larger lesions. Touch-up treatments are usually required, as there is a tendency for recurrence.[2]

Pitted Keratolysis

Maceration of the skin under conditions of sweat and heat create the ideal environment for a condition known as *pitted keratolysis*. A bacterial micro-organism infiltrates the horny layer of the skin, causing a superficial infection on the soles and under surfaces of the feet. These circular, pitted lesions may blend to produce large irregular margins. Because the condition is largely asymptomatic, individuals may be unaware that they have it, although repetitive trauma, such as running, may cause tenderness. The lesions may take on a green or brown discoloration and may be responsible for a foul odor of the feet (Figure 19-13).

Application of a topical antibiotic, such as sodium fusidate cream or mupirocin ointment, twice daily for 10 days will rapidly resolve this problem in most cases. Soaking the soles of the feet for 10 minutes a day in a mixture of 1 tablespoon of formalin and 18 tablespoons of water will help reduce sweat production and odor.

Conditions of Communal Contact

The interactive nature of sports places most athletes in an environment of communal contact. Even the cleanest facilities afford an opportunity for the transfer of bacteria, fungi, and viruses. Although any part of the body is susceptible, the feet are most commonly involved.

Conditions of Communal Contact
• Dermatophytes (fungal infections)
- Tinea pedis
- Tinea unguium
- Tinea cruris
• Viral infections
- Herpes simplex (fever blisters, cold sores)
- Warts
- Molluscum contagiosum
• Bacterial infections
- Impetigo
- Pseudomonas
• Parasites

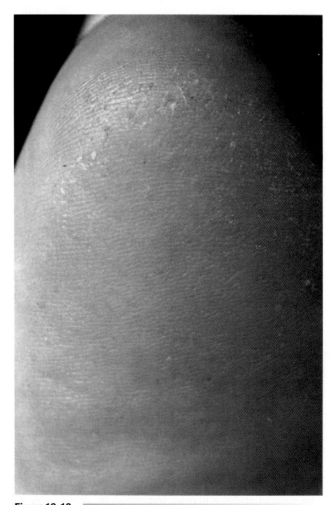

Figure 19-13
Pitted keratolysis (bacteria induced).

Dermatophytes

Dermatophyte is the medical term for ringworm, a fungus that causes keratin breakdown and inflammation of the skin. The moist, hot conditions created when an individual sweats during an athletic activity cause maceration of the stratum corneum, creating an ideal environment for fungal growth.

There are many different species and strains of dermatophytes, and the clinical features of the skin will vary somewhat depending on the type and size of the dermatophyte that is causing the problem. Variations in skin response also depend on the area of the body that has been infected and the immune response of the individual.[18]

Common areas of the body for dermatophyte infection, particularly among athletes, include the feet, the fingernails and toenails, the axillae, and the groin. Tinea pedis, fungal infection of the feet, is commonly referred to as "athlete's foot." If the nail plates of the feet or hands are involved, the condition is called *onychomycosis* or *tinea unguium*.

"Jock itch" is the lay term for *tinea cruris,* or fungal infection of the groin. Ringworm may also be found in other areas of the body: *tinea corporis* involves the entire body; *tinea capitis,* the scalp; *tinea barbae,* the beard; *tinea faciei,* the face; and *tinea manuum,* the hands.[19]

Tinea Pedis

Tinea pedis (athlete's foot) generally begins in the toe clefts, but may spread to other areas of the foot, particularly the sole. Scaling, peeling, and fissuring of the skin are clinical features of tinea pedis. Itchiness and an unpleasant foot odor are common. The condition may be aggravated by secondary bacterial infection (Figure 19-14).

Walking barefoot in communal areas such as locker rooms, showers, and along the sides of swimming pools is one of the most common means of dermatophyte transfer. Wearing protective footwear, such as thongs, in these areas is recommended. Keeping the foot dry, particularly between the toes, to prevent maceration of the skin so that it does not become a breeding ground for infection is important. Towel drying after cleansing followed by blow drying with cool air from a hair dryer is helpful. Absorbent socks and foot powders, such as Zeasorb cellulose powder, are recommended.

Tinea Unguium

Onychomycosis refers to fungal infection of the nail plate, whereas *tinea unguium* refers more specifically to the ringworm dermatophytes. In either case, fungal invasion of the nail plate presents a major therapeutic challenge. The nails of athletes play an important protective role in sports requiring either the hands or the feet. Yet trauma and the environmental conditions to which athletes are exposed—heat, sweat, occlusion, and communal exposure—make the nails of the athlete more susceptible to fungal infections.

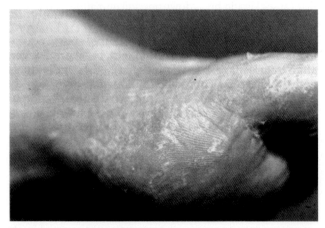

Figure 19-14
Tinea pedis (athlete's foot).

Fungal infection of the nail plate usually begins with a single digit. The typical early warning sign is a small area of discoloration, white or yellow, at the lateral free edge of the nail plate. It is at this point that treatment should be instigated to prevent damage to the nail plate and involvement of the other digits. As the fungus spreads inward and to the base of the nail, the discoloration may become darker and the nail plate becomes thicker. Subungual hyperkeratosis (thick scale under the nail) will cause the nail plate to lift and crack. Discomfort may accompany gross involvement of the nail plate.

Avoiding communal exposure by wearing protective footwear in sports facilities is the first step in prevention. The sharing of sports equipment such as gloves and footwear should also be avoided. Absorbent cotton socks, glove linings, and powders will help control the conditions that support the growth of fungi.

Tinea Cruris

Tinea cruris ("jock itch") is more common among men than women. This is probably due to the fact that men perspire more than women. Furthermore, the skin is more occluded in the groin area of men because the scrotum is in contact with the skin of the thighs and because of the type of undergarments that men wear.[18] It is an interesting fact that jock itch usually appears in the left groin crease first, because the left testicle descends lower than the right. Raised erythematous (red) plaques with distinct margins characterize tinea cruris. These plaques appear in the groin, extending down the thigh and onto the scrotum, giving a butterfly-like appearance. The condition is very itchy.

The fungus may be transferred from the feet to the groin, particularly when toweling off. Sharing of sports equipment, clothing, or towels contributes to the transfer of dermatophytes from one individual to the next.

To prevent the spread of tinea cruris, sports equipment, including towels, should not be shared (even after towels have been laundered). Also, individuals with athlete's foot should be cautioned to dry the body before drying the feet to avoid autoinfection of other areas, particularly the groin. Loose-fitting, absorbent undergarments are essential to the control of this condition, as dermatophytes thrive in occlusive, tropical environments.

The treatment of fungal infections including tinea pedis, tinea unguium, and tinea cruris is very similar. A topical antifungal cream, such as terbinafine (Lamisil), miconazole (Micatin), ketoconazole (Nizoral), or clotrimazole (Canesten), is applied after thorough cleansing and drying of the affected area, twice daily for 2 to 6 weeks. In resistant cases, systemic medication, such as ketoconazole, griseofulvin (Fulvicin), or terbinafine, taken orally may be required.

Common Dermatophyte Areas

- Fungal infections
  - Tinea pedis (feet)
  - Tinea unguium (nails of feet or hands)
  - Tinea cruris (groin)
  - Tinea corporis (entire body)
  - Tinea capitis (scalp)
  - Tinea barbae (beard)
  - Tinea faciei (face)
  - Tinea manuum (hands)
- Viral infections
  - Herpes simplex
  - Verruca (warts)
  - Molluscum contagiosum
- Bacterial infections
- Parasites

Viral Infections

Herpes Simplex (Fever Blisters, Cold Sores)

Herpes simplex, one of the most common viruses (Figure 19-15), has two classifications. Type 1 generally occurs on the face but may occur in the genital region. Type 2 is more often a genital condition, although oral genital contact has somewhat changed the distinction of type 1 and type 2 herpes by location. Type 2 herpes generally occurs after puberty, whereas type 1 herpes may occur at any age.

Herpes simplex is passed through skin-to-skin contact and can be aggravated by an increase in body temperature, exposure to sunlight, menstruation, ingestion of certain spicy foods, and a depression in the immune system caused by illness. Blunt trauma may also activate the virus owing to an increase in the body temperature and local immune deficiency at the site of the injury. Herpes may also result from exposure to infected saliva.

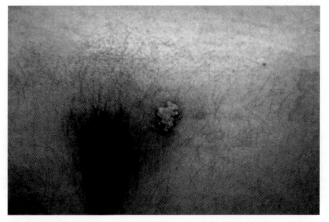

Figure 19-15
Herpes simplex (recurrent viral infection).

The primary herpes infection is characterized by painful, raised, erythematous lesions of the skin, known as *vesicles*. The vesicles contain intra- or intercellular fluid, giving the lesion a blisterlike appearance. Erosion of the skin and the mucous membrane in the area of the lesion is common and may be quite extensive. The infection may last from 2 to 6 weeks before healing spontaneously. Recurrence of the infection tends to be less traumatic. The lesions are smaller, less painful, and last on average 1 week.[11] Avoiding contact with an individual with an active herpes virus infection is the best means of prevention.

Acyclovir (Zovirax) or valacyclovir (Valtrex) are systemic treatments for herpes simplex. They are most effective when taken orally in the very early stages of the infection. A sensation of tingling at the site of a previous infection is an indication of a recurring episode. Treatment with acyclovir or valacyclovir should be initiated immediately.[11] If the medication has not been taken early enough to abort the lesion, the infection will generally run its course. During its active stage the lesion must be kept clean and dry. Some physicians recommend the use of a topical antibiotic to prevent secondary bacterial infection in the area. Other topical agents for the treatment of herpes have not proved to be effective. However, it has been shown that the use of topical acyclovir (Zovirax ointment) reduces the contagious nature of the herpes.

Warts

Verruca is the medical term for "wart." It is a virus that infiltrates the epidermal layer of the skin and susceptible mucosal membranes. Because the virus is made of deoxyribonucleic acid, it mimics the body's genetic makeup. This confuses the immune system, rendering the virus resistant to the body's natural defense mechanisms.

Athletes are particularly susceptible to the wart virus because of exposure through communal facilities and the role that trauma plays in the inoculation of the virus into the epidermal cells. Autoinfection, whereby the virus is transferred from one part of the body to another, is common. For example, warts may be transferred from the hands to the shaft of the penis or from the feet to the hands. Skin-to-skin contact with an individual with warts will also spread the infection. Verrucae may appear on any part of the body but are most common on the hands and feet. Common verrucae are characterized by raised, firm papules that tend to be paler than the surrounding tissue and have a rough, horny surface.[11]

Plantar warts commonly occur at pressure points on the bottom of the foot (Figure 19-16). They are characteristically flat or slightly raised, firm, circular lesions. A rough, keratotic surface is surrounded by a smooth, horny border. Plantar warts may vary from pale flesh tones to yellowish-gray lesions. These warts may be painful for some individuals.[11]

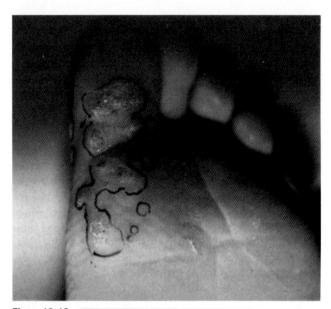

Figure 19-16
Plantar warts (outlined prior to laser removal).

Warts may spontaneously regress after a few weeks or may last for years. One school of thought is to leave the wart to follow its natural course. Owing to the contagious nature of warts and the social stigma attached to them, however, the authors advise seeking treatment as soon as possible.

Various topical agents are available for the treatment of warts. These include preparations of salicylic acid and lactic acid, formalin in water, glutaraldehyde in aqueous ethanol, and podophyllin. These preparations are generally applied daily to the wart under an occlusive dressing. Patience and determination are required.

If the warts are recalcitrant, more aggressive measures may be necessary to get rid of them. Cryotherapy, laser vaporization, and surgical removal are common strategies. Cryotherapy uses liquid nitrogen, which causes a localized frostbite that kills the virus. Alternatively, the liquid nitrogen may be applied less aggressively at 3-week intervals to stimulate the immune system to eradicate the wart. Vascular removal lasers such as the flash pump dye laser may be used to selectively compromise the supply of nutrients from the blood vessels and thereby cut off the wart's lifeblood. Another technique uses a vaporizing laser, such as the CO_2 laser, to heat the individual cells of the wart to 100°C (212°F), causing the lesion to disappear in a plume of steam and tissue particles.[1] The advantage of laser vaporization versus surgical removal is that the laser light seals the blood vessels, creating a better visual field for distinguishing the root of the wart from normal tissue. In this manner, the surgeon can be more certain that the entire wart has been removed with minimal disturbance of the surrounding tissue. This decreases the time required for healing, minimizes the amount of scar tissue formation, and reduces the likelihood of recurrence. Surgical removal involves an excision of the wart with a scalpel. This technique is rarely used today because of the formation of scar tissue and a high rate of recurrence.

Molluscum Contagiosum

Molluscum contagiosum is a pox virus that is common in children but can be transmitted sexually or through skin-to-skin contact in adults. Wrestlers are an example of athletes who might be susceptible to this condition. Small, discrete, dome-shaped, smooth papules can appear on any area of the body. They are translucent, flesh-colored lesions that may or may not be erythematous at the base of the dome. The papules have a core that, when expressed or opened, removes the virus. Therefore the treatment of choice usually involves curetting the lesions, although imiquimod 5% cream or liquid nitrogen in some cases may be recommended.

Bacterial Infection

Infections of the skin are caused by a multiplicity of bacteria that present with a variety of skin manifestations. This makes a definitive diagnosis challenging. Often they can only be differentiated by culture. These organisms may manifest in the skin as impetigo, folliculitis, furuncle (boil), carbuncle, or cellulitis. Of these, impetigo and folliculitis are most likely to appear in athletes and are due to the presence of the *staphylococcus aureus* or pseudomonas bacteria.

Impetigo is a superficial bacterial infection that may appear in athletes who sustain abrasions or lacerations as might be expected in contact sports. Folliculitis is an infection of the hair follicle that manifests as red, raised, pustules centered on the skin around the hair shaft.

Infections of the skin may be treated with antibacterial cleansers, topical antibiotics, or systemic antibiotics. The course of treatment is determined by the nature of the bacterial infection.

Of recent concern amongst athletes is the appearance of resistant strains of bacteria such as methicillin-resistant *Staphylococcus aureus* (MRSA) in otherwise healthy populations. As with other bacterial infections, athletes are particularly vulnerable because of skin-to-skin contact, the inherent risk of cuts and abrasions, and the use of communal facilities.[20] MRSA presents as sore, red bumps on the skin, which are swollen, infused with pus, and warm to the touch. They may give off a foul odor.[21] Descriptive terms like "pimples," "spider bites," or "boils" have been used when identifying these lesions. If unattended, these lesions may become abscessed, in which case surgical incision and drainage is necessary. In some cases the lesions may be accompanied by a fever. If such an infection goes unchecked, there is a risk that it could spread, resulting in life-threatening consequences.[21]

Treatment of MRSA skin infections with antibiotics may not be necessary if it is diagnosed in its early stages. Simply lancing the superficial lesion and expressing the pus may be enough to stop the infection. This should be done by a trained health care professional under sterile conditions. If antibiotics are indicated, vancomycin has proven effective. However, recent reports suggest that the bacterium is showing some signs of resistance to this treatment option. Broad-spectrum antibiotics such as fluoroquinolones or cephalosporins, which are normally used in the treatment of *Staphylococcus* infections, should not be used for the treatment of MRSA. Therefore, it is prudent when feasible to take a sample of the infected tissue and send it for analysis before prescribing antibiotics.[21]

Prevention is the key to the management of any bacterial infection and in particular MRSA.

Pseudomonas is an example of a common infection from an unexpected communal source. Many athletes find the tropical waters of a hot tub therapeutic. However, if the pH and chemicals of the water are not properly monitored, hot tubs become breeding grounds for the ubiquitous bacterium pseudomonas.[13] A diffuse rash occurs on areas of exposed skin. The rash may be tender and itchy and is characterized by red, raised papules. Of interest, these micro-organisms often give off a distinct fruity odor. Open sores may become infected, complicating the healing process. In the worst-case scenario, the bacterium may penetrate the internal organs, causing a systemic infection that may require hospitalization.

It is important to meticulously clean the hot tub with bleach and to find the proper chemical balance for the water to prevent further bacterial invasion. If the source of infection is a public facility, the maintenance staff should be informed and the facility should be avoided until it is properly cleaned.

Parasites

Swimmer's Itch

Vegetation in water may contain schistosomes, a parasite that enters the skin causing an inflamed, pruritic (itchy), papular eruption over the body. Any athlete who participates in water sports, whether in fresh or salt water, may experience this condition. If contact is suspected, immediate, vigorous

---

Personal Care for Prevention of Bacterial Infection

- Wash hands regularly and vigorously with soap and water. Avoid bar soaps. Dry with disposable towels, then turn the faucet off with a separate towel. If soap and water is not available, a hand sanitizer that has at least 62% alcohol in it can be used as an alternative.[21]
- Shower immediately after sports participation and before entering communal water facilities. Use a clean towel to dry off.
- Personal care items such as towels, bar soaps, roll-on deodorants, and razors should not be shared.
- Personal athletic equipment should not be shared.
- Wash and dry athletic wear after each use in hot water with detergent and if possible bleach. Dry in dryer using hot temperatures.
- Open cuts, abrasions, and sores should be covered with sterile, dry bandages until they heal. This is to protect the athlete from contracting methicillin-resistant *Staphylococcus aureus* in vulnerable lesions and to stop the spread of bacteria if the wound is infected. Seek advice from a professional health care provider if a lesion appears to be infected.
- Protective clothing should be worn to avoid skin-to-skin contact and communal facility contact. For example, wear flip-flops in the shower, a towel in saunas, and bathing suits in spas.

---

toweling of the exposed skin will prevent the cercariae from taking hold. Once the rash appears, it generally takes a couple of weeks to subside. At this stage, management of the symptoms is the general course of treatment as the cercariae is generally dead within 24 hours of entering the skin. Calamine lotion can help to control the itch and dry up the papules. In extreme cases, cortisone creams may be recommended.

Conditions of Environmental Exposure

The skin is one's protective covering from the harsh realities of the environment, yet it cannot stand alone or it will break down under the volley of destructive forces. The onus is on the athlete to take the necessary preventive measures to protect the skin from ultraviolet light, chemicals, and temperature fluctuations in the environment.

Facility Maintenance for Prevention of Bacterial Infection

- Disinfectants should be used to clean communal equipment after each use
- Locker rooms should be constantly monitored and cleaned daily
- Communal water facilities such as swimming pools and hot tubs should be carefully monitored for chemical and pH balance
- Persons with open cuts, abrasions, or sores should be discouraged from using communal swimming pools and spas until the lesions have healed

---

Skin Conditions from Environmental Exposure

- Photo injury
- Cold temperature cutaneous injury
  - Cold urticaria
  - Chilblains
  - Frostbite
  - Exostosis
- Chemical damage
- Asteatotic eczema

Photo (Sun Exposure) Injury

The sun is like a double-edged sword. It provides individuals with light and warmth. It stimulates the production of essential nutrients to sustain life on earth. It stimulates the metabolism of vitamin D, which is necessary for the development of a strong skeletal structure. It has the capacity to heal. Yet excess amounts of sun exposure can at the very least contribute to aging of the skin; at most, through invasive skin cancers, sun exposure can kill. The sun emits three types of radiation: visible, infrared, and ultraviolet. It is overexposure to ultraviolet light that can be harmful to the skin. Ultraviolet light consists of three basic wavelengths: the longest is ultraviolet A (UVA), the mid-range is ultraviolet B (UVB), and the shortest is ultraviolet C (UVC).

The effect of UVC rays is controlled by the ozone layer in the atmosphere, where these rays are absorbed. The epidermis is able to provide a protective barrier from the small amount of UVC light that may filter through the atmosphere. However, if larger doses reach individuals as a result of deterioration of the ozone layer, the UVC rays will be a major contributing factor in the formation of skin cancers.

UVB was at one time thought to be the major cause of sun damage to the skin because it is visible in the form of a sun burn. However, it is now known that UVA rays are absorbed into the epidermis and the dermis more efficiently and in much greater amounts than UVB rays, posing an even greater threat to the health of the skin. This is particularly important given that tanning parlors claim that the ultraviolet A light that they use is safe. UVA and UVB rays may also damage the eyes and the immune system. Damage to the lens and retina of the eye may cause cataracts and visual acuity problems. Ultraviolet light may also interfere with the functioning of the Langerhans cells of the skin. These cells play an important role in recognizing infections and setting the defense mechanism of the immune system in motion. Therefore, damage to these cells reduces the effectiveness of the immune system, increasing susceptibility to viral and other diseases.[2]

UVA and UVB rays stimulate a change in the normally well-organized cells of the epidermis, resulting in skin cancers. There are three basic types of skin cancers: squamous cell, basal cell, and malignant melanomas. The name reflects the level of cell involvement.

Basal cell and squamous cell carcinomas generally arise in individuals older than the age of 40 years who have experienced long-term exposure to ultraviolet light. Common areas of the body for these tumors to appear include the face, the outer rim of the ears, the lower lip, the neck, the upper chest, the forearms, and the back of the hands.

Clinically, a basal cell carcinoma begins as a small red, brown, or light flesh tone spot on the skin. It has a distinct pearly appearance and raised borders. Basal cell carcinomas enlarge steadily at one site but tend not to spread to other areas of the skin or metastasize to internal tissue. Without early intervention, the tumor will continue its slow, insidious growth. As the lesion grows larger, it may become scaly and may bleed and crust in a repetitive fashion.[20] Surgical removal is the treatment of choice. Early intervention is recommended, as the small tumour can generally be scooped out with a curette, leaving a cup-shaped lesion that heals with little or no residual scar tissue. Although a recurrence after removal is rare (less than 4%), this technique allows a recurring cancer to surface rather than being trapped under scar tissue. The larger the lesion, the more invasive the surgery becomes, increasing the risk of a cosmetically unacceptable scar.

Squamous cell carcinomas pose a greater threat than basal cell carcinomas because they grow quickly, spread rapidly, and are more likely to metastasize. Initially, a squamous cell carcinoma may appear as a raised, red or white, scaly sore on the skin that tends not to heal. It may bleed and may rapidly evolve into a large, ulcerated tumour.[22] Early diagnosis is important in nipping this potentially dangerous cancer in the bud, and surgical removal is the treatment of choice. An early warning sign of the potential development of squamous cell carcinomas is the appearance of actinic keratoses or sunspots. Although it is rare that these red, scaly spots change into squamous cell carcinomas, they indicate the extent to which the skin has been damaged by solar radiation and suggest that regular examination of the skin for more sinister lesions be performed.

A melanoma is the most dangerous type of skin cancer and if it is not removed in a timely fashion, a melanoma may metostasize resulting in death. It is alarming to note that the incidence of melanomas continues to rise on an annual basis. These cancers develop in and around moles and are less likely to be associated with sun exposure. They are commonly found on the trunks of ages of 25 and 50 years, although melanomas have been reported in individuals younger than the age of 20 years.[22]

Persons with a family history of melanoma; numerous moles on their body; excessively large moles; or moles that are unusual in color, texture, or shape are at greater risk for the development of the disease. If a mole or pigment spot suddenly appears on the skin or an existing mole shows signs of change in shape, color, size, or surface texture, it should be checked for malignancy. Variations of color within the mole and seepage of color beyond the border of a mole also serve as important indicators of malignancy. Itching and bleeding moles are cause for concern. Melanomas may go through a period of slow growth prior to entering a rapid growth phase during which they quickly metastasize to underlying tissue and spread throughout the body. Early intervention is absolutely essential for a successful outcome. In fact, the most significant breakthrough in the treatment of melanomas has been the identification and removal of nonmalignant moles known as *dysplastic nevi*. Research has demonstrated that 20% to 35% of malignant melanomas developed from nonmalignant dysplastic nevi; it has been suggested that these figures are an underestimate, because many melanomas overgrow the pigmented lesion to which they attach.[22] In comparison with normal nevi, a dysplastic nevus tends to be variable and asymmetric in color. It is also likely to be much larger (1 to 2 cm [0.4 to 0.8 inches]) than a normal nevus and to have irregular margins. Over time, normal nevi stop growing outward and become raised, soft, and devoid of pigment; dysplastic nevi, on the other hand, continue to spread out from the center, remain pigmented, and are flat. It is not uncommon for people to have more than one lesion. The removal of dysplastic nevi significantly reduces the risk of developing a malignant melanoma in the future.[23]

If the threat of skin cancer is not enough to encourage an athlete to use protective measures, it may help to be aware that exposure to ultraviolet light contributes significantly to the aging of the skin. Photo-aging is characterized by wrinkles and dilated blood vessels as well as by pigment and texture changes. Although much can be done to rejuvenate the skin through medicated creams, chemical peels, and laser resurfacing (lasabrasions), it is far easier and less costly to prevent the problem from occurring in the first place.

Staying out of the sun is probably the best protective measure, however unrealistic for most athletes. Therefore, the next best alternative for preventing sun damage is the liberal and frequent use of a broad-spectrum sunscreen as well as wearing protective clothing. In the event that adequate precautionary measures have not been taken and a sunburn occurs, steps should be taken to minimize the damage to the skin. In the early stages of a burn, the body releases the chemical prostaglandin into the skin. This chemical is responsible for the red, irritated tenderness of a burn. Acetylsalicylic acid (aspirin) is an antiprostaglandin. Therefore, if taken in high doses prior to the onset of inflammation and redness, acetylsalicylic acid will inhibit prostaglandin release. Two adult aspirin three times daily for 2 days will suffice, if the individual's digestive system can take it. Enteric-coated aspirin is less irritating to the stomach. Acetaminophen (Tylenol or Tempra) is effective in reducing the discomfort of the sunburn, but it does not have the beneficial effect of inhibiting prostaglandin release, which will prevent the sunburn from occurring.

Sun Protection

1. Minimize the amount of sun exposure that you receive, particularly in the middle of the day, when ultraviolet radiation is most intense. Be aware that a light cloud cover does not protect against the damaging rays of the sun and that reflective surfaces such as water, snow, sand, and concrete are sources of ultraviolet radiation, as they will reflect up to 85% of the sun's rays.
2. Apply a broad-spectrum sunscreen that protects against ultraviolet A (UVA) and ultraviolet B (UVB) wavelengths daily to sun-exposed areas of the skin. The sun protection factor (SPF) should be 15 or more. *SPF* refers to the time greater than normal that it takes for ultraviolet light from the sun's rays to burn the skin. For example, if the unprotected skin burns in 1 minute, an SPF 60 sunscreen allows 15 minutes of sun exposure before a sunburn will occur.
3. Apply adequate amounts of sunscreen, one ounce for one body for one application, and be thorough in covering the exposed areas of the skin.
4. Apply sunscreen to a cool body, ½ hour before sun exposure, so that it will bind more effectively to the skin.
5. Wear sunscreen under loosely woven clothing or wet clothing. The ultraviolet radiation can penetrate through cloth.
6. Reapply sunscreen throughout the day according to the amount of sun exposure. Water and sweat will wash away the sunscreen, so reapplication every hour is important. Sunscreen should be applied to dry skin 20 minutes before exposure to more moisture.
7. Wear protective clothing: tightly woven cloth, sun hats, and sunglasses.
8. Avoid tanning salons. Exposure to UVA light from a tanning bed for 15 minutes is equivalent to 3 days of sitting in the sun. The UVA rays penetrate deep into the skin, so that superficial burning does not occur unless the skin is exposed for long periods.[1]

Photo injury is a major factor in the aging of the skin. Many individuals seek help after the damage has been done. There are many alternatives available to rejuvenate the skin.

Cold Temperature Cutaneous Injury

With exposure to extremely cold environmental conditions, severe tissue damage will ensue. Skiers, skaters, bobsledders, snowmobilers, rock and ice climbers, horseback riders, and sailors are some of the sports-minded individuals who are susceptible to skin injury caused by cold weather conditions.

Cold Injuries to Skin

- Cold urticaria
- Chilblains
- Frostbite

Cold Urticaria

Urticaria is synonymous with "hives," which is an edematous swelling of the dermis or subcutaneous tissue in response to stimuli such as drugs, foods, food additives, inhalants, infections, heat, sweat, and cold, to name a few. Cholinergic (sweat-induced), cold, and mechanical urticaria are common among athletes. Accurate diagnosis is crucial to therapeutic success. Cholinergic urticaria is best treated with agents that reduce production of the chemical mediator acetylcholine. People who have a high level of cold proteins in their blood, which may be a reflection of systemic disease such as lupus erythematosus or a viral illness, are more prone to develop hives when exposed to a cold environment. In these cases, the underlying cause must be addressed therapeutically. Otherwise, avoidance of cold exposure is the best prophylaxis. Antihistamines may be helpful when cold conditions are unavoidable. Mechanical urticaria is best treated by avoiding direct pressure to the skin, as in the case of properly fitting equipment.

Chilblains

Chilblains or perniones develop when conditions are cold and damp. To preserve heat, vasoconstriction is the body's defense against the cold. However, this defensive action may compromise the tissue of the skin, making it a pawn in the battle against the cold. Chilblains appear on protruding extremities such as the fingers, toes, nose, and ears. The heels of the feet, the lower legs, and the thighs may also be involved. The skin and subcutaneous tissue swell, becoming itchy and red. Blistering may occur and, in more severe cases, ulceration.[24]

Chilblains are self-limiting. Once the humid, cold conditions disappear, so do the chilblains. Keeping the extremities warm and dry, even when indoors, is the first step to manage this problem. Vasoconstriction can be controlled by wearing properly fitting footwear and gloves. If treatment is required, topical corticosteroids may be prescribed to control the inflammation, and systemic vasodilators may be necessary to monitor the vasoconstriction.[13]

Frostbite

Frostbite is a paramount concern of winter sports athletes. Extremely cold conditions, especially at high altitudes or combined with a severe wind chill, will cause the tissue of the skin to freeze. In the initial stages, the individual experiences a very painful burning sensation. At this point individuals should remove themselves from the cold conditions, because once the pain subsides, freezing of the tissue has begun. As the temperature of the skin drops to 2°C (35.6°F), metabolism at the cellular level stops, causing destruction of enzymes and proteins.[24] Ice crystals begin to form inside and outside the cell.

A white patch on the skin is the first sign of freezing. The patch will spread as more tissue becomes involved and will remain devoid of color until removed from the cold. In mild cases, the skin may simply be red and inflamed for several hours. In more severe cases, blistering may occur. Frostbite may extend beyond the skin to involve the muscles, nerves, vascular structures, and bones. Extensive loss of tissue (gangrene) may result. In cases in which loss of tissue does not occur, the involved areas may be numb and hypersensitive to cold for several months owing to the damage to blood vessels and nerves.[24] Once removed from the cold, the affected body part should be rapidly warmed by immersing it in circulating water of 38°C to 44°C (100°F to 110°F),[25] and further exposure to extreme cold should be avoided.

Ensuring that all exposed skin is properly covered prior to venturing into the cold is the first step in prevention. The face is generally of greatest concern; face masks help. By not shaving, men can take advantage of the natural protection offered by their beards. Not washing prior to taking part in outdoor activities will allow the natural oils of the skin to provide a protective film against the cold. The use of sunscreens will provide double protection against two environmental hazards: the cold and the sun.[6]

Avoiding restrictive clothing prevents vasoconstriction. Wearing layers of lightweight clothing helps monitor temperature fluctuations. Inner garments should be such that they draw moisture away from the skin.[26] Preserving and managing changes in body heat and moisture will help protect against the dangers of chilblains, frostbite, and hypothermia.

Exostosis

Chronic wet and cold conditions, such as those experienced by surfers, may lead to the growth of bony spurs in the ear canal known as *exostosis*. Some serious surfers consider these lesions to be a kind of status symbol. These lesions may be removed surgically; however, they are generally considered to be asymptomatic.

Chemical Damage

Pigment changes of the hair may result from long-term exposure to chemically treated waters. It is not the chlorine or bromine but the copper in chemically treated pools that is responsible for the change in hair color. When the copper ions of a chemically treated pool become integrated into the hair matrix, the hair takes on a greenish coloration. A bathing cap should be worn in chemically treated waters to prevent the problem. Another alternative is to wet the hair and apply a moisturizing conditioner before entering the pool, although most public facilities frown on this practice. Specialized shampoos and conditioners, such as Ultra-Swim chlorine combating shampoo and conditioner and Le Remouver shampoo, are available to help remove some of the green discoloration from the hair.

Chemicals in swimming pools also contribute to hair shaft fragility, resulting in split ends and hair breakage. Thorough rinsing of the hair after shampooing helps control the problem. Conditioners contain proteins that help to temporarily mend damaged hair by binding hair shaft cells. Oils in conditioners also replenish the natural oils that have been stripped from the hair by exposure to chemicals and shampooing. They also contain quaternary compounds that help to control "fly-away" hair, a common problem in dry, cold climates and air-conditioned rooms.[1] In the case of severe damage, the only alternative is to cut the hair. To prevent the problem, a bathing cap should be worn.

Asteatotic Eczema

When dryness caused by lipid depletion results in irritated, inflamed skin, the condition is referred to as *asteatotic eczema* (Figure 19-17). This is a particularly common condition in athletes who are exposed to environmental conditions that strip the skin of its natural oils. Such environmental factors may include wind, chemicals in swimming pools, and deodorant soaps.

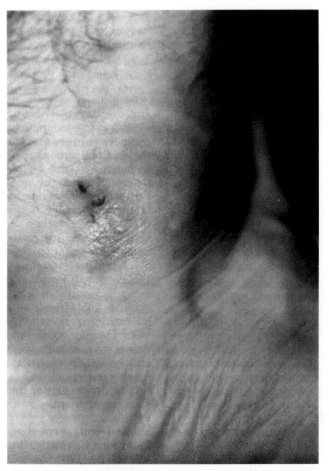

Figure 19-17
Asteatotic eczema (long-distance chlorine pool swimmer).

The skin is dry, itchy, scaly, and irritated. This can be particularly annoying to the athlete. The best treatment option for eczema is prevention. A soap that contains a high concentration of fat (animal, glycerin, or resin) should be used when bathing or washing the face. A deodorant or antiperspirant should be used separately. In severe cases, Cetaphil lotion is a good soap substitute. The skin should be thoroughly rinsed and patted dry, and then a moisturizer should be applied to slightly moist skin. Moisturizers with perfumes should be avoided, as they irritate the skin. The moisturizer does not replenish the natural oils but prevents the oil and moisture in the skin from escaping. Chemically enhanced moisturizers contain agents such as urea, glycolic acid, and lactic acid that improve the entrapment of the skin's natural oils, for example, Uremol 10 and Lac-Hydrin lotions. Calmurid cream is particularly useful for cracked and fissured heels. Apply the cream before going to bed, wrap the feet in a plastic wrap, and cover them with socks to maximize effectiveness.[2] In severe cases, topical cortisone or a course of treatment with controlled ultraviolet light may be required.

Scar Revision

Scar formation is inevitable when damage from an injury enters the deeper layers of the skin. The causes of scar formation are many and varied, and include external trauma such as abrasions, cuts, or burns, and internal trauma from disease entities such as acne, chicken pox, and shingles.

The appearance of a scar may vary according to intrinsic and extrinsic factors. Heredity and nutrition are intrinsic factors that may affect the way a wound heals. Infection, compromised blood supply, use of a topical or systemic steroid, foreign materials in the wound, and poor surgical technique are examples of extrinsic factors that contribute to the appearance of a scar.

Treatment Options for Scars

Scar revision requires an observant eye and a creative multidimensional approach to be successful. Component analysis of the scar is the first step. A scar may be linear, raised, thick, depressed, uneven, vascular, hyperpigmented (brown discoloration), or hypopigmented (devoid of color). By treating each of the components of the scar, the overall improvement is greatest. Cortisone injections, medicated creams, W-plasty, resurfacing lasers, vascular removal lasers, pigment removal lasers, and micropigment implantation are techniques that are used in isolation or in combination to improve the appearance of a scar. Multiple treatment sessions are usually required to achieve the best results.[27,28]

In most cases, the ideal time to begin scar revision is 6 to 12 weeks after the wound has occurred. This allows the surgeon to direct the body's natural healing process to an improved cosmetic result. In certain cases, re-excision of an old scar is performed prior to laser treatments in order to re-establish the 6- to 12-week window of opportunity for laser scar revision.[29]

Raised Scars

If a scar is simply raised, injecting it with cortisone will cause it to flatten, making it less obvious in appearance.

Linear Scars

Scars that are linear attract attention because we naturally tend to follow a straight line with our eyes. To break up the linearity of a scar, a W-plasty is performed in which the scar is excised and sutured in a zigzag fashion. This creates an optical illusion so the new scar appears less obvious. Also, the new scar is easier to remodel with lasers because the window of opportunity for taking advantage of the body's natural healing process has been re-established.

Thick, Irregular Scars

Scars may also be irregular, thick, and lumpy. Resurfacing with a CO_2 laser will smooth out a lumpy scar and blend the edges into the adjacent normal tissue. The CO_2 laser uses a very high-energy beam of light to heat the water in the scar tissue cells to 100°C (212°F), causing them to be vaporized away. The laser light penetrates to a very precise, controlled depth, making the procedure safe and predictable. To achieve the best results, this procedure often requires more than one session to gradually remove the layers of scar tissue.

Regular use of medicated creams containing tretinoin or glycolic acid are often used in combination with laser resurfacing. These creams help to realign the collagen building blocks of the skin as well as smoothing out irregular texture that is common to most scarring.

Keloid Scars

Keloid scars are a problematic form of raised, lumpy scarring. The tendency to form keloid scars is often hereditary. Keloid forms when the body produces an excessive amount of scar tissue in response to an injury of the skin. It is usually treated with cortisone injections, which flattens the scar, but in some cases keloids may be improved with lasers. Even after the scar has been flattened, the body continues to lay down scar tissue. Therefore, repeat treatments are usually required.

Depressed Scars

Depressions in the skin may take different forms. Ice pick scars and split pores are common postacne problems in which small pits or splits form in place of an oil gland. They are best treated with punch transfers or microsurgery. Punch transfers involve the removal of the pit with a circular scalpel. A small piece of skin from behind the ear is then transferred into the space where the pit was removed. Microsurgery is a technique in which a very small incision is made around the scar. The scar tissue is removed and the margins of the normal skin are sutured together. Laser resurfacing is often used after the punch transfer or microsurgery has healed to blend the edges into the normal surrounding tissue.

Saucer-shaped depressions in the skin require a different approach. To elevate the skin, implant therapy is generally the treatment of choice. Another option for the treatment of saucer-shaped depressions is to vaporize the elevations around the depression with a CO_2 resurfacing laser. This helps the depression to look less obvious.

Vascular Discoloration

Many scars are very vascular, resulting in a red discoloration to the scar. The vascularity can be removed with one of the target-specific lasers, such as the flash lamp dye or long-pulse Nd:YAG laser.

These lasers are effective because the wavelength of light that penetrates the skin has a selective affinity for blood vessels. It passes harmlessly through the top layer or epidermis of the skin, leaving it essentially intact. When it hits the targeted blood vessels, the flash lamp dye causes a microscopic fragmentation of the blood cells. The dispersed blood cells, in the form of a bruise, are then carried away by the body's debris collecting cells (macrophages) leaving behind normal skin. The Nd:YAG laser seals the blood vessels and does not leave a bruise after the treatment.

Changes in Pigment

Brown discolorations may occur in scars because of an excess amount of melanin or imbedded foreign material such as asphalt into the scar. In some cases, this can be effectively removed by using a bleaching cream containing hydroquinone or kojic acid. In other cases, laser treatment may be necessary.

The Q-switched Nd: YAG or Alexandrite lasers work in a similar fashion to the dye laser. The intense light from the laser passes harmlessly through the top layer of the skin and is selectively absorbed by brown, black, or blue pigment in the skin. The energy emitted by the laser light when it is absorbed causes the melanin or foreign material to break into miniscule particles that are removed by the body's immune system.

Hypopigmentation or the lack of color in a scar can be very difficult to change. It may be improved by the meticulous injection of flesh-colored pigment into the scar with a technique known as *microimplantation*. The other option is simply to cover the scar with cosmetics such as Derma Color.

Conclusion

Throughout this chapter, the authors have touched on some of the common skin problems encountered by the athlete. The protective role the skin plays in maintaining one's health cannot be overemphasized. As in any other area of medicine, some simple yet effective precautions may prevent skin diseases that can interfere with training and performance.

References

1. Lever WF, Schaumburg-Lever G: *Histopathology of the skin,* Philadelphia, 1983, JB Lippincott.
2. Groot DW, Johnston PA: *Young as you look,* Edmonton, Canada, 1993, InForum.
3. Groot DW, Johnston PA, Miller P, Sather G: Skin problems of a professional hockey club: A season in review, *Cont Derm* 2:13–22, 1988.
4. Lynch PJ, Boyer JT: Clotting disorders in the skin (purpura). In Fitzpatrick TB, Eisen AZ, Wolff K, et al, editors: *Dermatology in general medicine,* New York, 1971, McGraw-Hill.
5. Wilkinson DS: Cutaneous reactions to mechanical and thermal injury. In Rook A, Wilkinson DS, Ebling FJ, et al, editors: *Textbook of dermatology,* Volume 1, Oxford, 1986, Blackwell Scientific.
6. Basler RSW: Skin injuries in sports medicine, *J Am Acad Dermatol* 21:1257–1262, 1989.
7. Johnston PA, Groot DW: Tattoos: art or injury, *Pulse* 7(2):14–15, 1993.
8. Groot DW, Johnston PJ: A review of sports-related skin problems, *Can J CME* 2:19–27, 1990.
9. Ryan TJ, Wilkinson DS: Diseases of the veins and arteries—Leg ulcers. In Rook A, Wilkinson DS, Ebling FJ, et al, editors: *Textbook of dermatology,* Volume 2, Oxford, 1986, Blackwell Scientific.
10. Oxman MN: Varicella and herpes zoster. In Fitzpatrick TB, Eisen AZ, Wolff K, et al, editors: *Dermatology in general medicine,* New York, 1971, McGraw-Hill.
11. Nagington J, Rook A, Highet AS: Virus and related infections. In Rook A, Wilkinson DS, Ebling FJ, et al, editors: *Textbook of dermatology,* Volume 1, Oxford, 1986, Blackwell Scientific.
12. Evans JG: Recurrent aphthous stomatitis: Management of a patient, *Oral Health* 8:27, 1993.
13. Basler RSW: Skin problems in winter sports. In Casey MJ, Foster C, Hixson EG, editors: *Winter sports medicine,* Philadelphia, 1989, FA Davis.
14. Resnick SS, Lewis LA, Cohen BH: The athlete's foot, *Cutis* 20:351–355, 1977.
15. Sher RK: Jogger's toe, *Int J Dermatol* 17:719–720, 1978.
16. Gibbs RC, Boxer MC: Abnormal biomechanics of feet and their cause of hyperkeratosis, *J Am Acad Dermatol* 6:1061–1069, 1982.
17. Levit P: Jogger's nipples, *N Engl J Med* 297:1127, 1977.
18. Champion RH: Disorders of the sweat glands. In Rook A, Wilkinson DS, Ebling FJ, et al, editors: *Textbook of dermatology,* Volume 3, Oxford, 1986, Blackwell Scientific.
19. Roberts SOB, Mackenzie DWR: Mycology. In Rook A, Wilkinson DS, Ebling FJ, et al, editors: *Textbook of dermatology,* Volume 2, Oxford, 1986, Blackwell Scientific, 1986.
20. Centers for Disease Control and Prevention: *Frequently asked questions about methicillin-resistant staphylococcus aureus (MRSA) among athletes,* November 2008. http://www.cdc.gov/ncidod/dhqp/ar_MRSA_AthletesFAQ.html
21. Mayo Clinic: *MRSA: Understand your risk and how to prevent infection.* http://www.mayoclinic.com/health/mrsa/ID00049.
22. The Canadian Dermatology Association: "Dermatologists - Your Skin Experts," Kingston, 2009, The Canadian Dermatology Association.
23. McLean D: Dysplastic nevus: Precursor to melanoma, *Med North Am* 32:4460–4462, 1986.
24. Champion RH: Cutaneous reaction to cold. In Rook A, Wilkinson DS, Ebling FJ, et al, editors: *Textbook of dermatology,* Volume 3, Oxford, 1986, Blackwell Scientific.
25. D'Ambrosia RD: Cold injuries encountered in winter sport, *Cutis* 20:365–368, 1977.
26. Washburn B: Frostbite, *N Engl J Med* 266:974–989, 1962.
27. Groot DW, Johnston PA: An approach to laser therapy, *J Cutan Med Surg* 3(Suppl 4):S7–S13, 1999.
28. Groot DW, Johnston PA: Advances in cutaneous laser therapy, *Can J Cl Med* 4(8):4–8, 1997.
29. Yarborough JM: Ablation of facial scars by programmed dermabrasion, *J Derm Surg Oncol* 14:292–294, 1988.

PROTECTIVE EQUIPMENT IN SPORTS

Michael R. Mirabella and Timothy F. Tyler

Introduction

Protective equipment is clearly one of the most important aspects of sports medicine as well as care for athletes in general. The proper selection and fitting of athletic equipment is essential in preventing many sports injuries.[1] One of the main duties of the sports medicine clinician is to aid in the prevention of injuries and to protect existing injuries from further harm. Protective equipment plays a key role in this process. *Protective equipment* is any device or material that protects the athlete from injury or protects an existing injury from becoming worse during competition. This equipment can range from a simple foam pad to a highly sophisticated football helmet with the latest concussion-reducing technology. Materials may include neoprene, closed- or open-cell foam, plastic, metal, casting material or any combination of these. Protective equipment must provide protection while allowing the athlete to fully function on the field. It must also not pose a danger to the athlete, teammates, or to opposing players.[1]

History

As technology and individual sports have evolved, so too has protective equipment. As athletes have become bigger and stronger, so too has media interest and public demand for safety equipment for sports and athletics. Need and desire for protective equipment has continued to grow and evolve. Since the advent of the football helmet in 1896 and its continued development through the early 1900s, there has been a sharp decline in the number of head injuries in football. As technology has became more advanced, so too has the helmet and other forms of equipment. These advances have also aided in the sharp decline of injuries suffered while participating in sports.[2]

Standards for Sports Equipment

The evolution of sports and rule changes governing equipment has also had an effect in reducing injuries.[2] Standards for athletic equipment have become a major concern over the years. Durability of materials used in the manufacture of equipment, maintenance, and the handing down of equipment are primary concerns. Strict standards are needed when deciding whether equipment can be reconditioned or whether it needs to be thrown away. Equipment that is worn and poorly fitted should never be handed down to lower-level players, because to do so increases the chances of injury.[3] Concerns such as these led to the formation of the National Operating Committee on Standards for Athletic Equipment (NOCSAE). NOCSAE was commissioned in 1969 to develop research studies directed toward injury reduction. The need for such an organization had become evident in 1968 when there were 32 fatalities during organized football. Because of low funding, the committee concentrated mainly on the football helmet and its effectiveness on reducing injury. A standard test was published in 1973, and all helmets had to be certified beginning with the National Collegiate Athletic Association (NCAA) in 1978. All helmets also had to be reconditioned and recertified every year. This is an effective practice that continues today.[4]

Note: This chapter includes content from previous contributions by Ethan Saliba, PhD, ATC, PT, SCS; Susan Foreman, MEd, MPT, ATC; and Richard T. Abadie Jr., BA, EMC, as it appeared in the predecessor of this book—Zachazewski JE, Magee DJ, Quillen WS, editors: *Athletic injuries and rehabilitation*, Philadelphia, 1996, WB Saunders.

NOCSAE Warning to be Placed on the Exterior of All Football Helmets

- Do not strike an opponent with any part of this helmet or face mask. This is a violation of football rules and may cause you to suffer severe brain or neck injury, including paralysis or death.
- Severe brain or neck injury may also occur accidentally while playing football.
- **No helmet can prevent all such injuries.**
- **You use this helmet at your own risk.**

Legal Concerns Regarding Protective Equipment

Increased litigation related to protective equipment has come with increased participation in sports. Anyone who purchases equipment must be aware of the intended uses associated with such products. They must also be made aware of the risks involved in misusing equipment. The coach or sports medicine clinician must make the athlete aware of the proper uses for the equipment being issued and the consequences of its misuse.[4] If an injury occurs to an athlete using a piece of equipment, and the piece of equipment is deemed defective or inadequate, then the manufacturer is liable. If modifications are made to a piece of equipment by the athlete, coach, or sports medicine clinician then the liability of the manufacturer becomes void, and the individual who made the modification then becomes liable. Modifications range from painting a football helmet to removing and cutting padding from football pads.

Factors to Consider in Equipment Testing

- Limitations of size, weight, shape, materials, and durability of the device, with respect to the athletic performance, injury to other players, aesthetics, and cost
- Injury mechanisms—compression, tension, shearing
- Single- or multiple-impact protection
- Mechanisms of injury and the ability of tissues to withstand that injury at the protected location
- Equipment reassessment for weakness

If a sports medicine clinician modifies a piece of equipment and it results in injury to the athlete, the clinician can be found liable. Any lawsuit would involve the sports medicine clinician and the employing institution. To avoid a situation such as this, the sports medicine clinician, equipment manager, and coaches must follow the manufacturer's instructions.[3]

Degree of Contact

Football is not the only sport that requires protection. Each individual sport must be considered for the amount and severity of contact. For example, football and basketball have a high degree of contact. Contact is not only player-to-player. It also includes player and playing surface and equipment to player. This happens when a heavily protected body part comes in contact with another player's unprotected area and can result in injury. Hard and rigid materials may come in contact with the unprotected body part of an opposing player. The sports medicine clinician, equipment manager, coach, and athlete must be aware of the dangers that some protective equipment may pose to other players, and take steps to protect opposing players.[1] A cast, for example, is sometimes allowed to be worn on the forearm of a player who has suffered a fracture. Padding must be applied to protect other players from harm when coming into contact with the cast. This padding can also dissuade the player from using the cast as a weapon on the field, thus avoiding further injury. League regulations also play a role and may dictate which protective equipment is required for participation. These rules should not only dictate use but also misuse of equipment. An example of misuse is "spearing," in which the helmet is used as a weapon in football. The defender launches himself head-first into an opposing player, hitting him with the helmet. League rules are also created to protect the athlete wearing the equipment. High school–level ice hockey players are required to wear a full face shield, mouthguard, and throat protection as protection from injury to the head, face, teeth, and throat. This type of protection not only protects the athlete from opposing players but also from the puck. Projectiles such as pucks and balls can cause injury in sports. One such common projectile is the baseball. Competitive baseball leagues require that a helmet be worn by all batters. The catcher is also completely protected. Some batters even elect to wear a small shin guard to protect against foul balls.

Stock versus Custom Protection

There are two different types of equipment. Stock and custom equipment are both used in sports to protect a body part. Stock items are prefabricated and come ready to use. Custom items are constructed specifically for an individual athlete.

Custom-made items have definite advantages versus stock items in that they can be constructed and customized for a specific body part, injury, and athlete. Some problems with off-the-shelf equipment can include proper fit and comfort.[1] A customized pad must fit exactly as intended and must provide the protection or support specified for the injury or body part. The sports medicine clinician must be knowledgeable about the properties and uses of all of the materials used in the construction of custom padding or supports. For example, what materials have the ability to be heated and molded into a specific shape? These materials must also perform their purpose, and be safe for the athlete and opponents. Also, what are the methods used in heating and molding these materials? An example is the use of a hydrocollator to heat a thermomoldable plastic so it can be shaped. The sports medicine clinician must also possess some form of creativity or mechanical skill to create the pad or support needed by the injured athlete. Mechanical skill includes the ability to use the tools necessary to shape the materials, including scissors, flat knives, scalpels, or whatever the sports medicine clinician feels comfortable using.[1] The most common purpose for a custom-made pad is to absorb shock and deflect forces away from the injured area.

Protective Materials

Numerous materials are used in the manufacture of modern sports protective equipment. Every material of a given density, thickness, and temperature has certain properties that help define that material's use.[5] Soft materials usually have a lower density and are lightweight because air is incorporated into the material. Soft materials protect optimally at low levels of impact intensity.

Resilience or *memory* is another property of materials used in protective equipment. *Resilience* is the ability of a material to regain its shape quickly after impact. Highly resilient materials are used when protection from repeated impacts is required.[5] Nonresilient materials can be used when one-time or occasional impact is expected, although the protective equipment may be ruined by that impact. These materials must be checked to ensure that the athlete does not continue to use the equipment if the material is crushed or compacted by repeated impacts. For example, the polystyrene foam inside bicycle helmets is lightweight and will crush on impact to protect the skull. When the material has been altered because of impact, it no longer offers adequate protection and should be replaced. Nonresilient materials are tested by an independent company to determine whether deformation and energy absorption occurs below levels that would cause injury.

Silicone, fiberglass, polyethylene foam, thermoplastic materials (e.g., Orthoplast, Aquaplast), neoprene, moleskin, felt, and adhesive foams are among the materials used in fabricating customized splints or equipment.[6] Each has a unique protective ability to conform to the body, deflect impact, absorb shock, or immobilize a body structure. Lightweight plastics and foams can be combined to optimize the products' ability to absorb or deflect an impact. Most equipment companies combine materials, depending on the function of the particular piece of gear. This provides comfort and cushion close to the body, and firmer, nonyielding materials are placed on the outside to transfer the stresses over a broad area.[7] Sports medicine clinicians should be familiar with various materials and how they react on impact so that combinations of materials can be used effectively to prevent injury or reinjury.

Foam

Foam is one of the most common products used in constructing custom protective padding. It is available in an array of types, thicknesses, and densities, depending on what is needed for the particular device. The primary consideration in choosing foam padding is the energy and shock-absorbing capabilities of the material. These energy absorbing capabilities depend on the thickness and density of the foam. The foam should absorb shock and be light enough to be worn comfortably. The two main types of foam are open-cell and closed-cell. Open-cell foams (Figure 20-1, *A*) are low-density materials in which the cells are connected to allow air passage from cell to cell. Similar to a sponge, these materials have the capacity to absorb fluids and are commonly used to pad bony prominences or hard edges of protective equipment and custom-fabricated pads. Open-cell foams generally do not have good shock-absorbing qualities because they deform quickly under stress. Closed-cell foam (Figure 20-1, *B*) is preferred because of its superior shock-absorbing abilities, and its resilience to absorption of fluid such as perspiration.[8] Closed-cell foams should also rebound quickly after being compressed to maintain protection.

Dual-density foam is also available. This consists of high- and low-density foam that has been glued together by the manufacturer. This can be useful when creating a pad quickly on the field.

Some high-density foam is also thermomoldable. This means that when heated, it becomes flexible, allowing it to be shaped and modified as needed to a variety of shapes and sizes (Figure 20-2). After it has cooled it holds its final shape until reheated. Cramer High Density Foam is an example of foam that can be heated and molded into the shape needed.

Air Management Pads

Air management pads are a relatively new type of protective padding and are often used when maximal shock absorption is required in lightweight gear. These pads are constructed of various open- and closed-cell foam pads encased in polyurethane or a nylon material.[8] This encasement is airtight,

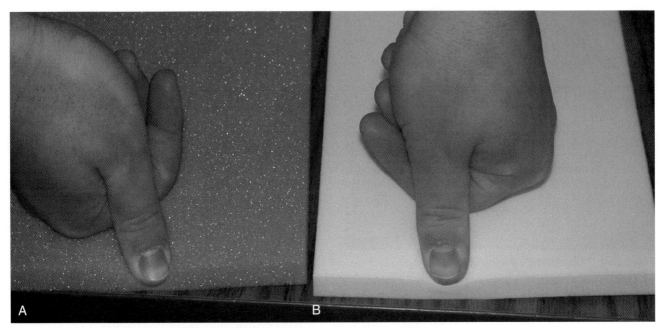

Figure 20-1
Demonstrating different densities of open-cell *(A)* and closed-cell foam *(B)*.

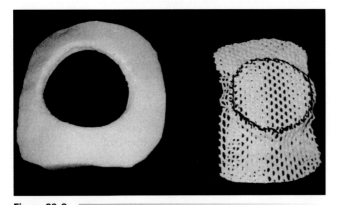

Figure 20-2
A custom-fabricated pad. A donut pad is cut from Thermoplast, and firmer Hexalite is molded and attached to the donut to give better protection. This pad is used to protect the acromioclavicular joint.

which prevents quick deformation of the foam so that the energy is dissipated over a broad area. Air pads are frequently used in football shoulder pads, and various companies incorporate different designs of foam placement within the nylon encasement. These pads are more expensive than traditional equipment, and the linings must be replaced or patched if the nylon is torn because this allows too much air to escape on impact. Nylon prevents fluids from entering the pads, which helps avoid adding significant weight to the equipment. Body fluids such as sweat and blood are easily cleaned from the nylon material with a weak bleach solution. Sanitation of traditional padding is more difficult because even closed-cell foam absorbs some fluids.

Gel

Another material that is useful in absorbing shock is gel. Many companies manufacture a variety of gels with different capabilities. An example of a gel-based shock absorbing material is Johnson and Johnson's product Orthogel (Figure 20-3). Orthogel comes in varying thicknesses and can be cut into different shapes. Because of the consistency of the gel, it can conform to bony areas of the body. Gel is useful for protecting bony areas such as the foot, hand, and acromioclavicular (AC) joint of the shoulder. Another quality is that the gel can be cut and used as a horseshoe pad when treating an acute ankle sprain. This horseshoe can be cooled and used for cryotherapy as it provides compression and reduces and prevents swelling in an acutely injured ankle. A drawback to using gel-based materials is the lack of longevity associated with such products. Gel has a tendency to absorb heat from the athlete's body often resulting in the pad losing its shape. This reduces the ability of the material to provide protection over a long period. For gel-based pads to last, an athlete must care for the material properly (e.g., allow to dry in a cool place). This is a drawback because the sports medicine clinician should be able to provide protection with minimal care. Because of the short lifespan of gel padding, the material should be reserved for protecting difficult bony areas. Gel is extremely useful in

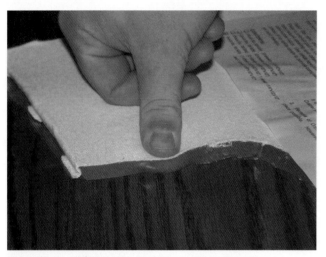

Figure 20-3
Shock-absorbing gel.

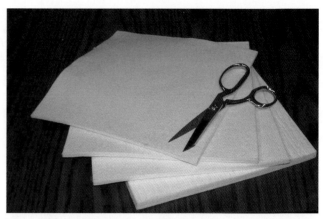

Figure 20-4
Sheets of felt demonstrating different thicknesses.

providing protection to the ankle, foot, and hand because it molds itself to these difficult body parts. Sorbothane is a self-adhesive viscoelastic polymer padding that dissipates and absorbs impact forces. This material is available in sheets or in prefabricated pads that can be placed in ball gloves, shoes, or splints.

Felt

Felt, which comes in different thicknesses, is another widely used material to create protective devices (Figure 20-4). For years, felt has been used to create protective padding.[1] Foam has surpassed felt in providing protection because of its superior shock-absorption qualities and felt's tendency to absorb water. Felt is extremely useful for creating various types of supports and protective pads. It can be cut into different shapes to provide the support needed and to relieve pressure on areas. Felt is also very durable and maintains its shape well. Felt is often used for arch supports and can be cut and sized to fit an athlete's foot. Another common use for felt is a horseshoe used to reduce edema while treating an acute ankle sprain. Lastly, it can be used to reduce pressure in high-friction areas such as the heel.

Thermomoldable Plastics

There are various thermoplastic materials that can be used for splint or custom pad fabrication. Thermoplastics, which were developed in the 1960s, become moldable when heated.[9] When hardened, the material gives rigid support to help restrict motion at a joint, such as on the hand. The material can also be used to relieve impact to an area when used in conjunction with a softer, more shock-absorbing material such as foam. The number of companies producing

thermoplastics has substantially increased, and the types of materials vary considerably. Different thermoplastic materials have unique characteristics such as moldability, durability, and thickness, which may make one material more suitable for a problem than another. Several of the available materials are identical in composition but are offered by various distributors under different names.

Thermoplastics can be divided into two basic categories: plastic and rubber. Subclassifications, which include plastic–rubber-like and rubber-like, exhibit characteristics of both groups.[9] The plastic group uses a polycaprolactone base with varying amounts of inorganic filler, resins, and elastomers. These agents act as modifiers that affect the memory, stiffness, and durability of the material. The base of the rubber group is composed principally of polyisoprene, which also has varying amounts of fillers and therefore demonstrates different characteristics.

The plastic category tends to be more conforming than the rubber-type materials. Therefore, plastic is more appropriate for small splints such as on the hand. Plastics include materials such as Aquaplast Bluestripe, Orfit, Multiform I and II, and Orthoplast II. Rubberlike materials include Ultraform Traditions, Orthoplast, Aquaplast Greenstripe, and Synergy.

The working temperatures of these materials range from 150°F to 180°F (65.5°C to 82.2°C). Most thermoplastics should be heated for approximately 1 minute with the material flat to minimize distortion or stretching. Most can then be manipulated for 3 to 4 minutes before resuming their hardened form. Some changes can be made with a heat gun. This should *not* be done while the splint is on the athlete.

Thermoplastic materials come in varying thicknesses and degrees of perforation. Perforation allows for ventilation in the material but can compromise its durability, especially when subjected to the forces associated with athletic competition.[10] Table 20-1 summarizes the various qualities

Table 20-1

Comparison of Thermoplastics

	Working Temperature (°F)	Rigidity	Shrinkage	Stretch	Drapability	Moldability	Bond	Memory	Comments
Plastic									
NCM Clinic (Precision Splint/RS 3000) North Coast/Polymed	160-170	3	1	3	3	3	3	2	Easy to work and contour
Polyform/Kay Splint-Rolyan/Sammons	150-160	2	1	2+	2+	3	3	1	Easy to mold; do not overheat
Ultraform (Sammons)	160	2	2	2	2	2	2	1	Nice feel/texture
Aquaplast, Blue-stripe (WFR/Aquaplast)	160-180	2	2	3+	3+	3	3	2	Better cut pattern when translucent; highly moldable
Orthoplast II (Johnson & Johnson)	150-170	2	1	3	3	2	3	1	Looks, behaves like multiform
Multiform I & II (AliMed)	150-180	3	2	3	3	2	3	1	Inexpensive; easy to mold and work
Plastic and rubberlike									
NCM Preferred/Custom Splint/JU1000 North Coast/Polymed	160-170	3	1	2	3	2	2	1	Versatile; skin rash with perspiration
Ultraform 294 (Sammons)	160	3	1	1	1	1	2	2	Difficult to form
Polyflex II/Kay Splint, Isoprene	160	2	1	3	3	3	2	1	Good for small/large orthoses; scraps recyclable
Aquaplast (WFR/Aquaplast)	160-180	2	3	3	3	3	3	3	Needs work with edges — for experienced splint makers
Orfit Soft (North Coast)	160-180	2	2	3	3	3	3	3	Similar to Aquaplast — shrinks less when allowed to cool on patient
Rubberlike									
NCM Spectrum/Ultrasplint/MR 2000 North Coast/Polymed	170	2	1	1	1	2	2	1	Reshapes and edges roll easily; Good for large orthoses; easy trim edge
Ezeform/Kay SplintIII Rolyan/Sammon	170	3	1	1	1	2	3	1	Great colors; contours nicely; easy to work
Aquaplast (Aqua-plast)	160-180	2	2	2	2	3	3	3	Less conforming but more rigid for larger orthoses
Aquaplast Greenstripe (WFR Aquaplast)	160-180	2	2	2	1	2	2	3	Increased thickness good for large orthoses
Ofit Stif (North Coast)	135	3	2	2	1	2	3	3	Attractive/nice feel; takes effort to contour
Synergy (Rolyan)	160	1	1	2	1	2	1	2	
Rubber									
Orthoplast (Johnson & Johnson)	160	1	1	1	1	3	2	1	Good edges, worse contour
Ultraform Traditions (Sammons)	160	2	2						Not tested

From Breger-Lee DE, Burford WL: Properties of thermoplastic splinting materials, *J Hand Ther* 4:202-211, 1992.
Range of scores is 1 (least) to 3 (most).

associated with some of the thermoplastic materials. Shelf life also affects the quality of these materials.

There are also high-temperature thermoplastics that become malleable at temperatures of 325°F to 350°F (163°C to 177°C). These can be vacuum-molded or shaped over plaster models. Heat guns can be used to make modifications. These materials can be transparent and are useful, for instance, if a full-contact face mask is desired to allow protection of a facial injury (e.g., W-Clear).

Plastics have come into their own in custom-made padding. The most widely used is Johnson and Johnson's Orthoplast. Orthoplast comes in sheets that are solid or perforated. These sheets can be heated and molded to fit a specific body part and form a hard protective shell (Figure 20-5). The sports medicine clinician can use a hydrocollator to heat the material before molding. When the material cools it maintains its shape and remains rigid until it is reheated. Plastazote

is a heat-activated, lightweight, closed-cell foam that is heated for 5 to 10 minutes in a convection oven at 285°F (140°C). This polyethylene material can be formed to the part to be protected and provides lightweight padding and support.[11] These protective devices can be extremely useful in protecting a quadriceps contusion to prevent repeated blows and possible subsequent development of myositis ossificans (see Chapter 18, "Medical Conditions in Sport").

Casting Material

Scotchcast fiberglass-polyurethane splints soften at room temperature (70°F to 75°F [21°C to 24°C]) and provide a one-step, easily moldable splint that sets in 3 to 4 minutes. Functional strength in the material is attained in 20 minutes. Scotchwrap has 25% of the fiberglass resin of Scotchcast, which causes it to be less rigid when dry. This could be an alternative to RTV 11 rubber in high school athletes, because it is easier to apply. However, a referee may require the material to be covered with soft padding during participation to avoid injury to other players.

Hexcelite or X-Lite is a low-temperature thermoplastic with an open-weave design that allows fabrication of lightweight, highly ventilated splints. This material becomes malleable with warm tap water and is self-bonding, so multiple layers can be used to increase the rigidity of the device.

Silicone elastomer has been popular in fabricating soft splints. This material is used when a more rigid material is considered illegal in sporting competition. Silicone elastomer casting is appropriate with certain types of hand or wrist injuries or when a fracture has reached a healing state that would not be compromised with less rigid protection. The liquid-style elastomer is reinforced with layers of gauze bandaging when used for casting. The set-up time is controlled by a separate catalyst that is added to the silicone when the cast is made. Because the silicone cast is nonporous in its finished form, it is typically worn only during competition. Skin maceration can occur if the cast is worn for too long. The athlete should wear a bivalved cast or splint at all other times until the injury has healed.

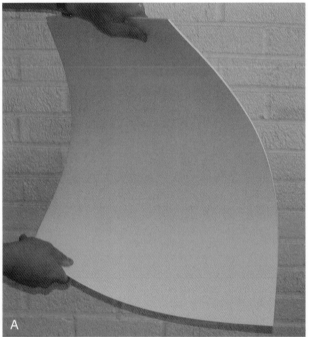

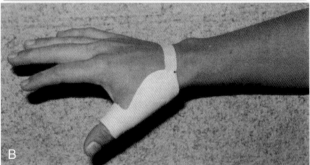

Figure 20-5
A, Orthoplast comes in stiff, bindable sheets that become malleable when heated. **B,** A thermoplastic splint. Depending on the league and sport, this splint may be used in a game to help stabilize the thumb. Athletic tape is often used to hold the device in place.

Legality of Hard Casts in High School Football

- The cast or splint must be constructed of approved material (no metal or plaster)
- The cast or splint must be covered by a minimum of ½-inch (1.3 cm) closed-cell foam
- A written authorization form must be signed and available to the officials at the beginning of the competition that indicates that the athlete may participate in football with the cast or splint
- The officials should check and approve the paperwork and the padded cast or splint prior to the game
- The referee has the authority to eject a player if he or she is using the cast or splint as a weapon

Another rigid form of protection is casting material such as Orthoglass (Figure 20-6). Orthoglass uses a fiberglass-type resin that, when combined with tap water, becomes rigid. This material combined with foam and tape can make a resilient pad. This technology is extremely useful when one needs to make a protective shell or splint quickly and only the material and water is available, such as on the sideline of a football game.

Miscellaneous Items

Off-the-shelf items can also be used in creating custom-made protection. The extremely durable plastic insert can be cut out of a thigh pad and used to create a custom pad. These plastics are known to be durable and are also thermo-moldable. Care must be taken when using these products especially if the sports medicine clinician does not have experience working with these materials. These materials should be researched to verify their safe use.

Tools Used for Customizing

Adhesives. A number of glues and adhesives can be used to create custom padding by holding different materials together to help form different shapes.

Adhesive Tape. Adhesive tape is one of the most commonly used tools in creating custom padding. Tape can be used to hold foam onto a hard shell, and can be used to cover up sharp edges on customized hard materials.

Heat Sources. The most common sources of heat to aid in the construction of protective padding include hot pack machines (i.e., hydrocollator), hot air guns, or hair dryers, and a conventional oven with temperature control.

Shaping Tools. The most commonly used tool used to create custom pads are heavy-duty scissors. Other tools include sharp knives or scalpels and cast saws.

Fastening Materials. Once created, custom pads are commonly held in place by tape adherent such as Tuff Skin and a simple wrap made of elastic and tape. Other methods include using hook-and-loop fastener straps, tensor bandages, and leather straps and buckles; even laces can be slipped through eyelets that are drilled into whatever hard material is being used. This process can be used to create pads for different body parts using simple modifications. For example, athletic tape can be used to create a higher dome when constructing a pad for an AC joint injury to provide greater protection (Figure 20-7). Off-the-shelf items can also be used in conjunction with these custom-made pads to help provide proper fit and comfort for the athlete. For example, shock pads, which are foam pads placed under standard football pads to absorb shock, can be used to keep a custom-made AC pad in place. Also, a snug-fitting football girdle can be used to help keep a custom-made thigh pad in place comfortably.

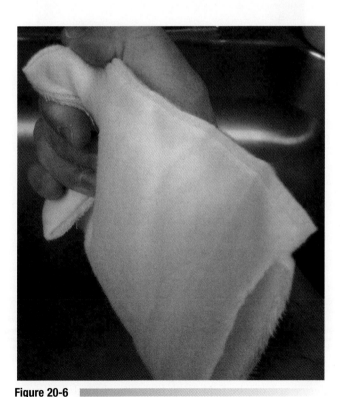

Figure 20-6
Orthoglass casting material used to cast thumb.

Creating a Custom Hard-Shell Pad

1. Select the proper tools and materials.
   - Thermomoldable plastic (e.g., Orthoplast)
   - Scissors
   - Felt material
   - High-density foam
2. Mark the margin of the tender area that needs protection.
3. Cut a felt piece or tape roll to fit in the outlined area (see Figure 20-7, *A*).
4. Heat plastic material until malleable as shown (see Figure 20-7, *B*).
5. Place heated plastic over felt and wrap in place with an elastic wrap.
6. When cooled (usually after 5 minutes) remove elastic wrap and felt pad or tape roll.
7. Trim plastic to desired shape. A domed shell has now been created (see Figure 20-7, *C*).
8. High-density foam can be cut to fit inside the shell. This foam is used to absorb and distribute force. The felt used to create the "bubble" can be used to outline the inside of the foam to create a donut.

Head Protection

Sports Requiring Helmets

- Amateur boxing
- Baseball
- Cycling
- Football
- Ice hockey
- Mens' lacrosse
- Softball
- Whitewater sports (e.g., kayaking)

Football Helmet

The football helmet has evolved from a simple leather cap to a technological achievement in head injury prevention. Not only are the materials used in creating the helmet important, but the design itself is imperative in preventing head injuries. These designs, NOCSAE standards, and rule changes have dramatically reduced injury since its creation in 1896.[2]

A NOCSAE–approved helmet must resist against concussive forces to the head that may injure the brain; however, the helmet is not a guaranteed fail-safe against injury.[3] The athlete (and, in the case of student athletes, the athlete's parents) must be made aware of the proper fitting and use of the helmet.

Suggested Daily Helmet Inspection Checklist by NOCSAE

Each player should inspect his helmet before each usage, as follows:
1. Check foam padding for proper placement and any deterioration.
2. Check for cracks in vinyl or rubber covering of air-, foam-, or liquid-padded helmets.
3. Check that protective system or foam padding has not been altered or removed.
4. Check for proper amount of inflation in air-padded helmets. Follow manufacturer's recommendations for adjusting air pressure at the valves.
5. Check all rivets, screws, Velcro, and snaps to ensure that they are properly fastened and holding protective parts.

Note: If any of these inspections indicates a need for repair or replacement, notify the equipment manager. This is the player's responsibility.

PLAYERS SHOULD BE ADVISED TO NEVER WEAR A DAMAGED HELMET.

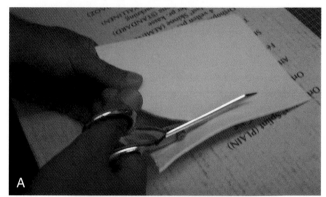
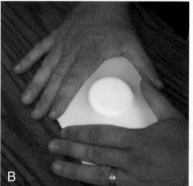
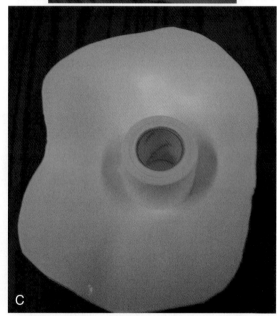

Figure 20-7

Using a roll of tape to make a hard shell pad to protect the acromio-clavicular joint. **A,** Cutting orthoplast. **B,** Molding warm orthoplast over roll of tape. **C,** Roll of tape used to mold orthoplast.

To make this clear to everyone involved in the use of football helmets, NOCSAE has adopted a warning label to be placed on all helmets. A helmet is not legal for use if this label is not visible. The label must be placed on the helmet by the manufacturer and the reconditioner.[3]

More recent technology has improved the effectiveness of the helmet. The most recent innovation is the Revolution helmet created by Riddell (Figure 20-8). Studies performed in the laboratory setting have concluded that there has been a 20% reduction in concussion risk during simulated National Football League game collisions.[12] In studies performed on the field using high school football players, the Revolution helmet has also been shown to reduce the risk of concussion by as much as 31%.[13] Figure 20-9

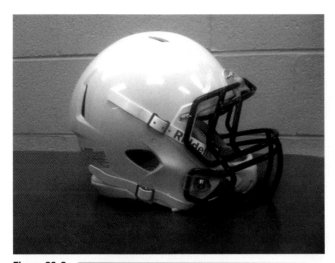

Figure 20-8
Riddell Revolution helmet.

shows various helmet linings, which vary from sport to sport.

Football Helmet Fitting

The coach, equipment manager, and sports medicine clinician must ensure that every athlete has a properly fitted helmet (Figure 20-10). The athlete should wet the hair or wear the hair the way it will be worn during the season. This will ensure that the proper fit will be maintained. Also, various accessories such as chin straps and different-sized cheek pads are available to make sure that the helmet fits snugly.

Helmet Fitting

- The athlete should wet the hair or wear hair the way it will be worn during the season.
- The helmet should fit snugly around all parts of the player's head. There should be no gaps (see Figure 20-10, *A*).
- It should cover the base of the skull (see Figure 20-10, *B*).
- It should not come down over the eyes. It should sit approximately ¾ inch (1.9 cm) or two finger widths above the eyes (see Figure 20-10, *C*).
- The ear holes should line up with the external ear canals (see Figure 20-10, *D*).
- It should not shift when manual pressure is applied.
- The chin strap should be properly aligned and keep the helmet from moving up and down or side to side (see Figure 20-10, *E*).
- The cheek pads should fit snugly against the sides of the face (see Figure 20-10, *E*).
- The face mask should allow a full field of vision and be approximately three finger widths from the nose (see Figure 20-10, *D*).
- The face mask should not move with external force; if it moves, the helmet is fitted too loosely.
- Air bladders can be adjusted easily but one must ensure to do so correctly. To inflate the bladder, the bulb is held with an arch in the hose and bulb (see Figure 20-10, *E*). To deflate, the bulb is in a straight position (see Figure 20-10, *F*).

Chin straps are important to help maintain a proper fit. They differ in many ways including number of snaps and padding for comfort. The most popular snap configuration is the four-snap chin strap that keeps the helmet from tilting forward and backward.[3]

Another accessory used in fitting a football helmet is the jaw pad, which fits inside the helmet. The jaw pads aid in reducing lateral motion of the helmet. They should fit snugly against the cheekbones.[3] Most helmets also come equipped with removable air bladders or have air bladders mounted into the helmet. These air bladders help with fitting and aid in shock absorption.

Ice Hockey Helmets

Ice hockey helmets have improved dramatically during the past 10 years. The hockey helmet, unlike the football helmet, usually must only absorb singular as opposed to multiple impacts. In addition to being able to protect the head during falls and body checks (high mass, low velocity), the helmet must absorb and protect the head from low-mass, high-velocity impact forces such as being hit with a stick or a puck. These helmets must be certified by the Canadian Standards Association (CSA). The use of the face shield has also reduced severe facial injuries. However, one study compared the use of a full-face shield with a half-face shield used

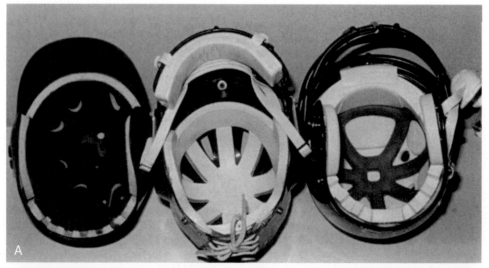

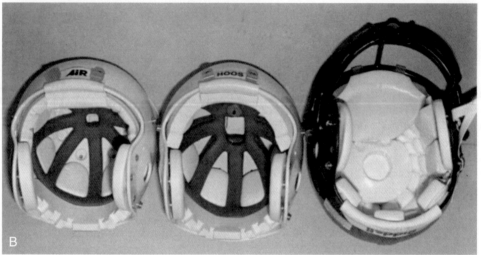

Figure 20-9

Helmet linings. **A,** Baseball, lacrosse, and football air helmets *(left to right)*. **B,** Various types of air helmets; AHI (Athletic Helmets, Inc.) single-bladder, AHI double-bladder, and Riddell air helmets *(left to right)*.

by intercollegiate ice hockey players. These results suggested that use of a full-face shield resulted in reduction of playing time lost because of concussion. It was also found that use of a full-face shield reduced the number and severity of facial injuries.

Baseball Helmets

Baseball helmets must be able to absorb high-velocity impacts. The baseball helmet's ability to prevent head injury is questionable. It is possible that the baseball helmet does little to prevent head injury. One possible solution that has been suggested is to add additional padding to absorb greater shock.[14] Baseball and softball helmets are required to have a NOCSAE seal similar to the stamp found on football helmets.

Face Protection

Face Guards

Face guards exist for a variety of sports. Their main purpose is to protect against projectiles, carried objects, and collisions with other players. Since the adoption of face guards in football, the incidence of facial injuries has dramatically decreased. Unfortunately concussions in football have increased. This has been attributed to athletes using the helmet as a weapon as a result of increased face protection.[3] A variety of bar configurations exist for football depending on the position played (Figure 20-11, Table 20-2). The bars should be secured into holes that have been drilled by the manufacturer. Drilling holes into a helmet or attaching unapproved bars can void the manufacturer's warranty.

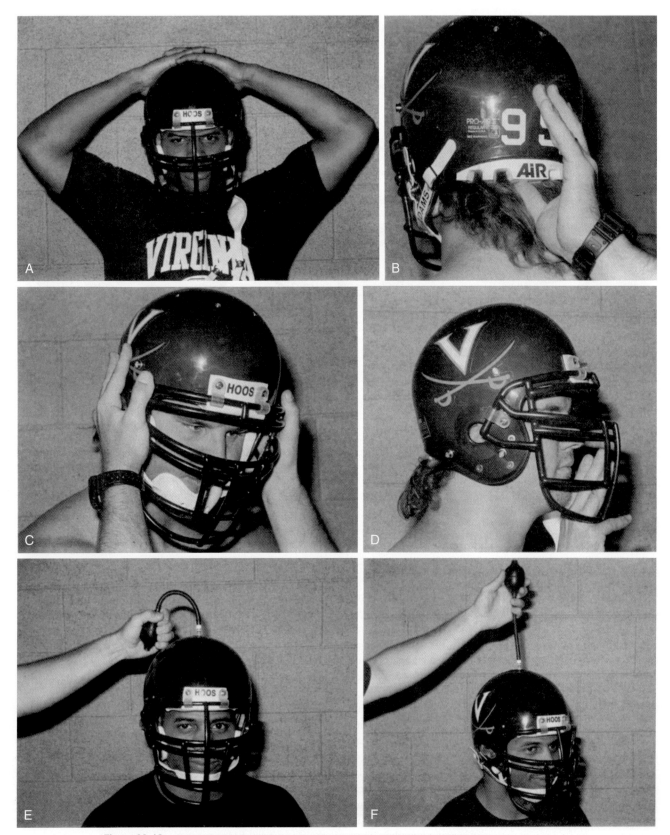

Figure 20-10

Fitting a football helmet (see box *Helmet Fitting* for explanation).

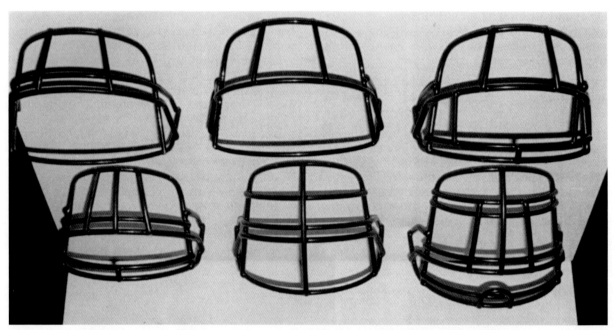

Figure 20-11
Different face mask configurations.

Table 20-2
Face Mask Type by Position Played in Football

Face Mask	Playing Position
Oral protection only	Quarterback(s), running backs, defensive backs, kickers, wide receivers
Nose and oral protection	Fullbacks, linebackers, tight ends
Jaw and oral protection (with or without nose protection)	Quarterbacks, linebackers, linemen

Ice hockey face visors and masks have been shown to reduce the number of facial injuries. Junior A hockey players wearing no face visor were 4.7 times more likely to suffer eye and face injuries compared with players who wore a visor or cage. It has also been suggested that both full and partial face protection significantly reduces the incidence of eye and face injuries without increasing neck injuries and concussions.[15] High school and NCAA ice hockey players are required to wear face protection. Helmets must be equipped with wire face masks. The openings in the wire guard must be small enough so that a hockey stick cannot fit through the holes and cause injury. Face guards used in hockey are approved by multiple agencies such as the Hockey Equipment Certification Council and the CSA. The National Federation of High School Athletic Associations and the NCAA require that goalkeepers wear throat protection as well as face protection. They also require that all players wear full-face protection.

Lacrosse face masks protect the face from impact of either the stick or the ball (Figure 20-12). Men's lacrosse

rules mandate helmets and face masks with a NOCSAE standard. The strength of the steel wire is intermediate compared with that required in football and ice hockey. The face mask is well off the face, but padding around the chin area protects the athlete if the face mask is driven backward in a collision.[16] Four-point chin straps are used on all helmets (Figure 20-13).

Face masks are now available that protect the jaw area and can be attached to baseball and softball batting helmets. These devices can also be used for players on the field. American Society for Testing and Materials (ASTM) standards have been developed, and progress is being made to require face masks on batters in Little League baseball. The prototypes are a wire-cage or a clear, plastic guard that is attached to the batting helmet and shields the mouth and jaw area, with an opening at the mouth to prevent fogging. The eyes are not covered, but are well protected from impact because the ball will not fit between the helmet's visor and the jaw protector (see Figure 20-12, *B*).

Chin Straps

Chin straps help secure a helmet on the head. Certain sports such as cycling and kayaking use a single strap that is hooked under the chin. A single strap allows some rotation of the helmet but is usually adequate in maintaining the appropriate position of the helmet on the top of the head. Football and lacrosse use four-point chin straps to prevent rotation of the helmet.

Chin straps are connected to the helmet with metal grommets that must be replaced occasionally. There are many companies that produce similar chin straps. Different

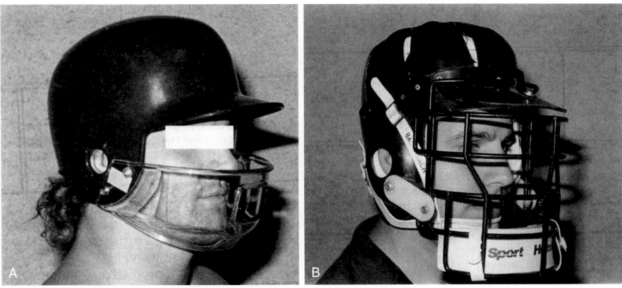

Figure 20-12
Face masks used in other sports. **A,** Plastic face mask used on baseball batting helmets. **B,** Lacrosse face mask.

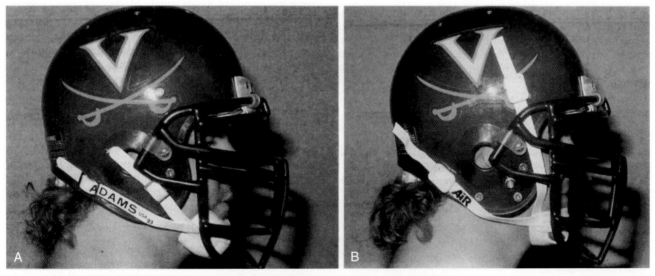

Figure 20-13
Chin straps. **A,** Low-hookup chin strap (hard-cup). **B,** High-hookup chin strap.

styles include the hard shell lined with a vinyl-dipped foam or a soft cup made of leather or vinyl. The hard cup gives the athlete added padding on the chin, whereas the soft cup primarily functions to hold the helmet in place. Some chin straps are available in different cup sizes.

In football, the four-point chin straps are secured by either the high hookup or the low hookup (see Figure 20-13). The Riddell helmets are drilled for low hookup, and the AHI (Athletic Helmets, Inc.) helmets are drilled for high hookup. Either helmet can be modified by punching through a marked area on the helmet and attaching a grommet. Some equipment managers have found that the decreased angle of the low hookup means that there is less chance of the chin strap rotating off the chin.

Eye Protection

Special precautions must be taken to protect athletes' eyes, especially in projectile sports such as ice hockey, men's and women's lacrosse, and handball. Besides these obvious sports, racquet sports pose serious risk to the eye. Eye guards should be made from polycarbonate to prevent shattering (Figure 20-14).[3]

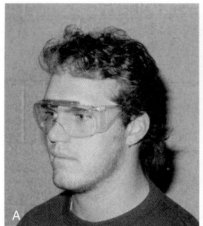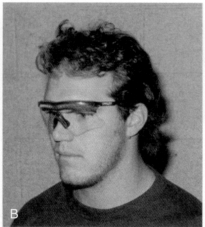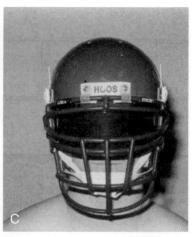

Figure 20-14

Examples of eye protectors. **A,** Plastic and lens are all one piece. **B,** Separate plastic lens. **C,** Polycarbonate shield attached to football face mask.

Types of Eye Protectors

- A *total head protector* is a helmet or face protection used in high-energy sports (football, lacrosse, hockey) that shields the entire face and head.
- A *full-face protector* is used in sports that threaten the face but not the brain, such as fencing, catching, or umpiring. Additional eye protection can also be worn with this type of protector.
- On a *helmet with a separate eye protector,* the eye protector is attached to the helmet in many cases. This type of protection is used in ski racing, auto racing, cycling, and horseback riding.
- A *Helmet only* provides partial eye protection, such as in boxing.
- *Sports eye protectors* are available in different designs and provide protection to the eyes only. These are recommended for sports that do not use other head gear, such as baseball or softball (fielders), soccer, and cross-country skiing. Participants in racquet sports should always wear some form of protective eye gear. The different classifications of these protectors are:
  - Class I—a molded single-unit lens and frame (see Figure 20-14, *A)*
  - Class II—lens mounted in a separate frame (see Figure 20-14, *B)*
  - Class III—protector that contains no lens that is used alone or over eyeglasses

The actual number of eye injuries in athletics is relatively low.[17,18] During a 16-year period at a Division III institution, 10 ocular injuries were sustained in five different sports.[17] Eye injuries can be a common problem in baseball, basketball, squash, and women's lacrosse.[18-20] It has been shown that this is especially true for women's lacrosse players.[20,21] Injury to the head, face, and eye in women's lacrosse is 1.76 times more likely than in the men's game and usually results from a stick or ball strike. Although only incidental contact is permitted, women suffer more face and

orbital injuries than men.[21] It has been shown that women's lacrosse goggles can reduce the incidence of eye injury.[22] Among varsity and junior varsity players, the rate of injury to the eye during games was 51% lower among goggled players than players who did not use goggles. The use of goggles in women's lacrosse became mandatory in 2004.[23]

Eyeglasses versus Contact Lenses

Properly constructed eyeglasses provide some inherent protection, although they have several disadvantages compared with contact lenses during sports participation. The disadvantages include difficulty in keeping them in place, perspiration or dirt that may distort vision, fogging, decreased peripheral vision, and difficulty fitting under head protection. Everyday eyeglasses are not safe in racquet or contact sports because glass or hardened plastic lenses may shatter on contact, resulting in serious eye injuries. Eye protectors with shatterproof polycarbonate or CR 39 prescription lenses give good protection during sports activities. Some prescriptions, however, are unavailable in the plastic.

Contact lenses do not provide protection from contact with an object or another player, but they are less cumbersome, do not fog, and do not decrease peripheral vision. Soft contacts are generally preferred over hard contacts because there is less chance of breaking, and soft contacts have a higher survival rate when they fall out of the eye.

"One-Eyed" Athletes

An athlete is considered to be "one-eyed" if the corrected vision is 20/200 or less in one eye.[24] These individuals should wear appropriate eye protectors at all times to ensure protection of the good eye. One-eyed athletes should not participate in extremely high-risk sports (e.g., boxing) and should be hesitant to engage in collision or contact sports because of the possibility of eye injury even with proper protection. The decision to play is up to the athlete, the athlete's parents if he or she is a minor, and the physician. Legal counsel may be necessary if handicap discrimination is an issue. A signed waiver may be indicated, stating the necessity of using protective eyewear and the possibility of injury to the good eye. Class I or II sports eye protectors should be worn at all times during athletic endeavors, with an additional face shield if there is a significant potential for injury.

Mouthguard

Many high school organizations and the NCAA require that participants in certain sports, such as football, wear mouthguards, whereas the American Dental Association recommends that all athletes wear mouthguards.

The most common types of mouthguards are the stock variety often referred to as "boil and bite" (Figure 20-15). These mouthguards are placed in hot water and then molded to the athletes' teeth by the athlete biting on the heated mouthguard. Another type is the custom-made mouthguard that is fitted to the athlete's maxillary arch by a dentist. Custom-made mouthguards are produced from molds made of the athlete's teeth. These devices are preferred by athletes because they make it easier to breathe and talk during play and generally feel more comfortable. However, cost may inhibit the use of custom mouthguards. Simple boil-and-bite mouthguards are as effective as custom pads and can be bought in bulk to fit an entire team.

The majority of dental trauma can be prevented by using a correctly fitted mouthguard. Mouthguards should never be cut down or modified. This would void the manufacturer's warranty and might create an obstructed airway. Mouthguards have also been shown to reduce shock from blows to the chin. Testing of the neurocognitive abilities of athletes who had suffered a concussion showed no difference between athletes who used mouthguards and those who did not. This suggests that mouthguards do not prevent or reduce the incidence of concussions.[25] Despite these findings, some manufacturers of different types of mouthguards have made claims that wearing their mouthguards can prevent concussions. The Brain Pad, manufactured by WIPSS, is an example of one of these mouthguards. It has been shown that there is no significant difference in the rate of concussion among football and rugby players using standard boil-and-bite mouthguards and the Brain Pad.[26]

Ear Protectors

The ears are protected from shearing forces and contusions by most helmets. Even though helmets are not used in boxing, wrestling, and water polo, ear protection is required because of the high incidence of ear injury in these sports. "Cauliflower ear," a hematoma in the outer ear, may occur without the use of appropriate equipment. This hematoma often requires aspiration, and a splint is applied to maintain pressure and prevent the hematoma from returning. If adequate pressure is not maintained, the blood and exudate collect between the skin and cartilage and may solidify, causing a permanent deformity. This type of injury is preventable with appropriate ear protection (Figure 20-16).[6]

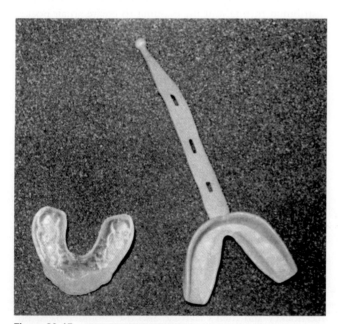

Figure 20-15
Examples of mouthguards; custom *(left)* and heat-molded *(right)*. Note that the heat-molded mouthguard has a face-guard attachment to attach the mouthguard to the face guard to prevent the mouthguard from being swallowed and to make it easier to remove.

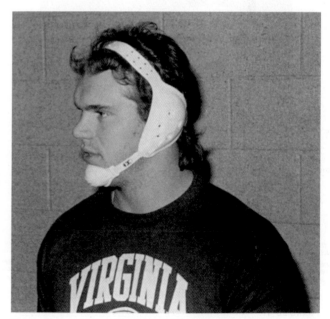

Figure 20-16
Example of ear protector: wrestling head gear.

Neck Protection

The effectiveness of neck protection is debatable. It has been shown in the laboratory setting that most neck protection does not protect from cervical injuries such as "burners."[27] Most neck protectors serve as more of a reminder to use proper technique while tackling (Figure 20-17). The anterior neck or larynx must be protected in sports that use a high-velocity projectile such as a baseball, hockey puck, or lacrosse ball and from sharp objects such as skates. Goalies and catchers are especially susceptible to injuries in this area and should wear hanging plastic shields from their face masks (Figure 20-18).

Upper-Extremity Protection

Football Shoulder Pads

Football shoulder pads are split into two types—cantilevered and noncantilevered—and are issued to players in different positions. A channel system has been incorporated into both the cantilever and the flat pads. The channel system uses a series of long, thinner pads that are attached by hook-and-loop fasteners into the shoulder pads. The pads are fitted to the athlete so that there is air space at the AC joint.[8] The

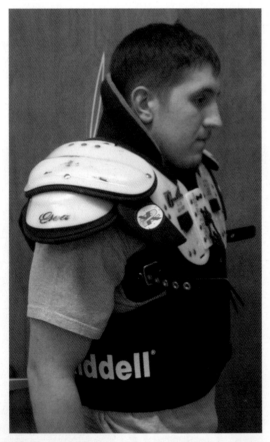

Figure 20-17
Neck protector used in football to prevent cervical extension and side flexion.

pressure is placed entirely on the anterior and posterior aspect of the shoulder. Many think that this system provides maximal protection when the pads are properly fitted and the inner pads are aligned to the individual (Figure 20-19).

Players who perform primarily tackling and blocking are given cantilevered pads (Figure 20-20). Cantilever pads are so named because of the hard plastic bridge they make over the superior aspect of the shoulder to protect the AC joint. They are now built to be lightweight, allow maximum range of motion, and distribute the force and pressure of a blow throughout the entire shoulder, chest, and back. Cantilever pads come in three types: inside, outside, and double cantilever. The inside cantilever fits under the arch of the shoulder pads and rests against the shoulder. It is more common because it is less bulky than the outside cantilever. The outside cantilever sits on top of the pad, outside of the arch. It provides a larger blocking surface and affords more protection to those who are in constant contact, such as linemen. The double cantilever, which is a combination of both the inside and the outside cantilever, affords a player the greatest amount of protection but is not feasible for all positions because of its bulk.

Players such as quarterbacks are given noncantilevered pads because they provide more freedom of movement. Flat pads (see Figure 20-19) do not use the cantilever struts and generally allow greater mobility. These pads are different from the earlier generation of flat pads because they use the "air management" system. The air management system is a combination of both open- and closed-cell foam pads encased in nylon, which are placed under the protective hard plastic. When contact is made with the shoulder, air is distributed throughout the padding to create an air pocket between the athlete and the shoulder pads. Flat pads are generally used by receivers and quarterbacks because they are lightweight and less restricting. However, they are becoming more popular for offensive linemen who principally use their hands to block. The flat pads must use the belt buckle strapping to create an archlike effect in the pads and to minimize pad displacement. The elastic webbing straps typically used in shoulder pads are inadequate for proper stabilization of flat pads.[28]

Football shoulder pads are generally made of lightweight yet hard plastic on the exterior that can effectively deflect a blow. The inner lining of the shoulder pads is composed of closed-cell or open-cell padding that absorbs the shock and distributes it over a broad area. Football pads provide the ultimate protection for the shoulder, clavicle, sternum, and scapula. Attachments can be added to the equipment to provide protection to the cervical spine, upper extremity, abdomen, ribs, flank, and back (Figure 20-21 and Figure 20-22). Ice hockey and men's lacrosse also use shoulder pads, but they are not as extensive or as protective as the football pads (Figure 20-23).

In addition to the cantilever, the football shoulder pads consist of an arch, two sets of epaulets, shoulder

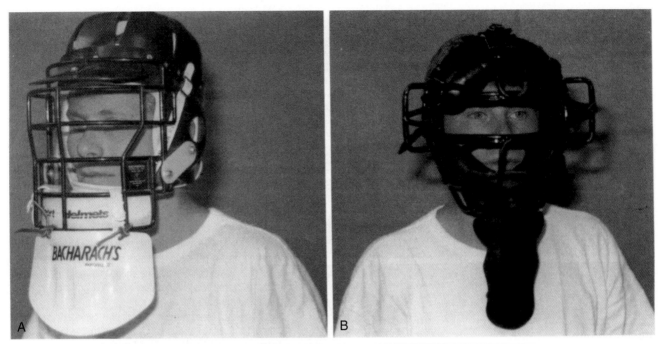

Figure 20-18
Examples of throat protectors. **A,** Throat protection for lacrosse goalie. **B,** Larynx extension for baseball catcher.

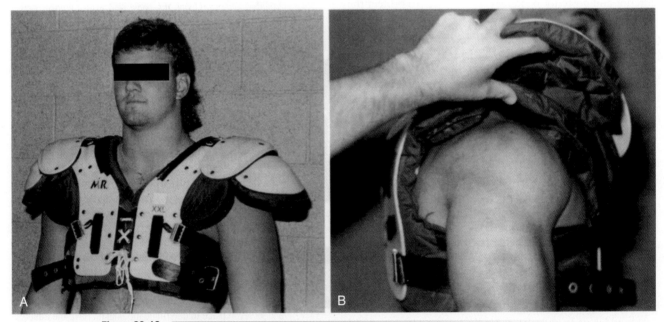

Figure 20-19
Examples of flat pads. **A,** Flat pad with belt attachment to help maintain an "air" pocket at the top of the shoulder on impact. **B,** Channel system features wedges of hook-and-loop fasteners on the inside of pads to protect the AC joint.

cups, and anterior and posterior pads. The arch around the cantilever is shaped to fit the contour of the upper body. The shoulder flaps (also called *epaulets*) extend from the edge of the arch over the shoulder caps. These further protect the top of the entire shoulder area. The shoulder cups also attach to the arch and are located just below the epaulets and should cover the deltoid. The posterior pads cover the trapezius and other posterior muscles in addition to covering the scapula and spine. The anterior pads cover the pectoral muscles as well as the sternum and clavicle. Anterior pads may be slanted forward or even built up in pads made for linebackers and

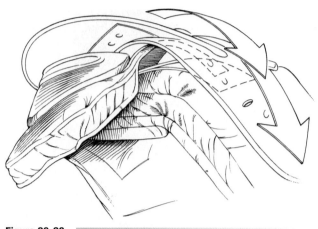

Figure 20-20
Schematic of cantilever pads.

others who routinely receive blows anteriorly or from an upright position.

Pads should be selected based on the athlete's position, body type, and history of injury.[28,29] Playing position often determines what style of shoulder pad is used. For example, anterior and posterior padding extends lower to protect the sternum and ribs of linemen, linebackers, and fullbacks, whereas defensive ends require the greater protection of larger cups and flaps for tackling. Offensive backs and receivers require smaller shoulder cups and flaps to allow them greater mobility when passing and catching. Cantilevers also come in different sizes so that quarterbacks and receivers who need more glenohumeral movement are not restricted. Linemen, who require little glenohumeral movement but need more protection against constant contact, use larger cantilevers. The shoulder pad can be customized by the equipment manager in many ways to give greater protection from injury or to make the pads lighter and more mobile. For example, a drop-back passer may not need as much padding as a running quarterback. A speed receiver who does not catch balls in the middle of the field requires less padding than a receiver who blocks or catches in the middle of the field. A fullback needs enhanced protection because of his constant hitting with or without the ball.

Shoulder pads must be correctly fitted and be in good condition to provide optimal protection for an athlete.[28,29] Each athlete must be fitted with quality equipment by knowledgeable personnel (Figure 20-24). Many injuries are caused by improper fit of the equipment rather than design flaws. Consultation with an athletic trainer or sports physical medicine clinician may be necessary to address unique medical conditions and whether additional padding may be necessary. A foam underpad, sometimes known as "shock pads," can be fitted underneath shoulder pads to provide extra protection.

Fitting Protocol for Football Shoulder Pads

1. Check pads for possible damage.
2. Review personal and medical history (e.g., history of acromioclavicular joint sprains, burners).
3. Fit without a T-shirt to allow visualization of body parts.
4. Use the chest girth measured at the nipple line or measure the distance between shoulder tips to determine size. Body weight is used by some manufacturers to determine initial size.
5. Select pads for player's position.
6. Place the shoulder pads on the player and tighten all straps and laces. The laces should be pulled together until touching. Tension on straps should be equal on both sides and as tight as functionally tolerable to ensure proper force distribution of the pads. Check to see that the clavicle is covered completely and that the neck opening is large enough for comfort but not too large, as this will allow exposure of the clavicles when the arms are raised. There should be enough room on either side of the neck roll to allow comfort when the arms are raised fully (see Figure 20-24, *A*).
7. *Anterior view:* Make sure the laces are centered over the sternum and that there is no gap between the two halves. There should be full coverage of the acromioclavicular joint, clavicles, pectoral muscles, and trapezius muscles. Caps should cover the deltoid muscles. The medial aspects of the clavicles should not be exposed. If the clavicles can be palpated without moving the pads, refit with a smaller pad. The inner padding (under the deltoid caps) should align with the tips of the shoulders. This fit can be confirmed by placing a ruler vertically on the lateral aspect of the deltoid muscle. The pads should align with the vertical ruler within half an inch (see Figure 20-24*B*).
8. *Lateral view:* The acromioclavicular joint is protected by the channel or cantilever system. Raise the deltoid cap and visualize if the channel or air space is in the proper location. This can be assessed by running a hand along the clavicle. The deltoid should be adequately covered by the deltoid cap (see Figure 20-24*C*).
9. *Posterior view:* There should be full coverage of the scapulae and rhomboid muscles. The latissimus should be adequately covered. The laces should be pulled together slightly and should be centered over the spine.
10. The axillary straps or belts should be secured so that the pads do not shift. The straps should be tight enough to allow only two fingers to be inserted under the strap. The strap is not tight enough if the hand can be slid under the straps or pad.
11. *Final inspection:* Check the shoulder pads with the helmet and jersey in place to determine the final fit. Have the athlete raise his arms to ensure comfort and no impingement in the cervical region.

Additional Shoulder Protection in Case of Injury
Acromioclavicular Sprain

An injured AC joint can be protected in a number of ways. An off-the-shelf item, known as the "Impact Pad," is currently available. It is constructed of plastic and high-density foam. The plastic is thermomoldable and can be

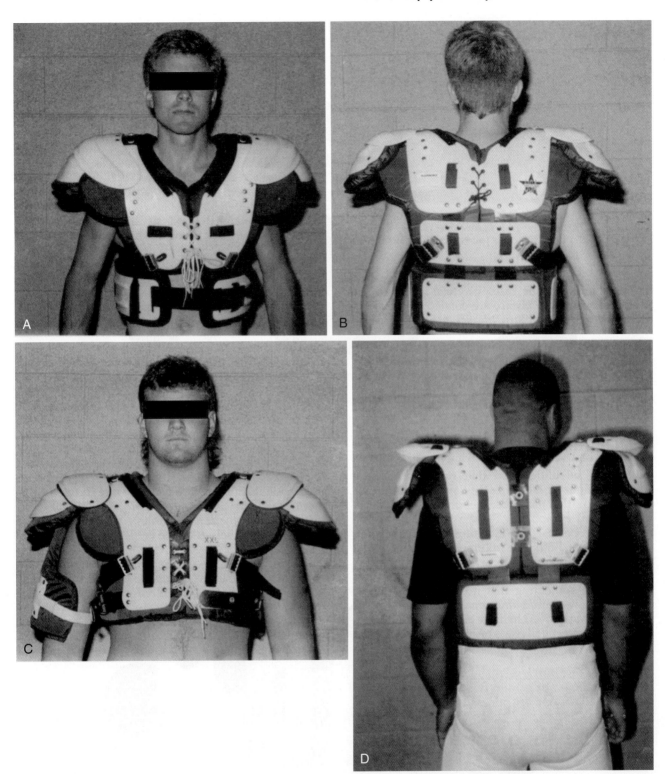

Figure 20-21

Standard extensions to football shoulder pads. **A,** Rib combination often used with football
quarterbacks. **B,** Posterior aspect of rib combination. **C,** Lateral arm protector, deltoid extension.
D, Back extension "kick plate."

ANTERIOR VIEW

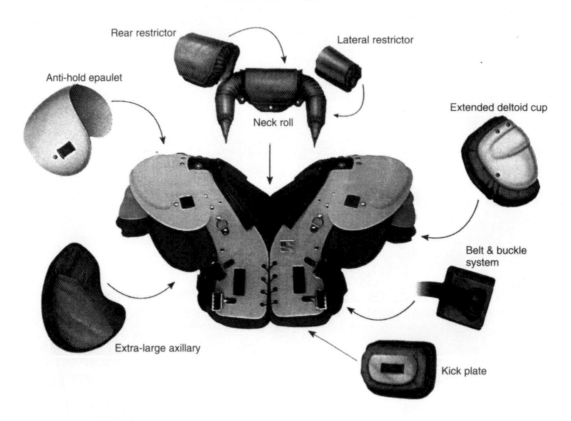

Rear restrictor

Lateral restrictor

Anti-hold epaulet

Extended deltoid cup

Neck roll

Belt & buckle system

Extra-large axillary

Kick plate

POSTERIOR VIEW

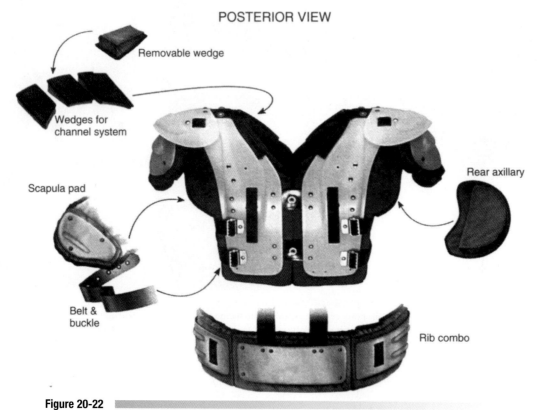

Removable wedge

Wedges for channel system

Rear axillary

Scapula pad

Belt & buckle

Rib combo

Figure 20-22
Shoulder pad components and common attachments.

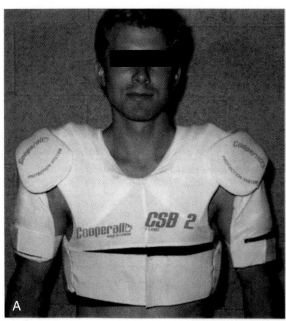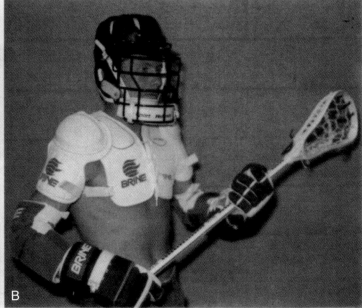

Figure 20-23
Examples of hockey and lacrosse shoulder pads. **A,** Ice hockey shoulder pads. **B,** Lacrosse shoulder pads.

fitted to the athlete and is held in place by hook-and-loop fasteners.

A protective shell such as this can be created by modifying the process described previously (see box "Creating a Custom Hard-Shell Pad"). A role of tape can be used to create a high dome. Once created, the shell can be held in place by attaching it to a pair of shock pads or strapping it to the athlete's body.

Shoulder Instability

Many different types of shoulder harnesses are commercially available. They are popular among athletes in collision-type sports. One example of a commercially available harness is the Sully Stabilizer. It has been shown that shoulder harnesses can limit the shoulder's range of motion. These devices are designed to limit external rotation and abduction.[30]

Elbow, Wrist, and Hand Protection

Injuries to the hands or fingers are among the most common injuries in sports—and the most neglected. These injuries often cause minimal functional disability, and adequate protection with splinting materials may disqualify the athlete. In collegiate and professional football, no rigid material can be worn at the elbow or below unless it is adequately padded with closed-cell foam. Rules vary regarding the legality of protective equipment on the hand, usually depending on the sport and league. Clinicians should consult an authority about specific rules for individual cases before making custom-fabricated pads or splints to be used at the elbow or below.

To prevent injury to the hand, gloves are often worn in addition to many types of foam or neoprene pads for the distal aspect of the upper extremity. Gloves with silicone gel or foam padding are used in football, baseball, hockey, and lacrosse (Figure 20-25).

The elbow, wrist, and hand also require protection from injury. Many of these injuries are from blunt trauma and many off-the-shelf neoprene-type sleeves and pads are available to provide protection.[3] Injuries to these body parts are often trivialized, but can be debilitating. This is especially true for throwing and catching sports. In sports such as ice hockey and lacrosse, gloves are essential to preventing injury to the wrist, hand, and fingers.

Custom-made protection can also be useful for protecting injuries to the hand. In the case of the ulnar collateral ligament of the thumb, a hard splint can be constructed using thermomoldable plastic to protect the injured ligament during play.

Splint for Ulnar Collateral Ligament Sprain

- Cut thermomoldable plastic to desired size and heat for 60 seconds.
- Cut to desired shape .
- Mold plastic to hand using elastic wrap to hold in place.
- Add padding and moleskin to provide comfort and protect opponents.
- Tape to athlete's hand to provide protection to the thumb.

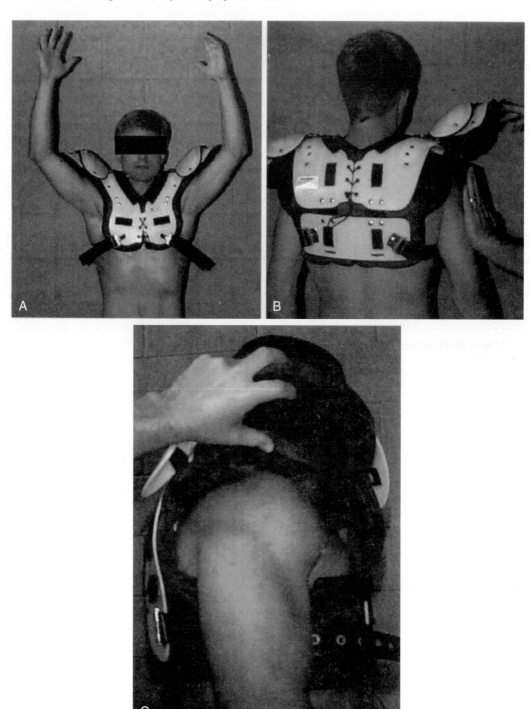

Figure 20-24
Fitting of shoulder pads.

Chest Protection

Chest and Rib Protection

Trunk and thorax protection including the chest and ribs are essential in many contact and projectile sports. Rib protection is commercially available and is most often used in football and lacrosse. These rib guards are easy to fit and can be used by athletes in other sports to protect an existing injury (Figure 20-26, *A*).

Body suits made of mesh with pockets to hold rib and hip pads can be used to add protection to the sides and back (see Figure 20-26, *B*). Although these suits are manufactured for football, they are easily adapted to other sports when additional protection is needed to prevent reinjury.

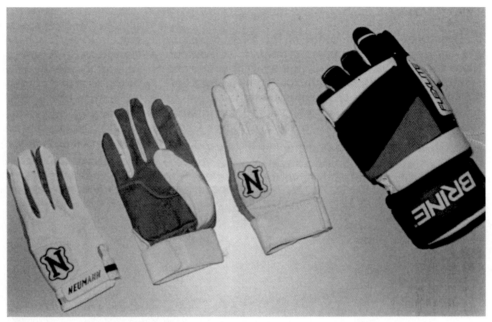

Figure 20-25
Examples of gloves for football and lacrosse. Varying amounts of dorsal and palmar padding are used, depending on the amount of contact.

Chest protection is also very commonly used. Baseball catchers at every level of play are required to wear a chest protector (Figure 20-27, *A*). Lacrosse and ice hockey goalies also wear a chest guard to absorb the shock of a lacrosse ball or puck shot on goal (see Figure 20-27, *B*). Most of these chest guards do nothing more than prevent mild contusions. It has been hypothesized that chest protectors can prevent sudden death; however, it has been shown in an animal model that commercially available baseball and lacrosse chest wall protectors were ineffective in preventing ventricular fibrillation triggered by blows to the chest.[31] Improved technology and materials may improve the effectiveness of such devices.

Bras

Sports bras are designed to restrict excessive movement of the breasts during exercise, which can cause bruising and stretching of the suspensory ligaments. The bra should have wide elastic straps to prevent friction or binding, and all metal should be covered. There should be no seams in the cup area. Sports bras should be constructed of a firm, compressive material and should allow for absorption of perspiration.

Lower-Extremity Protection

Thigh and Hip Protection

Thigh and hip protection is necessary in contact sports such as football and hockey. These pads, made of foam and plastic, are held in place by a girdle worn underneath the pants

(Figure 20-28). Protection can also be custom made to protect an existing injury as described previously. A simple donut can be added to a commercially available thigh pad for extra protection. Muscle strains to the quadriceps, groin, and hamstring are also common in sports. Neoprene sleeves are commercially available to help add extra support to strained muscles.

Properly fitting football pants are essential in maintaining proper placement of thigh and knee pads. Thigh pads should be centered over the quadriceps muscle group approximately 6 to 7 inches (15 to 17 cm) above the kneecap. When using asymmetrical thigh pads, the larger flare should be placed on the lateral aspect of the thigh to avoid injury to the genitalia.

Deep quadriceps contusions are common in all contact sports, although only football and hockey require thigh pads. Athletes in other sports may benefit from wearing football thigh pads in a girdle (see Figure 20-28, *B*) to protect a healing contusion. Some athletic trainers suggest that basketball players, especially those who frequently drive the lane, wear thigh pads in practice. Stromgren has produced a girdle with thigh pads sewn in place; these are easily used with the equipment of any other sport.

Jocks

Sports that use a high-velocity projectile such as a baseball, lacrosse ball, or hockey puck require protection of the genitalia for male participants.[6] A hard plastic shell fits into an opening in the athletic supporter to deflect forces.

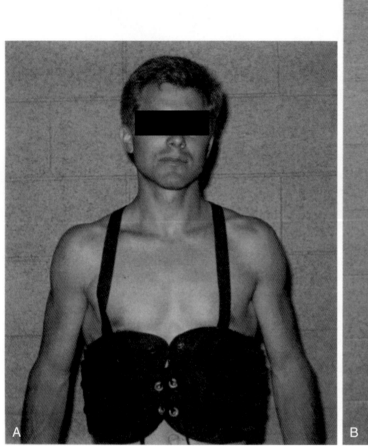

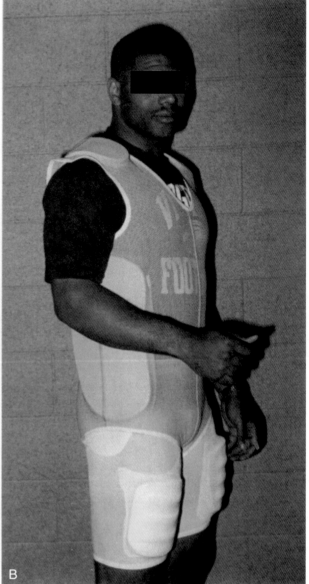

Figure 20-26
Rib protectors. **A,** "Flack jacket." **B,** Body suit worn under the pants and shoulder pads to give protection to the ribs and flanks.

Knee Protection

The knee is one of the most often injured and studied joints of the body. There are many commercially available products to help protect the knee joint. Some sports require knee protection. Knee pads are fit into football pants to help provide extra protection. These are also used by volleyball players to protect their knees while diving on a hard gym floor (Figure 20-29). These pads help to dissipate blunt force trauma but do nothing against twisting or medial and lateral forces.

Knee Braces

Braces are often used in sports to protect the knee from both compression forces and torsional stress. Knee braces are categorized according to their function: prophylactic, functional, or rehabilitative.[32] A *prophylactic brace* is used to reduce the incidence or severity of injury to uninjured normal anatomy or to a fully rehabilitated injury. A *functional brace* provides protection against reinjury following rehabilitation or surgical reconstruction of an injured knee. A *rehabilitative brace* provides protection of healing structures by limiting mobility following injury or surgery. The proper selection of a brace depends on the goal of the brace, the athlete's sport, position played, the cost, and the player's acceptance of the device.

Prophylactic knee braces are commonly seen as hinged braces on the lateral aspect of knees of football linemen (Figure 20-30). Some programs require interior linemen to wear the braces because of the high forces that can be

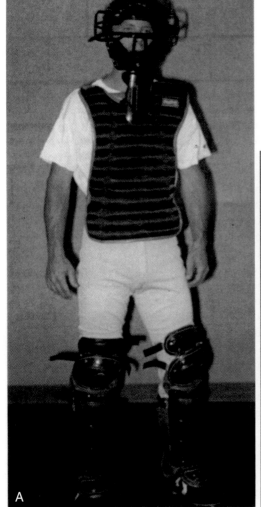
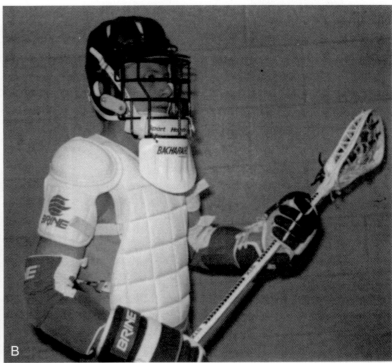

Figure 20-27
Examples of chest protectors. **A,** Chest protector for baseball catcher. **B,** Chest protector for lacrosse goalies.

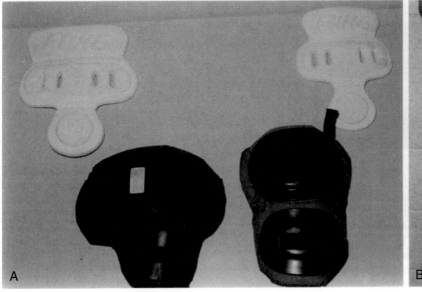
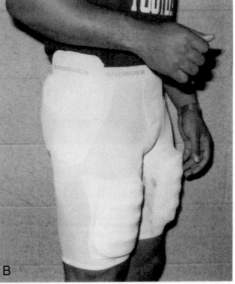

Figure 20-28
Examples of hip pads. **A,** Various types and sizes of hip pads for football. **B,** Girdle with pockets to hold hip and thigh pads can be used in many sports such as basketball to protect an injury.

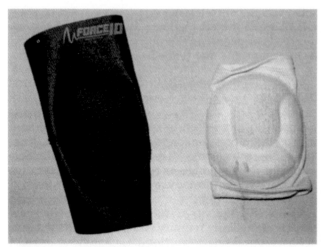

Figure 20-29

Examples of knee pads to protect the knees from impact.

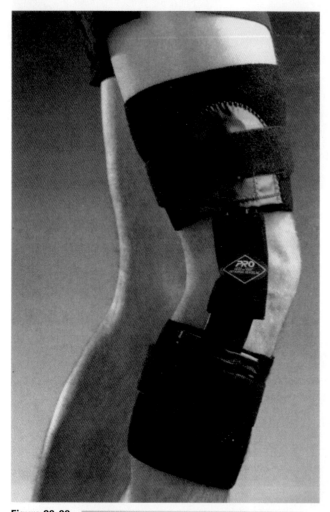

Figure 20-30

Example of prophylactic knee brace. (Courtesy PRO Orthopedic Devices, Inc., Tucson, AZ.)

imparted to the knee during games and practices. Some studies have shown a reduction in the number of knee injuries and fewer surgical interventions when athletes wear these braces.[33] However, other investigators have shown an increase in knee injuries in a Division I college football team during a period when players were required to wear lateral knee braces.[34]

There are various factors that make these epidemiological studies inconclusive. For example, there have been seven rule changes in college football since 1981, when these and other studies were conducted. The rule changes include penalties for blocking below the waist, chop blocking below the knee, running into the kicker, and executing crackback blocks. A *crackback block* is a play in which a receiver runs downfield and comes back to block behind the defensive secondary on a running play. These rule changes were designed specifically to reduce the incidence of knee injuries.[33] In addition to the rule changes, there were inconsistencies in the approach toward medial collateral ligament (MCL) injury management. Some physicians prefer conservative management rather than surgical intervention for grade III MCL injuries. Therefore, the number of knee injuries requiring surgery may not be consistent among testers.

The American Academy of Orthopaedic Surgeons presented a position statement on prophylactic knee braces in 1987 that reiterated the lack of conclusive evidence that knee braces reduce the incidence or severity of knee injury.[6] Prophylactic knee braces should not be required equipment. Functional knee braces are designed to restore functional stability to the knee after an athlete has suffered a ligamentous disruption.[35] Most functional braces on the market today are made for persons who have an anterior cruciate ligament (ACL)–deficient knee (Figure 20-31).

Clinical Note

The decision to wear braces should be made on an individual basis, and lateral knee stabilizers should be available if they make the athlete feel more confident.

The Anterior Cruciate Ligament–Deficient Knee

The Lenox Hill–type derotation brace has been widely used to provide stability in the ACL-deficient or reconstructed knee (Figure 20-32). It has been shown that 69% of patients have reported that the brace provided a significant reduction in episodes of "giving way" in the nonelite athlete.[36] This subjective report is promising, but the main function of the ACL is to provide stability in the knee as it provides 86% of primary restraint against anterior tibial translation. Bracing has been said to reduce this anterior translation of the tibia. It has been shown that bracing the ACL-deficient knee does reduce anterior translation during

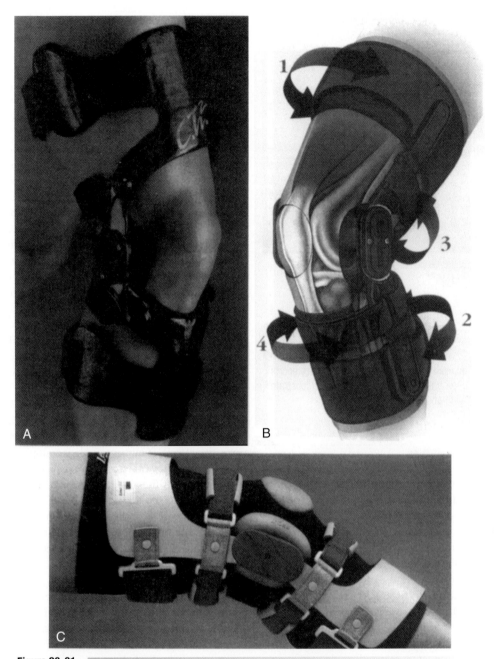

Figure 20-31
Examples of functional knee braces. **A,** CTi2 brace. **B,** Don Joy Defiance four-point brace. **C,** Lennox Hill precision-fit brace.

nonweightbearing and weightbearing activity.[37] However, during the transition from nonweightbearing to weight-bearing, or during high-impact loading, bracing has not been shown to stop anterior tibial translation.[38]

When dealing with the reconstructed knee, it is the authors' opinion that physicians seem to be prescribing braces to patients less often than in the past. Surveys given to physicians regarding whether to brace or not are varied. This suggests that there is a lack of consistency and scientific basis for bracing of the ACL-deficient or reconstructed knee.[39] This being said, it has been shown that skiers who do not wear a derotation brace after ACL reconstruction are 2.74 times more likely to suffer a recurrent tear than skiers who are braced. This positive effect of bracing reconstructed knees has not yet been shown to translate into other high-velocity or high-impact sports.

Functional knee braces can be used during rehabilitation to give an athlete added security and stability with early activity. It should be reiterated to the athlete that the brace can help control stability, but it does not replace strengthening of the limb, and the brace cannot prevent all injury.

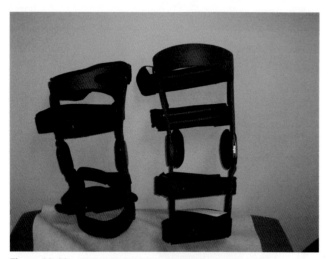

Figure 20-32
Lennox Hill derotation braces.

Clinical Note

No athlete should be allowed to participate fully in contact sports unless he or she has been fully rehabilitated and can demonstrate functional activity both with and without the brace.

The disadvantages of knee bracing during competition include cost; weight; difficulty in sizing; and breakdown of hook-and-loop fasteners, buckles, and elastic straps. Migration of the brace during vigorous activities severely affects its ability to stabilize the knee. In addition, psychological dependency may adversely affect an athlete in competition. Braces should not create a threat to other players and should be well padded on all metal surfaces. Many braces are now fabricated so that no metal is exposed, eliminating the need for additional padding.

Rehabilitative knee braces have three functions: to provide rigid immobilization at a selected angle, to permit controlled range of motion through predetermined arcs, and to provide protection from accidental loading in non-weightbearing patients.[35] When choosing a rehabilitative knee brace, accurate control of range of motion, limited migration, and edema control should be considered. The brace should be able to conform to various leg sizes and shapes. This is important, because muscular atrophy usually occurs postoperatively.

Lateral Knee Support and the Medial Collateral Ligament

Studies using both cadaveric models and human volunteers have shown that lateral knee bracing (see Figure 20-30) provides no significant protection to the MCL. This is especially true in cadaveric models in which it was shown that the brace tended to preload the MCL.

Prophylactic Knee Bracing in Football

A variety of knee braces are commercially available to help prevent or to protect from injuries. Protective knee braces such as functional braces and lateral hinge braces have been used prophylactically to prevent injury. This is especially true in football. There is some controversy surrounding the use of prophylactic braces. There has been concern over how effective such bracing is in preventing collateral ligament damage. Several studies conducted during the past 10 years have offered varying views on the effectiveness of prophylactic knee protection.[40-42] Studies in the past have suggested that prophylactic knee bracing has some inconsistent effect on reducing knee injury.[40] Among 1396 cadets at the United States Military Academy, there was no significant reduction in the severity of MCL or ACL injuries. Any reduction in the frequency of injury was specific to the position played in football. Defensive players had statistically fewer knee injuries than the control group, whereas there was no difference in offensive players.[40] More recent studies have also suggested that there is consistent injury reduction that is not statistically significant.[43] The research showed reduction in injuries to the linemen, linebackers, and tight-end groups. Bracing tended to offer some protection to assaults on the MCL resulting from direct contact such as a valgus blow. There may also be some negative effects. Symptoms such as cramping and fatigue have been reported by athletes wearing braces.[41,42] A more recent examination of the available research states that prophylactic knee bracing should neither be discouraged nor recommended for use by college football players.[43] More research studies using better methods are needed to determine if bracing is truly effective in preventing knee injuries in football.[43]

Neoprene

Neoprene is the nylon-coated rubber material used in wet suits. One or both sides of the material can be covered with nylon, which allows better absorption of sweat and less skin breakdown (Figure 20-33). Neoprene gives firm compression and retains body heat, which may increase local circulation. Many neoprene braces have hinged medial and lateral stays that provide support for the collateral ligaments of the knee and elbow. Neoprene sleeves can also be used to treat patella femoral conditions. Many of these braces have lateral patella stays that are advertised to prevent lateral translation or subluxation of the patella. A modification can also be made to functional braces in the form of an attachment that will prevent lateral subluxation of the patella.[44]

Shin Guards

Soccer, ice hockey, and field hockey players as well as baseball catchers are required to wear shin guards in intercollegiate play (Figure 20-34). Most shin guards are constructed of a

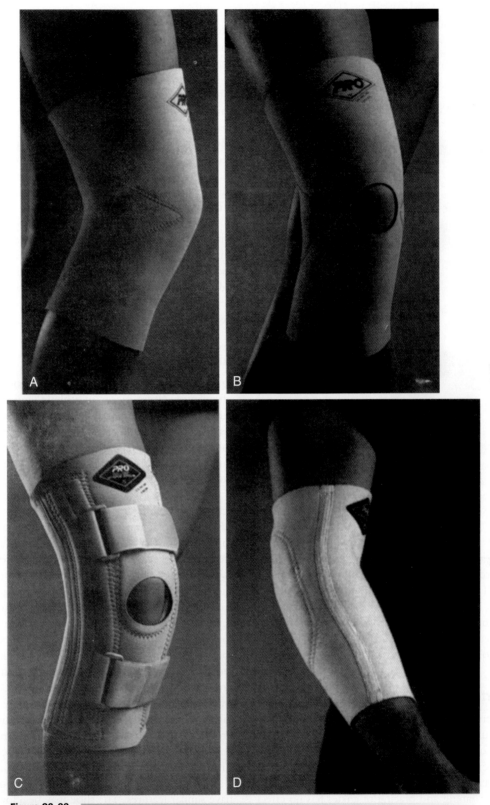

Figure 20-33

Neoprene braces. **A,** Neoprene knee sleeve. **B,** Knee sleeve with opening at the patella. **C,** Knee sleeve with patella stabilizers and felt buttresses sewed inside. **D,** Neoprene elbow sleeve with extra padding at the olecranon.

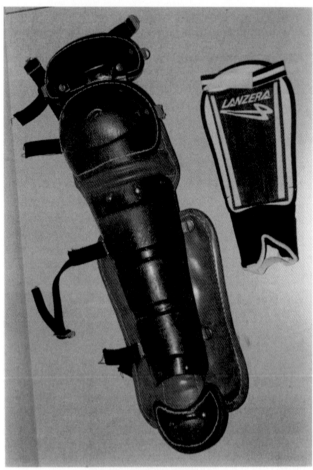

Figure 20-34

Shin guards. Baseball catcher's shin guard (also incorporates a knee guard) *(left);* soccer or field hockey shin guard *(right).*

hard, deflective outer layer and an inner layer of thin foam. Other shin guards are constructed with plastic stays sewn into a felt material. This design gives the athlete a more comfortable fit, because it conforms easily to the leg. Hook-and-loop straps and stirrups help stabilize the device inside the sock. Shin guards can also incorporate padding or plastic shells over the ankle malleoli, which is also a site for contusions.

Ankle Support

Ankle stabilizers, both rehabilitative and functional, are extremely popular in athletics. There are many different types of braces on the market and is usually chosen through personal preference (Figure 20-35).

The effectiveness of ankle bracing is in question. Studies have shown that taping and bracing of ankles has no effect on ankle instability.[45] Still other studies have shown that bracing can be effective in preventing ankle sprains.[43,44,46,47] Several laboratory studies have found that ankle bracing can reduce the forces inflicted on the ankle during sudden inversion and axial loading.[46,47] These studies also find that

a lace-up brace does decrease the forces placed on the ankle during sudden inversion, but a semiridgid brace provides the best protection and was more effective in preventing rearfoot motion.[46,47]

Studies also show that laboratory testing of braces translates into the real world. A systematic review of the literature has found that semirigid ankle bracing does reduce the incidence of ankle sprains, and reduces recurrent sprains.[48] More specifically, it has been shown that semirigid bracing reduced the occurrence of ankle sprains over a single collegiate volleyball season. These athletes wore double-padded, hinged, upright ankle braces at all times. Bracing was effective for this group of athletes.[49]

Bracing of ankles can also be more economic compared with taping. In one study, 83 athletes were followed for an entire season. Six ankle sprains occurred, three in each treatment group (bracing versus taping), and there was no statistically significant difference in the incidence of ankle sprains between the two groups. It appears that bracing ankles can help save time and money and be just as effective as taping.[50]

Footwear

Appropriate footwear is one of the most important and often intimidating pieces of athletic equipment. There are numerous shoe manufacturers producing hundreds of models. The principal concern for sports medicine clinicians is the possibility of an injury resulting from an improper selection. The shoes should be comfortable, prevent injury, and not deter performance.

It is not necessary to have a sport-specific shoe for all activities. Individuals may benefit from wearing shoes specific to their activities if they perform their sports more than three times a week.[51] Sport-specific shoes attempt to provide extra protection for stresses particular to that activity or to accommodate conditions unique to the surface on which the sport is played (Figure 20-36). Running shoes generally have extra flexibility in the forefoot region to accommodate the necessity for toe-off. Walking shoes have a more rigid forefoot to prevent the bending stress placed through the forefoot and toes. Court shoes such as those for tennis, racquetball, and basketball provide extra lateral support to protect the ankle from excess side-to-side motion. Cross-trainer shoes attempt to combine flexibility and lateral stability, but are not advisable for extensive running. Cleats are produced for various field sports and are designed for different surfaces and field conditions, including artificial turf, natural grass, and wet conditions.

There are numerous manufacturers of football shoes that have similar features. The shoe may be a low-top (come up to the ankle) or a high-top (cover the ankle) with different soles, depending on the type of playing surface. Low-top shoes are typically used on the running-intensive positions (e.g., running backs, defensive backs, or quarterbacks). The use of low-top shoes is often discouraged because of the loss

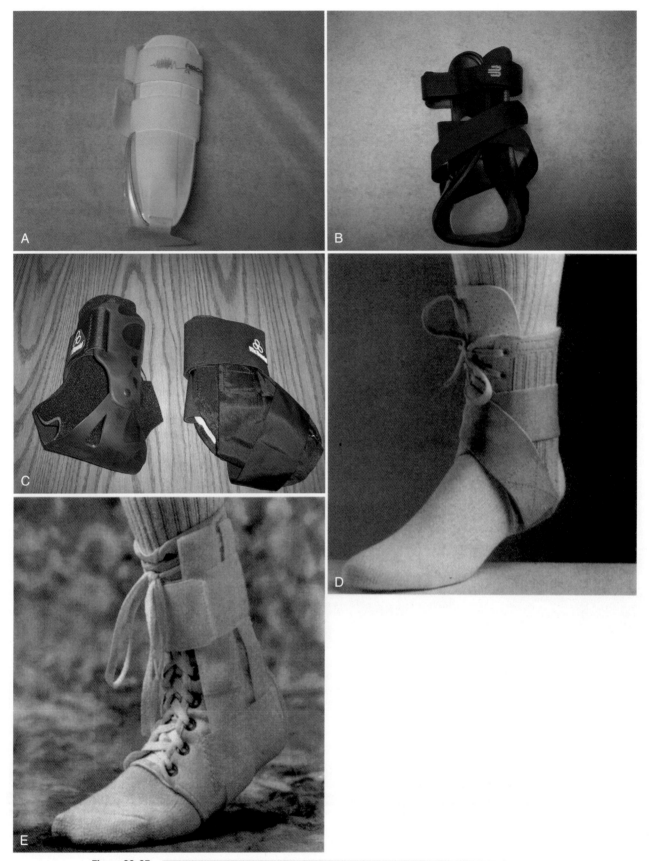

Figure 20-35

Types of ankle braces. **A,** Air cast. **B,** Lace-up figure-8. **C,** Hinge type. **D,** Pro ankle brace. **E,** Rocketsoc by Don Joy.

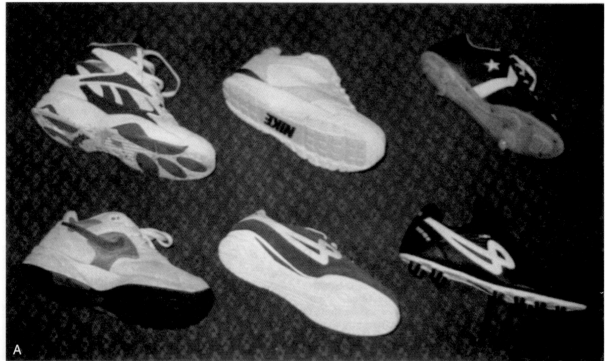

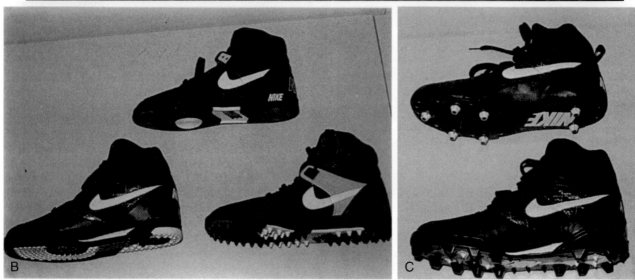

Figure 20-36
Various types of shoes. **A, left to right,** Basketball shoes, low-top court shoes, metal cleats for baseball, running shoes, flat soccer shoes, molded rubber cleats on soccer shoes. **B,** Dry-weather football shoes: flat and "turf." **C,** Football shoes for grass: seven screw-in studs for optimal traction *(top);* molded cleats on outer sole *(bottom).*

of additional ankle support that high-top shoes provide. The use of athletic tape over the shoe (i.e., spatting) to provide additional support is discouraged because of the difficulty in accessing the foot or ankle should an injury occur. The types of soles available for different playing surfaces include:

1. Artificial surfaces (see Figure 20-36, *B*). A *basketball sole* is a flat-bottom sole with small grooves to enhance

traction. Football players, especially linemen, wear this type of shoe on dry, artificial surfaces. *Multi-cleated soles* have 150 molded cleats ("turf shoes") used for dry-weather activity. *Molded cleats* have a molded sole with cone-shaped cleats of varying heights for increased traction in wet weather.

2. Grass (see Figure 20-36, *C*). *Seven-studded soles* have seven removable, or "screw-in," cleats on the bottom

of the sole. This shoe gives better traction on wet surfaces. These shoes are poorly tolerated for everyday use because they provide minimal foot support. *Molded cleats* have a molded sole with large cleats on the perimeter of the shoe and smaller cleats located centrally. This shoe cradles the foot, therefore providing adequate support and comfort.

It is difficult to stay current with the numerous brands and models of shoes available. Finding an athletic shoe store that employs serious recreational athletes can be helpful in selecting appropriate shoes. This selection process should include knowledge of certain orthopedic concerns, such as over- or underpronation, presence of a flat (flexible) or cavus (rigid) foot and bunions, as well as an athlete's physical characteristics and activity goals.

When selecting the size of the shoe, one should not rely on sizing to be standardized. Sizes can vary considerably among manufacturers, and even within the same model and company. The "last" of the shoe can affect sizing, as can the factory where a particular shoe was manufactured. Women with wide feet may consider using a boy's or man's shoe for a better fit. Women's sizes run 1.5 sizes larger than men's sizes (e.g., a 9.5 woman's size is equal to a man's 8.0).

Running Shoe Selection

For runners, the most important piece of protective equipment is the running shoe. A key to remember when considering a new purchase is that if one has a shoe that is working well, do not change models. Changing to the latest model or a different brand is frequently a factor in running injuries.

1. *Comfort.* There should be no pressure spots on any part of the foot. The athlete should not assume that the shoe will stretch out.
2. *Toe clearance.* There should be a thumb's breadth (½ inch/1.3 cm) between the longest toe and the end of the shoe. The toes should be able to fully extend. Make sure that the longer foot is used to determine the size. One foot is longer than the other in 75% of the population.
3. *Shoe width.* Eyelets should be at least 1 inch (2.5 cm) apart with normal lacing. If thumbs are pushed together over top of shoe, only a small "ripple" should be produced. The forefoot is typically the widest part of the foot and usually increases with activity. Shoe should not extend beyond sole on sides when weight bearing.
4. *Heel cup.* Shoes should give firm support at the heel and should not allow heel slippage.
5. *Heel height.* The running shoe should position the heel at least ½ inch above the outsole to minimize stretch on the Achilles tendon. Heel height is varied by the use of a wedge placed between the midsole and the heel counter of the shoe.
6. *Heel (sole) flare.* The sole of the heel of the shoes should not extend beyond the malleoli; if it does, it can cause pronation to occur too quickly.
7. *Forefoot cushioning.* This area should be firm and well cushioned, as most of the vertical force occurs just behind the metatarsal heads.
8. *Arch support.* Provides support along the medial aspect of the shoe. This area should resist compression as the foot progresses through the footflat phase when pronation occurs. The arch support is typically provided by the insole or molded sock liners. The upper of the shoe can provide some support if adequate reinforcement is part of the design of the shoe.
9. *Sole.* The midfoot region should have moderate support, but should not be rigid. Soles that are too rigid can transmit too much stress to the heel and leg, but if the sole is too flexible, forefoot and midfoot injury can result. Hold the heel of the shoe in one hand and with the index finger of the other hand, push the sole up. The sole should bend ("breaking point"), with moderate resistance (less than 10 lb/4.5 kg.) If the shoe bends easily into a U shape, it is considered too flexible.
10. *Sole tread.* The tread of running shoes comes in the horizontal bar or waffle design. The horizontal bar is generally considered appropriate for asphalt or concrete, and the waffle tread is more appropriate for off-road work, where traction is more important.
11. *Midsole.* This region provides shock absorption and motion control. The midsole is composed of ethylene vinyl acetate (EVA), polyurethane, or a combination of the two. The firmness of EVA can vary and is recognized as having good cushioning qualities, but it will break down over time. Polyurethane has minimal compressibility and therefore has good durability and stabilizing qualities. The use of a combination of these materials allows the shoe to provide good stability and motion control from the polyurethane and good shock absorption from the EVA.
12. *Heel counter.* This part of the shoe is considered critical in controlling rearfoot motion. Thermoplastic or fiberboard materials are used, the latter being found in lower-priced shoes. Thermoplastics are preferred, as they maintain their shape much longer, especially in adverse weather conditions. The heel counter should be firm, not collapsing when compressed. A heel counter stabilizer helps prevent heel counter breakdown.
13. *Control shoe.* A control shoe is designed for a person who has a mobile or pronated foot. Shoe helps to control motion from rigid heel strike to mobile foot flat to rigid toe off.
14. *Cushioned shoe.* A shoe designed for a person who has a rigid or cavus foot. Foot provides cushioning during the foot flat to toe off phase because foot is unable to fully pronate.
15. Shoes lose approximately 40% of their shock absorption qualities after 500 miles of running or less.
16. *Shoe last.* The shoe last is the shoe form on which the shoes are made. Most training shoes are made on a curved last.
17. When buying shoes, buy them at the time of day you plan to wear them, and with the socks you plan to use with them.

Orthotics

Orthotic devices such as shoe inserts can be used to accommodate for or help correct certain lower-extremity postural malalignments (Figure 20-37). Small modifications in the subtalar joint position can affect the stresses placed throughout the kinetic chain, such as at the ankle, knee, hip, or vertebra. Orthotic devices attempt to balance the foot in a subtalar neutral position to help the foot and ankle complex

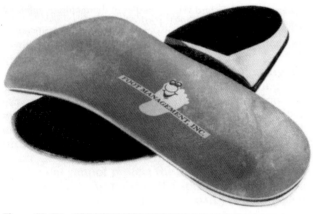

Figure 20-37
Examples of orthotic devices for shoe insertion. (Courtesy Foot Management, Inc., Salisbury, MD.)

undergo normal pronation and supination at the appropriate phases of gait. Orthotics can be used to help control excessive motion of the foot or to allow for limitations in range of motion. Various types of orthotics can be used as part of the total management of stress fractures, arch pain, plantar fasciitis, bunions, shin splints, and patellofemoral problems.

Temporary orthotics can be fabricated by sports medicine clinicians by cutting pads from orthopedic felt or closed-cell foam and placing the pad inside the shoe. Some manufacturers produce prefabricated pads such as arch supports and heel lifts that are easily added to the sock liner of the shoe. Custom orthotics are made from a cast or impression of the athlete's feet in a neutral position. The shoe insert is fabricated from a positive of this mold, and variations are made depending on the postural malalignments of the lower extremity or the symptoms. Posts or wedges are secured to the insert. The sock liner of the shoe is removed before positioning the custom orthotic. The athlete should be encouraged to "break in" the new orthotic as he or she would break in a new pair of shoes.

New Innovations

New technology and new innovative ideas will pave the way for new protective equipment that will hopefully aid in reducing the number and severity of sports injuries.

New Football Helmet Technology

Schutt has developed a new innovative design that is gaining popularity in NCAA and professional football. The new helmet, known as the *Ion 4D*, uses the Skydex cushioning system, which sits between the outer shell and the inner lining. The company claims that this system absorbs up to 55% more impact forces than the Revolution helmet. Other than winning "Best of Show" at the National Athletic

Trainers' Association national meeting in St. Louis, there seems to be no independent literature available to support their claims at the present time.

Football Shoulder Pads

One interesting addition to football shoulder pads is seen in the new Ridell shoulder pads. These shoulder pads are held in place by hook-and-loop fasteners and are now available in three thicknesses to protect the clavicle and AC joint. This change intuitively appears to be a great idea that hopefully will reduce the number of AC joint injuries in football.

Protective Apparel

McDavid seems to be at the forefront of new protective apparel. This apparel features McDavid's "hexpad" technology. Hexpads are available in three thicknesses, depending on the needs of the athlete. The thickest available is dual-density and is ideal for football. Apparel is available in many different configurations. Some of these include shorts with dual-density hip and thigh protection. Also available are shirts that protect different areas and are configured for different sports. For example, a shirt made for lacrosse has padding in the ribs, sternum, upper arms, upper back, and clavicle area. These areas are known to be high-impact areas in the game of lacrosse. Many of these configurations are available for both men and women.

Soccer Helmets

Like football and hockey players, soccer players have started to don helmets on the field to protect their heads. With evidence of long-term neurological damage among some soccer players, some soccer officials, parents, and physicians around the nation have recently been pushing for more safety measures for young players, including an outright ban on heading.

A 2007 study demonstrated that concussions represented 8.9% of all high school athletic injuries and 5.8% of all collegiate athletic injuries. Among both groups, rates of concussions were highest in the sports of football and soccer. In high school sports played by both sexes, girls sustained a higher rate of concussions, and concussions represented a greater proportion of total injuries than in boys.[51] A recent study using high-resolution T1-weighted magnetic resonance imaging scans from college-level soccer players found that soccer players showed decreased gray-matter density and volume in portions of the anterior temporal cortex bilaterally. The study concluded that the damage probably was a result of repeated heading.[52] Currently, this piece of equipment is optional for these athletes but may be warranted.

Conclusion

Protective equipment and its effect on injury and reinjury have greatly evolved during the past 100 years. New and exciting innovations in protective equipment and apparel continue to improve how athletes, coaches, and sports medicine clinicians prevent and treat injuries. The sports medicine clinician must not only know the correct use of this equipment, but also educate the athlete, coach, and parents about the equipment's safe use. The sports medicine clinician must also ensure that the piece of equipment fits comfortably. Athletes should be able to play their position without restriction. They must also remember to care for the equipment properly. This includes inspecting and cleaning the equipment daily. Any damage should be reported as soon as it is noticed. The athlete must also be made aware that protective equipment is only a part of injury prevention and care. The importance of conditioning to prevent initial injury and rehabilitation of existing injuries must be made clear to the athlete in question. The sports medicine clinician must also be sure that the athlete does not use the equipment as a weapon. If these issues are kept under consideration then the rate of injury can be greatly reduced.

References

1. Reese RC Jr, Burruss TP, Patten J: Athletic training and protective equipment. *The upper extremity in sports medicine*, St Louis, 1995, Mosby.
2. Levy ML, Ozgur BM, Berry C, et al: Birth and evolution of the football helmet, *Neurosurgery* 55(3):656–661, 2004.
3. Arnheim DD, Prentice WE: *Principles of athletic training*, ed 8, St Louis, 1993, Mosby.
4. Hodgson VR: National Operating Committee on Standards for Athletic Equipment football helmet certification programs, *Med Sci Sports* 7(3):225–232, 1975.
5. Hodgson VR: Athletic equipment and injury prevention. In Mueller FO, Ryan AJ, editors: *Prevention of athletic injuries: The role of the sports medicine team*, Philadelphia, 1991, FA Davis.
6. Arnheim DD: *Modern principles of athletic training*, St Louis, 1989, Times Mirror/Mosby College Publishing.
7. Rovere GD, Curl WW, Brownig DG: Bracing and taping in an office sports medicine practice, *Clin Sports Med* 8:497–515, 1989.
8. Miller R: *Presentation on protective padding*, NATA National Convention and Symposium, Columbus, OH, 1987.
9. Breger-Lee DE, Buford WL: Properties of thermoplastic splinting materials, *J Hand Ther* 4:202–211, 1992.
10. Mayer V, Gieck J: Rehabilitation of hand injuries in athletics, *Clin Sports Med* 5:783–793, 1986.
11. Gieck J: Protective equipment for sport. In Ryan AJ, Allman FL, editors: *Sports medicine*, New York, 1989, Academic Press.
12. Viano DC, Pellman EJ, Withnall C, Shewchenko N: Concussion in professional football: performance of newer helmets in reconstructed game impacts—Part 13, *Neurosurgery* 59(3):591–606, 2006.
13. Collins M, Lovell MR, Iverson GL, et al: Examining concussion rates and return to play in high school football players wearing newer helmet technology: A three year prospective cohort study. *Neurosurgery* 58(2):275–286, 2006.
14. Goldsmith W, Kabo JM: Performance of baseball headgear, *Am J Sports Med* 10(1):31–37, 1982.
15. Stuart MJ, Smith AM, Malo-Ortiguera SA, et al: A comparison of facial protection and the incidence of head, neck, and facial injuries in Junior A hockey players. A function of individual playing time, *Am J Sports Med* 30(1):39–44, 2002.
16. American Society for Testing and Materials, Philadelphia, 1994.
17. Youn J, Sallis RE, Smith G, Jones K: Ocular injury rates in college sports, *Med Sci Sports Exerc* 40(3):428–432, 2008.
18. Heimmel MR, Murphy MA: Ocular injuries in basketball and baseball: What are the risks and how can we prevent them? *Curr Sports Med Rep* 7(5):284–288, 2008.
19. Eime R, McCarty C, Finch CF, Owen N: Unprotected eyes in squash: Not seeing the risk of injury, *J Sci Med Sport* 8(1):92–100, 2005.
20. Livingston LA, Forbes SL: Eye injuries in women's lacrosse: Strict rule enforcement and mandatory eyewear required, *J Trauma* 40(1):144–145, 1996.
21. Lincoln AE, Hinton RY, Almquist JL, et al: Head, face, and eye injuries in scholastic and collegiate lacrosse: A 4-year prospective study, *Am J Sports Med* 35(2):207–215, 2007.
22. Webster DA, Bayliss GV, Spadaro JA: Head and face injuries in scholastic women's lacrosse with and without eyewear, *Med Sci Sports Exerc* 31(7):938–941, 1999.
23. Dick R, Lincoln AE, Agel J, et al: Descriptive epidemiology of collegiate women's lacrosse injuries: National Collegiate Athletic Association Injury Surveillance System, 1988–1989 through 2003–2004, *J Athl Train* 42(2):262–269, 2007.
24. American Academy of Ophthalmology: *The athlete's eye*, San Francisco, 1982, American Academy of Ophthalmology.
25. Mihalik JP, McCaffey MA, Rivera EM, et al: Effectiveness of mouthguards in reducing neurocognitive deficits following sports-related cerebral concussion, *Dent Traumatol* 23(1):14–20, 2007.
26. Barbic D, Pater J, Brison RJ: Comparison of mouth guard designs and concussion prevention in contact sports: A multicenter randomized controlled trial, *Clin J Sport Med* 15(5):294–298, 2005.
27. Gorden JA, Straub SJ, Swanik CB, Swanik KA: Effects of football collars on cervical hyperextension and lateral flexion, *J Athl Train* 38(3):209–215, 2003.
28. *American Equipment Manager's Certification Manual*, Health Care Forum, Inc. Athletic Equipment Managers Association, 1992.
29. Gieck J, McCue FC: Fitting of protective football equipment, *Am J Sports Med* 8:192–196, 1980.
30. Weise K, Sitler MR, Tierney R, Swanik KA: Effectiveness of glenohumeral-joint stability braces in limiting active and passive shoulder range of motion in collegiate football players, *J Athl Train* 39(2):151–155, 2004.
31. Weinstock J, Maron BJ, Song C, et al: Failure of commercially available chest wall protectors to prevent sudden cardiac death induced by chest wall blows in an experimental model of commotio cordis, *Pediatrics* 117(4):56–62, 2006.
32. Hald RD, Fandel D: Taping and bracing. In Mellion MB, editor: *Office management of sports injuries and athletic problems*, Philadelphia, 1988, Hanley & Belfus.
33. Hansen BY, Ward JC, Diehl RC: The preventive use of the Anderson knee stabler in football, *Phys Sports Med* 13:75–81, 1985.
34. Rovere GD, Haupt HA, Yates CS: Prophylactic knee bracing in college football, *Am J Sports Med* 15:111–116, 1987.
35. Cawley PW: Postoperative knee bracing, *Clin Sports Med* 9:763–769, 1990.

36. Colville MR, Lee CL, Ciullo JV: The Lenox Hill brace. An evaluation of effectiveness in treating knee instability, *Am J Sports Med* 14(4):257–261, 1986.

37. Beynnon BD, Good L, Risberg MA: The effect of bracing on proprioception of knees with anterior cruciate ligament injury, *J Orthop Sports Phys Ther* 32(1):11–15, 2002.

38. Millet CW, Drez DJ: Principles of bracing for the anterior cruciate ligament-deficient knee, *Clin Sports Med* 7(4):827–833, 1988.

39. Decoster LC, Vailas JC: Functional anterior cruciate ligament bracing: A survey of current brace prescription patterns, *Orthopedics* 26(7):701–706, 2003.

40. Sitler M, Ryan J, Hopkinson W, et al: The efficacy of a prophylactic knee brace to reduce knee injuries in football. A prospective, randomized study at West Point, *Am J Sports Med* 18(3):310–315, 1990.

41. Albright JP, Powell JW, Smith W, et al: Medial collateral ligament knee sprains in college football. Effectiveness of preventive braces, *Am J Sports Med* 22(1):12–18, 1994.

42. Najibi S, Albright JP: The use of knee braces, part 1: Prophylactic knee braces in contact sports, *Am J Sports Med* 33(4):602–611, 2005.

43. Pietrosimone BG, Grogaard JB, Grindstaff TL, et al: A systematic review of prophylactic braces in the prevention of knee ligament injuries in collegiate football player, *J Athl Train* 43(4):409–415, 2008.

44. Garrick JG, Requa RK: Prophylactic knee bracing, *Am J Sports Med* 16(S1):118–123, 1988.

45. Tyler TF: Risk factors for noncontact ankle sprains in high school athletes: The role of hip strength and balance ability, *Am J Sports Med* 34(3):470–475, 2006.

46. Tohyama H: Stabilizing effects of ankle bracing under a combination of inversion and axial compression loading, *Knee Surg Sports Traumatol Arthrosc* 14(4):373–378, 2006.

47. Cordova ML: Prophylactic ankle bracing reduces rearfoot motion during sudden inversion, *Scand J Med Sci Sports* 17(3):216–222, 2007.

48. Gross MT, Liu HY: The role of ankle bracing for prevention of ankle sprain injuries, *J Orthop Sports Phys Ther* 33(10):572–577, 2003.

49. Pedowitz DI, Reddy S, Parekh SG, et al: Prophylactic bracing decreases ankle injuries in collegiate female volleyball players, *Am J Sports Med* 36(2):324–327, 2008.

50. Mickel TJ, Bottoni CR, Tsuji G, et al: Prophylactic bracing versus taping for the prevention of ankle sprains in high school athletes: a prospective, randomized trial, *J Foot Ankle Surg* 45(6):360–365, 2006.

51. Gessel LM, Fields SK, Collins CL, et al: Concussions among United States high school and collegiate athletes, *J Athl Train* 42(4):495–503, 2007.

52. Adams J, Alder CM, Jarvis K, et al: Evidence of anterior temporal atrophy in college-level soccer players, *Clin J Sport Med* 17(4):304–306, 2007.

TAPING FOR ATHLETICS AND REHABILITATION

Robert C. Manske and Justin Rohrberg

Introduction

The prevention of injuries has been a longstanding initiative in the area of sports medicine and taping has been around since the beginning. The use of bracing and taping has been and continues to be the choice for many clinicians and coaches involved in the care of athletes. The effects of taping have been reported to have numerous therapeutic benefits. As taping continues to be used by those caring for athletes and their injuries, a true understanding of the evidence as a support mechanism, muscle enhancement technique, and passive restraint for joint structures is imperative. The goal of this chapter is to critically review and discuss the literature regarding the use of taping and provide evidence to support or refute its use in the field of sports medicine and rehabilitation. It must be noted that a review of the literature found a significant variety of taping methods, especially in the ankle. Particular methods of ankle taping were not researched individually as the method of taping can vary greatly and is often left to the discretion of the sports therapist or athletic trainer providing the service. Although the sports clinician should have mastery in the actual taping process, this chapter does not detail multiple methods for taping various joints. Complete instruction on taping techniques can be found in other sources[1,2] and is beyond the scope of this chapter. The focus of this chapter is on the evidence for or against taping for sports medicine and rehabilitation.

Uses of Taping

- Joint stabilization
- Alteration of joint position
- Inhibition of muscle activity
- Reduction of pain
- Altering motoneuron excitability
- Increasing joint torque

Taping for Support

The Ankle

The ankle complex is probably the joint most commonly taped for prevention of injury in athletics. Because of the inherent instability of the ankle, taping is used to provide a passive restraint to the joint in an effort to prevent injury. The theoretical aim of prophylactic ankle taping is to support externally a ligamentous structure without limiting normal range of motion (ROM) or function.[3] Limiting ROM to prevent injury may sound like the best option; however, athletes quickly realize the limits of their functional performance if the correct form of prevention is not used. The most common ankle injury is the lateral ankle sprain resulting from less ligamentous support, lack of bony stability, and lack of dynamic stability often provided by the muscle surrounding the joint.

Meta-Analysis and Systematic Reviews—Ankle Taping

Cordova and colleagues[4] examined 19 studies that included the effect of different prophylactic ankle stabilizers. Adhesive taping was evaluated for pre- and postexercise ROM restriction. Standardized effect sizes were calculated for taping as well as for lace-up and semirigid braces. Table 21-1 demonstrates effect sizes comparing control subjects receiving no taping interventions with those receiving taping interventions. These values reflected both pre- and postexercise limitations of movement. Taping interventions proved to provide 12° of restriction for pre- to postexercise measurements, which is clinically significant. This analysis supports the use of ankle taping as an effective method to limit ankle ROM both before and after exercise.

In another meta-analysis, Cordova and colleagues[5] analyzed 17 studies for the effect of three ankle stabilizing systems on functional performance. Vertical jump height, agility, and speed were all factors in the analysis. Negative effect

Table 21-1

Effect Size Comparing Interventions (Taping to No Taping)

Effect Sizes	Inversion	Eversion	Dorsiflexion	Plantar Flexion
Pre-exercise	-2.33 ± 0.38	-1.14 ± 0.24	-0.98 ± 0.29	-1.71 ± 0.33
Postexercise	-1.07 ± 0.20	-0.85 ± 0.32	0.89 ± 0.18	-1.24 ± 0.16

Data from Cordova ML, Ingersoll CD, LeBlanc MJ: Influence of ankle support on joint range of motion before and after exercise: A meta-analysis, *J Orthop Sports Phys Ther* 30(4):170-182, 2000.

sizes indicated a detriment in performance. Ankle taping had an effect size of -0.14 (90% confidence interval [CI] $-0.36–0.08$) for sprint speed, -0.01 (90% CI $-0.24–0.21$) for agility, and -0.14 (90% CI of $-0.37–0.09$) for vertical jump. The authors noted that effect sizes of 0.2 or greater were trivial and were equivalent to a 1% change in performance for the three functional tasks. Taping in most cases therefore has a small influence on increasing performance, and more likely inhibits it.

One of the earliest and most often referenced studies regarding ankle taping was performed by Myburgh and colleagues.[6] Tape was used as a mechanical restraint to passive ROM measured before and after play in two squash matches. Measurements were taken of 11 players before play began and at specific intervals during and after the two matches. Ankle ROM was measured using a digital goniometer. Tape provided significant restrictions in ROM values before exercise and continuing until up to 10 minutes into match play. The authors noted that the ROM restrictions prior to competition ranged between 30% and 50%. Restriction provided by the tape fell beyond 10 minutes of match play. It was also determined that nonelastic tape provided the most restriction among all types of ankle prophylaxis tested at each time interval.

Garrick and Requa[3] assessed the effects of ankle taping and shoe (high top versus low top) on more than 2500 intramural basketball players during the course of 2 years. Results concluded that ankle taping is an effective intervention in the prevention of ankle injury and ankle reinjury. Players wearing high-topped basketball shoes along with ankle taping had an ankle injury and sprain incidence of 6.5 per 1000 player-games. When compared to the high topped shoe without taping, an increase of almost five times was found at 30.4/1000 games. Low top shoes with ankle taping also found similar results in 17.6/1000 games versus 33.4/1000 games for the no tape condition. An interaction was noted between those with a previous history of ankle sprain and a decreased rate of re-injury. In addition to using athletic tape, elastic tape was found to have a positive effect on stability giving an injury rate of 6.9/1000 player-games. The authors also concluded that, given the rates of ankle injury among this group of athletes, ankle taping was effective in reducing the number of injuries.

Ankle Bracing Compared with Ankle Taping

Martin and Harter[7] used a treadmill tilted 8.5° to simulate the inversion stress to the right ankle of 10 subjects. Active ROM was measured on all subjects prior to testing, followed by application of taping or bracing intervention. The bracing interventions used were the Swede-O Universal lace-up ankle brace and the Aircast sport stirrup orthosis (Figure 21-1 and Figure 21-2). The preactivity ROM was then taken before subjects walked and ran on the slanted treadmill with video observation. Subjects performed 20 minutes of exercise with movements simulating those of athletic competition. Postexercise motion was measured along with a final walk or run on the treadmill that was again videotaped for analysis. Differences were found in walking and running average inversion restraint provided the taping and bracing interventions. When walking on the treadmill, the sport stirrup provided the most restriction both before and after exercise to inversion motion. While running on the treadmill, the Swede-O lace-up brace and sport stirrup provided the most restriction to inversion motion. Taping was not as effective in limiting inversion active ROM as the two bracing interventions. The authors compared overall effectiveness of the three interventions by averaging the restrictive properties of the interventions. Although the Swede-O lace-up brace and Aircast sport stirrup had identical rankings, the authors noted that they believed the sport stirrup provided the most restriction to motion. Taping was found to be the least effective method of limiting inversion ROM.

Measurements were taken before and after activity in a study by Paris and colleagues[8] that evaluated 30 male subjects without a history of ankle instability. The subjects were evaluated under three support conditions: the Swede-O lace-up ankle brace, the SubTalar Support brace, and taping.[8] Preactivity measurements were taken without support interventions for all subjects. When compared with the control group, preactivity values were significantly restricted for all four ankle motions (inversion, eversion, plantar, and dorsiflexion) under all conditions. Measurements were taken at 15-minute intervals with the subjects repeating the exercise activity between measurements. After 15 minutes of activity, all three interventions had lost some effectiveness preventing inversion. The SubTalar Support brace showed additional loosening between 15 and 30 minutes of activity. Eversion

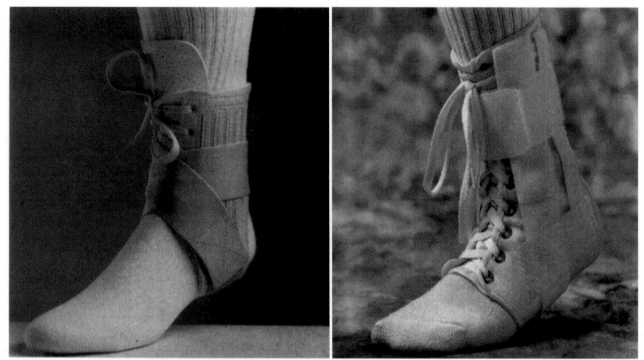

Figure 21-1

Lace-up ankle braces comparable to the Swede-O ankle brace. (From Saliba E, Foreman S, Abadie RT: Protective equipment considerations. In Zachazewski JE, Magee DJ, Quillen WS, editors: *Athletic injuries and rehabilitation,* p 928, Philadelphia, 1996, WB Saunders Company. Courtesy PRO Orthopedic Devices Inc., Tucson, AZ.)

motion restriction was lost in the taping intervention after 15 minutes, whereas the Swede-O brace took 60 minutes to lose its effectiveness. The SubTalar brace did not lose its effectiveness at limiting this motion. Plantar flexion–limiting capabilities for the SubTalar brace and taping interventions were lost after the first 15 minutes of activity, and taping continued to lose effectiveness at 30, 45, and 60 minutes of exercise. The Swede-O brace showed a significant increase in plantar flexion at 30 minutes. Taping was the only condition to lose dorsiflexion ROM limitations, which happened at 45 minutes of activity. The authors concluded that the Swede-O ankle brace and SubTalar brace were equally effective at limiting plantar-flexion ROM. The Swede-O ankle brace was seen to be more effective than taping and the SubTalar brace in limiting inversion ROM.

Passive inversion and eversion ROM was measured in a study by Gross and colleagues[9] using the Cybex II isokinetic dynamometer. Eleven subjects were tested before ankle taping or bracing, after application of tape or a brace, and following exercise with taping or bracing intervention. A conventional form of taping was compared with the Aircast air stirrup. Exercise consisted of 10 minutes running a figure-8 course and 20 toe raises. Analysis revealed significant restrictions in ROM after tape and brace application when compared with control measurements. After exercise, the taping and bracing interventions still provided significant restrictions in the total range of inversion and eversion,

as well as for inversion and eversion ranges separately. The limitations provided by the Aircast brace were more significant than those provided by the tape. Although the limitations of ranges were significant, there was a significant loss of restriction for the taping intervention between the second and third bouts of exercise for total ROM. The same loss of restriction was not noted in the bracing intervention.

Gross and colleagues assessed taping along with the Aircast sport stirrup and the Swede-O ankle brace on the ability to restrict eversion and inversion motions at the ankle.[10] In a design similar to the study by Gross and colleagues,[9] measurements were taken for 16 subjects before application of tape, after application, and again after running on a figure-8 course for 10 minutes and performing 20 unilateral toe raises. Each subject was positioned on a Biodex dynamometer system to assess passive ROM. Each of the three conditions were effective in limiting eversion range after application, each showed significant loss of effectiveness at limiting eversion with exercise, and each was determined to provide significant restriction after exercise when compared with preapplication eversion range. The taping and Swede-O brace interventions provided equal restriction in preactivity eversion motion, whereas the Aircast stirrup provided the most restriction. Inversion limitations were similar to eversion limits in that all three conditions provided for significant restriction following

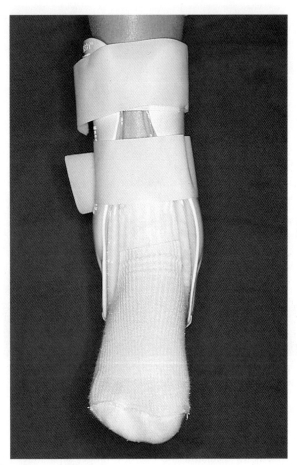

Figure 21-2
Aircast air splint. (From Turner WA, Merriman LM: *Clinical skills in treating the foot,* ed 2, p 335, Edinburgh, 2005, Elsevier–Churchill Livingstone.)

application. Taping did not hold up as well as the two bracing conditions with exercise; it was the only condition to significantly lose its restrictive properties. Both the Aircast and Swede-O braces did not loosen significantly. All three conditions were successful in limiting inversion ranges after exercise when compared with preapplication measurements. Prior to activity, taping provided the most restriction to inversion ROM. After activity the Aircast stirrup and taping provided equal amounts of restriction to inversion ROM, with the Swede-O ankle brace providing the least. A subjective assessment following the testing showed that the Aircast stirrup was the most comfortable for test subjects, followed by the Swede-O ankle brace, and then taping. Subjective assessments of perceived support by the three interventions showed that taping was believed to provide the most support; the Aircast and Swede-O braces had equal rankings. A limiting factor of this study was the use of the Biodex dynamometer system to measure passive ROM. Subjects were asked to remain relaxed during testing, which was assessed by asking the subjects if they were, indeed, relaxed. A more objective measurement may have been the

use of electromyographic (EMG) activity to ensure muscle relaxation. In addition, a passive ROM assessment by a researcher may have been able to assess end feels of the tape better than the Biodex assessing resistance to movement.

Clinical Point

Ankle taping can reduce the number of ankle injuries but its effectiveness decreases with activity.

Karlsson and Andreasson[11] found an insignificant decrease in mechanical instability for subjects with a unilateral ankle injury. Although the authors found that taping interventions did not significantly reduce talar tilt and anterior talar translation when assessed using stress radiography, they did note that the effect of taping may be more restricting at the extreme end ROM, and therefore advocated taping as a possible means of injury prevention.

The effects of two different taping methods were used by Wilkerson[12] to evaluate the stability of the subtalar joint in 30 college football players. Both ankles were taped, with one ankle wearing the conventional method of taping and the other wearing a modified version to enhance subtalar stability. The enhanced version used additional elastic tape to apply a subtalar sling to the traditional method of taping. Measurements were taken prior to tape application, immediately after taping, and after exercise, which included 2 to 3 hours of football practice for four motions: plantar flexion, supination, and a downward and inward complex movement referred to as *complex plantar flexion and inversion*. No significant difference was noted between the two methods after application in sagittal plane restriction. The modified taping method did provide significantly more restriction in the sagittal plane after activity and provided more initial restriction to supination and inversion both after application and activity.

Neuromuscular and Mechanical Effects

A recent study by Purcell and colleagues[13] tested three taping conditions on 20 subjects. The taping conditions used were white cloth athletic tape, self-adherent tape, and no tape. Each taping intervention used a version of the basket weave technique applied to the dominant ankle of each subject. ROM measurements were taken for inversion and eversion and plantar flexion and dorsiflexion using an ankle electrogoniometer before application of tape, immediately following application, and following 30 minutes of exercise activity that included a 5-minute warm-up and cool down. Exercise activities included lateral shuffles, running, figure-8 exercises, agility ladder, and jumping, among others. Analysis revealed the white tape restricted ROM after application of tape but before activity for eversion and inversion ROM. The self-adherent tape also restricted ROM after application for the same motions, and its restrictions of ROM lasted through the exercise bout. Both the white tape and self-adherent tape provided significantly restricted motion after application and exercise for dorsiflexion and plantar flexion motions. There were significant differences found between the two taping materials. The self-adherent tape provided more restriction for longer periods than did the white tape. The white tape lost 99% of its effectiveness for inversion and eversion restriction after exercise, whereas the self-adherent tape lost only 50%. Plantar flexion and dorsiflexion ranges for both taping materials maintained 65% of its pre-exercise ROM restriction.

The effect of ankle taping on mechanical stability and the influences on neuromuscular control of the ankle were studied by Alt and colleagues.[14] Two taping methods were tested using two different taping materials: Leukotape and Porotape. Twelve individuals without a history of ankle injury took part in five trials (control, standard or long-taping method with the two materials, and short-taping method with the two materials). Each trial was assessed for ankle inversion ROM, velocity of inversion, and the EMG activity of selected muscles (anterior tibialis, peroneus longus, and medial head of gastrocnemius) before and after an exercise bout. The exercise bout included injury simulations on a tilt platform, jumping from height, and jumping on oblique surfaces. Results for the mechanical stability of ankle taping revealed 42% and 41% decreases in inversion for the long-taping techniques and 27% and 30% decreases for the short methods before exercise, respectively, for both taping materials. After exercise, 38% and 37% decreases in inversion were found with the long methods and 16% and 22% for the short methods. The only statistically significant difference was found to be the short-taping method using Porotape when comparing scores before and after exercise. An overall decrease of 35% inversion was found prior to exercise. As reported in many studies, the loosening effect was also found in this study; however, it was not statistically significant for Leukotape. Porotape did have a statistically significant loss of ROM when applied in the short method. EMG activity demonstrated no significant difference between taping method and material used. Overall, the taping interventions decreased EMG activity approximately 18% across all conditions prior to exercise. This reduction in activity was also noted after exercise.

As described earlier, Karlsson and Andreasson[11] also examined the effect of taping on peroneal muscle reaction times. Twenty subjects, all of whom had a unilateral chronic lateral ankle injury, were tested with and without a taping intervention, while the activity of the peroneus longus and brevis were monitored. Testing was done on an inversion platform that would simulate an inversion ankle sprain. Both ankles were tested (both stable and unstable ankles) with and without tape. Unstable ankles had a significantly shortened peroneal muscle reaction time when compared with those without tape. This shortened reaction time was not present in all subjects, however; it appeared the ankles with the more stability did not show a significant difference in reaction time, whereas ankles with more instability had lengthened reaction times. In addition to these findings, the authors also noted that taped ankles reduced the reaction time, although this was not noted in all cases, with the most significant reductions coming from the more unstable ankles.

Dynamic Testing

Ankle taping along with the Swede-O ankle brace and the Kallassy brace were examined for their effects on four dynamic events. Burkes and colleagues[15] tested 30 subjects twice on each of four events—vertical jump height, broad jump, 10-yard shuttle run, and 40-yard sprint—without an ankle support and with the three support conditions. The results revealed that taping significantly decreased performance values on all but one of the events. Vertical jump, shuttle run, and sprint performance were all decreased by 4%, 1.6%, and 3.5%, respectively. The Swede-O ankle brace showed similar trends that decreased performance of the vertical jump, broad jump, and sprint by 4.6%, 3.6%, and 3.2%, respectively. The Kallassy brace reinforced the findings of the other conditions of the vertical jump, decreasing performance by 3.4%. In the shuttle run, the taping condition significantly impaired performance when compared with the Kallassy brace. A similar result was found for the broad jump when comparing the Swede-O brace with the Kallassy brace, which significantly limited distance. In addition, it must be noted that the application of any taping or bracing intervention decreased performance, although not all of the results were significant. The effectiveness of mechanical stability provided by the tape and other braces was not evaluated in this study; only the effect on performance was evaluated. Subjective assessments of the three conditions found that athletes felt most supported by tape, with the two braces lower but approximately equal. The Swede-O was found to be the least comfortable, with taping and Kallassy braces equal in comfort.

Future research on the effect taping has on ankle stability should focus on measurements of ankle movements during dynamic activities. The category of research may be more helpful in determining the actual dynamic ranges of motion involved with competitive movements in athletic competition. Meana and colleagues[16] examined the effect of taping on restricting static and dynamic movements of the ankle both before and after a 30-minute exercise bout on an agility course. The course performed by the athletes required changes of direction, moving from a straight run to a defensive slide. These movements were chosen to mimic the motions seen at the ankle during competitive sports competition. The researchers focused on two movements at the ankle complex: supination and plantar flexion static ROMs. Measurements were taken before applying tape, after applying tape, before the agility course, and after the course had been run. High-speed cameras measured the dynamic motions at a particular point in the exercise course. Static ROM values for supination and plantar flexion were found to be restricted by 64.5% and 49.6% respectively. For dynamic ROM values during the course, the effectiveness of the restriction was only significant for supination (13.5%) during the braking phase. For all four ankle motions (plantar flexion, dorsiflexion, supination, and pronation), there was significant loss in the effectiveness of the tape. Supination and plantar flexion revealed 49.3% and 47.6% respectively for static measurements, whereas the effectiveness during dynamic movements were not significant for either movement.

The effects of taping on inversion ROM was tested dynamically by Ricard and colleagues.[17] Dynamic inversion was measured in three different groups before and after exercise. Groups included taping (Figure 21-3) over prewrap, taping to skin, and control (no taping). Four variables were measured using an electric goniometer and an inversion trapdoor that simulated the effects of a dynamic inversion ankle sprain mechanism. The four variables included total inversion, time to maximal inversion, average inversion velocity, and maximum inversion velocity. The analysis revealed no significant difference between taping-over-prewrap and taping-to-skin interventions. However, additional analysis revealed that the two taping interventions did provide significant differences on all four variables. Again, as echoed by previous research, taping did provide for restriction in inversion ROM before and after exercise. Also interesting to note was the decrease in maximal inversion velocity and increase in time to maximal inversion. The authors support the notion that taping interventions, whether accompanied by prewrap or not, may provide for increased effectiveness of the dynamic stabilizers by increasing the amount of time available to react to an inversion ankle sprain mechanism.

Clinical Point

Taping may enhance the effectiveness of the dynamic stabilizers of the ankle.

Ankle Taping and Placebo

The placebo effect of taping has recently been investigated by Sawkins and colleagues[18] who tested 30 participants with a history of ankle injury. The subjects were tested under three conditions: true taping, placebo taping, and control taping (no taping). The subjects were to perform two functional tests (hopping and modified star-excursion balance test) in a random order, each being tested under all three tape applications, along with a practice trial that included no taping intervention. Subjects were blinded to their placement during and after tape application by a skirt that was to cover the applied tape during functional testing. No significant difference in performance in either the hopping test or the modified star-excursion balance test for the three taping applications occurred. A secondary analysis of perceptions held by the participants was completed to measure the stability, confidence, and reassurance of each taping application: 97% of those with the true taping felt more stability on the hopping test and 80% found the same on the modified star-excursion balance test. Placebo taping also showed increases in the three perception categories, with 17% of participants communicating improvements. A side note to this study was that there did not appear to be any functional deficits noted by the taping interventions when comparing the performance of taping with control taping.

FRONT & INSIDE VIEW	OUTSIDE VIEW	OUTSIDE VIEW	OUTSIDE VIEW
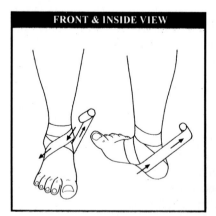	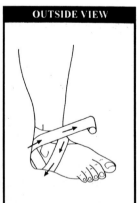	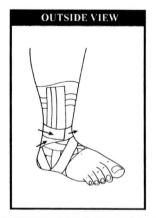	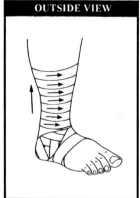

Figure 21-3

The Gibney basketweave taping mehtod, as an example. (From Kennedy R: *Mosby's sport therapy taping guide*, p 16, St Louis, 1995, Mosby.)

The Ankle and Proprioception

Robbins and colleagues[19] examined the effect of ankle taping and exercise on ankle proprioception. With the use of sloped blocks ranging from 0° to 25° in 2.5° increments, the researchers tested the effect of taping before and after exercise on the ability of 24 subjects to determine the slope of the blocks they were standing on. Ankle taping improved proprioceptive capabilities when the slope of the block was great than 10°. Measurements were taken as a percentage of absolute mean estimate error. Subjects in the taped group had an average increase in error of 7% after exercise, whereas those without tape averaged 39%. The effect of modern athletic footwear on position sense was also evaluated, and it was determined that this footwear significantly impaired the ability to distinguish foot position. The authors made strong claims about the role of footwear in ankle injuries, stating, "The inescapable conclusion is that footwear use is ultimately responsible for ankle injury."[19] Citing statistics from earlier work,[20] the authors compared shoe wearing with barefoot position sense and taping.

Refshauge and colleagues[21] investigated the effects of ankle taping on proprioceptive capabilities in subjects with recurrent ankle sprains and found no difference between control and ankle-taping groups when examining motions of dorsiflexion and plantar flexion. They tested 43 subjects at velocities of 0.1°, 0.5°, and 2.5° per second, none of which found a significant difference for the taped and untaped groups. There was no proprioceptive benefit to taping in the sagittal plane of movement at the ankle (Table 21-2). There was, however, an interaction between increasing speeds of movement for taped and untaped ankles. Expanding on this idea may show that increased cutaneous stimulation of ankle taping combined with faster movement may provide increased proprioceptive input, thereby improving ankle control and a resultant decrease in ankle injury.

Table 21-2
Proprioception and Movement Perception

	Inversion	Eversion
0.1 deg/sec		
Untaped	4.71 ±0.78	4.92 ±0.80
Taped	5.18 ±0.67	5.09 ±0.55
0.5 deg/sec		
Untaped	3.40 ±1.05	3.49 ±1.15
Taped	4.02 ±0.86	4.04 ±0.89
2.5 deg/sec		
Untaped	1.49 ±0.62	1.42 ±0.71
Taped	1.65 ±0.81	1.42 ±0.76

Data from Refshauge KM, Kilbreath SL, Raymond J: The effect of recurrent ankle inversion sprain and taping on proprioception at the ankle, *Med Sci Sports Exerc* 32:10-15, 2000.

Refshauge and colleagues[22] studied the effects of taping interventions on 16 subjects with a history of recurrent ankle sprains. An inelastic tape was compared with no tape in the ability of the subjects to detect passive movements of the ankle into eversion and inversion. Three different speeds were used to test for movement perceptions. The results demonstrated that not only did the taping not provide for enhanced proprioception, it actually decreased perception significantly.

Ankle and Postural Control

The effect of ankle taping on postural control was examined by Bennel and Goldie[23] using 24 subjects and a force platform plate system. Ankle taping, along with lace-up braces and elastic bandages, were investigated for their influence on postural control. Each subject was tested under each condition, along with the control. Subjects stood on the force platform with eyes closed and hands on hips. Measurements were taken for 5 seconds and data was analyzed for mediolateral ground reaction forces along with nonsupporting limb touchdowns. Tape, when compared with the control condition, was found to significantly inhibit postural control. The number of nonstance limb touchdowns was greatest for the ankle taping and bracing conditions, with taping having the most. It should be noted that the subjects in this study did not actively exercise between the application of the taping or bracing and the testing procedures. This was done to rule out any variations that might be caused by loosening of the tape and braces, therefore reducing their effect on the postural control.

In a similar study[24] on the effect of ankle taping on postural steadiness, which was performed using a force platform and taping, subjects with eyes open experienced no differences between taped and untaped ankle conditions. However, when tested with eyes closed, there was a significant difference in that taping adversely affected postural control. Conclusions were that during single-leg stance with eyes open, the visual inputs may have been able to counteract the decreased postural awareness found with the taping. A synopsis of all ankle studies can be seen in Table 21-3.

The Foot

Franettovich and colleagues[25] studied five subjects on the effect of low-dye taping (Figure 21-4) on arch height and muscle activity. The subjects were selected for the study because of the low medial longitudinal arch height with the stance phase of walking. The examiners took baseline measurements of arch height in standing and EMG readings of the tibialis anterior, tibialis posterior, and peroneus longus muscles while walking at the selected testing speed on a treadmill for 10 minutes. The low-dye taping intervention was then applied and arch height was reassessed along with the muscle activity of the participants as they walked again on the treadmill for an additional

Table 21-3
Ankle Taping Article Synopsis

Article	Population	Description	Results
Alt et al.[14]	12 subjects	Two taping techniques/materials	Decreased EMG activity and loosening of tape
Bennell and Goldie[23]	24 subjects	Postural control with tape	Taping inhibited postural control
Burkes et al.[15]	30 subjects	Functional performance	Taping decreased functional performance
Cordova et al.[4]	Meta-analysis	19 studies	Taping effective to limit ROM before and after exercise
Cordova et al.[5]	Meta-analysis	17 studies	Taping most likely decreases physical performance
Garrick and Requa[3]	2500+ basketball players	Taping and shoe height	High-top shoes and taping provided best protection against sprain
Gross et al.[9]	11 subjects	Pre- and postmeasurements	Tape had significant ROM restriction losses while maintaining significant overall ROM restrictions
Gross et al.[10]	16 subjects	Pre- and postmeasurements	Total ROM restrictions significant
Karlsson and Andreasson[11]	20 subjects	EMG activity and taping	Taping decreased reaction time of peroneals
Martin and Harter[7]	10 subjects	Running and walking with inversion stress and tape	Taping provided inversion restraint that faded after exercise
Meana et al.[16]	15 athletes	Static and dynamic ROM	Taping decreased ROM values with loosening after exercise
Myburgh et al.[6]	11 squash players	Pre- and postmeasurements	Significant restriction before exercise until 10 minutes into exercise
Paris et al.[8]	30 males	Pre- and postmeasurements	Tape had significant ROM restriction loss
Refshauge et al.[22]	43 chronic ankle sprain subjects	Proprioception with tape	No benefit provided with tape
Ricard et al.[17]	30 subjects	Taping to skin vs. prewrap	No significant difference in inversion restriction
Robbins et al.[19]	24 subjects	Proprioception with tape	Enhanced proprioception with taping when inversion slopes > 20°
Sawkins et al.[18]	30 subjects	Placebo taping	More stability with real taping
Wilkerson[12]	30 football players	Two taping methods	Modified method provided increased restrictions

EMG, Electromyography.

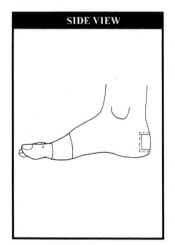
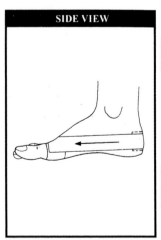
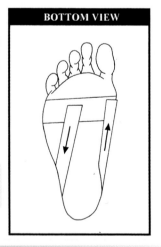
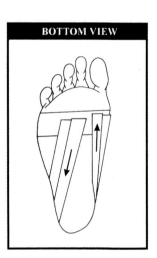

Figure 21-4
Medial longitudinal arch taping. (From Kennedy R: *Mosby's sport therapy taping guide,* p 45, St Louis, 1995, Mosby.)

10 minutes. Analysis revealed that the arch taping increased arch height by an average of 8 mm or 12.9% after tape application. Walking for 10 minutes reduced the average arch height to 5 mm or 8.5%. The taping intervention significantly reduced the activity of the tibialis anterior and tibialis posterior in both peak and average activity. There was also an earlier onset of tibialis anterior activity with taping. There were no significant findings for the peroneus longus muscle. The authors were not able to identify the reason or relationship of the increased arch height with taping and the decrease in EMG activity, only that the changes were induced by the taping.

A study[26] to examine the effects of four interventions of subjective reports of pain and activity limitation included 42 individuals with a history of plantar fasciitis–type foot pain. The four interventions included a control group who received no intervention, a stretching group receiving triceps surae stretching, calcaneal taping to pull the foot into inversion, and sham taping. The subjects received their interventions twice over the course of 1 week. Significant differences were found for all groups except for the control group in pre- and postintervention reports of pain relief. Although there were significant finding for reductions in pain for these three groups, the calcaneal taping proved to have significantly greater results in pain reduction.

The Elbow

Vincenzino and colleagues[27] investigated the effect of taping on grip strength and pain threshold in patients with lateral epicondylitis and demonstrated that a diamond-shaped (real) tape procedure was more effective in increasing pain-free grip strength than sham diamond taping or control. The study examined 16 subjects, who were treated with three conditions: no tape (control), sham taping, and diamond-shaped taping (real). The patients were treated with each of the taping conditions and tested for grip strength and the threshold of pain. Testing occurred at pretreatment, 10 minutes after treatment, and 30 minutes after treatment. The results revealed that true taping increased pain-free grip strength both immediately after and 30 minutes after treatment. The average score for grip strength increased 24%. The results for the pain threshold testing, although not significant, did reveal positive changes of 19.2%.

The Wrist

A study to determine the effectiveness of tape on increasing grip strength was performed by Rettig and colleagues.[28] This study included 20 Division I and 5 National Football League players. Grip strength was measured using a handheld dynamometer. Each player was measured without tape and with a self-taping intervention to the wrist or fingers. Testing occurred in varying combinations of dominant and nondominant hands, along with wrist or finger taping. The dominant hand with fingers taped had strength differences that were not significant, as did the nondominant hand with and without tape. There was a significant finding in that the untaped dominant hand was stronger that the dominant hand with finger and wrist taping.

The Finger

Warme and Brooks[29] studied the effect of taping on tendon pulley failure. Nine pairs of freshly frozen cadaver hands were used in combination with a jig simulating the "crimp grip" used in the sport of rock climbing. The A2 pulley (part of the flexor tendon sheath meant to anchor the flexor tendons of the fingers to the proximal phalanx of each digit) of selected fingers was reinforced with three wraps of cloth adhesive tape. Of the successful tests, the results revealed that the fingers reinforced with tape provided no deterrence to the pulley failure, and did not affect the order in which the other flexor pulleys failed. Also, in 55% of the successful tests, the A2 pulley failed at the same time as the A3 and A4 pulleys (A3 and A4 are additional parts of the flexor tendon sheaths that are more distal on the finger).

Cost Management of Taping

In a numbers-needed-to-treat (NNT) analysis by Olmsted and colleagues,[30] three studies were used to determine the effectiveness and cost of ankle taping versus bracing. The NNT analysis used the following estimations:

- Cost of one roll of tape: $1.37
- Cost of one lace-up brace: $35.00
- Taping interventions: 13 weeks per season with six interventions per week for a total of 78 interventions

Using the data from Garrick and Requa,[3] the authors[28] determined that to prevent one ankle sprain for a person with ankle instability, taping interventions had to be performed on 26 athletes. For those without an instability issue, ankle interventions had to be performed on 143 athletes. Again citing Garrick and Requa,[3] the cost of taping 26 athletes with a history of ankle sprains would be $2778. The cost of taping 143 athletes for one season would be $15,281. This cost was more than three times more expensive than bracing (no history of ankle injury: $5005; bracing those with history of ankle trauma: $910).

Citing data from Sitler and colleagues,[31] Olmsted and colleagues[30] found a similar trend, with the bracing being more cost-effective than taping. The analysis found the cost of treating 18 athletes with a history of ankle sprains to be $1923, whereas bracing the same group would cost $630. For the 39 athletes with no history of ankle injury, the cost came to $4168. Bracing in this same group was only $1365.

Similar findings continued when analyzing data from Surve and colleagues.[32] Taping five athletes with a history of ankle trauma or instability over the course of one athletic season would cost $4534 compared with $175 for bracing. Bracing was most cost-effective for athletes with no history of ankle sprains, with a cost of $1995 compared with the $6091 for taping the same group. The authors[30] concluded that ankle bracing was more cost-effective and required less time for sports medicine personnel during the course of one season. They were also able to conclude that application of taping and bracing is more effective from an NNT analysis and cost perspective in athletes with a history of ankle sprain. These cost numbers did not include the supply costs for use of a heel and lace pad, skin lubricant, spray-on tape adhesive, or underwrap.[30]

Clinical Point

Ankle bracing is more cost-effective than taping.

Patellofemoral Taping of the Knee

One of the most frequent uses of taping is for the evaluation and subsequent treatment of patients with patellofemoral pain. A thorough and consistent physical examination should precede any form of treatment for anterior knee pain.[33] Despite the fact that patellar taping has been used for the treatment of anterior knee pain for more than 30 years, debate still exists regarding the mechanism for its success or failure. McConnell originally described patellar taping techniques that were used to improve patellar tracking within the patellofemoral groove (Figures 21-5 through 21-8).[34,35] Tape is placed over the anterior knee in an attempt to correct patellar static position of tracking by enhancing medial stabilization and/or movement of the patella.

Numerous studies have looked at the effects of patellar taping for a variety of reasons. These studies appear to have tremendous inconsistencies resulting from many variables. The use of multiple taping techniques, different amounts of force used when taping, patients with different forms of patellofemoral pain, use of normal subjects, multiple

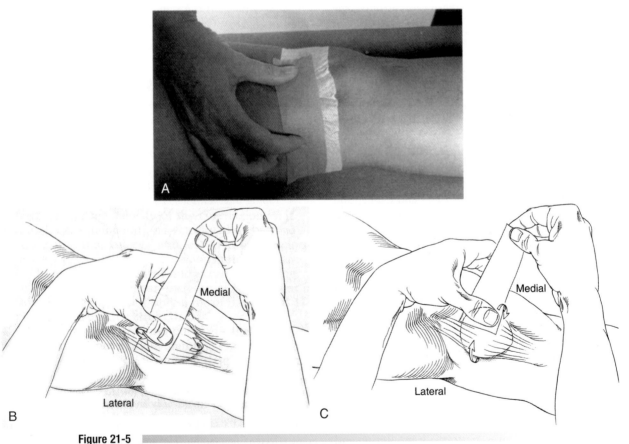

Figure 21-5

Correction of posterior and lateral tilt of patella. **A** and **B,** To correct an inferior tilt, tape is placed on the superior half of the patella. An anteroposterior force is exerted on the superior half of the patella to lift the inferior pole away from the femur and infrapatellar fat pad. **A** and **C,** To correct a lateral tilt, anteroposterior pressure is placed on the medial half of the patella to lift the lateral border away from the femur. (From McConell J, Fulkerson J: The knee: Patellofemoral and soft tissue injuries.)

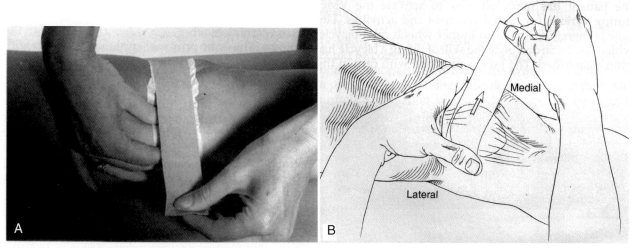

Figure 21-6

Correction of patellar glide. **A** and **B,** Tape is placed just lateral to the lateral border of the patella and is used to glide the patella medially on the femur. The thumb assists in gliding the patella medially, if necessary, while the fingers pull the skin toward the patella, creating a "wrinkle." Tape is anchored on the posteromedial aspect of the medial femoral condyle. Tape is *not* brought into the popliteal fossa, because this may irritate the skin in this area. (From McConnell J, Fulkerson J: The Knee: Patellofemoral and soft tissues injuries.)

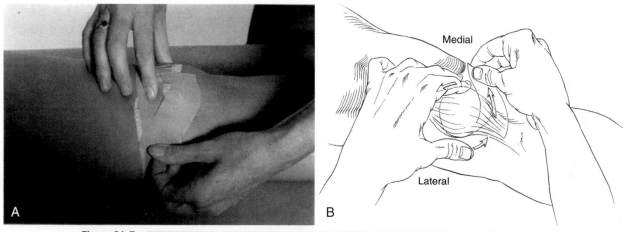

Figure 21-7

Correction of patella lateral-external rotation. **A** and **B,** Tape is initially placed at the inferior patella pole. The patella is grasped with the opposite hand and turned to decrease lateral-external rotation. Tape is anchored as depicted. (From McConnell J, Fulkerson J: The Knee: Patellofemoral and soft tissues injuries.)

outcome measures (visual analog scales, subjective forms, surface EMG, indwelling EMG, EMG of quadriceps muscles, quadriceps muscle ratios) have all contributed to these inconsistencies.

Altered Patellar Position

McConnell first described her results of using a patellar taping technique for the treatment of chondromalacia patella in 1986.[34] The purpose of the taping technique was to correct abnormal patellar tracking to allow a patient to engage in pain-free exercise and physical therapy. Excessive mechanical overload to the undersurface of the patella can be caused by both intrinsic and extrinsic means. Intrinsic factors include a patella alta or baja, deficiency of the lateral femoral condyle, and quadriceps muscle atrophy.[36] Extrinsic factors include hip retroversion or anteversion, hip muscle weakness, lateral tibial torsion, or excessive pronation of the foot.[36] It is purported that this strapping technique is critical for physical activity to promote quadriceps strengthening.[34] Several studies have attempted to assess patellar taping's ability to actually cause patellar positional changes using various techniques including radiographs, computed tomography (CT), and magnetic resonance imaging (MRI).

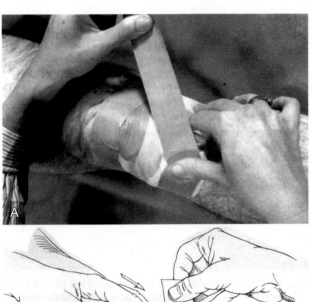

Figure 21-8

Fat pad taping. **A** and **B,** To "unload" the fat pad, tape is initiated at the tibial tubercle. Tape is pulled superiorly as the skin is pulled toward the patella, toward the joint line. Unloading strips are placed both medially and laterally. (From McConnell J, Fulkerson J: The Knee: Patellofemoral and soft tissue injuries.)

Altered Patellar Position—Positive Findings

Herrington recently examined lateral patella displacement (LPD) in eight subjects with a history of patellofemoral pain.[37] MRI scans of knees were performed before and after taping at 0°, 10°, and 20° of knee flexion. The taping was found to significantly reduce LPD at all joint angles. The changes found were 0.4, 1.1, and 0.7 mm at the 0°, 10°, and 20° angles, respectively. These changes are deemed small, but presently it is unknown what amount of decrease in LPD is needed to bring normal alignment to the patellofemoral joint. The small amounts of medialization of the patella could create a significant difference in symptoms according to the "envelope of function" theory and therefore could be clinically significant. According to the "envelope of function" theory, small changes can help the patient overcome an initial metabolic homeostatic crisis by taking normal activities of daily living out of the supraphysiological loading zone, and offloading it to a more tolerable level.[38,39]

Pfeiffer and colleagues[40] assessed a medial patellar taping procedure via kinematic MRI at knee flexion angles of 0°,

12°, 24°, and 36° in three conditions—no tape, McConnell taping for medial glide, and same taping followed by exercise. The exercise after taping was running an agility task around a rectangular course that was 60 feet by 20 feet. The 18 healthy female participants ran around the course for five sets of three repetitions with a 1-minute rest in between. Immediately following the task, the women were taken back to the laboratory, where the follow-up MRI was performed. The authors concluded that at all knee angles tested, the taping resulted in a significant movement medially when comparing the taping with the no-taping condition. However, following the exercise task, it was found that the taping procedure did not maintain the significant movement of the patella medially at any of the angles measured. Several important notices should be made with this study. Pfeiffer only assessed the medial glide technique in asymptomatic, healthy women. In addition, their subjects were examined in the nonweightbearing position with thigh muscles relaxed, which could have been a contributing factor to their findings.

Somes and colleagues[41] assessed the effects of patellar taping on patellar position in both the open and closed kinetic chain via radiography. The authors examined nine subjects with patellofemoral pain via x-ray examination in the open kinetic chain and closed kinetic chain at 45° of knee flexion with and without tape application. Results revealed a significant increase in lateral patellofemoral angle with patellar taping in the closed kinetic chain, indicating a more medially tilted patella. They also found a decrease in subjective complaints of anterior knee pain in this position.

Altered Patellar Position—Negative Findings

Gigante and colleagues[42] used CT and found that patella taping did not create an effect on patella position in 0° and 15° of knee flexion with the quadriceps contracted. Worrell, Ingersoll, and colleagues,[43] in a single-report case study, found that patella taping did not improve patellar position. The authors did find that taping increased LPD at angles less than 25°. Using a larger sample size, Worrell, and colleagues[44] were able to report that taping improved patellar position at the early knee flexion angle of 10°, but not at a variety of angles up to 45°.

In a similar study, Larsen and colleagues[45] examined the ability of patellar taping via use of medial glide technique to maintain a medial patellar position after exercise. Larsen used a standard radiologic technique via the "Merchant view" of the patellofemoral joint.[46] Larsen and colleagues performed radiographical assessment after taping before exercise and following exercise. Their determination was that patellar taping for a medial glide was able to have an effect on moving the patella medially, but was not able to maintain patellar position once subjected to physical exercise. The authors believed that this is probably due to tape breakdown or loosening during and following exercise.

Muscle Recruitment

Using patellar taping methods to increase muscle recruitment has been done primarily in an attempt to increase vastus medialis oblique (VMO) muscle firing in those with patellofemoral pain syndrome (PFPS). Either a weakness of the VMO or asynchronous firing patterns between the vastus lateralis (VL) and the VMO is thought to cause lateral tracking.[47,48]

Muscle Recruitment—Positive Findings

Recently Ryan and Rowe[49] assessed the effects of various taping techniques on the VM/VL ratio in 24 asymptomatic healthy students. Surface EMG recordings were collected during four single-legged squats under four tape conditions: (1) medial glide, (2) lateral glide, (3) neutral, and (4) no tape. What is interesting to note regarding this study is the use of a lateral-glide technique. Usually patellar taping dictates use of a medial glide instead of lateral. The lateral-glide procedure produced small (~5%) but significantly greater VM/VL ratios than medial and neutral, but not the no-tape condition. The reason this occurred was due to a nonsignificant increase in VMO and a nonsignificant decrease in VL during the procedure. The combined effects reached statistical significance. Because this study used a non symptomatic population, extrapolation of this data to a symptomatic population must be done with caution.

Christou[50] examined EMG activity of 30 women of whom half had PFPS. Participants performed maximal isokinetic leg presses at 30° per second for the following tape conditions: (1) no tape (control), (2) no glide (placebo), (3) medial glide, and (4) lateral glide. Christou also found that the experimental taping increased the VMO activity and decreased the VL activity in those with PFPS. Coincidentally, the taping had the opposite effects on the healthy, unimpaired subjects by increasing the VL and decreasing VMO activity. Christou reports that, because the placebo procedures also caused changes in VMO activity, the changes were probably not the result of an altered patellar position, but rather the result of enhanced support or cutaneous stimulation.

Cowan and colleagues[51] report that there is EMG evidence that patellar taping alters temporal characteristics of the VMO and VL. The authors assessed 10 participants with PFPS and 12 asymptomatic subjects using one of three conditions: (1) no tape, (2) therapeutic tape, and (3) placebo tape. Onset of VMO and VL were assessed during concentric and eccentric phases of stair stepping. When there was no taping performed, those with PFPS had the EMG onset of VL occur before that of the VMO. In those without PFPS (control), the VMO fired prior to VL during the concentric phase and simultaneously in the eccentric phase. However, when those with PFPS performed the task with therapeutic tape, EMG was altered so that the VMO fired before the VL during the concentric phase, whereas it fired simultaneously in the eccentric phase. The asymptomatic subjects observed no change in timing and onset of VMO and VL between taping procedures.

Although not using EMG, Powers and colleagues[52] examined the effects of patellar taping on functional outcomes. Their study of 15 female subjects, all with PFPS, assessed stride characteristics and sagittal plane motion via a motion analysis system. Outcomes were assessed while free walking, fast walking, and ascending and descending a ramp and stairs, and differences were noted between taped and untaped conditions. Taping resulted in an increased knee-loading response, which permitted increased shock absorption and increased quadriceps activity. In addition, using a functional activity, Ernst and colleagues[53] examined 14 women with PFPS while performing a single-leg vertical jump and lateral step-up, and collected data with a force plate and motion analysis system. Performance of these activities was performed using four conditions: (1) patellar tape, (2) placebo tape, (3) no tape, and (4) uninvolved knee with no tape (as control). Patellar taping resulted in greater knee extensor moment and power than did the nontaped and placebo taped conditions. The taped condition did not show a different vertical jump height than the placebo or no-tape condition.

Muscle Recruitment—Negative Findings

Bennell and colleagues[54] used surface EMG to determine activity of VMO compared with that of VL during stair stepping and normal-pace and fast-pace walking. Subjects included 12 patients with a history of PFPS, all of whom were asymptomatic at the time of the study. Conditions included (1) no tape, (2) control tape, and (3) therapeutic tape. Neither therapeutic tape nor control tape had any effect on VMO-VL onset timing via EMG. The authors suggest that tape-induced effects on neuromotor control of the vasti seen in other studies may be the result of reductions in pain rather than changes in a baseline motor timing issue.

Ng and Cheng[55] found a decrease in VM/VL ratio with a medial taping technique when assessing 15 patients with a history of PFPS. Their theory for this finding was the fact that the tape procedure might mimic the stabilizing effect of the VM itself. If the patella is already medialized, there is less need for VM to work as a medial stabilizer; therefore, the overall ratio would be decreased. This could be problematic for those with weakness of the VMO in that a medial-glide tape procedure would actually cause less activity, although the prevailing theory is that what is needed is more activity, which imparts a strengthening effect. A similar finding was seen by Mungovan and colleagues,[56] who found a decrease in VMO/VL ratio following application of a medial patella taping procedure. This conflicts with the presumed theory that taping in a medial glide will facilitate VMO activation in those with PFPS.

Salsich and colleagues[57] assessed EMG using a functional task of ascending and descending stairs either in the taped or nontaped condition in a pool of 10 subjects with PFPS. Unfortunately, this study only assessed EMG of the VL.

Subjects in this study did not demonstrate a change in VL EMG with the application of tape during either the stair ascent or descent.

Proprioception

Patellofemoral Joint

Callaghan and colleagues[58] found that the application of patellar tape significantly improved the active and passive joint position sense in healthy subjects whose proprioceptive levels were graded as "poor," whereas those with a good proprioception grade saw no improvement in scores. This would lead one to believe that patellar taping may enhance proprioception in the patellofemoral joint.

More recently, Callaghan and colleagues[59] assessed the ability to increase joint position sense through patellar taping in those with patellofemoral pain. The study tested 32 subjects with a history of patellofemoral pain before and after the introduction of patellar taping. Their study at first glance did not seem to show an enhancement of joint position sense following patellar taping. But, when the authors placed the subjects into a proprioception status according to their error, the "poor" proprioception cohort scores were enhanced at all angles tested; however, when looking at absolute error, scores were enhanced only to a significant level at 20° of knee flexion.

Decreased Patellar Pain

An obvious reason for patellar taping is that of reducing anterior knee pain. Despite conflicting evidence regarding various aspects of patellar taping, a large number of articles have emphatically found that patellar taping reduces anterior knee pain. Many authors have reported decreases in pain following patellar taping[48-50,53,55,60-65] and report that using both the medial glide and a placebo technique reduced perceived patellofemoral pain by 70% to 80% in those with symptoms.

> **Clinical Point**
>
> In most patellofemoral pain syndrome patients, medial taping decreases pain.

Systematic Reviews and Meta-Analysis

Recent reviews and meta-analysis have reported conflicting findings regarding the use of tape for those with PFPS. Aminaka and Gribble[66] identified and reviewed 16 studies with an average Physiotherapy Evidence Database (PEDro) score of 4.25 out of 10 and determined that although patellar taping appeared to reduce pain and improve function in patients with PFPS during activities of daily living and rehabilitation exercise, strong evidence to identify the underlying mechanisms is still not available. This is in contrast to the findings of Warden and colleagues,[67] who used 13 investigative trials to examine the effects of patellar taping or bracing. Through a meta-analysis, the authors concluded that on a 100-mm scale, tape applied to exert a medially directed force on the patella decreased chronic knee pain compared with no tape by 16.1 mm (95% CI −22.2, −10.0; $p < 0.001$). Coincidentally, sham taping applied to exert a medially directed force on the patella decreased chronic knee pain compared with no tape by 10.9 mm (95% CI −18.4, −3.4; $p < 0.001$).

Limitations of studies examining the effects of taping on patellofemoral pain appear to occur when evaluating varying results. Variations in sample populations and sample sizes reduce the ability to determine differences. Most studies are underpowered and the ability to detect statistical power is hampered. In addition, a lack of long-term follow up potentially limits generalizations of taping.[68]

A synopsis of all patellar taping articles can be seen in Table 21-4.

Patellofemoral Taping Clinical Prediction Rule

Lesher and colleagues[69] described a clinical prediction rule developed to determine which patients would respond favorably to patellar taping. Their study involved 50 volunteers with patellofemoral pain who received treatment with a medial-glide taping technique. Of these patients, 26 had immediate pain relief with patellar taping. Two of their examination items, (1) positive patellar tilt greater than 5° or (2) tibial varum greater than 5°, composed the clinical prediction rule for success. Application of these two items improved the probability of a successful outcome from 52% to 83%. This clinical prediction rule is useful in identifying characteristics of patients with PFPS who may benefit from taping. This was not a randomized controlled clinical trial, however, so they were unable to determine if the patient's response was solely the result of the taping technique.

Although there appears to be consensus that taping does relieve patellar pain in the short term, it is still presently unknown how or why this occurs. There continues to be inconsistencies regarding patellar taping and its ability to alter patellar mechanics, vasti inhibition, vasti muscle recruitment, and recruitment timing of vasti muscles. Further study is warranted in these inconsistent areas of knowledge.

Taping for the Shoulder

Although a multitude of studies exist for taping of the knee, the scientific literature is limited in regard to tape for shoulder conditions. Shoulder taping may be useful for some of the same reasons that knee taping is thought to benefit patient populations, such as stimulating greater proprioceptive

Table 21-4

Patellofemoral Taping Article Synopsis

Article	Population	Description	Results
		Pain	
Bockrath et al.[60]	PFPS—12 subjects	Assessment of congruence angle radiographically with isometric quadriceps contraction; VAS pain during step down (1) taped (2) untaped	No change in congruence; 50% reduction in pain
Christou[50]	PFPS—15 women Normal—15 women	Pain, force production, and EMG of VMO and VL—(1) taped medial glide, (2) taped lateral glide, (3) placebo during leg press	In PFPS, medial glide and placebo reduced pain; PFPS and tape did not alter leg press force; PFPS increased VMO, decreased VL; opposite in normal
Clark et al.[61]	PFPS—81 subjects	Pain, patient satisfaction, quadriceps strength, subjective scale scores (1) exercise, tape, and education; (2) exercise and education; (3) tape and education; (4) education alone	Taping was not associated with discharge; all exercise groups showed decrease in pain
Cowan et al.[51]	PFPS—10 subjects Normal—12 subjects	EMG of VMO and VL during stair ascent and descent	PFPS with taping changed temporal characteristics of VMO and VL; no increased EMG onset in asymptomatic patients.
Harrison et al.[62]	PFPS—113 subjects	Pain via VAS; subjective scores; step test (1) home exercise alone; (2) physical therapist monitored exercises program; (3) patellar taping, exercise, and biofeedback	PFPS with taping (group 3) showed significant improvement at 1 month. Groups 2 and 3 showed more improvement than group 1, but not at a significant level.
Herrington[63]	PFPS—14 subjects	Pain via VAS; concentric and eccentric quadriceps peak torque (1) taped, (2) un-taped	PFPS taping decreased pain and increased peak torque.
Kowall et al.[64]	PFPS—25 subjects	Pain via VAS; EMG activity; isokinetic strength testing (1) standard physical therapy, (2) standard physical therapy plus patellar taping	Both groups had decreased pain, taping was not significantly more than untaped subjects; both groups had greater strength and EMG activity.
Ng and Cheng[55]	PFPS—15 subjects	Pain and EMG VMO/VL ratio during single-legged semisquat (1) tape, (2) untaped	Taping significantly decreased pain and VMO/VL EMG ratio during single-legged semisquat.
Powers et al.[52]	PFPS—15 women	Stride characteristics and sagittal plane motion (1) taped; (2) untaped; free walking, fast walking, ascending and descending ramp and stairs	78% pain reduction with tape; only significant change was stride length increased during ramp ascent.
Salsich et al.[57]	PFPS—10 subjects: 5 women, 5 men	PFPS kinematics, ground reaction forces and EMG ascending and descending stairs (1) taped, (2) untaped	92.6% reduction in pain with taped condition; improved cadence, knee flexion angles, and moments with tape; no change in vastus EMG with tape.
Whittingham et al.[65]	PFPS—30 subjects: 24 men, 6 women	VAS for pain; functional scores (1) patellar taping and exercise, (2) placebo tape and exercise, (3) exercise alone	Improvements in pain and function for all groups; tape and exercise demonstrate better pain function scores.
		Neuromuscular Control, Muscle Recruitment, and Knee Joint Kinematics	
Bennell et al.[54]	Normal—12 with history of PFPS	Kinematics and EMG—stair stepping, normal gait, fast gait—(1) no tape, (2) control tape, (3) ther tape	Neither ther tape or control tape had an effect on EMG onset timing; ther tape increased stance knee flexion angles; initial ground reaction force decreased with tape.
Christou[50]	PFPS—15 women Normal—15 women	Pain, force production and EMG of VMO and VL—(1) taped medial glide, (2) taped lateral glide, (3) placebo during leg press	In PFPS medial glide and placebo reduced pain; PFPS and tape did not alter leg press force; PFPS increased VMO and decreased VL; opposite in normal.

Continued

Table 21-4

Patellofemoral Taping Article Synopsis—cont'd

Article	Population	Description	Results
Neuromuscular Control, Muscle Recruitment, and Knee Joint Kinematics				

Article	Population	Description	Results
Neuromuscular Control, Muscle Recruitment, and Knee Joint Kinematics			
Cowan et al[51]	PFPS—10 Normal—12	EMG of VMO and VL during stair ascent and descent	PFPS with taping changed temporal characteristics of VMO and VL; no change in EMG onset in asymptomatic.
Ernst et al.[53]	PFPS—14 women	Lower extremity kinetics during lateral step up and vertical jump—(1) taped, (2) untaped; (3) placebo tape, (4) uninvolved knee	Taping provided greater extensor moment and power than no tape and placebo; vertical jump was greater in uninvolved than taped, placebo or no tape; no difference in vertical jump height with tape.
Herrington[36]	Normal—10 women	Normals will see suboptimal firing with patellar taping; EMG and kinematics two conditions: (1) taping, (2) control	Taping significantly decreased VMO and VL EMG; taping significantly decreased peak stance knee flexion, knee flexion angular velocity.
Ng and Cheng[55]	PFPS—15 subjects	Pain and EMG VMO/VL ratio during single-legged semisquat (1) tape, (2) untaped	Taping significantly decreased pain and VMO/VL EMG ratio during single-legged semisquat
Powers et al.[52]	PFPS—15 women	Stride characteristics and sagittal plane motion (1) taped, (2) untaped; free walking, fast walking, ascending and descending ramp and stairs	78% pain reduction with tape; only significant change was increased stride length during ramp ascent.
Ryan and Rowe[49]	Normal—25 students 17 female, 8 male	Normal patients' EMG during performance of four single-leg squats with four taping conditions: (1) medial, (2) lateral, (3) neutral, (4) control	Lateral taping caused a small but significant increase in VM/VL ratios versus medial, but not no tape; no difference in medial taping.
Salsich et al.[57]	PFPS—10 subjects: 5 women; 5 men	PFPS kinematics, ground reaction forces and EMG ascending and descending stairs (1) taped, (2) untaped	92.6% reduction in pain with taped condition. Improved cadence, knee flexion angles, and moments with tape; no change in VL EMG with tape.
Patellar Position			
Gigante et al.[42]	PFPS—16 women	PFPS CT: (1) taping; (2) control; assess PF congruence angle; muscles relaxed, muscles contracted	Taping did not affect PF lateralization or tilt; findings do not support use of taping for passive correction of incongruence.
Herrington[37]	PFPS—8 subjects: 5 women; 3 men	PFPS MRI taken at 0°, 10°, 20° of knee flexion	Taping resulted in significant reduction of lateral patellar distance at all angles.
Larsen et al.[45]	20 asymptomatic men	Radiographs of modified Merchant view (1) pretape, (2) taped, (3) after exercise	Taping resulted in medial glide, but was ineffective after exercise.
Pfeiffer et al.[40]	18 asymptomatic women	MRI (1) taping, (2) no taping, (3) after exercise measured at 0°, 12°, 24°, and 36°	Significant difference in lateral displacement at all angles (taped and untaped condition). Significant differences in tape before and after exercise.
Somes et al.[41]	PFPS—9 subjects: 7 women; 2 men	Radiographs in open kinetic and closed kinetic chains at 45° knee flexion: (1) tape, (2) untapped conditions	Increased lateral PF angle with tape in CKC; no change in PF congruence angle; pain reduced 45% with tape.
Worrell et al.[44]	PFPS—12 subjects	PFPS MRI: (1) taping, (2) bracing, (3) control at eight different angles	Taping and bracing significantly decrease PF congruence at an angle of 10° only.
Joint Proprioception			
Callaghan et al.[59]	PFPS—32 subjects	Normal subjects performed active-angle reproduction, passive-angle reproduction, and threshold to detect passive movement	No statistically significant differences between taped or untaped conditions.

CKC, Closed kinetic chain; *CT,* computed tomography; *EMG,* electromyography; *MRI,* magnetic resonance imaging; *PF,* patellofemoral; *PFPS,* patellofemoral pain syndrome; *ther,* therapeutic; *VAS,* visual analog scale; *VL,* vastus lateralis; *VMO,* vastus medialis oblique.

feedback, improving scapulohumeral rhythm, improving joint position, and muscle length-tension relationships.

Ackerman and colleagues[70] looked at upper trapezius EMG activity in professional violinists. This is one of the few shoulder taping studies that actually assessed EMG during a true functional activity, in this case playing the violin. The authors used a taping technique to move the scapula away from excessive protraction in an effort to enhance muscular length-tension relationships. In addition, the violinist's music quality was independently assessed between taped and untaped conditions. Compared with the no-tape condition, scapular taping actually increased upper trapezius muscle activity by 49%. The raters, who were blinded to performance and taping condition, rated the musical pieces of the taped condition as of lower quality. It was believed that the mechanical restriction to movement during the taped condition and the violinist straining against this was the reason for the deterioration in musical performance quality.

Host[71] described a case study of a 40-year-old male patient with an 8-month history of anterior subacromial impingement who was able to return to full overhead sports activity following scapular taping. By using a scapular taping technique, the patient was able to return to full activities, including tennis and racquet ball, without symptoms after approximately 10 physical therapy visits.

Morrissey has reported that taping under tension in the line of a muscle's fiber direction facilitates muscle recruitment.[72] This has since been disputed, at least for muscle activity of the lower trapezius. Alexander and colleagues[73] were able to dispute that taping the lower portion of the trapezius would facilitate motor activity. In assessing the Hoffman reflex to determine motoneuron pool excitability, they found that using the application of cover tape inhibited the upper trapezius by 4%, and applying more pressure via a top tape layer inhibited the muscle by 22%. In addition, Cools and colleagues,[74] following a taping procedure across the muscle belly of the upper trapezius and parallel to the direction of the lower trapezius, were unable to find changes in EMG activity in any of the scapular muscles.

In direct contrast to these studies, Morin and colleagues[75] found significant alterations in the upper trapezius and middle trapezius with taping procedures. In their study, the upper trapezius was taped across the belly and resulted in muscle inhibition during an isometric contraction, whereas the middle and lower trapezius demonstrated an increase in EMG activity. Morin and colleagues studied the proposed effect on normal patients without pathological conditions. They recommended future studies be performed to see if the same effects would occur for those with pathological conditions of the shoulder. More recently, Selkowitz and colleagues[76] attempted to determine if upper trapezius EMG activity could be decreased with an upper trapezius inhibitory taping technique. Surface EMG of the shoulder girdle muscles was assessed while lifting overhead with and

without tape. Scapular taping decreased upper trapezius and increased lower trapezius activity in people with suspected shoulder impingement during an overhead reaching task. Taping also decreased upper trapezius activity during lifting into shoulder abduction in the scapular plane. The authors speculate the load used may not have been enough to affect the other muscles assessed because their EMG activity was not altered with the tape or no-tape procedures.

Joint Position Sense

Zanella and colleagues[77] quantified the effects of scapular taping on shoulder joint repositioning during motions of shoulder flexion and abduction. Assessing 30 subjects with no pathological conditions of the shoulder, they determined absolute error in joint reposition and scapular position via lateral scapular slide testing using a plumb line and winging. The authors found no difference for taped or untaped conditions in joint position sense or winging of the scapula.

Stabilization After Stroke

Hanger and colleauges[78] performed shoulder strapping with patients who had experienced a stroke. It was hoped that strapping in the hemiplegic shoulder would reduce pain, preserve ROM, and improve functional outcomes. In their study, Hanger and colleagues[78] randomized shoulder strapping with standard physical therapy for 6 weeks compared with standardized physical therapy alone. Intervention with strapping showed no differences for pain, ROM, or functional outcome after the intervention phase. It appeared that the presence of neglect or sensory loss, but not subluxation, at baseline was independently associated with a poor outcome.

Posture

Lewis and colleagues[79] objectively assessed postural changes and symptoms of those with subacromial impingement before and following scapular taping, and placebo scapular taping. Postural taping produced significant effects for all postural measures, including measurements for forward head, kyphosis, scapular displacements, and pain-free ROM. Visual analog pain scores for shoulder flexion and scapular plane abduction were not altered. These authors concluded that changing one or more components of posture may have a positive effect on those with subacromial impingement syndrome.

Although there is limited evidence to support taping for posture and muscle recruitment in the shoulder, it does appear that this form of treatment may be useful as an adjunctive therapy. As such, several precautions are advised. The taping procedure used should not restrict the athlete's ROM. When taped, the athlete should be able to move the shoulder through motions that were previously more painful. The amount of pain relief is generally variable, with the best outcome occurring with total or near-total relief of symptoms. It must also be stressed that this is generally not an isolated technique used all by itself. This is most often an intervening modality to allow athletes to perform their given activities. Once the athlete can perform normal activities, the taping should slowly be diminished.

At the present time, there continues to be ample evidence that a clear consensus cannot be met regarding recommendation of shoulder taping procedures. Differences in studies include surface versus indwelling EMG recordings, injured versus uninjured populations, dominant versus nondominant arm, isometric versus isotonic muscle contractions, and the use of various forms of tape and taping procedures.

Kinesio Tape

Kinesio tape (KT) procedures and techniques have been purported to improve a variety of physiological problems, including ROM and strength (Figure 21-9).[80] Kase and colleagues[81] proposed several benefits, depending on the amount of stretch applied to the tape during application: (1) provide positional stimulus through the skin, (2) align fascial tissue, (3) create space by lifting fascia and soft tissue above the area of pain and inflammation, (4) provide

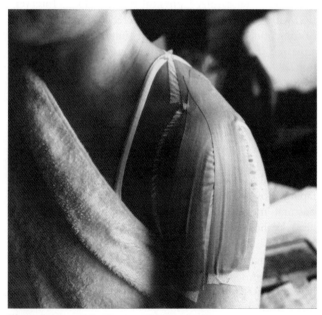

Figure 21-9
Shoulder Kinesio tape procedure. This is the anterior view of the tape application used to assist a member of the 2000 U.S. Olympic Team after she dislocated her shoulder on the floor exercise mat. (From Andrews JR, Wilk KE, Reinold MM: *The athlete's shoulder*, ed 2, Philadelphia, 2009, Churchill Livingstone.)

sensory stimulation to assist or limit motion, and (5) assist in the removal of edema by directing exudates toward a lymph duct. None of these claims, however, have been shown to be true. KT differs from traditional white athletic tape in that it is elastic and can be stretched to 140% of its original length before being applied to the skin.[82] In addition, KT is latex-free and the adhesive is 100% acrylic and heat-activated.[81] Because the tape is 100% cotton, it can be worn in the pool or shower and has a single-application wear time of approximately 3 to 4 days.[83]

Thelen and partners[83] assessed the clinical efficacy of KT compared with sham KT when applied for 2 days to college-age students with shoulder pain and diagnosis of shoulder impingement. The therapeutic KT group demonstrated immediate improvements in pain-free shoulder abduction, but were unable to show any differences between the sham treatment KT with regard to ROM, pain, or disability scores at any time interval.

Yoshida and Kahavov[84] were able to find an increase in trunk flexion ROM when compared with a group that was not taped. They were not able to find any differences for trunk extension and lateral flexion motions when evaluating taped versus untaped conditions.

Application of KT in an effort to increase reproduction of joint position sense of the ankle demonstrated no change in constant or absolute error as compared with no taping in a healthy, uninjured population.[82]

Finally, Fu and colleagues[83] looked at the immediate and delayed effects of KT on muscle strength in the quadriceps and hamstrings when tape was applied to the anterior thigh of healthy, young athletes. Their results revealed no significant difference in muscle power via isokinetic testing compared with no tape, immediately after taping, and 12 hours after taping.

At the present time, the studies on the effects of KT have been mostly empirically based rather than evidence-based, and come from case series, case studies, and small pilot studies. Unfortunately, these forms of evidence are at the lower end of the evidence-based hierarchy. At the present time, there is limited evidence regarding benefits for the use of KT techniques in athletic or general populations. Future studies are greatly needed to ultimately decide if this form of taping has a place in sports and orthopedic rehabilitation.

Conclusion

After a thorough review of the literature, one still wonders about the effects of taping in efforts to prevent injury or stabilize injured joints of the body. Conflicting or limited evidence seems to predominate. Clearly high level I and II randomized controlled clinical trials should be undertaken to determine efficacy of these procedures. There appears to be limited clinical evidence that ankle taping can be used to limit abnormal motion for brief periods. It has been consistently shown that patellar taping does provide a mechanism for pain relief in most studies, although it is still unclear exactly what mediates this favorable response. Newer techniques such as KT have yet to be scientifically proven effective. In this era of cost containment, clinicians should critically look at the use of taping for athletic musculoskeletal injury prevention and treatment approaches.

References

1. Perrin DH: *Athletic taping and bracing,* ed 2, Champaign, IL, 2005, Human Kinetics.
2. Prentice W: *Modern principles of athletic training,* St Louis, 1989, Mosby.
3. Garrick JG, Requa RK: Role of external support in the prevention of ankle sprains, *Med Sci Sports Exerc* 5:200–203, 1973.
4. Cordova ML, Ingersoll CD, LeBlanc MJ: Influence of ankle support on joint range of motion before and after exercise: A meta-analysis, *J Orthop Sports Phys Ther* 30(4):170–182, 2000.
5. Cordova ML, Scott D, Ingersoll CD, LeBlanc M: Effects of ankle support on lower-extremity functional performance: A meta-analysis, *Med Sci Sports Exerc* 37:635–641, 2005.
6. Myburgh KH, Vaughan CL, Isaacs SK: The effects of ankle guards and taping on joint motion before, during, and after a squash match, *Am J Sports Med* 12:441–446, 1984.
7. Martin N, Harter RA: Comparison of inversion restraint provided by ankle prophylactic devices before and after exercise, *J Athl Train* 28:324–329, 1993.
8. Paris DL, Kokkaliaris J, Vardaxis V: Ankle ranges of motion during extended activity periods while taped and braced, *J Athl Train* 30:223–228, 1995.
9. Gross MT, Bradshaw MK, Ventry LC, Weller KH: Comparison of support provided by ankle taping and semirigid orthosis, *J Orthop Sports Phys Ther* 9:33–39, 1987.
10. Gross MT, Lapp AK, Davis M: Comparison of Swede-O-Universal ankle support and Aircast Sport-Stirrup orthoses and ankle tape in restricting eversion-inversion before and after exercise, *J Orthop Sports Phys Ther* 13:11–19, 1991.
11. Karlsson J, Andreasson GO: The effect of external ankle support in chronic lateral ankle joint instability. An electromyographic study, *Am J Sports Med* 20:257–261, 1992.
12. Wilkerson GB: Comparative biomechanical effects of the standard method of ankle taping and a taping method designed to enhance subtalar stability, *Am J Sports Med* 19:588–595, 1991.
13. Purcell SB, Schuckman BE, Docherty CL, et al: Differences in ankle range of motion before and after exercise in 2 tape conditions, *Am J Sports Med* 37:383–389, 2009.
14. Alt W, Loher H, Gollhofer A: Functional properties of adhesive ankle taping: Neuromuscular and mechanical effects before and after exercise, *Foot Ankle Int* 20:238–245, 1999.
15. Burkes RT, Bean BG, Marcus R, Barker HB: Analysis of athletic performance with prophylactic ankle devices, *Am J Sports Med* 19:104–106, 1991.
16. Meana M, Alegre LM, Elvira JL, Aguado X: Kinematics of ankle taping after a training session, *Int J Sports Med* 29:70–76, 2008.
17. Ricard MD, Sherwood SM, Schulthies SS, Knight KL: Effects of tape and exercise on dynamic ankle inversion, *J Athl Train* 35:31–37, 2000.
18. Sawkins K, Refshauge K, Kilbreath S, Raymond J: The placebo effect of ankle taping in ankle instability, *Med Sci Sports Exerc* 39:781–787, 2007.
19. Robbins S, Waked E, Rappel R: Ankle taping improves proprioception before and after exercise in young men, *Br J Sports Med* 29:242–247, 1995.
20. Gregory JE, Morgan DL, Proske U: Changes in size of the stretch reflex of can and man attributed to after effects in muscle spindles, *J Neurophysiol* 58:628–640, 1987.
21. Refshauge KM, Kilbreath SL, Raymond J: The effect of recurrent ankle inversion sprain and taping on proprioception at the ankle, *Med Sci Sports Exerc* 32:10–15, 2000.
22. Refshauge KM, Raymond J, Kilbreath SL, et al: The effect of ankle taping on detection of inversion-eversion movements in participants with recurrent ankle sprain, *Am J Sports Med* 37:371–375, 2009.
23. Bennell KL, Goldie PA: The differential effects of external ankle support on postural control, *J Orthop Sports Phys Ther* 20:287–295, 1994.
24. Watson L, Bennel KL: The effect of ankle taping on postural steadiness, *Proceedings of the 10th International Congress of the World Confederation for Physical Therapy,* Sydney, Australia, 1987.
25. Franettovich M, Chapman A, Vincenzino B: Tape that increases medial longitudinal arch height also reduces leg muscles activity: A preliminary study, *Med Sci Sport Exerc* 40:593–600, 2008.
26. Hyland MR, Webber-Gaffney A, Cohen L, Lichtman PT: Randomized controlled trial of calcaneal taping, sham taping, and plantar fascia stretching for the short-term management of plantar heel pain, *J Orthop Sports Phys Ther* 36(6):364–371, 2006.
27. Vincenzino B, Brooksbank J, Minto J, et al: Initial effects of elbow taping on pain-free grip strength and pressure pain threshold, *J Orthop Sports Phys Ther* 33:400–407, 2003.
28. Rettig AC, Stube KS, Shelbourne DK: Effects of finger and wrist taping on grip strength, *Am J Sports Med* 25:96–98, 1997.
29. Warme WJ, Brooks D: The effect of circumferential taping on flexor tendon pulley failure in rock climbers, *Am J Sports Med* 28:674–678, 2000.
30. Olmsted LC, Vela LI, Denegar CR, Hertel J: Prophylactic ankle taping and bracing: A numbers-needed-to-treat and cost-benefit analysis, *J Athl Train* 39:95–100, 2004.
31. Sitler M, Ryan J, Wheeler B, et al: The efficacy of a semirigid ankle stabilizer to reduce acute ankle injuries in basketball: A randomized clinical study at West Point, *Am J Sports Med* 22:454–461, 1994.
32. Surve I, Schwellnus MP, Noakes T, Lombard C: A fivefold reduction in the incidence of recurrent ankle sprains in soccer players using the Sport-Stirrup orthoses, *Am J Sports Med* 22:601–606, 1994.
33. Manske RC, Davies GJ: A nonsurgical approach to examination and treatment of the patellofemoral joint, Part 1: Examination and treatment of the patellofemoral joint, *Crit Rev Phys Rehabil Med* 15:141–166, 2003.
34. McConnell J: The management of chondromalacia patellae: A long-term solution, *Aust J Physio* 32:215–223, 1986.
35. McConnell J, Fulkerson J:: The Knee: Patellofemoral and soft tissue injuries. In Zachazewski JE, Magee DJ, Quillen WS, editors: Athletic Injuries and Rehabilitation, Philadelphia, 1996, WB Saunders.
36. Herrington L: The effect of patellofemoral joint taping, *Crit Rev Phys Rehabil Med* 12:271–276, 2000.
37. Herrington L: The effect of corrective taping of the patella on patella position as defined by MRI, *Res Sports Med* 14:215–223, 2006.
38. Dye S: The pathophysiology of patellofemoral pain, *Clin Orthop* 436:100–110, 2005.
39. Dye S, Staubli H, Biedert R, Vaupel G: The mosaic of pathophysiology causing patellofemoral pain: Therapeutic implications, *Op Tech Sports Med* 7:46–54, 1999.

40. Pfeiffer RP, DeBeliso M, Shea KG, et al: Kinematic MRI assessment of McConnell taping before and after exercise, *Am J Sports Med* 32:621–628, 2004.

41. Somes S, Worrell TW, Corey B, Ingersol CD: Effects of patellar taping on patellar position in the open and closed kinetic chain: a preliminary study, *J Sport Rehabil* 6:299–308, 1997.

42. Gigante A, Pasquinelli F, Paladini P, et al: The effects of patella taping on patellofemoral incongruence, *Am J Sports Med* 29:88–92, 2001.

43. Worrell T, Ingersoll C, Farr J: Effects of patellar taping and bracing on patellar position: An MRI case study, *J Sports Rehabil* 3:146–153, 1994.

44. Worrell T, Ingersoll C, Bockrath-Pugliese K, Minis P: Effect of patellar taping and bracing on patellar position as determined by MRI in patients with patellofemoral pain, *J Athl Train* 33:16–20, 1998.

45. Larsen B, Andreasen E, Urfer A, et al: Patellar taping: A radiographic examination of the medial glide technique, *Am J Sports Med* 23:465–471, 1995.

46. Merchant AC, Mercer RL, Jacobsen RH, Cool CR: Roentgenographic analysis of patellofemoral congruence, *J Bone Joint Surg Am* 56:1391–1396, 1974.

47. Manske RC, Davies GJ: A nonsurgical approach to examination and treatment of the patellofemoral joint, Part 2: Pathology and nonsurgical management of the patellofemoral joint, *Crit Rev Phys Rehabil Med* 15:253–293, 2003.

48. Davies GJ, Manske RC, Slamma K, et al: Selective activation of the vastus medialis oblique: What does the literature really tell us? *Physiotherapy Canada* 53:136–151, 2001.

49. Ryan CG, Rowe PJ: An electromyographical study to investigate the effects of patellar taping on the vastus medialis/vastus lateralis ratio in asymptomatic participants, *Physiother Theory Pract* 22:309–315, 2005.

50. Christou EA: Patellar taping increases vastus medialis oblique activity in the presence of patellofemoral pain, *J Electromyography Kines* 14:495–504, 2004.

51. Cowan SM, Bennell SL, Hodges PW: Therapeutic patellar taping changes the timing of vasti muscle activation in people with patellofemoral pain syndrome, *Clin J Sports Med* 12:339–347, 2002.

52. Powers CM, Landel R, Sosnick T, et al: The effects of patellar taping on stride characteristics and joint motion in subjects with patellofemoral pain, *J Orthop Sports Phys Ther* 26:286–667, 1997.

53. Ernst GP, Kawaguchi J, Saliba E: Effect of patellar taping on knee kinetics of patients with patellofemoral pain syndrome, *J Orthop Sports Phys Ther* 29:661–667, 1999.

54. Bennell K, Duncan M, Cowan S: Effect of patellar taping on vasti onset timing, knee kinematics, and kinetics in asymptomatic individuals with a delayed onset of vastus medialis oblique, *J Orthop Res* 24(9):1854–60, 2006.

55. Ng GYF, Cheng JM: The effects of patellar taping on pain and neuromuscular performance in subjects with patellofemoral pain syndrome. *Clin Rehabil* 16:821–827, 2002.

56. Mungovan SF, Henley EC, Renton AL, Turner GR: The effect of patellofemoral taping on EMG activity and torques produced about the knee joint during standing up from a seated position. *Proceedings of World Confederation of Physical Therapy*, London, 1991.

57. Salsich GB, Brechter JH, Farwell D, Powers CM: The effects of patellar taping on knee kinetics, kinematics, and vastus lateralis muscle activity during stair ambulation in individuals with patellofemoral pain, *J Orthop Sports Phys Ther* 32:3–10, 2002.

58. Callaghan MJ, Selfe J, Bagley P, Oldham JA: The effect of patellar taping on knee joint proprioception, *J Athl Train* 37:19–24, 2002.

59. Callaghan MJ, Selfe J, McHenry A, Oldham JA: Effects of patellar taping on knee joint proprioception in patients with patellofemoral pain syndrome, *Man Ther* 13:192–199, 2008.

60. Bockrath K, Wooden C, Worrell T, et al: Effects of patellar taping on patella position and perceived pain, *Med Sci Sports Exerc* 25:989–992, 1993.

61. Clark DI, Downing N, Mitchell J, et al: Physiotherapy for anterior knee pain: a randomized controlled trial, *Ann Rheum Dis* 59:700–704, 2000.

62. Harrison EL, Sheppard MS, McQuarrie AM: A randomized controlled trial of physical therapy treatment program in patellofemoral pain syndrome, *Physiother Canada* 51:93–106, 1999.

63. Herrington L: The effect of patellar taping on quadriceps peak torque and perceived pain: A preliminary study, *Phys Ther Sport* 2:23–28, 2001.

64. Kowall MG, Kolk G, Nuber GW, et al: Patellar taping in the treatment of patellofemoral pain: A prospective randomized study, *Am J Sports Med* 24:61–66, 1996.

65. Whittingham M, Palmer S, Macmillan R: Effect of taping on pain and function in patellofemoral pain syndrome: A randomized controlled trail, *J Orthop Sports Phys Ther* 34:504–510, 2004.

66. Aminaka N, Gribble PA: A systematic review of the effects of therapeutic taping on patellofemoral pain syndrome, *J Athl Train* 40:341–351, 2005.

67. Warden SJ, Hinman RS, Watson MA, et al: Patellar taping and bracing for the treatment of chronic knee pain: A systematic review and meta-analysis, *Arthritis Rheum* 59:73–83, 2008.

68. Fagen V, Delahunt E: Patellofemoral pain syndrome: a review on the associated neuromuscular deficits and current treatment options, *Br J Sports Med* 42:489–495, 2008.

69. Lesher JD, Sutlive TG, Miller GA, et al: Development of a clinical prediction rule for classifying patients with patellofemoral pain syndrome who respond to patellar taping, *J Orthop Sports Phys Ther* 36(11):854–866, 2006.

70. Ackerman B, Adams R, Marshall E: The effect of scapula taping on electromyographic activity and musical performance in professional violinists, *Aust J Physio* 48:197–203, 2002.

71. Host HH: Scapular taping in the treatment of anterior shoulder impingement, *Phys Ther* 75:803–812, 1995.

72. Morrissey D: Proprioceptive shoulder taping, *J Bodywork Mov Ther* 4:189–194, 2000.

73. Alexander CM, Stynes S, Thomas A, et al: Does tape facilitate or inhibit the lower fibres of trapezius? *Man Ther* 8:37–41, 2003.

74. Cools AM, Witvrouw LA, Danneels LA, Cambier DC: Does taping influence electromyographic muscle activity in the scapular rotators in healthy shoulders? *Man Ther* 7:154–162, 2002.

75. Morin GE, Tiberio D, Austin G: The effect of upper trapezius taping on electromyographic activity in the upper and middle trapezius region, *J Sports Rehabil* 6:309–319, 1997.

76. Selkowitz DM, Chaney C, Stuckey SJ, Vlad G: The effects of scapular taping on the surface electromyographic signal amplitude of shoulder girdle muscles during upper extremity elevation in individuals with suspected shoulder impingement syndrome, *J Orthop Sports Phys Ther* 37:694–702, 2007.

77. Zanella PW, Willey SM, Seibel SL, Hughes CJ: The effect of scapular taping on shoulder joint reposition, *J Sport Rehabil* 10:113–123, 2001.

78. Hanger HC, Whitewood P, Brown G, et al: A randomized controlled trial of strapping to prevent post-stroke shoulder pain, *Clin Rehabil* 14:370–380, 2000.

79. Lewis JS, Wright C, Green A: Subacromial impingement syndrome: The effect of changing posture on shoulder range of movement, *J Orthop Sports Phys Ther* 35:72–87, 2005.

80. Yoshida A, Kahavov L: The effect of kinesio taping on lower trunk range of motion, *Res Sports Med* 15:103–112, 2007.

81. Kase K, Wallis J, Kase T: *Clinical therapeutic applications of the kinesio taping method*, Tokyo, Japan, 2003, Ken Ikai Co Ltd.

82. Halseth T, McChesney JW, DeBeliso M, et al: The effects of kinesio taping on proprioception at the ankle, *J Sports Sci Med* 3:1–7, 2004.

83. Thelen MD, Dauber JA, Stoneman PD: The clinical efficacy of kinesio tape for shoulder pain: A randomized, double-blinded, clinical trial, *J Orthop Sports Phys Ther* 38:389–395, 2008.

84. Yoshida A, Kahavov L: The effect of kinesio taping on lower trunk range of motion, *Res Sports Med* 15:103–112, 2007.

85. Fu TC, Wong AMK, Pei YC, et al: Effect of kinesio taping on muscle strength in athletes—a pilot study, *J Sci Med Sport* 11: 198–201, 2008.

Sports-Related Concussion

Alex M. Taylor and Michael W. Collins

Introduction

Approximately 1.6 to 3.8 million individuals sustain sport- or recreation-related concussions each year, with mild traumatic brain injury (mTBI) accounting for up to 6.2% of all collegiate injuries and 5.5% of all high school injuries.[1-3] Although clearly a significant patient population, there is a large degree of variation in the definition and diagnostic criteria for sports-related concussion. Currently, there are no clinically applicable neuroanatomical or physiological measures that can determine the presence of such injuries. Assessment measures and grading scales frequently rely on loss of consciousness (LOC) to classify injury severity despite little evidence to suggest that it reliably determines accurate diagnosis or recovery. It is presumed that up to 90% of sports-related concussion may be undetected or unreported.[4] Although symptoms often resolve completely in time and are likely to reflect neuronal dysfunction rather than cell death, recent investigations purport longer recovery than previously indicated and demonstrate the potential for long-term physical, cognitive, and emotional sequelae when concussive injuries are not managed appropriately.[5-7] This chapter, which uses the terms *sports-related concussion* and *mTBI* synonymously, focuses on the diagnosis and evaluation of concussion at all levels of sports participation with the aim of identifying the signs and symptoms of injury, managing recovery, and safely returning athletes to play.

Definition

No definition of concussion has been universally accepted. Literature often cites the Committee on Head Injury Nomenclature of Neurological Surgeons who defined the injury as "a clinical syndrome characterized by the immediate and transient post-traumatic impairment of neural function such as alteration of consciousness, disturbance of vision or

equilibrium, etc., due to brain stem dysfunction."[8] Realizing the anatomical limitations of this definition, the American Academy of Neurology defined concussion as "any trauma induced alteration in mental status that may or may not include a loss of consciousness."[9] Although suggesting that concussion may involve other brain structures (i.e., cortical), this definition also served to emphasize the presence of concussion without LOC.

The Concussion in Sport Group, which is composed of experts in the field of sport-related concussion, recently proposed a definition of concussion that has been endorsed by health care practitioners. It states, "Sports concussion is a complex pathophysiological process affecting the brain, induced by traumatic biomechanical forces."[10] This definition recognizes the complexity of concussion as reflected by its inclusion of several common features, including:

1. Concussion may be caused by a direct blow to the head, face, neck, or elsewhere on the body with an "impulsive" force transmitted to the head.
2. Concussion typically results in the rapid onset of short-lived impairment of neurological function that resolves spontaneously.
3. Concussion may result in neuropathological changes, but the acute clinical symptoms largely reflect a functional disturbance rather than structural injury.
4. Concussion results in a graded set of clinical syndromes that may or may not involve loss of consciousness. Resolution of the clinical symptoms typically follows a sequential course.
5. Concussion is typically associated with grossly normal structural neuroimaging studies.[10]

Although clearly more descriptive than those previously reported, this definition also recognized the complexity of concussion as reflected by its widely variable criteria. It also argues for more individualized treatment and conservative management of mTBI.

Biomechanics and Pathophysiology

It is generally accepted that concussion occurs when linear or rotational forces are applied to the head or body. A linear impact is characterized by a force that imparts acceleration or deceleration to the body or head in a straight line. A rotational injury is the result of force, usually lateral, that causes an angular acceleration or deceleration of the body or head. Although both linear and rotational impacts are associated with the occurrence of injury, rotational impacts are presumed to be more instrumental in sports-related concussion than linear and are associated with shearing or stretching rather than compression of brain tissue.[11,12] In sports-related concussion, neither type of impact causes perceptible structural injury in computed tomography or magnetic resonance imaging studies. However, recent literature suggests that mTBI affects the physiological and metabolic functioning of the brain.[13,14]

Using a rodent concussion model, researchers have demonstrated that cellular and vascular changes take place following mTBI, including ionic flux, metabolic disruption, and reduced cerebral blood flow (CBF). It is hypothesized that a trauma to the brain through a rotational or translational impact causes an indiscriminate release of excitatory amino acids, a massive efflux of potassium into the extracellular space, and an influx of intracellular calcium ($Ca2^+$). To restore normal homeostatic functioning, there is increased activation of the sodium-potassium pump and a greater demand for adenosine triphosphate that results in a state of hyperglycolysis and lactic acid accumulation. This process is accompanied by a decrease in CBF that is not well understood. It is presumed to be secondary to accumulation of $Ca2^+$, which is thought to cause widespread cerebral vascular constriction. The resulting "metabolical mismatch" between energy demand and the available energy supply may propagate a cellular vulnerability that is particularly susceptible to even minor changes in CBF, increases in intracranial pressure, and apnea. This metabolic dysfunction is theoretically related to *second impact syndrome* (SIS) and may form the basis for the less severe, although potentially incapacitating, *postconcussion syndrome*. Experimental models have shown that this dysfunction may last for up to 2 weeks and that homeostasis takes longer to achieve in younger rodents. Although there is no clear evidence that the findings from animal models generalize to humans, the processes involved may be the same and can exist with relatively asymptomatic individuals.[15]

Imaging and Physiological Studies

Traditional neuroimaging techniques, although useful in ruling out more serious pathological conditions, are almost always unremarkable following sports-related concussion.[16] However, several newer neurodiagnostic techniques are being investigated for the potential utility in identifying mTBI. For example, both positron emission tomography and single-photon emission computed tomography have demonstrated temporal and frontal hypometabolism at rest and during working memory tasks in mTBI patients. It is presumed that these changes correlate with decreased memory functioning.[17,18]

Changes in brain activation have also been observed following sports-related concussion.[19-22] These findings are based upon investigations with functional magnetic resonance imaging, a method of brain imaging that detects neuronal activation in cortical matter through blood oxygenation changes. In one investigation that compared concussed athletes with a nonconcussed control group during a working memory task, the concussed group demonstrated areas of decreased activation relative to controls in the prefrontal cortex, but increased activation in more posterior areas of the frontal lobe. Results showed that activation patterns in the only asymptomatic concussed subject were similar to those in the control group.[19] Studies have also found an association between postconcussion symptoms and brain activation in concussed athletes.[21,22] In one investigation comparing athletes diagnosed with "complex concussions" with athletes reporting low or moderate levels of postconcussion symptoms, differences in task performance and functional activation were found at least 1 month, and on average 5 months, after injury. Specifically, athletes with complex concussions (characterized by persistent symptoms, history of multiple concussions, or sequelae including LOC greater than 1 minute, prolonged cognitive impairment, or convulsions), were less accurate and slower on cognitive tasks. They also demonstrated reduced activation in the frontal lobes while performing working memory tasks when compared with athletes with moderate levels of postconcussion symptoms.[16,21] Even when concussed athletes' performance on cognitive tasks is equivalent to that of control athletes, research has found differential activation patterns, diffusely and within specific regions of interest.[19-21] In addition, the extent of hyperactivation in concussed athletes may be related to clinical recovery time.[22] Overall, this research suggests that sports-related concussion is associated with attenuated brain functioning, and that atypical patterns of brain activation may be related to a compensatory strategy for frontal lobe dysfunction.

Recording electrical activities in the brain where increased activity is associated with greater signal strength, the electroencephalogram (EEG) has also been used to study concussion in athletes. Standard clinical EEG assessments have revealed abnormalities associated with several years of participation in sports including boxing and soccer.[23-25] There is also evidence of decreased EEG signal intensity in concussed athletes during postural exercises. These decreases are most notable during standing as opposed to seated postures and may reflect the postural instability reported by concussed patients.[26] Similar findings were observed in a sample of concussed athletes involved in a motor control and coordination task.[27]

More recently, researchers have started to examine brain functioning with variants of traditional EEG: evoked potentials and event-related potentials (ERPs). The latter is presumed to be associated with cognitive rather than sensory processing.[28] Recent findings suggest that these techniques may be of considerable benefit for the assessment of a single concussive event and research has shown significantly decreased signal intensities in concussed athletes that are associated with severity of postconcussive symptoms.[29] Investigations focusing on the P300 response, which is a specific component of a ERP in which positive or negative amplitudes are associated with different cognitive processes, have shown attenuated signal amplitudes and longer reaction time in symptomatic concussed athletes when compared with an asymptomatic group and nonconcussed controls.[29,30] In addition, longer visual P300 peak latencies have been correlated with self-reported attention and memory deficits in athletes with three or more concussions.[29,30] However, two separate investigations of boxers found no unusual P300 latencies.[31,32] The discrepancy argues for continued research in this area to further explore the sensitivity of electrophysiological techniques to detect brain functioning abnormalities in concussed athletes.

Assessment of Concussion

There is evidence to suggest that many athletes do not regularly report concussive injuries to team physicians, sports physical therapists, certified athletic trainers, family members, or others.[33,34] In a study of Canadian Football League players, only 19% of those diagnosed with concussion realized they had sustained an injury.[35] Injuries also go unreported because athletes may not understand the seriousness of their injury or purposely deny symptoms to continue playing.[34]

Clinical Point

Up to 90% of concussions are undetected and most are not reported to health care practitioners.

In addition to under-reporting, the variable presentation and severity of mTBI makes it a difficult injury to recognize and assess. Athletes may present with only one or several symptoms, any and all of which are important from a diagnostic and management standpoint. There may be neither a direct trauma to the head nor LOC. Clumsiness, confusion, or obvious amnesia may not be evident. Many symptoms can reflect other causal factors, including dehydration, lack of sleep, or overtraining. There may also be concomitant or pre-existing disorders including anxiety, depression, learning disabilities, or anemia that complicate accurate diagnosis.[36,37] Athletes should be educated to a thorough knowledge of all potential signs and symptoms.

Symptoms of Concussion Reported by Athlete

- Headache
- Change in sleep pattern
- Feeling fatigued
- Feeling "foggy" or groggy
- Nausea
- Balance problems or dizziness
- Double vision or fuzzy or blurry vision
- Sensitivity to light or noise
- Feeling sluggish or slowed down
- Concentration or memory problems

Data from University of Pittsburgh Medical Center's Sideline Concussion Card.

It is helpful, although not always possible, to gain information from multiple informants (e.g., athlete, teammates, athletic trainer, parents, and coach) across multiple time points (e.g., immediately following injury, a few hours later, at 24 hours after injury, 48 hours after injury) to determine the severity of the injury and track recovery.

Sideline Assessment

As with any serious injury, assessment begins with the athlete's level of consciousness, and airway, breathing, and circulation. The attending medical staff must always be prepared with an emergency action plan in the event that the evacuation of a critically head- or neck-injured athlete is necessary. This plan should be familiar to all staff, be well delineated, and frequently rehearsed.

Loss of Consciousness

Although the dramatic on-field presentation of LOC can make concussion easy to detect and calls for the immediate removal from play, it is relatively uncommon in sports-related injury. In most studies, it is identified in less than 10% of all patients.[5-7] In addition, research has shown that the brief LOC (< 1 minute) typically associated with sports-related concussion may not reliably predict recovery time or neuropsychological outcome.[38-41] Despite these findings, most grading scales rely on the presence and duration of LOC to determine the severity of injury and make return-to-play decisions. Regardless of its prognostic value, a patient experiencing extended LOC (typically defined as greater than 1 minute) requires immediate neurological evaluation. Most practitioners agree that athletes who lose consciousness should not return to play immediately following their injury.

Amnesia

Amnesia is characterized by a loss of memory. It can take two forms: retrograde amnesia, which is difficulty recalling events prior to a trauma, and anterograde (post-traumatic) amnesia, which is difficulty recalling events following an injury. Either or both can be present following a concussion and evidence suggests this symptom may be related to worse acute cognitive difficulties and longer recovery time.[40-44] Moreover, its assessment is sometimes made difficult because of its similarity to confusion. The two are distinguished by the fact that confusion is not necessarily associated with difficulty recalling events, whereas amnesia is only diagnosed if there is a loss of memory.

The length of amnesia is variable and determined by the duration of time between a head trauma (e.g., an ice hockey player's forehead striking the boards) and the point at which the athlete reports a return of normal continuous memory functioning (e.g., remembering the athletic trainer asking orientation questions in the locker room). It may span a few seconds or minutes, but sometimes longer.

Anterograde amnesia should be assessed on the field or sidelines through immediate and delayed recall for three words (e.g., girl, dog, green). Additional questions should focus on the injured athlete's ability to recall any events that occurred immediately following the trauma.

Retrograde amnesia is defined as the inability to recall events preceding the trauma. Medical personnel should determine the athlete's memory of the injury (e.g., seeing a linebacker charge toward him with his helmet down, then falling backward and striking the back of his head to the ground) with additional questions probing for events increasingly remote from the injury (e.g., the score at the beginning of the first quarter, coming onto the field for stretching exercises, and getting dressed in the locker room). The length of retrograde amnesia typically declines or shrinks as the time since injury increases, although there is the potential for permanent memory loss. The presence and duration of retrograde amnesia has been associated with worse initial presentation and with slower recovery, suggesting that any positive findings should preclude a return to play.[40,44,45]

Confusion

Characterized by impaired awareness and orientation to surroundings, with intact memory, an athlete with postinjury confusion typically appears stunned, dazed, or "glassy-eyed" on the sideline or playing field. For athletes who do not remove themselves from play, confusion can be inferred by observing an athlete's failure to correctly execute their positional assignments, problems with appropriate playcalling, or difficulty in communicating game information to teammates or coaches. Within the context of competition, teammates are often the first to recognize that an injury has occurred. On the sideline, an athlete experiencing confusion may answer questions slowly or inappropriately, ask "what is going on" or "what happened," and may repeat things during the evaluation. Some may be temporarily disoriented to person, place, or time. Assessment should focus on responses to orientation questions such as the date and the names of the stadium, city, and opposing team.

Symptoms

As with the immediate signs of concussion, symptoms are variable both in severity and duration. Although an athlete may perceive one or several different symptoms, difficulties are typically categorized as somatic, cognitive, emotional, or sleep-related.

Somatic

Previous investigations have shown that headache is the most commonly reported symptom of concussion. It has been reported in up to 86% of concussed athletes and has been associated with longer-term outcomes.[6,46,47] Assessment may be complicated by the presence of myofascial headaches and other pre-existing syndromes including migraines, tension headaches, and sinus conditions. Moreover, headaches resulting from a concussion may not develop immediately after the injury, underscoring the need to assess patients across multiple time points.

Clinically, headaches following concussion are often described as a pressure sensation that can be localized to one region of the head or generalized in nature. Their severity and frequency have been shown to increase with exertion and more conservative management is indicated when headaches worsen with increased levels of either cognitive or physical activity. Notably, although headaches following a concussion usually do not constitute a medical emergency, a severe or progressively severe headache, particularly when accompanied by vomiting or rapidly declining mental status, may signal a subdural hematoma or other intracranial bleed. This should prompt immediate transport to a hospital and brain imaging.

Clinical Point

Progressively severe headaches especially with vomiting or rapidly declining mental status may indicate an intracranial bleed.

Given the prevalence of headaches reported by patients with sports-related concussion, this symptom has been examined extensively in the literature and some findings demonstrate its prognostic utility. For example, one investigation compared a group of concussed high school athletes who reported headaches to a concussed group with no headaches at an assessment occurring approximately 1 week after injury. Results indicated that athletes with headaches performed significantly worse on computerized neurocognitive measures of reaction time and memory. The athletes experiencing headaches also reported more overall symptoms on a postconcussion symptom scale than the nonheadache group.[46] Building on this study, another investigation determined that the type of headache reported is related to outcomes in concussed athletes. Specifically, concussed

athletes who presented with no headaches or with headaches that did not meet the criteria for post-traumatic migraine (PTM), including headache with nausea and sensitivity to light or noise, were compared with a group of athletes reporting PTM. Overall, the PTM group demonstrated worse outcomes with more pronounced difficulties at postinjury testing than did either the headache or non-headache group on computerized measures of neurocognitive functioning.[47] These findings suggest that concussed athletes presenting with symptoms of PTM may need to be managed more conservatively and that they may be more vulnerable to greater neuropsychological deficits and postinjury symptoms than athletes with no headaches or athletes reporting headaches without migrainous features.

In addition to headaches, health care practitioners should be aware of many other symptoms that may emerge as a result of concussive injury. Fatigue may be prominent in concussed athletes in the days following injury and in one study it was reported in 44% of injured athletes at follow-up evaluation.[48] Balance problems, lack of coordination, or dizziness may also be reported. There is also some objective evidence that postural instability can effectively discriminate concussed from nonconcussed athletes following injury, implicating the value of its assessment.[41] Athletes may report "feeling a step slow," or sluggish. There may be visual changes, including blurred vision, peripheral abnormalities, or seeing "spots," "lines," or other visual disturbances. Although less common, nausea and vomiting are also reported.

Cognitive

Following a concussion, athletes may report problems with attention, concentration, short-term memory, learning, and multitasking. These symptoms often become more noticeable when the athlete returns to school or work. Many athletes also experience a sense of mental fogginess. In a recent study, a sample of concussed high school students who reported feeling "foggy" on a symptom inventory were compared with concussed high school athletes who did not endorse this sensation. At 1 week after injury, the group experiencing subjective feelings of fogginess demonstrated significantly slower reaction times, attenuated memory performance, and slower processing speed on a computerized measure of neurocognitive functioning. In addition, the athletes with persistent fogginess endorsed a significantly higher number of other postconcussion symptoms when compared with the group that did not endorse fogginess.[49] Although this symptom is not well understood, its association with neurocognitive difficulties cautions against return to play when reported.

Emotional

Emotional changes are also commonly reported or observed following sports-related concussion. Most often, athletes will report increased irritability or having a "shorter fuse." Other emotional changes may occur such as sadness or depression, nervousness or anxiety, and less commonly, silliness or euphoria. Affect may be described by the athlete or parent as flattened or labile. Emotional changes may be very brief or may be prolonged in the case of a more significant injury such as when an athlete reports persistent depression.

Sleep Disturbances

Hypersomnia has been reported in athletes following sports-related concussion. Normal sleep-wake patterns can become dysregulated and some athletes experience difficulties initiating or maintaining sleep. These difficulties may contribute to daytime fatigue and decreased levels of energy. Proper sleep hygiene is advocated, including going to bed and waking at the same time, limiting caffeine intake, reducing naps, and eliminating reading or watching television in bed.

Neuropsychological Outcomes

In addition to reported symptoms, previous investigations have shown that concussed athletes perform worse on objective measures of neurocognitive functioning when compared with their own baseline (preinjury) scores or nonconcussed controls. With group data, most findings suggest that recovery occurs within 2 to 14 days, but some patients demonstrate significantly longer recovery.[7,37,41,42,50,51] In addition, studies have shown that injured athletes who report no symptoms demonstrate worse performance than uninjured controls, suggesting that subtle neurocognitive sequelae may linger beyond reported symptoms.[52,53]

The benefits of neuropsychological testing within the context of sports medicine were first recognized in the mid-1980s when employed as part of a 4-year prospective study of mTBI in college athletes.[54] Aiming to estimate the incidence of head injuries in football and to determine the neuropsychological sequelae of mTBI, recovery time, risk factors for injury, and potential for longer-term effects, results demonstrated the presence of acute deficits for up to 10 days in injured athletes and provided a framework for the future study of sports-related concussion. Subsequent studies have replicated initial findings in this area. For example, one investigation examined 1631 university football players. In addition to assessment of symptoms and postural stability, participants were evaluated before and after injury on traditional paper-and-pencil measures of neuropsychological functioning. Concussed athletes' balance problems resolved within 3 to 5 days, self-reported postconcussion symptoms gradually resolved by day 7, and neuropsychological functioning improved within 5 to 7 days.[5]

The utility of neuropsychological measures in documenting cognitive recovery following concussion in sports, even in the absence of reported symptoms, has prompted more widespread use as a clinical tool in concussion

management. Moreover, concussive injuries in well-known professional athletes raised awareness and resulted in mandated implementation of baseline computerized neuropsychological testing by the National Football League (NFL). Similarly, after career-ending concussive injuries in the National Hockey League (NHL), the NHL mandated baseline neuropsychological testing for all athletes. In addition, several large-scale studies of professional, collegiate, and high-school athletes have continued to demonstrate neurocognitive sequelae of concussion, and some have demonstrated longer recovery times than previously recorded. For example, in a 3-year prospective study of high school and college athletes, concussed high school athletes demonstrated more prolonged memory impairment than college athletes, and worse performance than age matched controls 7 days after injury. Neuropsychological functioning in the sample of injured college athletes was equal to age-matched controls by 3 days after injury.[55] In addition, a study of 2141 high school athletes found that a percentage of the concussed athletes continued to demonstrate difficulties on cognitive tasks 3 weeks after injury.[56] These results were in contrast to the findings of a 6-year prospective study involving the NFL. The latter investigation comprised a total of 887 concussions recorded in 650 players.[57] Recovery, as determined by return to play, was as follows: 56% recovered on the day of injury, 35.9% recovered 1 to 6 days after injury, 6.5% recovered 7 to 14 days after injury, and 1.6% recovered more than 14 days after injury. Those athletes who returned to play in the same game had fewer and briefer signs and symptoms of concussion, and they did not appear to have significantly increased risk for a second injury either in the same game or during the remainder of the season. In a subset of the concussed NFL players who underwent baseline neuropsychological evaluations and then completed a second evaluation within a few days following their concussion, there was no statistically significant decline on any traditional paper and pencil measures of neuropsychological functioning.[58] That these data contrast findings of studies examining younger athletes suggests that age and developmental factors may play a role in recovery from concussion.

Clinical Point

Neurocognitive assessment should be performed prior to the start of the season to determine "normal" or baseline level of cognitive functioning.

Variable findings in research investigating neuropsychological recovery following concussion have lead to more individualized management of concussion regardless of age. Initially, testing was mostly composed of traditional (e.g., paper-and-pencil measures) to assess baseline and postinjury levels of cognitive functioning. However, as an increasing number of sports organizations have recognized the utility of these measures, many limitations to traditional testing emerged, including the cost and availability of trained neuropsychologists to administer and interpret the data, leading to the development and increased use of computer-based neurocognitive testing.

Computer-based testing procedures have a number of advantages. First, the use of computers allows a large number of athletes to be tested with fewer resources. An entire football team may be baseline tested in one or two sessions. The data can easily be saved and accessed remotely, and with some systems data are summed into a clinical report that can be interpreted by an appropriately trained sports concussion specialist. The use of computers may provide a more accurate measurement of cognitive processes such as reaction time and information processing speed. This increased accuracy may increase the validity of test results in detecting subtle changes in neurocognitive processes. In addition, computerized testing allows for the randomization of test stimuli, which should improve reliability across multiple administration periods by minimizing practice effects.

Several computer-based tests currently exist, including Immediate Post-Concussion Assessment and Cognitive Testing (ImPACT), CogState, Headminders, and Automated Neurocognitive Assessment Matrices (ANAM).[59-62] Most have published manuals describing their psychometric properties, and studies have demonstrated their reliability, validity, sensitivity, specificity, and added value when compared with self-reported symptoms alone.[52,63,64] However, none should be used as a standalone measure and instead should be part of comprehensive assessment that includes a clinical interview, evaluation of symptoms, and overall medical history.

In ideal situations and as recommended by current guidelines, baseline neuropsychological assessment should be administered prior to the start of the season to determine "normal" individual cognitive functioning. Following injury and to assess the severity of injury as well as other management considerations, including return to school and exertion, the first evaluation is often performed while the athlete remains symptomatic. Subsequent testing is performed 7 to 10 days after injury and then as recommended by the treating clinician. A score significantly lower than baseline, defined by statistical reliable change, or premorbid estimates of functioning reflects ongoing sequelae and precludes return to play.

In summary, neuropsychological deficits associated with concussion are reported in the literature, and cognitive testing appears to be a highly valuable tool in documenting impairment and tracking recovery from concussive injury. As the diagnosis of concussion can be a difficult process and athletes at all levels of competition may minimize symptoms,

neuropsychological testing also provides practitioners with objective evidence to support their treatment plans.

Cumulative Effects

Although data concerning the longer-term effects of repetitive concussion vary, there is some evidence that a history of concussion is associated with changes in neurophysiology, subjective symptoms, and neuropsychological test performance.[65,66] However, the number or severity of previous injuries has not been shown to conclusively predict longer-term sequelae or increased vulnerability. In general, studies of athletes with three or more concussions suggest an increased risk of sustaining additional concussive injuries, worse on-field presentations with subsequent concussion, slowed recovery, and greater acute changes in memory performance.[66-68] Research examining athletes who have sustained one or two previous concussions have mixed results.[37,69-71]

In contrast with most studies of repetitive injuries, research evaluating the pathophysiology and neuropsychological functioning of boxers reveals the potential for significant longer-term sequelae.[72-78] At their worst, the neurological deficits affecting boxers may potentially resemble Parkinson disease and include a progressive pattern of difficulties characterized by confusion, loss of coordination, problems with speech, and upper-body tremors. Often referred to as *dementia pugilistica* or *chronic boxer's encephalopathy,* the neurological changes observed in boxers are associated with cerebral atrophy, cortical and subcortical neurofibrillary tangles, and cellular loss in the cerebellum.[79-81] Research has shown that genetic protein apolipoprotein E (APOE) with the ε4 allele may be a risk factor for development of neurological dysfunction and progressive disease in this population.[82,83]

There is also evidence demonstrating a relationship between boxing and neurocognitive impairment. Although the results have varied depending on the level of participation (e.g., amateur or professional), findings suggest that the extent of neuropsychological impairments may be associated with the number of bouts fought.[84,85]

Recovery and Return to Play

Although significant individual variability exists in recovery from concussion, previous group studies have indicated that a single concussion typically resolves in less than 2 weeks. More recent studies, however, have suggested even longer recovery times, especially at the high school level of participation.[43,55,56] Most sports medicine researchers and professionals agree that returning an athlete to contact sport participation prior to complete recovery might increase the risk of poor outcome. Authors have also indicated that retirement from sport should be considered when less biomechanical impact or indirect blows result in symptoms of concussion or when duration of symptoms is significantly increased with successive injuries.[86] Thus, the most important step a practitioner can take toward a positive prognosis is proper assessment and management of concussion in the acute and follow-up stages of injury.

Clinical Point

Any presentation of symptoms, cognitive deficits, balance difficulties, or other symptoms associated with cerebral concussion should preclude a return to sport participation until a completely asymptomatic status is achieved.

Management Guidelines and Grading Scales

More than 20 concussion management guidelines have been published during the previous 30 years with the aim of assisting physicians in classifying both the severity of the injury and when an athlete is safe to return to play. Most were developed by panels of experts in the field and are based on popular beliefs or clinical impressions rather than empirical evidence. A majority of management guidelines also rely on grading scales to reflect and characterize the severity of injury. Although these guidelines have very likely resulted in improved care of the athlete, their variable criteria have also created significant confusion as to the most effective management strategy.

In very general terms, guidelines typically classify concussions across a three-point scale with severity being determined by duration of symptoms and LOC. However, there is significant variability between the various guidelines with equally variable criteria for return to play. As a result, there has been a movement toward more individualized management protocols indicating that no athlete should return to play while symptomatic.

In 1999, the American Orthopaedic Society for Sports Medicine (AOSSM) published a report detailing the state of the classification systems and established possible practical alternatives. Although the AOSSM guidelines did not differ substantially from prior grading systems and classifications, the report was one of the first to stress individual management of injury, rather than applying a numeric grading system relying on a general set of standards and protocols to all injuries. Soon after, the Federation Internationale de Football Association (FIFA) in conjunction with the International Olympic Committee (IOC) and International Ice Hockey Federation (IHF) assembled a group of physicians, neuropsychologists, and sports administrators in Vienna, Austria, to explore methods of reducing morbidity and improve outcomes secondary to sports-related concussion. Perhaps the most important agreement to emerge from the meeting was that none of the previously published guidelines were adequate to ensure proper clinical care management of concussed athletes. In their consensus statement published in 2002, the group emphasized more individualized management and implementation of postinjury neuropsychological testing as a "cornerstone" of proper postinjury management and decisions regarding return to play.[10]

Clinical Point

Each concussion must be managed individually and should involve postinjury neurocognitive testing.

Second Impact Syndrome (SIS)

SIS is presumed to be related to an *extraordinarily rare* cascade of events. In all reported cases (approximately 35 in the past decade), athletes sustained an initial concussive injury, returned to sports or other activities, and sustained a second, typically milder, concussive event resulting in catastrophic brain injury. Although the injury is not well understood, SIS is thought to reflect cerebrovascular congestion or a loss of cerebrovascular autoregulation leading to considerable brain swelling and edema. When it occurs, morbidity is 100% and mortality is reported to occur in up to 50% of cases. To date, most cases of SIS have been reported in children or adolescents, and it appears that younger, "immature" brains may be more vulnerable to the effects of this condition.[87,88] There is significant debate regarding SIS, and some question its existence, but there is agreement that athletes should be removed from play until all symptoms have resolved to prevent its occurrence.[87]

Current Return-to-Play Criteria

Realizing that the variable criteria composing previous management guidelines and grading scales may not adequately prevent injured athletes from return to play, treatment and return-to-play decisions involve multiple factors. History of concussion, severity and duration of symptoms, and medical and psychiatric history, as well as neuropsychological performance should be considered. Current international standards of care require an athlete to satisfy three conditions before returning to play: athletes should be asymptomatic at rest, asymptomatic with both physical and cognitive exertion, and also demonstrate normal or baseline levels of performance on measures of neurocognitive functioning.

Return to Play Following Concussion

- Individual should be asymptomatic at rest
- Individual should be asymptomatic during physical and cognitive exertion
- Neurocognitive testing should show normal/baseline values

Asymptomatic Status at Rest

Before progressing to any significant level of physical exertion, the athlete should report being asymptomatic at rest for at least 24 hours. This is best determined through careful clinical assessment, completion of a symptom inventory, or both. It is important that it be determined whether the athlete is denying or minimizing symptoms and parents, sports physical therapists, certified athletic trainers, and teammates should be included to clarify symptom status.

Asymptomatic Status with Physical and Cognitive Exertion

Following a period of symptom-free status (at least 24 hours), athletes should undergo a graduated return to physical exertion. Given the pathophysiology of concussion, symptoms can develop with increased metabolic demands and the International Conference on Concussion in Sport recommends progression through the following exertional steps in 24-hour periods: (1) light aerobic exercise (walking, stationary biking), (2) sport-specific training (ice skating in hockey, running in soccer—typically moderately exertional), and (3) noncontact training drills (usually heavily exertional). If the athlete's previously resolved postconcussion symptoms return at any point during exercise, the athlete should return to the previous asymptomatic level of exertion.[10,16] Moreover, given the similar response to increased symptoms with cognitive exertion (e.g., school, studying), all athletes, particularly at the grade school, high school, or university level should be completely asymptomatical after a day of school or other cognitively demanding activity. It is important to achieve a completely asymptomatic status after both physical and cognitive activities.

Intact Neurocognitive Functioning

Neurocognitive recovery from concussion is assumed when the athlete's performance returns to baseline levels. If no preinjury data are available, recovery is assumed when results are consistent with premorbid estimates of functioning in which test data are compared with normative values. In ideal situations, clinicians will have access to norms that match the demographic and even sport-specific characteristics of the examinee.

Once symptom-free at rest and with physical exertion, and within expected levels on cognitive testing, athletes may return to graded contact training and activity, and then to competition. At all stages of recovery, very close monitoring of symptoms is indicated. If any symptoms emerge with return to contact participation, the athlete should return to a noncontact, asymptomatic level of physical exertion. The one uniform agreement among experts is that any athlete known to be exhibiting signs or symptoms of concussive injury should not return to play, given general issues surrounding increased neurological vulnerability to a second injury and that less biomechanical force may result in more severe postconcussion presentation.

Potential Risk Factors

Making the return-to-play decision following sports-related concussion is an individualized and dynamic process. A general awareness that concussion symptoms can evolve in time or worsen with exertion are critical factors to help guide health care practitioners in their assessment strategy and treatment plan. In addition, multiple factors have been identified that may contribute to an athlete's recovery.

Age

When recovery is defined as a return to baseline levels of cognitive functioning, research has demonstrated that pediatric athletes may recover more slowly from concussion than older athletes.[55,56] Results from one investigation comparing concussed college and high school athletes with uninjured controls found that the high school athletes took longer to recover than college-age subjects despite reporting less prior incidence of concussion and less severe in-season injury.[55] Moreover, a study examining mild concussions or "bell ringers," found that high school athletes with less than 15 minutes of on-field symptoms exhibited difficulties with memory and reported symptoms several days after their injury.[89] Results from these age-specific research studies provides support for removing all pediatric athletes from events in which they sustained a concussion until further assessment is completed.

Clinical Point

Pediatric patients are more vulnerable to the effects of concussions and tend to recover more slowly so should be treated more conservatively than adults.

Although no published research is available to document an age-based physiological or developmental vulnerability to concussion, it is presumed that children may undergo more prolonged and diffuse cerebral swelling. As a result, there may be increased risk for secondary intracranial hypertension and ischemia, which potentially increases the likelihood of permanent or severe neurological deficit should reinjury occur during recovery.[87-89] Researchers have also suggested that the developing brain may be 60 times more sensitive to glutamate-mediated N-methyl-D-aspartate excitotoxic brain injury. This hypersensitivity may render the child or adolescent more susceptible to the ischemic and injurious effects of excitatory amino acids after mTBI.[90,91] Regardless of the physiological process, current findings suggest more conservative management of younger athletes and that further research is warranted in this area.

Gender

Most of the research on sports-related concussion has focused on male athletes and demonstrates an equal or greater injury rate in this population.[92] However, there is some evidence to suggest that the injury rate is greater for females.[2,93] Females have also been shown to report more symptoms at baseline, greater postinjury symptoms, and longer recovery on measures of neuropsychological functioning.[93-96] Moreover, in TBI studies unrelated to sports, results have demonstrated worse outcomes in females. For example, in a meta-analysis of eight studies, outcome was worse for females than males across 85% of identified variables.[97] Research has also shown that when compared with controls, females are more likely to report sleep disturbances and headaches up to a year after injury, are less likely to be employed or in school 1 year after mild head injury, and report significant decrease in grade point average. There were no similar findings for males.

In contrast to these findings, animal models suggest that female sex hormones may actually protect neurons in the brain following concussive injury. Progesterone is thought to reduce cerebral edema and potentially facilitate cognitive recovery. Studies examining the role of estrogen have yielded mixed results, with one study demonstrating that estrogen can assist in maintaining normal CBF and actually decrease mortality when administered acutely.[98-101] Conversely, estrogen has been shown to play a protective role in males although increasing mortality in females.[102] More research in this area is necessary to better understand gender differences in sports-related concussion.

Learning Disability

Learning disability (LD) refers to a heterogeneous group of disorders characterized by difficulties in the acquisition and use of listening, speaking, writing, reading, reasoning, or mathematical abilities that are diagnosed in early childhood. There is evidence demonstrating that athletes with a previous history of concussion and a diagnosed LD perform worse on tests of neurocognitive functioning at baseline and after injury than athletes with multiple prior concussions, but no LD. In addition, athletes with a history of concussion and LD perform worse than athletes with LD, but no history of concussion.[37] These findings may reflect an additive effect of concussion and underscore the importance of a comprehensive clinical evaluation to determine any factors that may complicate diagnosis and return-to-play decisions.

Genetics

The apolipoprotein ε4 allele has been associated with poor outcomes in patients with moderate to severe TBI.[103,104] However, far fewer studies have sought to determine a relationship between APOE ε4 and concussion, and most of these have focused on boxers and are limited by variable findings. Yet there is evidence to suggest that APOE ε4 may increase risk of acute and longer-term neurocognitive sequelae of concussion.[82,83]

Conclusion

Current estimates find that the incidence of concussion is greater than previously reported. Complicating the diagnosis, athletes may be reluctant to report their injury. Guidelines that rely on LOC do not reliably determine severity of injury and there is no consensus on the amount of time required to achieve recovery from sports-related concussion. Thus, the treatment of sports-related concussion has moved toward an individualized, empirically driven approach with return-to-play decisions based on athletes' perceived symptoms and performance on objective measures of neurocognitive functioning. By these guidelines, most athletes recover from concussion and are returned to competition 2 weeks after injury, but recent evidence suggests that recovery is potentially longer for younger individuals. In addition to age, prior history of concussion, a previously diagnosed LD, gender, and a pre-existing history of headaches or migraines may negatively influence recovery. A recent study also demonstrated that higher levels of exertion during the acute phase of recovery moderated neurocognitive performance and symptom reports. Although the exact nature of the factors associated with concussion continues to be examined, evidence suggests they may affect recovery time and the concurrent period of increased vulnerability, highlighting the importance of an individualized approach to managing sports-related concussion. Continued research is necessary to delineate other potential contributing factors, including potential genetic, serum marker, sport-specific or other risk factors to better elucidate management considerations. This information will help to guide the therapies aimed at preventing and treating sports-related concussion.

References

1. Langlois JA, Rutland-Brown W, Wald MM: The epidemiology and impact of traumatic brain injury: A brief overview, *J Head Trauma Rehabil* 21:375–378, 2006.
2. Covassin T, Swanik CB, Sachs ML: Epidemiological considerations of concussions among intercollegiate athletes, *Appl Neuropsychol* 10(1):12–22, 2003.
3. Powell JW, Barber-Foss MS: Traumatic brain injury in high school athletes, *JAMA* 282:958–963, 1999.
4. NIH Consensus Development Panel on Rehabilitation of Persons with Traumatic Brain Injury: Consensus Conference: Rehabilitation of persons with traumatic brain injury, *JAMA* 282:974–983, 1999.
5. McCrea M, Guskiewicz KM, Marshall SW, et al: Acute effects and recovery time following concussion in collegiate football players: The NCAA concussion study, *JAMA* 290(19):2556–2563, 2003.

6. Guskiewicz KM, Weaver NL, Padua DA, Garrett WE Jr: Epidemiology of concussion in collegiate and high school football players, *Am J Sports Med* 28(5):643–650, 2000.

7. Macciocchi SN, Barth JT, Alves W, et al: Neuropsychological functioning and recovery after mild head injury in collegiate athletes, *Neurosurg* 39(3):510–514, 1996.

8. Congress of Neurological Surgeons: Committee on head injury nomenclature: Glossary of head injury, *Clin Neurosurg* 12:386–394, 1966.

9. American Academy of Neurology: Practice parameter: The management of concussion in sports (summary statement). Report of the Quality Standards Subcommittee, *Neurology* 48(3):581–585, 1997.

10. Aubry M, Cantu R, Dvorak J, et al: Summary and agreement statement of the First International Conference on Concussion in Sport, Vienna 2001. Recommendations for the improvement of safety and health of athletes who may suffer concussive injuries, *Br J Sports Med* 36(1):6–10, 2002.

11. Ommaya AK, Gennarelli TA: Cerebral concussion and traumatic unconsciousness. Correlation of experimental and clinical observations of blunt head injuries, *Brain* 97(4):633–654, 1974.

12. Gaetz M: The neurophysiology of brain injury, *Clin Neurophysiol* 115(1):4–18, 2004.

13. Katayama Y, Becker DP, Tamura T, Hovda DA: Massive increases in extracellular potassium and indiscriminate release of glutamate following concussive brain injury, *J Neurosurg* 73:889–900, 1990.

14. Giza CC, Hovda DA: The neurometabolic cascade of concussion, *J Athl Train* 36:228–235, 2001.

15. Giza CC, Hovda DA: The pathophysiology of traumatic brain injury. In Lovell MR, Echemendia RJ, Barth JT, Collins MW, Editors: *Traumatic brain injury in sports,* Lisse, Netherlands, 2004, Swets & Zeitlinger.

16. McCrory P, Johnston K, Meeuwisse W, et al: Summary and agreement statement of the 2nd International Conference on Concussion in Sport, Prague 2004, *Br J Sports Med* 39(4):196–204, 2005.

17. Chen SHA, Kareken DA, Fastenau PS, et al: A study of persistent post-concussion symptoms in mild head trauma using positron emission tomography, *J Neurol Neurosurg Psychiatry* 74:326–332, 2003.

18. Umile EM, Sandel ME, Alavi A, Plotkin RC: Dynamic imaging in mild traumatic brain injury: Support for the theory of medial temporal vulnerability, *Arch Phys Med Rehabil* 83:1506–1513, 2002.

19. Chen JK, Johnston KM, Frey S, et al: Functional abnormalities in symptomatic concussed athletes: An fMRI study, *Neuroimage* 22(1):68–82, 2004.

20. Jantzen KJ, Anderson B, Steinberg FL, Kelso JA: A prospective functional MR imaging study of mild traumatic brain injury in college football players, *Am J Neuroradiol* 25(5):738–745, 2004.

21. Chen JK, Johnston KM, Collie A, et al: A validation of the post concussion symptom scale in the assessment of complex concussion using cognitive testing and functional MRI, *J Neurol Neurosurg Psychiatry* 78:1231–1238, 2007.

22. Lovell MR, Pardini JE, Welling JS, et al: Functional brain abnormalities are related to clinical recovery and time to return to play in athletes, *Neurosurg* 61:352–360, 2007.

23. Kaplan HA, Browder J: Observations on the clinical and brain wave patterns of professional boxers, *JAMA* 156(12):1138–1144, 1954.

24. Kross R, Ohler K, Barolin GS: Cerebral trauma due to heading—Computerized EEG analysis of football players, *EEG-EMG* 14:209–212, 1983.

25. Tysvaer AT, Storli OV: Soccer injuries to the brain. A neurologic and electroencephalographic study of active football players, *Am J Sports Med* 17(4):573–578, 1989.

26. Thompson J, Sebastianelli W, Slobounov S: EEG and postural correlates of mild traumatic brain injury in athletes, *Neurosci Lett* 377(3):158–163, 2005.

27. Slobounov S, Sebastianelli W, Simon R: Neurophysiological and behavioral concomitants of mild brain injury in collegiate athletes, *Clin Neurophysiol* 113(2):185–193, 2002.

28. Mendez CV, Hurley RA, Lassonde M, et al: Mild traumatic brain injury: Neuroimaging of sports-related concussion, *J Neuropsychiatry Clin Neurosci* 17(3):297–303, 2005.

29. Dupuis F, Johnston KM, Lavoie ME, et al: Concussion in athletes produce brain dysfunction as revealed by event-related potentials, *NeuroReport* 11(18):4087–4092, 2000.

30. Lavoie ME, Dupuis F, Johnston KM, et al: Visual p300 effects beyond symptoms in concussed college athletes, *J Clin Exp Neuropsychol* 26(1):55–73, 2004.

31. Breton F, Pincemaille Y, Tarriere C, Renault B: Event-related potential assessment of attention and the orienting reaction in boxers before and after a fight, *Biol Psychol* 31(1):57–71, 1991.

32. Murelius O, Haglund Y: Does Swedish amateur boxing lead to chronic brain damage? 4. A retrospective neuropsychological study, *Acta Neurologica Scandinavica* 83(1):9–13, 1991.

33. Erlanger DM, Kutner KC, Barth JT, Barnes R: Neuropsychology of sports-related concussion: Dementia pugilistica to post concussion syndrome, *Clin Neuropsychol* 13:193–209, 1999.

34. McCrea M, Hammeke T, Olsen G, et al: Unreported concussion in high school football players: Implications for prevention, *Clin J Sports Med* 14(1):13–17, 2004.

35. Delaney JS, Lacroix VJ, Leclerc S, Johnston KM: Concussions during the 1997 Canadian Football season, *Clin J Sports Med* 10:9–14, 2000.

36. Iverson GL, Brooks BL, Collins MW, Lovell MR: Tracking neuropsychological recovery following concussion in sport, *Brain Inj* 20:245–252, 2006.

37. Collins MW, Grindel SH, Lovell MR, et al: Relationship between concussion and neuropsychological performance in college football players, *JAMA* 282(10):964–970, 1999.

38. Iverson GL, Lovell MR, Smith SS: Does brief loss of consciousness affect cognitive functioning after mild head injury? *Arch Clin Neuropsychol* 15(7):643–648, 2000.

39. Lovell MR, Iverson GL, Collins MW, et al: Does loss of consciousness predict neuropsychological decrements after concussion? *Clin J Sports Med* 9(4):193–198, 1999.

40. Collins MW, Iverson GL, Lovell MR, et al: On-field predictors of neuropsychological and symptom deficit following sports-related concussion, *Clin J Sports Med* 13(4):222–229, 2003.

41. Guskiewicz KM, Ross SE, Marshall SW: Postural stability and neuropsychological deficits after concussion in collegiate athletes, *J Athl Train* 36(3):263–273, 2001.

42. McCrea M, Kelly JP, Randolph C, et al: Immediate neurocognitive effects of concussion, *Neurosurg* 50(5):1032–1040, discussion 1040–1042, 2002.

43. Lovell MR, Collins MW, Iverson GL, et al: Recovery from mild concussion in high school athletes, *J Neurosurg* 98(2):296–301, 2003.

44. Pellman EJ, Powell JW, Viano DC, et al: Concussion in professional football: Epidemiological features of game injuries and review of the literature—Part 3, *Neurosurg* 54(1):81–94, discussion 94–96, 2004.

45. Asplund CA, McKeag DB, Olsen CH: Sport-related concussion: Factors associated with prolonged return to play, *Clin J Sports Med* 14(6):339–343, 2004.

46. Collins MW, Field M, Lovell MR, et al: Relationship between postconcussion headache and neuropsychological test performance in high school athletes, *Am J Sports Med* 31(2):168–173, 2003.

47. Mihalik JP, Stump JE, Collins MW, et al: Posttraumatic migraine characteristics in athletes following sports-related concussion, *J Neurosurg* 102(5):850–855, 2005.

48. Erlanger D, Kaushik T, Cantu R, et al: Symptom-based assessment of the severity of a concussion, *J Neurosurg* 98:477–484, 2003.

49. Iverson GL, Gaetz M, Lovell MR, Collins MW: Relation between subjective fogginess and neuropsychological testing following concussion, *J Int Neuropsychol Society* 10:904–906, 2004.

50. Barr WB, McCrea M: Sensitivity and specificity of standardized neurocognitive testing immediately following sports concussion, *J Int Neuropsychol Society* 7:693–702, 2001.

51. Warden DL, Bleiberg J, Cameron KL, et al: Persistent prolongation of simple reaction time in sports concussion, *Neurology* 57(3):524–526, 2001.

52. Fazio VC, Lovell MR, Pardini JE, Collins MW: The relation between post concussion symptoms and neurocognitive performance in concussed athletes, *NeuroRehabil* 22:207–216, 2007.

53. Erlanger D, Saliba E, Barth J, et al: Monitoring resolution of postconcussion symptoms in athletes: Preliminary results of a web-based neuropsychological test protocol, *J Athl Training* 36(3):280–287, 2001.

54. Barth JT, Alves WM, Ryan T, et al: Mild head injury in sports: Neuropsychological sequelae and recovery of function. In Levin HS, Eisenberg HM, Benton AL, Editors: *Mild head injury,* New York, 1989, Oxford.

55. Field M, Collins MW, Lovell MR, Maroon J: Does age play a role in recovery from sports-related concussion? A comparison of high school and collegiate athletes, *J Pediatrics* 142(5):546–553, 2003.

56. Collins MW, Lovell MR, Iverson GL, et al: Examining concussion rates and return to play in high school football players wearing newer helmet technology: A three-year prospective cohort study, *Neurosurg* 58(10):275–286, 2006.

57. Pellman EJ, Viano DC, Casson IR, et al: Concussion in professional football: Injuries involving 7 or more days out—Part 5, *Neurosurg* 55(5):1100–1119, 2004.

58. Pellman EJ, Viano DC, Casson IR, et al: Concussion in professional football: Repeat injuries—Part 4, *Neurosurg* 55(4):860–873, discussion 873–876, 2004.

59. Lovell MR, Collins MW: *ImPACT: Immediate post-concussion assessment and cognitive testing,* Pittsburgh, PA, 1998.

60. *CogSport,* accessed January 26, 2008, from http://cogstate.com/go/sport.

61. Erlanger DM, Feldman DJ, Kutner K: *Concussion resolution index.* New York, 1999, Headminder, Inc.

62. Reeves D, Thorne R, Winter S, Hegge F: *The united tri-service cognitive performance assessment battery, (UTC-PAB), Report 89-1,* San Diego, 1989, US Naval Aerospace Medical Research Laboratory and Walter Reed Army Institute of Research.

63. Schatz P, Pardini JE, Lovell MR, et al: Sensitivity and specificity of the ImPACT test battery for concussion in athletes, *Arch Clin Neuropsychol* 21:91–99, 2006.

64. Van Kampen D, Lovell MR, Pardini JE, et al: The "value added" of neurocognitive testing in managing sports concussion in athletes, *Am J Sports Med* 34(10):1630–1635, 2006.

65. Gaetz M, Goodman D, Weinberg H: Electrophysiological evidence for the cumulative effects of concussion, *Brain Inj* 14(12):1077–1088, 2000.

66. Iverson GL, Gaetz M, Lovell MR, Collins MW: Cumulative effects of concussion in amateur athletes, *Brain Inj* 18(5):433–443, 2004.

66. Collins MW, Lovell MR, Iverson GL, et al: Cumulative effects of concussion in high school athletes, *Neurosurg* 51(5):1175–1179, discussion 1171–1180, 2002.

67. Guskiewicz KM, McCrea M, Marshall SW, et al: Cumulative effects associated with recurrent concussion in collegiate football players: The NCAA Concussion Study, *JAMA* 290(19):2549–2555, 2003.

68. Moser RS, Schatz P, Jordan BD: Prolonged effects of concussion in high school athletes, *Neurosurg* 57(2):300–306; discussion 300–306, 2005.

69. Moser RS, Schatz P: Enduring effects of concussion in youth athletes, *Arch Clin Neuropsychol* 17(1):91–100, 2002.

70. Macciocchi SN, Barth JT, Littlefield L, Cantu RC: Multiple concussions and neuropsychological functioning in collegiate football players, *J Athl Training* 36(3):303–306, 2001.

71. Iverson GL, Brooks BL, Lovell MR, Collins MW: No cumulative effects for one or two previous concussions, *Br J Sports Med* 40(9):802–805, 2006.

72. Jordan BD, Zimmerman RD: Computed tomography and magnetic resonance imaging comparisons in boxers, *JAMA* 263(12):1670–1674, 1990.

73. Zhang L, Ravdin LD, Relkin N, et al: Increased diffusion in the brain of professional boxers: A preclinical sign of traumatic brain injury? *Am J Neuroradiol* 24(1):52–57, 2003.

74. Rabadi MH, Jordan BD: The cumulative effect of repetitive concussion in sports, *Clin J Sports Med* 11(3):194–198, 2001.

75. Dale GE, Leigh PN, Luthert P, et al: Neurofibrillary tangles in dementia pugilistica are ubiquitinated, *J Neurol Neurosurg Psychiatry* 54(2):116–118, 1991.

76. Roberts GW, Allsop D, Bruton C: The occult aftermath of boxing, *J Neurol Neurosurg Psychiatry* 53(5):373–378, 1990.

77. Miele VJ, Carson L, Carr A, Bailes JE: Acute on chronic subdural hematoma in a female boxer: A case report, *Med Sci Sports Exerc* 36(11):1852–1855, 2004.

78. Lampert PW, Hardman JM: Morphological changes in brains of boxers, *JAMA* 251:2676–2679, 1984.

79. Serel J, Jaros O: The mechanisms of cerebral concussion in boxing and their consequences, *World Neurol* 3:351–358, 1962.

80. Corsellis JA, Bruton CJ, Freeman-Browne D: The aftermath of boxing, *Psychol Med* 3(3):270–303, 1973.

81. Jordan BD: Neurologic aspects of boxing, *Arch Neurol* 44:453–459, 1987.

82. Jordan BD, Relkin NR, Ravdin LD, et al: Apolipoprotein E epsilon4 associated with chronic traumatic brain injury in boxing, *JAMA* 278(2):136–140, 1997.

83. Stewart WF, Gordon B, Selnes O, et al: Prospective study of central nervous system function in amateur boxers in the United States, *Am J Epidemiol* 139(6):573–588, 1994.

84. Kemp P, Houston A, Macleod M, Pethybridge RJ: Cerebral perfusion and psychometric testing in military amateur boxers and control, *J Neurol Neurosurg Psychiatry* 59:368–374, 1995.

85. Heilbronner RL, Bush SS, Ravdin LD, et al: Neuropsychological consequences of boxing and recommendations to improve safety: A National Academy of Neuropsychology education paper, *Arch Clin Neuropsychol* 24(1):11–19, 2009.

86. Echemendia RJ, Cantu R: Return to play following cerebral head injury. In Lovell MR, Echemendia RJ, Barth JT, Collins MW, Editors: *Traumatic brain injury in sports: A neuropsychological and international perspective,* Netherlands, 2004, Swets & Zeitlinger.

87. Cantu RC: Second-impact syndrome, *Clin Sports Med* 17(1):37–44, 1998.

88. McQuillen JB, McQuillen EN, Morrow P: Trauma, sport, and malignant cerebral edema, *Am J Forensic Med Pathol* 9(1):12–15, 1988.

89. Lovell MR, Collins MW, Iverson GL, et al: Grade 1 or "ding" concussions in high school athletes, *Am J Sports Med* 32(1): 47–54, 2004.

90. Bruce DA, Alavi A, Bilaniuk L, et al: Diffuse cerebral swelling following head injuries in children: The syndrome of "malignant brain edema." *J Neurosurg* 54(2):170–178, 1981.

91. Pickles W: Acute general edema of the brain in children with head injuries, *New Engl J Med* 242(16):607–611, 1950.

92. Barnes BC, Cooper L, Kirkendall DT, et al: Concussion history in elite male and female soccer players, *Am J Sports Med* 26(3):433–438, 1998.

93. Covassin T, Schatz P, Swanik CB: Sex differences in the neuropsychological function and post-concussion symptoms of concussed collegiate athletes, *Neurosurg* 61:345–350, 2007.

94. Broshek DK, Kaushik T, Freeman JR, et al: Sex differences in outcome following sports-related concussion, *J Neurosurg* 102: 856–863, 2005.

95. Covassin T, Swanik CB, Sachs M, et al: Sex differences in baseline neuropsychological functioning and concussion symptoms of collegiate athletes, *Br J Sports Med* 40:923–927, 2006.

96. Lovell MR, Iverson GL, Collins MW, et al: Measurement of symptoms following sports-related concussion: Reliability and normative data for the post-concussion scale, *Appl Neuropsychol* 13(3):166–174, 2006.

97. Farace E, Alves W: Do women fare worse: A meta-analysis of gender differences in traumatic brain injury outcome, *J Neurosurg* 93:539–545, 1998.

98. Roof RL, Duvdevani R, Stein DG: Gender influences outcome of brain injury: Progesterone plays a protective role, *Brain Res* 607:333–336, 1993.

99. Roof RL, Hall ED: Estrogen-related gender differences in survival rate and cortical blood flow after impact acceleration head injury in rats, *J Neurotrauma* 17:367–388, 2007.

100. Rogers E, Wagner AW: Gender, sex steroids, and neuroprotection following traumatic brain injury, *J Head Trauma Rehabil* 21(3):279–281, 2006.

101. Stein DG, Hoffman SW: Estrogen and progesterone as neuroprotective agents in the treatment of acute brain injuries, *Pediatr Rehabil* 6(1):13–22, 2003.

102. Emerson CS, Hadrick JP, Vink R: Estrogen improves biochemical and neurologic outcome following traumatic brain injury in male rats, but not females, *Brain Res* 8:95–100, 1993.

103. Teasdale G, Nicole J, Murray G: Association of apolipoprotein E polymorphism with outcome after brain injury, *Lancet* 350: 1069–1071, 1997.

104. Gross R: APOE epsilon 4 allele and chronic traumatic brain injury, *JAMA* 278:2143, 1997.

TRAUMATIC SPORTS INJURIES TO THE CERVICAL SPINE

James E. Zachazewski, Brant D. Berkstresser, Gary J. Geissler, Francis Wang, and Lars C. Richardson

Introduction

Millions of people participate each year in organized and recreational sports, placing themselves at risk for possible injury. The majority of individuals participate without suffering from significant injury or disability. Most injuries that do occur are relatively minor, allowing the participants to return to their desired recreational activities and lifestyle without incident. Unfortunately, catastrophic injuries do sometimes occur from participation in organized or recreational athletic activity. Such catastrophic, and potentially fatal, injuries involve fractures and fracture-dislocations of the cervical spine.

Current epidemiological data from the National Spinal Cord Injury Information Network[1] reveals that approximately 12,000 new traumatic spinal cord–injured patients each year require medical intervention (or 40 cases/million in the U.S. population). Involvement in athletic activity has accounted for 7.4% of all spinal cord injuries yearly since 2005. This recent data demonstrates a decrease in incidence caused by athletic competition compared with data from Keenen and Benson,[2] published in 1992, who reported that 15% of spinal cord injuries were a result of sports (Figure 23-1).

Sports medicine clinicians of all disciplines have always been actively involved in seeking improvements to athletic equipment, strength and conditioning programs, rules changes, coaching standards, and techniques that could affect injury rates in a positive manner. Advocacy of clinicians for these changes have focused on sports that place participants at high risk for spinal cord trauma, such as football and hockey. The change in the incidence of injury attributable to sports may speak to how clinicians involved in sports medicine may be in a position to influence the prevention, management, and outcome of these injuries. The role that providers play differs depending on the level of organization of the sport (i.e., youth league, interscholastic, intercollegiate, or professional), and the clinician's level of involvement with the team or athlete.

The makeup of the sports medicine team varies depending on the situation. In organized sports, physicians, athletic trainers, physical therapists, paramedics, and emergency medical technicians (EMTs) specifically trained in the management of acute cervical injuries are often present when an injury occurs and are available to assist. However, in recreational sports, a paramedic or EMT is often called on to manage an acute cervical injury after it has occurred.

Clinical Point

In organized sports, the overall responsibility of the sports medicine team is to establish and practice an effective emergency plan. This includes any policies and procedures necessary for the emergency management of catastrophic injuries prior to the occurrence of any injury.[3,4] All personnel must be appropriately trained and aware of their role and must practice to maintain proficiency. Communication links and an agreed-on chain of command within the sports medicine team and with all other appropriate medical personnel, such as paramedics and emergency medical technicians are pivotal to the successful management of any emergency. If catastrophic injury occurs, an effective emergency management plan can successfully be implemented in an efficient, expedient manner.

Note: This chapter includes content from previous contributions by James E. Zachazewski, MS, PT, SCS, ATC, Gary Geissler, MS, PT, SCS, ATC, and Donald Hangen, MD, as it appeared in the predecessor of this book—Zachazewski JE, Magee DJ, Quillen WS, editors: *Athletic injuries and rehabilitation*, Philadelphia, 1996, WB Saunders.

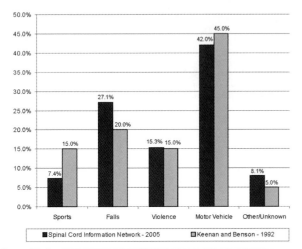

Figure 23-1

Causes of spinal cord injuries. (Data from the National Spinal Cord Injury Statistical Center: *Spinal cord information network: Facts and figures at a glance—Update January 2008*, University of Alabama Birmingham, available at www.spinalcord.uab.edu; and Keenen TL, Benson DR: Initial evaluation of the spine injured patient. In Browner BD, Juputer JB, Levine AM, Tafton PG, editors: *Skeletal trauma*, Philadelphia, 1992, WB Saunders.)

Tracking and Surveillance Methods

Tracking and understanding the incidence and patterns associated with any injury are critical to successfully reducing that injury's incidence and severity. This is certainly evidenced by the reduction of catastrophic cervical spine injuries since the 1960s. The National Football Head and Neck Injury Registry (NFHNIR) was established in 1975 in Philadelphia by Joseph S. Torg to determine whether injuries sustained by 12 players in 1975 reflected a national trend toward catastrophic neurotrauma related to football.[5] The purpose of the registry was to track sports-related head and neck injuries in the United States. The registry has built on the pivotal work initiated by Schneider from the years 1959 through 1963.[6,7] Retrospective data was compiled from 1971 through 1975, and data continued to be collected through the mid and late 1980s. Injuries continue to be tracked and reported on through the National Center for Catastrophic Sport Injury Research at the University of North Carolina.[8]

Through this tracking and surveillance mechanism, recommendations have been made for changes in rules, coaching and training practices, and equipment that have resulted in a decrease in the incidence of cervical spine injuries. The most apparent of these rules changes was adopted in 1976. Preliminary data analysis in 1975 demonstrated that the majority of serious cervical spine football injuries were caused by cervical flexion and axial loading. Because of the outcomes of this data, a rule change was implemented by the National Collegiate Athletic Association (NCAA) and the National Federation of High School Athletic Associations (NFHSAA) that prohibited spearing,

or using the crown of the helmet as the initial contact point when tackling. This change has resulted in a significant decrease in the incidence of cervical spine injury and quadriplegia (Figure 23-2).[9] Since that time, rules have been further strengthened eliminating the word *intentional* from the spearing rule. In addition, a recent "point of emphasis" to game officials in the rules of American Football at both the NCAA and National Football League (NFL) levels initiated in 2007 prohibits contact to the head of a player who cannot properly defend himself.

Data from 1977 to 2007 is presented in Figure 23-3 and is based on information from the National Center for Catastrophic Sport Injury Research. As can be seen in Figure 23-3, of the 282 total catastrophic injuries to the cervical spine that occurred in this 20-year period, 233 occurred in the high school age group. However, to fully understand the incidence data, rates must be compared based on

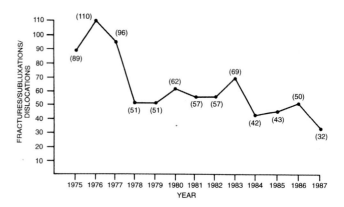

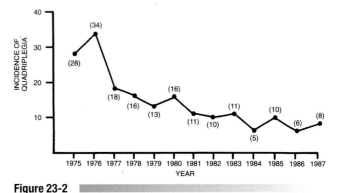

Figure 23-2

A, Yearly incidence of cervical spine fractures, dislocations, and subluxations for all levels of participation (1975-1987) decreased markedly in 1978 and continued to decline during the remaining 9 years as a direct result of the rule changes instituted in 1976 banning headfirst blocking, tackling, and spearing. **B,** Yearly incidence of permanent cervical quadriplegia for all levels of participation (1975-1987) decreased dramatically in 1977 after initiation of rule changes prohibiting use of head first tackling and blocking techniques. The number of injuries continued to decline until 1984, after which the dramatically lowered levels were maintained. (From Torg JS, Vgso JJ, O'Neil J et al: The epidemiologic, pathologic, biomechanical and cinematographic analysis of football-induced cervical spine trauma, *Am J Sports Med* 18:50-57, 1990.)

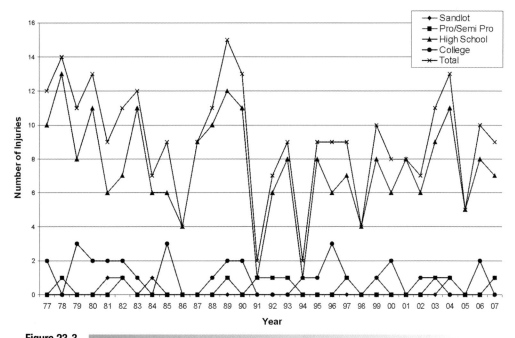

Figure 23-3

Catastrophic football injuries by year, 1977-2007. (Data from Mueller FO, Cantu RC: *Annual survey of catastrophic football injuries,* National Center for Catastrophic Sport Injury Research, University of North Carolina, Chapel Hill, NC; available at http://www.unc.edu/depts/nccsi/.)

incidence per participant. When Table 23-1 and Table 23-2 are reviewed, it can be seen that, although a greater number of high school football players have suffered catastrophic cervical spine injuries, the incidence is much higher in the collegiate athlete. This data has been fully reviewed and reported by Boden et al.[10]

Tracking of these devastating injuries should continue to allow the sports medicine community to continue to recognize patterns of injury and advocate for appropriate rules, technique, and equipment changes to minimize their effect.

Epidemiology

Types of Injury

Brachial Plexus Injuries

Brachial plexus injuries, often termed *burners* or *stingers,* are most commonly incurred in collision sports such as football (Figure 23-4). The football rules change instituted in 1976 as a result of the efforts of the NFHNIR required a return to shoulder blocking and tackling. Because of this change, an increase in the frequency of brachial plexus injuries might have been anticipated, because a common mechanism causing these injuries in football is shoulder depression during blocking and tackling. However, a review of data collected on collegiate athletes from 1975 through 1978 by the National Athletic Injury Reporting System did not demonstrate this to be the case.

The signs and symptoms of all types of brachial plexus injuries usually sustained in sports include sharp, burning pain in the shoulder that may shoot down toward the hand. Complaints of neck pain are infrequent. These symptoms are usually unilateral and transient in nature, lasting seconds to minutes. Pain and paresthesia may radiate into the upper extremity. Shoulder or arm weakness may be present as an additional symptom. Signs and symptoms are usually unilateral. If significant neck pain exists, if these symptoms include two or more extremities, or if any of the symptoms mentioned previously last beyond a few minutes, clinicians should consider the possibility of a more significant injury and initiate cervical spine injury precautions.

Statistically these injuries are infrequent in sports, with the exception of American football.[11,12] The *burner* or *stinger* is the most common neural injury sustained by football players. Burners or stingers most commonly affect defensive backs, linebackers, and lineman because of the most common mechanism of injury, tackling.[13] Clancy and colleagues,[14] Clancy,[15] Markey and colleagues,[16] and Sallis and colleagues[17] have reported that up to 65% of collegiate football players have sustained at least one burner during their collegiate careers. These injuries and other nerve peripheral nerve injuries about the shoulder and cervical spine have been thoroughly reviewed and discussed by Safran in 2004.[18,19]

Sprains and Strains

Minor injuries to the cervical spine that are a result of trauma are usually termed *sprains* (collagen tissue) or *strains* (contractile tissue). Trauma is imposed by some means of acceleration, deceleration, or contact with an object such as the ground, an opponent, or the ball. This is probably the most common type of injury to the cervical spine in sports, although no reports are available in the literature detailing the specific incidence of this injury.

Table 23-1

Catastrophic Cervical Spine Injuries per 100,000 Participants 1997-2007*

Year	High School	College
1977	0.77	2.67
1978	1.00	0.00
1979	0.62	4.00
1980	0.85	2.67
1981	0.46	2.67
1982	0.54	2.67
1983	0.85	1.33
1984	0.46	0.00
1985	0.46	4.00
1986	0.31	0.00
1987	0.69	0.00
1988	0.77	1.33
1989	0.80	2.66
1990	0.73	2.66
1991	0.07	0.00
1992	0.40	0.00
1993	0.53	0.00
1994	0.07	1.33
1995	0.47	1.33
1996	0.40	4.00
1997	0.47	1.33
1998	0.27	0.00
1999	0.53	1.33
2000	0.40	2.66
2001	0.53	0.00
2002	0.33	1.33
2003	0.60	1.33
2004	0.67	0.00
2005	0.20	0.00
2006	0.53	2.66
2007	0.40	0.00

From Mueller FO, Cantu RC: *Annual survey of catastrophic football injuries,* National Center for Catastrophic Sport Injury Research, University of North Carolina, Chapel Hill, NC; available at http://www.unc.edu/depts/nccsi/.
*From 1977-1988 based on 1,300,000 high school and junior high school players and 75,000 college players. In 1989, high school and junior high school figure increased to 1,500,000.

Clinically, the athlete may complain of "jamming" his or her neck. Pain is most often localized to the area of the upper trapezius and cervical spine. Pain may radiate down one or both upper extremities if a nerve root is involved or inflamed, but this is not usually the case. Symptoms usually consist of pain, with or without radiation or paresthesia. Cervical range of motion may be limited. The clinical neurological examination is usually negative for reflex or sensory changes. Weakness of the cervical musculature may be present as a result of pain and spasm. If the injury was a result of contact, a radiographical examination should be performed as a precaution to rule out a fracture. Noncontact injuries without radicular symptoms do not necessarily mandate radiological examination. The injured or involved structures may include the muscles, tendons, ligaments, intervertebral disc, or intervertebral joints.

Treatment considerations vary based on the stage of healing and the symptoms present. In the very acute period, the goal is to reduce the inflammatory response. The athlete should be instructed to use ice and counseled on appropriate positions of comfort. Nonsteroidal anti-inflammatory agents or analgesics may be used as indicated based on symptoms. Soft cervical collars are of no biomechanical use in restraining motion; however, they may serve as a "reminder" that injury has occurred and that the head and neck should not be moved too vigorously during various activities of daily living. Therapeutic modalities may be used as appropriate to assist in providing symptomatic relief. As the athlete's condition improves, various forms of therapeutic exercise and manual therapy techniques may be initiated to facilitate range of motion and strength. The athlete should not be allowed to return to participation until full range of motion and strength of the neck has returned. Individuals participating in collision sports should not be allowed to return until they are able to hold their body weight in all directions when positioned at a 45° angle (Figure 23-5).

Fractures, Subluxations, and Dislocations

Fractures, subluxations, and dislocations constitute the type of injury that may result in the greatest degree of morbidity. They may be divided into injuries that occur in the upper

Table 23-2

Epidemiological Summary

	High School		College		Combined	
Annual Average: 1998-2002	Mean	SD	Mean	SD	Mean	SD
Direct catastrophic football cervical spine injuries	11.54	4.24	3.54	1.61	15.08	4.7
Annual Average: 1998-2002	Mean	95% CI	Mean	95% CI	Mean	95% CI
Incidence/100,000 players	1.10	(0.92-1.27)	4.72	(3.35-6.08)	1.34	(1.15-1.53)

Data from Boden BP, Tacchetti RL, Cantu RC et al: Catastrophic cervical spine injuries in high school and college football players, *Am J Sports Med* 34:1223-1232, 2006.
CI, Confidence interval; *SD,* standard deviation.

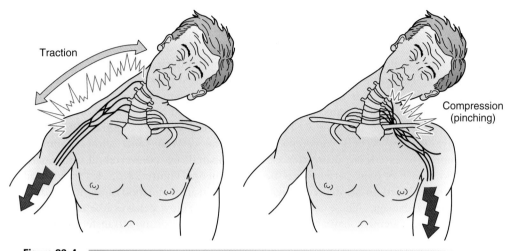

Figure 23-4

Mechanism of injury for brachial plexus (burner or stinger) pathological conditions. (From Magee DJ: *Orthopedic physical assessment*, ed 5, p 139, St Louis, 2007, Saunders.)

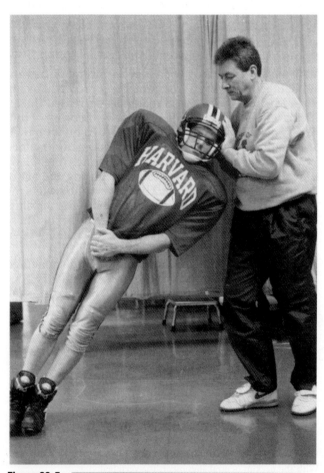

Figure 23-5

Athletes involved in collision sports such as football should be able to support their body weight in a neutral position in all directions when positioned at a 45° angle without pain, compromise in position, or discomfort.

(C1-C2), middle (C3-C4), or lower (C5-C7) cervical spine. A full description of the pathomechanics involved in fractures and fracture-dislocations will be presented later in this chapter.

Upper Cervical Spine (C1-C2). Upper cervical spine injuries are rare in sports but their proximity to the brain, cranial nerves, and vascular tissues in addition to the spinal cord requires special care and consideration if injury is suspected. Injuries in this region of the cervical spine include fractures of the atlas and the odontoid.[20] Injuries to both of these anatomical structures occur as a result of a vertical compressive force to the head. A burst fracture of the atlas may occur as force is transmitted to the occipital condyles and lateral masses of C1. A flexion or extension force associated with this vertical compressive force may result in fractures of one or more of the arches of the atlas (anterior, posterior, or both) or a fracture of the odontoid. The mechanism of odontoid fractures is less well understood. Atlantoaxial dislocations may occur as a result of ruptures of the transverse and alar ligaments. These injuries may be associated with a flexion mechanism of injury. Reporting on catastrophic cervical spine injuries sustained in players between 1989 and 2002, Boden and colleagues state that 8.2%, or 16, of the 196 injuries suffered during that period involved the C1-C2 levels. Of the 16 injuries, 3 resulted in quadriplegia. Of the 16 injured players, 12 (75%) were playing defense, 3 (19%) were playing offense, and 1 (6%) was on special teams.[10]

Middle Cervical Spine (C3-C4). Traumatic injuries to the middle cervical spine associated with sports were rare and infrequently reported until documented by NFHNIR in 1979 and 1986.[21,22] These injuries are the result of axial loading. The frequency of bony fracture is low, which makes these injuries unique.[23] From 1971 through 1988, the NFHNIR documented 1062 cervical injuries in sports that resulted in a fracture, subluxation, or dislocation. of these, 25, or 2.4%, involved the C3-C4 level.[24]

Lower Cervical Spine (C5-C7). Injuries at the lower cervical spine account for most of the fractures and dislocations seen in sports. The most common level of injury is C5-C6.[25] Again, axial loading is the most common mechanism of injury, although six common patterns of injury have been reported in the literature.[26] These patterns are compressive flexion, vertical compression, distractive flexion, compressive extension, distractive extension, and lateral flexion. Each of these patterns may be further subdivided into stages based on the degree of ligamentous injury and osseous damage. These stages and their medical and surgical management have been fully reviewed by Leventhal.[27]

Mechanism of Injury to the Cervical Spine
• Vertical (axial) compression (upper, middle, and lower)
• Compressive flexion (upper and lower)
• Distractive flexion (lower)
• Compressive extension (upper and lower)
• Distractive extension (lower)
• Lateral flexion (lower)

Banerjee and colleagues provide an excellent summary of unstable fractures and dislocations of the lower cervical spine.[28] The axial force that most often causes these catastrophic injuries is a result of the cervical spine being compressed between the mass of the oncoming body versus the instant deceleration of the head. The position of the head and cervical spine often dictate the effect of this compressive force. Neutral alignment or slight lordosis of the cervical spine allows compressive forces to be dissipated by paravertebral musculature and vertebral ligaments (Figure 23-6, *A*). Slight head and neck flexion result in an elimination of cervical lordosis (Figure 23-6, *B*). The spine now behaves like a column, energy from compressive forces is now transferred directly to the vertebrae as opposed to the soft tissues, causing buckling of the column and potentially catastrophic injury (Figure 23-6, *C*). Most commonly, slight flexion occurs with this compressive force. The compressive failure of the vertebral body, in conjunction with lengthening of the posterior column often results in a "flexion teardrop" injury (Figure 23-7, *A*). This injury is highly unstable and often associated with spinal cord injury.[29] Pure compressive force results in a burst type fracture with retropulsion of osseous material into the spinal canal causing cord compromise (Figure 23-7, *B*).

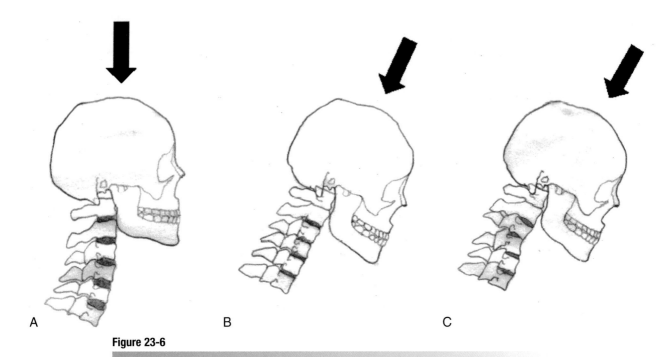

A   B   C

Figure 23-6

Response of the cervical spine to applied axial load. **A,** With the neck in neutral alignment, the vertebral column is extended. The compressive force can be dissipated by the spinal musculature and ligaments. **B,** With the neck in a flexed posture, the spine straightens out and becomes collinear with the axial force. **C,** At the time of impact, the straightened cervical spine undergoes a rapid deformation and buckles under the compressive load. (From Banerjee R, Palumbo MA, Fadale PD: Catastrophic cervical spine injuries in the collision sport athlete, Part I—Epidemiology, functional anatomy and diagnosis, *Am J Sports Med* 32:1081, 2004.)

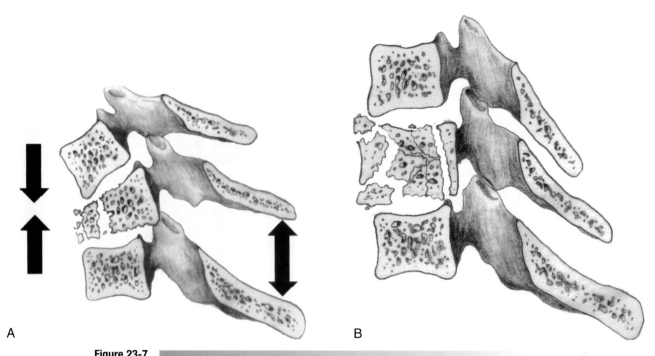

A   B

Figure 23-7

Compression injuries of the lower cervical spine. **A,** Compressive-flexion pattern. The "teardrop" fracture variant is characterized by compressive failure of the anterior column with a coronal plane fracture extending through the vertebral body. Tensile forces cause the disruption of the posterior spinal ligaments. **B,** Vertical compression pattern. In the "burst" fracture variant comminution of the vertebral body can be associated with retropulsion of osseous fragments into the spinal canal. (From Banerjee R, Palumbo MA, Fadale PD: Catastrophic cervical spine injuries in the collision sport athlete, Part I— Epidemiology, functional anatomy and diagnosis, *Am J Sports Med* 32:1082, 2004.)

Cervical Spine Stenosis with Cord Neurapraxia and Transient Quadriplegia

This syndrome was originally reported by Torg and colleagues in 1986[30] and reviewed by Torg and Fay in 1991.[31] Torg and colleagues estimate the incidence rate for transient quadriplegia to be 7.3 per 10,000 exposures in football,[30,32] and the rate for paresthesia associated with transient quadriplegia was 1.3 per 10,000 exposures in the survey of a single season.[30] Athletes with cervical stenosis, whether acquired or developmental, appear to be predisposed to this condition.[33] Neck pain is usually not present and cervical range of motion is uncompromised. Symptoms of transient paresthesia ("tingling") or loss of sensation) may be associated with motor deficits ranging from no motor deficit to mild quadriparesis or complete quadriplegia involving both arms, both legs, all four extremities, or an ipsilateral arm and leg. Signs and symptoms are temporary and function returns during a wide time frame ranging from 15 minutes to 48 hours.[34]

This very acute, transient neurologic episode is of cervical spinal cord origin. This diagnosis should not be confused with nerve root or brachial plexus injuries, which are unilateral. This syndrome may follow forced hyperflexion, hyperextension, or axial loading of the spine. Routine radiographs are negative for fracture or dislocation. Developmental cervical spine narrowing is often apparent, either as an isolated finding or associated with congenital fusion, disc disease, or ligamentous instability.[30]

The diagnosis of cervical spinal stenosis is based on the size of the vertebral canal relative to the vertebral body, as originally described in 1986 by Torg and colleagues.[30] For this initial study, a group of 24 football players with transient quadriplegia attributed to neurapraxia of the cervical spinal cord was studied. All demonstrated vertebral canal/vertebral body ratios of less than 0.80 (Figure 23-8). This ratio was thought to indicate significant spinal stenosis, as the ratio in a group of controls was 0.98.[35]

Since the original description and the development of the Torg "ratio," other conflicting studies have questioned the use of this ratio as an absolute value to be used as criteria for significant spinal stenosis.[36,37] Odor and colleagues demonstrated that 74 of 224 asymptomatic professional and rookie football players (33%) demonstrated a Torg ratio of less than 0.80 at one or more levels between C3 and C6,[36] whereas Herzog and colleagues examined 80 symptomatic professional football players and reported an abnormal Torg ratio in 49%.[37] Although demonstrated to be highly sensitive at 93%, unfortunately the Torg ratio demonstrates a positive predictive value of only 0.2%.[38] Thus, the Torg ratio may be abnormal in individuals with and without a transient quadriplegic episode. These

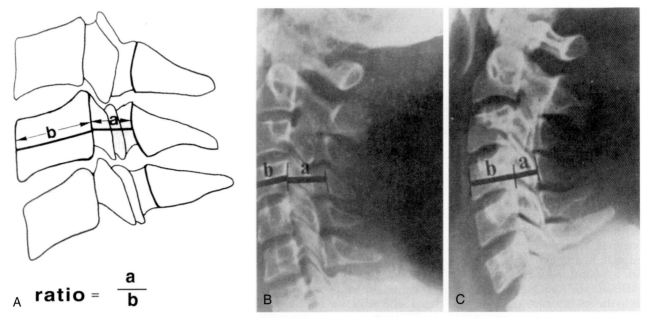

$$A \quad \mathbf{ratio} = \frac{a}{b}$$

Figure 23-8

A, The spinal canal/vertebral body ratio is the distance from the midpoint of the posterior aspect of the vertebral body to the nearest point on the corresponding spinolaminar line *(a)* divided by the antero-posterior width of the vertebral body *(b)*. **B** and **C,** Comparison between the spinal canal/vertebral body ratio in a "normal" control subject with that in a stenotic patient demonstrated on lateral radiographs of the cervical spine. The ratio is 1:1 (1) in the control subject **(B)** compared with 1:2 (0.50) in the stenotic patient **(C)**. (From Torg JS, Pavlov H, Genuario S et al: Neurapraxia of the cervical spinal cord with transient quadriplegia, *J Bone Joint Surg Am* 68:1354-1370, 1986.)

factors make the use of this ratio a poor screening tool for sports participation.

Ratios and tools such as these, however, are of assistance in return to play decisions that the medical team must make if injury with cervical cord neurapraxia has occurred. The recurrence of cervical cord neurapraxia, and the sensory and motor symptoms that occur with it, are more predictable. Based on logistic regression analysis by Torg and colleagues,[34] there is a strong inverse correlation between the risk of recurrence and the disk-level canal diameter and the ratio of the spinal canal to the vertebral body (Figure 23-9). Using this graph, it can be seen that the risk of recurrence is predictable and the clinician can accurately counsel athletes, coaches, and parents regarding return to play.

The Torg ratio and other factors may have to be considered prior to diagnosing a significant spinal stenosis and determining whether an athlete may continue to play. It is important, however, that each case is evaluated on an individual basis.

Sport-Specific Incidence of Cervical Trauma
Football
Trauma to the cervical spine in football that produces significant injuries is infrequent but often catastrophic. Torg, in a retrospective review of the years 1971 through 1975,[39] demonstrated that the rate of fractures, subluxations, or

> ### Clinical Caution
>
> The presence of a canal/vertebral body ratio of 0.8 or less (see Figure 23-8) is not a contraindication to participation in contact sports for asymptomatic individuals. However, for individuals with a ratio of less than 0.8 who do experience a cervical cord neuropraxia, there is a relative contraindication to return. The risk of recurrence is strongly and inversely correlated with the sagittal diameter of the canal. In this case, the diameter is useful in the prediction of future episodes of neuropraxia ($p < 0.001$) (see Figure 23-9).[34]

dislocations of the cervical vertebrae *increased* 204% to 4.14 per 100,000 exposures, and the rate of cervical injuries associated with quadriplegia *increased* 116% to 1.58 per 100,000 exposures compared with data reported by Schneider and Kahn for the years 1959 through 1963.[40] During this same period, a *decrease* in the rate of intracranial hemorrhages (66%) and craniocerebral deaths (42%) was noted (Figure 23-10).[39] This shift in injury patterns—a decrease in significant head injuries and an increase in cervical spine injuries—is probably attributable to changes in protective equipment used from the early 1960s to the early 1970s. During this period, better protection of the face and head were afforded by a change in face mask designs and helmet technology. The protection provided by improved

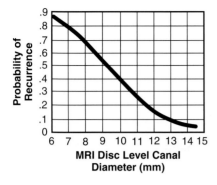

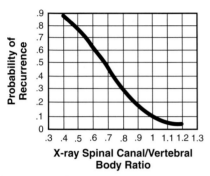

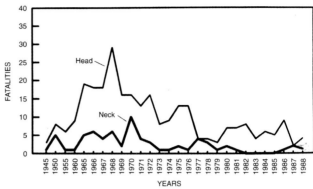

Figure 23-10

Intracranial and cervical spine injury fatalities, 1945-1988. (From Clarke KS: An epidemiologic view. In Torg JS, editor: *Athletic injuries to the head, neck and face,* ed 2, St Louis, 1991, Mosby.)

Figure 23-9

Graphs developed using logistic regression analysis in which the risk of recurrence can be plotted as a function of the disc-level diameter measured on magnetic resonance imaging *(upper)* and the spinal canal/vertebral body ratio calculated on the basis of x-ray films *(lower).* The construction of these plots is based on the result that increased risk of recurrence is inversely correlated with the canal diameter. Future cervical cord neurapraxia patients can be counseled regarding their individual risk of recurrence based on the particular size of their spinal canal. (From Torg JS, Corcoran AT, Thibault LE et al: Cervical cord neurapraxia: Classification, pathomechanics, morbidity and management guidelines, *J Neurosurg* 87:847, 1997.)

helmet designs and materials decreased the incidence and severity of head injury. However, because of the perceived increase in protection felt by football players, they may have believed they were at greater liberty to hit with their head as the initial point of contact, increasing the incidence of catastrophic cervical spine injuries (Figure 23-11).

Most cervical spine injuries occur during the act of tackling an opposing player. The player who suffers the injury is usually the player who is in the act of tackling (see Figure 23-11). Consequently, the highest percentage of these injuries are suffered by defensive players making open-field tackles.[21]

Because of the rise in cervical injuries documented and reported in several studies by Torg the NCAA and NFHSAA adopted rule changes that stated "no player shall intentionally strike a runner with the crown or the top of the helmet or deliberately use his helmet to butt or ram a player." These rule changes decreased the use of the head as the initial point of contact in blocking and tackling in football. This rule has been further changed,

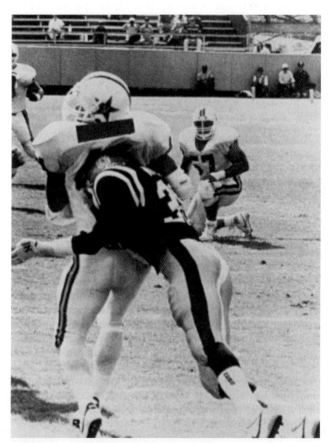

Figure 23-11

Inappropriate tackle that resulted in a catastrophic cervical spine injury. Note the position of slight cervical flexion, which enables axial loading to be produced when a tackler is spearing. (From Torg JS, Sennett B, Pavlov H et al: Spear tackler's spine, *Am J Sports Med* 21:640-649, 1993.)

striking the word *intentionally* so that now all contact with the head as the initial point of contact is illegal for high school and college football.[8] In addition, it was made a "point of emphasis" by the American Football Coaches Association in 2007 that game officials should call a foul when such incidences occur.

Traumatic cervical spine fractures, subluxations, and dislocations have continued to progressively decrease since the 1976 rule change. Between 1976 and 1987, the rate of severe cervical spine injuries decreased 70% at the high school level and 65% at the collegiate level. The largest rate change took place in 1977 and 1978, the 2 years after the rule change took effect. Injuries continued to decline until approximately 1984 and remained the same during the next 3 years.[41] Data for subsequent years, available through the National Center for Catastrophic Sports Injury Research, can be viewed in Figure 23-3.[8]

Ice Hockey

In Canada, spinal cord injuries incurred as a result of playing ice hockey were rare until approximately 1980. Prior to 1980, there was an average of two to three injuries per year. From 1982 to 1987, approximately 15 injuries per year were reported. Tator reviewed the literature available and documented a total of 117 cervical spine and spinal cord injuries between 1966 and 1987 in Canada.[42] In a subsequent publication encompassing a longer period, reviewing the years 1966 to 1993, Tator and colleagues[43] reported a total of 241 spinal fractures and dislocations, 90% involving C1 to T1. Between the years 1982 and 1993, an increased rate of spinal column injury occurred equal to 16.8 per year. A total of 207 players had good medical documentation. Based on this documentation, it has been reported that 8 players died, 108 sustained permanent spinal cord injury, and the cord lesion was complete in 52 players. It has been reported that the incidence of spinal cord damage and paralysis is three times greater in Canadian ice hockey than American football.[8,43]

Of these injuries, 70% occurred when a checked player collided headfirst with the boards; 73% of these injuries occurred during games, when the intensity of competition and checking from behind were the highest. Tator also attributed the increase in incidence since 1980 to better reporting mechanisms, physical factors related to players (e.g., increased weight and speed of skating), social and psychological factors among young hockey players (e.g., increased aggression and willingness to take risks), coaching attitudes and techniques (e.g., insufficient emphasis on conditioning, the risks of hockey, and methods of protecting the spine from injury; overemphasis on body contact), and small rinks with rigid boards. In an effort to prevent these injuries, rule changes have been instituted prohibiting checking from behind and checking an opponent who does not have control of the puck.[44] Unlike in football, Tator has stated that he has found no evidence that the increased use of helmets and face masks,

which have decreased the incidence of facial injuries, has increased the incidence of cervical spine injury.

Winter Sports

Considering the number of individuals who participate in winter sports, the incidence of injury is surprisingly low. Reid and Saboe have reviewed spine injuries specific to sports in Canada. Of 202 injuries reviewed, 25% ($n = 48$) occurred from participation in winter sports.[45] In their study, done in 1991, snowmobiling accounted for 10%, tobogganing for 6%, alpine skiing for 6%, and ice hockey for 3% of the cervical spine injuries.

Cervical spine injuries account for approximately 25% of all spine fractures that occur in relation to snowmobiling. Injuries are often related to driving a snowmobile at night; being under the influence of alcohol; being unfamiliar with the terrain; or various operator errors, such as becoming airborne, colliding with objects, or tipping over. Toboggan injuries frequently involve younger individuals. Approximately one third of the cervical spine fractures in tobogganing occur in individuals younger than the age of 15. Collisions with objects, becoming airborne, and demonstrating poor judgment account for most mechanisms of injury.

It has been estimated that spinal injuries account for between 4% and 17% of all injuries to alpine skiers and snowboarders. Although this is low in comparison with other orthopedic trauma, the catastrophic factor can be much higher. The incidence of significant spinal injury (lumbar and cervical) is reported to be 1 for every 100,000 skier days for skiing and 4 for every 100,000 snowboarder days.[46,47] During the course of two seasons (1994-1996), Tarazi and colleagues detailed 14 fractures associated with the cervical spine out of a total of 56 skier or snowboarders with spinal related injuries. A total of eight fractures were reported in skiers and six in snowboarders, with jumping being attributed as the major cause of injury.[46] In a longer-term retrospective review during 11 ski seasons, Floyd reported a total of 12 cervical fractures or dislocations out of a total of 57 significant spinal injuries.[47] The most common mechanisms of injury include attempting a jump and landing poorly or losing control and hitting a tree. Other factors are collisions with other skiers or objects. All of these factors are related directly or indirectly to errors in judgment and control, which often cannot be influenced by the health care professional.

Water Sports

Between 1964 and 1974, 152 of 1600 patients (9.5%) admitted to the Spinal Cord Injury Service at Rancho Los Amigos Hospital were injured during recreational activities. Of these patients, 82 (54%) had been injured while diving. The average depth of water into which these individuals were diving was 5 feet (1.5 m). Surfing accounted for 29 injuries, and water skiing for seven.[48] All of these individuals were injured by striking the head on the bottom of the pool, lake, river, or ocean. As the head struck, the body continued to progress forward, resulting in an axial loading or compressive flexion injury. A typical vertical compression load may result, although opinions vary.[49]

Rugby

Rugby is gaining popularity in North America, as evidenced by club- and varsity-level competition for men and women at universities and numerous recreational leagues. Injury data must be drawn from the British Commonwealth countries, where it is played on a large scale.

Retrospective data available for Australia and England between the years 1960 and 1985 demonstrates that 107 injured patients were admitted to spinal cord centers in Australia[50] and 82 injuries occurred in England from 1959 through 1987.[51] Injuries usually occurred from a collapsing scrum or from tackling. Hookers were the most often injured players in amateur play because of their position and its requirements during play. A rule change was initiated in England in 1983 that reduced injuries from 10 the previous season to 5 between 1986 and 1987. This change kept players on their feet and in a more upright position in the scrum and the maul. Silver and Gill described the mechanisms of injury during rugby as the head being driven into the ground or a blow to the head.[51] Retrospective data published in the United States details similar results. Wetzler and colleagues[52] report that between 1970 and 1996 of the 62 significant cervical spine injuries that occurred in U.S. rugby, 36 (58%) happened during the scrum. During this portion of the rugby match, the head and neck of a player involved in the scrum is in a flexed position and may have a compressive load imposed upon it. Wetzler and colleagues[52] provide great detail regarding the method of injury and possible explanation of the mechanism of failure in their review.

Gymnastics, Trampoline, and Cheerleading

Significant cervical spine injuries associated with gymnastics are predominantly associated with the use of the trampoline as a training device. Of permanent spinal cord injuries to female gymnasts from 1973 through 1975, 70% were associated with the trampoline. Other pieces of apparatus may be involved, however. During the same period, 33% of men's injuries were associated with the trampoline, 22% with the floor exercise and high bar, and 11% with the rings and mini-trampoline.[53] More than 114 catastrophic injuries have been attributed to the use of a trampoline since the initial report by Ellis in 1960.[54] These injuries are usually associated with a somersault and an uncontrolled landing.[55]

The incidence of injury led to a position paper by the American Academy of Pediatrics in 1977.[56] This paper caused the American Alliance for Health, Physical Education and Recreation and the NCAA Committee on Competitive Safeguards and Medical Aspects of Sports to issue guidelines making use of the trampoline optional and voluntary, and specifically detailing safety and maintenance standards. Since 1978, a distinct decrease has been observed in all catastrophic gymnastic injuries and, more specifically, in injuries resulting from the use of trampolines and mini-trampolines.[55]

Cheerleading injuries have risen significantly since 1980 as this activity has become more popular in the United States and has increased in complexity and danger. The Consumer Product Safety Commission reported an estimated 4954 hospital emergency room visits in 1980 caused by cheerleading injuries. By 1986 the number had increased to 6911, to approximately 16,000 in 1994, to 21,906 in 1999, and to 28,414 in 2004.[8] Data from the National Center from Catastrophic Sports Injury Research between 1982 and 2002 report 1.95 catastrophic injuries (0.6/100,000 participants). Of the 39 catastrophic injuries reported, 8 involved cervical fractures or major ligament injuries and 3 involved spinal cord contusions. Injury rates for college versus high school cheerleaders demonstrate a 5:1 ratio.[8]

Recent rule changes by the American Association of Cheerleading Coaches and Administrators (AACCA) were put in place in an effort to reduce the number of injuries. In 2006, the AACCA College Rules Committee restricted 2½-high pyramids, basket tosses, and other select skills to be performed only on grass or matted surfaces. High school teams, which were already restricted from performing 2½-high pyramids at all, were also restricted from performing basket tosses without a mat by the AACCA and National Federation of High Schools. In addition, The NCAA introduced legislation in 2006 requiring all collegiate cheerleading coaches to be safety-certified for their teams to qualify for the NCAA's catastrophic insurance plan. Additional rules were added in 2008 to both the AACCA College and National Federation of High School Rules Committees standardizing basketball court rules for these age levels, prohibiting released twisting skills and inverted skills on this surface.

Mechanics and Pathomechanics

Mechanism of Injury

Multiple mechanisms of injury may be responsible for cervical fractures, subluxations, or dislocations. Numerous theories have been proposed regarding the mechanism of injury that is usually associated with sports. Purported mechanisms of injury must withstand the scrutiny of research and critical review. Although mechanisms such as hyperflexion and hyperextension are feasible, they have not withstood such scrutiny. Even though injury may be possible from hyperflexion, hyperextension, or lateral bending and rotation, most of the force of these energies is absorbed by the cervical spine range of motion, strength of the musculature, intervertebral discs, and, to a lesser extent, the ligaments. Injuries that occur from these forces are most often sprains, strains, or brachial plexus injuries, generally not fractures, subluxations, or dislocations.

Attempts have been made to associate equipment specific to football with these mechanisms. It has been stated that the face mask may cause hyperflexion with the ground or an opponent; however, this was not reported to be the factor in the more than 200 injuries that occurred between 1971 and 1975.[57] Various authors and researchers have also demonstrated that the so-called guillotine effect of the helmet (the posterior rim of the helmet impacts the cervical spine during tackling or contact with another player) is not implicated in football-related cervical spine fractures and dislocations.[22,23,58,59]

Clinical Point

Current theory and evidence demonstrate that the most commonly acknowledged mechanism responsible for fracture-dislocation of the cervical spine in sports is that of axial loading in flexion. The factor of axial loading is a common thread presented earlier in this chapter concerning the sport-specific incidence of injury.

When the cervical spine is placed in a position of slight flexion, there is a reduction of cervical lordosis, and the cervical spine is straightened (Figure 23-12). When an axial load is applied in this position (as may be the case with spearing in football or diving into a shallow pool) (Figure 23-13), the energy-absorbing and energy-dissipating mechanisms afforded to the cervical spine through flexion, extension, and lateral bending and rotation are reduced. Load thus occurs on a segmented vertical column. When this load exceeds the energy-absorbing capacity of the vertebral bodies, intervertebral discs, posterior elements or ligaments, failure and injury result. Injuries incurred may be crush fractures of the cervical vertebrae, buckling (which produces an acute flexion dislocation at one level), or a combination of these two modes. The numerous anatomic and analytical modeling studies confirming this mechanism of injury have been reviewed by Otis and colleagues.[57]

Because of the mechanics just described, it should be obvious that the majority of cervical spine injuries in sports that produce cervical fracture or fracture-dislocation, with or without neurological involvement, are caused by cervical flexion with axial loading. Proper technique is critical in the prevention of injury. Tackling or contact with the head in any collision sport (e.g., football, rugby, ice hockey) or diving into shallow water and striking the crown of the head may produce catastrophic injury. These injuries are prevented not by equipment, but by adherence to appropriate technique, following the rules, and common sense.

Legal Considerations

Catastrophic injuries to the cervical spine impose a severe emotional shock, pain and suffering, potential financial ruin, and anger on the injured athlete and family. A desperate need to shift responsibility outside the family is often felt. A member of the medical team often becomes the target of this shift. Any time members of the team are in a position to manage a catastrophic and potentially fatal injury, they may be at risk of being accused of incompetence or negligence. Patterson[60] and Heck and colleagues[61] provide an excellent, concise discussion of the legal aspects of athletic injuries to the cervical spine.

General claims against the athletic or sports medicine staff usually concern instruction in proper technique, the condition and appropriateness of equipment, the matching of participants based on size and skill, supervision, or postinjury care. Defensive responses to these claims include the assumption of risk by the competitor, statutory immunity, a release or waiver signed by the participant or parents, and the standard of reckless disregard.[61] Whether such defenses are successful in exonerating the medical team of legal liability depends on the facts of each particular case and the law of the state in which the legal action is brought.

To be better positioned to both avoid and defend such legal claims, the medical team must take reasonably prudent precautions to minimize the risk of injury for the participant during practice or competition and to minimize their own risk should catastrophic injury and the possibility of litigation occurs. To minimize the athlete's risk, all equipment should be in good repair, comply with standards set by the National Operating Committee on Standards for Athletic Equipment, and be fit by appropriately trained personnel only (e.g., athletic trainer, equipment manager, coach). All athletes should undergo a preseason physical examination that specifically includes questions relevant to previous cervical spine injuries and examination and screening of the cervical spine if the athlete is involved in a collision sport. The medical staff must make sure that a well-defined and well-communicated emergency plan is in place. Education, training, continuing practice and preparation are key elements to the successful management of a true emergency situation. Recognized policies and procedures should be in place and agreed on by all medical personnel, athletic administrators, coaches, and outside emergency medical personnel such as EMTs or paramedics who will assist the sports medicine staff. The appropriate equipment must be available, readily positioned, and in good repair to allow for appropriate management of catastrophic cervical spine injuries.[3,62] Practice and competition venues should be easily accessible to all emergency personnel.

Clinical Note

All personnel involved in caring for the injured athlete must be properly trained and practice regularly. Training in the management of catastrophic injuries should be reviewed yearly.

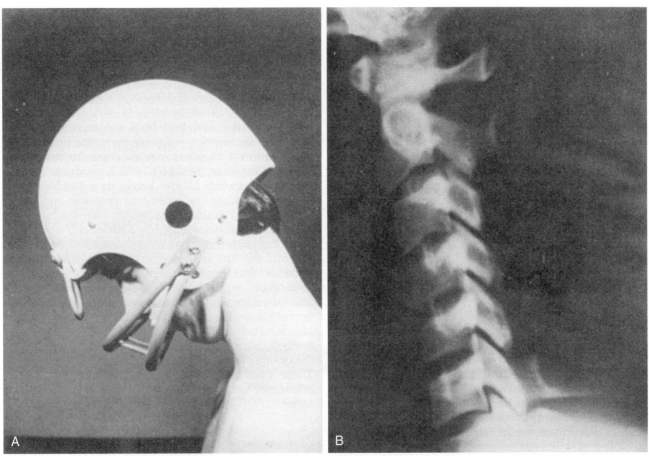

Figure 23-12
When the neck is flexed approximately 30° **(A),** the cervical spine becomes straight from the standpoint of force, energy absorption, and effect on tissue deformation and failure. The straightened cervical spine, when axially loaded, acts as a segmented column **(B).** (From Torg J: National Football Head and Neck Injuries Registry: Report on the cervical quadriplegia from 1971-1975, *Am J Sports Med* 7:127, 1979.)

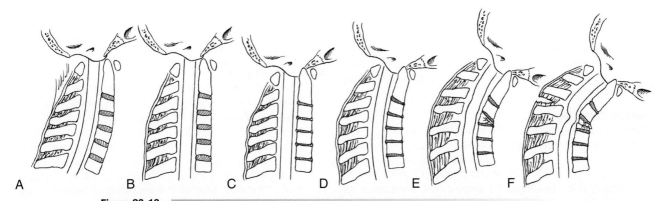

Figure 23-13
Axial load applied to a segmented column initially results in deformation by compression. If the axial load is large enough, more marked deformation occurs. Absorption of excessive amounts of energy during this axially applied load may result in buckling, with resultant fracture or dislocation of the segmented column.

In addition, consideration should be given to the use of acknowledgment of risk, informed consent, and medical release questionnaires and statements. These forms should be on file prior to the start of any practice or competition. The ability to use these types of documents will vary depending on the situation (e.g., recreational youth league versus interscholastic versus intercollegiate versus professional team) and recommendations provided by the governing legal counsel. Legal review should occur before these types of documents are considered. If used, both coaches and athletes (or parents if the athlete is a minor) should sign statements to document that (1) correct techniques outlining the dangers of initial contact with the head while involved in a collision sport have been reviewed, understood, and implemented; (2) rules and procedures to minimize exposure will be enforced continuously; and (3) appropriate strength and flexibility programs are included in conditioning drills.

Emergency Management

Practice and Competition Sites

In 1998 the National Athletic Trainers Association formed the Inter Association Task Force for Appropriate Care of the Spine-Injured Athlete to develop guidelines for the appropriate management of the catastrophically injured athlete.[3] The guidelines and recommendations developed by this task force are presented in Box 23-1 and Box 23-2. Box 23-3 details the NCAA Sports Medicine Handbook's guidelines to use during a serious player injury.[63] These recommendations are widely used in sports and are adapted from guidelines developed in 1999 by the NFL for the management of serious on-field player injuries.[64] Banerjee and colleagues have also recently published a review article with an online appendix showing appropriate emergency management techniques.[65]

Box 23-1 Guidelines for Appropriate Care of the Spine-Injured Athlete

General Guidelines
- Any athlete suspected of having a spinal injury should not be moved and should be managed as though a spinal injury exists.
- The athlete's airway, breathing, circulation, neurological status, and level of consciousness should be assessed.
- The athlete should not be moved unless absolutely essential to maintain airway, breathing, and circulation.
- If the athlete must be moved to maintain airway, breathing, and circulation, the athlete should be placed in a supine position while maintaining spinal immobilization.
- When moving a suspected spine-injured athlete, the head and trunk should be moved as a unit. One accepted technique is to splint the head to the trunk.
- The Emergency Medical Services system should be activated.

Face Mask Removal
- The face mask should be removed prior to transportation, regardless of current respiratory status.
- Those involved in the prehospital care of the injured football players should have the tools for face mask removal readily available.

Football Helmet Removal
The athletic helmet and chin strap should only be removed:
- If the helmet and chin strap do not hold the head securely, such that immobilization of the helmet does not also immobilize the head
- If the design of the helmet and chin strap is such that, even after removal of the face mask, the airway cannot be controlled nor ventilation provided
- If the face mask cannot be removed after a reasonable period
- If the helmet prevents immobilization for transportation in an appropriate position

Helmet Removal
- Spinal immobilization must be maintained while removing the helmet.
- Helmet removal should be frequently practiced under proper supervision.
- Specific guidelines for helmet removal need to be developed.
- In most circumstances, it may be helpful to remove cheek padding and deflate air padding prior to helmet removal.

Equipment
- Appropriate spinal alignment must be maintained.
- There needs to be a realization that the helmet and shoulder pads elevate an athlete's trunk when in the supine position.
- Should either the helmet or shoulder pads be removed—or if only one of these is present—appropriate spinal alignment must be maintained.
- The front of the shoulder pads can be opened to allow access for cardiopulmonary resuscitation and defibrillation.

Additional Guidelines
- The Inter-Association Task Force for the Appropriate Care of the Spine-Injured Athlete encourages the development of a local emergency plan regarding the prehospital care of an athlete with a suspected spinal injury. This plan should include communication with the institution's administration and those directly involved with the assessment and transportation of the injured athlete.
- All providers of prehospital care should practice and be competent in all of the skills identified in these guidelines before they are needed in an emergency situation.

From Kleiner DM, Almquist JL, Bailes J et al: *Prehospital care of the spine-injured athlete: A document from the Inter-Association Task Force for Appropriate Care of the Spine Injured Athlete*, p 30, National Athletic Trainers Association, Dallas, TX, March 2001.

Box 23-2 Recommendations for Appropriate Care of the Spine-Injured Athlete

The Inter Association Task Force for the Appropriate Care of the Spine-Injured Athlete:
- Commends the current and on-going commitment of helmet and face guard manufacturers for integrating safety in the development of their products.
- Encourages manufactures to continue to support research promoting helmet and face guard safety.
- Recommends that manufacturers provide information to purchases on the best methods for the emergency removal of the face guard.
- Recommends that the National Operating Committee on Standards for Athletic Equipment (NOCSAE) develop equipment standards that would allow for the emergency removal of helmets and face guards.
- Recommends that helmets and face guards that meet current NOCSAE standards be worn by all football, lacrosse, baseball, and softball players.
- Recommends that football helmet face guards be attached by loop straps and not bolted on to facilitate appropriate emergency management by medical personnel.
- Recommends that loop straps be made of material that is easily cut, and that the producers of loop straps provide appropriate tools to cut and remove the loop straps that they manufacture.

From Kleiner DM, Almquist JL, Bailes J et al: *Prehospital care of the spine-injured athlete: A document from the Inter-Association Task Force for Appropriate Care of the Spine Injured Athlete,* p 31, Dallas, TX, 2001, National Athletic Trainers Association.

Box 23-3 National Collegiate Athletic Association Sports Medicine Handbook—Guidelines to Use During a Serious On-Field Player Injury

These guidelines have been recommended for National Football League officials and have been shared with National Collegiate Athletic Association championships staff.
- Players and coaches should go to and remain in the bench area once medical assistance arrives. Adequate lines of vision between the medical staffs and all available emergency personnel should be established and maintained.
- Players, parents, and nonauthorized personnel should be kept a significant distance away from the seriously injured player or players.
- Players or nonmedical personnel should not touch, move, or roll an injured player.
- Players should not try to assist a teammate who is lying on the field (i.e., removing the helmet or chin strap or attempting to assist breathing by elevating the waist).
- Players should not pull an injured teammate or opponent from a pile-up.
- Once the medical staff begins to work on an injured player, they should be allowed to perform services without interruption or interference.
- Players and coaches should avoid dictating medical services to the athletic trainers or team physicians or taking up their time to perform such services.

From National Collegiate Athletic Association: *2007–08 NCAA Sports Medicine Handbook 2007-08,* p 11, Indianapolis, IN, 2007, National Collegiate Athletic Association.

Clinical Point

The emergency medical management of any athlete who has suffered a catastrophic cervical spine injury is the responsibility of the sports medicine team present at the practice or competition site. The makeup of this team may vary depending on the setting (professional, college, high school, or recreational). Regardless of the setting, an action plan should be developed and agreed on prior to the start of the season. Teamwork is critical to ensure safe, efficient management of these injuries.

In the organized athletic setting, the medical team usually comprises the team physician(s), athletic trainers, sports physical therapists, and emergency medical services (EMS) personnel. In the well-organized, well-funded settings (such as collegiate or professional), there may often be a greater number of physicians, athletic trainers, and sports physical therapists in comparison with EMS personnel making up this team. In many other settings (such as high school or recreational and youth league sports), EMS personnel may make up a greater percentage of this team, and carry more responsibility for the overall management of this type of injury.

Duties and lines of communication should be determined prior to the start of the season. Members of the sports medicine staff should meet with local EMS personnel to work out specific logistics of access to facilities, transport, and responsibilities. Not all EMS agencies are capable of delivering advanced life support measures, and 911 service may not be available in all regions of the United States or Canada.[66] To facilitate the most appropriate handling of these injuries during "home" contests, additional meetings should be held with the local emergency department's medical staff, and guidelines developed to determine proper management and facility transport of these potential catastrophic injuries. Prior to the start of the season, it should be decided who has primary responsibility to direct all facets of emergency care, immobilization, and transport of the athlete who has suffered a cervical spine injury—the physician, the athletic trainer, or EMS personnel. Scenarios should be put in place in regard to who is going to assume emergency responsibilities if one member of the medical team mentioned previously is not in attendance. If responsibilities cannot be predetermined, trauma triage guidelines and legal regulations must be followed regarding lines of authority.

Clinical Point

In any emergency situation, communication is the key factor. All professionals involved in this situation have the same primary goal: the safe, efficient management of a traumatic situation.

Prior to the start of the season, all protective equipment and emergency care equipment must be checked to make sure that it is in good operational condition. Some members of the team may be uncomfortable with the evaluation and management of the cervical spine owing to the severity of the consequences of significant injury or the potential for further damage if mishandled. Training sessions should be scheduled with all members of the sports medicine staff, and local EMS personnel if possible. These training sessions should assist in easing lack of confidence in handling specific

situations. Hypothetical injury situations should be used so that techniques of immobilization and transport may be practiced and everyone knows his or her role. Ensuring proper training of staff and communication among all personnel involved is the best way to guarantee appropriate management of this type of injury. *On-the-job training at the time of the emergency is inappropriate.*

On-field management consists of injury recognition and triage, situation management and immobilization of the cervical spine, and transport.[62] Only a small percentage of sports-induced cervical spine injuries are significant and result in permanent neurological deficit. Figure 23-14 and Figure 23-15 summarize and present algorithm-based action plans for significant cervical spine injury.

Clinical Caution

A cervical lesion without neurological deficit can easily become one with a neurological deficit if it is improperly handled.[28,67]

Suspicion of cervical spine injury may occur through observation of the position of the head and neck at the time of the injury. If the mechanism of injury was not observed, observing whether the athlete is moving immediately following the injury will provide significant information

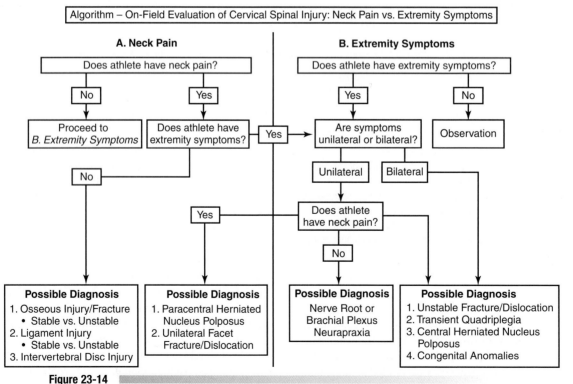

Figure 23-14

Algorithm for on-field evaluation of cervical spine injury: neck pain versus extremity symptoms. (From Banerjee R, Palumbo MA, Fadale PD: Catastrophic cervical spine injuries in the collision sport athlete, Part I—Epidemiology, functional anatomy and diagnosis, *Am J Sports Med* 32:1077-1087, 2004.)

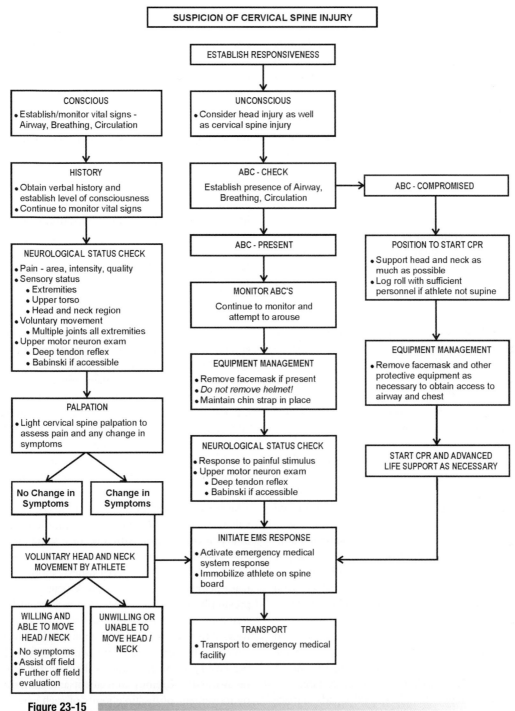

Figure 23-15

Algorithm for suspicion of cervical spine injury.

about the severity of the injury. Most athletes will move after injury if they are able. An athlete lying completely still following injury is an indication that a potentially significant injury has occurred. Teammates of the injured athlete should be instructed not to move or touch the athlete until the clinician has determined exactly what is wrong.

The clinician's initial duty is to establish the responsiveness of the athlete while stabilizing the athlete's cervical spine. It is imperative that the athlete not be moved while checking for

responsiveness. Responsiveness and consciousness determine the next sequence of events (see Chapter 18 in *Orthopedic Physical Assessment*, 5th edition, another book in this series).

Clinical Note

On reaching the injured athlete, responsiveness, airway, breathing, and circulation must be always be established.

Unconscious Athlete

In an unconscious athlete, the possibility of cervical injury as well as head injury must be considered. All unconscious athletes must be treated as if a significant cervical injury has occurred until determined otherwise. Establishing a viable airway, breathing (respiration), and pulse (circulation) are critical. This is known as the *ABCs* of cardiopulmonary resuscitation (CPR). If the athlete is not breathing or does not have a pulse, the local EMS system should be activated and the athlete placed in a supine position appropriate for the administration of rescue breathing or CPR. If possible, care should be taken to attempt to logroll the individual to minimize trauma to the cervical spine. If the athlete is wearing a face mask, as is common in sports such as football, ice hockey, or lacrosse, it should be removed as soon as possible.[3] Face masks may be removed without significant motion of the cervical spine by cutting the plastic pieces or loops that commonly hold the mask in place while stabilizing the head and neck (Figure 23-16). All loops that hold the mask in place should be cut to allow for full removal of the face mask. Multiple tools have been marketed and studied that allow the loops of a face mask to be cut. These different tools have been reviewed and summarized by Kleiner and colleagues.[3] The most efficient tool for cutting loop straps associated with face masks of those reviewed was found to be the anvil pruner, a common garden tool.

However, some of the new helmet designs recently on the market do not adequately allow for the cutting of the plastic straps. The face masks on these helmets may be removed by unscrewing the screws that attach the plastic straps to the face mask and helmet. This may be performed with the use of an electric screwdriver. However, it is highly recommended for emergency personnel to maintain a stub nose screwdriver for back up purposes in case the electric screwdriver malfunctions. One may recommend that emergency personnel carry all three types of face mask removal tools to be properly prepared for all types of helmet and face mask removal procedures.

The best type of tool for the helmet-face mask system used by the team should be determined prior to the start of the season and the staff should practice removal while maintaining stability of the head and neck during the procedure.

The uniform and straps that hold shoulder pads in place may also have to be cut to allow access to the chest if the administration of CPR is required. *The helmet should not be removed.* This will be discussed in depth later in this chapter. CPR and advanced life support should be started when and if appropriate. The athlete should be immobilized and then transported to an appropriate emergency medical facility.

If the athlete is unconscious but is breathing and has a pulse, members of the sports medicine team should continue to monitor the injured athletes' vital signs and attempt to gently arouse the athlete without movement of the athlete. If a face mask is present, it should be removed at this time without moving the athlete and while stabilizing the head and neck. (Removal of the face mask at this time will allow access to the airway if necessary. The helmet should not be removed, as stated earlier.) If the face mask cannot be removed without moving the athlete, this step is delayed until one is ready to immobilize the athlete. The ABCs are continuously monitored. A neurological check is then initiated.[62] This check incorporates a response to painful stimuli (e.g., a sharp or dull instrument or pulling on extremity hair) and assessment of deep tendon reflexes related to C5-C7 and L5-S1. The Babinski sign may be elicited if the sole of the foot is readily accessible. Once the examination is completed, the athlete should be immobilized and transported. Immobilization will be described in detail later in this chapter.

Conscious Athlete

In the conscious athlete, the clinician must continue to monitor his or her vital signs. Removal of the face mask is recommended in the event the athlete's vital signs change. A history should be obtained from the athlete in a slow, firm, confident voice. Composure by the physician, athletic trainer, sport physical therapist, or EMS personnel at the scene will assist the injured athlete in maintaining his or her composure, reduce anxiety, and help to control the situation. During this portion of the examination, the athlete should not be moved and should be kept calm and quiet. Memory and recollection of the event of the injury should be established. The athlete may be able to describe the mechanism of injury and what he or she felt at the time of injury. Attention should be paid to the quickness, comprehensiveness, and confidence of the athlete's response and the clarity of his or her speech, as this will assist the clinician in determining the possibility of head injury in conjunction with a cervical spine injury. While one member of the sports medicine team monitors the athlete's vital signs and level of consciousness, another member of the team begins a neurological check. Pain is assessed as stated previously. Dermatome sensation is assessed for all four extremities, as well as for exposed areas of the face, neck, and torso. Attention is paid to the ability of the athlete to perceive which body part or parts are being touched. The ability to perceive light touch as well as sharp or dull sensation should be assessed. Extremity movement and strength are assessed by movement of multiple joints of each extremity. The athlete's ability to follow directions and comprehension are also important at this time. If sensation and movement are compromised in any extremity or dermatome, a complete neurological examination, including assessment of deep tendon reflexes and the Babinski sign as described earlier, should be completed. On completion of the neurologic check, light, gentle palpation of the cervical spine and upper shoulders is performed. Pain, spasm, and any type of asymmetry of the cervical musculature or spinal erector muscles are noted. Particular attention is paid to any finding of point tenderness and abnormal alignment of the spinous processes of the

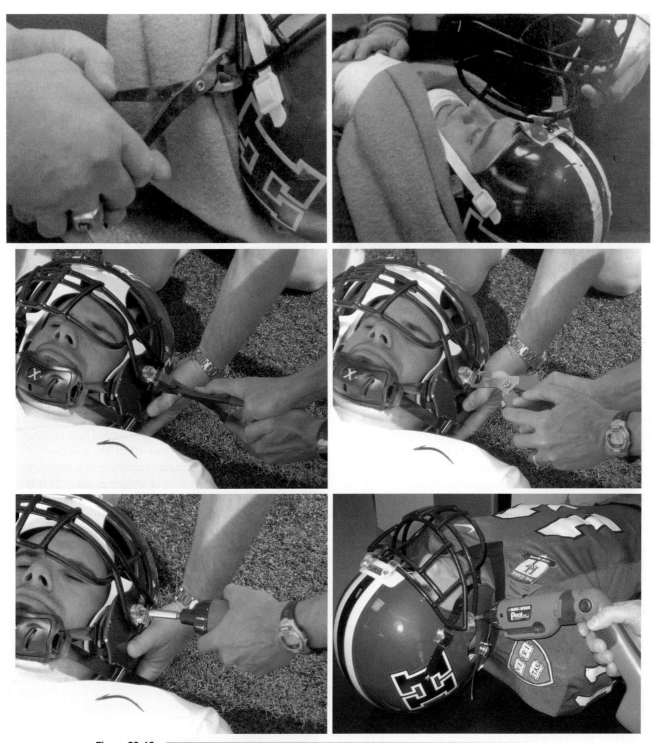

Figure 23-16

Plastic pieces that hold face masks in place may be cut with a razor knife or other commercially available products, or may require the use of an electric screwdriver to allow the face mask to swing out of the way, enabling access to the athlete's airway without removal of the helmet.

Continued

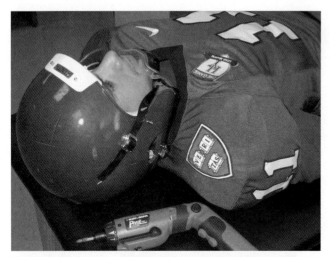

Figure 23-16, cont'd

cervical spine. The examiner and other members of the team should be continually assessing if this palpation examination creates any alteration in the athlete's current symptoms, sensation and ability to move. If there is any alteration in these factors, spine stabilization should proceed immediately.

If all components of the examination described previously are normal, the athlete may then attempt to move his or her head and neck. If there is any unwillingness or hesitancy of the athlete to move the head and neck, or any perception by the athlete, or member of the sports medicine team that symptoms, sensation, or the ability to move are altered, the athlete is immobilized immediately. If the athlete is willing to move the head and neck, and there are no symptoms or complaints of extremity numbness, painful dysesthesias or paresthesias, weakness or neck pain consideration may be given to assisting the athlete off the field without spine board immobilization.

Spine Board Immobilization

A well-coordinated group effort is required to safely and efficiently immobilize an athlete with a suspected cervical spine injury. As mentioned previously, the specific technique to be used should be repeatedly practiced prior to the start of any season. If members of the sports medicine team have not had the opportunity to practice these techniques or are not familiar with them, only trained EMS personnel should be involved with the immobilization procedure.

Clinical Caution

When dealing with spinal injury, the sports medicine team should always err on the side of caution. If any doubt exists, immobilize the athlete on a spine board.

Having the appropriate equipment readily available to immobilize the cervical spine is mandatory for collision sports such as football, ice hockey, or lacrosse, or other sports in which there is significant risk, such as gymnastics. Immobilization of the spine traditionally has been carried out by using a full-length spine board. Spine boards are usually fabricated from plastic or aluminum and may be purchased commercially from various emergency medical equipment manufacturers. The board must be designed to allow multiple positions for using strap systems to immobilize the injured athlete (Figure 23-17). Vacuum form splinting and immobilization systems have been developed that allow total body immobilization (e.g., Med Tech Sweden, Inc., http://www.medtechsweden.com). Although these systems offer the advantage of being lightweight and easily transportable, they tend not to be commonly found in most sports medicine settings for cervical spine immobilization. However, they are commonly used for extremity immobilization. There are advantages and disadvantages of all equipment and systems for spinal immobilization following injury. The correct system and equipment should be chosen by the sports medicine team for the particular team and sport. This equipment should be available for the team's athletes at home and away contests.

For sports that require helmets (i.e., football, lacrosse, ice hockey) there is disagreement in the literature regarding whether the helmet should be removed. These differences are based on how removal can affect the position of the head and neck, and potentially create cervical spine movement that places the spinal cord at further risk.[67-80] It is the recommendation of the Inter Association Task Force for the Appropriate Care of the Spine-Injured Athlete that the helmet and shoulder pads, if present, should remain on when immobilizing the injured athlete on some type of spine board.[3]

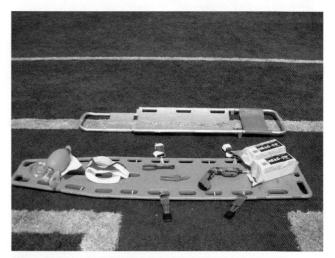

Figure 23-17
Plastic backboard and scoop stretcher.

Because helmets are usually used in conjunction with shoulder pads in sports, removal of the helmet without removal of all other protective padding from the chest up may alter head and neck position when immobilizing the spine on a backboard. The removal of the helmet and shoulder pads should be an "all-or-none" proposition. Any attempt to remove the helmet should be delayed until both the helmet and shoulder pads can be removed in a controlled setting such as the emergency department.

After establishing vital signs and responsiveness, preventing further injury is the single most important objective. The member of the medical team who is at the head of the injured athlete and who established vital signs and responsiveness is responsible for directing the emergency management of the injured athlete. At this time, the head should be immobilized by holding it in the position in which it lies. Once the head is immobilized manually, it is not released until the body and head are fully immobilized on the spinal board.[72] Because this may be a lengthy process, the individual who is manually immobilizing the head and neck should choose his or her position of comfort carefully.

The Inter Association Task Force for Appropriate Care of the Spinal-Injured Athlete only recommends that stabilization of the head and spine be maintained; they do not specify position—neutral in line or in the position that the injured athlete lies. This is due to controversy regarding whether the athlete whose head is in less than an anatomically correct position should be repositioned,[3] because there is the possibility of conversion of an unstable injury causing more damage if the athlete is mishandled.[81] In most cases, an injured athlete's head and neck is repositioned into a neutral in-line position. This is most often done so stabilization can occur with the equipment available.

If the injured athlete is in a face-down position, he or she must be rolled to a face-up position. If the athlete is not breathing, this must be done immediately. Conscious or unconscious, if the athlete is breathing, rolling should be delayed until all the personnel and equipment necessary are available; the athlete should be monitored at all times.

A logrolling technique is demonstrated in Figure 23-18. The leader of the team is at the head of the injured athlete and is responsible for maintaining the head and neck complex in the position in which it was found. The leader has responsibility for controlling and stabilizing the head and neck position, directing the team, and monitoring the injured athlete's breathing and heart rate throughout the spine board process. When feasible, depending on the equipment the athlete is wearing and his or her position, a rigid immobilization collar should be applied. If this is not possible until the athlete is turned, the leader has responsibility for controlling the position of the head and neck throughout the logroll. An adequate number of assistants (a minimum of three) is required to logroll the injured athlete without compromising the athlete's condition or safety. These assistants should be stationed at the shoulders, pelvis, and legs. A greater number of assistants may be required to roll a larger or heavier athlete. The leader who is controlling the position of the cervical spine is responsible for coordination of the logroll procedure through direct commands. A smooth coordinated roll is accomplished by the assistants stationed as just described. The assistants should *always* roll the injured athlete toward them.[67,72] The injured athlete may be rolled directly onto the spine board. Any face mask, if not already removed, is removed once the athlete is in the supine position.

Often it is difficult to logroll an injured player who is wearing protective equipment such as a helmet and shoulder pads directly onto a spine board for immobilization. It is not as difficult to obtain the correct position with athletes who are not wearing protective equipment. If the player must be moved from his or her initial position to obtain proper immobilization, it must be done with extreme caution. A well-coordinated effort is required to lift the injured athlete and reposition the spine board or vacuum mattress. The three or more assistants should be stationed on this

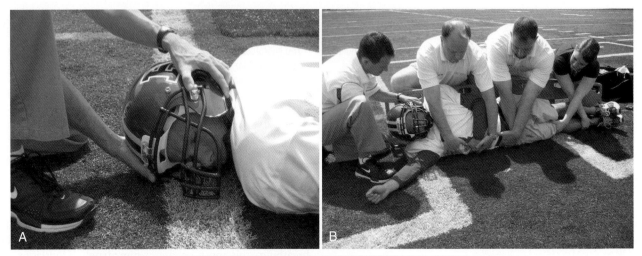

Figure 23-18

A, Appropriate grasp and immobilization of the athlete's head and neck. The member of the team immobilizing the head and neck must make sure that when the athlete is rolled into a supine position, the hands are not crossed and the team member is able to maintain appropriate support for the duration of the time required to fully immobilize the athlete. **B,** Appropriate logrolling technique. Sufficient support of the entire body with assistance in placing the backboard in the best position is needed to prevent moving the athlete a second time to place him or her in the center of the board.

same side of the injured player. The team leader is still responsible for immobilization and control of the head and neck. A fourth assistant is responsible for repositioning the board under the athlete. The athlete is lifted and lowered on command of the leader to a height sufficient to allow the spine board or vacuum mattress to be repositioned under the athlete.

Clinical Caution

The spine board or vacuum mattress is moved relative to the athlete. The athlete is not moved in any direction other than vertically. This minimizes movement of the athlete and the potential for complications.

The athlete's vital signs, level of consciousness, and neurological status are monitored by the team leader throughout the procedure of positioning the athlete on the spine board. At this time, extrication or other type of rigid collar should be applied to assist in immobilization of the head and neck if the athlete is not wearing a helmet (Figure 23-19).[72] Commercially available cervical collars may not fit if an athlete is wearing a helmet or shoulder pads. In this situation the head is blocked with foam blocks that may be incorporated as part of the backboard immobilization. If these are not available, a towel or blanket roll should be substituted when immobilized on the spine board.[68] The towel roll or blanket is slid under the athlete's neck and the ends are brought together and secured. After some type of cervical support is applied as described earlier, the athlete's torso is secured to the spine board prior to securing the head.[72] Areas around the athlete's legs and in the lumbar area are padded to remove any room between the athlete and strapping system when using a spine board. This minimizes any movement of the athlete's torso relative to the board. After the athlete's torso is secured, the head and neck are secured. A foam block, a rolled-up blanket, or towels are placed around the head when securing the athlete to a spine board to assist in immobilization (Figure 23-20).

If a vacuum splint or mattress system is being used, the head may be sufficiently immobilized without use of the towel or blanket roll. This additional padding is not necessary when using the vacuum mattress system and vacuum cervical collar, as they may be brought in close proximity to the athlete prior to removing the air from the system. Together these create a rigid support (Figure 23-21). As with any system of spine immobilization, sufficient personnel are required to carry out the task, minimizing the chances of further injury to the athlete. Care is taken to maintain appropriate access to the athlete's airway, should it be required.

Throughout the procedure of applying an extrication collar, blanket roll, or vacuum immobilization system, longitudinal support and control of the head are maintained by the team leader. Only after the athlete's head and neck are secured to the immobilization device does the team leader relinquish control of the head and neck. Once the athlete has been secured, he or she is lifted

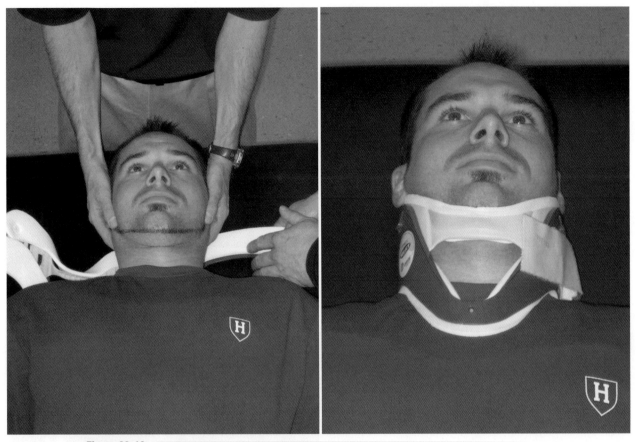

Figure 23-19
Application of an extrication collar with the athlete in a supine position. This type of collar cannot usually be used if the athlete is wearing a helmet.

using the immobilization device and transported to the appropriate emergency medical facility for further management.

Emergency Department Management

The goals of emergency department management of athletes with suspected cervical spine trauma are to (1) avoid, if present, further damage to the spinal cord; (2) prevent injury to uninjured tissues; (3) assess the athlete for neurological injury; and (4) image the cervical spine for the presence of fractures, dislocations, instability, or disc herniations. The dictum of "do no harm" certainly applies. Early pharmacological treatment can be instituted and the appropriate neurosurgical and orthopaedic consultations obtained for definitive treatment and stabilization.

It is important to maintain a high suspicion for cervical spine injury and obtain a prompt diagnosis. In one series,[82] a delay in diagnosis of spine trauma led to a 10% incidence of secondary neurological deficits. Patients with a spine injury diagnosed on initial evaluation had a much lower (1.5%) incidence of secondary neurological injury. Reasons for a delay in diagnosis included failure to obtain a radiograph, missing a fracture on a radiograph, or failure of the

athlete to seek medical attention. Other reasons included polytrauma and altered levels of consciousness. The incidence of a delay in diagnosis of trauma in the cervical spine is estimated to be approximately 30%. It should also be noted that approximately 50% to 60% of spine-injured patients have an associated nonspinal injury.[83]

It has been estimated that 5% to 10% of spinal cord injuries occur in the immediate postinjury period.[84] Extreme care must be exercised when moving and transporting athletes with possible cervical trauma. Immobilization of the cervical spine must be maintained during examination and imaging until an unstable cervical spine injury is ruled out. This immobilization includes a spine board, cervical collar, or other appropriate stabilization devices. If a helmet is in place, it should remain on during transport; however, the face mask must be removed as previously discussed. The helmet can be useful in assisting with stabilization of the cervical spine during transport. In addition, removal of the helmet requires significant motion of the cervical spine. Therefore, it is best to exclude unstable fractures prior to removal, if possible. In the presence of cervical spine injury, the helmet should be removed only in the emergency department setting by personnel trained in the care of such injuries.

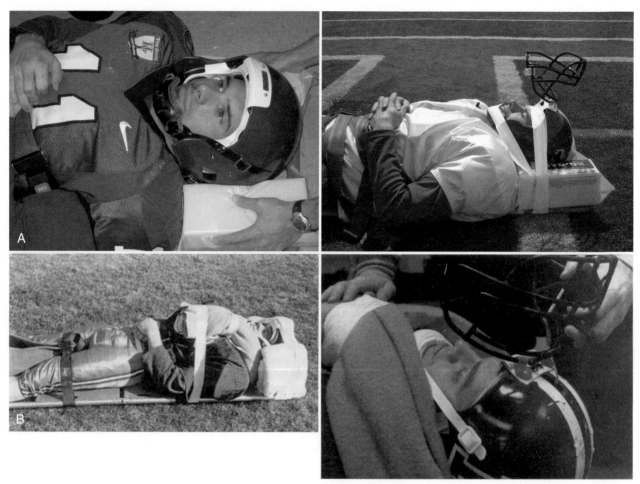

Figure 23-20
A, Athlete secured to backboard with a foam block incorporated into the backboard system. **B,** A towel or blanket roll appropriately placed around the head and neck for immobilization if other types of material for securing the head and neck are not available.

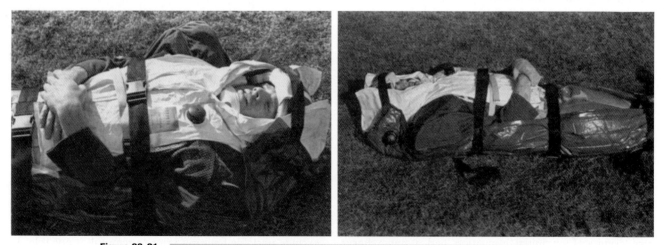

Figure 23-21
Athlete immobilized in a vacuum cervical collar and mattress.

Physical Examination

Cervical spine–injured athletes should be considered trauma patients and undergo a trauma evaluation, including the ABCs and cervical spine as part of the initial survey. A complete physical examination should be performed that literally involves an examination from head to toe. The entire spine should be inspected for wounds and ecchymosis and palpated for any point tenderness or any step deformity. A thorough neurological examination is necessary and includes motor testing of the upper and lower extremities. Motor testing is conducted by nerve root level and is graded using the 0-to-5 Oxford scale, in which 0 is no contraction, 1 is a trace contraction without motion, 2 is motion with gravity eliminated, 3 is motion against gravity, 4 is motion against resistance but diminished strength, and 5 is normal motor strength. With cervical spine injuries, diaphragm motion indicates function to the C4 root level, and patients with complete injuries proximal to this level generally do not survive. Injury to the C5 level is indicated by altered deltoid and biceps function, to C6 by weakness of the short and long radial wrist extensors, to C7 by weakness of the triceps and finger extensors, to C8 by weakness of the finger flexors, and to T_1 by intrinsic hand muscle weakness.

Sensory examination of all dermatomes is completed using pin-prick sensation and proprioception. Care is used in examining the anal and perineal regions. The skin in these regions is innervated by sacral nerve roots, and sensation in these areas may indicate an incomplete lesion in an otherwise insensate patient. Deep tendon stretch reflexes at multiple nerve root levels should be assessed. Reflexes involving cervical nerve roots include the biceps (C5), brachioradialis (C6), and triceps (C7). Additional important reflexes include the Babinski reflex (a pathological reflex) in the foot and the bulbocavernosus reflex. The bulbocavernosus reflex involves contraction of the bulb of the penis (males) or bulbus vestibule (females) when the dorsum of the penis is tapped or the bulb is compressed. If the latter reflex is absent, the patient may be in spinal shock, and the neurological level of injury cannot be determined until the reflex returns. The unconscious athlete presents a more difficult examination problem, although much information can be obtained from examination of rectal tone, reflexes, and responses to painful stimuli.

There are various patterns of neurological injury in spinal cord–injured athletes based on anatomical areas of injury. Not all athletes fit into a single category, but it is important to document the patterns as accurately as possible because of the prognostic importance that various patterns have for neurological recovery and return to function. The end of spinal shock is determined by return of the bulbocavernosus reflex, and it is at this time that the degree of spinal cord injury can be evaluated. Injuries can be classified as either complete (no function below the level of injury) or incomplete (some neurological function persists caudal to the level of injury). Incomplete injury patterns include the *central cord syndrome*, the most common type of incomplete injury, which presents with sacral sparing (i.e., perianal sensation, rectal motor tone, and great toe flexor activity) and carries a relatively good prognosis for the return of functional activity. The *anterior cord syndrome*, which presents with complete motor and sensory loss (with the exception of some retained deep pressure and proprioception), carries a poor prognosis. The *posterior cord syndrome*, a rare injury, presents with the loss of only deep pressure, pain, and proprioception. The *Brown-Séquard syndrome* presents with an ipsilateral motor deficit and a contralateral pain and temperature deficit, indicating unilateral cord injury.

Clinical Note

Spinal shock is defined as a nonstructural dysfunction of the spinal cord that occurs soon after injury and usually ends within 24 hours.

Radiological Examination

The standard plain film radiological examination of the cervical spine is made up of five views: a cross-table lateral, an anteroposterior view of the atlantoaxial segments done through an open-mouth projection, an anteroposterior view of the remainder of the cervical spine, and left and right oblique projections. *The cross-table lateral view, anteroposterior views, and open-mouth projections should be completed prior to removal of the helmet, if possible.* Completion prior to helmet removal allows the physician to visualize obvious trauma and deformity and make an initial assessment of the extent of trauma. Football helmets and shoulder pads have been demonstrated to interfere with radiographical imaging of the cervical spine, especially in the area of the cervicothoracic junction.[85-87] If complete visualization of the spine is not possible with the helmet or any other protective equipment on, then the helmet and other protective equipment (shoulder pads) should be removed and the radiological examination repeated.

Standard Radiological Examination Following Trauma to the Cervical Spine

- Cross-table lateral
- Anteroposterior of C0-C2 (open mouth)
- Anteroposterior of C2-C7
- Oblique (left and right)

The cross-table lateral cervical spine radiograph should show the entire cervical spine from the occiput to the top of T1. It should be remembered that a normal lateral view does not "clear" the cervical spine but rather serves to identify or exclude grossly unstable cervical spine fractures and to check for the presence of prevertebral soft tissue swelling. Cervical spine alignment is determined by four parallel lines running along the anterior surface of the vertebral bodies, the posterior border of the vertebral bodies, the posterior surface of the facet joints, and the spinolaminar interfaces.[88] The lateral view is also used to assess vertebral body height and disc spaces, as well as the spinal canal diameter and the atlas-dens interval.

The open-mouth view is used specifically to examine the atlantoaxial vertebrae for fractures or abnormal relationships that may indicate rotary subluxation. The other anteroposterior view is used to visualize from C3 to C7. This view demonstrates the tracheal air shadow (which should be in midline) and the alignment of the pedicles, spinous processes, and articular masses. Oblique projections are used to give additional information about the facet joints and to image neural foramen. Readers are referred to the text by Harris for a complete description of evaluation cervical spine films, which is beyond the scope of this chapter.[89]

Other imaging studies include tomograms, which can be used to look for subtle fractures in areas of super-imposed bony structures. Computed tomography (CT) provides axial images that can be used to better evaluate subtle fractures and to image areas not well visualized on plain radiographs. In addition to axial images, three-dimensional reconstructions can be done to image complex fractures. Myelography alone or in combination with CT scans can be used to evaluate for any cord or nerve root compression. Magnetic resonance imaging techniques can be used to obtain sagittal, axial, and coronal views of bony elements, intervertebral discs, the spinal cord, cerebrospinal fluid, ligaments, and other anatomical structures.

Flexion and extension lateral views of the cervical spine can be obtained to look for ligamentous instability. These views should be obtained only after an unstable fracture pattern has been excluded and should be done with voluntary motion. They are contraindicated in patients with neurological injury and those with altered states of consciousness. These views are useful in assessing not only acute ligamentous instability, but also late cervical spine instability following traumatic injury. White and Punjabi have defined stability of the lower cervical spine as "the ability of the spine to limit the patterns of displacement under physiologic stress so as not to damage or irritate the spinal cord or nerve roots."[90] Radiographically, this displacement has been defined as angular displacements of 11° more than visualized in adjacent vertebral segments, or sagittal plane displacements of one segment in relationship to another of greater than 3.5 mm.

Helmet and Shoulder Pad Removal

Helmet and shoulder pad removal is often required to obtain full radiographic evaluation and has been well-summarized by Denegar and Saliba.[68] Manual stabilization

of the player's head and neck should be reapplied as the head is released from the spine board. This is accomplished by having an assistant place his or her fingers on each side of the mandible around the helmet. At this time the head and neck are stabilized by placing one hand behind the athlete's neck and exerting pressure along the occiput, and placing the other hand along the mandible. The helmet is removed by unsnapping the cheek pads and expanding it laterally to clear the ears. After it is removed, longitudinal manual stabilization should be maintained by placing one hand on each side of the head with the fingers under the angle of the mandible and in the proximity of the mastoid process (Figure 23-22). The shoulder pads may then be removed by cutting all straps and slipping them off the athlete, being careful not to disturb the position of the head and neck. Cervical spine films are repeated if appropriate visualization was not obtained with the helmet and shoulder pads in place.

Intervention

When spinal cord injury is present, prompt consideration should be given to early pharmacological treatment.[3] Although there has been much controversy about the safety and efficacy of various treatments, animal studies and clinical trials have demonstrated the value of some agents. A randomized controlled clinical trial of methylprednisolone, a corticosteroid, demonstrated some efficacy of this agent following acute spinal cord injury.[91] Patients in this study were given a 30-mg/kg dose of methylprednisolone, followed by 5.4 mg/kg/hr given by continuous drip for a total of 23 hours. Theoretically, steroids will reduce the degree of edema in injured spinal cord tissues. Other drugs that may be of possible benefit to spinal cord–injured patients include opiate antagonists such as thyrotropin-releasing hormone and opiate receptor antagonists such as naloxone.

Once an unstable cervical spine injury is detected, prompt involvement of specialists trained in definitive management of such injuries is instituted. Although the individuals involved vary among institutions, generally an orthopaedic surgeon manages further stabilization and a neurosurgeon is involved if significant neurological injury is present. Stabilization procedures completed in the emergency department include applying traction through either a halo ring or the more rapidly applied Gardner-Wells tongs. In some cases traction may be the definitive treatment, or it may be preliminary to surgical stabilization. The halo ring can also be connected to a vest apparatus for long-term immobilization.

Return-to-Play Considerations and Contraindications

Following a cervical spine injury the sports medicine staff is often asked by the athlete "When can I return to play?" Whether or not an athlete can return to play and assume the risk of potential recurrence of what could be a

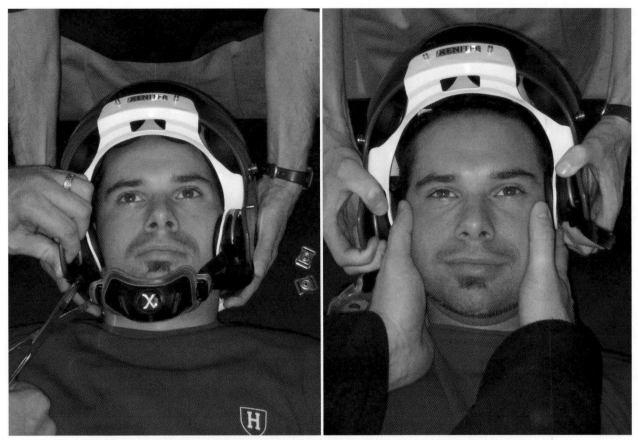

Figure 23-22
Helmet removal. Care is taken to manually support and immobilize the head and cervical spine. The cheek pads are carefully removed and the helmet is spread laterally prior to removal.

catastrophic injury is not an easy question to answer. The over-riding factor relative to return to play following cervical spine injury has been that the individual is neurologically intact, asymptomatic, pain free, and has full strength and range of motion. Although these physical examination factors may be present, there may continue to be an underlying risk for recurrence. Providing the best advice for the indications and contraindications relative to return to play based on evidence has been, and continues to be, difficult.

Until recently, the literature concerning cervical spine injuries has centered around diagnosis and treatment. Comprehensive guidelines regarding the return to sports that place an athlete at risk for a potentially catastrophic cervical spine injury have been lacking. Torg has recently published a report to describe the developmental and post-traumatic conditions of the cervical spine that might present as no contraindication, a relative contraindication, or an absolute contraindication to continued participation.[92] Torg defines *no contraindication* as a condition in which no recognized risk factors are documented in the literature or known on the basis of anecdotal evidence, *relative contraindication* as a condition in which permitting return to play is predicated

on less than unequivocally substantiated data regarding risk as documented in the literature or by anecdotal evidence, and *absolute contraindication* as a condition in which recognized factors are documented in the literature or known on the basis of experience. However, clinicians should keep in mind at all times Torg's statement: *"The criteria for return to contact activities in the presence of cervical spine abnormalities or post injury are intended as guidelines only. Owing to the lack of credible scientific evidence, they are for the most part predicated on anecdotal experience at best."*[92] Tables 23-3 to 23-8 provided by Torg, a leading authority in the area of cervical spine trauma in athletics, provide a valuable resource for sports medicine clinicians who must provide advice to athletes regarding to play.

Conclusion

Injuries to the cervical spine associated with sports have the potential to cause severe spinal cord trauma or quadriplegia; they may even prove to be fatal. It is therefore imperative that the sports medicine team be well skilled in on-field emergent care management, immobilization, transportation, and emergency department management of these

Table 23-3

Congenital Conditions: Contraindications to Return to Athletic Activity

Congenital Condition	Contraindication		
	None	Relative	Absolute
Odontoid agenesis			X
Odontoid hypoplasia			X
Os odontoideum			X
Spina bifida occulta	X		
Atlanto-occipital fusion			X
Klippel-Feil anomaly			
Type I:			X
Mass fusion of the cervical and upper thoracic vertebrae			
Type II:	X		
Fusion of only one or two interspaces at C3 and below with full cervical range of motion and not occipitocervical abnormalities, instability, disc disease, or degenerative changes			

From Torg JS: Cervical spine injuries and return to football, *Sports Health* 1:376-383, 2009.

Table 23-4

Developmental Conditions: Contraindications to Return to Athletic Activity

Developmental Condition	Contraindication		
	None	Relative	Absolute
Stenosis of the cervical spine (i.e., one or more vertebrae with a canal-vertebral ratio of < 0.8)			
Spinal Stenosis of the cervical spine and no other symptoms	X		
Spinal Stenosis of the cervical spine and motor or sensory manifestations of cervical cord neurapraxia		X	
Spinal Stenosis of the cervical spine and documented episode of cervical cord neurapraxia associated with ligamentous instability, magnetic resonance imaging evidence of neurological damage lasting longer than 36 hours, or multiple recurrence			X
Spear-tacklers spine: Developmental stenosis of the cervical canal; persistent straightening or reversal of the normal cervical lordotic curve; pre-existing post-traumatic roentgenographic abnormalities of the cervical spine; a history of prior root or cord neurapraxia and documentation of the patient's using the spear-tackling technique			X

From Torg JS: Cervical spine injuries and return to football, *Sports Health* 1:376-383, 2009.

Table 23-5

Traumatic and Ligamentous Injuries of the Upper and Middle/Lower Cervical Spine: Contraindications to Return to Athletic Activity

Upper Cervical Spine: Traumatic Injuries	Contraindication		
	None	Relative	Absolute
Almost all injuries of C1-C2 that involve fracture or ligamentous laxity			X
Healed, nondisplaced Jefferson fractures in patients who are pain free, have full range of cervical motion, and have no evidence of neurological injury		X	
Healed type I and type II odontoid fractures in patients who are also pain free and have full range of cervical motion and have no evidence of neurological injury		X	
Healed lateral mass fractures of C2 patients who are pain free, have full range of cervical motion, and have no evidence of neurological injury		X	

Middle and Lower Cervical Spine: Ligamentous Injury			
> 3.5 mm of horizontal displacement of either vertebra in relation to the other			X
< 3.5 mm of horizontal displacement of either vertebrae in relation to the other and depending on the patient's level of performances, physical habits, and position played		X	
> 11° of rotation of either adjacent vertebrae			X
< 11° of rotation of either adjacent vertebrae and depending on the patient's level of physical performances, physical habits, and position played		X	

From Torg JS: Cervical spine injuries and return to football, *Sports Health* 1:376-383, 2009.

Table 23-6

Fractures: Contraindications to Return to Athletic Activity

Fractures	Contraindications		
	None	Relative	Absolute
Healed, stable compression fractures of the vertebral body in an asymptomatic patient with no evidence of neurologic-injury and full, pain-free range of cervical motion: These fractures can settle and cause increased deformity. Patients with this type of fracture should be carefully observed.	X		
Healed, stable end plate fractures without involvement of the ligamentous or posterior bony structures in asymptomatic patients with no evidence of neurologic-injury and full, pain-free range of cervical motion	X		
Healed, stable spinous process "clay shoveler" fractures in an asymptomatic patient with no evidence of neurologic-injury and full, pain-free range of cervical motion	X		
Healed, stable fractures involving the elements of the posterior neural ring in asymptomatic patients with no evidence of neurologic-injury and full, pain-free range of cervical motion: Because a rigid ring cannot break in one location, healing of paired fractures of the ring must be evident on x-ray and imaging studies		X	
Acute fractures of the vertebral body or posterior bony structures with or without associated ligamentous laxity			X
Vertebral body fractures with evidence of a sagittal component on anteroposterior radiographs			X
Vertebral body fractures with or without displacement associated with posterior arch fractures or ligamentous laxity			X
Comminuted vertebral body fractures with displacement into the spinal canal			X
Any healed fracture of the vertebral body or the posterior bony structures; in patient with associated pain, evidence of neurologic injury and limitation of cervical motion			X
Healed, displaced fractures involving the lateral masses with resulting facet incongruity			X

From Torg JS: Cervical spine injuries and return to football, *Sports Health* 1:376-383, 2009.

Table 23-7

Intervertebral Disc Injuries: Contraindications to Return to Athletic Activity

Injury	Contraindication		
	None	Relative	Absolute
Healed anterior or lateral disc herniation that is treated conservatively in patients who are asymptomatic; have no evidence of neurological injury; and have full, pain-free range of cervical motion	X		
Lateral or central disc herniation that has been treated with intervertebral diskectomy and interbody fusion in patients who have a solid fusion; are asymptomatic; have no evidence of neurological injury; and have full, pain-free range of cervical motion	X		
Acute or chronic cervical disc herniation in patients with associated neurological findings, pain, or significant limitation of cervical motion			X

From Torg JS: Cervical spine injuries and return to football, *Sports Health* 1:376-383, 2009.

Table 23-8

Status Following Cervical Fusion: Contraindications to Return to Athletic Activity

Status	Contraindication		
	None	Relative	Absolute
Stable single-level anterior or posterior fusion in patients who are asymptomatic; have no evidence of neurological injury; and have full, pain-free range of cervical motion	X		
Stable two- or three-level fusion in patients who are asymptomatic; have no evidence of neurological injury; and have full, pain-free range of cervical motion		X	
Anterior or posterior fusion of four or more levels; because of the increased stresses on the articulations of the adjacent vertebrae and the propensity for the development of degenerative changes at these levels, these patients (with only rare exception) should not be permitted to return to athletic activity			X
Any fusion for instability of C1 regardless of roentgenographic evidence of successful fusion			X

From Torg JS: Cervical spine injuries and return to football, *Sports Health* 1:376-383, 2009.

injuries. Management of the injury by the sports medicine team, in whom the injured athlete is placing his or her trust, must be efficient and flawless to minimize the consequences of traumatic cervical spine injuries. Policies, procedures, and protocols for the management of these injuries should be in place for all organized athletic teams and organizations. The sports medicine team should practice techniques involved in on-field emergent care, immobilization, and transportation at least once each year.

References

1. National Spinal Cord Injury Statistical Center: *Spinal cord information network: Facts and figures at a glance—Update January 2008,* University of Alabama Birmingham; accessed at www.spinalcord.uab.edu.
2. Keenen TL, Benson DR: Initial evaluation of the spine injured patient. In Browner BD, Juputer JB, Levine AM, Tafton PG, editors: *Skeletal trauma,* Philadelphia, 1992, WB Saunders.
3. Kleiner DM, Almquist JL, Bailes J, et al: *Prehospital care of the spine-injured athlete: A document from the Inter-Association Task Force for Appropriate Care of the Spine Injured Athlete,* Dallas, TX, 2001, National Athletic Trainers Association.
4. Banerjee R, Palumbo MA, Fadale PD: Catastrophic cervical spine injuries in the collision sport athlete—Part 2, *Am J Sports Med* 32:1760–1764, 2004.
5. Torg JS, Quedenfeld TC, Bustein A, et al: National Football Head and Neck Injury Registry: Report on cervical quadriplegia 1971–1975, *Am J Sports Med* 7:127–132, 1979.
6. Schneider RC: Serious and fatal neurosurgical football injuries, *Clin Neurosurg* 12:226–236, 1966.
7. Schneider RC: *Head and neck injuries in football,* Baltimore, 1973, Williams & Wilkins.
8. Mueller FO, Cantu RC: *Annual survey of catastrophic football injuries,* National Center for Catastrophic Sport Injury Research, University of North Carolina, Chapel Hill, NC; accessed at http://www.unc.edu/depts/nccsi/).
9. Clarke KS: An epidemiologic view. In Torg J, editor: *Athletic injuries to the head, neck and face,* St Louis, 1991, Mosby.
10. Boden BP, Tacchetti RL, Cantu RC, et al: Catastrophic cervical spine injuries in high school and college football players, *Am J Sports Med* 34:1223–1232, 2006.
11. Hirasawa Y, Sakakida K: Sports and peripheral nerve injury, *Am J Sports Med* 11:420–426, 1983.
12. Takazawa H, Sudo N, Akoi K, et al: Statistical observation of nerve injuries in athletes (in Japanese), *Brain Nerve Injury* 3:11–17, 1971.
13. Hershman EB: Brachial plexus injuries, *Clin Sports Med* 9:311–329, 1990.
14. Clancy WG, Brand RL, Bergfeld JA: Upper trunk brachial plexus injuries in contact sports, *Am J Sports Med* 5:209–214, 1977.
15. Clancy WG: Brachial plexus and upper extremity peripheral nerve injuries. In Torg JS, editor: *Athletic injuries to the head, neck and face,* Philadelphia, 1982, Lea & Febiger.
16. Markey KL, Di Bennedetto M, Curl WW: Upper trunk brachial plexopathy: The stinger syndrome, *Am J Sports Med* 21:650–655, 1993.
17. Sallis FE, Jones K, Knopp W: Burners: Offensive strategy for an under-reported injury, *Phys Sports Med* 20:47–55, 1997.
18. Safran MR: Nerve injury about the shoulder in athletes, Part I—suprascapular nerve and axillary nerve, *Am J Sports Med* 32:803–819, 2004.
19. Safran MR: Nerve injury about the shoulder in athletes, Part II—Long thoracic nerve, spinal accessory nerve, burners/stingers, thoracic outlet syndrome, *Am J Sports Med* 32:1063–1076, 2004.
20. Glasgow SG: Upper cervical spine injuries (C1–C2). In Torg J, editor: *Athletic injuries to the head, neck and face,* St Louis, 1991, Mosby.
21. Torg JS, Treux R, Quedenfeld TC, et al: The National Football Head and Neck Injury Registry: Report and conclusions 1978, *JAMA* 241:1477–1479, 1979.
22. Torg JS, Vegso JJ, Sennett B, et al: The National Football Head and Neck Injury Registry: 14 year report on cervical quadriplegia, 1971–1984, *JAMA* 254:3439–3443, 1986.
23. Torg JS, Treux RC, Marshall J, et al: Spinal injury at the third and fourth cervical vertebrae from football, *J Bone Joint Surg Am* 59:1015–1019, 1977.
24. Torg JS, Pavlov H: Middle cervical spine injuries (C3 and C4). In Torg JS, editor: *Athletic injuries to the head, neck and face,* St Louis, 1991, Mosby.
25. Shields CL, Fox JN, Stauffer ES: Cervical cord injuries in sports, *Phys Sports Med* 6:71–76, 1978.
26. Allen BL, Ferguson RL, Lehmann TR, et al: A mechanistic classification of closed, indirect fractures and dislocations of the lower cervical spine, *Spine* 7:1–5, 1982.
27. Leventhal MR: Management of lower cervical spine injuries. In Torg J, editor: *Athletic injuries to the head, neck and face,* St Louis, 1991, Mosby.

28. Banerjee R, Palumbo MA, Fadale PD: Catastrophic cervical spine injuries in the collision sport athlete, Part I—Epidemiology, functional anatomy and diagnosis, *Am J Sports Med* 32:1077–1087, 2004.

29. Torg JS, Pavlov H, O'Neil MJ, et al: The axial load teardrop fracture: A biomechanical, clinical and roentgenographic analysis, *Am J Sports Med* 19:355–364, 1991.

30. Torg JS, Pavlov H, Genuario SE, et al: Neurapraxia of the cervical spinal cord with transient quadriplegia. *J Bone Joint Surg Am* 68:1354–1370, 1986.

31. Torg JS, Fay CM: Cervical stenosis with cord neurapraxia and transient quadriplegia. In Torg J, editor: *Athletic injuries to the head, neck and face*, St Louis, 1991, Mosby.

32. Torg JS, Guille JT, Jaffe S: Injuries to the cervical sine in American football players, *J Bone Joint Surg Am* 84:112–122, 2002.

33. Torg JS, Pavlov H: Cervical spinal stenosis with cord neurapraxia and transient quadriplegia, *Clin Sports Med* 6:115–133, 1987.

34. Torg JS, Corcoran AT, Thibault LE, et al: Cervical cord neurapraxia: Classification, pathomechanics, morbidity and management guidelines, *J Neurosurg* 87:843–850, 1997.

35. Pavlov H, Torg JS, Robie B, et al: Cervical spinal stenosis: Determination with vertebral body ratio method, *Radiology* 164:771–774, 1987.

36. Odor JM, Watkins RG, Dillin WH, et al: Incidence of cervical spinal stenosis in professional and rookie football players, *Am J Sports Med* 18:507–509, 1990.

37. Herzog RG, Wiens JJ, Dillingham MF, et al: Normal cervical spine morphometry and cervical spinal stenosis in asymptomatic professional football players, *Spine* 16:178–186, 1991.

38. Torg JS, Naranja RJ, Pavlov H, et al: The relationship of developmental narrowing of the cervical spinal canal to reversible and irreversible injury of the cervical spinal cord in football players, *J Bone Joint Surg Am* 78:1308–1314, 1996.

39. Torg JS: Epidemiology, biomechanics and prevention of cervical spine trauma resulting from athletics and recreational activities, *Oper Tech Sports Med* 1:159–168, 1993.

40. Schneider RC, Kahn EA: Serious and fatal neurosurgical football injuries, *Clin Neurosurg* 12:226–236, 1966.

41. Torg JS, Vegso JJ, O'Neill J, et al: The epidemiologic, pathologic, biomechanical and cinematographic analysis of football induced cervical spine trauma, *Am J Sports Med* 18:50–57, 1990.

42. Tator CH: Injuries to the cervical spine and spinal cork resulting from ice hockey. In Torg J, editor: *Athletic injuries to the head, neck and face*, St Louis, 1991, Mosby.

43. Tator CH, Carson JD, Edmonds VE: Spinal injuries in ice hockey, *Clin Sports Med* 17:183–194, 1998.

44. Tator CH, Edmonds VE, Lapczak L. Spinal injuries in ice hockey: A review of 182 North American cases and analysis of etiologic factors. In Castalki CR, Bishop PJ, Hoerner ER, editors: *Safety in ice hockey*, Vol 2, Philadelphia, 1993, American Society for Testing and Materials.

45. Reid DC, Saboe LA: Spine injuries resulting from winter sports. In Torg J, editor: *Athletic injuries to the head, neck and face*, St Louis, 1991, Mosby.

46. Tarazi F, Dvorak MF, Wing PC: Spinal injuries in skiers and snowboarders, *Am J Sports Med* 27:177–180, 1999.

47. Floyd T: Alpine skiing, snowboarding and spinal trauma, *Arch Orthop Trauma Surg* 121:433–436, 2001.

48. Shields CW, Fox JM, Stouffer ES: Cervical cord injuries in sports. *Phys Sports Med* 6:71–76, 1978.

49. Torg JS: Injuries to the cervical spine and cork resulting from water sports. In Torg J, editor: *Athletic injuries to the head, neck and face*, St Louis, 1991, Mosby.

50. Taylor TKF, Coolican MRJ: Spinal cord injuries in Australia football, 1960–1985, *Med J Aust* 147:112–118, 1987.

51. Silver JR, Gill G: Injuries of the spine sustained during rugby, *Sports Med* 5:328–334, 1988.

52. Wetzler MJ, Akpta T, Laughlin W, et al: Occurrence of cervical spine injuries during the rugby scrum, *Am J Sports Med* 26:177–180, 1998.

53. Clarke K: Survey of spinal cord injuries in schools and college sports, 1973–1975, *J Safety Res* 9:140, 1977.

54. Ellis WG, Green D, Holzaepfel NR, Sahs AL: The trampoline and serious neurological injuries: A report of five cases, *JAMA* 174(13):1673-1676, 1960.

55. Torg JS: Trampoline induced cervical quadriplegia. In Torg J, editor: *Athletic injuries to the head, neck and face*, St Louis, 1991, Mosby.

56. American Academy of Pediatrics, Committee on Accident and Poison Prevention: *Trampolines*, Evanston, IL, 1977, American Academy of Pediatrics.

57. Otis JC, Burstein AH, Torg JS: Mechanisms and pathomechanics of athletic injuries to the cervical spine. In Torg J, editors: *Athletic injuries to the head, neck and face*, St Louis, 1991, Mosby.

58. Virgin H: Cineradiographic study of football helmets and the cervical spine, *Am J Sports Med* 8:310–317, 1980.

59. Carter DR, Frankel VH: Biomechanics of hyperextension injuries to the cervical spine in football, *Am J Sports Med* 8(5):302–319, 1980.

60. Patterson D: Legal aspects of athletic injuries to the head and cervical spine. In Torg J, editor: *Athletic injuries to the head, neck and face*, St Louis, 1991, Mosby.

61. Heck FJ, Weiss MP, Gartland JM, et al: Minimizing liability risks of head and neck injuries in football, *J Athl Training* 29:128–139, 1994.

62. Bailes JE, Petschauer M, Guskiewicz KM, et al: Management of cervical spine injuries in athletes. *J Athl Training* 42:126–134, 2007.

63. National Collegiate Athletic Association: *2007-08 NCAA Sports Medicine Handbook 2007–08*, Indianapolis, IN, 2007, National Collegiate Athletic Association.

64. National Football League: *Guidelines for game officials to use during a serious on-field player injury*, New York, 1999, National Football League.

65. Banerjee R, Palumbo MA, Fadale PD: Catastrophic cervical spine injuries in the collision sport athlete, *Am J Sports Med* 32:1760–1764, 2004.

66. Feld F: Management of the critically injured football player, *J Athl Training* 28:206–212, 1993.

67. Vegso JJ, Torg JS: Field evaluation and management of cervical spine injuries. In Torg J, editor: *Athletic injuries to the head, neck and face*, St Louis, 1991, Mosby.

68. Denegar C, Saliba E: On field management of the potentially cervical spine injured athlete, *J Athl Training* 24:108–111, 1989.

69. Feld F, Blanc R: Immobilizing the spine injured football player, *J Emerg Med Serv* 12:38–40, 1987.

70. Feld F: Management of the critically injured football player, *J Athl Training* 28:206–212, 1993.

71. Segan RD, Cassidy C, Bentkowski J: A discussion of the issue of football helmet removal in suspected cervical spine injuries, *J Athl Training* 28:294–305, 1993.

72. Heckman JD: *Emergency care and transportation of the sick and injured*, ed 5, Rosemont, IL, 1993, American Academy of Orthopaedic Surgeons.

73. DeLorenzo RA, Olson JE, Boska M, et al: Optimal positioning for cervical immobilization, *Ann Emerg Med* 28:301–308, 1996.

74. Tierney RT, Mattacola CG, Sitler MR, et al: Head position and football equipment influence cervical spinal-cord space during immobilization, *J Athl Training* 37:185–189, 2002.

75. La Prade RF, Schentzler KA, Broxterman JR, et al: Cervical spine alignment in the immobilized hockey player: A computed tomographic analysis of the effects of helmet removal, *Am J Sports Med* 28:800–803, 2000.

76. Metz CM, Kuhn JE, Greenfield ML: Cervical spine alignment in immobilized hockey players: Radiographic analysis with and without helmets and shoulder pads, *Clin J Sports Med* 8:92–95, 1998.

77. Donaldson WF, Laureman WC Heil B, et al: Helmet and shoulder pad removal from a player with suspected cervical spine injury, *Spine* 23:1729–1733, 1998.

78. Prinzen RK, Syrotuik DG, Reid DC: Position of the cervical vertebrae during helmet removal and cervical collar application in football and hockey, *Clin J Sports Med* 5:155–161, 1995.

79. Swenson TM, Lauerman WF, Donaldson WF, et al: Cervical spine position in the immobilized football player—radiographic analysis before and after helmet removal, *Med Sci Sports Exerc* 26(suppl):S148, 1994.

80. Hulstyn MS, Palumbo MA, Fadale PD, et al: The effect of protective football equipment on alignment of the injured cervical spine: Radiographic analysis in a cadaveric model. Presented at *American Orthopaedic Society of Sports Medicine*, Toronto, Canada, July 1995, Abstracts, p 27.

81. Shriger DK: Immobilizing the cervical spine in trauma: Should we seek an optimal position or an adequate one? *Ann Emerg Med* 28:351–353, 1996.

82. Reid DC, Henderson R, Saboe L, et al: Etiology and clinical course of missed spine fractures, *J Trauma* 27:980–986, 1987.

83. Benson DR, Keenen TL, Antony J: Unsuspected associated lesions in the fractured spine, *Presented at the Orthopaedic Trauma Association Meeting*, Dallas, TX, October 1988.

84. Castelano V, Bocconi FL: Injuries of the cervical spine with spinal cord involvement (myelic fractures): Statistical considerations, *Bull Hosp Joint Dis* 31:188–194, 1970.

85. Davidson RM, Burton JH, Snowise M, et al: Football protective gear and cervical spine imaging, *Ann Emerg Med* 38:26–30, 2001.

86. Hollengerg GM, Beitia AO, Tan RK, et al: Imaging of the cervical spine in sports medicine, *Curr Sports Med Rep* 2:33–40, 2003.

87. Waeckerle FJ, Kleiner DM: Protective athletic equipment and cervical spine imaging, *Ann Emerg Med* 38:26–30, 2001.

88. Pavlov H, Potter HG: Imaging techniques applicable to athletically induced cervical spine trauma, *Oper Tech Sports Med* 1:169–182, 1993.

89. Harris JH: *The radiology of acute cervical spine trauma*, ed 2, Baltimore, 1987, Williams & Wilkins.

90. White AA, Punjabi MM: *Clinical biomechanics of the spine*, Philadelphia, 1978, JB Lippincott.

91. Bracken MB, Shepard MJ, Collins WF, et al: A randomized controlled trial of methylprednisolone or naloxone in the treatment of spinal cord injury, *N Engl J Med* 322:1405–1411, 1990.

92. Torg JS: Cervical spine injuries and return to football, *Sports Health* 1:376–383, 2009.

MAXILLOFACIAL INJURIES

John P. Kelly

Introduction

Even though the widespread use of improved protective devices, such as helmets, face masks, eye shields, and mouthguards, has significantly reduced the incidence of injury to the head and neck region, such use has not eliminated the common occurrence of both major and minor injuries to the critical structures of this anatomical area. In fact, concerns have been expressed that in some sports, improvements in protective headgear have given athletes a false sense of invulnerability, leading to more dangerous play and transference of the site of injury from the face to the central nervous system or the cervical spine, as discussed in the preceding chapters. Nevertheless, the large numbers of athletes participating in sports in which facial protection is not customary or is not complete and the occurrence of injuries despite full headgear make a thorough knowledge of maxillofacial trauma important to physicians, sport physical therapists, and athletic trainers who work with such athletes.

Initial Management Priorities

Fortunately, most maxillofacial injuries in sports occur as isolated injuries. However, the potential for serious injury must not be overlooked. The types of trauma suffered in athletic competition (excluding auto racing) tend to be "low-energy" wounds with relatively few associated injuries. However, both the apparently trivial bruise to the chin and the dramatically bleeding scalp laceration can be indicative of potential serious injury to the intracranial vault or the cervical spine. Injuries such as these must always be suspected and ruled out.

As with major trauma, the highest priority must be given to the adequacy of the patient's airway. Blows to the neck resulting in a fracture of the larynx are most likely to produce serious compromise of the airway and require emergency treatment, as discussed later. Difficulty with breathing as a result of oral, nasal, or pharyngeal bleeding is rarely a problem in low-energy trauma, but positioning the patient on his or her side or in a prone position may be necessary for comfortable air exchange until hemorrhage is controlled.

Maxillofacial Management Priorities

- Ensure adequate airway and breathing
- Control bleeding
- Confirm patient's medical history

After management of the airway and breathing, control of bleeding is the next priority in the initial treatment. Direct pressure applied with sterile gauze sponges or any clean, absorbent cloth is the mainstay of primary therapy for wounds of the head, face, and neck. Rarely in athletic injuries will the amount of blood loss result in acute circulatory embarrassment. It is generally not necessary or desirable to attempt ligation of bleeding vessels in the field. Specific management of bleeding will be covered in the discussion of particular injuries in the following pages.

The athlete's pertinent past medical history must be confirmed. Of particular importance to those responsible for emergency care are the existence of drug allergies, current use of medications, and the history of tetanus immunization. The Centers for Disease Control and Prevention (CDC) currently recommends use of a new tetanus, reduced diphtheria, and pertussis vaccine for wound management in adolescents and adults; for children aged 7 or younger, the diphtheria, tetanus, and acellular pertussis vaccine is recommended. Table 24-1 summarizes the 2008 CDC recommendations.

Table 24-1

Prophylaxis Against Tetanus: 2008 CDC Recommendations

History of Previous Tetanus Immunization	Clean, Minor Wounds	All Other Wounds
Uncertain or fewer than three doses	Give vaccine (< 7 years old: DTaP; 10-64 years old: Tdap)	Give vaccine and tetanus immune globulin
Three or more previous doses	No need to vaccinate (unless > 10 years since last dose)	Give vaccine if > 5 years since last dose

Data from Centers for Disease Control and Prevention: Prevention of specific infectious diseases. In *CDC Travelers' Health,* Atlanta, GA, Centers for Disease Control and Prevention. Accessed at http://wwwn.cdc.gov/travel/yellowBookCh4-Tetanus.aspx.
CDC, Centers for Disease Control and Prevention; *DTaP,* diphtheria, tetanus, and acellular pertussis; *Tdap,* tetanus, diphtheria, and acellular pertussis.

Airway Injuries

The most dangerous of all maxillofacial injuries encountered in athletics is that resulting from a blow to the neck by a hockey stick, puck, or other such equipment (Figure 24-1). Careful attention and observation of even seemingly minor injury to the larynx is critical because of the potential for progressive worsening to life-threatening airway obstruction as edema progresses in the postinjury period.[1]

For a patient with a history of blunt trauma to the neck, the significant signs and symptoms of laryngeal injury include hoarseness, difficulty breathing, pain (including pain on swallowing), tenderness, subcutaneous emphysema, hematoma, and hemoptysis (coughing up blood). On examination, the voice quality may be described as muffled, hoarse, or "breathy," depending on the specific location of injury in the laryngotracheal area. At the scene of injury it is primarily important to recognize a *change* in voice quality. Fracture of the thyroid or cricoid cartilage may be suggested by a flattening or loss of normal prominence in the anterior neck, although these structures may be difficult to evaluate if there has been sufficient time for edema or hematoma to obscure the anatomical features. A critical finding is the presence of subcutaneous emphysema, which signifies loss of integrity of the upper aerodigestive tract and requires urgent attention.

Signs and Symptoms of Laryngeal Injury

- Hoarseness
- Difficulty breathing
- Pain (especially on swallowing)
- Tenderness around larynx
- Subcutaneous emphysema
- Hematoma
- Hemoptysis

All patients with suspected laryngeal injury, based on these signs and symptoms, should be referred immediately for endoscopic examination and definitive therapy. Minor airway symptoms will usually require only observation, and return to full activity can be anticipated in several days. When airway compromise is present, obtaining a clear airway is critical. Some controversy exists as to whether endotracheal intubation or tracheostomy is the preferred emergency measure for such patients. The preponderance of opinion favors tracheostomy, as intubation may cause additional trauma to the already injured larynx. An emergency tracheostomy in the field is an extremely uncommon event in the context of athletic injuries.

Soft Tissue Injuries

The most common injuries to the head and face involve trauma to the soft tissues, resulting in contusions, abrasions, or lacerations.

In all locations, a contusion from contact with a blunt object requires attention to the possibility of injury to a deeper, bony structure. In the absence of such damage, the bruised area needs little more than ice for comfort and pressure to inhibit the development of a hematoma. Special consideration, however, must be given to a contusion to the external ear. In such an injury, any accumulated blood beneath the skin surface should be aspirated or drained to prevent permanent deformation of the underlying auricular cartilage ("cauliflower ear") (Figure 24-2). This condition is quite common in wrestlers and is easily prevented with the use of appropriate protective headgear. With trauma, fluid accumulates between the skin and the cartilage. If the fluid is not evacuated, fibrosis and keloid formation result.

Aspiration can usually be carried out without anesthesia, but formal incision and drainage may require infiltration of local anesthesia. A small amount of lidocaine with

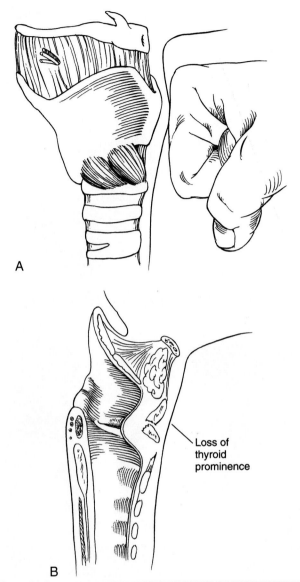

Figure 24-1

A, External trauma to larynx over prominence of thyroid cartilage ("Adam's apple"). **B,** Fracture of the larynx, as seen on the lateral view, produces narrowing of airway and disruption of the vocal cords. Airway compromise is worsened as tissues become edematous.

such material must be meticulously removed so as to prevent permanent "tattooing" of the abraded area. Small areas of abrasion are readily treated immediately and require only a simple antibiotic ointment dressing. Larger areas or areas with deeply embedded foreign material may require local or general anesthesia for adequate debridement. Flushing the affected area with sterile saline under pressure, using a 30-mL syringe, is an effective method of cleansing for all abrasions. Scrubbing the area with a sterile brush is usually reserved for deeper wounds or those with extensive foreign material.

Lacerations of the face, scalp, and neck may be accompanied by brisk bleeding initially, which reflects the area's rich blood supply. This blood supply is greatly beneficial in terms of quick healing and resistance to infection. Control of acute bleeding is the first priority and is accomplished by simple pressure over the wound with sterile gauze. Placement of absorbable cellulose gauze (Surgicel) into the wound may assist with hemostasis until definitive treatment can be accomplished.

Lacerations

Types

Simple *linear lacerations* result from contact of the skin with sharp objects such as skates or sticks. *Stellate lacerations* have the appearance of a bursting of the skin and usually result from a blunt object striking skin that overlies bone (Figure 24-3). In either case, it is not uncommon for large lacerations to give the appearance of tissue loss owing to retraction of the wound edges along the lines of skin tension; however, careful inspection and reapproximation of the wound edges will frequently reveal no loss of tissue. *Avulsive wounds* actually do result in loss of tissue and require more complex methods of repair.

Types of Lacerations

- Linear
- Stellate
- Avulsion

Cleansing and Debridement

The most favorable repair of lacerations occurs when early cleansing is carried out and debridement of all foreign material is accomplished. This is particularly important for wounds that are grossly contaminated with dirt, grass, gravel, and the like, as foreign material may promote subsequent wound infection. Effective cleansing, debridement of foreign material, and prompt skin closure are the most effective means of promoting good healing in the absence of infection, making antibiotic use rarely necessary for simple facial lacerations.

epinephrine is injected into the hematoma, and the area is gently massaged. The lidocaine and hematoma are then removed. A form-fitting compression dressing is applied after the procedure and left in place for 48 to 72 hours. Return to activity is strictly a matter of the athlete's comfort.

Abrasions occur when the integrity of the skin surface is lost as a result of falls or collisions with hard or rough surfaces. Careful, gentle cleansing of the abraded surface should be carried out, and particular attention must be paid to any embedded foreign bodies, such as dirt or asphalt;

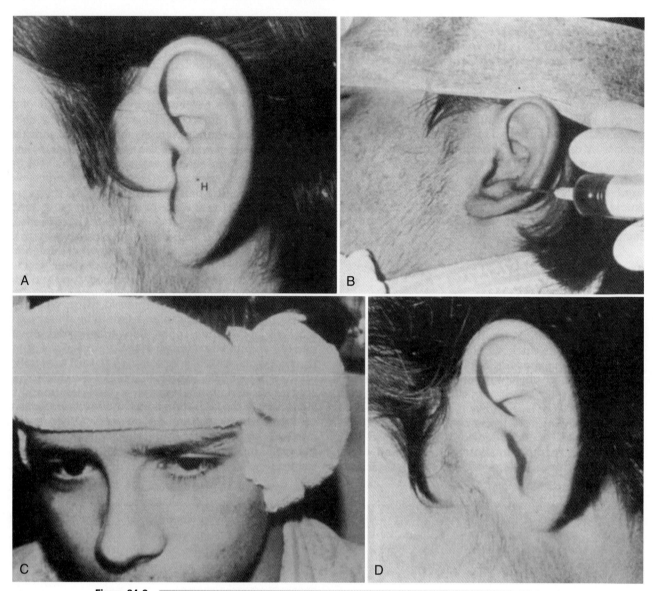

Figure 24-2

"Cauliflower ear." **A,** Hematoma *(H)* of the auricle caused by a wrestling injury. **B,** Hematoma being aspirated. **C,** Contoured head dressing to force perichondrium back against auricular cartilage. **D,** Good result 4 weeks after injury. (From Handler SD: Diagnosis and management of maxillofacial injuries. In Torg J, editor: *Athletic injuries to the head, neck and face,* pp 611–634, St Louis, 1991, Mosby.)

Inspection of the wound prior to closure is essential for identification of devitalized tissue whose retention will contribute to the promotion of later wound infection. However, the excellent blood supply of this region allows the physician to be very conservative in the debridement of tissue. Compromised tissue, whether it is contused or jagged, can and should be preserved in most facial wounds; only skin that is definitively necrotic should be sacrificed at the time of initial repair. It is not necessary to shave hair at the site of a laceration on the scalp or face. In fact, shaving of the eyebrows is contraindicated, both because a vital landmark for alignment of the laceration is lost and because regrowth of the eyebrow cannot be ensured. Other specific anatomical landmarks for the alignment of lacerations are the gray line of the eyelid and the vermillion border of the lip (Figure 24-4).

Anesthesia

For all but the most extensive lacerations, local anesthesia is the preferred method of management. Although regional nerve blocks of the supraorbital, infraorbital, or mental

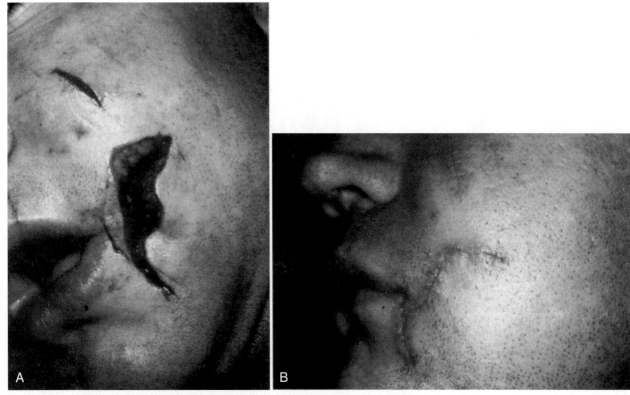

Figure 24-3
Linear and stellate type lacerations before (**A**) and after (**B**) skin closure.

nerves may be employed, infiltration of the wound edges with a solution of 2% lidocaine containing 1:100,000 epinephrine will provide excellent anesthesia and aid in hemostasis of the wound. However, care must be taken not to distort the wound by excessive infiltration, as vital clues to perfect alignment of the skin edges can be lost.

Special Structures

The specialized anatomy of facial structures requires careful attention in the course of treatment of lacerations. Both deep and surface structures must be taken into account.

Structures Requiring Special Care and Consideration when Suturing

- Facial nerve
- Parotid duct
- Eyebrows
- Eyelids
- Ears
- Nose
- Lips
- Tongue

Facial Nerve. Deep lacerations of the cheek, posterior to a vertical line from the lateral canthus of the eye, place the main branches of the facial nerve at risk (Figure 24-5). Examination of a patient with such an injury requires that attention be paid to the patient's ability to raise the eyebrow, furrow the forehead, close the eyes tightly, and smile and pucker the lips. Any deficit in these facial animations in the presence of a laceration in the described location suggests an injury to a branch of the facial nerve, which can and must be repaired primarily. For lacerations occurring anterior to that line, facial nerve reanastomosis is not necessary, because the nerve has branched sufficiently that animation of the involved muscles can be anticipated to return without surgical intervention. Facial nerve repair generally requires that the athlete be transferred to a hospital where an operating microscope is available.

Parotid Duct. The salivary duct from the parotid gland, which opens into the mouth through the buccal mucosa adjacent to the upper molar teeth, runs along a course externally identified by a line from the tragus of the ear to the alar base of the nose. Any deep laceration of the posterior cheek that traverses this line must be inspected carefully for identification of the duct. If the duct is severed, it will require direct suture repair along with placement of a plastic catheter within its lumen for a period of 7 to 10 days.

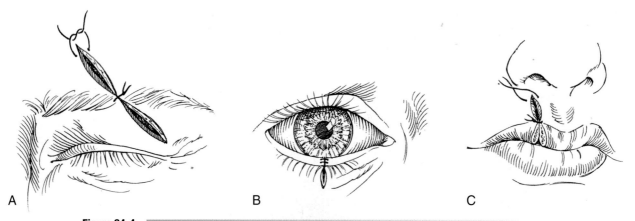

Figure 24-4

Anatomical landmarks for alignment of lacerations. **A,** Eyebrow. **B,** Gray line of eyelid. **C,** Vermillion border of lip.

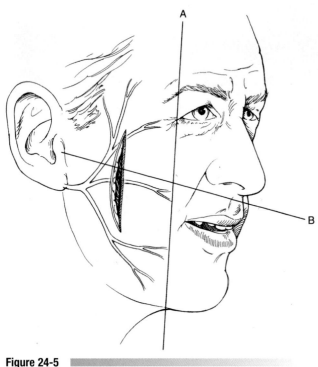

Figure 24-5

Landmarks for identification of critical area for facial nerve injury *(A)* and parotid duct laceration *(B).*

Eyebrows. As mentioned earlier, the eyebrows provide an excellent cue to proper alignment of lacerations in that area. Failure to repair the wound with excellent alignment of the eyebrow will result in a very noticeable cosmetic deformity that is difficult to repair at a later date.

Eyelids. As will be discussed shortly, a through-and-through laceration of the eyelid requires careful examination to rule out injury to the globe itself. Repair of the eyelid must be carried out with attention to alignment and repair of the deep structures (the orbicularis oculi muscle, the levator muscle of the upper lid, the orbital septum, and the tarsal plate) and the surface anatomy (the lashes and the "gray line" of the lid edge) (see Figure 24-4, *B*). Both cosmetic and functional impairment can be the result of inattention to the anatomical details in this area.

Ears and Nose. Deep lacerations of the ear and nose share the common problem of laceration of underlying cartilage, which must be repaired or debrided prior to skin closure, lest the cosmetic result be unfavorable.

Lips. Like the eyelid, the lips must be carefully repaired after lacerations to preserve function and appearance. Through-and-through lacerations of the lips, which are frequently the result of external blows that drive the teeth through the lip, must be inspected for the presence of any tooth fragments that may have been dislodged by the external blow. The circumferential muscle of the lip, the orbicularis oris, must be repaired with sutures prior to closure of the skin or the mucosa. Any laceration that crosses the vermilion border of the lip, where the mucosa meets the skin, requires precise alignment of the vermilion border before any other sutures are placed (Figure 24-6).

Tongue. Most lacerations of the tongue result from external force that causes the patient's teeth to bite the tongue. Most tongue lacerations are minor and do not necessitate suture closure. However, if there is persistent bleeding or there is a large flap defect of the tongue, suturing is recommended and will allow for prompt return to full activity.

Suturing

Although many minor facial lacerations might be managed successfully by approximating the wound edges with adhesive strips, such indirect measures may not be adequate for the athlete seeking a quick return to activity. Suture repair of even small lacerations provides hemostasis and skin integrity to allow the athlete to return to competition immediately. A dressing of collodion is often more effective than

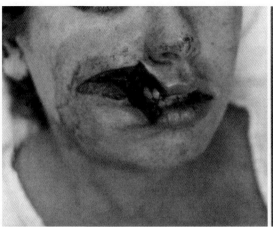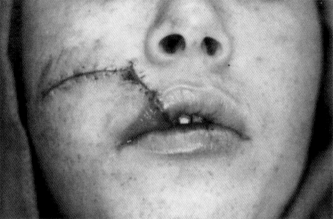

Figure 24-6
Laceration of the lip that involves the orbicularis oris. This structure must be repaired prior to closure of the skin. Note how the vermillion border of the lip is precisely aligned following repair.

any attempts to protect the facial or scalp wound with bandaging; small areas may simply be dressed with an antibiotic ointment. Facial sutures can be safely removed in 4 or 5 days, with the longer time being favored for the athlete whose wound will be at risk for reopening by continued competition.

Tissue Adhesives

The use of tissue adhesives (various types of cyanoacrylates) has become widespread in emergency departments and primary care facilities for management of acute, linear lacerations in which the wound length, width, and depth allow for tension-free approximation of the wound edges. No differences in ultimate cosmesis is seen after use of the adhesives when compared with standard wound closure techniques, and the use of adhesives is associated with decreased procedure time. However, the increased incidence of wound dehiscence following adhesive closure, even in an "unstressed wound," must be considered in choosing the closure technique for an athlete who is returning to competition right away.

Antibiotics

Systemic antibiotics are not generally indicated for treatment of facial or scalp lacerations that have received prompt attention and careful cleansing and debridement. The exception to the rule may be the common use of penicillin (or erythromycin for those allergic to penicillin) for intraoral lacerations of the tongue, lips, or cheeks and for through-and-through wounds involving the lips and cheeks. Such use is not universally accepted, however, and many clinicians reserve it for severe wounds or for wounds in which there is high risk of contamination by external debris. There is no evidence that the use of antibiotics adds to the success of treatment when the wound has been properly cared for.

Ocular Injuries

An estimated 100,000 ocular injuries occur annually in the United States as a result of athletic activities.[2] The use of protective equipment in sports such as football and amateur hockey has caused a significant reduction in such injuries, but the large number of players who are unprotected—in baseball, basketball, racquet sports, and professional hockey, for example—results in a significant risk for devastating injury. Even an apparently trivial injury can be vision threatening, making early recognition, appropriate emergency care, and prompt referral for definitive ophthalmological treatment essential priorities for all who care for athletes.

Anatomy

Knowledge of the anatomy of the eye is fundamental to the evaluation of injuries (Figure 24-7 and Figure 24-8).

The visible anatomy of the eye consists of the *cornea* through which light must pass to reach the retina. This outermost layer of the eye is fully translucent and allows visualization of the iris and pupil beneath it. Continuous with the cornea is the *sclera,* the tough, white, fibrous outer layer of the globe that surrounds the entire eye to become continuous with the dura overlying the optic nerve posteriorly. The junction of the cornea and the sclera is the *limbus.* Anteriorly, the sclera is covered by the loose layer of tissue known as the *conjunctiva,* which attaches to the upper and lower lids. Posteriorly, the loose covering over the sclera is known as *Tenon capsule.* The *iris,* the colored part of the eye that opens and closes as a diaphragm, allows light to pass through the pupil. The *ciliary body* produces the aqueous fluid of the anterior chamber of the eye and regulates the focusing of the lens within the eye. The *choroid* carries the blood supply to the *retina,* the inner coating of the eye and a highly specialized tissue that converts light impulses to

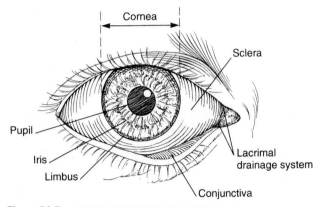

Figure 24-7
Landmarks of surface anatomy of the globe.

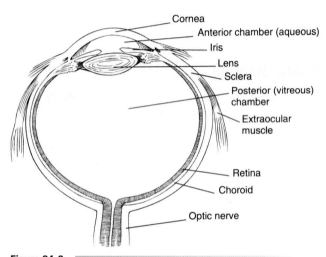

Figure 24-8
Cross-sectional anatomy of the globe.

electrical signals, which are then transmitted by the optic nerve to other portions of the brain.

The anatomy of the eye must further be understood in terms of the compartments or chambers into which it is organized. The anterior chamber, containing aqueous fluid, extends from the cornea to the iris. The posterior chamber contains the lens by which light is focused and extends from the iris to the vitreous space. The latter is the largest compartment of the eye and is filled with a clear gel that maintains the shape of the eye and the retina while transmitting focused light to the retina.

External to the eye are the six extraocular muscles, which extend from the orbit to the sclera and move the eyes in coordinated fashion in all directions. The lacrimal system, which is responsible for the production of tears that lubricate and cleanse the anterior surface of the cornea, consists of the lacrimal gland in the upper lateral portion of the orbit and the collecting ducts at the lower, inner side of the lid.

Any alteration in the integrity of this delicate system can result in loss of vision. Alteration may involve loss of clarity of the light-transmitting portions of the visual tract, loss of alignment of the focusing elements, loss of shape of the light-receiving retina, loss of blood supply to the retina, or loss of integrity of the transmitting optic nerve.

Examination

In the absence of effective prevention of eye injury, the priorities for those with initial responsibility for management involve recognition of the injury, limitation of progression of the injury's severity, and arranging for prompt referral for specialized care.[3]

Priorities in Management of Eye Injuries

- Recognize degree of injury, especially visual acuity
- Limit the injury's severity
- Arrange, as appropriate, prompt specialized care

Evaluation begins with a pertinent history of how the injury occurred, what struck the eye, the symptoms experienced by the patient, and the patient's use of contact lenses or corrective eyewear.

Visual acuity is the most important aspect of assessment of any traumatized eye. Any deviation from normal must be documented, as must any progressive change in acuity over time. The athlete's best visual response is recorded concerning his or her ability to read, count fingers, detect hand motion, and perceive light. Partial loss of vision and the visual field defects that may be produced are also recorded. More sophisticated evaluation of acuity is reserved for the ophthalmological setting.

The lids and orbital rims are palpated to assess any irregularities that might suggest fractures or foreign bodies. Gentle palpation of the globe through the lid allows for gross assessment of elevated intraocular pressure or softening.

A simple penlight examination can be carried out to determine normal pupillary response and clarity and gross integrity of the cornea, the anterior chamber, and the lens. Visual inspection of the conjunctiva and the sclera is also done at this time. Protrusion of the eye (a result of increased pressure behind the globe) or retraction of the globe (resulting from increased orbital volume with fractures into the adjacent sinuses) should also be noted.

When complaints of pain and foreign body sensation suggest the possibility of corneal abrasion, examination of the eye with a blue light after instillation of fluorescein dye on moistened strips is essential in this initial evaluation.

In the field, examination of the posterior chamber and the vitreous is usually confined to observation of a red reflection (the "red reflex") seen when light is shone onto the retina. Absence of such a reflection from the retina may indicate bleeding into the vitreous fluid or detachment of the retina. In either case, ophthalmological consultation is essential for full examination of the retina with dilation of the pupils.

By asking the patient to move the eye in all directions, assessment of the functions of the extraocular muscles can be readily carried out. Impairment in motion may be the result of direct injury to the muscles or injury to the cranial nerves supplying the muscles.

Anterior Eye Segment Injuries

Anterior Eye Injuries

- Foreign bodies
- Corneal abrasion
- Subconjunctival hemorrhage
- Hyphema

Foreign Bodies. Foreign bodies, including displaced contact lenses, are probably the most common and the most benign of the emergency problems that athletes encounter. Care must be taken not to allow the athlete to rub the eye, because this may cause a corneal abrasion. The simple sensation of a foreign body, occasionally accompanied by tearing and scleral redness in the area of the foreign object, requires that the lids be everted to search for the object. Copious irrigation with normal saline is usually sufficient to remove the offending agent, and the athlete can return to activity immediately. If the article is embedded such that it cannot be flushed away, referral for ophthalmological consultation is preferable to attempted instrumentation and risk of corneal abrasion. If the athlete must be transported for consultation, *both eyes* should be covered to minimize any movement of the injured eye.

Corneal Abrasion. When there has been a glancing blow to the eye, a scratch, or a persistent foreign body, the likelihood of corneal abrasion is high. The patient usually has exquisite pain; photophobia and tearing are common accompaniments. A fluorescein-impregnated strip can be moistened and touched to the conjunctival fold between the sclera and the lower lid. Examination with a blue light will then demonstrate the corneal defect as a green stain or streak. Once the diagnosis is made, the eyelid should be closed and patched and the patient sent for ophthalmological referral. Definitive care usually includes cycloplegic eyedrops, topical antibiotics, and patching for several days. In the absence of other accompanying injury, the athlete can return to full competition as soon as the patch is removed.

Subconjunctival Hemorrhage. Bright red blood overlying the sclera in the plane beneath the conjunctiva may occur spontaneously (often in scuba divers) or as the result of a minor blow to the eye. In the absence of other symptoms or signs, no treatment is required, and the individual can return to full activity immediately, with the expectation that the bloody discoloration will resolve in a week or two.

Chemosis, or edema of the conjunctiva, which is seen in association with subconjunctival hemorrhage, mandates a thorough investigation for more significant injury either to the orbit or to the globe itself. Diffuse chemosis and subconjunctival hemorrhage may indicate actual corneal laceration or perforation of the globe; such serious injury may have no other signs or symptoms initially but must be suspected. Should these findings be made after trauma, a plastic or metal shield should be placed over the eye while prompt referral for ophthalmological care is made.

Hyphema. Bleeding into the anterior chamber of the eyes, ranging from small streaks visible beneath the cornea to complete filling of the anterior chamber that obliterates the view of the iris and pupil, is known as *hyphema*. This type of injury is vision threatening, even with the smallest amount of blood, not only because of the high risk of rebleeding within 3 or 4 days and the significant risk of developing post-traumatic glaucoma (i.e., increased intraocular pressure), but also because one third of patients with hyphema have other significant eye injuries that must be diagnosed and treated. Such injuries may occur readily in sports such as squash and hockey in which small, hard projectiles or sticks can injure the unprotected eye. Suspicion or evidence of this injury demands prompt referral, with the eye protected by a shield in the interim. Patients with sickle cell disease are at higher risk for the secondary complications of hyphema.

Posterior Eye Segment Injuries

Even in the absence of grossly visible injury to the anterior portions of the eye, blunt trauma can result in severe damage to the posterior segments of the eye. Such injuries include lens dislocation, retinal edema, retinal tears or detachment, vitreous hemorrhage, choroidal rupture, and optic nerve injury. Various degrees of alteration of vision, ranging from minor blurring to loss of visual fields to complete loss of vision, signify the presence of such injuries after trauma. The absence of a red reflex when a light is shone through the pupil may be noted with such injuries, but the symptoms of visual loss alone are sufficient to warrant that the athlete be withdrawn from activity and referred for specialized examination and treatment. Again, a shield that protects the eye from pressure should be placed while the patient is in transit.

Clinical Point

Alteration in vision suggests injury to the posterior eye segment following trauma.

Prevention of Eye Injuries

As noted earlier, most eye injuries in sports can be prevented by appropriate equipment. The virtual elimination of serious eye injuries in hockey with the use of full face shields has been well documented; in contrast, the use of visors to protect the eye has resulted in several serious injuries when sticks have been lodged between the visor and the eye. Similarly, an awareness of the value of eye protection has increased in those who play racquet sports or sports such as baseball and basketball, which theoretically do not involve contact.[4] Those involved in the care of athletes must continue to campaign for prevention of eye injuries by insisting on the use of effective protective gear at all levels of sports.

Facial Fractures

Nasal Fractures

Given its "leading" position on the face, the nose is frequently traumatized in any sport involving contact.

Simple nosebleed, or *epistaxis,* is the most common result of blunt trauma to the nasal area. External compression of the nose performed by squeezing the nostrils shut is usually successful in stopping the bleeding. Persistence or recurrence of hemorrhage may require the placement of intranasal petrolatum gauze packs or the use of silver nitrate cauterization under direct vision. Careful intranasal examination must be carried out to rule out a septal hematoma with accumulation of blood beneath the mucosa overlying the septal cartilage of the nose. Such hematomas must be drained and evacuated because of the high risk of infection and septal necrosis associated with this injury if it is not treated promptly.

Examination of the traumatized nose is directed first at the external appearance to determine the presence of deviation of the tip or the dorsum of the nose (Figure 24-9). Next the nose is palpated to determine whether crepitus, step deformities, or bony asymmetries are present. Finally, the patency of each nostril is assessed by having the patient breathe through each nostril separately. Visual inspection of the interior nasal anatomy is performed to evaluate whether there is deviation of the septum.

This physical examination of the traumatized nose, focusing on external deformity and airway patency, will

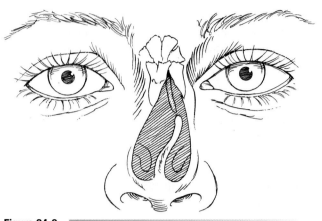

Figure 24-9

Nasal bone fracture with deviation of septum and obstruction of the airway.

usually determine the need for any treatment. X-ray studies are rarely of significant help in the management of isolated nasal fractures.

Treatment of nasal fractures requiring reduction is usually carried out right away, using local anesthesia in most instances. If edema prevents adequate evaluation of the deformity, treatment may be delayed by as much as 7 days without compromising the outcome. Beyond that time, a formal rhinoplasty procedure will usually be required to correct the post-traumatic deformity.

Closed reduction of the nasal fracture generally requires placement of intranasal packing and application of an external splint. The packing is left in place for 3 to 7 days; during this time the athlete's breathing ability is significantly compromised, and exertion is not recommended. The external splint is removed in 7 to 10 days, although it can be left in place longer for protection of the nose of the athlete who is returning to competition. When return to full activity is not crucial, a period of 2 to 3 weeks away from endangering competition is prudent. Athletes who return to competition should wear some type of protective face mask.

Zygomatic Fractures

Collisions involving heads, fists, elbows, racquets, and projectiles are so common in athletic competition that fractures of the cheeks are frequently seen (Table 24-2).

Table 24-2

Location and Cause of Injury Resulting in Facial Bone Fractures for a Professional Hockey Team, 1991-1994

Location of Fracture	Cause
Mandibular symphysis	Errant puck
Mandibular symphysis	Penalized high stick
Mandibular body/condyle	Penalized elbow contact
Zygoma/orbit	Errant puck
Nose	Penalized punch
Nose	Legal check
Zygomatic arch	Errant puck (practice)

The zygoma is the most likely of the midfacial bones to be fractured in the context of injuries related to athletics. The more complicated midfacial fractures (Figure 24-10) are high-energy injuries and are rarely seen in ordinary athletic trauma. Blows to the cheeks or the orbit, on the other hand, frequently result in fracture of the zygoma and its attachments to the frontal, temporal, sphenoid, and maxillary bones; because of the zygoma's important contribution to the structure of the orbital rim and floor, fractures involving this bone may have significant consequences relative to vision. An additional important relationship is that of the arch of the zygoma, which forms the lateral portion of the cheek, to the underlying temporal muscle and the coronoid process of the mandible to which the muscle attaches.

Diagnosis of maxillary or zygomatic fractures by physical examination can be difficult shortly after the injury because of the development of edema. Prompt physical examination is necessary. Possible physical findings from this examination are listed in Box 24-1 and illustrated in Figure 24-11.

When the fracture involves the floor of the orbit, double vision *(diplopia),* inability to move the eye in an upward gaze, and *enophthalmos* or "sunken eye" may be observable. Fractures confined to the arch of the zygoma present with localized depression of the cheek over the arch and painful limitation of motion of the mandible owing to impingement of the arch on the temporal muscle as it attaches to the mandible. Observation of cerebrospinal fluid leaking from the nose or ear or blood coming from the ear often signifies a major LeFort-type fracture and requires specialized study and treatment.

Nondisplaced zygomatic fractures do not require treatment, but careful ocular examination is essential to rule out associated injury to the globe.

The indications for surgical repair of displaced fractures of the zygomatic complex are related to functional problems (e.g., visual disturbance, limitation of mandibular motion, or infraorbital nerve dysfunction) or to cosmetic deficits. Evaluation of the latter often requires waiting several days for edema to subside. Repair can safely be delayed for 7 to 10 days without compromising the result.

Return to full athletic activity after midfacial fractures depends on resolution of double vision, pain, and edema. The resolution of double vision is of most obvious importance. Participation without protective headgear should be avoided for at least 6 weeks when there is high likelihood of repeated trauma.

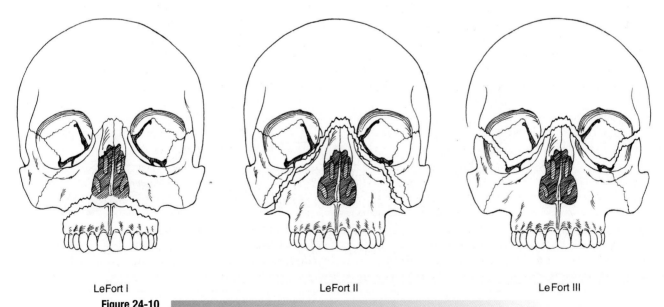

LeFort I   LeFort II   LeFort III

Figure 24-10

LeFort classification for midface fractures. **LeFort I,** A horizontal maxillary fracture at the level of the nasal floor. **LeFort II,** A pyramidal fracture, with the base of the pyramid being the palate and upper teeth and the apex of the pyramid at the nasal bone. **LeFort III,** Complete separation of the midface from the base of the skull.

Box 24-1 Physical Examination Findings: Maxillary and Zygomatic Fractures

1. Facial asymmetry
2. Loss of cheek prominence
3. Palpable steps
   - Infraorbital rim (zygomaticomaxillary suture)
   - Lateral orbital rim (frontozygomatic suture)
   - Root of zygoma intraorally
   - Zygomatic arch between ear and eye (zygomaticotemporal suture)
4. Hypoesthesia/anesthesia
   - Cheek, side of nose, upper lip, and teeth on the injured side
   - Compression of infraorbital nerve as it courses along floor of the orbit to exit into the face via the foramen beneath the orbital rim

Mandibular Fractures

Fractures of the lower jaw may be seen in any sport with the possibility of collision of bodies or equipment. Even athletes with apparent facial protection (i.e., with helmet and face mask) are subject to mandibular fractures from blows directed from below the face mask.

The key symptoms of such fractures are *malocclusion* (inability to bring the teeth easily into the preinjury position, as subjectively reported by the injured athlete) and pain on movement of the jaw. Signs for the examiner include deviation of the jaw, visible malocclusion (occlusion that differs from the patient's normal bite, as indicated by wear facets on the teeth), crepitus (palpable steps along the inferior border of the jaw), mobility of segments of the tooth-bearing portions of the jaw relative to one another (as distinct from mobility of individual teeth or segments of teeth that are mobile independent of the jaw), and the presence of bleeding or bruising between teeth or in the floor of the mouth adjacent to the jaw (Figure 24-12).

Key Indicators of a Mandibular Fracture

- Inability to bring teeth into preinjury position (malocclusion)
- Pain on moving jaw

Particular attention must be paid to examination of the condyles, especially when the trauma has been directed at the point of the chin. Neither pain in the joints nor malocclusion can be used to definitively diagnose a condylar fracture, because traumatic effusion (bleeding into the joint as a result of a blow to the chin) can produce either finding without the presence of a fracture. On the other hand, a fracture usually produces both preauricular pain and malocclusion and is accompanied by limitation of jaw motion and deviation of the jaw on mouth opening in the direction toward the fractured side. On physical examination, palpation of the condyle by placing a finger just anterior to the ear or in the ear canal will reveal an absence of movement by the fractured condyle when the jaw is opened.

Fracture of the mandible must be distinguished from traumatic dislocation or subluxation of the jaw. Dislocation is accompanied by a fixed opening of the jaw, with the

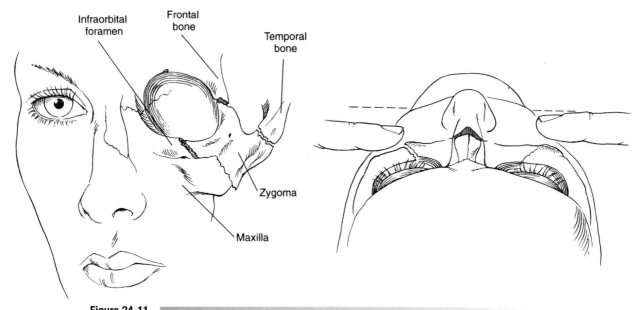

Figure 24-11

Zygomatic fractures. Inspection from above with palpation of the cheek demonstrates asymmetry and depression of the fractured zygoma.

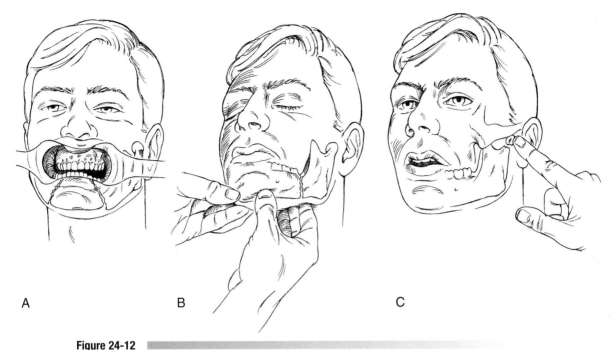

Figure 24-12
Mandibular fractures. **A,** Malocclusion. **B,** Palpation of the inferior border of the mandible. **C,** Palpation of the mandibular condyle.

patient unable to close. Palpation of the condyles will show an absence of condyles in the usual position immediately anterior to the tragus of the ear and the presence of a bony prominence 1 to 2 cm (0.4 to 0.8 inches) anterior to the normal position of the joint.

Early reduction of the dislocated jaw is most effective, as delayed reduction is complicated by the development of pain and muscle spasm, which may necessitate pharmacological muscle relaxation or anesthesia. In the acute phase, the jaw is relocated as follows:

1. The clinician faces the patient, who is seated in a sturdy chair.
2. The clinician's thumbs are placed in the mouth lateral to the posterior teeth (never on the teeth), with the fingers grasping the lower border of the jaw externally.
3. A rotational force is applied to bring the posterior jaw downward while the chin is brought forward.
4. When the condyle is rotated sufficiently to clear the anterior margin of the joint, the jaw will passively retrude, and the teeth can gently be brought together.

The athlete must be cautioned to limit jaw-opening width for several days, and anti-inflammatory medication is recommended to reduce the joint effusion that follows such an injury.

When a jaw fracture is diagnosed, referral for specialty care is required. Treatment ranges from a soft diet and analgesics for patients with undisplaced or incomplete fractures to surgical reduction and fixation for patients with more significant injuries. Although many fractures of the lower jaw can be treated successfully with closed reduction, such treatment requires immobilization of the jaw by wiring the upper and lower teeth to one another for a period of 4 or more weeks. This treatment clearly compromises the athlete's ability to compete, both because of nutritional difficulties and because of the inability to engage in mouth breathing during exertion. An alternative to closed reduction is surgical repair with rigid plating of the fractured bone (Figure 24-13). Although this is more complex surgically, the patient's jaw can be mobilized early, nutrition and breathing are greatly improved, and early return to competition (based on resolution of pain and swelling and the use of protective headgear) can be anticipated.

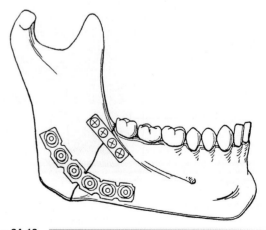

Figure 24-13
Rigid plating of a mandibular fracture.

Dental Injuries

The mandatory use of mouthguards by high school and college football players (since 1962 and 1973, respectively) has significantly reduced the incidence of oral injuries for these athletes, but injuries to the teeth remain a significant problem for players of most other sports.[5]

The simplest trauma to teeth is a concussive injury. The tooth is neither loosened nor fractured, but the blow may lead to necrosis of the pulp and a subsequent need for endodontic (root canal) therapy. Only discoloration and darkening of the tooth give a clue to the developing abnormality.

Common Tooth Injuries in Sports

- Concussive Injury
- Fracture
- Avulsion

Direct trauma to a tooth may result in a fracture of the substance of the tooth (Figure 24-14). A simple chip of the enamel will be asymptomatic, but any sharp edges will have to be smoothed or recontoured to avoid uncomfortable abrasion of the lip or tongue. When the fracture involves a deeper layer of tooth structure and dentin is exposed, there may be sensitivity to thermal changes or to touching of the exposed surface with the tongue, but routine restorative dentistry can salvage the tooth.

A tooth with pulp exposed as a result of coronal fracture will be exquisitely tender to touch and to exposure to cold air. On inspection, the pulp is visible as a pink area within the white surrounding dentin. Acute dental treatment is required and involves either "capping" of the exposed pulp or extirpating the pulp in preparation for root canal treatment.

When the fracture line of the crown extends below the gingival level, consultation with a dentist is necessary to determine whether the tooth can be restored or must be removed.

A tooth that is loosened by trauma must be carefully evaluated to differentiate a tooth with a fractured root from one that is partially dislodged from its socket. Repositioning of the tooth and splinting it to adjacent teeth is the preferred treatment in either case.

When several teeth are loosened as an independent segment, fracture of the alveolar bone is to be expected (Figure 24-15). Radiographic evaluation is essential, and splinting of the segment to adjacent stable teeth is required after repositioning of the segment.

Indirect injury to teeth, as when a blow from below the chin forces the teeth sharply together, can cause vertical fracture of posterior teeth. Diagnosis is made by visual inspection and palpation of a split tooth or by extreme tenderness to biting pressure on the tooth. Referral for dental treatment is necessary.

Occasionally a vertical force on an anterior tooth will intrude the tooth beneath the gingiva. This is particularly likely to occur in younger patients with immature root formation. No treatment is necessary, as the tooth will normally re-erupt.

Avulsion or loss of a tooth from its socket is a common injury among athletes of all ages. The success of replantation of the tooth is directly related to the length of time that

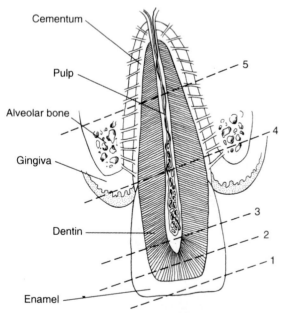

Figure 24-14

Anatomical classification of dental injuries. *1,* Enamel fracture. *2,* Fracture exposing the dentin. *3,* Fracture exposing the pulp. *4,* Fracture extending below the gingiva. *5,* Root fracture.

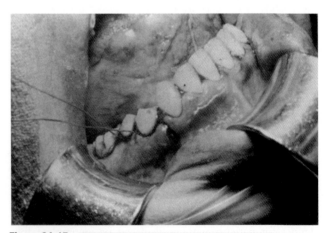

Figure 24-15

Multiple teeth loosened as an independent segment as a result of blunt trauma.

the tooth is out of its socket. Hence, the tooth should be recovered and replaced promptly. Only gentle rinsing of the tooth with saline or water should be performed before replantation. The root surface should be handled minimally and should not be scrubbed. If the tooth cannot be replaced in its socket immediately, the best transport vehicle is the patient's mouth. Obviously, the patient must be conscious and capable of holding the tooth in the cheek without swallowing it while awaiting definitive dental care. If necessary, the tooth may be transported in media listed in Box 24-2. After replantation, the tooth requires splinting to adjacent teeth for a period of 1 week. Dental follow-up is necessary to determine whether such a tooth will require root canal treatment (see Box 24-2).

Clinical Point

Survival of the avulsed tooth decreases quickly after 1 hour.

Both custom-made and self-adapted mouthguards afford significant protection against dental injury in athletes, and their use should be strongly encouraged, if not mandated. Custom-made mouthguards are easily constructed by the patient's dentist, and such appliances offer more comfort and better acceptance for the wearer, although self-adapted guards have the advantage of lower cost.

Conclusion

Prevention of maxillofacial injuries in athletics remains the best treatment. Wearing of protective eyewear, mouthguards, and effective face masks and enforcement of the rules of play will reduce even further the incidence of injuries. Effective treatment and prompt rehabilitation of the facially injured athlete are a function of effective initial diagnosis and treatment, as outlined here, and prompt referral for consultation with the appropriate maxillofacial, ophthalmological, or dental specialist.

References

1. Schaefer SD: The treatment of acute external laryngeal injuries: State of the art, *Arch Otolaryngol Head Neck Surg* 117:35–39, 1991.
2. Stock JG, Cornell FM: Prevention of sports-related eye injury, *Am Fam Physician* 44:515–520, 1991.
3. Shingleton BJ: Eye injuries, *N Engl J Med* 325:408–413, 1991.
4. Zagelbaum BM, Hersh PS, Donnenfeld ED, et al: Ocular trauma in major league baseball players, *N Engl J Med* 330:1021–1023, 1994.
5. DeYoung AK, Robinson E, Godwin WC: Comparing comfort and wearability: Custom-made vs. self-adapted mouthguards, *J Am Dent Assoc* 125:1112–1118, 1994.

Box 24-2 Guidelines for Initial Treatment of an Avulsed Tooth

Extraoral Time
1. Extraoral time is one of the most critical factors affecting prognosis.
2. If possible, replant the tooth immediately at the time of injury. If contaminated, rinse with water before replanting.
   - If notified by telephone, instruct patient, parent, or involved party on replantation technique.
   - Stress importance of seeing a dentist immediately for follow-up splinting and treatment.

Transport Media
When immediate replantation is not possible, place tooth in the best transport medium possible.
1. Buccal vestibule (in saliva between cheek and gum, but patient must be conscious because of the possibility of aspiration or swallowing, especially if a small child)
2. Hanks' Balanced Salt Solution
3. Milk
4. Saline
5. If none of these are readily available, water

SECTION III MANAGEMENT OF SPORTS INJURY AND ILLNESS

ABDOMINAL AND THORACIC INJURIES

Benjamin M. J. Thompson and Brian D. Busconi

Introduction

Abdominal and thoracic injuries are common occurrences in athletic competition. The sports medicine clinician must be vigilant in the recognition of these injuries to avoid the significant morbidity and mortality that is often associated with them. The abdomen is predisposed to soft tissue injury because of its lack of circumferential bony protection. According to a recent study, abdominal wall injuries in athletes are actually reported much less than they occur.[1] Of all athletic injuries, 7% to 10% affect the abdomen, the most commonly injured abdominal organs being the spleen, liver, and kidney.[2,3]

Clinical Point

Abdominal injuries typically are not immediately life-threatening, unless a major exsanguination (loss of blood) has occurred.

One quarter of all trauma-induced deaths result from chest injuries. The thoracic cavity is circumferentially protected by the rib cage, making low-energy injuries more uncommon occurrences. Injuries to the thoracic cavity are more often the result of high-velocity sports, accidents, or the use of inadequate protective equipment. The severity of these injuries may escalate rapidly and become life-threatening if not accurately assessed and treated.

Note: This chapter includes content from previous contributions by Andrew W. Nichols, MD, as it appeared in the predecessor of this book—Zachazewski JE, Magee DJ, Quillen WS, editors: *Athletic Injuries and Rehabilitation*, Philadelphia, 1996, WB Saunders.

Abdominal Injuries

Injuries of the Abdominal Wall

Abdominal Wall Contusion

Abdominal wall muscular contusion is a common injury affecting athletes involved in contact sports. As a result of intramuscular and subcutaneous bleeding, the athlete will often present with pain, swelling, and ecchymoses.[4] This injury is rarely serious because of the compressive, blow-cushioning effect of the soft abdominal contents. Early diagnosis is crucial because it may be difficult to differentiate the symptoms of contusion from intra-abdominal injury.

Injuries to the Abdominal Wall

- Abdominal wall contusion
- Blow to solar plexus
- Abdominal muscle strain
- Hernia
- Obturator nerve entrapment
- "Stitch" in the side
- Surgical wounds

Abdominal wall contusions tend to manifest clinically with localized tenderness over the area of impact. Pain is exacerbated by actively contracting the underlying muscles and relieved by relaxing them. Referred pain is normally absent. "Hip pointers" are contusions of the abdominal muscles at their insertion on the iliac crest. This condition may adversely affect athletic performance to a much greater extent than would be expected by the degree of injury. Ice and oral analgesics are normally sufficient to relieve symptoms. Once the athlete is pain free he or she may return to sport.[4] The presence of any contusion of the upper abdominal wall should prompt consideration of concurrent injury to the lower floating ribs (Figure 25-1).

Blow to the Solar Plexus. The condition commonly known as "having the wind knocked out of you" is caused by a traumatic blow to the abdomen of an athlete whose abdominal muscles are not tensed. The athlete will normally report an inability to catch his or her breath. The initial management includes ruling out airway obstruction by objects such as the mouth guard, tongue, or turf from the field. If symptoms persist once a clear airway is confirmed, the hip belt should be loosened and an attempt to relax the athlete made by placing the athlete in the supine crook lying (the knees and hips flexed with feet on ground). Having the athlete take a repeated deep breath and hold it often restores the athlete's breath more quickly. A cold towel may be applied to the forehead, and the athlete should be assured that symptoms will be short-lived. Because of the

lack of circumferential protection to the abdomen, the sports medicine clinician must be aware of the possibility of intra-abdominal injury in the patient who has had a blow to the solar plexus. Table 25-1 helps to differentiate among the signs and symptoms of a blow to the solar plexus, an abdominal wall injury, and an intra-abdominal injury.

Abdominal Muscle Strain

Strains of the abdominal muscles are extremely common athletic injuries. Symptoms depend on the size and location of injury. The most commonly injured abdominal muscle, the rectus abdominis, may be damaged at the musculotendinous junction adjacent to the lower anterior rib origin, at the pubic insertion, or at the horizontal fibrous bands within the muscle itself.

The potential mechanisms of injury include a sudden, violent muscular contraction or recurrent microtrauma

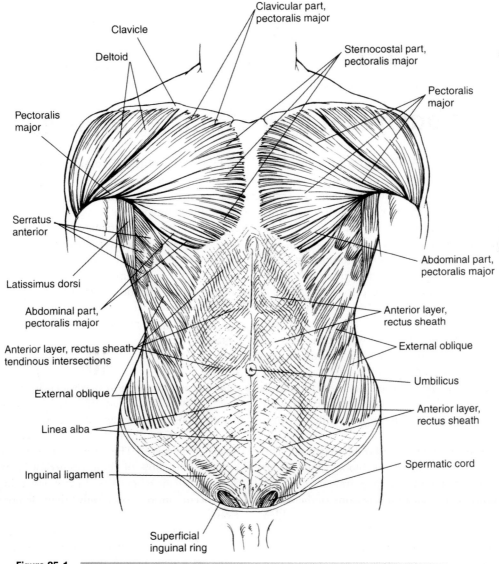

Figure 25-1

Superficial anatomy of the abdominal and thoracic wall.

Table 25-1

Differentiation of Intra-Abdominal Injury from Abdominal Wall Injury from Blow to the Solar Plexus

	Intra-Abdominal Injury	Abdominal Wall Injury	Blow to Solar Plexus
Mechanism	Blunt or penetrating trauma	Direct trauma	Blow to untensed abdominal muscle
Pain location	Initially localized, often becomes diffuse	Localized	Minimal pain
Symptoms	Pain that increases	Steady pain	Inability to catch breath
Duration	Prolonged	Moderate to prolonged	Brief
Pain with tensing muscles	Often	Yes	No
Referred pain	Often	No	No
Physical examination	Guarding, rebound, rigidity, quiet bowel sounds	Localized tenderness	Minimal to no tenderness
Laboratory studies	Abnormal	Normal	Normal

from overuse, such as commonly occurs in soccer or other sports requiring repetitive abdominal contractions. Physical examination reveals localized tenderness and muscle spasm at the site of injury and pain during active muscle contraction or stretching. It is vital that this injury be differentiated from damage to the intra-abdominal organs.

Certain forms of abdominal muscle strain, especially those that occur at the ribs, pubis, or the iliac crest, may result in chronic symptoms. Initial treatment should include relative rest and protection of the injured muscle. Activity should be limited by pain. An avulsed fragment of iliac crest is often reattached surgically, although surgery has little role in the treatment of proximal or midsubstance tears. Rectus abdominis muscle strains have been identified as an extremely common occurrence in competitive tennis players. The injury mechanism was felt to be eccentric overload, followed by forced contraction of the nondominant rectus during the cocking phase of the service motion. A tennis-specific rehabilitation program stressing eccentrics and plyometric strengthening of the abdominal wall muscles was introduced to prevent recurrences.[5,6] A different study identified a group of soccer players with chronic groin pain and the absence of preoperatively identifiable inguinal hernias, who at the time of surgical exploration were found to have various irregularities of the abdominal wall, including inguinal hernias, and microscopic tears or avulsions of the internal oblique muscle. These individuals were successfully treated with herniorrhaphy and were able to return to play within 3 months.[6]

Rectus Abdominis Intramuscular Hematoma. The rectus abdominis muscle receives its blood supply from branches of the underlying inferior epigastric arteries. Sudden severe motions, such as an abrupt twisting of the trunk, a sudden contraction of the abdominal muscles, or a sudden extension of the spine, may produce a tear in the rectus abdominis muscle. The resultant shearing forces may rupture the supplying epigastric artery or vein, resulting in intramuscular hematoma formation.

The onset of symptoms is generally abrupt, with localized pain, muscle guarding, nausea, and vomiting. Pain may be provoked by straight-leg raising or hyperextension of the back. A palpable mass, which becomes fixed when the muscle is contracted, is often identifiable. A bluish discoloration of the periumbilical area, known as the Cullen sign, may appear. Computed tomography (CT) helps to confirm the diagnosis and outline the extent of hematoma formation.[7]

Most cases of rectus abdominis hematoma may be treated nonoperatively. Treatment includes application of ice during the first 48 hours after injury, followed by heat. Strengthening of the abdominal muscles should be instituted with isometric exercises and should progress to sit-ups, crunches, and other exercises as pain permits. If active bleeding persists, surgical ligation of the inferior epigastric artery and hematoma evacuation may be required. Because a relatively small approach that spares the abdominal fascia can be used for this drainage, surgery may actually speed up return to sport. High-speed and contact sports may be resumed as soon as the area is pain free, usually in 1 to 2 weeks.[4] Percutaneous drainage of the hematoma is rarely successful because of early clot organization.

Hernia

A *hernia* is a protrusion of an anatomical structure via a passageway or weakened area of the body wall. Approximately 1.5% of Americans are estimated to have hernias.[8] Table 25-2 lists the relative occurrence rates of various forms of hernias.[9] The groin is the location of 81% of hernias, with 86% of these occurring in men. Although 84% of all femoral hernias affect women, inguinal hernias still occur more commonly than femoral hernias in women.[9]

It seems unlikely that hernias are ever exclusively caused by athletic participation, although they may be aggravated by activities that increase intra-abdominal pressure such as weightlifting and rowing. Hernias should always be considered in the

Table 25-2

Frequency of Various Types of Hernias

Hernia Type	Frequency (%)
Indirect inguinal	50
Direct inguinal	25
Ventral	10
Femoral	6
Umbilical	3
Epigastric	3
Esophageal	1
Miscellaneous	2

Types of Hernia

- Direct inguinal
- Indirect inguinal
- Athletic pubalgia (sports hernia)
- Femoral
- Ventral
- Umbilical
- Epigastric

differential diagnosis of the athlete complaining of groin pain (Table 25-3).

In one study of 78 athletes, herniography diagnosed a hernia in 84%.[10] Kluin performed diagnostic endoscopy on 14 athletes with undiagnosed groin pain. Nine of these patients were found to have an inguinal hernia that was subsequently repaired, allowing them to return to full activity.[11] It is often difficult to diagnose the exact source of groin pain in the athlete, so magnetic resonance imaging (MRI) has been used to determine the exact injury site, extent, and characteristics. MRI findings have also been used to predict the amount of time that the athlete may miss from sports.[12]

Nonoperative management of hernias in athletes is not recommended. Some surgeons believe that the earlier a hernia is detected and repaired, the stronger the repair will be.[13] Early repair is also advocated to avoid the potentially serious complications of hernia incarceration and strangulation. *Incarceration* occurs when a loop of bowel becomes swollen and edematous before becoming trapped outside the abdominal cavity. Incarceration is the most common cause of bowel obstruction in a patient who has not had prior abdominal surgery.[14] Reduction of incarcerated hernias is successful 60% to 70% of the time and may prevent strangulation. *Strangulation* results from a compromise of blood flow to the incarcerated bowel segment, which ultimately leads to bowel necrosis (Figure 25-2). Loops of bowel and omentum may remain incarcerated for months to years without proceeding to strangulation.[14] Absolute recommendations as to the appropriate timing of surgery

Table 25-3

Differential Diagnosis for Groin Pain

Orthopaedic Etiologies	Nonorthopaedic Etiologies
Muscle	*Hernia*
Adductor strain/tendonitis	Inguinal hernia
Rectus femoris strain/tear	Femoral hernia
Iliopsoas strain/tear	Preperitoneal lipoma
Rectus abdominis strain/tear	
Muscle contusion	*Urological*
Gracilis syndrome	Prostatitis
Athletic hernia	Epididymitis
	Urethritis/UTI
Bone/Joint	Testicular neoplasm
Osteitis pubis	Ureteral colic
Degenerative joint disease: hip	- Testicular torsion
Avascular necrosis: hip	- Hydrocele/
Labral tear: hip	varicocele
Femoral neck fracture/stress fracture	
Pubic ramus stress fracture	*Gynecological*
Myositis ossificans, adductors	Endometriosis
Slipped capital femoral epiphysis	Pelvic inflammatory disease
Avulsion fracture: ASIS/AIIS/ Ischium	Ovarian cyst
	Surgical/GI
Nerve	Rectal/colon neoplasm
Lumbar radiculopathy	Inflammatory bowel disease
Ilioinguinal neuropathy	Diverticulitis
Obturator neuropathy	
Other Orthopaedic	
Bone/soft tissue neoplasm of hip/pelvis	
Seronegative spondyloarthropathy	

From Swan KG, Wolcott M: The athletic hernia, *Clin Orthop Relat Res* (455):78-87, 2007.

for hernias are difficult. Decisions are best made on a case-by-case basis, depending on the type of hernia, the presence of symptoms, and the level of sports participation. Individuals with symptomatic hernias should undergo immediate surgical repair or cease the activity that is exacerbating their symptoms. Generally, athletes at the nonprofessional level should undergo immediate repair of even asymptomatic hernias. Elite athletes who wish to delay repair must be made aware of the potential complications associated with continued participation in sports. These athletes should be followed throughout the season with serial physical examinations for the development of symptoms. They should be instructed to avoid wearing a truss, because this may mask worsening symptoms while providing little protection from injury. A *truss* is a ball made out of rubber, leather, or fabric that is positioned over the bulge and kept in place with straps. Truss use has been shown to have the potential to

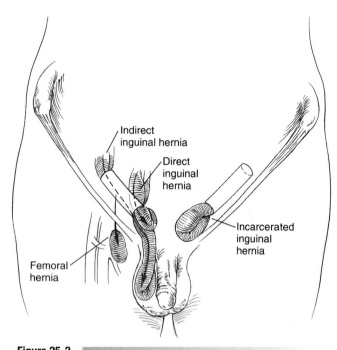

Figure 25-2

Diagram showing courses of inguinal hernias and incarcerated inguinal hernia.

increase the risk of scarring and incarceration.[14] Participants in contact sports must have additional padding to the area, and hernia repair should be performed as soon as the season ends. Return to sport after hernia repair depends just as much on the motivation and conditioning of the athlete as it does on the type of hernia and surgical approach performed. Newer open repairs using mesh provide for a tension-free repair, whereas laparoscopic repair often affords the athlete the potential to incur less pain and allow for earlier return to full activity.[14] Both open-mesh and laparoscopic repairs have the added advantage of extremely low recurrence rates. Some authors have reported return to exercise after laparoscopic repair at only one week.[15] Open repair may delay return to vigorous activity for an additional 1 to 2 weeks.[4]

Inguinal Hernias. Inguinal hernias are the most common type of hernia in young athletes and are often discovered on routine physical examination. As many inguinal hernias are asymptomatic, their identification requires a thorough history and examination by the physician. The examination is performed by checking for an inguinal bulge, followed by insertion of the examiner's finger into the patient's inverted scrotum and through the external ring of the inguinal canal. If present, an inguinal hernia will tap against the examiner's finger when the athlete is asked to cough.

Childhood indirect inguinal hernias are extremely common. Treatment is via high ligation of the hernia sac. The treatment of adult indirect hernias is more difficult, usually requiring sac ligation in addition to repair of the inguinal canal floor. Direct inguinal hernias, which represent protrusions

through the weakened floor of the inguinal canal, require more extensive repairs than indirect hernias. Direct hernias do not involve a hernia sac and are more likely to be acquired as a result of pressure on the muscle and fascia over time.[14] The recurrence rate of direct hernias is 13% compared with less than 5% for indirect hernias.[13]

Inguinal hernias may produce groin pain in the absence of an identifiable inguinal hernia on physical examination. In one study, eight such individuals were treated with herniorrhaphy, and all were able to return to full activity by 12 weeks postoperatively.[6] Inguinal hernia must be considered as a potential source of chronic groin pain, even in the absence of hernia on physical examination.

Athletic Pubalgia: "Sports Hernia". Groin pain is an extremely common complaint in athletes involved in sports that involve kicking and rapid changes of direction such as soccer, Australian rules football, hockey, and tennis. A rate as high as 5% to 8% in soccer players has been reported.[16,17] The cause of athletic groin pain is often difficult to assess because of the complex anatomy and the multitude of possible differential diagnoses (Figure 25-3). Meyers defines *athletic pubalgia* as a series of disorders relating to the musculoskeletal region surrounding the pelvis outside of the ball-and-socket joint of the hip, not including the sacrum or the spine.[18] He discredits the use of the term *sports hernia* because true hernias are rarely found in these patients who are suffering pain that involves what he describes as the *pubic joint.*

Clinical Point

During the last 20 years the diagnosis of athletic pubalgia or sports hernia for the athlete with groin pain of unknown cause has gained popularity. There has, however, been an extremely inconsistent explanation as to the exact definition and cause of this elusive injury.

Patients are generally male,[19-21] although recently the literature has shown an increase in the number of women suffering from pubalgia.[18] Usually the athlete has suffered a prolonged course of groin pain with nonspecific symptoms that have been resistant to nonoperative intervention. A tear of the posterior inguinal wall or the transversalis fascia has been postulated as a cause of the chronic groin pain found in athletic pubalgia, with one study finding a deficiency in 85% of athletes who underwent surgical exploration (Figure 25-4).[22] Meyers, however, has defined 18 or 19 distinct syndromes of athletic pubalgia involving up to 17 different musculoskeletal structures.[18] Several studies have looked at shearing across the pubic symphysis from thigh hyperabduction and trunk hyperextension as a cause of athletic pubalgia.[23,24] These shearing forces have been shown to be much stronger in athletes with an imbalance between the strong thigh adductor muscles and the weaker lower abdominal musculature.[25]

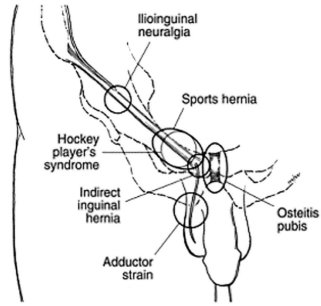

Figure 25-3

Typical sites of pain from multiple causes in the same general anatomical region. (From Lacroix VJ: A complete approach to groin pain, *Phys Sportsmed* 28:66-86, 2000.)

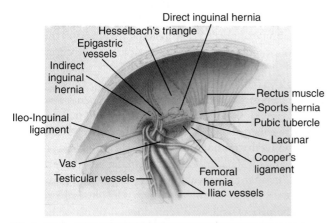

Figure 25-4

Anatomy of the posterior inguinal area *(left side)*. (From Genitsaris M, Goulimaris I, Sikas N: Laparoscopic repair of groin pain in athletes, *Am J Sports Med* 32:1238-1242, 2004.)

A thorough history and physical examination is crucial for the patient who is suspected of having a sports hernia. The history of athletic pubalgia will typically show pain that is insidious, unilateral, and deep.[21,26] Timing of the onset of groin pain is important, as acute pain is typically the result of a more common injury such as a hip adductor strain or a bony avulsion from the ischial tuberosity or anterior inferior or superior iliac spines.[27] Symptoms of athletic pubalgia are only present with activity and pain is typically severe and debilitating, often prohibiting the athlete from returning to sport.[21,26,28] Sudden movements such as sneezing, coughing, kicking, pivoting, or sprinting may exacerbate the groin pain.[21,25,28] A thorough review of systems is extremely important to rule out more serious pathological conditions. The athlete should be asked if he or she is suffering from back pain or radiculopathy, and pathological conditions of the bowel and bladder should be ruled out. Constitutional symptoms such as weight loss, rest pain, and night pain should alert the sports medicine clinician to the possibility of neoplasm.

The importance of the physical examination in the patient with athletic pubalgia cannot be overstated as it is the best opportunity for the clinician to narrow the differential diagnosis. During the physical examination, the abdomen, pelvis, hips, thighs and lumbosacral spine should be palpated. The hallmark of the physical examination in the patient with athletic pubalgia is that no inguinal hernia is palpated[21,26]; however, a thorough hernia examination should still be performed on the athlete. Gentisaris and colleagues found tenderness and dilation of the superficial inguinal ring in 94% of patients with athletic hernia.[29] Physical examination findings in sports hernia may also include tenderness over the conjoined tendon, the pubic tubercle, and the posterior wall of the inguinal canal.[21,26] Pain is often elicited with resisted sit-ups, as well as resisted hip flexion and adduction.[19,21,25] Resistance testing should also be performed on the rectus abdominis, rectus femoris, and iliopsoas to attempt to provoke the athlete's symptoms.

Diagnosis via diagnostic imaging is an emerging topic of discussion in the sports medicine literature. Even though they are likely to be negative, hip, pelvis, and lumbar spine radiographs should all be performed as a matter of routine to rule out any pathological condition. Bone scans have also been used by sports medicine clinicians to attempt to diagnose athletic pubalgia. Although the results have been nonspecific, bone scans have been useful diagnostic tools to rule out other conditions such as osteitis pubis or tumor.[30]

MRI has seen increased usage in recent years to assess pathological conditions of the soft tissue, as well as to rule out other sources of groin and pelvic pain such as osteitis pubis, avascular necrosis, and stress fractures.[31] Albers looked at MRIs from 32 patients with confirmed sports hernia and found that the most common MRI findings were increased signal in one or both pubic bones or within one or more of the abdominal muscles. Bulging or attenuation of the musculofascial layers of the abdominal wall was also noted. There was a 95% correlation rate between surgical findings and attenuation of the abdominal wall musculofascial layers.[32] In recent studies, Meyers has used new techniques in MRI to further clarify the pathological condition diagnosed by physical examination. Pathological conditions of the adductors in combination with the rectus abdominis were the most common findings in patients with athletic pubalgia. There was a 91% correlation between these MRI findings and what was found intraoperatively.[18,33-35] MRI may be an extremely useful technique to determine if bilateral athletic hernia repairs need to be performed or if any repair needs to be done at all.[32]

Ultrasound has been suggested as a less expensive alternative to MRI in the diagnosis of athletic pubalgia. Some authors have shown a strong correlation between ultrasound findings of posterior abdominal wall insufficiency and intraoperative findings.[36] Herniography involves plain radiographs that are obtained after injection of a radio-opaque dye into the peritoneal cavity. It is commonly employed in Europe to determine if a patient with chronic groin pain will benefit from a herniorrhaphy. Limitations of herniography include a high false-positive rate,[37] as well as the possibility of hollow viscus perforation, vasovagal reactions, allergic reactions to contrast dye, and infections.[38-40] The high complication rate of 3% to 6% has made herniography a rarely used diagnostic tool in the United States.

The treatment of athletic pubalgia is normally surgical because nonoperative treatment with rest, anti-inflammatories, massage, and heat or ice is rarely successful.[6,21,23] Physical therapy with a focus on core strengthening may actually resolve the imbalance between the hip and pelvic muscle stabilizers.[21] If all other sources of groin pain have been ruled out and 6 to 12 weeks of nonsurgical management have failed, surgical repair should be considered.[6,11,20] Laparoscopic or open surgical repair of the weakened posterior inguinal wall has been shown to have excellent results with an 80% to 97% success rate.[11,20,21,24,26] Meyers has been a proponent of pelvic floor repair with reattachment of the inferolateral edge of the rectus abdominis to the pubic bone with or without adductor longus release.[18] Regardless of the type of repair that is done, laparoscopic repair has shown a more rapid return to sport with an average of 2 to 6 weeks in comparison with 1 to 6 months with open repair.[41] Laparoscopic repair also has the benefit of better visualization of the involved structures and ability to perform repair of bilateral hernias through the same incision.[42]

Another common cause of groin pain is a pathological condition of the intra-articular hip such as from a labral tear or cartilage defect. The history and physical findings of the patient with a labral tear is often very similar to that of the patient with sports hernia and thus should always be included in the differential diagnosis. Pain is typically activity-related and exacerbated by passive rotation of the hip. MRI and magnetic resonance arthrogram are excellent diagnostic tools to rule out pathological conditions of the hip in the patient with chronic groin pain. Intra-articular corticosteroids into the hip can be used as both a diagnostic and therapeutic modality.[43]

Other Abdominal Hernias. Femoral hernias, which occur far more commonly in women, are often difficult to detect. The hernia protrudes through the femoral ring, beneath the inguinal ligament, just medial to the femoral vein at the fossa ovalis. Surgical repair should be carried out as early as possible so as to avoid incarceration or strangulation, which are common sequelae of this hernia type.

Umbilical hernias are common in infants and children. Of white newborns, 10% are born with umbilical hernias, as are 40% to 90% of black newborns. The great majority are small and close spontaneously by the age of 2 years, thus requiring no specific treatment. If surgical repair is necessary, the procedure is relatively simple in children, but is more complicated in adults. In adults, the surrounding walls of the linea alba are rigid and thus predispose patients to strangulation and incarceration of intra-abdominal structures that may protrude.[14]

Epigastric hernias are located in the linea alba, or abdominal midline, superior to the umbilicus, and generally contain only a small amount of preperitoneal fat. Epigastric hernias are often asymptomatic and not recognized; autopsy studies reveal their presence in 5% of normal adults.[9] Surgery is indicated only if enlargement or pain develops, in which case repair is relatively simple.

Ventral hernias, which are typically complications of previous midline abdominal surgery, are uncommon in athletes. Repair of ventral hernias may be quite difficult, especially when they are of large size, occur in obese individuals, or are associated with vertical incisions. The recurrence rate is high at 15%.[13] Table 25-4 provides useful guidelines for the timing of return to activity after the surgical repair of various hernia types and other abdominal surgical procedures.

Obturator Nerve Entrapment. A frequently recognized cause of chronic groin pain in athletes is entrapment of the obturator nerve as it enters the thigh within the fascia of the short adductor muscle. Obturator nerve entrapment pain is insidious in nature and characteristically noted around the pubic bone, where the adductor muscle has its origin. Pain may be referred to the anterosuperior iliac spine on the same side as the nerve entrapment and often radiates down the medial thigh toward the knee.[44] Exercise commonly exacerbates the pain and it is relieved by rest. Incomplete adductor muscle weakness or spasm in the affected leg may occur after exercise along with numbness or paresthesia if the entrapment is long-standing. On physical examination, the patient will have reproduction of his or her pain with resisted internal hip rotation or by passively externally rotating and abducting the affected hip while standing.[44]

Imaging studies are rarely useful in the diagnosis of obturator nerve entrapment, although MRI may show atrophy of the short and long adductor muscles as well as the gracilis muscle. Electromyography (EMG) studies are commonly used in the workup of neuropathy and often reveal chronic denervation in the short and long adductor muscles. When trying to determine the diagnosis and the need for surgical intervention, a selective anesthetic block of the obturator nerve may be performed. A successful nerve block will alleviate pain brought on by provocative maneuvers and reproduce any postexercise weakness.[44]

Treatment of obturator nerve entrapment is initially conservative with rest, nonsteroidal anti-inflammatory drugs (NSAIDs), physical therapy involving adductor muscle and pelvic strengthening exercises, and groin stretches. Conservative therapy is more effective in patients without EMG evidence of denervation or with a short duration of

Table 25-4

Hernia Repair and Abdominal Surgery: Return-to-Activity Guidelines

Procedure	Return to Classes	PRE* and Conditioning	Noncontact	Full Activity
Inguinal hernia				
Indirect (children)	1 wk	2 wk	3 wk	4 wk
Indirect (adult)	1 wk	3 wk	7 wk	8-10 wk
Direct	1 wk	3 wk	8 wk	12 wk
Femoral hernia	1 wk	3 wk	8 wk	12 wk
Umbilical hernia				
Children	1 wk	2 wk	3 wk	3 wk
Adults	1 wk	2 wk	4-6 wk	8 wk
Epigastric hernia	1 wk	2 wk	3-4 wk	6 wk
Ventral hernia	2 wk	8 wk	3-6 mo	?avoid
Appendectomy	1 wk	3 wk	4 wk	6 wk
Other uncomplicated abdominal operations	2 wk	4 wk	8 wk	12 wk

*Progressive resistance exercise

From Nichols AW: Abdominal and thoracic injuries. In Zachazewski JE, Magee DM, Quillen WS, editors: *Athletic injuries and rehabilitation*, p 489, Philadelphia, 1996, WB Saunders. Adapted from Haycock CE: How I manage hernias in the athlete, *Phys Sports Med* 11:77-79, 1983; Olsen WR: Abdominal trauma in the athlete. In Schneider RC, Kennedy JC, Plant ML, editors: *Sports injuries — mechanisms, prevention, and treatment*, pp 809-817, Baltimore, 1985, Williams & Wilkins.

symptoms. In more chronic cases of entrapment, surgical intervention with obturator nerve release may be necessary. After surgery, return to sport is normally delayed for 3 to 6 weeks.[44]

"Stitch" in the Side

A "stitch" in the side, or "side-ache," is characterized by sharp pains in the runner's upper abdominal side behind the lower ribs. Potential causes include trapped colonic gas bubbles, localized diaphragmatic hypoxia with spasm, liver congestion with stretching of the liver capsule, and poor conditioning. Poorly conditioned athletes commonly experience stitches, with a reduction in their frequency as fitness improves. An athlete may be able to "run through" a stitch by exhaling steadily and forcefully through pursed lips. Alternative means of relieving stitches include lying on the back with the arms extended overhead or flexing the trunk so that the chest nears the thighs. Once the discomfort of a stitch has abated, a workout may usually be completed without further recurrences.

Surgical Wounds

Physical activity produces an increase in intra-abdominal pressure, which may exert stress on surgical wounds and consequently delay or prevent healing. Skin wounds heal rapidly, whereas deep tissues heal much more slowly, increasing the risk of wound dehiscence. Douglas has demonstrated that aponeurosis tissue regains only 50% of its previous tensile strength at 2 months after surgery (Figure 25-5).[45] Table 25-4 provides useful guidelines for the timing of returning athletes to various levels of physical activity after abdominal surgery.[13,46]

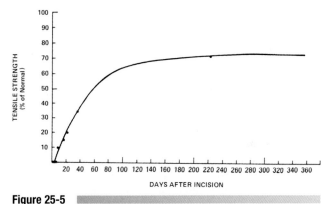

Figure 25-5

Tensile strength of healing wounds versus time. (From Olsen WR: Abdominal trauma in the athlete. In Schneider RC, Kennedy JC, Plant ML, editors: *Sports injuries—Mechanisms, prevention, and treatment*, Baltimore, 1985, Williams & Wilkins.)

Intra-Abdominal Injuries

Evaluation of the Injured Athlete

Abdominal injuries occur in two forms: penetrating trauma and blunt trauma. Common forms of penetrating injury include knife, gunshot, and impalement wounds, which may occur accidentally in certain sporting events such as the javelin throw. Penetrating injuries caused by large foreign objects should initially be managed by leaving the impaled object in place during transport to a surgical operating room unless the airway is compromised.[47] If the size of the object interferes with transport, a portion of the exposed object may be cut away. The application of direct pressure around the impaled object will help control bleeding from the entrance and exit wounds.[47] Traction should never be applied to the impaled object. Removal of the object should take place only after large-bore needle intravenous access has been obtained and blood is available for emergent transfusion in the case of major exsanguination (blood loss) at the time of removal.

> ### Clinical Caution
>
> Large, penetrating foreign objects should only be removed in a surgical operating room except when the airway is compromised.

Blunt trauma is by far the most common type of athletic abdominal injury. The same blows that produce abdominal muscle contusions and rectus sheath hematomas may lead to severe intra-abdominal trauma.[4] At the onset of the traumatic event, the unprotected abdomen is struck by an opposing force, and the abdominal organs are compressed against the vertebral column. The severity of symptoms resulting from blunt abdominal trauma varies widely, ranging from severe pain in the presence of significant bleeding and peritoneal irritation to only mild tenderness. Peritoneal irritation may occur after injury to the stomach, gallbladder, pancreas, small intestine, or colon as a result of bacterial or chemical contamination. Initially the only symptom that may be present is localized tenderness, but soon the peritoneal signs, including abdominal rigidity, guarding, referred pain, and loss of bowel sounds, may ensue. Diaphragmatic irritation caused by an injury to the liver or spleen, or a subdiaphragmatic fluid collection may produce pain that is referred to the corresponding shoulder. Table 25-1 helps to differentiate the signs and symptoms of intra-abdominal visceral injury from abdominal wall injury and a solar plexus blow.

The initial evaluation of an awake and alert individual who has sustained acute, blunt abdominal injury begins with a careful history of injury and complete physical examination, including abdominal palpation, auscultation, and hemodynamic evaluation.[4] Figure 25-6 illustrates the major organs of the abdominal cavity. Depending on the findings, it is often possible to avoid extensive laboratory, radiographic, and invasive procedures. Suspicion must be maintained, because up to 43% of individuals who have a significant intra-abdominal injury initially present with a negative findings on physical examination (Table 25-5).[46,48] Moreover, it has been reported that 20% of subjects with a retroperitoneal hematoma appear to have an initially benign abdominal examination.[49]

> ### Clinical Caution
>
> With abdominal injuries, the presence of pain out of proportion to the injury, peritoneal pain, referred pain to the back and shoulder, tachycardia, hypotension, multiple body system injuries, or an impaired ability to respond to painful stimuli should prompt the clinician to perform additional diagnostic studies.

Prior to the advent of faster and more precise CT scans, diagnostic peritoneal lavage (DPL) was a useful test in the initial evaluation of an individual with multiple system injuries or an impaired level of consciousness. The procedure involves paracentesis with abdominal cavity saline lavage. DPL has fallen out of favor because of its inability to specify the location or extent of intra-abdominal injury, high sensitivity which overpredicts the need for surgery,[4] poor results in the detection of retroperitoneal bleeding, risk associated with its invasiveness, and controversy over the management of intermediate results. CT has gained widespread acceptance in the initial evaluation of intra-abdominal trauma. It is noninvasive and extremely accurate in the identification of the location and extent of significant intra-abdominal injury, including liver, spleen, and kidney lacerations, as well as retroperitoneal hematomas.[50] CT is also particularly valuable in avoiding unnecessary exploratory laparotomies and potential organ removal,[4] which may have previously been performed on the basis of equivocal DPL results. Overall, CT has increased the nonoperative management of blunt abdominal trauma.[51] Shortcomings of CT include its limited ability to detect hollow viscus injuries, and the expertise required to accurately interpret subtle findings.

The initial treatment decision in the presence of intra-abdominal injury is whether to operate. The presence of obvious intra-abdominal bleeding, penetrating trauma to the abdomen or the thorax, or a mechanism and physical findings in an injury that is strongly suggestive of a "surgical abdomen" indicates the need for urgent laparotomy. Such individuals should not be observed for an extensive period, because these injuries may result in sudden and rapid deterioration.

An approach to the initial evaluation of the acutely injured abdomen begins with observation of the entire exposed anterior and posterior abdomen, flanks (side of individual between rib and hip), lower chest, buttocks, and perineum for evidence of contusions, abrasions, lacerations, and penetrating wounds. Contusions may not appear for several hours after trauma has occurred. The abdomen should then be auscultated to assess the frequency and quality of bowel sounds. The presence of bacteria, blood, or chemical irritants in the abdomen may result in an ileus, or paralysis of the intestines, manifested by absent or reduced bowel sounds. This finding, however, is extremely nonspecific and should prompt further evaluation. The abdomen should then be examined for physical signs of peritoneal irritation, including rebound tenderness, muscle guarding, tenderness with percussion, or pain with coughing.

The complete examination of the abdomen must include careful evaluation of the three regions of the abdomen: the intrathoracic abdomen, the "true" abdomen, and the retroperitoneal abdomen. The organs

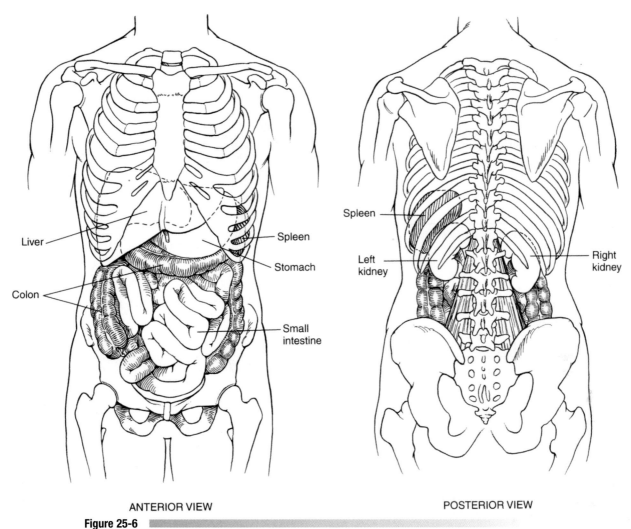

ANTERIOR VIEW   POSTERIOR VIEW

Figure 25-6
Anatomy of the abdominal cavity.

Table 25-5

Physical Examination of the Abdomen After Blunt Trauma Frequently is Misleading

Signs of Visceral Injury on Initial Abdominal Examination	Percent of Patients	Incidence of Significant Intra-Abdominal Injury (%)
Obvious	22	80
Equivocal	46	35
Negative	12	43
Unreliable because of head or spine injury	19	35

From Olsen WR: Abdominal trauma in the athlete. In Schneider RL, Kennedy JC, Plant ML, editors: *Sports injuries — mechanisms, prevention, and treatment,* pp 809-817, Baltimore, 1985, Williams & Wilkins.

located in each region are listed in Table 25-6. The intra-thoracic abdomen, which is difficult to palpate because it lies protected by the bony thorax, is susceptible to injury from blows to the lower or middle abdomen, which direct forces upward. The true abdomen is more accessible to examination by palpation, whereas the retroperitoneal abdomen is often extremely difficult to evaluate by physical examination. Hematomas are a common finding in the retroperitoneal space, and CT is often required for a diagnosis. Table 25-7 summarizes the usefulness of the various diagnostic modalities in the evaluation of each abdominal region.

Table 25-6

Organs of the Three Abdominal Regions

Intrathoracic Abdomen	"True" Abdomen	Retroperitoneal Abdomen
Spleen	Small intestines (most of)	Retroperitoneal colon
Liver	Colon (most of)	Retroperitoneal duodenum
Diaphragm	Bladder (most of)	Pancreas
	Uterus	Kidneys
	Fallopian tubes	Retroperitoneal bladder
	Ovaries	

From Nichols AW: Abdominal and thoracic injuries.

Table 25-7

Usefulness of Diagnostic Evaluation Methods by Abdominal Region

Region	Palpation	DPL	CT
Intrathoracic	1+	2+	3+
"True"	3+	2+	3+
Retroperitoneal	1+	1+	3+

CT, Computed tomography; *DPL,* diagnostic peritoneal lavage.
From Nichols AW: Abdominal and thoracic injuries.

Intra-Abdominal Structures that Could Be Injured in Sport

- Spleen
- Liver
- Intestinal tract
- Kidney
- Urethra
- Bladder
- Pancreas

Splenic Injury

The spleen, located deep to the left ninth through eleventh ribs, is the most commonly injured organ in the abdomen[4] and a recent review of the national pediatric trauma registry found that the spleen is also the most commonly injured organ in team and contact sports.[52] Laceration or rupture may occur as a result of blunt trauma to the left upper abdomen or lower chest wall, sudden deceleration tearing the hilum[4] or secondary to overlying lower rib fractures (Figure 25-7). The clinical features of splenic injury are often insidious in onset, because symptoms develop secondary to bleeding. Significant and rapid bleeding occurs in as much as 85% of

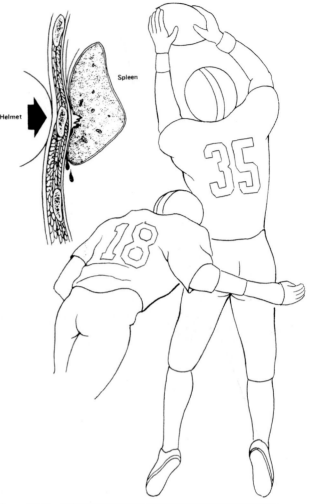

Figure 25-7

Mechanism of spleen injury by direct blunt trauma. (From Olsen WR: Abdominal trauma in the athlete. In Schneider RC, Kennedy JC, Plant ML editors: *Sports injuries—Mechanisms, prevention, and treatment,* Baltimore, 1985, Williams & Wilkins.)

cases of frank rupture. Subcapsular hematoma formation results in less bleeding, although rupture with resumption of bleeding may occur from even minor recurrent trauma up to several weeks later. On physical examination, the athlete with a splenic injury may have left upper quadrant tenderness, abrasions or contusions, rib tenderness, and hypotension or shock. Kerr sign, which is shoulder pain that is referred from the diaphragm when it is irritated by blood from a splenic injury, is often present.[4]

Splenic injury may be fatal if not promptly diagnosed or if appropriate treatment is delayed. The diagnosis may be readily confirmed by CT, which has the advantage versus diagnostic peritoneal lavage in its greater than 95% accuracy, information provided regarding the location and severity of the splenic damage, quantity of hemoperitoneum, and ability to identify associated injuries. Affleck[53] and Buntain and colleagues[54] have provided a useful classification of splenic injury based on CT appearance to assist with management decisions (Figure 25-8).

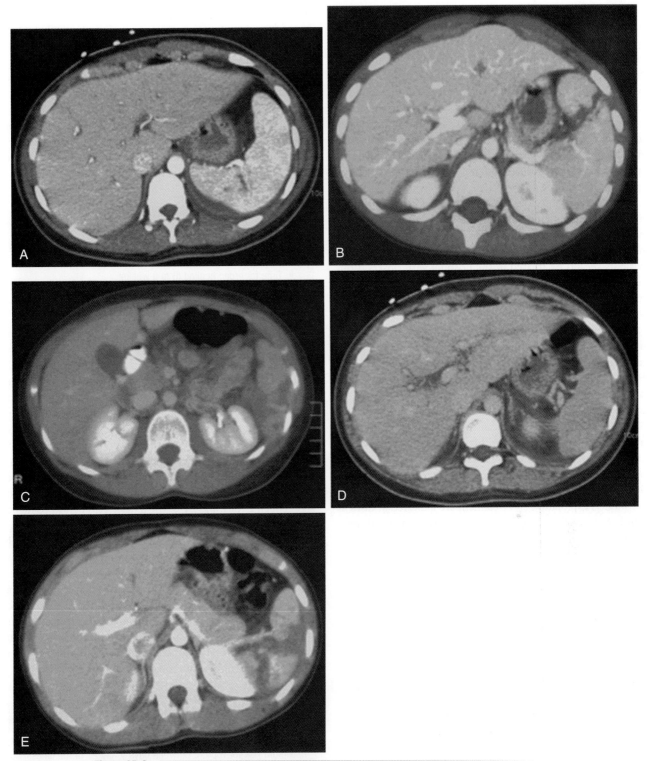

Figure 25-8
Computed tomography–based classification of splenic injury:
Class 1, Subcapsular hematoma or localized capsular disruption without significant parenchymal injury.
Class 2, Single or multiple capsular and parenchymal disruptions, transverse or longitudinal, that do not extend into the hilum or involve major blood vessels. Intraparenchymatous hematoma may or may not coexist.
Class 3, Deep fractures, single or multiple, transverse or longitudinal, extending into the hilum and involving the major blood vessels.
Class 4, Completely shattered or fragmented spleen, or separated from its normal blood supply at the pedicle (may or may not have associated intra- or extra-abdominal injury). (Text from Buntain WL, Gould HR, Maull KI: Predictability of splenic salvage by computed tomography, *J Trauma* 28(1):24-34, 1988. Illustrations from Afflect TP: Severe sports-related spleen injury, *Phys Sports Med* 20:109-123, 1992.)

The spleen was once considered an expendable organ that played little physiological role in adults. The treatment of splenic injuries has now taken a major shift toward the preservation of splenic tissue. Splenectomy results in the loss of an invaluable reticuloendothelial filter of the blood, reduced immune function with lowered levels of immunoglobulin G and immunoglobulin M and T-cells, and an increased risk of overwhelming bacterial infection. The encapsulated organisms *Streptococcus pneumoniae, Haemophilus influenzae* type B, and *Neisseria meningitides* are particularly virulent for splenectomized individuals and are often the cause of postsplenectomy sepsis.[4]

The criteria for nonoperative management of splenic injuries include hemodynamic stability with an adequate hematocrit, a nonenlarging splenic defect, no evidence of head injury, and stable peritoneal findings. All nonoperative patients should be treated in the hospital with observation, serial examinations, and hematocrit levels to detect any hemodynamic instability. Strict bedrest is necessary. Up to 90% of class 1 and 2 injuries can be treated nonoperatively, without blood transfusions, and can be ready for discharge in less than 7 days.[53] Hospitalization is particularly important, given the risk of delayed rupture or hemorrhage. Failure of nonoperative management is normally noted at 48 to 72 hours, but there may be ruptures as late as 2 months after injury.[4] A repeat CT should be performed 5 to 7 days after the initial scan to look for stabilization or improvement. If the injury to the spleen seems to be worse at this point, then operative management is needed. Nonoperative management has been shown to be effective in 90% of children and 70% of adults.[4]

Surgical exploration and treatment are indicated in cases in which conservative management fails or is deemed inappropriate. After surgery, the athlete generally spends 5 to 7 days in the hospital. Strenuous activity should be avoided for 6 to 8 weeks and contact sports returned to in 3 months.[4]

Return-to-play decisions after splenic injury require great prudence. Class 1 and 2 injuries (see Figure 25-8) may heal completely within 6 to 8 weeks without surgery.[53] Two weeks of endurance training should be instituted before return to even noncontact sports. Return to contact sports should be delayed for another 2 to 3 weeks following the healing period and may take more than 4 months total. If the athlete is trying for an earlier return to contact sports, a careful evaluation of radiographic evidence via CT must be performed to assess the spleen and liver score. There is no single parameter to predict safe return to sport. In general, the patient must be evaluated at the 1-month mark to make sure that he or she is afebrile (no fever), well hydrated, and asymptomatic without any evidence of a palpable liver or spleen. Even when all of these conditions are met, there is no guarantee that the spleen may not rupture with trauma.[55] It is important that each athlete treated nonoperatively be taken on a case-by-case basis looking at both physical and radiographic criteria.[4] Severe injuries may be followed with serial CT scans or ultrasonograms on a monthly or bimonthly basis until complete healing is con-

firmed. Endurance training for 2 to 3 weeks is advised, followed by return to noncontact sports and ultimately to contact sports; however, this is not always followed. A recent journal article reported on the case of a competitive college football player who suffered a grade 3 splenic injury that required surgery. A laparoscopic splenectomy was performed on the patient and he was discharged from the hospital 20 hours later. He was able to play football 12 days later. The authors stressed that although most consider minimally invasive surgery for the treatment of splenic injuries contraindicated, there may be a role in select patients.[56]

Clinical Point

Generally, return-to-play criteria following intra-abdominal injuries should include:
- Time for organ healing (6 to 8 weeks)
- Endurance training before noncontact sports (2 weeks)
- Radiographic evidence organ has healed
- Normal laboratory results for that organ

Infectious Mononucleosis and Splenic Damage. Infectious mononucleosis, a viral infection caused by the Epstein-Barr virus, commonly affects adolescents and young adults and is found in 3% of all college students.[57] Clinical manifestations include sore throat, fever, cervical adenopathy (enlarged cervical glands), splenomegaly (enlarged spleen), and hepatomegaly (enlarged liver). Splenic enlargement occurs in up to 70% of individuals with infectious mononucleosis between days 4 and 21 of the illness. This period coincides with the time of maximal risk for splenic rupture, which complicates 0.1% to 0.2% of cases. Individuals with splenomegaly who participate in contact sports are at increased risk for splenic rupture. Vigorous physical activity should be curtailed until splenomegaly resolves. A spleen that is palpable during abdominal physical examination is at least two to three times its normal size. It may take as long as 3 weeks from the time that the splenic tip is no longer palpable for splenomegaly to completely resolve. There have been no reports in the literature of splenic rupture in mononucleosis after 3 weeks.[57]

Clinical Caution

In individuals with infectious mononucleosis, the spleen is at maximum risk for rupture between days 4 and 21 of the illness, so high-impact activity and contact sports should be avoided.

The management of mononucleosis-induced splenomegaly includes examinations of the abdomen on at least a weekly basis. Radiographs, ultrasonograms, and CT scans may also be helpful to confirm resolution of splenomegaly before allowing the athlete to return to activity. Low-impact endurance training should be resumed initially, whereas high-impact activity and contact sports should be avoided for an additional 2 to 3 weeks.[58,59] Corticosteroids may be useful in the treatment of upper airway obstruction, which is often associated with infectious mononucleosis, although they have not been shown to reduce the prevalence or severity of splenomegaly.

Liver Injury

With the advent of the CT scan, the ability of the clinician to diagnose minor liver injuries has been greatly increased.[4] The liver now accounts for 4.4% to 4.9% of athletic injuries.[1] It is especially at risk because of its large size and unprotected position. Athletes with hepatomegaly should not engage in contact sports until the liver has returned to normal size.[4] The most common mechanism of injury is a blunt blow to the right abdomen or lower chest, but liver injuries can also occur by a sudden deceleration or displacement of a lower right rib fracture. A case report has also described liver injury after a blow to the left abdomen.[60] Symptoms of liver injury vary with the severity of damage but may include right upper quadrant pain, diffuse abdominal pain, or peritoneal irritation signs, if heavy bleeding is present. Liver injuries, unlike splenic injuries, rarely progress to serious hemorrhage.

Hepatic contusions result in mild right upper quadrant abdominal pain, occasional nausea and vomiting, hemodynamic stability, and an absence of peritoneal signs. Treatment includes bed rest with observation and avoidance of athletic activities for at least 2 to 3 weeks, at which time endurance activities may be gradually reintroduced.[61]

Hepatic lacerations range from minor tears producing little bleeding, to more severe, deeper parenchymal bleeding. Hemodynamic instability caused by parenchymal bleeding will require surgical intervention and repair. Of all liver injuries, 80% involve the right hepatic lobe because of its larger volume, proximity to the lower ribs, and the location of the falciform ligament.[61] Most liver lacerations result in subcapsular hematoma formation or intraparenchymal tears. Associated hemorrhage is typically minimal, with 70% having stopped bleeding by the time of laparotomy.[62,63] The American Association for the Surgery of Trauma organ injury scale is used to classify hepatic injuries on as scale from I to VI. Unfortunately this grading system does not have applicability to guiding thereapy.[4] The amount of hemoperitoneum detected by CT scan, rather than the degree of liver damage, correlates well with the need for operative intervention.[60] Liver trauma may be managed nonoperatively in the presence of hemodynamic stability and the absence of peritoneal signs or significant extrahepatic injury. Nonoperative management consists of bedrest, careful hemodynamic monitoring and frequent physical and laboratory evaluation.[4] If the patient remains stable, then a CT should be repeated 5 to 7 days after the injury. If, at this time,

the symptoms or appearance are worsened then operative intervention is necessary. Surgical management is indicated if hemodynamics are unstable, the abdomen distends, and the hematocrit continues to fall or fails to respond to blood transfusions. After surgery, the patient may require a long hospital stay. Clinical recovery is best assessed by the use of serial CT scans, which will demonstrate early healing within 2 to 4 weeks. Complete healing must be confirmed before permitting an athlete to return to full activity under careful monitoring. The process of complete healing usually takes 3 to 6 months.[64]

Intestinal Tract Injury

Ruptured Hollow Viscus. Rupture of a hollow viscus is an uncommon injury, but has been reported in athletes who have sustained blunt abdominal trauma.[60,65,66] The specific segments of bowel that are fixed to the abdominal wall appear to be most susceptible to rupture. These include the duodenum, proximal jejunum, terminal ileum, and any areas attached by adhesions. The mechanism of injury is not known, although it is suspected that the bowel is crushed against the spine, resulting in rupture or hematoma formation.[66] The duodenum seems to be particularly vulnerable to injury where it crosses the spine.

The symptoms of bowel rupture include severe abdominal pain, nausea, vomiting, and muscle spasm. The quality of abdominal pain is typically diffuse, and "gripping" or "crampy" in nature. Injury to various portions of the intestinal tract may refer pain to other locations in the abdomen as follows: stomach or duodenum to the epigastrium, small bowel to the umbilical area, and colon to the suprapubic region. The physical examination may reveal rebound tenderness consistent with peritoneal irritation, an absence of bowel sounds, and abdominal rigidity.

The diagnosis of bowel rupture may be suspected by the presence of free air under the diaphragm on an upright abdominal radiograph and may be confirmed by CT with contrast, MRI scan, or exploratory laparotomy. The treatment of a ruptured hollow viscus is surgical, with immediate repair of damage, irrigation of the abdominal cavity, and appropriate treatment of peritonitis.

Intramural Hematoma. Intestinal intramural hematoma has been reported as a result of contact in an adolescent football player.[65] The duodenum is particularly susceptible to injury, given the presence of a transitional area between the portion that is tightly anchored to the abdominal wall and the loosely tethered segment attached to mesentery. This area becomes particularly stressed during sudden deceleration, which commonly occurs in football, bicycling, and equestrian sports. The resultant forces may cause the submucosal vessels to be sheared against the muscularis mucosa, with bleeding into the duodenal wall, between the muscularis and submucosal layers. Partial to complete luminal obstruction may ensue. The mechanism of this injury is severe deceleration rather than blunt trauma.[65]

Intestinal Ischemia. Ischemic bowel disease can occur in the athlete and the team physician should be aware of the symptoms as well as the proper methods of diagnosis and management. Abdominal pain and diarrhea may actually be early symptoms of ischemia. The range of ischemic bowel disease is varied in severity and treatment. Gastritis caused by ischemia may be treated with acid blockade, whereas colitis may require volume repletion with intravenous fluids or even transfusion with blood products. Resection is rarely necessary. Severe infarctions caused by intestinal ischemia are rare but sometimes fatal.[67]

Kidney Injury

The kidney is the second most commonly injured intra-abdominal organ in sports participants after the spleen.[52] Glenn and Harvard found that renal trauma was the cause of hospitalization in 19% of all injured athletes who required hospitalization for sports trauma.[68] Two 2003 reviews of pediatric trauma registries revealed that although renal injuries do occur in sports, they happen at a much lower rate than from other causes. McAleer showed that out of 113 injuries incurred from team sports, only 6 sustained renal injuries.[69] Wan and colleagues performed a retrospective review of 81,923 cases, of which 5439 were sports-related.[52] Of the 42 total kidney injuries found in this review, 26 were associated with football. A recent study looking at renal injuries in professional football players showed an average of 2.7 renal injuries per season.[70] Most injuries are renal contusions that result from blunt blows to the flank or abdomen. The upper one third of the right kidney and the upper one half of the left kidney lie above the twelfth rib, within the thorax. Three layers of anterior abdominal muscles, retroperitoneal fat, the psoas muscles, and the paravertebral muscles provide further renal protection, particularly when the muscles are tensed. Kidney injury may be severely painful, particularly if damage has occurred within the substance of the kidney with resultant bleeding into the collecting system. Occult hematuria (blood in the urine) without radiographic evidence of injury is a common finding in boxers, football players, basketball players, and long-distance runners. A 1993 study looked at the urine of 45 male and female athletes after completing a long-distance race. On lab analysis, 24.4% were found to have red blood cells in their urine. The source of the blood was found to be the lower urinary tract and after 7 days, there was no sign of blood in the athletes' urine.[71]

Clinical Note

Children may be at increased risk of renal damage because of the absence of fatty anatomical padding, decreased rigidity of the rib cage, and the larger size of the pediatric kidney. A recent study showed that the size and maturity of the child may play a role in his or her potential for renal injury.[52]

Kidney damage must be suspected when an athlete has sustained a blow to the flank, abdomen, or lower chest. The most common sign of renal injury is hematuria, but kidney damage may be present without it in 25% of cases.[72,73] Other signs and symptoms of renal damage include flank pain, tenderness, and ecchymosis. The quantity of hematuria (blood in the urine) correlates poorly with the degree of renal injury, but if it persists longer than 48 to 72 hours, a more comprehensive workup for renal trauma must be performed.[73] An example of a susceptible body position for renal injury occurs when the body is extended, and the abdominal muscles are relaxed, as when a football player is leaping for a pass.[74] Hematuria may also occur secondary to repeated microtrauma from exercise, resulting in cumulative damage to the urinary tract. The source of exercise-induced hematuria may be the kidney, bladder, urethra, or prostate.[73] Long-distance runners are particularly prone to this condition as a result of shock transmission from repeated footstrikes, as are boxers who sustain recurrent punches to the torso.

Types of kidney injuries include contusion, subcapsular hematoma, parenchymal rupture into the renal pelvis, rupture across the capsule, and laceration (Figure 25-9).[3] Renal contusion, the most common type of kidney injury, typically

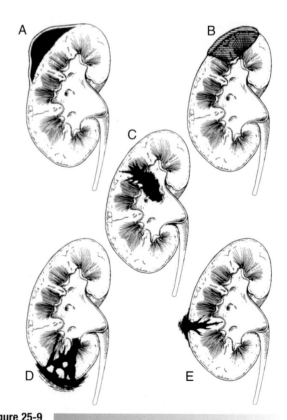

Figure 25-9

Common kidney injuries. **A,** Subcapsular hematoma. **B,** Contusion. **C,** Parenchymal rupture into renal pelvis. **D,** Rupture across capsule. **E,** Laceration. (From Diamond DL: Sports-related abdominal trauma, *Clin Sports Med* 1:91, 1989.)

results from a shock transmitted to the kidney after a blow to the torso. These injuries are usually self-limited, although extravasated blood under the capsule may be problematic if it becomes infected. Increasing forces may produce more serious kidney damage, such as capsular rupture, perirenal hematoma formation, and subcapsular hemorrhage with progression to kidney necrosis. The severity and clinical manifestations of renal rupture depend on the extent and area of injury. Extrinsic hemorrhage may trigger symptoms of localized pain, back and flank muscle spasm, and painful muscle functioning.

The issue of the athlete with only one functioning kidney is one that has arisen in the literature during the last few years. In 1986, Dorsen recommended that young patients with solitary kidneys only participate in noncontact sports to avoid the possibility of renal injury. Older patients with financial incentive or exceptional skill were taken on a case-by-case basis if they were able to give informed consent and sign a waiver if they wished to participate.[75] A 1994 survey to members of the American Medical Society for Sports Medicine revealed that 54.1% of those polled allowed athletes with a solitary kidney to participate in collision or contact sports as long as protective equipment was used, a waiver signed, and consultation with a urologist obtained.[76] In the pediatric patient, it is imperative that parents be counseled about the risk of renal injury caused by sporting injuries, especially in the child with a solitary kidney. Protective equipment should be offered and the parent made aware that modifications to the child's participation in high-risk sporting activities be made to decrease the risk of injury to the solitary kidney.[77] In a 2008 poll of National Football League (NFL) physicians and trainers, 61% of respondents would allow a professional athlete with one kidney to play, 50% would not allow a college athlete with one functioning kidney to play, and 60% would advise against a high school player with one kidney from participating in football.[70]

Clinical Caution

Athletes with one kidney should only be allowed to compete in collision sports if they understand the risk, wear extra protective padding over the kidney, sign a waiver, and consult a urologist.

The medical evaluation of an athlete with hematuria who has sustained trauma to the abdomen, back, or lower chest should include a complete history and physical examination, urinalysis, complete blood count, and a plain-film radiograph of the abdomen. Patients with gross hematuria, microscopic hematuria, hypotension, or a flank mass may require further evaluation with a CT scan or intravenous pyelogram (IVP).[4] Plain x-ray films may disclose associated injuries, such as lower rib or lumbar vertebral fractures, as well as loss of the psoas muscle and renal outlines, if retroperitoneal bleeding is present. Contrast-enhanced CT scan, if available, is generally preferable to IVP, because it is quicker to perform, noninvasive, and has greater accuracy in diagnosing a renal hilar injury, renal contusion or laceration, extravasation of urine, and possible retroperitoneal bleeding.[4] CT has the additional advantage of assessing damage to other organs.[78] IVP has a lower specificity, and is inadequate in the diagnosis of vascular injuries such as renal artery thrombosis, which may necessitate the use of arteriography.

Differential Diagnosis of Hematuria

- Trauma
- Infection
- Urinary tract stones
- "Runner's hematuria"
- Neoplasms (benign and malignant)
- Prostatitis (inflamed prostate)
- Glomerulonephritis (inflamed glomerulus of kidney)
- Analgesic nephropathy (kidney disorder)
- Sickle cell anemia
- Disorders of coagulation
- Thrombocytopenia (reduced number of platelets)

The absence of red blood cells on a single urinalysis does not exclude the possibility of renal damage. If the clinical presentation and mechanism of injury provide a strong suspicion of renal damage, successive urine specimens should be collected. If continued concern exists, contrast CT or IVP should be performed.

The treatment of renal injuries depends on the type and extent of damage. The great majority of cases without hemodynamic instability and a stable hematocrit will heal without complications when treated with monitoring and complete bed rest until hematuria clears. This approach has had the added benefit of decreasing the number of nephrectomies done when renal injuries are explored at the time of injury. Hospitalization is indicated to monitor for continued bleeding, development of shock, hematoma expansion, or continued free extravasation of urine on IVP or contrast CT scan. These conditions warrant surgical intervention. Prior to discharge, the renal injury should be documented by a repeat CT to determine stabilization and healing. The patient should also be told that microscopic hematuria may persist for 2 to 4 weeks after the injury. If hematuria persists longer than 4 weeks or reappears at a later point in time, re-evaluation is necessary.[4]

The athlete who has sustained a relatively minor renal injury should avoid strenuous sports activity for at least 4 weeks. This reduces the risk of rebleeding, because it takes 15 to 21 days for clots to dissolve. The recovery phase of more significant renal trauma should include serial monitoring of the blood pressure, urinalysis, and CT or IVP every 3 months for 1 year. These measures will help identify the late-developing complications of urinoma, hydronephrosis, transient hypertension, reduced renal function, infection, and renal calcification. The athlete who has sustained extensive renal laceration or contusion should be allowed to return to contact sports only after contrast CT confirms complete healing, which often takes 6 or more months.[79]

Ureteral Injury

The ureter is the least commonly injured portion of the urinary tract. Avulsion of the ureter has been reported after a severe blow to a hyperextended back, which may occur during a fall from a horse or during a motor vehicle accident. The most common symptom of ureteral rupture is nondescript back pain, often in conjunction with signs of severe abdominal injuries and peritoneal irritation. The diagnosis may be confirmed by contrast CT or IVP, and the treatment is surgical.

Bladder Injury

The urinary bladder is infrequently injured in sports because of its location deep to the pubic bones within the protective pelvic ring. The empty bladder's collapsed configuration also reduces its susceptibility to injury.

Clinical Caution

As a preventive measure for bladder injuries, it is wise to have contact-sport athletes use the bathroom to void prior to competition so the bladder is under less tension.

Bladder contusion, the most common bladder injury, typically results from abdominal or pelvic trauma. The presentation is hematuria with indefinite suprapubic tenderness and an absence of peritoneal signs, such as abdominal rigidity and rebound tenderness. Bladder rupture is a rare but extremely serious condition that necessitates prompt recognition and surgical treatment. The symptoms of bladder rupture include severe suprapubic pain, which often progresses rapidly to peritoneal signs and shock. An individual who is unable to void after abdominal or pelvic trauma should undergo a cystogram. Any extravasation of contrast on cystography accurately depicts the site of injury. If urethral damage is suspected, retrograde urethrography should precede blind catheterization to avoid inducing further damage to the urethra.

"Runner's hematuria" must be considered in the evaluation of an athlete with hematuria. Macrohematuria or microhematuria, often with dysuria (painful urination) and suprapubic pain, has been reported in up to 18% of runners at the conclusion of a marathon race.[80] Cystoscopic studies have identified the presence of a mucosal contusion at the bladder base that involves the trigone, from the internal meatus to the interureteric ridge, and a mirror image contusion lesion on the posterior bladder wall.[81] It is suspected that the repetitive impacts of running result in the bladder mucosal contusion, especially if the bladder is empty. Hematuria typically resolves rapidly with rest.

Pancreatic Injury

Sports-related injury to the pancreas is uncommon because of its relatively protected anatomical location, deep in the retroperitoneum. Injuries can result from atraumatic methods as well as blunt abdominal trauma.[82] An extremely forceful abdominal blow that compresses the organ against the spine is usually necessary to produce pancreatic damage. Because of the vital physiological nature of the pancreas, the severity of trauma necessary to induce damage to the pancreas, and the corrosive nature of pancreatic contents, injuries to the pancreas are often life-threatening. For this reason, pancreatic injury should always be included in the differential diagnosis of the athlete with abdominal pain.[82]

The signs and symptoms of pancreatic injury include mild to severe midabdominal pain that often radiates to the back, nausea and vomiting, signs of peritoneal irritation, and shock. Damage to the pancreas may occur in the form of a contusion with pseudocyst development, traumatic pancreatitis, laceration, or transection. Incidental pancreatitis, such as that occurring with excessive alcohol intake or cholelithiasis, must also be considered in the differential diagnosis of pancreatic abnormalities. The diagnosis is made by CT or MRI scan. Serum amylase determination may serve as a useful screening test, but a level in the normal range does not exclude the possibility of pancreatic damage. Atraumatic pancreas injury is treated via limitation of gastric stimulation, fluid replacement, analgesia, and metabolic stabilization. Traumatic injury to the pancreatic duct has been found in the recent literature to be the primary source of morbidity and mortality. Any treatment plan, whether nonoperative or surgical, should focus on serial clinical examinations, measuring pancreatic enzyme levels, and magnetic resonance cholangiopancreatography (MRCP) or endoscopic retrograde cholangiopancreatography (ERCP) to rule out ductal injury.[82] The treatment of a sports-related traumatic pancreatic injury is determined by the severity of the injury. Conservative care includes bed rest, bowel rest, and fluid replacement, whereas severe injury may require surgical intervention, including distal pancreatectomy.

Injuries to the Genitalia and Perineum

Genitalia and Perineum Structures That Could Be Injured in Sports

- Testicles
- Scrotum
- Penis
- Urethra
- Perineum

Testicular and Scrotal Injury

Groin trauma is relatively common in sports that use hard implements, such as ice hockey, baseball, softball, and lacrosse. Many of these sports use hard, protective cups to safeguard this area, and thus serious injury occurs only rarely. Interestingly, football players seldom, if ever, wear such protection. Testicular injury was actually found to have a relatively low incidence in a recent review of the National Pediatric Trauma Registry, with only 1 case out of 459 sports-related injuries reported.[52] The symptoms of testicular or scrotal injury, which include localized pain, scrotal swelling, and ecchymosis, are relatively nonspecific (Figure 25-10). The early identification of serious injuries, such as testicular rupture or torsion, however, is essential for the preservation of the injured testicle. Scrotal trauma can displace the testicles into the perineum, suprapubic area, or inguinal region.[4]

Testicular rupture, the most serious groin injury, is uncommon because of the mobility of the testes. Rupture usually results from high-velocity sports, such as bicycling, when a testis is compressed between the bicycle saddle and the pubic bones or when hit by a puck in ice hockey. The tunica vaginalis, which covers the tubular and vascular components of the testis, ruptures after impact. The symptoms include pain and bleeding into the scrotum with massive swelling. The treatment is emergent surgical testicular repair and drainage of the scrotum.

Blunt groin trauma may cause a rapid accumulation of blood in the scrotum, known as a *hematocele,* which is caused by rupture of the pampiniform plexus venous network of the spermatic cord. Treatment for a hematocele involves bed rest, application of ice, and elevation of the scrotum with the possibility of surgical ligation of bleeding vessels in case the hematoma continues to accumulate rapidly. Individuals with varicoceles, a condition characterized by chronic engorgement of the pampiniform plexus, seem to be at increased risk of developing a hematocele.

Contusions of the testicle or scrotum are the most common groin injuries. They are most accurately evaluated in the period immediately following the injury, before swelling develops. Initial treatment should include bed rest, the application of ice packs, scrotal elevation, and oral analgesics.

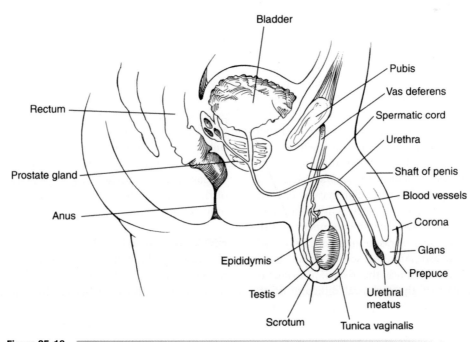

Figure 25-10
Anatomy of the male genitalia.

Ambulation is permitted once pain has resolved and swelling has stabilized. A scrotal support should then be worn for several days.[83]

Torsion of the spermatic cord may occur spontaneously, after a blow to the scrotum, or as a result of forceful contraction of the cremasteric muscle, which draws the testis superiorly over the pubis and twists the cord. Torsion is unlikely if a supporter is worn. This injury must be suspected, particularly in the young athlete who experiences sudden or slowly progressive abdominal or groin pain with no history of trauma. The physical examination may reveal poor definition of the scrotal structures. The diagnosis is suggested further by a radionuclide scan that shows reduced uptake in the involved testicle, an indication for prompt surgical intervention.

Other conditions that must be considered in the evaluation of an athlete with groin pain include epididymitis and neoplasms. *Epididymitis* (inflammation of elongated, cordlike structure along the posterior border of the testis) typically manifests with a gradual onset of scrotal pain in young males. A soft, nontender testis adjacent to a discretely tender, swollen epididymis, is noted on physical examination. Pyuria (pus in urine) may be apparent on urinalysis. Testicular carcinomas are relatively common neoplasms in young men and must be considered in the evaluation of any scrotal masses.

The workup and evaluation of scrotal and testicular injuries always should begin with a thorough history of injury. The physical examination may be best performed with the individual in the supine position so as to help relieve discomfort and reduce the tug of gravity on the testicle. The anatomical structures should be palpated systematically with an attempt to identify each testis, epididymis, and spermatic cord. The presence of scrotal swelling or fullness should prompt the use of transillumination to help differentiate between a hydrocele, which does transilluminate and produces a testicular shadow, and a hematocele or testicular mass that does not transilluminate. A Doppler probe evaluation is useful if one suspects torsion of the cord, and the presence of a spermatic artery pulse at the hilum of the testis helps to rule out torsion. Ultrasonography provides the most useful noninvasive imaging assessment of the scrotal contents. It helps to identify hematoceles, testicular masses, epididymal swelling, and testicular integrity. Ultrasonography may be limited, however, by available equipment and the expertise of the individual ultrasonographer. Diagnostic percutaneous needle aspiration of scrotal fluid should generally be avoided to reduce the risk of introducing infection and because of the technical difficulty of the procedure. Aspiration may be appropriate, however, in the presence of a tensely swollen scrotum.[83] As a general rule, if groin trauma results in a nonpalpable testicle and a scrotum in which transillumination is ineffective, testicular rupture must be considered, and urgent urological consultation should be sought.

Based on recent studies, testicle injuries are a relatively rare phenomenon in American sports, but do occur.[52,69] The athlete with a single testicle must be counseled as to the risk for a catastrophic injury should the remaining testicle be damaged. Protective equipment should always be used and appropriate activity modifications made to provide the best level of groin protection to the athlete.

Penile and Urethral Injury

The penis is rarely injured when the athlete wears an athletic supporter. Bicycle racers commonly experience a traumatic irritation of the pudendal nerve as a result of prolonged episodes of direct pressure from the hard bicycle saddle on the pudendal nerve. Symptoms, which may include localized penile numbness, priapism (erection of penis), and ischemic neuropathy, typically resolve after the bicycle race. The condition is usually preventable by using a longitudinally furrowed saddle and by the athlete avoiding squeezing the saddle during hill-climbing.

The urethra is rarely injured in athletics. Men are generally affected more commonly than women. The mechanism of injury is often a straddle injury, which most frequently occurs in bicycling, gymnastics, or equestrian events. The bulbous portion of the urethra is most often involved, because the penile urethra is usually protected by the supporter, and the posterior urethra by the pubic bones. A serious blow to the perineum, pelvic diastasis, or the presence of blood at the urethral meatus should prompt further diagnostic investigation with retrograde urethrography. Other symptoms of urethral injury may include penile or perineal hematoma, and an absent or high-riding prostate on rectal examination.[4] If urethral injury is suspected, retrograde urethrography should always be performed before passing a urethral catheter. Extravasation of contrast during the retrograde urethrogram accurately delineates the location and extent of urethral damage. The treatment is surgical repair, with a suprapubic cystostomy placed for urinary diversion. Catheterized stenting or cystostomy may be used for 8 to 10 days without further surgery depending on the extent of the injury to the urethra.[4] Urethral stricture is a common complication.

Perineum Injuries

Hematoma. Women athletes occasionally sustain sports-related trauma (e.g., straddle injury, fall in water skiing) to the vulva and labia, resulting in edema and hematoma formation. Appropriate treatment includes ice application, oral analgesics, and protection. Vulvar hematomas rarely require surgical intervention and athletes may return to sport once the pain and swelling have resolved.[4] Vaginal lacerations rarely accompany such injuries, but their prompt recognition and treatment are necessary to avoid infection or long-term dysfunction.

Vaginal Water Injection Injuries. The female reproductive organs are fortunately well protected by the pubis and thus not very frequently injured. Water skiing, however, may result in "water injection" damage to the vagina, uterus, and fallopian tubes. A novice skier may have difficulty standing and consequently assumes a squatting position, which may enable water to enter the vagina. Vaginal damage, incomplete abortions, and salpingitis (inflammation of the uterine tube) may occur. Salpingitis manifests with signs of an acute abdomen and sepsis. However, symptoms do not generally appear clinically until after 3 days, at which time the athlete may not associate the injury with the infection. Vaginal injection of water injuries may be avoided by wearing neoprene shorts or wetsuits.

Thoracic Injuries

Thoracic Structures that Could Be Injured in Sport

- Ribs
- Thoracic muscles
- Sternum
- Pectoralis major
- Breast
- Vascular tissue
- Lungs
- Heart
- Esophagus

Injuries of the Chest Wall

Rib Injuries

Twelve pairs of ribs articulate with the twelve corresponding thoracic vertebrae. Strong ligaments firmly attach each rib to its analogous vertebra and to those located immediately above and below. Ribs one, eleven, and twelve articulate with only one vertebra, and ribs two through ten articulate posteriorly via the costovertebral and costotransverse joints with the two adjacent vertebrae. Additional capsular ligaments hold each rib tightly against the vertebral body and transverse process at each level, whereas other ligaments extend vertically from the transverse process of the vertebrae above, to the upper aspect of the rib below. The strength of these ligamentous attachments makes sprains uncommon. The anatomy of the ribcage is presented in Figure 25-11.

Each rib-costocartilage pair, the corresponding vertebra, and the sternum form a ring structure that is smallest and most circular in the superior thorax and becomes progressively larger and more oval in shape inferior to the seventh rib. The orientation of the ribs is nearly horizontal at the top, gradually becomes increasingly oblique lower in the thorax, and approaches verticality at the inferior end. The upper seven "true" ribs articulate anteriorly with the sternum by costochondral cartilage. The costochondral cartilage of the so-called false eighth through tenth ribs does not attach immediately to the sternum, but instead joins the costocartilage of the adjacent rib above. The eleventh and twelfth ribs, known as the *floating ribs*, are engulfed by abdominal musculature anteriorly, with no bony attachment. The undersurface of each rib has a groove through which traverse the intercostal neurovascular structures. The intercostal nerves may refer pain to the chest and directly innervate the thoracic wall.

The ribs lie subcutaneously in the anterior chest. This places them at greater risk for damage from direct trauma than the deeper-positioned posterior aspects of the ribs, which are better protected by the heavy musculature of the back and paraspinal muscles. The ribs are elevated by the intercostal and other accessory muscles during inspiration, with a resultant increase in the anterior-posterior diameter of the lower thorax. Adjacent ribs are further secured by fascial extensions from the external intercostal muscles between ribs. The abdominal muscles stretch from the lower anterior ribs to the pelvic brim, providing the anterior connection between the thorax and the pelvis.

Contusion. A direct blow to the anterior chest often leads to contusion of the subcutaneously located ribs, whereas a similar blow to the posterior chest is more likely to cause paraspinal muscular injury. The most common symptom of a rib contusion occurring from direct trauma is localized pain during deep inspiration. The physical examination reveals localized tenderness over the injury without the crepitation that is sometimes noted with a rib fracture. In addition, manipulation of the affected rib at a site distant to the injury should not induce injury site pain. A rib contusion should be treated symptomatically. Once the possibility of an occult fracture has been eliminated, the athlete may be allowed to return to participation with padding over the injury site.

Clinical Note

The clinical differentiation of a rib fracture from a contusion is difficult, but injury site (localized) pain being elicited when the examiner compresses the chest by placing one hand on the back of the hemithorax and the other on the front is usually indicative of fracture.

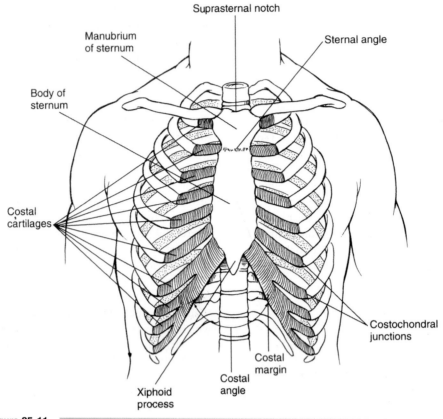

Figure 25-11

Anatomy of the ribcage, sternum, and costochondral joints.

Sprain, Subluxation, or Dislocation of the Vertebral Attachments. Damage to the ligaments and joints of the rib may occur posteriorly at the vertebral attachment (Figure 25-12) or anteriorly at the costochondral junction. Sprains of the vertebral attachment are uncommon, although they may be identified by point tenderness over the injured ligament complex. Costovertebral joint injuries may also refer pain to the anterolateral chest wall, as has been seen in rowers and swimmers who compete in the butterfly.[84] Mild sprain is characterized by an absence of discomfort during inspiration, whereas a more severe sprain results in pain on inspiration. The treatment of vertebral attachment sprains is symptomatic, including initial cold application, followed by heat, thoracic spine mobilization, and protection against motion at the injured joint by use of a rib belt or strapping of the lower chest. In some cases, the rib articulations may be hypomobile following trauma with the rib limited in motion being either an elevated rib (does not fall on exhalation) or a depressed rib (does not elevate on inspiration). Appropriate joint play mobilization can restore the rib motion.

Subluxation of the rib-vertebral attachment may occur, but dislocation is thought to be rare. Most cases of subluxation

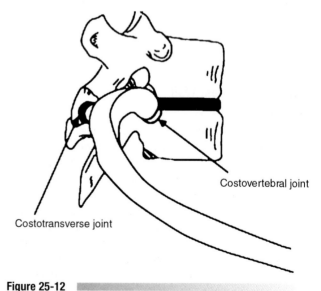

Figure 25-12

Articulations of a rib with the vertebrae. (From Gregory PL, Biswas AC, Batt ME: Musculoskeletal problems of the chest wall in athletes, *Sports Med* 32(4):238, 2002.)

have spontaneously reduced by the time a physician is consulted. The diagnosis of a rib-vertebral subluxation or reduced dislocation is made by the identification of a localized tender spot that corresponds to the site of injury and the complete resolution of symptoms when local anesthetic is injected into the joint. If the subluxation has reduced, the athlete may return to sports participation in 7 to 10 days with lower chest strapping.

Occasionally, dislocations remain unreduced at the time of evaluation. Pain is typically more severe, and physical findings reveal localized tenderness, muscle spasm, and joint motion. Associated damage to the neurovascular bundle often causes neuritis symptoms in the distribution of the costal nerve. Unreduced dislocations should be manually reduced to prevent complications of long-term degenerative joint disease. Reduction may be accomplished by hyperextending the spine and allowing the shoulders and arms to fall backward, and then applying direct pressure to the posterior dislocated segment while simultaneously applying pressure against the anterior chest.

Acute Costochondral Injuries. The anterior attachment of the rib is far more frequently injured than the vertebral junction. Direct sternal trauma or lateral compression of the chest may produce costochondral joint sprain, subluxation, or dislocation. The diagnosis is made based on the presence of tenderness at the costochondral junctions, which are located one to two finger-breadths lateral to the costosternal junctions. Occasionally a popping sensation or palpable step-off is felt with twisting of the torso. The severity of the injury is determined by the amount of tenderness, localized anterior chest wall swelling, and hematoma formation over the injury site. The patient will have full range of motion of the shoulder but active abduction may cause the swelling to become more prominent.[85] More severe sprains are associated with pain during deep inspiration. Persistent joint dislocation is readily apparent clinically as a step-off at the joint site, which may reduce with an audible click, as direct pressure is applied over the rib end. Radiographs are of little use in diagnosing costochondral separations, because the costocartilage is radiolucent. MRI may be used if there is significant clinical concern for the injury.

Acute costochondral separation without displacement or a palpable click involves an at least partially intact ligamentous complex. The treatment is to prevent further injury and relieve discomfort with injection of a long-acting local anesthetic. In the presence of a palpable step-off or audible click, the treatment should be directed toward preventing recurrence. A direct pressure pad should be applied over the anterior end of the rib rather than over the costochondral joint. A rib belt or strapping may be used to hold the pad in place. Union of acute costochondral separation occurs slowly (often longer than a rib fracture), typically taking 6 to 8 weeks. Participation in contact sports should be withheld for 3 to 4 weeks.

Chronic Costochondral Injuries. Costochondral subluxation becomes chronic when an athlete fails to seek medical evaluation until after multiple episodes of subluxation have occurred. The treatment of this condition is determined by the amounts of instability and pain. In the presence of joint stability, when pain is the major complaint, local injections with anesthetics and corticosteroids may be employed. If some degree of pain relief is not achieved after repeated injections during the first 3 to 4 days, it is unlikely that further injections will be effective. If pain is severe and disabling with or without instability, surgery may be considered. Surgery involves the resection of adequate opposing joint surfaces so that they no longer rub together. Given the inherent stability of the rib even after resection of the costochondral junction and the difficulty in fusing rib to cartilage, the rib end is generally not internally fixated. Chronic instability or dislocation alone does not justify surgery, but if localized pain, swelling, and muscle spasm occur, surgery may become necessary. Surgery in such cases involves the resection of a portion of chondral cartilage or the rib end to avoid painful impingement.

Fortunately, given the common occurrence of costochondral injuries, few are severe enough to require the discontinuation of sports. It is important, however, to treat acute injuries with reduction, pad application, and strapping to avoid chronic symptoms. Union of a separated costochondral junction takes 8 weeks, during which time contact sports should be avoided.

Costochondritis. It is important to recognize costochondritis (inflammation of the costal cartilage) as a source of chest pain in the athlete. Often, it presents as pain and tenderness over the second to fifth costochondral or chondrosternal joints. Swelling, heat, and erythema are normally absent. Inflammation has been suggested as the source of costochondritis because some patients show an elevated erythrocyte sedimentation rate (ESR) and morning stiffness.[86] Symptoms are often provoked by shoulder adduction with rotation of the arm to the same side. Radiographs are usually negative but can potentially show mild soft tissue swelling. CT and bone scan may also be used to make the diagnosis.[85] The treatment of costochondritis is with analgesia and reassurance, and symptoms usually resolve within 1 year.

Fracture. In both the athlete and nonathlete, a simple, nondisplaced rib fracture is the most common result of blunt thoracic trauma.[4] The first through third ribs are well protected by the shoulder girdles, making superior rib fractures rare. First and second rib fractures usually only occur from significant direct force or from deceleration. Therefore, the presence of these injuries should suggest the possibility of coexisting injuries to the aorta, great vessels, and airways. Arteriography may be considered if clinically appropriate. A special type of stress fracture of the first rib has also been reported (discussed later).

The fourth through ninth ribs are the most commonly fractured ribs, as a result of their greater exposure to direct trauma and rigid anterior and posterior fixations. The mechanism of such injuries may involve direct chest trauma, which may occur from a pitched baseball, or a blunt blow to the chest. The eleventh and twelfth ribs, or floating ribs, are extremely mobile, lacking anterior bony attachments, and thus are less susceptible to injury. The presence of a lower rib fracture (ninth to twelfth) is associated with splenic, hepatic, or renal damage, and therefore warrants a careful abdominal evaluation.

Fractures may be nondisplaced or displaced. Nondisplaced fractures are generally uncomplicated, whereas displaced fractures are often accompanied by complications that may be far more serious than the rib injury itself. The mechanisms of most rib fractures are either direct blows or compressive forces. Ribs typically break at the point of impact or at the rib's weakest point — the posterior angle. Potential complications of displaced rib fractures include penetration of the lung with development of a pneumothorax, hemothorax, or subcutaneous emphysema; penetration of the pericardium with development of a pericardial effusion or tamponade; damage to the internal mammary artery; and injury to the intercostal neurovascular bundle, which may produce marked swelling, hematoma, and neuritis symptoms. These complications are discussed later in the chapter.

The symptoms of a rib fracture include pleuritic pain aggravated by coughing, deep inspiration, and chest movement at the site of injury. Pain tends to be most severe during the first 3 to 5 days following injury, at which time it gradually subsides, and it ultimately disappears after 3 to 6 weeks. The physical examination discloses localized tenderness and may reveal crepitus if displacement is present. The diagnosis may be confirmed by a coned-down "rib detail" view shot obliquely to the suspected rib fracture site. Even with special radiographic views, however, up to 50% of rib

fractures are not apparent radiographically during the first 10 to 14 days after injury.[87] The subsequent formation of callus eventually results in the ability to identify most fractures on radiographic examination.[88] The early identification of acute rib fractures in a patient with trauma-induced chest pain has been shown not to affect medical management.[89]

The management of rib fractures should initially ensure full recovery from any associated dyspnea. If respiratory distress, cyanosis, or shock is present, a thorough investigation for underlying visceral injury should be undertaken.

Pain and muscle spasm of an uncomplicated fracture may be treated with oral analgesics and local anesthetic infiltration into the intercostal nerve region. The location of needle insertion should be at the inferior edge of the affected rib, at least one hands-breadth proximal (toward the spine) from the fracture. The syringe plunger should be drawn back prior to the injection, to avoid intravascular injection. In addition to the affected rib, the two ribs above and the two ribs below may also require intercostal nerve blocks to achieve complete pain control.

A rib fracture may cause the individual to "splint" during respiration, in an attempt to protect the injured area. As a consequence, respiratory function may be compromised, which predisposes to atelectasis (incomplete expansion of lungs) and pneumonia. Deep breathing exercises, incentive spirometry, and early ambulation should be encouraged to reduce the risk of such complications.

To prevent turning a nondisplaced rib fracture into a displaced one, it is recommended that contact sports and other high-risk activities be avoided until the rib fracture is completely healed, regardless of the time required. If an athlete is allowed to return to contact sports participation, a local rigid protective pad should be worn over the injured area for 4 to 6 weeks, at which time healing should be complete. The pad may be secured with a rib belt. Athletes who are involved in noncontact sports may return to play after their pain has returned to a manageable level, usually 1 to 2 weeks after injury.[91] Under no circumstances should an acute rib fracture be injected with anesthetics to allow sports participation.

More than 300 cases of stress fractures of the first rib in athlete participants in overhead or throwing sports have been described.[92] Golfers, baseball pitchers, rowers, tennis players, weightlifters, and gymnasts have all been reported with the condition.[36] Rib stress fractures occur in 2% to 12% of rowers and are the most common cause of time lost from competition.[93] First-rib stress fractures occur not from direct trauma, but as a result of contraction of the anterior scalene muscles against the subclavian sulcus. The scalene, intercostal, and serratus muscles exert repetitive indirect shearing forces during activities such as throwing, serving a tennis ball, and pressing a barbell overhead, which may result in a fracture. Rapid increases in training have also been shown as a possible cause for first-rib stress fractures in baseball players.[85] The symptoms of first-rib stress fractures range from dull, aching pain along the distribution of the first intercostal nerve to a pleuritic, knifelike shoulder pain radiating to the sternum or pectoral region. The pain may be acute or insidious in nature. Radiographs are typically negative until at least 14 days after the injury, although CT, MRI, and triple-phase bone scans may identify the fracture earlier. The treatment involves avoidance of the offending mechanism, analgesia, use of an arm sling, and a graduated exercise program. In rare cases, a surgical emergency may develop if the subclavian artery is acutely torn. The athlete should be assessed with serial radiographs for 6 months so as to avoid missing late complications. In a recent case report, a stress fracture of the first rib in a tennis player developed into a symptomatic pseudarthrosis. His symptoms presented as shoulder pain.[94]

Stress fractures of other ribs have been reported in elite female athletes who participate in rowing, tennis, golf, and gymnastics. Symptoms include pain in the posterolateral scapular region of the thorax. Clinical symptoms have typically been present for 2 to 6 months prior to the establishment of a diagnosis. Plain radiographs often fail to identify stress fractures, but triple-phase bone scans can provide an early diagnosis (Figure 25-13). The treatment is avoidance of the causative activity. Karlson has suggested that rowers could potentially decrease their chance for rib stress fractures by rowing with less scapula protraction as the oars enter the water and less retraction at the end of pull-through.[93]

Thoracic Muscle Strain

The muscles of the chest wall may be injured either by violent exertional forces or overstretching of the chest muscles. A discussion of thoracic muscle strains should

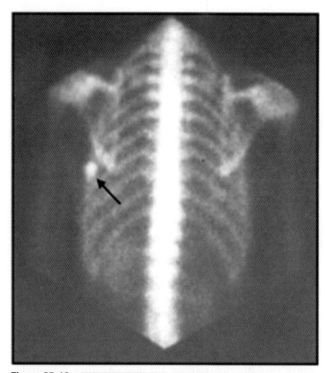

Figure 25-13

Triple-phase bone scan showing rib stress fracture. (From Gregory PL, Biswas AC, Batt ME: Musculoskeletal problems of the chest wall in athletes, *Sports Med* 32(4):241, 2002.)

actually be included in a review of shoulder injuries, because most of the injured thoracic muscles are associated with the upper extremity. However, given the location of pain and to aid in the differentiation from other chest injuries, these strains are included in this section (see also Chapter 4 of *Pathology and Intervention in Musculoskeletal Rehabilitation*, volume 3 in this series).

Thoracic muscle strains typically involve muscles that connect the chest to another body part. Examples include the rhomboids, which connect the scapula to the thorax; the serratus muscles, which connect the upper extremity to the chest; and the rectus abdominus muscles, which connect the pelvis to the thorax. The intercostal muscles rarely experience isolated injury, because they are protected by superficial muscular structures and are generally unable to contract with sufficient force to rupture muscle fibers.

Muscle strains occurring at the rib attachments are likely to be more painful than disabling. The often considerable muscle spasm that may accompany such injuries may result in respiratory "splinting," with the risk of pulmonary complications and decreased ability to train. The treatment of thoracic muscle strains is determined by the specific muscle or group of muscles that are injured. Local injection is often difficult because of the broad thoracic muscle insertions. Ice should be applied initially, followed by heat and gradual rehabilitation. If the injured muscle is attached to the scapula, a sling may be worn to promote rest and recovery. Similarly, if an abdominal muscle has been injured, bed rest, with the head of the bed and the knees elevated to completely relax the abdominal muscles, may be prescribed.

Sternum

The sternum, which protects the vital anatomical structures of the mediastinum, is made up of three bones: the upper manubrium, the middle body, and the lower xiphoid (see Figure 25-11). The first rib and the upper portion of the second rib usually inserts onto the manubrium. The lower portion of the second rib and the third through sixth (and sometimes seventh) ribs insert on the sternal body. The seventh rib usually inserts on the xiphoid. The newborn has six unfused sternal segments, which gradually fuse through the late teenage years to form the three-bone adult sternum. Persistent perfusion lines should not be mistaken for fractures when radiographically evaluating children and adolescents.

Contusion. The subcutaneous location of the sternum makes it susceptible to contusions. Participants in contact sports that do not require the use of protective sternal pads or that involve high-velocity objects are particularly vulnerable to sternal injury. A direct blow to the sternum typically produces superficial edema, ecchymosis, periosteal reaction, and a severe "shock reaction," in which the athlete transiently senses difficulty with respiration. Deep inspiration will not typically aggravate pain in the absence of complications.

Mild and moderate sternal contusions are treated with ice, followed by heat application. If pain is severe, however, the area of injury may be injected with local anesthetics. A protective pad should be applied before permitting the athlete to return to contact sports. Football shoulder pads generally provide excellent sternal protection.

Sprain, Subluxation, and Dislocation. A direct sternal blow may also result in sternal joint sprain, subluxation, or dislocation. The ligaments between the manubrium and body are quite firm and thus are rarely damaged. When joint subluxation or dislocation does occur, however, reduction is usually spontaneous. Clinical symptoms include pain and tenderness at the manubrium-body junction without pain during ordinary breathing. But severe pain is produced when direct compressive pressure is placed on the manubrium or sternal body.

The treatment of a sprain or spontaneously reduced subluxation entails avoidance of sports participation for a minimum of 7 to 10 days, followed by usage of a hollowed plastic sternal pad. If chronic pain symptoms persist, injections of local anesthetics with corticosteroids may be considered.

On rare occasions, sternal injury produces a complete dislocation. These injuries should be reduced as soon as possible. Closed reduction, under general anesthesia, may initially be attempted, although open reduction with wire loop internal fixation may be required. As with any severe chest injury, the presence of subluxation or dislocation should alert the clinician to the possibility of underlying visceral injury.

Sprains are uncommon at the junction of the sternal body and xiphoid as a result of the free anterior-posterior movement of this joint. Sternal body–xiphoid dislocations are rare.

Sternoclavicular Dislocation. Dislocation of the sternoclavicular joint is a relatively rare occurrence with an incidence of only 1% of all dislocations. Regardless of its low incidence, the sports medicine clinician should be wary of the potential complications of mediastinal hemorrhage, tracheal rupture, and esophageal perforation, which may be associated with this injury.[95-97]

Sternoclavicular dislocations have been found in athletes engaged in contact sports such as football and rugby. Patients tend to be males younger than 25 years old.[98] Anterior dislocations are seen much more commonly than posterior dislocations because of the weakness of the anterior sternoclavicular ligaments.[99]

Clinical Caution

Posterior dislocations of the sternoclavicular joint are much more dangerous because of the risk of injury to the great vessels and airway that lie directly beneath the sternoclavicular joint.

A thorough history and physical examination is normally all that is needed to make the diagnosis of sternoclavicular dislocation. The patient will have pain in the area of the sternoclavicular joint, which is exacerbated by motion of the arm. If the diagnosis is not obvious, an x-ray examination can be performed with a 40° cephalic tilt or a CT scan may be done.[100] CT has the added benefit of being able to diagnose injury to the retrosternal structures.[101]

Treatment of acute sternoclavicular dislocations depends on the direction of the dislocation. Anterior dislocations may be reduced acutely, whereas posterior dislocations must be reduced emergently in the operating room because of the possibility of compression of the mediastinal structures. A thoracic surgeon may be needed to assist with surgery in the case of vascular injury. Postreduction management is with sling immobilization for 4 to 6 weeks until healing is complete.[96,98] If the joint remains unstable, it may need to be repaired surgically. Athletes should avoid returning to play until they have pain-free range of motion with a stable sternoclavicular joint.

Fracture. Sternal fractures may also result from direct trauma. Most fractures occur in the upper portion of the sternal body, caused by direct pressure driving the body backward, relative to the first and second ribs, which are fixed to the manubrium. Fractures may be complete or incomplete and displaced or nondisplaced.

The history of injury is a direct sternal blow and immediate loss of breath. Severe pain is provoked only with deep inspiration if the fracture is incomplete, but pain occurs during normal respiration if the fracture is complete. The patient with this injury will often present with localized sternal tenderness on physical examination. The diagnosis may be confirmed with a sternal-view radiograph as well as a lateral view to establish the presence of displacement.[4]

Management of sternal fractures is very similar to that for rib fractures and is focused on pain control as well as recognizing and treating any potential pulmonary complications. The treatment of an undisplaced sternal fracture includes cold application, followed by heat. Chest compression with a rib binder may be used to provide comfort, but is not recommended because of the risk of worsening pulmonary complications. A displaced fracture typically results in fragments that are caught or locked on each other. Reduction usually must be accomplished under anesthesia. Participation in contact sports should be restricted for at least a few weeks after reduction, unless the athlete is completely pain-free during deep inspiration and with chest compression.

Significant amounts of force are required to cause a sternal fracture; therefore, there was once thought to be a high correlation with intrathoracic injuries such as pneumothorax, hemothorax, subcutaneous emphysema, damage to the great vessels, hemopericardium, and cardiac contusion. The current literature does not support this correlation, however, with a rate of only 1% to 5% for myocardial contusion,[102,103] less than 10% associated spine fracture,[104] less than 20% associated rib fracture,[104] no association with aortic rupture,[102,105,106] and an overall mortality rate of only 1%.[85] Because they take several hours to clinically develop, if mediastinal injuries are suspected, the athlete should be admitted to the hospital for bed rest, observation, and serial radiographic studies. Return to sport should occur when the athlete is pain free. Protective equipment such as a flak jacket should be worn when playing contact sports.

Stress fractures of the sternum may occur as the result of repetitive contraction of the muscles attached to the sternum especially in a deconditioned athlete. Sternal stress fractures are very rare, with a reported rate of only 0.5% of all sternal fractures. The patient will report a recent increase in physical activity or training with anterior chest pain that is worse with deep breathing and activity. CT or bone scan may be used to confirm the diagnosis in patients in whom there is a high level of suspicion. Treatment involves rest and analgesia followed by a structured physical therapy program prior to return to sport. Symptoms may take more than 15 months to fully resolve.[4]

Pectoralis Major Injury

Rupture of the pectoralis major muscle is a relatively uncommon event, although it has been reported with increasing frequency in male weight lifters.[107-109] Early reports of this injury occurred when an individual extended the arms to break a fall.[110]

The pectoralis major muscle has a dual origin with an upper clavicular and a lower sternocostal head. Laterally, the two parts of the muscle converge to insert over a 5-cm area of the lateral lip of the bicipital groove. The posterior lamina of the tendon is formed from the fibers of the sternocostal head as they pass under the fibers of the clavicular head. The posterior lamina then rotates 180° and inserts at the most proximal aspect of the humerus.[111] The anterior lamina of the tendon is formed by the clavicular fibers and will insert more distally (Figure 25-14). The primary action of the pectoralis major muscle is to adduct the humerus. It also contributes to forward flexion and internal rotation of the shoulder.

Pectoralis major muscle rupture may occur as a result of a direct blow to the chest or from a violent, eccentric contraction of the pectoralis muscle in activities such as weight lifting in the bench press or football.[107,108] Of all ruptures, 50% occur in athletes.[111] Most ruptures caused by direct trauma occur within the muscle itself, whereas those caused

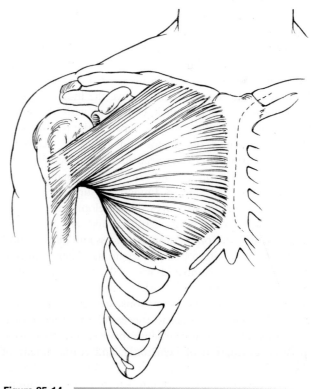

Figure 25-14
Anatomy of the pectoralis major muscle. (From Wolfe SW, Wickiewicz TL, Cavanaugh JT: Ruptures of the pectoralis major muscle, *Am J Sports Med* 21:475-477, 1992.)

by uncoordinated eccentric contraction occur at the musculotendinous junction, or as an avulsion of the tendon from the humerus.[74] Wolfe et al[108] and Kakwani and Matthews[111] demonstrated that the relatively short muscle fibers of the inferior portion of the sternocostal head of the pectoralis muscles must lengthen disproportionately during the final 30° of humeral abduction, external rotation, and extension as the weight is lowered during the bench press. These inferior fibers are placed at a mechanical disadvantage, which, in conjunction with the high-load eccentric forces of the lift, causes rupture.[108]

The symptoms of acute pectoralis major muscle rupture are a tearing sensation into the axilla; severe anterior chest pain, which may radiate to the shoulder or upper arm; a "snapping" or "popping" sound; ecchymosis; and swelling. The diagnosis may be difficult to confirm unless the injury is seen immediately after rupture, because of nonspecific swelling and extreme pain. Repeated physical examinations are often necessary. Characteristic physical findings include bruising and local tenderness accompanied by weakness of upper arm adduction, flexion, internal rotation and bulging of the torn pectoralis muscle during forced adduction. In addition, if the tear occurs with an avulsion of the tendon, a palpable defect may be noted in the anterior axillary fold. A tear localized at the musculotendinous junction may be inapparent to palpation and inspection because of the integrity of the fascial covering. A clue to the diagnosis is an absent pectoralis major shadow and a loss of the normal anterior axillary fold on the frontal chest radiograph.[111]

The treatment of complete pectoralis major rupture is generally nonsurgical for elderly or sedentary individuals. Incomplete tears are also typically treated nonoperatively. Injuries that go unrepaired will leave the individual with a significant strength deficit compared with the uninvolved side. Immediate surgical repair is the treatment of choice for young or athletic individuals.[109] Pectoralis major ruptures that are repaired surgically result in comparable muscular torques and work measurements relative to the uninvolved side.[108] Immediate surgical repair is optimal, because this reduces the development of adhesions, muscle retractions, atrophy, and any delays in return to athletic competition. A success rate of 90% good to excellent results for acute repair has been reported in the literature compared with 70% for nonoperative treatment.[110,112] Individuals with chronic tears, who may be identified by serial examinations, strength testing, and MRI scan, have undergone successful operative repair. The common surgical procedure involves a deltopectoral incision, evacuation of hematoma, and reattachment of the tendon to bone with a variety of techniques including direct suture to the periosteum, suture to the remaining tendon, drill holes, and suture anchors. A sling is generally used for 2 to 4 weeks postoperatively. Kakwani now

recommends an accelerated rehabilitation protocol for pectoralis major rupture starting with elbow range of motion from day 1. At 2 weeks, passive external rotation is introduced along with isometric strengthening exercises for the rotator cuff and pectoralis muscles with the shoulder in neutral rotation. It is imperative that the physical therapist be in contact with the surgeon so as to ascertain the proper "safe arc" for external rotation exercises as determined on intraoperative testing of the repaired pectoralis tendon.[111] The "safe arc" is determined by the surgeon after reattachment of the distal end of the pectoralis tendon in the operating room. By testing the stability of the fixation and determining a range of motion in which the repair is sound, the physical therapist can be given parameters within which he or she can successfully rehabilitate the patient without fear of rupturing the newly repaired tendon.

MRI is an excellent early diagnostic tool to assist in the diagnosis and management of pectoralis major ruptures and will allow for the identification of the exact location and extent of the rupture.[107,111] To help prevent ruptures, it seems sensible to change the arc of the bench press exercise to limit hyperextension of the arm and the resultant passive stretch of the muscle fibers. In addition, despite denials of anabolic steroid usage in weight lifters who had sustained pectoralis major ruptures, the possibility of an association must be considered.[107]

Breast Injury

Athletic female breast injury has become an increasingly common occurrence as the number of women participating in sports at all levels has increased. Breast injury may occur as a result of direct trauma or repetitive microtrauma from inadequate breast support. One report revealed that 56% of physically active female subjects had experienced previous sports-related breast discomfort or pain.[113]

Direct trauma to the breast may produce fat necrosis or hematoma formation, both of which are painful and may result in the formation of a focal breast mass. Mammographic appearance of these lesions is often indistinguishable from that of malignancy. The treatment of direct breast trauma is oral analgesics, cold application, followed by heat application, breast support, and protection with padding. NSAIDs are contraindicated because of the risk of increased bleeding.[4] Sports participation should be limited until inflammation has subsided.

Running causes the female breasts to bounce vertically and slap against the chest wall, producing breast contusions and soreness. Women with large breasts are especially at risk for running-induced breast injury. Inadequate breast support may also result in stretching of the Cooper ligaments, the structures that attach the breast to the chest wall. This has been called *runner's breast* and often results in pain. Chronic lack of breast support may exacerbate ptosis, or sagging, of the breasts. Sports brassieres have been shown to help prevent runner's breast and breast ptosis by limiting breast motion during running and by holding the breasts against the chest wall.

Many different sports bras are available to the consumer. Large-breasted women generally require more rigidity in the bra construction than do smaller-breasted athletes. Athletes who compete in sports that require overhead arm activities require elastic shoulder straps to avoid the bra's riding up. Runners who engage in little overhead activity are better served by wide, nonstretch shoulder straps. In addition to the shoulder straps, support should come from lift provided below the breasts. The bra fabric should contain adequate cotton to allow absorbency, whereas elasticity should be minimized but sufficient to permit easy respiration. Insertable protective cup pads are desirable for participants in contact sports. The bra design should avoid irritating seams or fasteners and should include nonslip shoulder straps; rounded cup shapes that hold the breasts firmly against the body; and firm, durable construction. Better support may be achieved, with breast motion reduced by 50%, when a 4-inch or 6-inch (10 to 15 cm) elastic binder wrap or tensor is worn over a sports bra.[114]

Injuries to the male breast are similar to those affecting female breasts, occurring in the form of contusions secondary to direct trauma. Symptoms include inflammation around the nipple and areola, erythema, tenderness, and a serous nipple discharge. Treatment is heat application and protective pads. On occasion a painful, fibrous nodule persists and may require surgical excision.[115]

Both female and male athletes may experience nipple skin friction, or "runner's nipples," from a running shirt. This may be avoided by wearing a noncotton synthetic shirt or by applying a protective Band-Aid or dab of petroleum jelly over the nipple.

Effort Thrombosis

Vascular injuries are an extremely rare cause of shoulder pain. Repetitive trauma to the subclavian or axillary vein from the motion of an overhead throwing athlete may lead to a condition known as *effort thrombosis* or *Paget-Schroetter syndrome*. In this condition the athlete will present with pain, swelling, heaviness, and fatigue in the affected extremity as well as numbness. Ultrasound or venogram may be used to confirm the diagnosis. A chest x-ray examination should always be performed to rule out a cervical rib. Treatment consists of rest, elevation, and anticoagulation with heparin with a transition to warfarin (Coumadin). The long-term use of warfarin for anticoagulation precludes the return to contact as well as many noncontact sports. Effort thrombosis often recurs if the athlete returns to the prior level of activity once off of warfarin therapy.[4]

Intrathoracic Injuries
Evaluation of the Injured Athlete

Tissue hypoxia is the critical pathological condition responsible for the high morbidity and mortality associated with chest injuries. Hypoxia and metabolic acidosis may result from various mechanisms, including hypoventilation, hypoxemia, respiratory alkalosis, reduced cardiac output, and pulmonary shunting. The clinician's initial evaluation of the athlete with an isolated chest injury should include assessments of the airway, breathing, and circulation. This should identify the presence of any acutely life-threatening conditions, such as airway obstruction, massive hemothorax, cardiac tamponade (acute compression of heart), tension pneumothorax, flail chest, open pneumothorax, and massive tracheoesophageal air leakage, and allow for their appropriate management.

Acute Life-Threatening Conditions Associated with Abdominal and Thoracic Injuries

- Airway obstruction
- Hemothorax
- Cardiac tamponade
- Tension pneumothorax
- Flail chest
- Open pneumothorax
- Tracheoesophageal air leakage

The airway should be checked for obstruction by listening for air movement at the mouth and nose, observing for intercostal and supraclavicular muscle retractions, monitoring the respiratory rate and pattern, and recognizing the presence of cyanosis. To properly assess breathing, the chest must be completely exposed, and respirations should be observed, palpated, and auscultated. Circulation is evaluated by monitoring the rate, regularity, and quality of the pulse and the width of the pulse pressure. The neck veins should be examined for distention, and the peripheral circulation must be judged by skin temperature and color.

Upper airway obstruction results in an ashen, gray, or cyanotic skin color; an absence of normal breath sounds, often with gurgling or stridor; and the use of accessory respiratory muscles. The presence of paradoxical respiratory chest movements may be due to a flail chest, which should be apparent if the chest has been properly exposed. Sucking wounds of the chest should be evident by their characteristic sound. A large hemothorax may be suspected by the presence of dullness to percussion over the affected lung field. A tension pneumothorax results in absent breath sounds on the affected side with tracheal deviation contralaterally. Cardiac tamponade produces a narrowed pulse pressure and distended neck veins.

Pulmonary Injuries

Contusion. Most cases of pulmonary contusion result from motor vehicle accidents, although athletes may experience blunt chest trauma of sufficient force to cause the condition. Trauma-induced alveolar capillary damage with interstitial and intra-alveolar hemorrhage leads to pulmonary parenchymal edema and hemorrhage, atelectasis, and copious tracheobronchial secretions, which may impair pulmonary function. Hypoxemia ensues because of the ventilation-perfusion mismatch that is created.[14]

Initial chest radiographs are often normal, but unilateral or bilateral, patchy, ill-defined pulmonary infiltrates may develop within 1 to 6 hours of injury.[14] Thus, if a pulmonary contusion is suspected, the athlete should be admitted to the hospital, and serial chest x-ray films should be obtained. CT scan has recently gained favor because of its high diagnostic sensitivity in the early stages of contusion.[116]

Clinical Caution

Patients with pulmonary contusions may have normal initial chest radiographs, but pulmonary infiltrates can develop within 1 to 6 hours of injury.[14] If the mechanism of injury is indicative of a pulmonary contusion, the athlete should be admitted to the hospital for serial chest x-ray examinations or a computed tomography scan.

The symptoms of a mild contusion include tachypnea, tachycardia, the presence of rales on auscultation of the lung fields, and a cough with abundant blood-tinged secretions (hemoptysis). Hemoptysis is present in 50% of all patients with pulmonary contusion.[90] The treatment of mild pulmonary contusion incorporates pulmonary physical therapy, nasotracheal suctioning, analgesics, humidified oxygen supplementation, bronchodilators as needed, and appropriate antibiotic therapy or prophylaxis. In general, mild pulmonary contusions are self-limited and the athlete may begin gradual training as soon as the symptoms resolve and there is radiographic resolution with the knowledge that both exercise tolerance and reserve will be greatly lowered.[14,117]

Clinical Note

The athlete who has suffered a mild pulmonary contusion may return to gradual training as soon as the symptoms resolve and there is radiographic resolution.

Severe pulmonary contusions often occur in conjunction with extrathoracic injuries, which may detract from the danger of the pulmonary damage. Children are prone to pulmonary contusions in the absence of rib fractures because the compressive nature of their rib cages allows the force of the impact to be primarily transmitted to the lungs.[117] A severe contusion results in an increased alveolar-to-arterial oxygen gradient and reduced arterial oxygen pressure while breathing 100% oxygen, in addition to the presence of frankly bloody tracheobronchial secretions and progressive respiratory failure. Despite aggressive treatment with mechanical ventilation, tracheobronchial suctioning, bronchodilators, and diuretics to reduce pulmonary edema, this condition may prove fatal.

Pneumothorax. Pneumothorax is the most common complication of rib fractures and the most common intrathoracic injury following blunt thoracic trauma.[117] A fractured rib edge may puncture the pleura and lung to cause a leakage of air into the intrapleural space (i.e., a pneumothorax). A simple pneumothorax may also occur in the absence of rib fractures. Mechanisms of injury include sudden compression of the chest while the glottis is closed with resultant alveolar blowout and spontaneous bleb rupture. Most episodes of simple pneumothorax are self-limited in that the apposition of the lung and pleural surfaces tends to seal the air leak. The findings of dyspnea, cyanosis, and progressive respiratory collapse are consistent with severe cases. Signs of pulmonary insufficiency may be absent, however, in young, athletic individuals because of their large functional cardiopulmonary reserve.

Clinical Caution

A young athletic individual who has suffered a thoracic injury resulting in a pneumothorax may not show the signs of pulmonary insufficiency such as dyspnea, cyanosis, and progressive respiratory collapse because of their large functional cardiopulmonary reserve.

The physical examination may reveal tachypnea, decreased breath sounds to auscultation, and hyperresonance to percussion. Chest radiography often confirms the presence of a pneumothorax, and the sensitivity is improved further by obtaining upright inspiration and expiration films (Figure 25-15).

The treatment of a simple pneumothorax depends on the percentage of lung volume that is lost, the severity of pulmonary compromise, and the need for general anesthesia to address associated injuries. The size of a pneumothorax is estimated as a percentage of volume loss within a hemithorax, by viewing the chest radiograph. Generally, a pneumothorax of 15% to 25% without respiratory distress or the need for general anesthesia may be treated without a chest tube.[117] Serial chest radiographs should be obtained to confirm improvement. A pneumothorax should resorb by

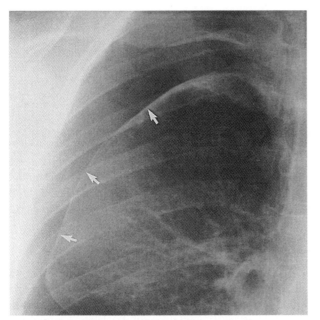

Figure 25-15
Pneumothorax on radiograph. *Arrows* point to edge of lung tissue that has collapsed. (From Fraser RS, Muller NL, Colman NC, Paré PD, editors: *Fraser and Paré's diagnosis of diseases of the chest,* ed 4, Philadelphia, 1970, WB Saunders.)

approximately 1% volume per day. Aspiration of small, apical pneumothoraces via serial catheterization has been done, with some authors reporting an earlier hospital discharge.[90] Physical activity should be restricted during recovery.

A pneumothorax occupying more than 30% of the hemithorax, associated with pulmonary compromise, or in conjunction with other injuries that may require general anesthesia for treatment should be treated with a chest tube. The chest tube is generally inserted in the third intercostal space at the anterior axillary line and is connected to underwater seal drainage, with or without suction. Re-expansion of the lung occurs relatively rapidly when a chest tube is placed, because the leak becomes sealed as a result of apposition of the visceral and parietal pleurae. The chest tube is removed once the leak has been eliminated for 24 hours. Return to vigorous athletic participation should be restricted for 3 to 4 weeks and contact sports avoided for 4 to 6 weeks.[118,119]

Clinical Note

A pneumothorax of 15% to 25% without respiratory distress may be treated without a chest tube, but if it occupies more than 30% of the hemithorax and is associated with pulmonary compromise, it should be treated with a chest tube.

Spontaneous pneumothorax, in the absence of trauma, may occur in individuals with a congenital predisposition for pulmonary bleb rupture. Usually these patients are tall,

thin males who are likely to be smokers. Onset of symptoms may be insidious to acute and there is a 20% to 50% recurrence rate.[120,121] Surgical resection of a nest of pulmonary apical blebs is often recommended after a third pneumothorax has occurred.[120]

Tension Pneumothorax. Tension pneumothorax is a severe, life-threatening form of pneumothorax. This may develop secondary to a rib fracture that produces a tangential tear in the pulmonary parenchyma, resulting in a flapvalve mechanism that permits air to enter the pleural space during inspiration. The evolution of positive intrapleural pressure relative to the atmosphere may cause the mediastinum to shift away from the injured side, compression of the vena cava, reduced cardiac diastolic filling, and decreased cardiac output. If untreated, a tension pneumothorax may rapidly progress to fatal hypoxia and acidosis. The symptoms of tension pneumothorax include acute respiratory distress, restlessness, and agitation. The physical examination reveals tachypnea, hypotension, tachycardia, respiratory distress, absent breath sounds to auscultation, hyperresonance to percussion of the involved hemithorax, and tracheal deviation toward the uninvolved side.

Signs of Tension Pneumothorax

- Tachypnea
- Hypotension
- Tachycardia
- Respiratory distress
- Absent breath sounds to auscultation
- Hyper-resonance to percussion of the involved hemithorax
- Tracheal deviation toward the uninvolved side

Early treatment of a tension pneumothorax is crucial, and thus confirmation with chest radiographs is usually not possible. The immediate treatment involves the insertion of a 14- to 18-gauge needle into the pleural cavity through the second intercostal space in the midclavicular line (Figure 25-16). The needle should pass over the superior edge of the third rib, so as not to damage the neurovascular bundle. If the correct diagnosis has been made, the puncture should produce a rush of air and immediate clinical improvement. This procedure converts a tension pneumothorax into a much less serious simple pneumothorax. It is far better to produce a pneumothorax while erring on the side of aggressiveness in relieving a tension pneumothorax than to allow the progression of respiratory collapse.

Hemothorax. Hemothorax, a collection of blood within the thoracic cavity, is a common sequela of blunt chest trauma. The source of bleeding may be from a rib fracture–induced lung laceration, or from a compression "blowout" injury. Bleeding from the lung tends to be selflimited because of the relatively low pulmonary vasculature pressure. If an intercostal artery is lacerated, however, the

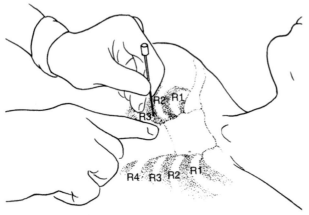

Figure 25-16

Emergent needle decompression of a tension pneumothorax is achieved by inserting a 14- to 18-gauge needle into the second intercostal space (at the level of the angle of Louis) in the midclavicular line. The needle should be inserted over the superior aspect of the rib to avoid injury to the intercostal vessels that course along the inferior edge of the rib. As extrapulmonary intrathoracic air under pressure is evacuated through the needle, the tension pneumothorax is converted to a simple pneumothorax, which is far better-tolerated physiologically and can then be treated with a chest tube.

bleeding may be brisk and severe. Symptoms associated with a large hemothorax (400 mL or more) may include hypotension, hypovolemia, reduced cardiac output, hypoxia, compression of the ipsilateral lung, and deviation of the mediastinum away from the involved side. A small hemothorax of less than 400 mL is often asymptomatic.

The physical examination reveals dullness to percussion over the hemothorax, reduced or absent breath sounds, less tactile fremitus (vibration of chest wall), and mediastinal shift toward the uninvolved side. A chest x-ray film will show blunting of the costophrenic angles with as little as 250 to 300 mL of fluid collection.

The treatment depends on the clinical condition. If the hemothorax is small, serial chest x-ray films may be obtained for several days to ensure blood resorption, which is usually completed within 2 weeks. If blood appears to occupy one third or more of the hemithorax (500 to 2000 mL), a large-bore chest tube should be placed in the sixth intercostal space at the anterior axillary line. If bleeding is noted to continue at a rate of at least 300 mL per hour or if serial chest x-ray films show a worsening radiographic appearance, emergency thoracotomy is indicated.

Mediastinal or Subcutaneous Emphysema. Fractured ribs may result in the leakage of air into the mediastinum with spread into the subcutaneous soft tissues of the upper chest and neck. Clinically, subcutaneous emphysema is apparent by swelling of the neck and characteristic crepitation under the skin. On rare occasions, mediastinal air may be under sufficient pressure to force collapse of the great veins, which restricts blood return to the right side of the heart and consequently causes cardiac decompensation.

Clinical Caution

Although the majority of subcutaneous emphysema caused by rib fractures resolves spontaneously, occasionally cardiac decompensation may occur as a result of pressurized mediastinal air, forcing collapse of the great veins and restricting blood return to the right side of the heart.

Subcutaneous emphysema typically resolves spontaneously. On occasion, however, the affected individual should be hospitalized for observation, and serial x-ray films taken to rule out progression of the condition.

Cardiac Injuries

Myocardial Contusion. Blunt trauma to the chest wall may produce cardiac contusion. The most common mechanism of this injury is compression of the sternum against the steering wheel, as occurs in a rapid-deceleration motor vehicle accident. Although cardiac contusion is not a common form of sports trauma, participants in sports that involve great velocities and forces may sustain this injury. Examples of these include car racing, cycling, skiing, sky diving, and rock climbing. The majority of patients with cardiac contusion will have associated injuries such as pulmonary contusion, pneumothorax, or damage to the great vessels.[122]

Sports Associated with Myocardial Contusion

- Car racing
- Cycling
- Skiing
- Sky diving
- Rock climbing

The degree of myocardial injury ranges from localized contusion of the anterior myocardium to complete myocardial rupture. Prompt recognition of even mild cardiac contusions is essential, because delayed ventricular rupture may occur for up to several months after the injury.

Clinical Caution

There is still the risk of ventricular rupture for months after sustaining a myocardial contusion.

Significant cardiac events tend to be rare in young patients who are the victim of blunt trauma to the chest,[14] but on occasion the coronary arteries may be damaged, resulting in thrombosis that may lead to myocardial infarction. Additional potential complications of cardiac contusion are right-sided heart failure, hypotension, arrhythmia, and rupture of the intraventricular septum, with a resultant acute left-to-right shunt.[14]

Cardiac contusion is diagnosed by maintaining suspicion based on the mechanism of injury and by the characteristic electrocardiographic changes that are consistent with myocardial damage. Of all patients with cardiac contusion, 70% show sinus tachycardia on electrocardiogram (ECG).[90] Other ECG findings include premature atrial and ventricular complexes. In addition to an ECG, the athlete suspected of having a myocardial contusion should have serial cardiac enzymes and an echocardiogram. Unfortunately, the available diagnostic tools are not specific for cardiac contusion and are unable to predict the risk of complications.

General Workup for an Athlete with Suspicion of Cardiac Contusion Should Include:

- Electrocardiogram
- Serial cardiac enzymes
- Echocardiogram
- Admission to hospital for 24 hours of observation
- Consultation with a cardiologist

The treatment of cardiac contusion is similar to that for acute myocardial infarction, including electrocardiographic monitoring in a hospital coronary care unit and cardiovascular support. The athlete with a mechanism suspicious for cardiac contusion should be admitted for 24 hours of observation even if the athlete is asymptomatic because dysrhythmias have been shown to develop in the first 12 hours after injury.[117]

Clinical Caution

Dysrhythmias are most likely to develop in the first twelve hours after suffering a cardiac contusion.

The presence of arrhythmia, heart failure, elevated creatine kinase myocardial band, or wall motion abnormalities requires a longer inpatient observation period. Decisions on return to play after cardiac contusion depend on the extent of the injury and the presence of associated injuries. Consultation with a cardiologist is recommended.[91]

Commotio Cordis. *Commotio cordis* is the commonly used term for ventricular fibrillation resulting from a sudden blow to the anterior chest wall during an extremely vulnerable time in the cardiac cycle.[123,124] Ultimately, commotio cordis may lead to sudden cardiac death. The automated external defibrillator (AED) should be used if an episode of commotio cordis occurs. If an AED is not available, a precordial "thump" can be given to start the heart.[123] Commotio cordis has been seen in such sports as youth baseball, lacrosse, hockey, cricket, and soccer.

Clinical Note

An automated external defibrillator should be kept with the trainer's equipment at athletic activities. In the unlikely event that one is not available or malfunctioning, a precordial thump may be used in the event of a witnessed episode of commotio cordis.

Pericardial Tamponade. Acute hemorrhage into the pericardial cavity, or pericardial tamponade, is an uncommon athletic injury. Blunt trauma of a force sufficient to rupture the myocardium or lacerate a coronary artery may give rise to this often fatal injury. The most common mechanism of injury is a penetrating wound to the chest, such as that inflicted by a knife. This type of injury is not expected to occur in most sporting events, but it may transpire accidentally in sports that use high-speed, sharp objects or missiles carrying a risk of impalement. Examples include arrows in archery, the javelin in field events, and the epée in fencing.

Clinical features of a small cardiac tamponade include neck vein distension, pulsus paradoxus (pulse becomes weaker with inhalation and stronger with exhalation), shock, and cyanosis. Prompt recognition of the diagnosis, with confirmation by echocardiography, if immediately available, should direct urgent pericardiocentesis. The definitive treatment is thoracotomy with pericardial decompression, and suture repair of the damaged myocardium. Massive cardiac tamponade almost always results in immediate death.

Physical Signs of Pericardial Tamponade

- Neck vein distension
- Shock
- Cyanosis
- Pulsus paradoxus (an abnormal decrease [< 10 mm Hg] in systolic pressure and pulse wave amplitude during inspiration)

Rupture of the Aorta. Rupture of the aorta is a rare complication of blunt chest trauma in which the descending aorta undergoes torsion, and the aortic wall is disrupted at the ligamentum arteriosum. Occasionally, damage occurs to the ascending aorta at the root of the heart. Most victims of aortic rupture die immediately from massive exsanguination, but a few survive as a result of the formation of a "false aneurysm" between the periaortic tissues and the pleura. The diagnosis may be suspected on the basis of widening of the cardiac silhouette on chest radiograph. CT scan, MRI scan, or retrograde aortography is confirmatory. The treatment is immediate surgical repair.

Esophageal Injury

Most injuries to the esophagus are the result of penetrating trauma rather than blunt injury. Esophageal perforation may manifest as extreme chest pain followed by the gradual onset of fever over several hours. Regurgitation of blood, hoarseness, dysphagia, and respiratory distress may also be present. The chest radiograph may show mediastinal air, widening, and a pleural effusion. The diagnosis is confirmed by water-soluble contrast radiography or esophagoscopy. The treatment is immediate surgical debridement, suture closure of damaged tissues, and drainage.

Conclusion

The abdominal cavity, by nature of its relative lack of bony protection, is quite susceptible to blunt trauma injury during athletics. The structures of the abdominal wall are often injured by direct compression forces, whereas the intra-abdominal organs are often damaged by compression against the spine. Injuries to the abdomen may become life-threatening, particularly if significant time passes without treatment. A major exsanguination from a ruptured blood vessel may rapidly progress to shock and death without prompt, appropriate treatment.

Thoracic injuries are more likely to be life-threatening because of a disruption of the cardiopulmonary systems. Most serious intrathoracic injuries result from shearing forces of deceleration that may disrupt vital structures. Penetrating trauma from objects such as a displaced rib fracture must also be considered as causes of thoracic injury. Injuries to the surface of the thorax typically manifest as muscle strains or ruptures, contusions, or bony fractures. The athletic health care professional must be well trained and knowledgeable in the early assessment, stabilization, and management of the various types of traumatic injuries that may involve the abdomen and chest.

References

1. Johnson R: Abdominal wall injuries: Rectus abdominis strains, oblique strains, rectus sheath hematoma, *Curr Sports Med Rep* 5(2):99–103, 2006.
2. Bergqvist D, Hedelin H, Karlsson G, et al: Abdominal injury from sporting activities, *Br J Sports Med* 16:76–79, 1982.
3. Diamond DL: Sports-related abdominal trauma. In Ray RL, editor: *Clinics in sports medicine—Emergency treatment of the injured athlete*, Philadelphia, 1989, WB Saunders.
4. Amaral JF: Thoracoabdominal injuries in the athlete, *Clin Sports Med* 16(4):739–753, 1997.
5. Maquirriain J, Ghisi JP, Kokalj AM: Rectus abdominis muscle strains in tennis players. *Br J Sports Med* 41(11):842–848, 2007.
6. Taylor DC, Meyers WC, Moylan JA, et al: Abdominal musculature abnormalities as a cause of groin pain in athletes, *Am J Sports Med* 19:239–242, 1991.
7. De Shazo WF: Hematoma of the rectus abdominis in football, *Phys Sports Med* 12:73–75, 1984.
8. US Department of Health, Education, and Welfare: *National health survey of hernias*, Series B, No. 25, Dec 1960.
9. Nyhus LM, Bombeck CT: Hernias. In Sabiston DC, editor: *Textbook of surgery—The biological basis of modern surgical practice*, ed 13, Philadelphia, 1986, WB Saunders.
10. Smedberg SGG, Broome AEA, Gullmo A, Roos H: Herniography in athletes with groin pain, *Am J Surg* 140:378–382, 1985.
11. Kluin J, den Hoed PT, van Linschoten R, et al: Endoscopic evaluation and treatment of groin pain in the athlete, *Am J Sports Med* 32(4):944–949, 2004.
12. De Paulis F, Cacchio A, Michelini O, et al: Sports injuries in the pelvis and hip: Diagnostic imaging, *Eur J Radiol* 27 Suppl 1:S49–59, 1998.
13. Haycock CE: How I manage hernias in the athlete, *Phys Sports Med* 11:77–79, 1983.
14. Lawrence PF, Bell RM, Dayton MT, Ahmed MI: *Essentials of general surgery*, ed 3, Philadelphia, 2000, Lippincott Williams & Wilkins.
15. Stoker DL, Spiegelhalter DJ, Singh R, Wellwood JM: Laparoscopic versus open inguinal hernia repair: Randomized prospective trial. *Lancet* 343:1243–1245, 1994.
16. Renstrom P, Peterson L: Groin injuries in athletes, *Br J Sports Med* 14:30–36, 1980.
17. Ekstrand J, Hilding J: The incidence and differential diagnosis of acute groin injuries in male soccer players, *Scand J Med Sci Sports* 9:98–103, 1999.
18. Meyers WC, McKechnie A, Philippon MJ, et al: Experience with "sports hernia" spanning two decades, *Ann Surg* 248(4):656–665, 2008.
19. Lovell G: The diagnosis of chronic groin pain in athletes: A review of 189 cases, *Aust J Sci Med Sport* 27:76–79, 1995.
20. Malycha P, Lovell G: Inguinal surgery in athletes with chronic groin pain: The "sportsman's" hernia, *Aust N Z J Surg* 62:123–125, 1992.
21. Ahumada LA, Ashruf S, Espinosa-de-los-Monteros A, et al: Athletic pubalgia: Definition and surgical treatment, *Ann Plast Surg* 55:393–396, 2005.
22. Polglase AL, Frydman GM, Farmer KC: Inguinal surgery for debilitating chronic groin pain in athletes, *Med J Aust* 155:674–677, 1991.
23. Larson CM, Lohnes JH: Surgical management of athletic pubalgia, *Oper Tech Sports Med* 10:228–232, 2002.
24. Meyers WC, Foley DP, Garrett WE, et al: Management of severe lower abdominal or inguinal pain in high performance athletes: PAIN (Performing athletes with Abdominal or Inguinal Neuromuscular Pain Study Group), *Am J Sports Med* 28:2–8, 2000.
25. Leblanc KE, Leblanc KA: Groin pain in athletes, *Hernia* 7:68–71, 2003.
26. Hackney RG: The sports hernia: A cause of chronic groin pain, *Br J Sports Med* 27:58–62, 1993.
27. Renstrom P: Tendon and muscle injuries in the groin area, *Clin Sports Med* 11:815–830, 1992.
28. Steele P, Annear P, Grove JR: Surgery for posterior wall inguinal deficiency in athletes, *J Sci Med Sport* 7:415–421, 2004.
29. Gentisaris M, Goulimaris I, Sikas N: Laparoscopic repair of groin pain in athletes, *Am J Sports Med* 32:1238–1242, 2004.

30. Farber AJ, Wilckens JH: Sports hernia: Diagnosis and therapeutic approach, *J Am Acad Orthop Surg* 15(8):507–514, 2007.

31. Verrall GM, Slavotinek JP, Fon GT: Incidence of pubic bone marrow edema in Australian rules football players: Relation to groin pain, *Br J Sports Med* 35:28–33, 2001.

32. Albers SL, Spritzer CE, Garrett WE, Meyers WC: MR findings in athletes with pubalgia, *Skeletal Radiol* 30: 270–277, 2001.

33. Shortt CP, Zoga AC, Kavanagh EC, Meyers WC: Anatomy, pathology, and MRI findings in the sports hernia, *Semin Musculoskelet Radiol* 12(1):54–61, 2008.

34. Zajick DC, Zoga AC, Omar IM, Meyers WC: Spectrum of MRI findings in the sports hernia, *Semin Musculoskelet Radiol* 12(1): 3–12, 2008.

35. Zoga AC, Kavanagh EC, Omar IM, et al: Athletic pubalgia and the "sports hernia": MR imaging findings, *Radiology* 247(3): 797–807, 2008.

36. Orchard JW, Read JW, Neophyton J, Garlick D: Groin pain associated with ultrasound finding of inguinal canal posterior wall deficiency in Australian rules footballers, *Br J Sports Med* 32: 134–139, 1998.

37. Joesting DR: Diagnosis and treatment of sportman's hernia, *Curr Sports Med Reports* 1:121–124, 2002.

38. Sutcliffe JR, Taylor OM, Ambrose NS, Chapman AH: The use, value and safety of herniography, *Clin Radiol* 54:468–472, 1999.

39. Hamlin JA, Kahn AM: Herniography: A review of 333 herniograms, *Am Surg* 64:965–969, 1998.

40. Ekberg O: Complications after herniography in adults, *Am J Roentgenol* 140:491–495, 1983.

41. Unverzagt CA, Schuemann T, Mathisen J: Differential diagnosis of a sports hernia in a high school athlete, *J Orthop Sports Phys Ther* 38(2):63–70, 2008.

42. Liem M, van der Graaf Y, van Steensel CJ, et al: Comparison of conventional anterior surgery and laparoscopic surgery for inguinal hernia repair, *N Engl J Med* 336:1541–1547, 1997.

43. Swan KG, Wolcott M: The athletic hernia, *Clin Orthop Relat Res* 455:78–87, 2007.

44. Bradshaw C, McCrory P, Bell S, Brukner P: Obturator nerve entrapment: A cause of groin pain in athletes, *Am J Sports Med* 25(3):403–409, 1997.

45. Douglas DM: The healing of aponeurotic incisions, *Br J Surg* 40:79, 1952.

46. Olsen WR: Abdominal trauma in the athlete. In Schneider RC, Kennedy JC, Plant ML, editors: *Sports injuries—Mechanisms, prevention, and treatment,* Baltimore, 1985, Williams & Wilkins.

47. Higgins GL: Penetrating trauma—Managing and preventing javelin wounds, *Phys Sports Med* 22:88–94, 1994.

48. Green GA: Gastrointestinal disorders in the athlete, *Sports Med* 11:453–470, 1992.

49. American College of Surgeons: Abdominal trauma. In *Advanced trauma life support student manual,* Chicago, 1989, American College of Surgeons.

50. Coant PN, Kornberg AE, Brody AS, Edwards-Holmes K: Markers for occult liver injury in cases of physical abuse in children, *Pediatrics* 89:274–278, 1992.

51. Fabian TC, Croce MA: Abdominal trauma, including indications for celiotomy. In Feliciano DV, Moore EE, Mattox KL, editors: *Trauma,* ed 3, Stamford, CT, 1996, Appleton & Lange.

52. Wan J, Corvino TF, Greenfield SP, DiScala C: Kidney and testicle injuries in team and individual sports: Data from the national pediatric trauma registry, *J Urol* 170:1528–1532, 2003.

53. Affleck TP: Severe sports-related spleen injury, *Phys Sports Med* 20:109–123, 1992.

54. Buntain WL, Gould HR, Maull KI: Predictability of splenic salvage by computed tomography. *J Trauma* 28:24–34, 1988.

55. Waninger KN, Harcke HT: Determination of safe return to play for athletes recovering from infectious mononucleosis: A review of the literature. *Clin J Sports Med* 15(6):410–416, 2005.

56. Mostafa G, Matthews BD, Sing RF, et al: Elective laparoscopic splenectomy for grade III splenic injury in an athlete. *Surg Laparosc Endosc Percutan Tech* 12(4):283–286; discussion 286–288, 2002.

57. Kinderknecht JJ: Infectious mononucleosis and the spleen, *Curr Sports Med Rep* 1(2):116–120, 2002.

58. Maki DG, Reich RM: Infectious mononucleosis in the athlete: Diagnosis, complications, and management, *Am J Sports Med* 10:162–173, 1982.

59. Rutkow IM: Rupture of the spleen in infectious mononucleosis, *Arch Surg* 113:718–720, 1978.

60. Stricker PR, Hardin BH, Puffer JC: An unusual presentation of liver laceration in a 13-yr-old football player, *Med Sci Sports Exerc* 25:667–672, 1993.

61. Mustalich AC, Quash ET: Sports injuries to the chest and abdomen. In Scott WN, Nisonson B, Nicholas JA, editors: *Principles of sports medicine,* Baltimore, 1984, Williams & Wilkins.

62. Hiatt JR, Harrier D, Koenig BV, Ransom KJ: Nonoperative management of major blunt liver injury with hemoperitoneum, *Arch Surg* 125:101–103, 1990.

63. Moon KL, Federele MP: CT in hepatic trauma, *Am J Radiol* 141:309–314, 1983.

64. Cywes S, Rode H: Blunt liver trauma in children—Non-operative management, *J Pediatr Surg* 20:14–18, 1985.

65. Henderson JM, Puffer JC: Abdominal pain in a football player, *Phys Sports Med* 17:47–52, 1989.

66. Murphy CP, Drez D: Jejunal rupture in a football player, *Am J Sports Med* 15:184–185, 1987.

67. Moses FM: Exercise-associated intestinal ischemia, *Curr Sports Med Reports* 4(2):91–95, 2005 Apr.

68. Glenn JF, Harvard BM: The injured kidney, *JAMA* 173:1189, 1960.

69. McAleer IM, Kaplan GW, LoSasso BE: Renal and testis injuries in team sports, *J Urol* 168:1805–1807, 2002.

70. Brophy RH, Gamradt SC, Barnes RP, et al: Kidney injuries in professional American football: Implications for management of an athlete with 1 functioning kidney, *Am J Sports Med* 36(1): 85–90, 2008.

71. Kallmeyer JC, Miller NM: Urinary changes in ultra long-distance marathon runners, *Nephron* 64(1):119–121, 1993.

72. Peterson NE: Genitourinary trauma. In Feliciano DV, Moore EE, Mattox KL, editors: *Trauma,* ed 3, Stamford, CT, 1996, Appleton & Lange.

73. Holmes FC, Hunt JJ, Sevier TL: Renal injury in sport, *Curr Sports Med Reports* 2(2):103–109, 2003.

74. Kulund DN: *The injured athlete,* Philadelphia, 1982, JB Lippincott.

75. Dorsen PJ: Should athletes with one eye, kidney, or testicle play contact sports? *Phys Sportsmed* 14:130, 1986.

76. Anderson CR: Solitary kidney and sports participation, *Arch Fam Med* 4:886, 1994.

77. Psooy K: Sports and the solitary kidney: How to counsel parents, *Can J Urol* 13(3):3120–3126, 2006.

78. Kenney P: Abdominal pain in athletes, *Clin Sports Med* 6: 885–904, 1987.

79. Stricker PR, Puffer JC: Case report: Renal laceration—A skateboarder's symptoms are delayed, *Phys Sports Med* 21:59–68, 1993.

80. Siegel AJ, Hennekens CH, Soloman HS, Van Boeckel B: Exercise-related hematuria, *JAMA* 241:391–392, 1979.

81. Blalock NJ: Bladder trauma in long-distance runners, *Am J Sports Med* 7:239–241, 1979.
82. Echlin PS, Klein WB: Pancreatic injury in the athlete, *Curr Sports Med Reports* 4(2):96–101, 2005.
83. Hoover DL: How I manage testicular injury, *Phys Sports Med* 14:127–129, 1986.
84. Thomas PL: Thoracic back pain in rowers and butterfly swimmers: Costo vertebral subluxation, *Br J Sports Med* 2(2):81, 1988.
85. Gregory PL, Biswas AC, Batt ME: Musculoskeletal problems of the chest wall in athletes, *Sports Med* 32(4):235–250, 2002.
86. Disla E, Rhim HR, Reddy A, et al: Costochondritis: A prospective analysis in an emergency department setting, *Arch Int Med* 154(21):2466–2469, 1994.
87. Thompson BM, Finger W, Tonsfeldt D: Rib radiographs for trauma: Useful or wasteful? *Ann Emerg Med* 15:261–265, 1986.
88. DeLuca SA, Rhea JT, O'Malley T: Radiographic evaluation of rib fractures, *Am J Roentgenol* 138:91–92, 1982.
89. De Lacey G: Clinical and economic aspects of the use of x-rays in accident and emergency departments, *Proc R Soc Med* 69:758–759, 1976.
90. Eckstein M, Henderson S, Markovchick V: Thoracic trauma. In Marx JA, Hockberger RS, Walls RM, editors: *Rosen's emergency medicine*, ed 5, St Louis, 2002, Mosby.
91. Perron AD: Chest pain in athletes, *Clin Sports Med* 22:37–50, 2003.
92. Sullivan JA: In Grana WA, Kalenak A, editors: *Clinical sports medicine*, Philadelphia, 1991, WB Saunders.
93. Karlson KA: Rib stress fractures in elite rowers: A case series and proposed mechanism, *Am J Sports Med* 26(4):516–519, 1998.
94. Mithofer K, Giza E: Pseudoarthrosis of the first rib in the overhead athlete, *Br J Sports Med* 38(2):221–222, 2004.
95. Cope R: Dislocations of the sternoclavicular joint, *Skeletal Radiol* 22:233–238, 1993.
96. Ferrera PC, Wheeling HM: Sternoclavicular joint injuries, *Am J Emerg Med* 18:58–61, 2000.
97. Jougon JB, Lepront DJ, Dromer CEH: Posterior dislocation of the sternoclavicular joint leading to mediastinal compression, *Ann Thorac Surg* 61:711–713, 1996.
98. Fererra PC, Williams CC: Posterior sternoclavicular joint dislocation, *Phys Sportsmed* 27:105–113, 1999.
99. Djerf K, Tropp H, Asberg B: Case report: Retrosternal clavicular dislocation in the sternoclavicular joint, *Clin Radiol* 53:75–76, 1998.
100. Lee FA, Gwinn JL: Retrosternal dislocation of the clavicle, *Radiology* 110:631–634, 1974.
101. Destout JM, Gilula LA, Murphy WA, et al: Computed tomography of the sternoclavicular joint and sternum, *Radiology* 138:123–128, 1981.
102. Chiu WC, D'Amelio LF, Hammond JS: Sternal fracture in blunt chest trauma: A practical algorithm for management, *Am J Emerg Med* 15:252–255, 1997.
103. Wright SW: Myth of the dangerous sternal fracture, *Ann Emerg Med* 22:1589–1592, 1993.
104. Jones HK, McBride GG, Mumby RC: Sternal fractures associated with spinal injury, *J Trauma* 29:360–364, 1989.
105. Hills MW, Delprado AM, Deane SA: Sternal fractures: Associated injuries and management, *J Trauma* 35:55–60, 1993.
106. Sturm JT, Luxenberg MG, Moudry BM, et al: Does sternal fracture increase the risk for aortic rupture? *Ann Thorac Surg* 48:697–698, 1989.
107. Miller MD, Johnson DL, Fu FH: Rupture of the pectoralis major muscle in a collegiate football player: Use of magnetic resonance imaging in early diagnosis, *Am J Sports Med* 21:475–477, 1993.
108. Wolfe SW, Wickiewicz TL, Cavanaugh JT: Ruptures of the pectoralis major muscle, *Am J Sports Med* 20:587–593, 1992.
109. Zeman SC, Rosenfeld RT, Lipscomb PR: Tears of the pectoralis major muscle, *Am J Sports Med* 7:343–347, 1979.
110. McEntire JE, Hess WE, Coleman SS: Rupture of the pectoralis major muscle, *J Bone Joint Surg Am* 54:1040–1046, 1972.
111. Kakwani RG, Matthews JJ: Rupture of the pectoralis major muscle: Surgical treatment in athletes, *Int Orthop* 31:159–163, 2007.
112. Park JY, Espinella JL: Rupture of the pectoralis major muscle: A case report and review of the literature, *J Bone Joint Surg Am* 52:577–581, 1970.
113. Lorentzen D, Lawson L: Selected sports bras: A biomechanical analysis of breast motion while jogging, *Phys Sports Med* 15:128–139, 1987.
114. Gehlsen G, Albohm M: Evaluation of sports bras, *Phys Sports Med* 8:89–98, 1980.
115. O'Donoghue DH: *Treatment of injuries to athletes*, Philadelphia, 1984, WB Saunders.
116. Brooks AP, Olson LK: Computed tomography of the chest in the trauma patient, *Clin Radiol* 40:127–132, 1989.
117. Richardson M: Injury to the lung and pleura. In Feliciano DV, Moore EE, Mattox KL, editors: *Trauma*, ed 3, Stamford, CT, 1996, Appleton & Lange.
118. Curtin SM, Tucker AM, Gens DR: Pneumothorax in sports, *Phys Sportsmed* 28:23–32, 2000.
119. Partridge RA, Coley A, Bowie R, et al: Sports-related pneumothorax, *Ann Emerg Med* 30:539–541, 1997.
120. Schramel FM, Postmus PE, Vanderschueren RG: Current aspects of spontaneous pneumothorax, *Eur Respir J* 10(6):1372–1379, 1997.
121. Abolnik IZ, Lossos IS, Gillis D, et al: Primary spontaneous pneumothorax in men, *Am J Med Sci* 305:297–303, 1993.
122. Fabian TC, Kram HB, Appel PL, Shoemaker WL: Increased incidence of cardiac contusion in patients with traumatic thoracic aortic rupture, *Ann Surg* 208:615–618, 1988.
123. Geddes LA, Roeder RA: Evolution of our knowledge of sudden death due to commotio cordis, *Am J Emerg Med* 23:67–75, 2005.
124. Fuchs T: Commotio Cordis in an athlete, *Heart Rhythm* 2(9):991–993, 2005.

THE FEMALE ATHLETE

Janice Loudon, Lori A. Bolgla, and Steven A. Greer

Introduction

The opportunity for women and girls to participate in sports has increased dramatically. According to statistics from the National Collegiate Athletics Association (NCAA), female participation in collegiate sports has increased 456% between 1971 and 2005.[1] At the high school level, roughly one in three girls participate in organized sports. Benefits from participating in sports are significant. It has been demonstrated that athletic women and girls have improved health, better grades, and increased confidence, and are less likely to use drugs.

Along with these benefits comes an increased chance of injury. In 2000, 10-year NCAA data showed increased risk of the female knee to injury when compared with the male knee in comparable sports of soccer and basketball.[2] Several articles have been written hypothesizing the reason for this injury trend and some of this research is discussed in this chapter.

This chapter focuses on issues related to the female athlete. The physiological and musculoskeletal differences between males and females are reported first. This is followed by a discussion of common musculoskeletal injuries, the female athlete triad, and issues related to the older woman athlete.

Physiological Differences Between the Sexes

When comparing absolute strength, adolescent males score considerably higher in strength than adolescent females in all muscle groups. These differences are dramatic for the upper body, with males exhibiting 40% to 50% greater strength than females. In the lower body, the strength difference is less. Females average 20% to 30% less strength than males. This strength discrepancy decreases when relative values based on lean body mass are reported. The strength difference between sexes is due to males' total muscle mass and the presence of testosterone. There is no difference between the muscle structure of males and females.[3]

Relative maximal oxygen uptake (VO_2 max) for untrained women typically averages 15% to 30% below scores for men. In trained women, the difference becomes less, but women still present with a 10% to 15% lower VO_2 max. The apparent gender difference in aerobic capacity has been attributed to lower oxygen carrying capacity, lower blood volume, fewer red blood cells, lower hemoglobin content, smaller hearts, lower stroke volume, and smaller muscle fiber area in women. It does not appear that lactate threshold or efficiency varies between men and women.[3] A summary of these changes can be seen in Table 26-1.

Musculoskeletal Differences Between the Sexes

Related to the musculoskeletal system, there are differences between males and females that may make the female athlete more susceptible to certain injuries. Figure 26-1 portrays differences between the sexes. In the lower extremity, females present with an increased quadriceps angle (Q-angle), wider pelvis, increased genu valgum, and increased tibial torsion. Other differences include an increase in joint flexibility in the female including genu recurvatum which may contribute to less knee control. In the upper limb, cubitus valgus is more common in females.

Musculoskeletal Injuries

Much attention has focused on the causes and management of musculoskeletal injuries in the female athlete. Four of the common areas of interest include anterior cruciate ligament (ACL) injury, patellofemoral pain syndrome (PFPS), medial tibial stress syndrome (MTSS), and spine injuries.

Table 26-1
Physiological Differences between Adult Males and Females

Variable	Difference
Upper extremity strength	Males are 40% to 50% stronger
Lower extremity strength	Males are 20% to 30% stronger
VO$_2$ max (untrained)	Males are 15% to 30% higher
VO$_2$ max (trained)	Males are 10% to 15% higher

VO$_2$ max, Maximum oxygen consumption.

The purpose of the following sections is to provide the best available evidence to guide clinical decision making when treating the female athlete.

Anterior Cruciate Ligament Injury

ACL injury is one of the most serious knee injuries experienced by physically active individuals. The average estimated annual cost associated with treatment (e.g., diagnostic testing, surgical reconstruction, and rehabilitation) in the United States has been estimated to exceed $2 billion.[4] Despite progressive treatment, a risk remains for the development of knee osteoarthritis.[5,6] These findings have led to the identification of risk factors and the development of ACL-injury prevention programs.[7]

Nearly 70% of ACL injuries occur from a noncontact mechanism during sports such as basketball and soccer.[8] A common mechanism of injury involves deceleration or a sudden change in direction such as a cutting movement.[9] This maneuver may apply excessive torsional force onto the ACL and result in rupture.[4] Noncontact ACL injuries also may occur when landing from a jump with the body positioned in minimal hip and knee flexion. DeMorat and colleagues[10] have shown that excessive quadriceps force relative to the hamstring muscles can cause excessive tibial forward translation, especially with the knee positioned in minimal flexion.

Following the passage of Title IX, researchers have reported a higher relative incidence of ACL injury in females who participate in basketball and soccer.[8,11-13] Prodromos and colleagues[14] recently examined the incidence of ACL injury across gender and sport. They reported that female basketball and soccer players were generally three times more likely to sustain an ACL injury than males.

During the past 25 years, researchers have identified both intrinsic and extrinsic risk factors that may account for the ACL injury gender bias (Table 26-2). Intrinsic factors include anatomical or physiological factors such as intercondylar notch width, ACL size, posterior tibial slope, physiological laxity, and hormonal influences.[45] Extrinsic influences include biomechanical or neuromuscular factors such as in nature. They are modifiable to change and are the basis for many injury prevention programs.[46-48]

Intrinsic Risk Factors

ACL injury is thought to occur when the ligament is stretched excessively over the femoral condyles. This mechanism may occur with the abutment of the ACL within the intercondylar notch when the knee is positioned close to full extension.[49] Therefore, individuals with a decreased intercondylar notch size may be more prone to an ACL injury. Based on this theory, many investigators[15-17] have

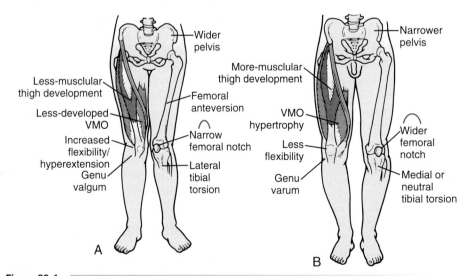

Figure 26-1
Musculoskeletal differences between the sexes. **A,** Female lower-extremity posture. **B,** Male lower-extremity posture. (From Griffin LY, editor: *Rehabilitation of the injured knee,* pp 298-299, St Louis, 1995, Mosby.)

Table 26-2

Summary of Intrinsic and Extrinsic Factors that May Contribute to Sex Differences Regarding Anterior Cruciate Ligament Injury

Intrinsic Factors	Extrinsic Factors
Intercondylar notch size[15-17]	Kinematics[31-38]
Anterior cruciate ligament size[16,18]	Quadriceps activation[33,39,40]
Tibial plateau slope[19-21]	Hip abductor strength[41,42]
Physiological laxity[22,23]	Fatigue[43,44]
Hormonal influences[24-30]	

examined a possible association between intercondylar notch size and ACL injury. To date, data have not supported an absolute relationship between decreased notch width and female ACL injury. Rather, it appears that both male and female athletes who have a smaller notch, and thus a smaller ACL, may be more susceptible to injury.[15,17]

Recently, Chandrashekar and colleagues[16] and Hashemi and colleagues[18] examined ACL sex differences using a cadaveric model (six male, mean age 34 years; six female, mean age 34 years). Ligaments from female specimens were smaller with respect to length, cross-sectional area, and volume, and had less stiffness. They attributed this sex difference to the amount of collagen fibrils present, because male specimens exhibited a higher percentage area filled with collagen fiber (e.g., area of collagen fibers/total area of the micrograph). These findings suggest that females who have a smaller intercondylar notch, in combination with a weaker ligament, may be more susceptible to injury.

A few investigators[19-21] have reported an association between an increased posterior tibial slope (the angle formed by the tibial plateau relative to the long axis of the tibia) and ACL injury. They have theorized that an increased posterior tibial slope would place the femur in a more posteriorly directed position and promote anterior tibial translation. Because of the limited scope of data, additional studies are needed to better understand this influence.

Increased ACL laxity has been identified as another risk factor for the female athlete.[22] Uhorchak and colleagues[23] found that females were 2.7 times more likely to sustain an ACL injury if they had ligamentous laxity values that were one or more standard deviations (SDs) above the mean value. The effect of the menstrual cycle on ligamentous laxity also has received much attention. Refer to the separate section in this chapter for additional information.

Extrinsic Risk Factors

Extrinsic risk factors include biomechanical and neuromuscular characteristics that are amenable to change. Researchers have identified gender differences in lower-extremity biomechanics during running,[31] cutting,[32,33,50]

and single-leg landing[34,35,37,51] tasks. Results from these studies infer that females perform these maneuvers with greater knee valgus, femoral internal rotation, femoral adduction, and tibial external rotation. Ireland[52] has described this pattern as the "position-of-no-return" (Figure 26-2). High knee valgus loads generated in this position, especially performed on a minimally flexed knee, are thought to significantly strain the ACL.[34,50,53]

Neuromuscular factors may further contribute to gender differences. The hamstrings play an important role in minimizing excessive anterior tibial translation caused by a strong quadriceps contraction. Females also have demonstrated increased quadriceps activation relative to the hamstrings during athletic maneuvers.[39] This activation pattern, when performed in limited knee flexion, may contribute to excessive anterior tibial translation and cause ACL injury.

Researchers have examined the influence of other muscle groups to better understand the gender bias. During single-leg landing[40] and cutting maneuvers,[33] females attenuate greater energy using the quadriceps and ankle plantar flexors, whereas males disperse more energy using the quadriceps and hip extensors.[40] Fleming and colleagues[54] have shown how co-contraction of the quadriceps and gastrocnemius result in greater ACL strain with the knee flexed at 15° and 30°. However, others[33] have postulated that gastrocnemius activation may reflect a means for increasing knee stiffness. Additional works are needed to better understand the interaction between these muscles.

Differences in lower-extremity strength also may contribute to the gender bias. Sex differences regarding general knee strength occur after puberty when males demonstrate greater increases in strength, power, and coordination compared with females.[55] Thus, differences in knee strength may contribute to the higher incidence of ACL injury in females. Hip weakness also may contribute to lower extremity injury.[56] Jacobs and colleagues[41] found a greater association between hip abductor weakness and knee valgus during a single-leg landing task in females. Lawrence and colleagues[42] reported that females with greater hip and knee strength attenuated ground reaction forces more effectively and generated smaller external knee adduction and flexor moments during a single-leg landing. These findings support the importance of strong hip muscles for maintaining good lower-extremity alignment. They also support findings from Decker and colleagues[40] that strong hip muscles may reduce some of the ground reaction forces applied to the knee during a drop landing task.

Limitations of prior studies have been the examination of subjects in controlled laboratory settings that do not replicate aspects of the field environment, such as fatigue and decision-making tasks.[57] Kernozek and colleagues[43] reported that females could not reduce anterior knee shear forces as effectively as males during a single-leg landing following a fatiguing program. Borotikar and colleagues[44] reported increased hip internal rotation, knee abduction, and knee internal rotation during anticipated and unanticipated

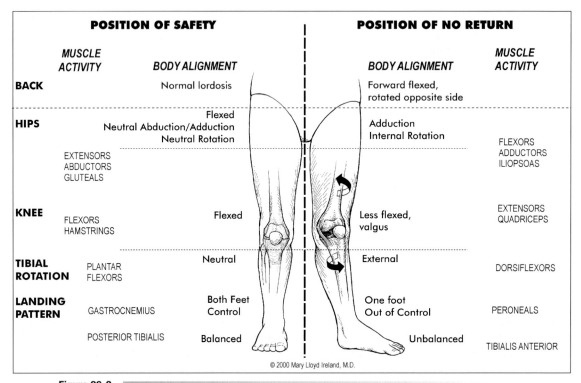

Figure 26-2

The position-of-no-return mechanism for anterior cruciate ligament injury in the female athlete.
(© 2000 Mary Lloyd ML Ireland, MD. Reproduced with permission.)

cutting maneuvers following a fatiguing protocol. Moreover, these differences were more pronounced during the unanticipated task. Together, results from these studies support the need for additional work that better depicts field conditions.

Menstrual Cycle and Anterior Cruciate Ligament Injury

Some believe that hormonal differences may contribute to the increased risk of ACL rupture in female athletes. This line of research is based on the premise that fluctuation in estrogen levels may contribute to ACL injury.

Beginning with the onset of menses, the menstrual cycle can be divided into the following phases: follicular, ovulatory, and luteal. Within this cycle, estrogen levels are lower during the follicular phase and rise dramatically during the ovulatory phase and throughout the luteal phase. Researchers[24,25] believe that increased estrogen levels may contribute to ACL laxity, thus predisposing the female athlete to injury. Although investigators[25-28] have examined the relationship between menstrual cycle and ligamentous laxity, conflicting results exist. Criticisms include small sample size and the reliance on subjective history for identifying the phase of menstrual cycle at the time of injury.[45]

Hewett and colleagues[58] recently conducted a systematic review of the literature regarding menstrual cycle and ACL injury risk. Based on this review, they concluded that a female is more likely to incur an ACL injury during the preovulatory phase (follicular and ovulatory phases). This conclusion contradicts the previous premise regarding increased estrogen and ACL laxity. Hewett and colleagues[58] suggested that reduced dynamic knee stability (e.g., decreased neuromuscular control) might contribute to ACL injury during earlier phases of the menstrual cycle based on earlier work by Sarwar and colleagues.[59] However, more recent works[29,30] have not found a relationship between fluctuating estrogen levels and knee neuromuscular control.

Oral contraceptives (OCs) increase and stabilize either levels of estrogen and progesterone, or just those of progesterone, and prevent the luteinizing hormone surge and resultant ovulation. Some believe that controlling fluctuations in estrogen levels may minimize the risk of ACL injury. Hewett and Myer[60] reported increased passive and dynamic knee stability in females who took OCs compared with those who did not take OCs. Although OC use may reduce female ACL injury rates,[61-63] further studies are needed to establish this association.

Prevention Programs

As described previously, extrinsic factors are modifiable and correction of these factors has been the focus on many ACL-injury prevention programs. Most programs[7,46,48,64] have included a combination of strengthening, neuromuscular training, and instruction in proper landing and cutting techniques. Although findings from these studies support the use of prevention programs, it remains elusive as to the most important element of each. Lephart and colleagues[65] reported favorable changes in neuromuscular and biomechanical parameters in healthy high school female athletes who completed an 8-week intervention of either plyometric or resistance exercise.

More recent studies[7,46] have prospectively followed female soccer players who have participated in the Prevent Injury and Enhance Performance (PEP) injury prevention program (www.aclprevent.com). This program is a combination of strengthening, stretching, plyometrics, agilities, and instruction in proper technique as part of a warm-up to play. Gilchrist and colleagues[7] recently reported that female soccer players who participated in the PEP program were 3.3 times less likely to sustain an ACL injury.

Grindstaff and colleagues[66] conducted a systematic review and support the use of ACL-injury prevention programs. Important aspects of a program include dynamic balance activities, agility skills, plyometrics with an emphasis on proper knee position (i.e., minimizing a knee valgus or varus alignment), and core and hip strengthening. Perhaps the most important aspect of a prevention program is attention to proper technique. Female athletes should be encouraged to land softly using a greater degree of hip and knee flexion to minimize external moments applied to the knee. They also should be instructed to avoid pivoting on a fixed foot and taught to decelerate using a multiple-step technique.

Although much attention has been focused on the causal factors and prevention of ACL injury, additional studies are needed to understand this enigma. Future investigations should be directed toward examining mechanisms of injury in an on-field setting and identifying the critical components of prevention programs. Furthermore, Prodromos and colleagues[14] recently found that injury prevention programs were more effective at preventing ACL injury in female soccer players than in those playing basketball. These findings infer the need for the development of prevention programs specific to a particular sport.

Patellofemoral Pain Syndrome

Patellofemoral pain syndrome (PFPS) is one of the most common pathological conditions of the knee. Unlike research regarding the incidence of ACL injury, limited data exist regarding the incidence and causes of PFPS in females. However, clinicians have anecdotally concluded a gender bias regarding causal factors of PFPS.

Causal Factors

PFPS may result from abnormal patella tracking that causes excessive compressive stress to the lateral patella facet. Clinicians routinely measure the Q-angle to quantify the degree of lateral patella tracking and consider a Q-angle greater than 20° as excessive.[67] Although females generally appear to exhibit higher Q-angles than males, studies have not supported the relationship between a higher Q-angle and PFPS.[68] A reason for this finding is that the Q-angle is a static measure that may not adequately depict patella movement during dynamic activities. Powers[69] has theorized that increased hip adduction and internal rotation can increase the Q-angle by moving the patella medial to the anterior superior iliac spine (referred to as an increase in the "dynamic" Q-angle). Based on this premise, a female with a "normal" static Q-angle may perform dynamic activities such as running, jumping, and stair descent with increased hip adduction and internal rotation. Prior works[31,70] have shown that females perform athletic maneuvers with greater hip adduction and internal rotation than males; these findings may support a relatively higher incidence of PFPS in females. Therefore, assessment of changes in the Q-angle during dynamic tasks might provide conclusive information regarding the relationship between PFPS and the Q-angle.

Hip Influences and Patellofemoral Pain Syndrome

An emerging body of work has focused on the influence of the hip on PFPS. To date, many researchers[71-75] have examined hip strength and consistently found hip abductor, external rotator, and extensor weakness in females with PFPS. Because these muscles primarily control hip adduction and internal rotation during dynamic activities, weakness or faulty timing could cause altered hip kinematics and possibly contribute to abnormal lateral patella tracking at the knee. Table 26-3 summarizes reference force values and test positions that clinicians may use for identifying hip weakness in females with PFPS.

A few studies have simultaneously examined the interrelationship between hip weakness and altered lower extremity kinematics in females with PFPS. Bolgla and colleagues[73] were the first to examine hip strength and hip and knee kinematics in this patient population. Although subjects with PFPS demonstrated significant hip abductor and external rotator weakness, they did not exhibit increased hip adduction, hip internal

Table 26-3

A Summary of Force Values (Expressed as a Percentage of Body Mass) for Females Diagnosed with Patellofemoral Pain Syndrome

	Hip Abductors	Hip External Rotators
Ireland et al.[71]	23.3 ± 6.9	10.8 ± 4.0
Robinson and Nee[72]	16.0 ± 8.0	16.0 ± 6.0
Cichanowski et al.[74]	29.0 ± 8.0	17.0 ± 4.0
Bolgla et al.[73]	22.5 ± 5.9	11.1 ± 3.1
Willson and Davis[75]	21.1 ± 6.0	9.1 ± 2.6

rotation, or knee valgus during stair descent. Although this task was representative of one that elicits patellofemoral joint pain, subjects might have used compensatory patterns to minimize knee pain when performing this lower demanding task.[76]

Others have examined hip and knee kinematics during more demanding activities such as running, single-leg squats, and single-leg jumping. Findings from Willson and colleagues[77] and Willson and Davis[78] showed that females with PFPS exhibited greater hip adduction, but less hip internal rotation, compared with controls during running, single-leg squatting, and repetitive single-leg jumping. They concluded that decreased hip internal rotation might have represented a means for reducing lateral patella stress. Dierks and colleagues[79] reported a strong correlation ($r = -0.74$) between hip abductor weakness and peak hip adduction following prolonged running. These results implied that patients with PFPS might not demonstrate altered kinematics until they achieve a certain threshold of weakness. In summary, females with PFPS commonly demonstrate hip weakness and use altered lower-extremity mechanics compared with controls. It remains elusive whether hip weakness was the cause of or the result from PFPS. Prospective studies are needed to understand associations between hip strength and lower extremity kinematics.

Foot and Ankle Influences and Patellofemoral Pain Syndrome

Tiberio[80] has theorized that excessive subtalar pronation may contribute to PFPS. From a biomechanical standpoint, increased subtalar joint pronation results in obligatory tibial internal rotation. Interestingly, tibial internal rotation brings the patella toward the tibial tubercle and decreases the Q-angle. However, during gait, the knee must extend during the latter phases of stance to propel the limb to the swing phase. To achieve knee extension, the tibia must be in an externally rotated position relative to the femur, a position accomplished via increased femoral internal rotation. As described previously, increased femoral internal rotation will cause an increase in the dynamic Q-angle and may contribute to PFPS.

Powers and colleagues[76] examined foot and lower-extremity rotation in subjects diagnosed with and without PFPS during gait. They did not find any between-group differences regarding the amount or timing of peak foot pronation or tibial internal rotation. However, subjects with PFPS exhibited significantly less hip internal rotation than controls. These authors concluded that subjects with PFPS might have reduced the Q-angle using this compensatory hip strategy.

Recently, researchers[81-83] have prospectively examined the influence of increased foot pronation on PFPS causes. Results from these studies have not supported an association between increased pronation and PFPS. Instead, data from these studies suggested that subjects who exhibited

foot function that impeded shock attenuation (e.g., gait patterns of greater pressure on the lateral aspect of the foot and running patterns of greater vertical peak force under the lateral heel) developed PFPS. It is important to note that few studies have examined the relationship between foot function and PFPS; additional studies are needed to better understand this interrelationship.

Interventions

Unlike ACL-prevention programs specifically aimed at reducing injury in the female athlete, the best treatment approach for females with PFPS remains elusive. However, more recent works[84] support the use of hip strengthening for the treatment of PFPS. Mascal and colleagues[85] reported positive outcomes for two female subjects who participated in a 14-week intervention that targeted the hip, pelvis, and trunk muscles. Tyler and colleagues[86] and Boling and colleagues[87] also reported improvements in pain and function in subjects with PFPS who participated in a program targeting the hip musculature. Limitations for these studies included use of a case report format,[85] inclusion of male and female subjects,[86,87] and use of hip exercise that also affect the quadriceps. Future works should examine the effects of isolated hip strengthening on improving impairments associated with PFPS.

Prior works[88,89] have supported the use of quadriceps strengthening for the treatment of PFPS. Although many clinicians prefer weightbearing (closed kinetic chain) exercise, studies have not supported the preferential use of weightbearing exercise over nonweightbearing (open kinetic chain) exercise.[84,90] Rather, quadriceps exercise performed in a pain-free manner appears to be the critical consideration.

Herrington and Al-Sherhi[91] recently conducted a controlled trial of weightbearing and nonweightbearing quadriceps exercises for a group of males with PFPS. Regardless of exercise group, males demonstrated significant improvements with knee pain, strength, and function. These findings support the primary use of quadriceps strengthening for males; however, it is unclear if females with PFPS will respond similarly. Although females with PFPS may respond well to quadriceps strengthening,[90] they may receive additional benefit from hip strengthening. Future works should focus on developing a clinical prediction rule for identifying a patient cohort that may respond more favorably to a combination of hip and knee strengthening exercise.

Evidence[92,93] supports orthosis use for the treatment of PFPS. Sutlive and colleagues[50] identified aspects of a physical examination to determine a cohort of subjects with PFPS that may benefit from orthosis prescription in combination with activity modification. They found that subjects with PFPS who exhibited a forefoot valgus greater than or equal to 2°, passive great toe extension less than or equal to 78°, and a navicular drop less than or equal to 3 mm responded favorably. These results inferred that subjects with a more rigid foot type received greater benefit from the orthosis intervention and suggested that shock attenuation may have reduced PFPS symptoms. These findings also are consistent with prospective etiological studies[81,82] that reported the development of PFPS in subjects who exhibited less pronation during gait.

In summary, PFPS is a multifactor problem with no clear cause or recommended best practice pattern. Prospective studies are needed to better understand the influences of the hip, knee, and foot-ankle complex on the cause of PFPS. Researchers also should strive to establish both classification systems and clinical guidelines[94,95] to further improve the management of patients with PFPS. More information on this topic can be found in Chapter 18, "Patellofemoral Joint" in *Pathology and Intervention in Musculoskeletal Rehabilitation*, volume III in this series.

Medial Tibial Stress Syndrome (MTSS)

MTSS is one of the most common causes of exercise-related leg pain.[96] The term sometimes referred to as *shin splints* describes a specific overuse injury producing pain along the posteromedial aspect of the distal two thirds of the tibia. The sports in which athletes are most commonly afflicted are cross-country, track, basketball, and volleyball. The incidence of MTSS in long-distance runners can be as high as 16.8% and is more prevalent in the female runner.[97,98]

The pathogeneses of MTSS is controversial. Some authors characterize the condition as a periostitis (inflammation of the periosteum) caused by strain of the medial tibial fascia. Others describe it as a tearing at the muscle-bone interface. Muscles that have been identified as possible culprits include the posterior tibialis,[99,100] soleus,[101,102] and flexor digitorum longus.[103] However, in a review of literature, Tweed and colleagues[104] concluded that MTSS "is not an inflammatory process of the periosteum but instead a stress reaction of the bone that has become painful." It is a condition that has the potential of developing into a stress fracture if not cared for properly.

The diagnosis of MTSS is based on clinical history and symptoms. Pain and tenderness is usually diffuse and located along the medial-distal two thirds of the tibia. Commonly, athletes will complain of pain at the beginning of a run. The pain may subside during the middle of the run but recurs at the end of the run. Provocative tests to rule in MTSS include pain with passive ankle dorsiflexion, resisted plantar flexion, toe raises, or single-leg hops. If the clinician suspects a tibial stress fracture, then a bone scan should be sought.

Potential biomechanical risk factors for MTSS include excessive foot pronation,[98,105] increased velocity of pronation, and increased compensated rear- and forefoot varus alignment.[106] Theoretically, the antipronation muscles fatiguing over time may increase the amount of force attenuated by the bone and periosteal tissue.

Bennett and colleagues[107] measured tibiofibular varum, weightbearing resting calcaneal position, and gastrocnemius length in 125 high school cross-country runners prior to their competitive season. All athletes were monitored for symptoms of MTSS. After 8 weeks, 15 runners (25 limbs) presented with MTSS compared with a randomly select 25 limbs. Navicular drop test (NDT) was compared in these 50 limbs. A T-test showed a significant difference in NDT between injured and uninjured limbs, with the injured limb having greater navicular drop (6.8 mm vs. 3.6 mm). Plisky and colleagues[108] examined bilateral NDT, foot length, height, body mass index, previous running injury, running experience, and use of orthoses or tape in a group of high school cross-country runners. Runners were followed during the season to determine athletic exposure and occurrence of MTSS. Overall injury rate was higher in females. Only gender and body mass index were significantly associated with the occurrence of MTSS. In addition, those runners with a previous running injury were more than two times as likely to develop MTSS.

Other contributing factors are repetitive overload, running on an unyielding surface, and shoe error (wrong type or wearing too long [i.e., shoe worn out]). It is also speculated that increasing training volume and hills contribute to MTSS.

Treatment should focus on relative rest in the acute phase. The athlete's biomechanics should be examined and an off-the-shelf orthotic device prescribed for the athlete with pes planus to minimize the amount of pronation. In those athletes who present with a rigid foot, shock absorbing shoes should be worn. Gastrocnemius and soleus length needs to be assessed and flexibility exercises given if the complex is tight. Strengthening of the hip musculature such as the gluteus medius is also advocated.

> ## Suggested Parameters for Safe Return-to-Running Program
>
> - Start at 50% of the preinjury state (intensity and duration)
> - Level surface
> - Appropriate warmup
> - Increase 10% per week
> - Progress duration prior to intensity

The last resort for treatment of MTSS is a fasciotomy. The decision for surgery is based on the failure of conservative measures. The literature presents positive outcomes following fasciotomy.[109] For more information on repetitive stress injuries see Chapters 21 and 22 on repetitive stress pathological conditions in *Pathology and Intervention in Musculoskeletal Rehabilitation*, volume III in this series.

Spine Injuries

An epidemiological study by Jackson and Mannarins[110] indicated that 55% of all athletes sustain at least one injury to the spine during their sports careers with recurrence at 42%. The highest incidence of spine injuries in females occurs in sports such as gymnastics, racquet sports, golf, equestrian skills, and weight lifting.[111] Compared with the general population, the athlete responds better to conservative management of musculoskeletal-related spine injuries and most will recover within 10 days.[112] If symptoms linger and the athlete cannot participate in her sport, it is likely that she has sustained substantial damage to either a bony or collagenous component of the spine. One must keep in mind that adolescents have a higher incidence of nonmuscular causes for low back pain, such as tumor.[113] The clinician needs to be aware of red flags when dealing with spinal injuries. Any one of the signs is an indication that further medical workup by a physician is required.

Red Flags Associated with Spinal Injury Indicating the Need for Further Medical Workup by a Physician

- Unrelenting back pain (worse at night)
- Progressive neurological deficits
- Unexplained weight loss
- Bladder or bowel paralysis (cauda equina)
- Positive Babinski sign

In addition, ankylosing spondylitis, an inflammatory disease, should be considered if the female athlete complains of a gradual onset of pain and stiffness in the thoracolumbar or sacroiliac (SI) area that is not associated with activity. Further workup including a bone scan and blood tests (human leukocyte antigen [HLA] B$_{27}$) deserve consideration.

Spondylolysis and Spondylolisthesis

Spondylolysis is the most common cause of low back pain in the active adolescent seeking medical attention (70%).[113] Spondylolysis is a stress fracture through the pars interarticularis of the posterior lumbar vertebra. Repeated axial loading of the pars interarticularis can cause the stress fracture,[114] but it also can occur developmentally.[115] Hyperextension of the normal lordosis alters the biomechanics of loading force distribution throughout the lumbar spine and creates abnormal stress upon the pars interarticularis region. This type of stress is common in sports such as weightlifting and gymnastics. A 32% incidence of spondylolysis has been found in female gymnasts, 63% in divers, and 12% to 15% in dancers.[116]

Spondylolisthesis is a bilateral fracture of the pars interarticularis with actual slippage forward of the superior vertebra on the inferior vertebra. Nerve root involvement is possible with the slippage of the vertebra. The most common level of occurrence is at the L5-S1 level (90%) followed by L4 then L3.[117] The anterior slippage is graded on the percent of the vertebral body that has slipped forward. A grade I spondylolisthesis indicates anterior slippage less than 25% of the vertebral body. A grade II is slippage between 25% and 50%, grade III is 50% to 75%, and a grade IV is anything greater than 75% slippage. For grade I treatment, see the following text. For grade II or greater, the athlete may be prohibited from playing in aggressive, collision sports such as rugby or repetitive-stress sports such as gymnastics and dance.[117,118]

Symptoms include a dull backache with or without buttock pain and possible sciatica. The back pain is aggravated by extension activity and may increase with prolonged standing. One should not forget that pain in the low back may be referred from the uterus, indicating the possible need for a gynecological consult.

The athlete usually presents with hyperlordotic posture and tight hip flexors. The erector spinae and hamstring muscles may present with spasm. The clinician may feel a step-off at the involved vertebral level. The single-leg standing hyperextension test (Stork test) may be positive (Figure 26-3). Neurological examination may be positive for changes in

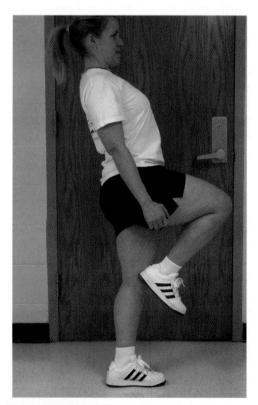

Figure 26-3

Single-leg standing hyperextension (Stork) test.

sensation, reflexes, or myotomes. A radiograph using an oblique view may identify a Scottie Dog sign (fracture through the pars). Stress fractures may not show-up initially with radiographs; therefore, a bone scan or magnetic resonance imaging (MRI) scan is recommended.

Spondylolysis and grade I spondylolisthesis are treated with training modifications to correct hyperextension during techniques.[119] The athlete should be trained to maintain a neutral spine with static and dynamic activities. Muscle imbalances, such as tight hip flexors, should be restored around the hip joint. An athlete with a grade II spondylolisthesis or higher should be cautioned about aggressive sporting activities that require hyperextension. Radiographs should be performed annually to check for a progression in the anterior slippage. External supports may provide stability and proprioceptive cuing. Joint mobilization of stiff segments above the fractured level is beneficial. Prognosis for a grade I and II spondylolisthesis is good. Surgical intervention may be required in a low percentage of athletes if neurological signs progress. Low grade slips can be addressed by direct fusion with return to noncontact sports.[120]

Pathological Conditions of the Sacroiliac Joint

The SI joint is inherently a stable joint with little motion.[121] However, injury can occur to this joint from excessive loading or from a fall onto the buttock. The female athlete may be particularly vulnerable to SI injury secondary to monthly cycling of hormones or increased ligamentous laxity during pregnancy. According to Marymont and colleagues,[122] most SI problems typically affect the young, skeletally immature female athlete. A sacral stress fracture also should be ruled out, especially in distance runners who report pain in the sacral region.

Symptoms associated with SI-related pathological conditions include joint pain that may refer to the groin. Pain is worse with extension and rotation to the side of dysfunction, compression or distraction of the SI joint, and loading activities such as hopping. Hip and trunk motion may be painful and should be evaluated. Special tests such as the flexion, abduction, and external rotation test (FABER or Patrick test) and specific joint techniques (i.e., shear, compression, distraction) should also be performed.

A thorough clinical examination may reveal SI joint, pelvic asymmetry, and leg length discrepancy. X-ray examinations of the pelvis and SI joint may be normal. An MRI can be helpful in detecting both soft tissue and stress fracture, although MRI for a typical SI joint dysfunction has low specificity. The gold standard is a diagnostic injection under fluoroscopic guidance to confirm a pathological condition of the joint. Blood work (HLA B_{27}) will help to differentiate between sacroiliitis or ankylosing spondylitis.

Exercises to help stabilize the SI joint should include the hip rotators, especially the posterior fibers of the gluteus medius and the single-joint hip extensors. Exercises such as wall sits with gluteal squeeze, lateral step-ups with gluteal

squeeze, isometric hip external rotation (Figure 26-4), and repetitive prone knee curls are helpful. An SI belt helps with instability and can be worn until muscle strength is adequate to stabilize the joint. Joint mobilization to hypomobile joints in the lumbar spine also may be indicated. Biomechanical analysis of running and sport techniques is appropriate.

Intervertebral Disc Lesion

The intervertebral disc has limited vascularity and therefore depends on mechanical pumping and movement for health and repair. Most disc lesions come on gradually and affect the levels of L4-L5 and L5-S1.[122] A woman who is older than 25 years old is more prone to disc lesions than the younger athlete, although the incidence in adolescents appears to be increasing.[123] The mechanism of injury usually involves some combination of lumbar hyperflexion, axial compression, and rotation. The disc injury may occur from a single episode or repetitive trauma. Repeated minor trauma, such as sustained compression in flexion and rotation, gives rise to circumferential fissures usually located along the inner portion of the annulus.[124] Weakening of the annular layers reduces the ability of the annulus to contain the nucleus, which can lead to disc protrusion. Disc injuries are found in athletes who participate in sports that require excessive torsion such as golf, racquetball, or tennis. In the event that the disc material impinges on the nerve root, neurological signs will be present. Sciatica has a high sensitivity (95%) for disc herniation.[125]

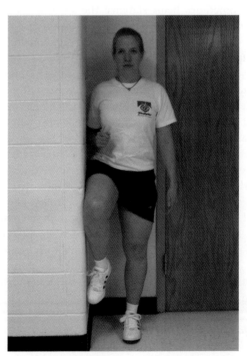

Figure 26-4
Gluteal strengthening exercises.

Discogenic pain can range from a minor complaint of back pain to severe disability. The athlete, in mild cases, may continue her activity but will notice a gradual increase in pain and stiffness. In single, acute incidences, the athlete may be stopped in her tracks by the pain. The lumbar discomfort often worsens at night and the athlete may awaken with morning stiffness.[97]

Physical examination may reveal a lateral shift, positive straight-leg raise, diminished reflexes, or radicular symptoms. Symptoms are usually aggravated by trunk flexion. If irritation of the nerve root sleeve is present, the athlete will present with a positive slump test or straight leg raise.[126] Other neurological symptoms include tingling, numbness, paresthesia, muscle (myotome) weakness, and altered reflexes.

Diagnostic testing should include anterior-posterior and lateral films with oblique views to visualize the pars interarticularis and findings should be correlated with physical signs and symptoms. MRI is the most sensitive test and will delineate the disc and nerve roots. Abnormal findings may not be the source of the athlete's pain. Disc degeneration and protrusion has been demonstrated on MRI in 20% to 25% of asymptomatic individuals.[127]

Fortunately, the symptoms of an acute disc injury often resolve without surgery. In acute stages, the goal is to minimize pain and muscle spasm. Unloading of the disc is performed by positioning the athlete in a side lying position to increase the size of the intervertebral foramen with the convex side up. Sustained lumbar traction may offer relief. Clinically, McKenzie's extension protocol seems to help a high percentage of patients with disc injury.[107] A corset sometimes helps stabilize the spine as the athlete recovers from acute symptoms, but its use should be closely monitored. In extreme cases, epidural injections are helpful.

For chronic disc injury, a more aggressive approach is indicated. Heavy mechanical traction has been proposed by Saunders and Saunders.[126] Joint mobilizations, including central techniques and rotations,[128] may also be effective. Clinical prediction rules have become increasingly available to the clinician to identify the appropriate candidate for manipulation.[49,129] In the presence of adverse neural tension, slump stretching and "flossing" is indicated (Figure 26-5). Once symptoms and signs are controlled, the athlete should be placed on a lumbar stabilization exercise program. Manipulation is contraindicated when neurological deficit is present or if the patient presents with ligamentous laxity. If joint instability is accompanied by neurological signs, the athlete may need to undergo surgical intervention (fusion).

Lumbar Spine Strain and Sprain

A *lumbar strain* or *sprain* or *low back pain* refers to injury in the musculotendinous or ligamentous tissue. Common mechanisms of injury include high-velocity torsion or twisting movements or repetitive overload. This loading creates

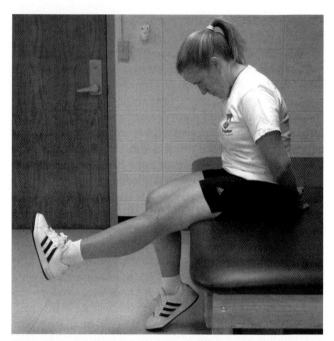

Figure 26-5
Slump stretching.

excessive and abnormal tension in collagen fibers causing microtearing.[130] An acute, violent torsion may be associated with avulsion of the transverse process by strong contraction of the quadratus lumborum or iliopsoas. Chronic overload strains are due to poor posture or faulty mechanics. Growth spurts may increase the incidence of back strain because of soft tissue inextensibility.[131]

The athlete will complain of local pain with trunk motion. Motion is usually restricted in flexion and rotation. Pain or weakness will be present with resisted trunk motion. In chronic situations, trigger points, localized areas of increased sensitivity, or irritability in soft tissue structure may cause referred pain.

In the acute stage, rest and local modalities will help with pain and muscle guarding. A brace or corset worn for 2 to 3 weeks will sometimes help with debilitating pain. Soft tissue mobilization including trigger point therapy along with posture correction is started on day 2 or 3 following injury. Improper body mechanics, poor conditioning, and poor warmup should all be addressed in chronic situations.

Structural Scoliosis

Scoliosis is defined as a lateral spinal curvature usually associated with rotation of vertebral body. Idiopathic adolescent scoliosis is relatively common in the general population and is unrelated to sporting activity. A *structural curve* as seen in idiopathic scoliosis refers to a fixed, bony deformity. A *functional curve*, as seen in a disc lesion, is reversible and is due to muscle imbalance. A mild idiopathic spinal deviation is usually well tolerated and the female athlete has no trouble participating in sports. However, if scoliosis progresses to a severe deformity (greater than 40° to 50°

Cobb angle), compromise of the cardiopulmonary system is probable. There appears to be an association between scoliosis and participation in sports such as gymnastics, ice skating, and dance. Smith and Micheli[116] found the prevalence of scoliosis to be 33% in female skaters compared with the general population.

In mild cases, the athlete may be asymptomatic. In other cases, the athlete will complain of back pain that may be aggravated by prolonged positioning or intense exercise. Radiographic evidence will reveal a scoliotic curve. Clinical signs include a lateral curvature of the spine, lateral shift, leg length discrepancy, and rib hump (structural scoliosis).

The key to managing scoliosis is early diagnosis and intervention. As well, the clinician must counsel the young athlete on sport participation. Although sports are not contraindicated, the athlete needs to alert the health professional of spine pain during activity. Rehabilitation focuses on maintaining trunk mobility, muscle balance, soft tissue techniques, and breathing exercises. In moderate cases, bracing may be appropriate. In contact sports, the brace must be padded to prevent lacerations and contusions. Surgery is indicated for severe progressive curves.

Costochondral Joint

The costochondral joint may be injured from direct impact or overuse.[132] Possible joint separation may occur when a force is applied to the chest, causing the costal cartilage to separate from the sternum. The athlete complains of pain and tenderness in one of the costochondral joints. A snapping sensation may also be present. Symptoms will be made worse by sudden movements, strain, and coughing. It appears that this condition is more common in young adults; is related to exercise; and is more common in sports such as golf, rowing, and throwing sports.[133] Radiological examination is normal. Effective treatment includes corticosteroid injections into the region and nonsteroidal anti-inflammatory drugs (NSAIDs). Modalities such as phonophoresis and electrical stimulation may be used initially for pain, followed by a progressive exercise program focusing on the pectoralis and serratus muscles. Joint mobilization and manipulation may be indicated for associated hypomobile joints in the thoracic spine or costal articulations.[134] Strapping or taping may help with pain or instability. Taping can be applied over the affected joint in a criss-cross or L-shaped manner to help stabilize the joint. Differential diagnosis includes cardiac involvement because Tietze disease is a condition involving the same area of the anterior chest, but is associated with swelling. Polyarthritis is characterized by inflammation of five or more joints.

Female Athlete Triad

The female athlete triad was first described in 1992 as a combination of disordered eating, amenorrhea, and osteoporosis in female athletes.[135] Each of these areas represents a spectrum of three interrelated aspects of women's

health: energy availability, menstrual function, and bone health. Therefore, alterations in one or more of these areas may adversely affect the health of the female athlete.[136]

Energy Availability

Bonci and colleagues[137] have stated that low energy availability is the hallmark factor contributing to the other aspects (amenorrhea and osteoporosis) of the triad. *Energy availability* is defined as the energy intake minus the exercise energy expenditure per kilogram of lean body mass.[136] An athlete may lessen energy availability by either decreasing intake (e.g., disordered eating or eating disorder) or increasing expenditure (e.g., excessive exercise).

Disordered eating refers to an entire spectrum of abnormal behavior such as fasting, restrictive consumption, or the use of laxatives or diuretics.[137] In contrast, *eating disorders*, such as anorexia and bulimia nervosa, represent clinical syndromes defined by strict diagnostic criteria.[137] However, both represent a means of reducing the available energy by reducing intake. Conversely, an athlete can reduce energy availability by increasing energy expenditure through excessive exercise. Therefore, an athlete need not necessarily present with disordered eating to be at risk for detrimental effects caused by low energy availability.

When energy availability decreases, the body attempts to maintain energy balance by disrupting reproduction, cellular maintenance, thermoregulation, and growth.[138] Decreased energy availability associated with disordered eating may further lead to an increased risk of depression and anxiety and adversely affect the cardiac, gastrointestinal, endocrine, reproductive, skeletal, renal, and central nervous systems.[139]

Menstrual Dysfunction

Menstrual function may be described as *eumenorrhea* (menstrual cycle at a 28-day median interval), *oligomenorrhea* (menstrual cycle at a 35-day or longer median interval), or *amenorrhea* (absence of a menstrual cycle),[136] with dysfunction resulting from altered hypothalamic regulation. Specifically, decreased secretion of gonadotropin-releasing hormone by the hypothalamus reduces the pulsatility of the luteinizing hormone produced by the pituitary.[140] Loucks and Thuma[141] and Loucks and colleagues[142] have reported a reduction in luteinizing hormone pulsatility when decreasing energy availability in females who have a regular menstrual cycle. These findings suggest that a loss in energy availability may contribute to amenorrhea.

Amenorrhea associated with a decrease in estrogen[143] may lead to anovulation (failure to ovulate), infertility, and decreased bone density. Although infertility is generally reversible with the restoration of menses, it is important to note that ovulation may return prior to menses restoration. Therefore, an athlete may become pregnant should she not use an adequate form of birth control during this time. Unfortunately, bone density loss may remain even after the restoration of menses.[144,145]

Other adverse effects associated with lack of estrogen include decreased oxidative metabolism in skeletal muscle, increased low-density lipoprotein (LDL) cholesterol levels,[146,147] and vaginal dryness.[148] Decreased oxidative metabolism translates to decreases in performance. Increased LDL levels may increase the risk of cardiac disease. Vaginal dryness can increase the prevalence of candidal infection and dyspareunia (abnormal pain during sexual intercourse). In summary, although reduced estrogen is commonly manifested with menstrual dysfunction, it adversely affects other systems.

Bone Mineral Density

Reduced bone mineral density (BMD) has important implications for the female athlete as it may lead to osteoporosis as well as the incidence of stress fracture. When associated with amenorrhea, the risk of incurring a stress fracture increases twofold to fourfold.[149]

In females, BMD normally increases until approximately age 30 and significantly tapers after menopause. Reduced BMD occurs when bone resorption exceeds bone formation. Risk factors associated with reduced BMD include female sex, low weight, and decreased estrogen.[136] Estrogen is needed to facilitate bone remodeling as it has an inhibitory effect on osteoclast activity in studies examining osteoporosis and decreased estrogen in postmenopausal females.[150]

Evidence has suggested a similar decrease in estrogen in response to low energy availability.[122,130] Ihle and Louks[151] have quantified a dose-response relationship between energy availability and bone turnover in young exercising females. They found that reduced energy availability suppressed estradiol and altered selected bone marker concentrations indicative of increased bone resorption. These findings suggest that low energy availability can adversely affect hypothalamic function, as manifested by reduced estrogen secretion, and lead to decreased BMD.

Evaluation

Up to 84% of athletes with disordered eating are asymptomatic.[152] This is particularly concerning given that the incidence of eating disorders in athletes may be as much as 20 to 30 times higher than age-matched peers.[153] Because of this, practitioners must be aware of the various aspects of the spectrum and be vigilant for clues to its presence when working with the female athletes. Interaction with the female athlete may occur during a preparticipation evaluation, an annual health visit, and or a health visit associated with one or more areas of the triad. Bonci and colleagues[137]

have recommended the use of self-report questionnaires to facilitate the detection of disordered eating as athletes are commonly less apt to disclose these behaviors. More important, health care providers and coaches should observe and monitor athletes for behavior changes such as excessive weight loss, fatigue, excessive exercise, and decreased performance.[137]

The medical history should focus on diet and energy intake, exercise, weight changes, menstrual history, fracture history, and the patient's satisfaction with current weight. Mental health practitioners should be consulted if disordered eating is discovered. Because early intervention is preferred, *Diagnostic and Statistical Manual* criteria need not be strictly observed.[154]

The physical examination should address signs of eating disorders, such as lanugo (fine soft hair covering body), bradycardia, and hypercarotenemia (high levels of carotene in blood giving the skin a yellow appearance). The practitioner also should assess height and weight. Fingernails should be examined for brittleness; the backs of the hands should be examined for signs of callus or abrasion from induced vomiting.[137] A pelvic examination may reveal vaginal atrophy. An electrocardiogram may show a prolonged QT interval.

Clinical Signs and Symptoms Associated with the Female Triad

- Lanugo (a soft, fine hair covering all parts of the body)
- Bradycardia (decreased heart rate)
- Hypercarotenemia (excessive carotene in blood—abnormal yellow skin)
- Low body weight
- Fingernail discoloration
- Vaginal atrophy
- Abnormal electrocardiogram (prolonged QT interval)

Laboratory tests should include a complete blood cell count with differential blood chemistries and electrolytes, thyroid stimulating hormone, erythrocyte sedimentation rate, and urinalysis to identify abnormalities indicative of malnutrition or its sequelae. Secondary amenorrhea should be evaluated by a pregnancy test, follicle stimulating hormone, leuteinizing hormone, prolactin, and cortisol levels. If these are normal, the physician should perform a progesterone challenge. In the presence of estrogen, withdrawal bleeding will occur in 7 to 10 days. Possible diagnoses will then include progesterone deficiency, polycystic ovarian syndrome, some medications and normogonadotropic hypogonadism. If the challenge fails, test for androgen excess caused by tumors, adrenal hyperplasia, or certain genetic disorders such as Turner syndrome should be performed. If all of the testing is normal, functional hypothalamic amenorrhea is diagnosed by exclusion. One exception is that an athlete in recovery may respond to the progesterone challenge.

BMD testing should be performed on any individual with a 6-month history of disordered eating or amenorrhea or after suffering multiple stress fractures.[155] The World Health Organization (WHO)[156] has established criteria based on BMD, as measured using techniques such as dual-energy x-ray absorptiometry, for diagnosing osteoporosis. The diagnosis is based on a T-score, which represents the number of SDs above or below the average BMD for young, healthy, white women.[157] The WHO[156] considers a person with a T-score more than 2.5 SD below the average BMD as having osteoporosis. A limitation of this classification system is that the WHO has based these criteria on studies using postmenopausal women.[158]

The International Society for Clinical Densitometry (ISCD) recommends comparing young individuals' bone density with that of age- and sex-matched controls to determine those with low bone density (defined as a *Z-score*).[158] The ISCD defines osteoporosis as a Z-score below −2, meaning that the BMD is less than that expected for a specified age range. This system may be more advantageous than that used by the WHO osteoporosis scale as it accounts for differences in age and sex. Refer to the National Athletic Trainers' Association Position Statement: Preventing, Detecting, and Managing Disordered Eating in Athletes[137] for comprehensive guidelines for additional information.

Treatment

Because bone density loss may not be fully recoverable, prevention is paramount. Prevention programs should include nutrition and exercise counseling and education. Once diagnosed, treatment of the triad should be comprehensive and include a variety of players. The primary team should include a physician, dietitian, and coach. When available, family members; an athletic trainer or sports physical therapist; an exercise physiologist; and a psychologist, psychiatrist, or clinical social worker also should be consulted. The initial intervention should focus on increasing energy availability to greater than 45 kcal/kg per day. Simply increasing body weight will promote bone density and restore normal menstruation for an athlete with low body weight.[136] Athletes with disordered eating also should enter into a contract with the treatment team and be allowed to participate only if they adhere to the treatment plan and show signs of improved health.

Antidepressants may assist in the treatment of eating disorders; however, medications have not been effective for improving bone density in young athletes. Prior research[159] has shown that hormone replacement therapy (HRT) and OCs are ineffective in individuals with eating disorders. In those without eating disorders, data are inconclusive. Although bisphosphonates are a mainstay of treatment in postmenopausal women, their benefit is unproven in premenopausal women. Evidence[160] suggests that use in a premenopausal female may adversely affect the growth and development of a fetus should she become pregnant. Therefore, bisphosphonates are contraindicated in athletes of childbearing age because of possible detrimental effects on a fetus. Given the time these drugs stay in human bone and their slow release, the detrimental effects are not assuaged by simply stopping when trying to become pregnant.[160]

Pregnancy and Exercise

The recommendations for exercising while pregnant have become clearer in the last decade. Most research has shown that females will benefit from aerobic exercise.[161-163] The level at which they exercise depends on prepregnancy fitness level and should be guided by their physicians. The American College of Obstetricians and Gynecologists (ACOG) has led the way in setting guidelines for exercising while pregnant, first with a statement in 1985 and subsequent updates in 1994 and 2002 (available at www.acog.org/publications/patient_education/bp119.cfm).[164]

Many physiological changes occur during pregnancy that have an effect on exercise. With regard to the cardiovascular system, there is a 50% increase in cardiac output, blood volume increases by 45%, and resting heart rate can increase up to 15 beats per minute.[165] The respiratory system responds to pregnancy with an increase in minute ventilation and breathing effort.[166] The required energy intake increases to approximately 3000 kcal/day and carbohydrates are the preferred fuel source. Related to the musculoskeletal system, there is an increase in joint laxity, weight gain ranges from 20 to 40 pounds (9 to 18 kg), and there is an increase in lumbar lordosis.[163] All these factors will affect the intensity and mode in which the pregnant woman can exercise.

The benefits of exercising while pregnant can be both physical and psychological. It has been shown that exercising women have improved strength and posture and there is a prevention of excessive maternal weight gain.[167] These factors undoubtedly help with a reduction in low back pain.[167] Related directly to birthing, Clapp[168] found that women who take part in some form of exercise on the average had a shorter active labor during vaginal births. Plasma glucose has been shown to be significantly reduced by 45 minutes of exercise a day at least three times per week, and it may help to control or prevent gestational diabetes.[169] Some of the psychological benefits of exercise include a reduction of depression[170] and improved self-esteem.[171]

The exercise prescription should be designed in conjunction with the woman's physician. Guidelines have been defined by both the American College of Sports Medicine (available at www.acsm.org/AM/Template.cfm?Section=current_comments1&Template=/CM/ContentDisplay.cfm&ContentID=8638)[172] and the ACOG (available at

---

Benefits of Exercising While Pregnant

Physical Benefits
- Improves posture
- Improves strength
- Improves endurance
- Prevention of excessive weight gain
- Reduces low back pain
- Shorter active labor
- Controls blood glucose levels

Psychological Benefits
- Improves self-image
- Reduces depression

Table 26-4
Exercise Prescription During Pregnancy

Sedentary	
Frequency	3 times per week
Intensity	Perceived exertion: moderately hard; HR: 65% to 75% max
Type	Low impact (walking, bicycling, swimming, aerobics)
Time/duration	30 minutes

Recreational Athlete	
Frequency	3 to 5 times per week
Intensity	Perceived exertion: moderately hard to hard, HR: 65% to 80% max
Type	Low impact (running, tennis, cross-country skiing)
Time/duration	30 to 60 minutes

Elite Athlete	
Frequency	Minimum 4 to 6 times per week
Intensity	Perceived exertion: hard, HR: 75% to 80% max
Type	As with recreational athlete, can include competitive activities
Time/duration	60 to 90 minutes

Adapted from Joy EA: Exercise and pregnancy. In Ratcliffe SD: *Family practice obstetrics*, ed 2, Philadelphia, 2001, Hanley & Befus. *HR*, Heart rate.

www.acog.org/publications/patient_education/bp119.cfm).[164] Both groups recommend aerobic exercise such as walking or swimming at moderate intensity (3-4 metabolic equivalent tasks). Running is appropriate only if the individual was running prior to her pregnancy. In general, peak heart rate should not exceed 140 beats per minute. Regarding duration and frequency of exercise, the 2002 position statement from the ACOG states that "in absence of either medical or obstetric complications, 30 minutes or more of moderate exercise a day on most, if not all days of the week is recommended for pregnant women."[173] For more specific guidelines based on prepregnancy training level see Table 26-4.

The effect of high-volume exercise during pregnancy in elite female athletes has been published in the literature.[162,172] The investigations found no detrimental results to the mother or fetus with the exercise program. Beilock and colleagues found that highly trained women who limited their aerobic and strength training during pregnancy did not significantly affect their postpartum training program.[175]

Further recommendations and warning signs are found in Table 26-5. There are few absolute and relative contraindications to aerobic exercise in pregnancy and these are found in Table 26-6. In conclusion, it appears that healthy females with uncomplicated pregnancy can continue to exercise at moderate levels without harm to themselves or their child.

Older Female Athlete

It has been reported that one of the fastest growing groups of exercisers is the middle-aged and older woman. Benefits of choosing a physically active lifestyle include a lower incidence of chronic degenerative disease, lower age-specific mortality rate, and the ability to live independently. The older athletic woman has unique challenges that may affect her ability to be active, including hormonal changes that influence tissue health and the cardiovascular system.

In addition, with aging, there is a decline in strength that can lead to injury and stress urinary incontinence (SUI).

Hormonal Changes

For women in their late 40s and early 50s, cessation of menstruation (menopause) will occur. Problems associated with menopause include an increase incidence of osteoporosis and a decline in cardiovascular health caused by diminishing estrogen levels.[145] In addition, after approximately age 30, women begin to lose muscle mass and strength. Age-related decline in lean body mass correlates with several alterations, including a decrease in endogenous growth hormone, a decrease in pituitary responsiveness to growth hormone–releasing hormone, and neuromuscular alteration.

Many of these detriments that occur with aging can be prevented or minimized with a consistent routine of aerobic exercise and strength training. Researchers have found that exercise along with proper calcium-rich diet can enhance bone density and reduce bone loss.[176] The increased mechanical stress associated with weightbearing exercise can increase bone mineralization. In addition, upper-extremity bone mass can be improved with strengthening exercise.

Table 26-5

Recommendations and Warning Signs Related to Exercise and Pregnancy[164,172]

Recommendations	Warning Signs to Stop Exercise and Seek Medical Evaluation
Drink plenty of water before, during, and after exercise	Vaginal bleeding
Eat small, frequent meals throughout the day	Dyspnea prior to exertion
Avoid exercises that require bouncing, jarring, leaping, risk of abdominal injury such as contact sports, downhill skiing, scuba diving, horseback riding	Dizziness
	Headache
Do not exercise on the back as this may reduce blood flow to the heart	Chest pain
Avoid heavy weightlifting and any activities that require straining	Muscle weakness
Avoid exposures to extremes of air pressure as in high altitude (unless you are accustomed) or scuba diving	Calf pain or swelling
	Preterm labor
Do not increase intensity of your workout beyond prepregnancy levels	Decreased fetal movement
	Amniotic fluid leakage

Table 26-6

Absolute and Relative Contraindications to Exercise during Pregnancy

Absolute Contraindications to Exercise during Pregnancy	Relative Contraindications to Exercise during Pregnancy
Hemodynamically significant heart disease	Severe anemia
Restrictive lung disease	Unevaluated maternal cardiac arrhythmia
Incompetent cervix or cerclage	Chronic bronchitis
Multiple gestation at risk for premature labor	Poorly controlled type I diabetes
Persistent second or third trimester bleeding	Extreme morbid obesity
Placenta previa after 26 weeks' gestation	Extreme underweight (body mass index < 12)
Premature labor during the current pregnancy	History of extremely sedentary lifestyle
Ruptured membranes	Intrauterine growth restriction in current pregnancy
Pre-eclampsia or pregnancy-induced hypertension	Poorly controlled hypertension
	Orthopedic limitation
	Poorly controlled seizure disorder
	Poorly controlled hyperthyroidism
	Heavy smoking

Data from the American College of Obstetricians and Gynecologists.

Regarding the risk of cardiovascular disease, exercise along with a low-fat diet may reduce this risk. Higher levels of physical activity are associated with lower blood pressure, heart rate, serum cholesterol, LDLs, body mass index, fasting insulin, and fasting insulin/glucose ratios.

Training-induced improvements in strength and balance may provide an added benefit by preventing the falls that cause a great number of fractures among the elderly.[177] Helping young women learn how to strength train (i.e., proper technique, proper loading) during the years when they are able to increase bone mass may help to prevent osteoporosis and related fractures.

HRT is a choice for some women following menopause. HRT will help to decrease vasomotor symptoms, urogenital atrophy, cardiovascular disease risk, and bone loss. Unfortunately, accompanying these benefits are side effects such as weight gain, headaches, leg cramps, and a potential increased risk of breast cancer. Natural hormones made from soy or yams are becoming more popular.

Stress Urinary Incontinence

As more women engage in regular exercise, the issue of bladder leakage has surfaced.[177-179] Nygaard and colleagues[178] reported 47% of women who exercise regularly have some degree of urinary incontinence. Complaints of SUI during physical activity have prompted greater attention to conservative management techniques that support a woman's goal of fitness and establishment of healthy pelvic muscles simultaneously, especially those of the pelvic floor.

Pelvic floor muscles form a hammock of muscular tissue that provides support for the pelvic organs in addition to sphincter control. These muscles are sensitive to hormonal status and are rich in estrogen receptor sites. High-impact physical activities, estrogen depletion,[180] and pelvic muscle weakness are among the risk factors associated with SUI.

Conservative treatment for SUI includes a pre-exercise routine of voiding prior to exercise and avoiding beverages that include caffeine and alcohol. It may be necessary to restrict fluids, although not to the point of dehydration, during the exercise session. While exercising, the athlete may need to wear a minipad or, in some cases, an intravaginal support such as a pessary or bladder neck support prosthesis. Strengthening exercises and muscle re-education should be a component of the woman's fitness routine. Physical therapists and other health care providers can ask women more questions about pelvic floor function, encourage women to exercise these muscles, and seek medical care when they exhibit problems such as SUI. Health care providers should promote preventative pelvic muscle exercises rather than restorative.

Conclusion

During the last 25 years, the opportunities for females in sports have grown tremendously. The high number of females participating in sports has been associated with an increase in a number of musculoskeletal injuries and other high-level activity problems. In some circumstances, there appears to be a predisposition of the female to injury. This chapter presented the most common musculoskeletal injuries, including ACL injury, PFPS, MTSS, and other problems common to the female athlete. Strategies and programs to prevent injury are also discussed. Along with musculoskeletal injuries, the existing knowledge on the female triad is summarized with information given on the symptoms, diagnosis, and treatment. The chapter concludes with unique issues facing the older woman athlete.

References

1. National Collegiate Athletics Association: *Gender equity in intercollegiate athletics. A practical guide for colleges and universities,* Indianapolis, IN, 2008, National Collegiate Athletics Association.
2. Griffin LY: Better understanding of ACL injury prevention, *The NCAA News,* October 9, 2000, http://www.ncaa.org/wps/ncaa?ContentID=26659.
3. McArdle WD, Katch FI, Katch VL: *Exercise physiology: Energy, nutrition, and human performance,* ed 6, Philadelphia, 2007, Lippincott Williams & Wilkins.
4. Silvers HJ, Mandelbaum BR: Prevention of anterior cruciate ligament injury in the female athlete, *Br J Sports Med* 41(Suppl I):i52–i59, 2007.
5. van der Hart CP, van den Bekerom MPJ, Patt TW: The occurrence of osteoarthritis at a minimum of ten years after reconstruction of the anterior cruciate ligament, *J Orthop Surg* 3:24, 2008.
6. Lohmander LS, Ostenberg A, Englund M, Roos H: High prevalence of knee osteoarthritis, pain, and functional limitations in female soccer players twelve years after anterior cruciate ligament injury, *Arthritis Rheum* 50(10):3145–3152, 2004.
7. Gilchrist J, Mandelbaum BR, Melancon H, et al: A randomized controlled trial to prevent noncontact anterior cruciate ligament injury in female collegiate soccer players, *Am J Sports Med* 36(8):1476–1483, 2008.
8. Griffin LY, Agel J, Albohm MJ, et al: Noncontact anterior cruciate ligament injuries: Risk factors and prevention strategies, *J Am Acad Orthop Surg* 8:141–150, 2000.
9. Renstrom P, Ljungqvist A, Arendt EA, et al: Non-contact ACL injuries in female athletes: An International Olympic Committee current concepts statement, *Br J Sports Med* 42:394–412, 2008.
10. DeMorat G, Weinhold P, Blackburn T, et al: Aggressive quadriceps loading can induce noncontact anterior cruciate ligament injury, *Am J Sports Med* 32(2):477–483, 2004.
11. Roush MB, Sevier TL, Wilson JK, et al: Anterior knee pain: A clinical comparison of rehabilitation methods, *Clin J Sport Med* 10:22–28, 2000.
12. Arendt EA, Dick RW: Knee injury patterns among men and women in collegiate basketball and soccer. NCAA data and review of the literature, *Am J Sports Med* 23:694–701, 1995.
13. Hootman JM, Dick RW, Agel J: Epidemiology of collegiate injuries for 15 sports: Summary and recommendations for injury prevention initiatives, *J Athl Train* 42(2):311–319, 2007.
14. Prodromos CC, Han Y, Rogowski J, et al: A meta-analysis of the incidence of anterior cruciate ligament tears as a function of gender, sport, and a knee-injury-reduction regimen, *Arthroscopy* 23(12):1320–1325, 2007.
15. Ireland ML, Ballantyne BT, Little K, McClay IS: A radiographic analysis of the relationship between size and shape of the intercondylar notch and anterior cruciate ligament study, *Knee Surg Sports Traumatol Arthrosc* 9:200–205, 2001.
16. Chandrashekar N, Slauterbeck J, Hashemi J: Sex-based differences in the anthropometric characteristics of the anterior cruciate ligament and its relation to intercondylar notch geometry, *Am J Sports Med* 33(10):1492–1498, 2005.
17. Shelbourne KD, Davis TJ, Klootwyk TE: The relationship between intercondylar notch width of the femur and the incidence of anterior cruciate ligament tears, *Am J Sports Med* 26(3):402–408, 1998.
18. Hashemi J, Chandrashekar N, Mansouri H, et al: The human anterior cruciate ligament: Sex differences in ultrastructure and correlation with biomechanical properties, *J Orthop Res* 26 (945–950), 2008.
19. DeJour H, Bonnin M: Tibial translation after anterior cruciate ligament rupture. Two radiological tests compared, *J Bone Joint Surg Br* 76:745–749, 1994.
20. Brandon ML, Haynes PT, Bonamo JR, et al: The association between posterior-inferior tibial slope and anterior cruciate ligament insufficiency, *Arthroscopy* 22(8):894–899, 2006.
21. Stijak L, Herzog RF, Schai P: Is there an influence of the tibial slope of the lateral condyle on the ACL lesion? A case-control study, *Knee Surg Sports Traumatol Arthrosc* 16(2):112–117, 2008.
22. Rosene JM, Fogarty TD: Anterior tibial translation in collegiate athletes with normal anterior cruciate ligament integrity, *J Athl Train* 34:93–98, 1999.
23. Uhorchak JM, Scoville CR, Williams GN, et al: Risk factors associated with noncontact injury of the anterior cruciate ligament: A prospective four-year evaluation of 859 West Point cadets, *Am J Sports Med* 31:831–842, 2003.
24. Wojtys EM, Huston LJ, Lindenfeld TN, et al: Association between the menstrual cycle and anterior cruciate ligament injuries in female athletes, *Am J Sports Med* 26(5):614–619, 1998.
25. Romani W, Patrie J, Curl LA, Flaws JA: The correlations between estradiol, estrone, estriol, progesterone, and sex hormone-binding globulin and anterior cruciate ligament stiffness, *J Women's Health* 12:287–298, 2003.

26. Belanger MJ, Moore DC, Crisco III JJ, et al: Knee laxity does not vary with the menstrual cycle before or after exercise, *Am J Sports Med* 32(5):1150–1157, 2004.

27. Shultz SJ, Kirk SE, Johnson MJ, et al: Relationship between sex hormones and anterior knee laxity across the menstrual cycle, *Med Sci Sports Exerc* 36(7):1165–1174, 2004.

28. Beynnon BD, Bernstein IM, Belisle A, et al.: The effect of estradiol and progesterone on knee and ankle joint laxity, *Am J Sports Med* 33(9):1298–1304, 2005.

29. Abt JP, Sell TC, Laudner KG, et al: Neuromuscular and biomechanical characteristics do not vary across the menstrual cycle, *Knee Surg Sports Traumatol Arthrosc* 15:901–907, 2007.

30. Chaudhari AMW, Lindenfeld TN, Andriacchi TP, et al: Knee and hip loading patterns at different phases in the menstrual cycle. Implications for the gender difference in anterior cruciate ligament injury rates, *Am J Sports Med* 35(5):793–800, 2007.

31. Ferber R, Davis IM, Williams DSI: Gender differences in lower extremity mechanics during running, *Clin Biomech* 18:350–357, 2003.

32. Ford KR, Myer GD, Toms H, Hewett TE: Gender differences in the kinematics of unanticipated cutting in young athletes, *Med Sci Sports Excer* 37(1):124–129, 2005.

33. Landry SC, McKean KA, Hubley-Kozey CL, et al: Neuromuscular control and lower limb biomechanical differences exist between male and female elite adolescent soccer players during an unanticipated run and crosscut maneuver, *Am J Sports Med* 35(11):1901–1911, 2007.

34. Ford KR, Myer GD, Hewett TE: Valgus knee motion during landing in high school female and male basketball players, *Med Sci Sports Exer* 35:1745–1750, 2003.

35. Lephart SM, Ferris CM, Riemann BL, et al: Gender differences in strength and lower extremity kinematics during landing, *Clin Orthop* 401:162–169, 2002.

36. McLean SG, Huang X, Su A, van den Bogert AJ: Sagittal plane biomechanics cannot injure the ACL during sidestep cutting, *Clin Biomech* 19:828–838, 2004.

37. Nagano Y, Ida H, Akai M, Fukubayashi T: Gender differences in knee kinematics and muscle activity during single limb drop landing, *The Knee* 14:218–223, 2007.

38. Schmitz RJ, Kulas AS, Perrin DH, et al: Sex differences in lower extremity biomechanics during single leg landings, *Clin Biomech* 22:681–688, 2007.

39. Wojtys EM, Ashton-Miller JA, Huston LJ: A gender-related difference in the contribution of the knee musculature to sagittal-plane shear stiffness in subjects with similar knee laxity, *J Bone Joint Surg Am* 84:10–16, 2002.

40. Decker MJ, Torry MR, Wyland DJ, et al: Gender differences in lower extremity kinematics, kinetics, and energy absorption during landing, *Clin Biomech* 18:662–669, 2003.

41. Jacobs CA, Uhl TL, Mattacola CG, et al: Hip abductor function and lower extremity landing kinematics: Sex differences, *J Athl Train* 42(1):76–83, 2007.

42. Lawrence III RK, Kernozek TW, Miller EJ, et al: Influences of hip external rotation strength on knee mechanics during single-leg drop landings in females, *Clin Biomech* 23:806–813, 2008.

43. Kernozek TW, Torry MR, Iwaski M: Gender differences in lower extremity landing mechanics caused by neuromuscular fatigue, *Am J Sports Med* 36(3):554–565, 2008.

44. Borotikar BS, Newcomer R, Koppes R, McLean SL: Combined effects of fatigue and decision making on female lower limb landing postures: Central and peripheral contributions to ACL injury risk, *Clin Biomech* 23:81–92, 2008.

45. Counts J, Bolgla LA, Ireland ML. Female issues in sport: Risk factors and prevention of ACL injuries. In: Johnson D, Pedowitz R, editors, *Practical orthopaedic sports medicine and arthroscopy*, Philadelphia, 2006, Lippincott Williams & Wilkins.

46. Mandelbaum BR, Silvers HJ, Watanabe DS, et al: Effectiveness of a neuromuscular training program in preventing anterior cruciate ligament injuries in female athletes, *Am J Sports Med* 33:1003–1010, 2005.

47. Hewett TE, Lindenfeld TN, Riccobene JV, Noyes FR: The effect of neuromuscular training on the incidence of knee injury in female athletes, *Am J Sports Med* 27(6):699–705, 1999.

48. Pollard CD, Sigward SM, Ota S, et al: The influence of in-season injury prevention training on lower-extremity kinematics during landing in female soccer players, *Clin J Sport Med* 16:223–227, 2006.

49. Cleland JA, Fritz JM, Whitman JM, et al: The use of a lumbar spine manipulation technique by physical therapists in patients who satisfy a clinical prediction rule: A case series, *J Orthop Sports Phys Ther* 36:209–214, 2006.

50. Sutlive TG, Mitchell SD, Maxfield SN, et al: Identification of individuals with patellofemoral pain whose symptoms improved after a combined program of foot orthosis use and modified activity: A preliminary investigation. *Phys Ther* 84(1):49–61, 2004.

51. Schmitz RJ, Riemann BL, Thompson T: Gluteus medius activity during isometric closed-chain hip rotation, *J Sport Rehabil* 11(3): 179–188, 2002.

52. Ireland ML: The female ACL: Why is it more prone to injury? *Orthop Clin North Am* 33:637–651, 2002.

53. Fung DT, Zhang LQ: Modeling of ACL impingement against the intercondylar notch, *Clin Biomech* 18:933–941, 2003.

54. Fleming BC, Renstrom PA, Ohlen G, et al.: The gastrocnemius muscle is an antagonist of the anterior cruciate ligament, *J Orthop Res* 19:1178–1184, 2001.

55. Hewett TE, Myer GD, Ford KR: Decrease in neuromuscular control about the knee with maturation in female athletes, *J Bone Joint Surg Am* 86(8):1601–1608, 2004.

56. Leetun DT, Ireland ML, Willson JD, et al: Core stability measures as risk factors for lower extremity injury in athletes, *Med Sci Sports Exer* 36(6):926–934, 2004.

57. McLean CL: The ACL injury enigma: We can't prevent what we don't understand, *J Athl Train* 43(5):538–540, 2008.

58. Hewett TE, Zazulak BT, Myer GD: Effects of the menstrual cycle on anterior cruciate ligament injury risk: A systematic review, *Am J Sports Med* 35(4):659–668, 2007.

59. Sarwar R, Niclos BB, Rutherford OM: Changes in muscle strength, relaxation rate and fatigability during the human menstrual cycle, *J Physiol* 493:267–272, 1996.

60. Hewett TE, Myer GD: The effects of oral contraceptives on knee stability and neuromuscular performance in female athletes, *Med Sci Sports Exerc* 32:S207, 2000.

61. Moller-Nielsen J, Hammar M: Women's soccer injuries in relation to the menstrual cycle and oral contraceptive use, *Med Sci Sports Exerc* 21:126–129, 1989.

62. Moller-Nielsen J, Hammar M: Sports injuries and oral contraceptive use. Is there a relationship? *Sports Med* 12:152–160, 1991.

63. Myklebust G, Engebretsen L, Braekken IH, et al: Prevention of anterior cruciate ligament injuries in female team handball players: A prospective intervention study over three seasons, *Clin J Sports Med* 13:71–78, 2003.

64. Zebis MK, Bencke J, Andersen LL, et al: The effects of neuromuscular training on knee joint motor control during sidecutting in female elite soccer and handball players, *Clin J Sport Med* 18:329–337, 2008.

65. Lephart S, Abt JP, Ferris CM, et al: Neuromuscular and biomechanical characteristic changes in high school athletes: A plyometric versus basis resistance program, *Br J Sports Med* 39:932–938, 2005.

66. Grindstaff TL, Hammill RR, Tuzson AE, Hertel J: Neuromuscular control training programs and noncontact anterior cruciate ligament

injury rates in female athletes: A numbers-needed-to-treat analysis, *J Athl Train* 41(4):450–456, 2006.

67. Livingston LA: The quadriceps angle: A review of the literature, *J Orthop Sports Phys Ther* 28:105–109, 1998.

68. Caylor D, Fites R, Worrell TW: The relationship between quadriceps angle and anterior knee pain syndrome, *J Orthop Sports Phys Ther* 17(1):11–16, 1993.

69. Powers CM: The influence of altered lower-extremity kinematics on patellofemoral joint dysfunction: A theoretical perspective, *J Orthop Sports Phys Ther* 33(11):639–646, 2003.

70. Lephart SM, Ferris CM, Riemann BL, et al: Gender differences in strength and lower extremity kinematics during landing, *Clin Orthop* 401:162–169, 2002.

71. Ireland ML, Willson JD, Ballantyne BT, Davis IM: Hip strength in females with and without patellofemoral pain, *J Orthop Sports Phys Ther* 33(11):671–676, 2003.

72. Robinson RL, Nee RJ: Analysis of hip strength in females seeking physical therapy treatment for unilateral patellofemoral pain syndrome, *J Orthop Sports Phys Ther* 37(5):232–238, 2007.

73. Bolgla LA, Malone TR, Umberger BR, Uhl TL: Hip strength and hip and knee kinematics during stair descent in females with and without patellofemoral pain syndrome, *J Orthop Sports Phys Ther* 38(1):12–18, 2008.

74. Cichanowski HR, Schmitt JS, Johnson RJ, Niemuth PE: Hip strength in collegiate female athletes with patellofemoral pain, *Med Sci Sports Exer* 39(8):1227–1232, 2007.

75. Willson JD, Davis I: Lower extremity strength and mechanics during jumping in women with patellofemoral pain, *J Sport Rehabil* 18(1):75–89, 2009.

76. Powers CM, Chen PY, Reischl SF, Perry J: Comparison of foot rotation and lower extremity rotation in persons with and without patellofemoral pain, *Foot Ankle Intern* 23(7):634–640, 2002.

77. Willson JD, Binder-Macleod S, Davis IS: Lower extremity jumping mechanics of female athletes with and without patellofemoral pain before and after exertion, *Am J Sports Med* 36(8):1587–1596, 2008.

78. Willson JD, Davis I: Lower extremity mechanics of females with and without patellofemoral pain across activities with progressively greater task demands, *Clin Biomech* 23:203–211, 2008.

79. Dierks TA, Manal KT, Hamill J, Davis IS: Proximal and distal influences on hip and knee kinematics in runners with patellofemoral pain during a prolonged run, *J Orthop Sports Phys Ther* 38(8):448–456, 2008.

80. Tiberio D: The effect of excessive subtalar joint pronation on patellofemoral mechanics: A theoretical model, *J Orthop Sports Phys Ther* 9(4):160–165, 1987.

81. Thijs Y, Van Tiggelen D, Roosen P, et al: A prospective study on gait-related intrinsic risk factors for patellofemoral pain, *Clin J Sport Med* 17(6):437–445, 2007.

82. Hetsroni I, Finestone A, Milgrom C, et al: A prospective biomechanical study of the association between foot pronation and the incidence of anterior knee pain among military recruits, *J Bone Joint Surg Br* 88(7):905–908, 2006.

83. Thijs Y, De Clercq D, Roosen P, Witvrouw E: Gait-related intrinsic risk factors for patellofemoral pain in novice recreational runners, *Br J Sports Med* 42(6):466–471, 2008.

84. Fagan V, Delahunt E: Patellofemoral pain syndrome: A review on the associated neuromuscular deficits and current treatment options, *Br J Sports Med* 42:489–495, 2008.

85. Mascal CL, Landel R, Powers CM: Management of patellofemoral pain targeting hip, pelvis, and trunk muscle function: 2 case reports, *J Orthop Sports Phys Ther* 33(11):647–660, 2003.

86. Tyler TF, Nicholas SJ, Mullaney MJ, McHugh MP: The role of hip muscle function in the treatment of patellofemoral pain syndrome, *Am J Sports Med* 34(4):630–636, 2006.

87. Boling MC, Bolgla LA, Mattacola CG, et al: Outcomes of a weight-bearing rehabilitation program for patients diagnosed with patellofemoral pain syndrome, *Arch Phys Med Rehabil* 87(11):1428–1435, 2006.

88. Natri A, Kannus P, Jarvinen M: Which factors predict the long-term outcome in chronic patellofemoral pain syndrome? A 7-yr prospective follow-up study, *Med Sci Sports Exerc* 30:1572–1577, 1998.

89. Bolgla LA, Malone TR: Exercise prescription and patellofemoral pain: Evidence for rehabilitation, *J Sport Rehabil* 14(1):72–88, 2005.

90. Witvrouw E, Danneels L, van Tiggelen D, et al: Open versus closed kinetic chain exercise in patellofemoral pain. A 5-year prospective randomized study, *Am J Sports Med* 32(5):1122–1129, 2004.

91. Herrington L, Al-Sherhi A: A controlled trial of weight-bearing versus non-weight-bearing exercises for patellofemoral pain, *J Orthop Sports Phys Ther* 37(4):155–160, 2007.

92. Eng JJ, Pierrynowski MR: Evaluation of soft foot orthotics in the treatment of patellofemoral pain syndrome, *Phys Ther* 73(5):62–68, 1993.

93. Johnston LB, Gross MT: Effects of foot orthoses on quality of life for individuals with patellofemoral pain syndrome, *J Orthop Sports Phys Ther* 34(8):440–448, 2004.

94. Wilk KE, Davies GJ, Mangine RE, Malone TR: Patellofemoral disorders: A classification system and clinical guidelines for nonoperative rehabilitation, *J Orthop Sports Phys Ther* 28(5):307–322, 1998.

95. Witvrouw E, Werner S, Mikkelsen C, et al: Clinical classification of patellofemoral pain syndrome: Guidelines for non-operative treatment, *Knee Surg Sports Traumatol Arthrosc* 13:122–130, 2005.

96. Andrish JT: Leg pain. In DeLee JC, Drez D, editors: *Orthopedic sports medicine,* Philadelphia, 1994, WB Saunders.

97. Clement DB, Taunton JE, Smart GW, McNicol KL: A survey of overuse running injuries, *Phys Sportsmed* 9:47–58, 1981.

98. Yates B, White S: The incidence of risk factors in the development of medial tibial stress syndrome among naval recruits, *Am J Sports Med* 32:772–780, 2004.

99. Saxena A, O'Brien T, Bunce D: Anatomic dissection of the tibialis posterior muscle and its correlation to medial tibial stress syndrome, *J Foot Surg* 29:105–108, 1990.

100. D'Ambrosia RD, Zelis RF, Chuinard RG, Wilmore J: Interstitial pressure measurements in the anterior and posterior compartments in athletes with shin splints, *Am J Sports Med* 5:127–131, 1977.

101. Beck BR, Osternig LR: Medical tibial stress syndrome. The location of muscles in the leg in relation to symptoms, *J Bone Joint Surg Am* 76:1057–1061, 1994.

102. Detmer D: Chronic shin splints: Classification and management of medial tibial stress syndrome, *Sports Med* 3:436–446, 1986.

103. Beck BR, Osternig LR: Medial tibial stress syndrome. The location of muscles in the leg in relation to symptoms, *J Bone Joint Surg Am* 76:1057–1061, 1994.

104. Tweed JL, Avil SJ, Campbell JA, Barners MR: Etiologic factors in the development of medial tibial stress syndrome, *J Am Podiatric Med Assoc* 98:107–111, 2008.

105. Ilahi OA, Kohl HW: Lower extremity morphology and alignment and risk of overuse injury, *Clin J Sports Med* 8:38–42, 1998.

106. Messier SP, Pittala KA: Etiologic factors associated with selected running injuries, *Med Sci Sports Exerc* 20:501–505, 1988.

107. Bennett JE, Reinking MF, Pluemer B, et al: Factors contributing to the development of medial tibial stress syndrome in high school runners, *J Orthop Sports Phys Ther* 31(9):504–510, 2001.

108. Plisky MS, Rauh MJ, Heidersheit B, et al: Medial tibial stress syndrome in high school cross-country runners: Incidence and risk factors, *J Orthop Sports Phys Ther* 37(2):40–47, 2007.

109. Slimmon D, Bennell K, Brukner P, et al: Long term outcome of fasciotomy with partial fasciectomy for chronic exertional compartment syndrome of the lower leg, *Am J Sports Med* 30:581–588, 2005.

110. Jackson DW, Mannarino F: Lumbar spine injuries in athletes. In Scott WN, Nisonson B, Nicholas JA, editors: *Principles of sports medicine*, Baltimore, 1984, Williams & Wilkins.

111. Hall SJ: Mechanical contribution to lumbar stress injuries in female gymnasts, *Med Sci Sports Exerc* 18:599–602, 1986.

112. Reid DC: *Sports injury assessment and rehabilitation*, New York, 1992, Churchill Livingstone.

113. Micheli LJ, Wood R: Back pain in young athletes: Significant differences from adults in causes and patterns, *Arch Pediatr Adolesc Med* 149(1):15–18, 1995.

114. Barash HL, Galante J, Lambert C, Ray R: Spondylolisthesis and tight hamstrings, *J Bone Joint Surg Am* 52(7):1319–1328, 1970.

115. Corrigan B, Maitland GD: *Practical orthopedic medicine*, London, 1983, Butterworth-Heinemann Ltd.

116. Smith AD, Micheli LJ: Injuries in competitive figure skaters, *Phys Sportsmed* 10:36–47 1982.

117. Congeni J, McCulloch J, Swanson K: Lumbar spondylolysis: A study of natural progression in athletes, *Am J Sports Med* 25(2):248–253, 1997.

118. Kirkaldy-Willis WH, Wedge JH, Yong-Hing K, Reilly J: Pathology and pathogenesis of lumbar spondylosis and stenosis, *Spine* 3:319–328, 1978.

119. Porterfield JA, DeRosa C: *Mechanical low back pain: Perspectives in functional anatomy*, Philadelphia, 1991, WB Saunders Co.

120. Debnath UK, Freeman BJ, Gregory P, et al: Clinical outcome and return to sport after the surgical treatment of spondylolysis in young athletes, *J Bone Joint Surg Br* 85:244–249, 2003.

121. Lee D: *Manual therapy for the thorax*, Delta, Canada, 1994, DOPC.

122. Marymont JV, Lynch MA, Henning CE: Exercise-related stress reaction of the sacroiliac joint, *Am J Sports Med* 14:320–323, 1986.

123. Gerbino II PG, Micheli LJ: Back injuries in the young athlete, *Clin Sports Med* 14:571–590, 1995.

124. Adams MA, Hutton WC: The mechanical function of the lumbar apophyseal joints, *Spine* 8:327–330, 1983.

125. Deyo RA, Diehl AK, Rosenthal M: How many days of bed rest for acute low back pain? A randomized clinical trial, *N Engl J Med* 315:1064–1070, 1986.

126. Saunders HD, Saunders R: *Evaluation, treatment, and prevention of musculoskeletal disorders*, Chaska, MN, 1993, Saunders Group.

127. Boden SD, Davis DO, Dina TS, et al: Abnormal magnetic-resonance scans of the lumbar spine in asymptomatic subjects: A prospective investigation, *J Bone Joint Surg Am* 72:403–408, 1990.

128. Maitland GD: *Vertebral manipulation*, ed 5, London, 1986, Butterworth-Heinemann Ltd.

129. Childs JD, Fritz JM, Flynn TW, et al: A clinical prediction rule for classifying patients with low back pain most likely to benefit from spinal manipulation: A validation study, *Ann Intern Med* 141(12):920–928, 2004.

130. Grieve GP: *Common vertebral joint problems*, Edinburgh, 1981, Churchill Livingstone.

131. Jull GA: Examination of the lumbar spine. In Grieve GP, editor: *Modern manual therapy of the vertebral column*, Edinburgh, 1986, Churchill Livingstone.

132. Gregory PL, Biswas AC, Batt ME: Musculoskeletal problems of the chest wall in athletes, *Sports Med* 32(4):235–250, 2002.

133. Rumball JS, Lebrun CM, Di Ciacca SR, Orlando K: Rowing injuries, *Sports Med* 35(6):537–555, 2005.

134. Aspegren D, Hyde T, Miller M: Conservative treatment of a female collegiate volleyball player with costochondritis, *J Manipulative Physiol Ther* 30(4):321–325, 2007.

135. Nattiv A, Agostini R, Drinkwater B, Yeager KK: The female athlete triad. The inter-relatedness of disordered eating, amenorrhea, and osteoporosis, *Clin J Sports Med* 13:405–418, 1994.

136. Nattiv A, Loucks AB, Manroe MM, et al: Position stand: The female athlete triad, *Med Sci Sports Exerc* 39(10):1867–1882, 2007.

137. Bonci CM, Bonci LJ, Granger LR, et al: National Athletic Trainers' Association position statement: Preventing, detecting, and managing disordered eating in athletes, *J Athl Train* 43(1):80–108, 2008.

138. Wade GN, Schneider JE, Li HY: Control of fertility by metabolic cues, *Am J Physiol* 270:E1–E19, 1996.

139. Romes ES, Ammerman S, Rosen DS, et al: Children and adolescents with eating disorders: The state of the art, *Pediatrics* 111:e98–e108, 2003.

140. Loucks AB, Mortola JF, Girton L, Yen SSC: Alterations in the hypothalamic-pituitary-ovarian and the hypothalamic-pituitary-adrenal axes in athletic women, *J Endocrinol Metab* 68:402–411, 1989.

141. Loucks AB, Thuma JR: Luteinizing hormone pulsatility is disrupted at a threshold of energy availability in regularly menstruating women, *J Clin Endocrinol Metab* 88(1):297–311, 2003.

142. Loucks AB, Verdun M, Heath EM: Low energy availability, not stress of exercise, alters LH pulsatility in exercising women, *J Appl Physiol* 84(1):37–46, 1998.

143. Zanker CL, Swaine IL: Relation between bone turnover, oestradiol, and energy balance in women distance runners, *Br J Sports Med* 32:167–171, 1998.

144. Keen AD, Drinkwater BL: Irreversible bone loss in former amenorrheic athletes, *Osteoporos Int* 7:311–315, 1997.

145. Warren MP, Brooks-Gunn J, Fox RP, et al: Osteopenia in exercise associated amenorrhea using ballet dancers as a model: a longitudinal study, *J Clin Endocrinol Metab* 87:3162–3168, 2002.

146. Friday KE, Drinkwater BL, Bruemmer B, et al: Elevated plasma low-density lipoprotein and high density lipoprotein cholesterol levels in amenorrheic athletes: Effects of endogenous hormone status and nutrient intake, *J Clin Endocrinol Metab* 77:1605–1609, 1993.

147. O'Donnel E, De Souza MJ: The cardiovascular effects of chronic hypoestrogenism in amenorrheic athletes: A critical review, *Sports Med* 34:601–627, 2004.

148. Hammar ML, Hammar-Henriksson MB, Frisk J, et al: Few oligo-amenorrheic athletes have vasomotor symptoms, *Maturitas* 34:219–225, 2000.

149. Bennell K, Matheson G, Meeuwisse W, Brikner P: Risk factors for stress fractures, *Sports Med* 28:91–122, 1999.

150. Hassager C, Colwell A, Assiri AMA: Effect of menopause and hormone replacement therapy on urinary excretion of pyridinium cross-links: A longitudinal and cross-sectional study, *Clin Endocrinol* 37(1):45–50, 1992.

151. Ihle R, Loucks AB: Dose-response relationships between energy availability and bone turnover in young exercising women, *J Bone Miner Res* 19:1231–1240, 2004.

152. Hinton PS, Kubas KL: Psychosocial correlates of disordered eating in female collegiate athletes: Validation of the ATHLETE questionnaire, *J Am Coll Health* 54(3):149–156, 2005.

153. Brownell KD, Rodin J, Wilmore JH: *Eating, body weight and performance in athletes: Disorders of modern society,* Philadelphia, 1992, Lea and Febiger.

154. American Academy of Pediatrics Committee on Adolescence: Identifying and treating eating disorders, *Pediatrics* 111: 204–211, 2003.

155. Khan AA, Hanley DA, Bilezikian JP, et al: Standards for performing DXA in individuals with secondary causes of osteoporosis, *J Clin Densitom* 9:47–57, 2006.

156. World Health Organization: Assessment of fracture risk and its application to screening for postmenopausal osteoporosis, *WHO Tech Report Ser* 843:1–129, 1994.

157. NIH Consensus Development Panel: Osteoporosis prevention, diagnosis, and therapy, *JAMA* 285(6):785–795, 2001.

158. International Society for Clinical Densitometry Writing Group for the ISCD Position Development Conference: Diagnosis of osteoporosis in men, women, and children, *J Clin Densitom* 7:17–26, 2004.

159. Falsetti L, Gambera A, Barbetti L, Specchia C: Long-term follow-up of functional hypothalamic amenorrhea and prognostic factors, *J Clin Endocrinol Metab* 87:500–505, 2002.

160. Patlas N, Golomb G, Yaffe P, et al: Transplacental effects of bisphosphonates on fetal skeletal ossification and mineralization in rats, *Teratology* 60:68–73, 1999.

161. Artal R, Sherman C: Exercise during pregnancy: Safe and beneficial for most, *Phys Sportsmed* 27:51–58, 1999.

162. Kardel KR: Effects of intense training during and after pregnancy in top-level athletes, *Scand J Med Sci Sports* 15:79–86, 2005.

163. Paisley TS, Joy EA, Price RJ: Exercise during pregnancy: A practical approach, *Current Sports Med Reports* 2:325–330, 2003.

164. Comittee on Patient Education of the American College of Obstetricians and Gynecologists: Excersise during pregnancy. American Congress of Obstetricians and Gynecologists, 2003. Accessed at www.acog.org/publications/patient-education/bp119.cfm.

165. Veille JC: Maternal and fetal cardiovascular response to exercise during pregnancy, *Semin Perinatol* 20:250–262, 1996.

166. Jaque-Fortunato SV, Wiswell RA, Khodiguian N, Artal R: A comparison of the ventilatory responses to exercise in pregnant, postpartum, and nonpregnant women, *Semin Perinatol* 20:263–276, 1996.

167. Dewey KG, McCrory MA: Effects of dieting and physical activity on pregnancy and lactation, *Am J Clin Nutrition* 59:446S–453S, 1994.

168. Clapp JF: The course of labour after endurance exercise, *Am J Obstet Gynecol* 163:1799–1805, 1990.

169. Dye TD, Knox KL, Artal R, et al: Physical activity, obesity, and diabetes in pregnancy, *Am J Epidemiol* 146:961–965, 1997.

170. Clarke PE, Gross H: Women's behavior, beliefs and information sources about physical exercise in pregnancy, *Midwifery* 20: 133–141, 2004.

171. Wallace AM, Boyer DB, Dan A: Aerobic exercise, maternal self-esteem and physical discomforts during pregnancy, *J Nurse-Midwife* 31:255–262, 1986.

172. Artal R, Clapp JF, Vigil DV: ACSM Current Comment: Exercise during pregnancy. American College of Sports Medicine. Acessed at www.acsm.org/AM/Template.cfm?section=current_comments18 Template=/CM/ContentDisplay.cfm8contentID=8638.

173. American College of Obstetricians and Gynecologists: Exercise during pregnancy and the postpartum period. American College of Obstetricians and Gynecologists Committee Opinion No. 267, *Obstet Gynecol* 99:171–173, 2002.

174. Kardel KR, Kase T: Training in pregnant women: Effects on fetal development and birth, *Am J Obstet Gynecol* 178:280–286, 1998.

175. Beilock SL, Feltz DL, Pivarnik JM: Training patterns of athletes during pregnancy and postpartum, *Res Quart Ex Sport* 72: 39–46, 2001.

176. Krolner B, Toft B, Nielson SP, Tondevold E: Physical exercise as prophylaxis against involutional vertebral bone loss: a controlled trial, *Clin Sci* 64:541–546, 1983.

177. Elia G: Stress urinary incontinence: Removing barriers to exercise, *Phys Sportsmed* 27(1):39–52, 1999.

178. Nygaard IE, DeLancey JO, Arnsdorf L, Murphy E: Exercise and incontinence, *Obstet Gynecol* 75(5):848–851, 1990.

179. Wallace K: Female pelvic floor functions, dysfunctions, and behavioral approaches to treatment, *Clin Sports Med* 13(2): 459–481, 1994.

180. Griebling TL, Nygaard IE: The role of estrogen replacement therapy in the management of urinary incontinence and urinary tract infection in postmenopausal women, *Endocrinol Metab Clin North Am* 26(2):347–360, 1997.

Musculoskeletal Dance Medicine and Science

Jeffrey A. Russell

Introduction and Objectives

Dance medicine and science is a specialized field concerned with studying and caring for a fascinating type of individual who is often overlooked as an athlete, that is, the dancer. Dancers in all genres of dance will benefit from a cadre of well-trained, compassionate health care clinicians and scientists. This chapter is not an exhaustive compendium of dance medicine and science. Rather, its primary aim is to present information about the musculoskeletal aspects of dance medicine and science so that musculoskeletal clinicians and scientists can:

1. Recognize the rigorous physical performance that is required of dancers.
2. Appreciate the psyche of dancers and how it relates to effective provision of care for dance injuries.
3. Understand some fundamental skills of dancers as they pertain to common dance injuries.
4. Gain insight into specific injuries that are common in dance so that, in consultation with the other volumes of the *Musculoskeletal Rehabilitation* series, the reader will be equipped to deliver excellent care to the multitude of dancers who need it.

Intertwining Science and Art

At first impression, the melding of something as artistic as dance with something as analytical as science may seem unusual. However, dance is an anatomical art, founded at its core in movement. As such, it actually lends itself well to an understanding through scientific study in much the same way sports movement does. Thus, dance medicine and science, as a field of expertise, is not unlike sports medicine and science.

Both fields are professional disciplines based on scientific and clinical principles. Both fields focus on studying the attributes and abilities of physically active people—many of whom are extraordinarily skilled—and applying the knowledge to improving performance and preventing and managing injuries and conditions suffered by participants in their respective domains. This chapter introduces musculoskeletal health care practitioners to concepts that will help them appropriately manage injuries in dancers and understand some of the idiosyncrasies that make dance medicine and science a challenging, yet rewarding, subspecialty in musculoskeletal practice.

Sports medicine and science in Western civilization can be traced to Herodicus in the fifth century BC.[1] In America, however, Dr. Edward Hitchcock is credited as the first sports medicine physician,[2] practicing at Amherst College in the 1850s. Although the first known published material about the benefits of therapeutic treatments and exercises for injuries were books by Avicenna, an Islamic medical practitioner in the tenth century AD,[1] the first report locatable in the medical literature that clearly shows an emphasis on dance medicine and science appeared in 1952 in the British journal *Physiotherapy*.[3] (It is important to note here that *dance medicine and science* is a distinctly different field from *dance therapy*, with the latter referring to psychoemotional interventions using dance as the medium.)

The most prominent professional society devoted exclusively to the medical and scientific aspects of dance is the International Association for Dance Medicine and Science (IADMS). Founded in 1990, by the following year its membership was 48 clinicians, scientists, educators, and dancers.[4] Today the group comprises more than 900 members from a wide variety of dance-related disciplines. The stated purpose of IADMS is to "enhance the health, well-being, training, and performance of dancers by cultivating educational, medical, and scientific excellence."[4] Worldwide, several other professional associations are either totally devoted to dance medicine and science or embrace this specialty as part of the broader performing arts medicine field. In addition, some national dance associations maintain subgroups focused on dance medicine and science. Table 27-1 identifies many of these organizations.

The relative newness of dance medicine and science compared with sports medicine and science, combined with the complex technical intricacies of dance means that there are many fertile areas for research to advance the field. Some of the demands of dance on the musculoskeletal system are inferred by supposition or anecdote rather than by scientific inquiry. However, an increasing number of researchers are accelerating the field's knowledge base. For example, a casual review of the Medline and the Cumulative Index to Nursing and Allied Health Literature (CINAHL) databases reveals that the number of articles therein containing either the word *dance* or the word *ballet* in their titles and that are devoted to some aspect of dance medicine and science has increased substantially in the last five decades; there were no such articles in 1959. This point, of course, excludes publications not indexed in those two databases, conference presentations, and similar dissemination avenues. Clearly, the discipline's breadth is increasing.

Dance as an Athletic Endeavor

Anyone who spends time in a dance teaching, rehearsal, or performance venue will have little doubt about the vigor and athleticism of dancers. Stretanski has called classical ballet a "full contact sport"[5] because of its potential for injury. Others corroborate the view that dancers as artists certainly possess characteristics associated with traditional athletes.[6-11] Any dissenting opinion is likely based solely in one's unwillingness to understand the extent to which aerobic and anaerobic power; flexibility; muscular strength, endurance, and power; proprioceptive function; coordination; agility; and other parameters commonly associated with sports participation are required for success in dance. Although typical dance training—without ancillary physical conditioning workouts—does not improve maximum oxygen consumption and other physiological variables to the same degree that sports training does,[7,12-17] dancers' bodies must withstand high physical stresses like those of their sports counterparts.[18] The daily regimen of training that is common in dance creates a level of exposure and movement repetition that increases susceptibility to injury when compared with nondancers.[19]

Differences in Working with Dancers versus Traditional Athletes

It is not required that the health care professional have dance experience to administer care to dancers, although it is helpful. Experience in sports medicine is generally useful for the clinician working with dancers, but there is not an automatic knowledge transfer. Understanding these points and motivating oneself to understand dancers in the context of their sphere of physical activity will prevent many misunderstandings and grievances.

Table 27-1

Representative Professional Organizations Wholly or Partially Devoted to Dance Medicine and Science*

Country	Organization
Organizations Primarily Focused on Dance (or Performing Arts) Medicine and Science	
France	Médecine des Arts (Arts Medicine)
Germany	Tanz Medizin Deutschland e.V. (TaMeD, Dance Medicine Germany)
Monaco	Association Danse Médecine Recherche (Dance Medicine Research Association)
The Netherlands	Nederlandse Vereniging voor Dans–en Muziek Geneeskunde (Dutch Performing Arts Medicine Association)
New Zealand	Arts Medicine Aotearoa New Zealand
Spain	Asociación Española de Medicina de la Danza (Spanish Association of Dance Medicine)
United Kingdom	British Association for Performing Arts Medicine
United States	International Association for Dance Medicine and Science
	Performing Arts Medicine Association
	National Athletic Trainers' Association, Clinical & Emerging Practices Athletic Trainers' Committee, Performing Arts Medicine Workgroup
	American Physical Therapy Association, Performing Arts Special Interest Group
National Dance Associations with Specific Focus on Dancer Health	
Australia	Ausdance
New Zealand	DANZ
United Kingdom	DanceUK
United States	DanceUSA

*Not an exhaustive list.

> ## Dance is an Athletic Activity
>
> - Dance is a rigorous physical performance activity that requires the same high levels of physical capacities as those required in sports
> - Dancers clearly are athletes in their own right
> - Because of its artistic component, dancers cannot and should not be forced into a traditional sports medicine model of care

It may be helpful to the clinician anticipating or wishing to work with dancers to first understand a small amount of background about dance. Dance is a multifaceted performing art that increasingly defies classification because there is such breadth in its practice and performance. Many different genres of dance are presented on stage and dancers train rigorously to participate in these. Although ballet and modern dance (also called *contemporary dance*) are two dominant genres, there is a vast assortment of others. Some of these include tap, jazz (including hip-hop and break dance), and ballroom. There also is a virtually limitless collection of world dance forms with rich national or cultural roots, such as flamenco, belly dance, Irish step dance, dances of India like *Bharatanatyam* and *Kuchipudi*, and many types of Latin American theatrical folk dances. In addition, public interest has been fueled by a number of television programs partly or fully devoted to competitive dance.

The accoutrements of dance differ markedly from the uniforms and equipment of sports. Overall, classical ballet is structured according to a codified movement vocabulary named in French. The clothing usually is tights and leotards for women and tights and close-fitting shirts for men. Footwear may be ballet slippers or *pointe* shoes. Modern dance is a more freeform genre with wider variability in choreography. Modern dancers typically do not wear shoes, and their attire may range from minimal clothing to casual street clothes to elaborate, very colorful costumes. Many of these features of modern dance also are seen in some contemporary ballet performances.

Injuries in ballet[20-29] and modern dance[29-32] have received the most attention in the orthopaedic and sports medicine literature. Although research about the demands on the musculoskeletal system of most of the other genres is scant at best, enough is known about some of them to indicate that substantial numbers of injuries do occur.[33-45] This suggests that there are many dancer-patients requiring musculoskeletal practitioners motivated to skillfully and compassionately care for them, a need that was identified as early as 1978 when Washington[46] encouraged orthopaedic surgeons to care for dancers because he foresaw an enlarging dance population—with a resulting proliferation of dance injuries—in the United States.

Health Care Access for Dancers

- Although ballet and modern dance are the most well-known genres in the United States, many varieties of dance are performed around the world
- In spite of a very high injury rate in dance, many dancers do not have access to necessary injury care
- There is a great need for musculoskeletal health care practitioners to gain expertise in dance medicine to increase proper care for dancers

---

The Dancer's Psyche

A cardinal rule for health care providers without a dance background who work with dancers is to understand and respect the dancer's psyche. This is related to the rigor of the physical regimen to which they apply themselves. Dancers are artists—athletically so, as previously described—and they approach their craft with intensity and fervor. They also are typically very grateful for well-delivered care. However, within any group of dancers, several will relate stories of well-meaning but ill-informed practitioners giving the poorly conceived advice to "stop dancing" as a standard cure for physical ailments. Sadly the prevalence of such episodes have frustrated many dancers and planted in them seeds of distrust toward allopathic health care[47] (although a notable contrast to this generality exists in the Netherlands[48]). Obviously there are injuries (e.g., stress fracture) when complete rest from dancing is the appropriate standard of care. Nonetheless, finding alternative methods to keep an injured dancer active and prevent deconditioning is important, as it is with any athlete. In cases in which some degree of dance can continue, the practitioner must work with the dancer—and his or her teachers and directors when possible—to develop a moderated activity plan that reduces the load on the compromised body region while still allowing the dancer to engage in as much of his or her usual activity as possible.

Another means of counteracting dancers' skepticism toward health care providers is judicious attention to the "history" portion of the commonly used injury evaluation methodology of history, observation, movement assessment, special testing, and palpation. Listening intently to symptom descriptions offered by the dancer-patient will yield valuable information as a foundation to the remainder of the evaluation, in part because dancers know their bodies very well. Furthermore, they will sense the practitioner's respect for dance and for the information they are providing and respond accordingly. Still another way for medical professionals to understand dance, and thereby demonstrate their interest to dancers, is attending dance performances. Dancers consider this to be a very important characteristic in their health care providers.[49]

Understanding how dancers approach pain is fundamental to success in caring for them. They possess both a higher threshold and a higher tolerance for pain than do nondancers.[50] That is, in comparison with nondancers, not only is more pain required for dancers to perceive it (threshold), they also can withstand greater levels of pain (tolerance). Experiencing pain as a dancer is so customary that it could be considered "normal."[51] However, dancers may not differentiate well between pain brought on by performing their usual dance activities and pain that results from injury.[52] The obsessive passion for dance (as opposed to harmonious passion) that many dancers exhibit has been associated with willful neglect of injuries.[53] "Dancing through" injuries is typical,[47] especially in dancers with more experience[48] or in those who believe that engaging in a treatment regimen will interfere with their ability to participate in dance.[49] Regardless of dancers' general propensity to tolerate pain, injuries create psychological stress that can adversely affect their ability to dance.[20,54,55] Furthermore, the psyche of the dancer that allows him or her to achieve excellence may be a contributor to injury incidence,[53] particularly in classical ballet.[22]

Dance Health Care

- Dancers are extremely diligent in their work ethic and they typically take dance classes and rehearse for many hours daily
- Dancers tend to "dance through" injuries rather than seek health care advice
- Although a sports medicine model is helpful in working with dancers, these athletic artists must be respected for their unique talents and abilities that require adaptation of sports medicine methods
- "Stop dancing" is injury care advice that is universally deplored by dancers

---

Environmental Differences

Athletes in typical sports environments are usually accustomed to the cadre of professionals who surround them: physicians, athletic trainers, physical therapists, and a variety of other specialists. In fact, it is unlikely in professional and Olympic sports and extremely unusual at the university level, and even at most large- to medium-sized high schools, for there to be no sports medicine provision whatsoever. In addition, American sports receive unprecedented public attention and they usually enjoy a financial state in which health care for their participants is both possible and presumptive. Virtually the opposite is true of most dance programs below the top echelon of professional companies; furthermore, many dancers are medically uninsured or underinsured.[56,57] This problem is particularly exacerbated for dancers in small professional companies or who dance part-time.[56] Ambegaonkar and Caswell[58] found that university-level dance students in the United States are woefully underserved by the medical profession. A discussion about the relative merits of funding either sports or dance is not the place of this chapter, but it seems indisputable that financial disparity exists between sports and the arts and one effect of this is a negative effect on dancers' access to health care. Moreover, because they have not progressed through systems in which specialized health care providers were readily available, dancers tend to be more independent when confronted by injuries. In light of this, it is important to note that management of injuries by qualified health care

practitioners has been shown to reduce both time loss from dancing and medical expenses.[31]

Limitations Imposed by Wardrobe and Performance

One of the most noticeable differences between dancers and traditional athletes is the amount of taping and bracing that is possible. While these prophylactic and protective measures are taken for granted as part and parcel of sports, the appearance requirements for dancers on stage and the range of motion necessary for their successful performance restrict some of the clinician's options. The aesthetic faux pas of a tutu-clad ballerina wearing a knee-stabilizing brace over her tights is obvious. Another common example is ankle taping; most dancers likely will reject taping such as that used for basketball or football players because it is too restrictive of plantar flexion and they do not wear socks plus sneakers or cleats that would hide the tape. When a dancer does permit taping, a reduced volume will be used; flesh-colored tape is preferable, or the dancer will apply makeup cream or powder to blend white tape into the skin. Modern dancers pose even greater challenges with their bare feet because foot pads, supports, and orthotics are not easily affixed, they detach easily, they change how the dancer senses the interface between the foot and the floor, and they may be evident to the audience.

The Panoply of Injuries in Dance

Dance participation is associated with a high frequency of injury.[20,21,27,29,31,46,51,59-72] The percentage of participants affected is high; 95% is not unheard of in a professional ballet company.[27,51] Table 27-2 provides overall injury rates reported by various authors. Although epidemiological correction is not made for the variety of possible definitions of "injury" that would aid comparisons among studies[73-78] and in spite of the fact that vast numbers of dancers lie outside the medical profession's sphere of data collection ability, it is clear that dancers sustain substantial numbers of injuries. The data on dance injuries are less sophisticated simply because dancers as a subpopulation have not enjoyed the same level of access to injury evaluation and recording processes compared with those available in a typical sports medicine setting; consequently, more systematic research is required.

Several reasons for such a high injury incidence are apparent. Chief among these, especially for amateur dancers, is their lack of the body structure (e.g., tissue strength, flexibility) and biomechanical capability that allows them to succeed in dance.[79] This is particularly true in ballet, in which the requirements are very regimented and can be unforgiving to the musculoskeletal system. Injurious technical errors may develop from inadequate dance training, maladaptation to choreography that is beyond the dancer's skill level, or neuromuscular compensation because of injury. If such errors are not corrected they may be carried

Table 27-2

Injury Data for Dancers Reported by Various Authors

Authors	Type of Dancer	Injury Data	Duration of Data Collection
Arendt and Kerschbaumer[67]	Professional ballet	7.4 injuries per dancer (567 injuries in 77 dancers)	5 years
Bowling[62]	Professional ballet and modern	84% of dancers injured (118 of 140) 12% had 5 or more injuries	Career
Byhring and Bø[20]	Professional ballet	75% of dancers injured (31 of 41) 3.2 injuries per dancer	5 months
Gamboa et al.[86]	Elite preprofessional ballet	42% of dancers injured (151 of 359) 1.3 injuries per dancer (198 injuries in 151 dancers)	5 years
Garrick[279]	Female preprofessional ballet	64% of dancers injured (38 of 59) 5.1 injuries per dancer (194 injuries in 38 dancers)	20 months
Garrick and Requa[21]	Professional ballet	2.97 injuries per dancer (309 injuries in 104 dancers) 23% of dancers accounted for more than 50% of all injuries	3 years
Kerr et al.[61]	Female university dance students	97% of dancers injured (38 of 39) 2.4 injuries per dancer	8 months
Laws[63]	Student and professional dancers, all genres	80% of all dancers injured more injuries in ballet than modern	1 year
Liederbach et al.[29]	Professional ballet and modern dancers	2.5 injuries per dancer per year (3721 injuries in 298 dancers)	5 years
Luke et al.[102]	Preprofessional dancers	112 self-reported injuries in 39 dancers 71 injuries in 39 dancers reported to and identified by a physical therapist 95% of dancers reported at least 1 injury during their careers	1 season
Nilsson et al.[27]	Professional ballet	95% of dancers injured (93 of 98) 3.8 injuries per dancer (390 injuries in 98 dancers)	5 years
Rovere et al.[65]	Dance students, all theatrical genres	85% of dancers 1.9 injuries per dancer (352 injuries in 185 dancers)	1 year
Solomon et al.[28]	Professional ballet	average of 84% of dancers injured per year 560 total injuries in 5 years in a company with an average size of 62 dancers per year	5 years
Thomas and Tarr[280]	Professional and student dancers, all genres	90% of 204 dancers injured at least once no dancer older than age 35 had not been injured in dancers younger than age 35, the number of uninjured dancers decreased with increasing age	Career

Note: Reported data is not the same for all authors because of differences in how the studies were done.

throughout a dancer's career, thus compounding their deleterious effects.

The inherent nature of dance requires countless repetitions of movements in the quest to perfect choreography to the satisfaction of the artistic director, teacher, and audience. Dancers usually spend far more hours daily in the studio than traditional athletes spend on the field, court, or track, and the lack of the well-defined season and off-season periods characteristic of most sports requires dancers to stay at peak performance continuously.[59] This creates not only increased exposure time in which injuries can occur, but it induces fatigue, a known contributor to injury.[80-83] Other factors associated with the high injury rate include poor training,[51] suboptimal lower body muscular power,[84] and low aerobic fitness.[85]

Injuries to the lower extremity account for the vast proportion of all dance injuries,[20,27,29,46,62,65,68,70,86] with most of these occurring in the ankle and foot. One factor reportedly contributing to this is low thigh torque and power.[87] A number of studies report that trunk or spine injuries compose 20% or more of all injuries in dancers.[21,51,61-63] Overuse injuries generally are more common than traumatic injuries simply because of the repetitive nature of dance rehearsal. Nilsson[27] found that incidences in overuse versus traumatic injuries were related to gender. In their study of professional ballet dancers, men suffered more lower-extremity traumatic injuries, whereas women suffered more overuse injuries in this region. Men also experienced more upper-extremity injuries than women because of the partner-lifting that is integral to their role in classical ballet. However, this difference may disappear in modern dancers because the nature of their partnering work is different and they perform more upper-extremity weightbearing maneuvers on the floor than do ballet dancers.[32]

Dancers and Injury

- Research suggests that the proportion of dancers who suffer injuries is 95% or higher
- The lower extremity is the most commonly affected body region, with the ankle being the joint most frequently injured
- The high injury rate in dance and the relatively low probability that dancers have adequate access to specialized health care (compared with traditional athletes) presents an opportunity for musculoskeletal health care providers to care for these athletic artists

---

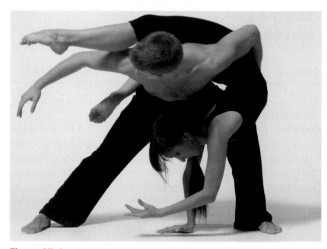

Figure 27-1

An example of partnering in modern dance. Note the requirement for special capacity in strength, flexibility, agility, balance, and other physical parameters. (© iStockphoto.com/Alexander Yakovlev.)

Clinically Relevant Concepts in Dance Kinesiology

There are some characteristics of dance movement that may predispose dancers to certain types of injuries and create an environment in which injuries are exacerbated or, at best, heal more slowly than usual. Long hours, repetitive motions, and unusual movement patterns are examples. Because most of these are generally ingrained in dance practice, a properly motivated health care worker will learn as much as possible about dance and dancers to deliver effective care and offer sound advice for reducing the likelihood of injury. A few clinically relevant aspects of dance technique are described in this section.

Different types of injuries are incurred in different dance genres. Classical ballet requires hundreds of repetitions of very prescriptive movements; thus, overuse injuries are more likely compared with other genres and these usually occur in the lower extremity in which the majority of weightbearing movements are performed. In ballet there also are differences between injury types in men and women,[27] largely because of differences in technique that include the male dancer lifting his female partner off the floor and even over his head. Male ballet dancers suffer more traumatic injuries and a greater percentage of knee, upper extremity, and lower back injuries than do their female counterparts. Male dancers also tend to jump higher because their thighs and legs typically are stronger than those of females. On the other hand, modern dance, with its freer movement patterns, heavy emphasis on floor work, and greater incorporation of the upper extremities in partnering and weightbearing (an example is shown in Figure 27-1) yields a greater proportion of traumatic injuries that are spread across both sets of extremities and the trunk.[29] Different still are the rapid percussive movements that subject the feet to significant repetitive forces in flamenco dance and Irish dance and the weightbearing contact between the head and the ground seen in break dance.

The *Pointe* Shoe

Dancing *en pointe* and wearing *pointe* shoes do not seem to be conducive to healthy feet. Nonetheless, *pointe* is a beautiful and integral part of classical ballet that will remain. All dancers need both support and the ability to sense the floor to execute their choreography. Therefore, health care practitioners must learn about the technique to best advise *pointe* dancers under their care. In the first two decades of the nineteenth century when dancing *en pointe* started gaining popularity,[88] *pointe* shoes did not exist; rather, dancers darned the soles of their soft ballet slippers with additional yarn to provide some further support.[89] The first use of stiff blocking in *pointe* shoes to offer a more stable platform on which to balance on the toe tips occurred in 1880,[90] an achievement accomplished by the use of paper, cardboard, and cloth stiffened by soaking them in glue and letting them dry. By the middle of the twentieth century *pointe* shoes were constructed with even greater stiffness to accommodate increasingly demanding choreography.[89] Most of today's *pointe* shoes retain the traditional satin, burlap, paper, leather, and glue construction (Figure 27-2 and Figure 27-3), but modern materials like thermoplastics and microfiber fabric have been incorporated by some shoe companies, including Gaynor Minden[91] and Bloch.[92] Every ballet dancer who dances *en pointe* engages in an individualized routine to break in a new pair of *pointe* shoes, something which often is a daily or every-other-day custom in professional ballet companies. A careful method of padding the toes in the shoe also is employed by many dancers. A prima ballerina—the most prominent female dancer in a

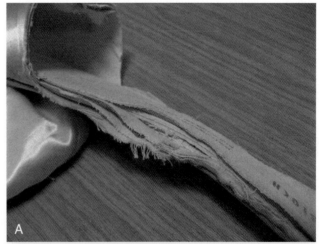

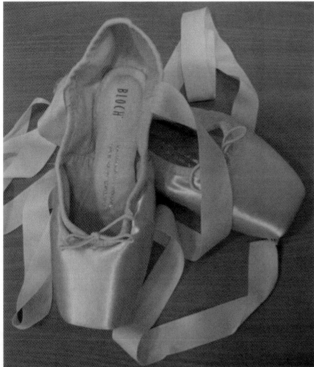

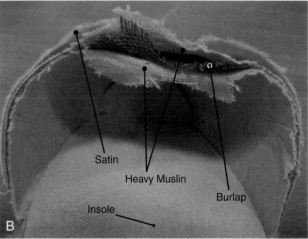

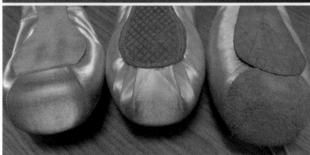

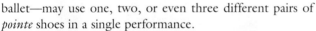

Figure 27-2

Typical *pointe* shoes, including a close-up of three different styles of the platform on which the dancer stands when *en pointe*. Ballet dancers select their shoes with specific features they prefer and then prepare the shoes for use by a customized conditioning process according to their personal taste.

Figure 27-3

A, A side view of a cutaway shank of a *pointe* shoe showing the layers of fabric and leather construction. **B,** A view directly into the toe box of a *pointe* shoe after the rest of the shoe has been cut away. The several layers of materials used in constructing *pointe* shoes are shown, as well. These are typically impregnated with glue to form and harden the toe box.

ballet—may use one, two, or even three different pairs of *pointe* shoes in a single performance.

The anatomy of a *pointe* shoe has been well described elsewhere,[89,93,94] and it is illustrated in Figure 27-4. Knowledge about the shoes is important when consulting with a dancer about foot injuries, or with parents about their youngsters beginning *pointe* work. *Pointe* shoes do not come in right and left; neither are their sizes related to women's street shoe sizes, although conversion charts are available.[89] Dancers and teachers have very particular preferences from both fitting and aesthetic perspectives. In general the shoes should fit closely about the foot and not unduly compress the sides of the forefoot. Subungual hematoma, hallux valgus, Morton's neuroma and other forefoot problems may result from poorly fitting shoes.

From an injury-prevention perspective, a properly fitting *pointe* shoe provides key support to the dancer; the shoe is especially important for stability of the midfoot as it augments the ligaments of the Lisfranc joints,[95] which include the dorsal tarsometatarsal, plantar tarsometatarsal, and interosseous ligaments.[96,97] Additional dependable information about *pointe* shoes is available from sources for both health care providers[93] and performers and teachers.[89]

The Ankle and Foot in *Demi-plié, Demi-pointe, and en Pointe*

Of all athletic activities, only classical ballet requires its participants to repeatedly move from full forced dorsiflexion (in the *demi-plié* position) to full forced plantar flexion (the

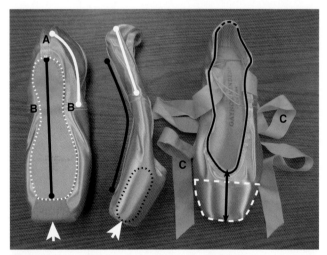

Figure 27-4

Left to right: Bottom, side, and top views of a *pointe* shoe showing its anatomy. *A*, Rear seam; *B*, waist seams; *C*, ribbons. *White lines with circle ends* = heel counter or heel quarter. *White dotted line* = outsole. *Black lines with circle ends* = shank, a rigid spine along the bottom of the shoe between the insole and outsole. *White arrowheads* = platform, the surface on which the dancer stands when *en pointe*. *White dashed line* = toe box or block. *Black line with arrowhead ends* = vamp. *Black dotted line* = wing (side of toe box). Black line coursing around the collar of the shoe indicates the drawstring casing, the posterior part of which is dashed to show the edge of the heel counter that compresses the Achilles tendon.

en pointe position). *Demi-pointe*—or half *pointe*—is distinguished from full *pointe* by hyperextended metatarsophalangeal joints. (These three positions are shown in Figure 27-5.) *Demi-pointe* essentially places the ankle in full plantar flexion, but to successfully stand in this position, at least 90° of hyperextension is required in the first metatarsophalangeal joint (Figure 27-6). Whereas the typical ankle range of motion for nondancers is 20° of dorsiflexion and 50° of plantar flexion,[98-100] dancers normally exhibit much greater motion.[101-106] This is especially true in plantar flexion for which dancers ideally need 90° to 100° of weightbearing plantar flexion; motion up to 113° has been reported in female professional ballet dancers.[101] Table 27-3 summarizes various authors' measurements of ankle range of motion in female dancers.

However, all such plantar flexion does not occur in the ankle—that is, the talocrural—joint. A substantial amount of plantar flexion in nondancers has been attributed to the joints of the foot; in other words, goniometry of the ankle includes movements in the foot joints.[101,103,106-109] Clinically measured ankle motion is greater than talocrural motion,[110] but clinical measurement of talocrural motion is difficult.[111] As much as 40% of plantar flexion motion occurs in the joints of the midfoot,[107,111] but the relative amounts attributable to each of these joints varies widely among subjects. These researchers reported mean talocrural motion as 23° of dorsiflexion and 28° of plantar flexion.[107] Russell and Shave developed an x-ray measurement technique to evaluate the motion of the tibia and bones of the foot relative to

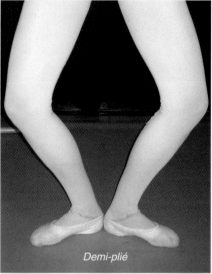

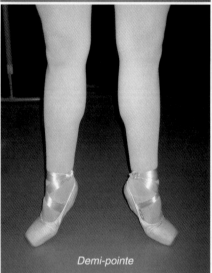

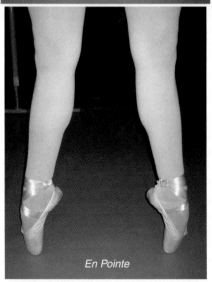

Figure 27-5

The lower extremity positions in ballet that require maximum range of motion: dorsiflexion in *demi-plié* and plantar flexion in *demi-pointe* and *en pointe*.

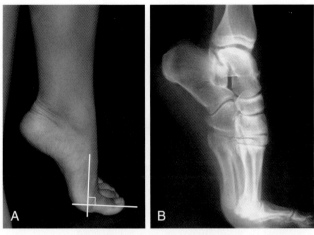

Figure 27-6

A, Modern dancer standing in *demi-pointe* showing the 90° of first metatarsophalangeal joint hyperextension required to attain this position. **B,** X-ray showing positions of the bones in *demi-pointe*. (**B** from Kennedy JG, Hodgkins CW, Columbier J-A et al: Foot and ankle injuries in dancers. In Porter DA, Schon LC, editors: *Baxter's the foot and ankle in sport*, ed 2, p 478, Philadelphia, 2008, Mosby.)

the talus in the *en pointe* positions of female professional ballet dancers.[112] They found a mean talocrural motion of 58° and motion of the navicular, second cuneiform, and first metatarsal ranging from 5° to 9° each. This translates to approximately 30% of the total *en pointe* plantar flexion occurring in the bones of the foot. The percentage likely varies depending on the foot flexibility of a given dancer and, perhaps, the age a dancer began training, the total number of years dancing, and the predominant genre. Additional research about dancers' ankle and foot ranges of motion certainly is warranted.

The laterally located anterior talofibular ligament and the calcaneofibular ligament are the most commonly injured ankle ligaments[113-115]; thus, it is important to gain an understanding of how they are situated during the ankle range of motion required for dance. These ligaments change position substantially between *demi-plié* and *en pointe*.[116] When the ankle is in anatomical position, the anterior talofibular ligament is approximately horizontal and the calcaneofibular is nearly vertical. Upon moving to *demi-plié*, the positions of the ligaments in space change very little, but their orientations relative to the fibula change. The anterior talofibular ligament's angle with the fibula becomes more acute and the calcaneofibular ligament becomes almost parallel to the fibula. When *en pointe*, the anterior talofibular ligament is nearly vertical while the calcaneofibular moves to a somewhat horizontal position. Figure 27-7 shows the relationships of the ligaments to the bones of the ankle and foot.

The anterior talofibular ligament is weaker than the calcaneofibular ligament.[108,117,118] Furthermore, as plantar flexion increases, the anterior talofibular ligament undergoes increasing strain[117,119-121] as it is stretched between its proximal and distal attachments. On superficial analysis, this would seem to predispose dancers to lateral ankle sprain, especially of the anterior talofibular ligament. However, in the *en pointe* position the ankle receives added stability from compressive "locking" of the posterior tibial plafond against the posterior talus and superior calcaneus[11,122-125] and from contraction of the leg, ankle, and foot musculature.[126] Therefore, although ankle sprains are common in dancers—as in most sports—the extreme plantar-flexed position *en pointe* is not necessarily an influencing factor for this.

Table 27-3

Ankle Range of Motion in Female Dancers Reported by Various Authors

Authors	Measurement Method	Mean Age of Participants	Mean ± SD Dorsiflexion	Mean ± SD Plantar Flexion
Bennell et al.[281]	Active WB inclinometry	9.6 yr	32.9° ± 6	NR
Bennell et al.[282]	Active WB inclinometry	10.7 yr	33.8° ± 6.2	NR
Hamilton et al.[101]	Active NWB goniometry	29.3 yr	10°	113°
Khan et al.[283]	Active WB inclinometry	16.9 yr	R: 33.7° ± 4.5 L: 34.2° ± 4.3	NR
Lin et al.[284]	Active five camera motion analysis *en pointe*	19.2 yr	NR	R: 52.9° ± 4.3 L: 53.8° ± 6.0
Luke et al.[102]	Active NWB goniometry	15.8 yr	R: 8.8° ± 3.7 L: 7.0° ± 4.9	R: 76.2° ± 7.0 L: 75.4° ± 8.0
Novella[285]	Active NWB inclinometry	23 yr	NR	98° ± 3
Steinberg et al.[104]	Passive NWB goniometry	16 yr	12°	87°
Wiesler et al.[105]	Active NWB goniometry	17.5 yr	R: 78.0° ± 2.3 L: 77.4° ± 2.2	R: 96.3° ± 2.7 L: 101.0° ± 2.5

NR, Not reported; *NWB,* nonweightbearing; *WB,* weightbearing.

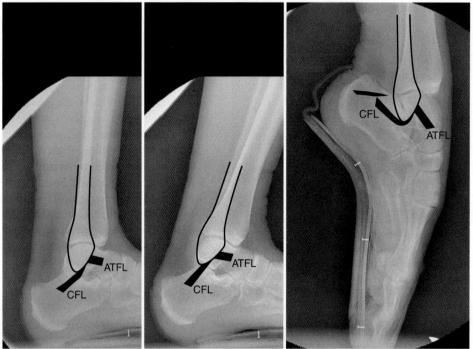

Figure 27-7

Orientations of the anterior talofibular (*ATFL*) and calcaneofibular ligaments (*CFL*) in different ankle positions. The ligament positions are based on investigations performed in nondancers[108,113,114,274-278] because these ligaments have not previously been studied in situ in a dancer population. The fibula is outlined for ease of visualization. (From Russell JA, McEwan IM, Koutedakis Y et al: Clinical anatomy and biomechanics of the ankle in dance, *J Dance Med Sci* 12(3):77, 2008. Reprinted with permission of J. Michael Ryan Publishing.)

Ballet Positions and Movements

- The position of *demi-plié* requires maximum weightbearing dorsiflexion
- The *en pointe* position requires maximum weightbearing plantar flexion
- Standing on *demi-pointe* requires maximum plantar flexion and approximately 90° of first metatarsophalangeal joint hyperextension
- *Relevé* is the movement of rising to the toes, such as is done to reach *demi-pointe*
- Classical ballet requires repetitive movement from maximum forced dorsiflexion to maximum forced plantar flexion and back again. This puts tremendous stress on the dancer's ankles and heightens the likelihood of injury

Of the three positions *demi-plié, demi-pointe,* and *en pointe,* the latter produces the greatest potential for injury to the forefoot and midfoot. It is crucial that dancers receive proper instruction in *pointe* work from the initial time they undertake training in this skill. The lengths of the toes relative to one another do not seem to have an effect on the pressure per unit area applied to the hallux *en pointe*[94]; that is, the hallux receives the same amount of pressure regardless of the length of the other toes. However, toe length is related to foot pain. Ballet dancers with their first and second toes of the same length or their first toe longer than the second toe reported lower pain scores and less first metatarsophalangeal joint inflammation.[127] Conversely, in ballet dancers with the second toe longer than the first (Morton's foot), more forefoot signs and symptoms were present. Additionally, unlike in ballet dancers, second-toe length has no bearing on forefoot problems in folk dancers.[127]

Dancing *en pointe* yields some generalized patterns of toe placement in the shoes.[128] This is simply related to the need to fit a variety of foot shapes into the toe box. When *en pointe,* force is exerted on the medial edge of the great toe[128,129] because of the truncated ellipsoid cone shape of the toe box (see Figure 27-3) that forces the hallux laterally and possibly hastens the development of hallux valgus and bunions. An undesirable "winging" of the foot *en pointe* aggravates this tendency. The force on the medial aspect of the great toe moves the forefoot into valgus as shown in Figure 27-8, *A.* The opposite of winging the foot is termed *sickling,* a position in which the force is directed laterally, the forefoot moves toward varus, and the heel inverts. Figure 27-8, *B-D* compare proper foot alignment with sickling and winging. Sickling and winging can be problematic whether a dancer is *en pointe* or *en demi-pointe,* so strong feet and ankles and proper instruction will help alleviate these technical faults, both of which can lead to stress injuries.

Appropriate Age at Which to Start Pointe Work

Few questions are as common among parents and teachers of girls in ballet than, "At what age can she start *pointe* work?" Although it may seem desirable to answer with a definite age,

this does not serve the dancer well. Ages most often proposed are 11 to 14. One study of ballet dancers with flexor hallucis longus (FHL) tendinopathy found the range of ages at initial training *en pointe* to be 4 to 16 years old, with a mean of 10.[130] Meck and colleagues[131] discovered that age was the most common parameter used by ballet schools to determine a student's ability to begin *pointe;* 96% of the schools studied incorporated age into their *pointe* readiness evaluation programs and the mean age when *pointe* was initiated was 11.2 years. Nonetheless, chronological age must not be the most heavily weighted variable informing the

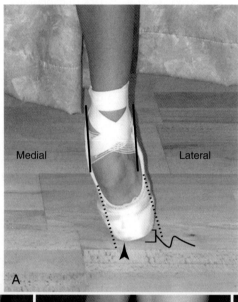

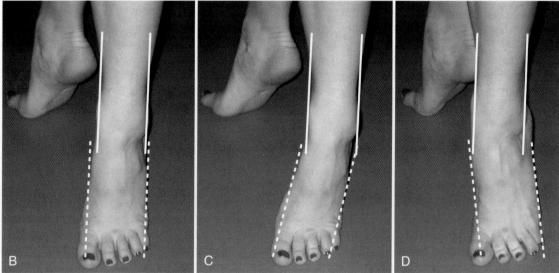

Figure 27-8

A, A ballet dancer standing *en pointe* with a winged foot, an alignment that places stress on the hallux and midfoot. Notice the angular difference between the hindfoot/ankle *(solid lines)* and the midfoot/forefoot *(dotted lines).* The *tailed bracket* marks the lift of the lateral toe box off the floor and the *arrowhead* identifies where this dancer's weight is being borne. **B,** Proper alignment of the ankle and foot. **C,** A sickled foot. Compared with **B,** notice the angle between the distal leg and ankle and the midfoot/forefoot. **D,** A winged foot, where the angle between the leg/ankle and the midfoot/forefoot is in the opposite direction as that in a sickled foot.

decision to allow a young dancer to commence *pointe* work. The consequences of starting too early are far greater than those of starting too late. The ability to succeed technically is improved and the risk of injury is reduced if the youngster waits until the skeleton and musculature are strong enough.[11,132-134]

Balance and coordination are additional important factors.[129] Strength in the ankles and feet are not the only important components; strong and well-controlled musculature in the trunk, hips, and thighs are equally important to dancing *en pointe,* and are even more critical for dancers with hypermobile feet and ankles.[132]

The attributes outlined in the following textbox offer a guideline that, although seemingly a "rule-of-thumb," must not be applied without careful evaluation of the individual dancer. If the student began serious ballet training at age 8 or later, participates in ballet class at least twice a week, and possesses adequate maturity in the areas listed previously, then *pointe* work is usually appropriate beginning in the fourth year of ballet training. Dancers taking instruction only once per week, who are not intending to engage in preprofessional ballet training, or who lack the necessary skeletal maturity and muscular strength must be discouraged from *pointe* work.[133] For further information, the reader is referred to a detailed history and physical examination for young dancers that is offered by Shah.[134]

Factors for Deciding When to Begin Training En Pointe[133]

- Stage of physical development
- Quality of trunk, abdominal, and pelvic control (i.e., core stability)
- Hip-knee-ankle-foot alignment
- Strength and flexibility of the feet and ankles
- Frequency and duration of the student's ballet training
- Age

The Lower Extremity and Turnout

Ballet is the dance genre in which turnout (i.e., the ability to laterally rotate the entire lower extremity) is exceedingly important and in which it receives the most attention (often excessively so, to the point of injury). The ideal ballet turnout is 180°; that is, in a fully turned-out position a dancer wishes to set his or her calcanei back-to-back with the longitudinal axes of the feet along a straight line. This is termed *first position,* one of six fundamental stances in ballet (Figure 27-9 and Figure 27-10). Functional turnout is the amount of turnout motion attained by a dancer in his or her usual studio setting. The vast majority of dancers are unable to achieve the desired 180°, although they try various methods to squeeze a few more degrees from their lower extremities. First-position turnout values reported in the

literature include 127° for university dancers[135] and 128° for preprofessional dancers.[70]

Turnout is not a simple movement of hip external rotation, even though that is its primary component. A ratio of 60% of turnout motion occurring above the knee and 40% of the motion occurring below the knee has been proposed as an appropriate guideline.[69,101] If the ideal 90° of turnout in one limb can be performed, this is accumulated from 60° to 70° of hip external rotation and 20° to 30° spread across the natural positioning of the knee, ankle, and foot.[136] Actual external rotation range of motion may be less of a limiting factor compared with the lack of experience and technical ability that prevents dancers from maximizing their turnout when dancing. In fact, improved neuromuscular coordination and strengthening the hip's external rotators can yield an additional 15° to 30° of turnout.[137]

Femoral neck version plays a role in a dancer's ability to attain turnout. An anteverted femoral neck may mechanically limit a dancer's potential for turnout, whereas a retroverted femoral neck allows greater turnout (Figure 27-11).[126,136,138,139] It has been postulated that dancers who begin their training early in life experience a "molding" of the femoral neck that accommodates to the turned out position by the time the skeleton solidifies. Some reports have indicated that those who started dance training by age 5 or 6 exhibit more clinical turnout than dancers who started later,[26] and after age 11, increases in turnout motion can only occur via hip capsule extensibility.[140] In another study, however, students who participated in at least 6 hours of ballet training per week between the ages of 11 and 14 showed less femoral neck anteversion than students who trained less than 6 hours per week.[141] Counterintuitively, these authors did not find an association between age of starting ballet training and femoral neck version, passive hip external rotation, nor functional turnout. Neither were these variables related to the number of years of training.

A "normal" version angle is between 8° and 15°.[142] Bauman and colleagues[143] calculated an average neck version angle of 11.4° using data from five studies containing a total of 1436 subjects; the range of measurements in these studies was 20° of retroversion to 50° of anteversion. Then Bauman's group compared this value with version angles in a contingent of professional ballerinas. The dancers exhibited a mean femoral version angle similar to the general population: 11.9° of anteversion (range = 4° to 24°). Practically speaking, the more a dancer tends toward femoral neck anteversion, the more potential turnout limitation he or she will have. Conversely, the more he or she tends toward retroversion, the easier it will be to achieve turnout. Longitudinal studies that periodically measure femoral version in a cohort of dancers from age of initiating ballet training (often age 4) through to adulthood are the only way to confirm the effect of ballet training on the femoral neck.

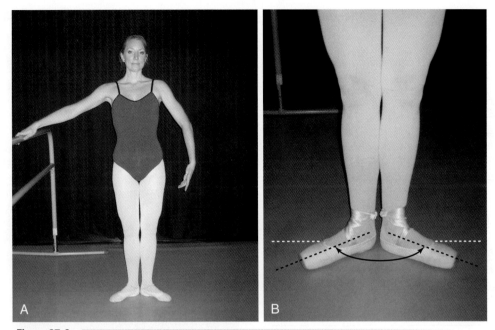

Figure 27-9
A, A dancer standing in first position. **B,** The close-up of turnout. The *white dotted line* indicates the 180° ideal, whereas the *black dotted lines* bisect the foot and represent this dancer's functional turnout.

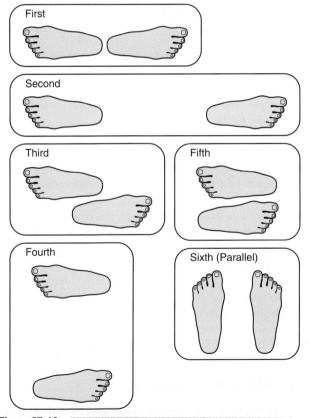

Figure 27-10
The six primary foot positions used in ballet. The dancer faces in the direction of the "first" diagram. These feet show ideal turnout of 180°. Other than the parallel position, these are achieved mainly by externally rotating the hips and placing the feet in the specified positions.

Turnout

- In turnout, 60% should occur above the knee (60° to 70° of hip external rotation) and 40% below the knee (20° to 30° at the knee, ankle, and foot)
- Strengthening the hip external rotators and improving neuromuscular coordination can add 15° to 30° to turnout
- Both bony and soft tissue limitations can restrict a dancer's ability to achieve his or her desired turnout
- Forcing one's turnout can lead to foot pronation, knee valgus stress, anterior pelvic tilt, and lumbar lordosis

Apart from femoral neck version, other factors contribute to the amount of turnout a dancer can attain, including tibial torsion[144,145] and soft tissue flexibility (especially of the anterior hip ligaments). Forcing turnout beyond a dancer's natural range of motion results in foot pronation, knee valgus stress,[126,130,136,146] anterior pelvic tilt, and lumbar lordosis.[137,147] One very unhealthy technique used by some dancers to maximize their functional turnout is setting the feet as close to the desired 180° turnout angle as possible with the knees flexed in *demi-plié* and then raising the body by straightening the knees and maintaining the feet in the set position. This puts undue stress on the knees as they are "screwed home" into extension. It also is likely to force the feet into pronation (Figure 27-12).

The difference between a dancer's hip external range of motion and his or her functional turnout angle may be related to injury. This difference was significantly larger in

With feet in Parallel   After turning out

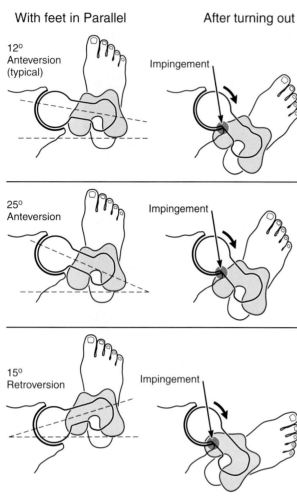

Figure 27-11

Schematic diagram showing the superior view of a transverse section through the right hip joint and indicating the relationship between femoral neck version angle and turnout. The *light gray* shape represents the position of the femoral condyles. Notice the differences in foot position among the neck version angles following external rotation to the point at which the femoral neck impacts the posterior lip of the acetabulum *(dark shaded circles)*. Dancers with greater anteversion will be more limited in their turnout ability, whereas retroverted femoral necks are favorable to attaining turnout.

dancers who were injured versus dancers who were not injured (25.4° vs. 4.7°), suggesting that forcing one's turnout is related to incidence of injury.[148] In a group of 28 elite professional ballet dancers[101] and another group of 29 preprofessional dancers,[70] those with less functional turnout experienced more injuries. It is speculated that the dancers with lower turnout were accustomed to forcing their turnout motion, which led to increased injury rates.

Selected Musculoskeletal Injuries in Dancers

Injuries in dancers are, in general, pathologically similar to injuries sustained by traditional athletes even though the exact mechanisms of injury may differ. That is to say, the

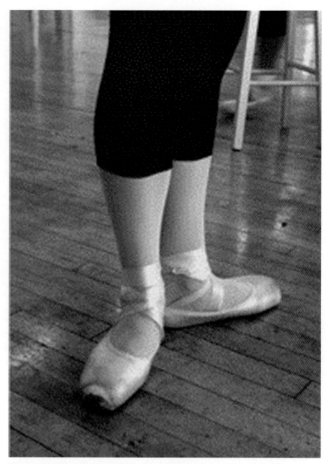

Figure 27-12

Pronation of the feet that is a consequence of forcing turnout. (From Kadel NJ: Foot and ankle injuries in dance, *Phys Med Rehabil Clin North Am* 17(4):815, 2006.)

pathological finding of posterior ankle impingement in a soccer player is not appreciably different from that of the same injury in a dancer even though the mechanism of onset and the kinesiology of the activities causing the problem are different. The same is true of ankle sprains, Achilles tendinopathy, and many other injuries. The following is not intended to be an exhaustive monograph describing all common dance injuries. A few injuries are highlighted here because of their prevalence in the dance population or because the circumstances surrounding their occurrence in dancers are particularly unique and interesting.

Ankle Impingement Syndromes

The requirement that dancers repeatedly plantar flex and dorsiflex the ankle in weightbearing can give rise to impingement syndromes on both the posterior and anterior aspects of the ankle. These types of injuries often are related to anatomical variations in the foot (e.g., os trigonum)[149-153] in addition to the pathomechanics of executing dance skills such as *demi-plié, demi-pointe,* and *pointe*.[150-152,154,155]

Posterior Ankle Impingement

The cause of posterior impingement most familiar to clinicians is os trigonum, an anatomical variation that appears in 5% to 25% of adults.[156-162] Closely related to this is a protruding lateral talar tubercle, or Stieda process.[132,163-166] Figure 27-13 illustrates three anatomical variations of the talus. Some debate exists about whether what appears to be an os trigonum in certain individuals may in fact be a Stieda process separated from the body of the talus by a compression fracture secondary to forced plantar flexion.[167-169] Soft tissue structures, including the FHL tendon,[149,170-175] deep posteromedial deltoid ligament,[176] posterior intermalleolar ligament,[177,178] and posterior tibiotalar ligament,[179] also can produce posterior impingement symptoms.

Peace and colleagues[153] used magnetic resonance imaging (MRI) scans to study ballet dancers with posterior impingement symptoms; 30% of the subjects exhibited os trigonum. This is higher than the prevalence reported in the general population, perhaps because of the forced plantar flexion of ballet during the years when the secondary ossification center of the lateral talar tubercle is adjoining the tubercle and the talar body. An os trigonum might be quiet for years until it becomes symptomatic following a sprained ankle or other traumatic episode.[149,180,181] This may be related to force created by the posterior talofibular ligament during ankle trauma because the ligament attaches to the lateral talar tubercle.

Additional anatomical variations have been shown to predispose dancers to pathological conditions of the ankle, especially posterior impingement syndrome.[149,153,154,167,168,182,183] Greater than 5 mm of downward protrusion of the posterior lip of the tibial plafond (posterior malleolus) and greater than 5 mm of upward protrusion of the superior calcaneal tuberosity both have been cited as contributory to pathological conditions resulting in posterior impingement.[153] These are depicted in Figure 27-14.

One other mechanism of posterior impingement bears mentioning. Lateral ankle sprains that lead to ankle instability also can produce a posterior impingement syndrome.[79,180] In a dancer with an unstable ankle, the foot moves forward from under the tibia during *relevé*, or rising on the toes. In this scenario, the talus slides anteriorly in the ankle mortise and the superior calcaneus similarly moves forward, impinging against the posterior edge of the tibial plafond and causing pain.

Regardless of the exact pathogenesis, any space-occupying structure in the posterior compartment of the ankle can create symptoms when the calcaneus and talus approach the posterior distal tibia during plantar flexion. Pain associated with posterior impingement, especially an os trigonum or Stieda process, most often occurs posterolaterally, thus differentiating these problems from FHL tendinopathy, a syndrome that produces pain at the posteromedial ankle.[180,184] Dancers with posterior impingement syndrome complain of posterior ankle pain and describe a limitation of motion in their *demi-pointe* or *en pointe* positions. During a clinical examination, forced plantar flexion of the ankle reproduces these symptoms. In cases of failed conservative measures, operative treatment has been shown successful.[168,173,182,185,186]

Anterior Ankle Impingement

As in the posterior ankle, impingement syndrome in the anterior region of the ankle can arise from bone or soft tissue. Symptoms originating in bone can be initiated by repetitive impact of the anterior edge of the tibial plafond and the dorsal talus that causes exostoses to form on either or both bones.[139,151,155,187-194] Although contact between the tibia and talus does not usually occur, dancers may experience impingement when they repeatedly force their ankles into maximum dorsiflexion during *demi-plié*.[151,155] Because of this required repetition, exostosis formation occurs more frequently in dancers than nondancers,[155,195] and both pes cavus[79,151] and limited subtalar motion[145] can increase the likelihood that a dancer will develop exostoses. Another possible result of repeated forced dorsiflexion in *demi-plié* is a deepened sulcus on the dorsal talar neck.[196]

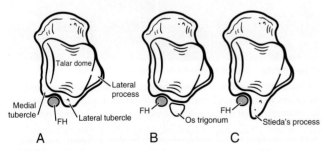

Figure 27-13

Superior view of three right tali, with posterior being toward the bottom of the diagram. Three different variations of the lateral talar tubercle are illustrated and the position of the tendon of flexor hallucis longus is indicated by the circle marked *FH*. **A,** A typical talus. **B,** A talus with an os trigonum. **C,** A talus with a Stieda process.

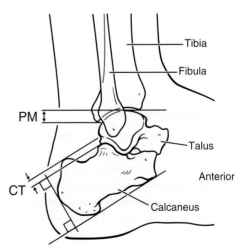

Figure 27-14

Lateral view of ankle anatomy showing a protruding posterior malleolus (*PM*) and calcaneal tuberosity (*CT*), either of which increases the likelihood of posterior ankle impingement in dancers.

Ankle Impingement

- Ankle impingement syndromes result from bony or soft tissue symptoms that have been irritated by compression during the extreme range of ankle motion required of dancers
- A lateral ankle sprain in a dancer can precipitate posterior impingement symptoms when an os trigonum is present or an anterior impingement when hypertrophic scar tissue develops in the region of the anterior talofibular ligament

The relative positions of tibial and talar exostoses usually preclude them impinging on one another.[188] Tibial spurs generally occur lateral to the sagittal midline of the ankle and talar spurs occur medial to the midline. The inner surface of the medial malleolus and the medial surface of the talus are common locations for exostoses in dancers because maximum weightbearing dorsiflexion generally forces the foot into pronation against the medial malleolus.[151] A lateral radiograph taken in full dorsiflexion may be helpful in assessing bony impingement[194,197] because this view improves the ability to see anterior exostoses; however, it is easy to underestimate their sizes if the spurs overlap.[197,198] Moreover, true lateral radiographs may be insufficient to identify the pathological condition in many cases.[18,191,199,200] Tol and colleagues[191] recommend a special oblique antero-medial impingement view they designed that improves the sensitivity of radiographic diagnosis from 40% to 85%.

Soft tissue causes of anterior impingement include thickened and inflamed soft tissue caught between the tibia and talus[189,190,192]; the anterior inferior tibiofibular ligament[169,190,192-194,201-204]; and inflamed, hypertrophic tissue in the lateral gutter following a typical lateral ankle sprain.[175,198,205-210] The lateral gutter is significant clinically because its anterior aspect is the site of most anterolateral soft tissue impingement.[197,206,211-213] Inasmuch as ankle sprains are a common occurrence in physical activity[77,214-216] and the ankle is the most frequently injured body region in dance,[63,65,102] it is wise to consider post-traumatic soft tissue impingement as a sequela that may hamper a dancer's return to activity following an ankle sprain.

Achilles Tendinopathy

Tendinopathy[217] or *tendinosis*[218] are the terms currently employed to describe tendon overuse injury because the classic signs of inflammation—denoted by the suffix in the word *tendinitis*—are generally not present in this type of condition.[217,219] The distinguishing difference between these two terms is the presence of intratendinous degeneration in tendinosis[218,220]; *tendinopathy* refers to any abnormal state of a tendon. The Achilles tendon is prone to injury in any genre of dance in which repeated dorsiflexion and plantar flexion are required; however, classical ballet presents a greater challenge to the tendon than other types of dance. One suggested cause of tendinopathy is variable force distribution across a tendon's diameter that creates abnormal frictional forces between the fibers[221] and disrupts the fibers' microstructure.[222] The Achilles tendon is compressed in ballet when the foot and ankle are maximally plantar flexed in the *en pointe* position. The posterior upper edge of the *pointe* shoe's heel counter, the shoe's ribbons tied around the distal leg and ankle, and the compressed skin folds over the tendon all create a fulcrum that forces the tendon into a curved path and creates indentations that exert pressure on it (Figure 27-15). Also, a drawstring encircles the shoe's opening, a feature that, when tightened, can further bind against the tendon and its insertion.

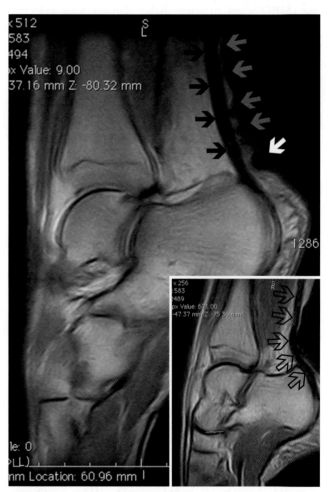

Figure 27-15

T1-weighted magnetic resonance images of ballet dancers standing *en pointe*. In the larger image, the *black arrows* indicate the band of hypointense signal of the Achilles tendon. The *white arrow* indicates the indentation made by the posterior lip of the *pointe* shoe and the *gray arrows* indicate the impressions of the shoe's ribbon. The inset image is a different dancer exhibiting an even more pronounced curve in the tendon substance, as indicated by the *open arrows*. To understand the components of the overlaying shoe, compare these images with the photo of the ankle and foot *en pointe* in Figure 27-5 and the *en pointe* x-ray image in Figure 27-7.

With very few exceptions (e.g., the men's ballet troupe *Les Ballets Trockaderos de Monte Carlo*), *pointe* dancers are women. Following exercise-induced collagen degradation, the rate of collagen synthesis is reduced in women compared with men,[223] a phenomenon possibly related to circulating estradiol levels,[224,225] but apparently independent of menstrual phase.[223,226] If a hormonal mediation of relative collagen strength exists, it may intimate a greater incidence of Achilles tendinopathy in women dancers, especially in conjunction with the potential for added insult to the morphological structure of the tendon that is elicited by the *en pointe* position as just described. Further insight into pathological changes in tendon can be found in "Tendon Pathology and Injuries: Pathophysiology, Healing, and Treatment Considerations," which is Chapter 3 in *Scientific Foundations and Principles of Practice in Musculoskeletal Rehabilitation*, another book in this series.

Flexor Hallucis Longus Tendinopathy

FHL tendinopathy, also known as "dancer's tendinopathy," is a very common dance injury, and the FHL tendon is the involved structure in nearly all medial ankle tendon problems that occur in dancers.[227] This is not surprising given the large number of dance movements requiring *relevé*. As they do with many injuries, dancers often try to "dance through" FHL tendinopathy—in one study, they tolerated the symptoms longer than did nondancers prior to seeking treatment.[130] Hamilton[227] calls this tendon the "Achilles' tendon of the foot" in dancers who work *en pointe*. The tendon courses from the FHL muscle in the deep posterior muscle compartment behind the tibia, along a groove between the medial and lateral talar tubercles that lie posterior to the talus, around a bend and through a tunnel that lies under the sustentaculum tali, then along the underside of the first ray to attach on the proximal plantar surface of the first distal phalanx. In particular, the bend in the tendon just before it enters the fibro-osseous tunnel under the sustentaculum tali (Figure 27-16) heightens the chance of injury from a nonhomogeneous force distribution through the tendon[221] during rising to and lowering from the toes, and when jumping. In an advanced stage, the FHL tendon and its synovial sheath may swell and develop adhesions, or the tendon may develop areas of degeneration. Any or all of these can cause a hallux saltans ("trigger toe") tenosynovitis when the tendon does not slide smoothly through its tunnel.[139,180,228,229]

FHL tendinopathy may be precipitated by the presence of an unstable os trigonum[171] because the trigonal bone is a nonunited protrusion of the lateral tubercle that creates the lateral border of the groove for the tendon. Several authors corroborate a strong, direct relationship between symptoms in these two structures[149,170,171,173-175,230,231] because of their proximity to one another.

Fracture of the Fifth Metatarsal

A spiral fracture of the distal shaft of the fifth metatarsal is termed a *dancer's fracture*[138,232-234] because of its association with an inversion mechanism of a dancer falling from *demi-pointe* or *en pointe*. An unstable landing from a jump can also induce a dancer's fracture.[146] Torsion of the foot exerts

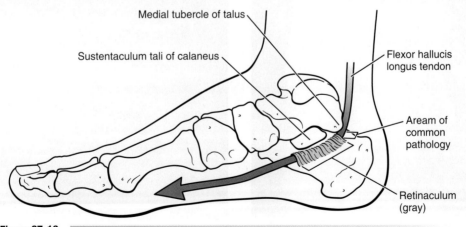

Medial tubercle of talus

Sustentaculum tali of calaneus

Flexor hallucis longus tendon

Aream of common pathology

Retinaculum (gray)

Figure 27-16
Medial view of the foot showing the path of the flexor hallucis longus tendon as it changes direction around the posterior talus and under the sustentaculum tali. The *grey arrow* indicates the usual position of pathological conditions of the tendon just proximal to the retinacular tunnel that can cause a triggering injury.[223]

the rotational force that results in this fracture's characteristic appearance (Figure 27-17).

A Jones fracture (Figure 27-18) occurs at the junction of the diaphysis and proximal metaphysis of the fifth metatarsal.[232,234,235] Named for the author who first described it in 1902, Jones[236] reported that this injury occurred in his own foot—recounting that he sustained it while dancing—and in patients seen in his practice. This particular fracture must be cared for surgically because of its propensity to proceed to malunion or nonunion, often because of a poor or disrupted blood supply.[235] Furthermore, those who participate in sports and dance are unlikely to accept an extended period of immobilization and the risk of nonunion that can complicate treatment of a Jones fracture.

Stress Fractures

Stress fractures are a common overuse injury in dance, especially in the foot.[237] The second metatarsal shaft is the most frequently affected; because of its length, it bears more force than the other metatarsals when a dancer stands in *demi-pointe*.[232] Cortical hypertrophy of the diaphyses in such areas is not unusual in response to arduous schedules of dance rehearsal and performance (Figure 27-19). Periosteal elevation indicates the presence of the reparative callus associated with stress fractures.[238] The second metatarsal can also exhibit a stress fracture at its base, an injury that is rare in nondancers because it is induced by the repetitive longitudinal forces through the foot that are sustained during dance.[239-242] Other common sites for stress fractures in dancers are the tibia (often related to later stages of shin splints), fibula, and lumbar spine.[232,237,243,244]

The rigors of dance training combined with intervals of amenorrhea have been suggested as risk factors for stress fractures in dancers.[237,243,245] Dancers may ignore the early symptoms of stress reactions and stress fractures because of the tenacity they possess for continuing their dance activity. However, this can be disastrous if the pathological condition proceeds through the cortex of the involved bone, particularly in a weightbearing bone like the tibia.[246] For more information on stress fractures, see "Repetitive Stress Pathology—Bone," Chapter 21, in *Pathology and Intervention in Musculoskeletal Rehabilitation,* another book in this series.

Anterior Cruciate Ligament Sprain

Injury to the anterior cruciate ligament (ACL) is much less common in dancers than in most traditional athletes,[29,30,247] yet it is debilitating when it occurs. Because of the sophisticated jumping and cutting maneuvers required of dancers, a dancer with a torn and unrepaired ACL would likely be unable to continue performing. Meuffels and Verhaar[30] reported the incidence of ACL tear in 253 Dutch professional ballet and modern dancers to be 1.6 per 100,000

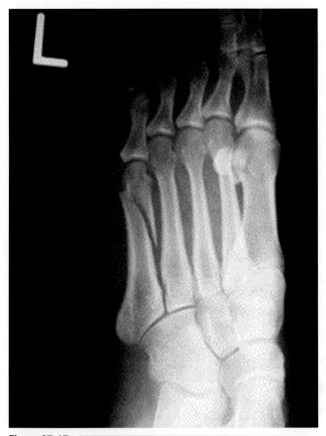

Figure 27-17
Spiral "dancer's fracture" of the fifth metatarsal shaft. (From Kadel NJ: Foot and ankle injuries in dance, *Phys Med Rehabil Clin North Am* 17(4):818, 2006.)

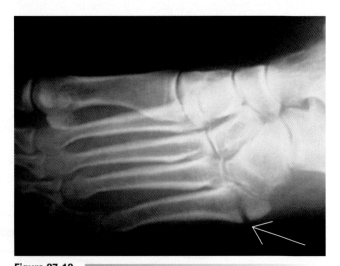

Figure 27-18
Jones fracture *(arrow)* of the proximal fifth metatarsal diaphysis. (From Kennedy JG, Hodgkins CW, Columbier J-A et al: Foot and ankle injuries in dancers. In Porter DA, Schon LC, editors: *Baxter's the foot and ankle in sport,* ed 2, p 474, Philadelphia, 2008, Mosby.)

dancing days, or 3.2 per 100,000 dancing days when considering classical ballet dancers only. In fact, in their 10-year study, the modern dancers experienced no ACL tears whereas the classical dancers sustained six. The left knee was involved in every case and, of these, four occurred in men and two occurred in women. All were treated operatively, but three dancers had to retire from dance because of post-surgical symptoms. These authors calculated the risk of a dancer suffering an ACL rupture of the left knee in a 10-year classical ballet career to be 7%.

In another study, Liederbach and colleagues[29] prospectively studied 298 professional ballet and modern dancers for 5 years. In this cohort, 12 ACL sprains occurred, 10 of which were in women. Contrasting with the data of Meuffels and Verhaar, in this study, modern dancers experienced a higher risk than did classical ballet dancers: 9 of the 12 injuries were in modern dancers. The ACL injury rate in ballet was 0.005 injuries per 1000 exposures and for modern dance, it was 0.012 injuries per 1000 exposures (an *exposure* was a single class, rehearsal, or performance in which a dancer participated). Overall, the injury rate of ACL injury in all dancers was 0.009 per 1000 exposures. It is important to note that Meuffels and Verhaar studied ACL *rupture,* whereas Liederbach and colleagues recorded ACL *injuries* (an *injury* being "a first-time partial or com-plete rupture of the ligament confirmed by clinical and radiological examination"[29]).

Substantial evidence exists that women athletes who participate in sports that elicit rotational forces across the knee—such as those requiring cutting and jumping—are much more likely than men to sustain an ACL injury.[215,248-250] Jump landings have been proposed as one mechanism for such injury.[251] Both studies of ACL injuries in dance outlined previously reported virtually identical injury mechanisms in their samples of dancers: knee valgus and external rotation forces upon landing from a jump (Figure 27-20). One set of investigators proposed this landing style as the single most important risk factor for ACL tear in dancers.[30] With the large proportion of dancers being women and the heavy emphasis on jumping in many dance genres, it is perhaps surprising that more ACL injuries are not reported. Although it does not appear that male and female dancers differ in their jump landing biomechanics,[252] several parameters about dance and dancers may account for the contrast of these results with ACL injuries in a sports environment. These include more forgiving shoe-to-floor or foot-to-floor interfaces, more controlled (i.e., choreographed) movements, and generally greater flexibility among dancers. Consistent exposure to balance training and jump training may also

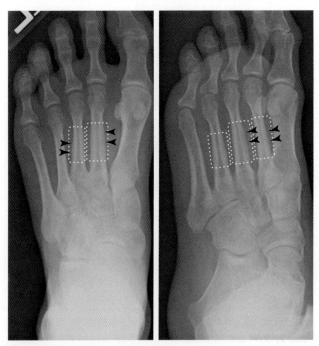

Figure 27-19

Anterior-posterior and oblique x-ray examinations of the left foot of a ballet dancer who presented with a clinical history of relentless rehearsals *en pointe* over several weeks, extreme midfoot pain, and exquisite point tenderness on the second and third metatarsals. *Dotted boxes* highlight second, third, and fourth metatarsal shafts with cortical thickening. *Arrowheads* indicate areas of periosteal elevation suggesting stress fractures of second and third metatarsals.

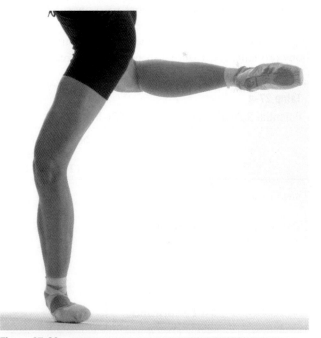

Figure 27-20

Characteristic landing pattern of a dancer that is associated with anterior cruciate ligament injury. Note the externally rotated hip and pronated foot with resulting valgus stress to the left knee. (From Meuffels DE, Verhaar JAN: Anterior cruciate ligament injury in professional dancers, *Acta Orthop* 79(4):516, 2008.)

play a role.[29,252] One more crucial factor to contemplate was identified by Liederbach and colleagues' study. As shown in Table 27-4, most ACL injuries occurred in the evening, at the end of a season, and during performances, suggesting that fatigue may play a role in these dance injuries.

Knee Ligament Injuries in Dancers

- Anterior cruciate ligament (ACL) rupture is not a common occurrence in dancers, but the nature of dance likely precludes participation by a dancer with a torn ACL
- Occurrence of ACL injuries in dancers seems to be associated with fatigue and related factors because research shows that most of the injuries occur late in the day, at the end of the season, and during performances

---

Internal Snapping Hip

Snapping hip, or coxa saltans, is a frequent finding in dancers; many will report it, although it may be neither painful nor necessarily restrictive. Of all dancers in a study by Winston and colleagues,[253] 91% reported snapping hip; in 80% of these cases the snap was bilateral. Although coxa saltans can encompass a number of pathological entities,[254] one customary way of categorizing the condition is as either external or internal snapping hip. The nature of hip motion in dance requires as large a range of motion in this joint as possible—this capability is integral to success. The varied movements along with the concentration on external rotation for turnout in ballet routinely draw soft tissues across bony prominences. External snapping hip is created by the posterior iliotibial band or anterior edge of the gluteus maximus muscle sliding across the greater trochanter.[254] On the other hand, the internal type may result—among several causes—from the iliopsoas tendon rubbing over the anterior ridge on the femoral head,[140] the iliopectineal ridge,[11] or a portion of the iliacus muscle belly.[253,255] Jacobs and Young[256] found certain kinesiological characteristics in dancers with a snapping hip compared with dancers without a snapping hip: narrow width between the pelvic ilia, increased hip abduction range of motion, decreased hip external rotation range of motion, and increased external rotation strength.

The iliopsoas is the most frequently involved anatomical structure in snapping hip.[253] This complex is a combination of the iliacus and psoas major muscles with their distal tendinous portions forming a common tendon that inserts at the lesser trochanter of the femur. Figure 27-21 illustrates the femoropelvic anatomy deep to the iliopsoas

Table 27-4
Potential Role of Fatigue in Dance ACL Injuries

		Number of ACL Injuries (Total = 12)
Time of Day	Morning	1
	Mid-day	3
	Evening	**8**
Time of Season	Off-season	2
	Early season	1
	End of season	**9**
Type of Activity	Class	1
	Rehearsal	4
	Performance	**7**

Data from Liederbach M, Dilgen FE, Rose DJ: Incidence of anterior cruciate ligament injuries among elite ballet and modern dancers: A 5-year prospective study, *Am J Sports Med* 36(9):1779-1788, 2008. *ACL,* Anterior cruciate ligament.
Note: Bold figures show greatest incidence of injury when dancers were most fatigued or under the most intense conditions.

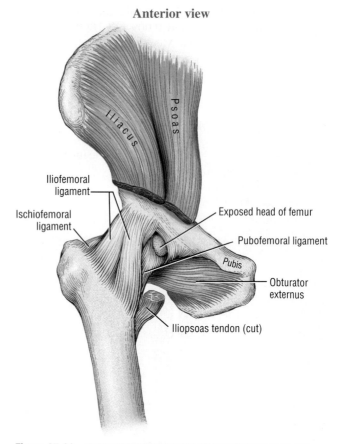

Anterior view

Figure 27-21

Deep anatomy of the anterior hip joint with a portion of the iliopsoas muscle and tendon resected. The area labeled *Exposed head of femur* is the location where the distal muscle belly and tendon of iliopsoas can snap across the anterior edge of the femoral head during hip movement. A bursa lies between the muscle-tendon and the femur and can become inflamed, as well. (From Neumann DA: *Kinesiology of the musculoskeletal system: Foundations for physical rehabilitation,* p 400, St Louis, 2002, Mosby.)

muscle and tendon. In addition to a snapping tendon, iliopsoas tendinopathy and iliopsoas bursitis often occur concurrently because the structures are so close anatomically.[257] Ultrasonography is helpful in establishing a pathoanatomical diagnosis.[253,255] If neither external nor internal snapping hip is suspected in a dancer presenting with pain and crepitus in the hip region, intra-articular injuries such as labral tears or loose bodies should be suspected.[258]

Joint Hypermobility

In dance parlance, the objective of training is to exhibit a good "line," meaning that the technical form of the body in its dance positioning should be aesthetically pleasing. A portion of executing a desirable line depends on the dancer's natural form, including the ranges of motion of the joints. It is customary for dancers to exhibit better flexibility than nondancers.[259] This is undoubtedly because of the nature of their training and the aesthetic requirements of dance, but there may also be some self-selection bias involved as presumably many individuals with less than desirable flexibility opt out of dance participation. Ballet dancers tend to be more flexible than modern dancers.[260] Nonetheless, this generally increased flexibility is often unbalanced between opposing joint motions (e.g., internal hip rotation versus external hip rotation), a characteristic that may predispose ballet dancers to injury in the knee and hip.[259] One reason for such imbalances is a flexibility emphasis based on the perceived need to accentuate a particular skill (e.g., turnout) and the concomitant neglect of the opposite motion.

One widely accepted and easily administered screening tool for joint hypermobility is the Beighton score.[261-263] This method is shown in Table 27-5 and is composed of four bilateral assessments plus trunk flexion, for a total of 9 possible points. A score of 4 or greater is suggestive of joint hypermobility[262-264] and may additionally point to benign joint hypermobility syndrome.[265,266] Interestingly, a longitudinal study of ballet dancers reported that their Beighton scores increased across a 4-year follow-up period.[267] This result appeared to stem from improvement in the trunk flexion component that was gained by training; the authors further suggested that trunk flexion ability in dancers develops over at least 4 years rather than being an innate quality of the body.

Several studies confirm that hypermobility can be a liability for dancers[262,263,267,268]; however, none suggest that the condition should preclude dance participation. Moreover, there appears to be no relationship between joint hypermobility and technical excellence.[267] The main challenges for the hypermobile dancer are an increased likelihood of injury,[262] increased rehabilitative time following injury,[263,268] and proprioceptive difficulty attaining proper positioning in technical training.[263] Hypermobility prevalence was found to be inversely proportional to rank within a professional

Table 27-5

Grading Scale for Determining Joint Hypermobility Based on Beighton's Criteria[261]

		Score	
Passive fifth metacarpophalangeal joint hyperextension ≥ 90°	Right	0	1
	Left	0	1
Passive wrist flexion to touch thumb to volar forearm	Right	0	1
	Left	0	1
Elbow hyperextension (cubitus recurvatum) ≥ 10°	Right	0	1
	Left	0	1
Knee hyperextension (genu recurvatum) ≥ 10°	Right	0	1
	Left	0	1
Trunk flexion to place both palms flat on floor		0	1
Total score (≥ 4 suggests hypermobility):		0 1 2 3 4 5 6 7 8 9	

A score of *0* = Not Present, *1* = Present.

ballet company,[263] suggesting that perhaps the dancers who are elevated to higher skill levels are not the hypermobile ones because they are not burdened by the detriments associated with hypermobility. Deficient collagen structure has been proposed as the root of many of the adverse consequences of joint hypermobility syndrome[265,266]; because this is unalterable, dancers who display hypermobility symptoms must be carefully educated about how best to adapt to the rigors of their training.

Hypermobility and Dancers

- Joint hypermobility is more common in dancers than in nondancers
- Hypermobile dancers are more prone to injury and have a greater challenge achieving proper positioning in their technical training compared with nonhypermobile dancers
- Hypermobility is not a contraindication for participating in dance

A study of female soccer players revealed an intriguing relationship between hypermobile (Beighton score ≥ 4) players and loading of the medial foot during barefoot walking.[264] Two factors about this research are worth noting when considering hypermobile dancers. First, the study was conducted with the subjects in bare feet; modern dancers usually wear no shoes and a ballet slipper provides little more substance than a bare foot. Second, although the subjects were soccer players the medial loading hypothesis is important to consider because of the tendency for dancers forcing turnout to pronate and, thus, load the medial foot (see Figure 27-12) and because a common mechanism of ACL injury involves landing from a jump with substantial medial loading (see Figure 27-20). Whether hypermobile dancers are more prone to injury because they also exhibit a proclivity to medially load the lower extremity warrants study.

Osteoarthritis

Based on the demanding activities and schedules of most dancers, it is often presumed that development of osteoarthritis is an inevitable consequence of participating in dance. As summarized in Table 27-6, this seems to be generally true,[196,269-272] but the extent of the symptoms associated with arthritic changes in dancers' joints is widely variable. The finding of degenerative joint disease is not, by itself, necessarily adverse to dancing.[271-273] Teitz and Kocoyne[271] found that radiographically confirmed hip capsule calcifications and knee, ankle, and first metatarsophalangeal joint changes occurred in young (late 20s to early 40s) retired dancers, yet did not correlate with the dancers' symptoms. Neither was the x-ray evidence associated with dancers' retirement from dance. Van Dijk and colleagues[272] studied retired dancers between 50 and 66 years old and found no clinical complaints among them in spite of a plethora of hip, ankle, subtalar, and first metatarsophalangeal arthroses on x-ray examination. Andersson and colleagues[269] studied the same joints in a cohort of former dancers ranging in age from 44 to 80 years and, although the prevalence of joint degeneration was greater in dancers than nondancers, only in the hips and knees were frequent symptoms reported. Only one study could be found that evaluated dancers with backgrounds other than just classical ballet. The long-term effect of other dance genres on joint degeneration represents a fertile field for research.

> ## Dancing and Osteoarthritis
>
> - Osteoarthritic changes seen on x-ray examinations are a typical finding in dancers
> - The first metatarsophalangeal joint is the most common site for osteoarthritis in dancers
> - Even among older, retired dancers, physical symptoms usually do not correlate with x-ray examination manifestations of osteoarthritis

Case Studies

The following two case studies illustrate the importance of careful diagnostics in dance medicine. In both of these cases, the dancers involved sought care for recalcitrant injuries, but sadly that care was not helpful and the dancers became frustrated with their injuries and their caregivers. However, once a dance medicine specialist established a correct diagnosis, the dancers were able to proceed toward recovery. Both of these are fairly recent cases. The intent is not to show the clinical progression to a successful resumption of activity, but, rather, to focus on how a health care provider's familiarity with the demands of dance and special attention to a dancer-patient's complaints can yield an appropriate diagnosis and treatment regimen.

Case Study 1: Posterior Ankle Pain

A 19-year-old female ballet and modern dancer presented to a dance medicine clinician complaining of persistent posterior left ankle pain. She reported a history of symptoms in

Table 27-6
Radiographic Findings of Arthroses in Dancers Reported by Various Authors

Author(s)	No. Subjects	Age of Subjects	Genre	General Presence of Degenerative				
				Hip	Knee	Ankle	Subtalar	First MTP
Ambré and Nilsson[273]	20 F	28 ± 7	Ballet	NR	NR	NR	NR	Yes (minor)
Andersson et al.[269]	29 F	44-80	Ballet	Yes	Yes	1 case	NR	Yes
	15 M							
Brodelius[270]	13 F	21-46	Ballet	NR	NR	Yes	NR	NR
	3 M							
Schneider et. al.[196]	39 F	12-41	Ballet	4 cases	2 cases	6 cases	NR	Yes
	13 M							
Teitz and Kocoyne[271]	9 F	27-46	Ballet and	Yes	5 cases	Yes	NR	Yes
	5 M		modern					
Van Dijk et al.[272]	19 F	50-66	Ballet	No	NR	Yes	Yes	Yes

F, Female; *M*, male; *MTP*, metatarsophalangeal joint; *NR*, not reported.
X-ray examination findings are indicated "Yes" or "No" for arthroses, or "NR" for not reported.

this ankle region of more than 2 years' duration. The working clinical impression given to her by a previous clinician was Achilles tendinopathy. This was the impetus for various treatments during the 2 years. In addition, she reported a history of lateral ankle injury, but indicated that her symptoms from two prior sprains were resolved except for the persistent pain that accompanied her current complaint. Interestingly, she connected the initial ankle sprain to her current condition. She also disclosed a prior visit to a primary care physician who had ordered an ankle x-ray examination and corroborated the diagnosis of Achilles tendinopathy. Conservative treatments did not ameliorate the symptoms; only rest from dance was beneficial in reducing her pain. The dancer reported that she continued to dance, interspersing periodic rest as necessary for pain relief. Her exasperation with being persistently unable to participate fully in dance was readily evident.

On examination, the dance medicine clinician found her Achilles' tendon was neither swollen nor markedly tender. The dancer reported that the greatest pain emanated from the posterolateral portion of the ankle, indicating that she felt it was down inside somewhere. She also described pain during *relevé* and a feeling that something was keeping her from fully plantar flexing to *demi-pointe* and *en pointe*. Edema was present between the posterior aspect of the lateral malleolus and the lateral border of the Achilles tendon. Tenderness was noted in this area, as well. Forced passive plantar flexion provoked pain and the dancer described crepitus and a firm, uncomfortable endpoint of the motion. Active maximum plantar flexion evaluation revealed that the involved side was slightly reduced in this ability compared with the uninvolved side.

The dance medicine clinician's clinical impression was os trigonum, so the patient was referred back to her primary care physician for a review of her previous radiographs. The os trigonum was confirmed based on the lateral x-ray view on which this accessory bone was originally missed (Figure 27-22). The dancer was scheduled for orthopaedic consultation and surgery for resection of the offending ossicle. Following this procedure, her healing was uneventful, and she has returned fully to dance.

This case study demonstrates the importance of two functions of the clinician: understanding what is required of the ankle in dance and carefully evaluating an injury in light of the history reported by the dancer. Of note is the dancer's belief that the origin of the intractable posterior pain seemed to coincide with a lateral ankle sprain. This is not an unusual mechanism by which a previously asymptomatic os trigonum can be disrupted. Furthermore, close attention to pathoanatomy is a must. In this instance, localizing the pain and swelling and coordinating these with the dancer's symptom description was an effective combination for developing an accurate clinical impression.

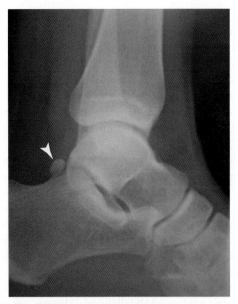

Figure 27-22

Lateral x-ray examination of the ankle of a 19-year-old ballet and modern dancer who complained of pain posterior to the ankle and limited plantar flexion. *Arrowhead* indicates an os trigonum.

Case Study 2: First Metatarsophalangeal Joint Pain

A 14-year-old female ballet dancer presented to a dance medicine clinician with the chief complaint of first metatarsophalangeal joint pain in her left foot. She was highly skilled in ballet, having participated in well-known training programs in New York City. She also had performed with a professional dance company. Her symptoms were several months in duration; the diagnosis provided on initial assessment by another clinician was first metatarsophalangeal joint sprain, or "turf toe," and the dancer was treated accordingly. Nonetheless, conservative treatment for this condition did not allow the dancer to return to full dance activity.

A visit to an orthopaedic surgeon did not reveal further insight. This spurred the dancer's mother to seek the advice of the dance medicine clinician. At this point in the case, the dancer's foot had been completely rested for 6 weeks. The dancer reported that *relevé* was painful and working in the *demi-pointe* position elicited more pain under the ball of the foot than did working *en pointe*. She felt an increase in pain as she moved through *relevé* to rise to her toes. Periods of rest had reduced the pain, but it returned when she resumed any substantial amount of dance. All methods of padding had not alleviated her symptoms.

On assessment, the dancer denied a traumatic onset. Her pain was plantar and slightly proximal to the first metatarsophalangeal joint rather than periarticular, such as would be expected in a turf toe injury. The lateral sesamoid was particularly tender. Dancing in a *pointe* shoe greatly exacerbated the symptoms because of the shoe's relatively hard and stiff sole. The dancer denied paresthesia in her toes and swelling was unremarkable in any part of the forefoot. As a result of the history and examination—and considering the concentration of symptoms at the lateral sesamoid—the dance medicine clinician's clinical impression was bipartite lateral sesamoid. Lateral sesamoiditis was a differential impression. The dancer was referred to her orthopaedic surgeon again, and radiographs confirmed a bipartite lateral sesamoid (Figure 27-23). The surgeon advised against surgery (surgery is contraindicated in the first metatarsophalangeal joint of dancers because of the likelihood that the joint's crucial hyperextension range will be compromised), but acknowledged a lack of expertise for working with dancers and referred the dancer back to the dance medicine clinician who consulted with a podiatrist specializing in injuries of elite dancers. MRI examination was undertaken to discern the extent of bone and soft tissue involvement. The MRI examination confirmed the diagnosis, demonstrating bone marrow edema and soft tissue inflammation, so the dancer was removed from participation to allow the greatest chance for healing. Following 6 months of rest, the dancer began to test her injured foot in a very controlled fashion, but *relevé* remained painful. Because the load on the sesamoids during ballet is substantial, she continued pursuing the conservative course of rest in the hope of being able to return to dance later. After a complete year of rest, she undertook a very gradual and methodical resumption of her dance activity, with hopefulness that her symptoms will not recur.

Significant to this case was the need to listen to the dancer's history to establish the probable mechanism. It was thought that, apart from trauma, a turf-toe type of injury that was so painful and persistent was unlikely. Furthermore, the intense focal pressure on the sesamoids during *demi-pointe*—especially considering how a *pointe* shoe's sole could amplify this—was deemed important and, in fact, this is what elicited the greatest pain. Point tenderness over the lateral sesamoid added further to the suspicion of bipartite sesamoid or sesamoiditis. Once again, careful attention to the injury history and to the dancer's equipment and regimen provided vital assistance to caring for her. Moreover, it is not a minor point that this case is saddled with the added emotional challenge of a very talented dancer requiring an extended period of discontinuance from dance.

Conclusion

Dancers certainly are athletes and dance injuries are commonplace. Unquestionably, working with dancers presents many challenges to the musculoskeletal health care provider; but the challenges are also what make the task enjoyable. Health care providers will find in dancers an extremely creative, interesting, and grateful group of patients. A traditional sports medicine model is helpful in working with dancers, yet it is not an ideal match because of several unique characteristics of a dance environment. These include the dancer's intense psyche, limitations imposed by wardrobe requirements, and unrelenting training regimens.

The majority of dance injuries are of the overuse variety. It is highly unlikely that a dancer will escape injury during his or her career; most musculoskeletal conditions are exacerbated by the very nature of dance training, and many of them are endemic to dance. Careful assessment and well-considered care plans are helpful, whereas advice to "stop dancing" as a categorical solution to injuries is quite the opposite and will only frustrate the dancer-patient, as it would any athlete. Dancers respond well to practitioners who show genuine interest in dance and at least a basic understanding of what dance entails as a physical and artistic activity.

Acknowledgments

I am grateful for three of my students at the University of California–Irvine who served as models for some of my figures: Ashley McConnell, Laura Obler, and Amy Quanbeck. Also, I deeply appreciate my former faculty colleagues and students in the Dance Department at Belhaven College and my current faculty colleagues and students in the Dance Department at UC-Irvine. They have taught me much more about dance and dance medicine than they realize. Two of my current colleagues, Dr. Lisa Naugle and Dr. Nancy Ruyter, provided invaluable reviews of portions of this chapter. Finally, my wife, Ruth, deserves a special accolade for the encouragement she gave me to undertake this writing project.

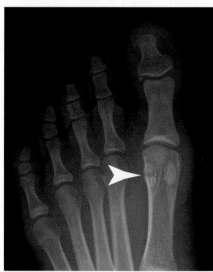

Figure 27-23

X-ray examination of the forefoot of a 14-year-old ballet dancer with pain and exquisite point tenderness over the lateral hallux sesamoid. *Arrowhead* points to the bipartite sesamoid that was the source of the dancer's symptoms.

References

1. Snook GA: The history of sports medicine. Part I, *Am J Sports Med* 12(4):252–254, 1984.
2. Welch JE: Pioneering in health education and services at Amherst College, *J Am Coll Health* 30(6):289–295, 1982.
3. Sparger C: Physiotherapy at the Sadler's Wells School of Ballet, *Physiotherapy* 38(1):8–13, 1952.
4. International Association for Dance Medicine and Science: *About IADMS*, 2009. Available at: http://www.iadms.org/displaycommon.cfm?an=8. Accessed November 21, 2009.
5. Stretanski MF: Classical ballet: The full contact sport, *Am J Phys Med Rehabil* 81(5):392–393, 2002.
6. Fitt SS: *Dance kinesiology*, ed 2, New York, 1996, Schirmer Books.
7. Koutedakis Y, Jamurtas A: The dancer as a performing athlete, *Sports Med* 34(10):651–661, 2004.
8. Koutedakis Y, Pacy PJ, Carson RJ, et al: Health and fitness in professional dancers, *Med Prob Performing Artists* 12(1):23–27, 1997.
9. Stretanski MF: Medical and rehabilitation issues in classical ballet, *Am J Phys Med Rehabil* 81(5):383–391, 2002.
10. Council of Arts Accrediting Associations: *Briefing paper: An overview of health issues for performing and visual arts students*, Reston, VA, 1991, Council of Arts Accrediting Associations.
11. Toledo SD, Akuthota V, Drake DF, et al: Sports and performing arts medicine. 6. Issues relating to dancers, *Arch Phys Med Rehabil* 85(Suppl 1):75–78, 2004.
12. Baillie Y, Wyon M, Head A: Highland dance: Heart-rate and blood lactate differences between competition and class, *Int J Sports Physiol Perf* 2(4):371–376, 2007.
13. Koutedakis Y, Hukam H, Metsios G, et al: The effects of three months of aerobic and strength training on selected performance- and fitness-related parameters in modern dance students, *J Strength Cond Res* 21(3):808–812, 2007.
14. Redding E, Wyon M: Strengths and weaknesses of current methods for evaluating the aerobic power of dancers, *J Dance Med Sci* 7(1):10–16, 2003.
15. Wyon MA, Abt G, Redding E, et al: Oxygen uptake during modern dance class, rehearsal, and performance, *J Strength Cond Res* 18(3):646–649, 2004.
16. Wyon MA, Deighan MA, Nevill AM, et al: The cardiorespiratory, anthropometric, and performance characteristics of an international/national touring ballet company, *J Strength Cond Res* 21(2):389–393, 2007.
17. Wyon MA, Redding E: Physiological monitoring of cardiorespiratory adaptations during rehearsal and performance of contemporary dance, *J Strength Cond Res* 19(3):611–614, 2005.
18. Conti SF, Wong YS: Foot and ankle injuries in the dancer, *J Dance Med Sci* 5(2):43–50, 2001.
19. Solomon R, Brown T, Gerbino PG, et al: The young dancer, *Clin Sports Med* 19(4):717–739, 2000.
20. Byhring S, Bø K: Musculoskeletal injuries in the Norwegian National Ballet: A prospective cohort study, *Scand J Med Sci Sports* 12(6):365–370, 2002.
21. Garrick JG, Requa R: Ballet injuries: An analysis of epidemiology and financial outcome, *Am J Sports Med* 21(4):586–590, 1993.
22. Hamilton LH, Hamilton WG, Meltzer JD, et al: Personality, stress, and injuries in professional ballet dancers, *Am J Sports Med* 17(2):263–267, 1989.
23. Hardaker WT Jr.: Foot and ankle injuries in classical ballet dancers, *Orthop Clin North Am* 20(4):621–627, 1989.
24. Khan K, Brown J, Way S, et al: Overuse injuries in classical ballet, *Sports Med* 19(5):341–357, 1995.
25. Milan KR: Injury in ballet: A review of relevant topics for the physical therapist, *J Orthop Sports Phys Ther* 19(2):121–129, 1994.
26. Miller EH, Schneider HJ, Bronson JL, et al.: A new consideration in athletic injuries: The classical ballet dancer, *Clin Orthop* 111:181–191, 1975.
27. Nilsson C, Leanderson J, Wykman A, et al: The injury panorama in a Swedish professional ballet company, *Knee Surg Sports Traumatol Arthrosc* 9(4):242–246, 2001.
28. Solomon R, Solomon J, Micheli LJ, et al: The "cost" of injuries in a professional ballet company, *Med Prob Performing Artists* 14:164–169, 1999.
29. Liederbach M, Dilgen FE, Rose DJ: Incidence of anterior cruciate ligament injuries among elite ballet and modern dancers: A 5-year prospective study, *Am J Sports Med* 36(9):1779–1788, 2008.
30. Meuffels DE, Verhaar JAN: Anterior cruciate ligament injury in professional dancers, *Acta Orthop* 79(4):515–518, 2008.
31. Bronner S, Ojofeitimi S, Rose D: Injuries in a modern dance company: Effect of comprehensive management on injury incidence and time loss, *Am J Sports Med* 31(3):365–373, 2003.
32. Sides SN, Ambegaonkar JP, Caswell SV: High incidence of shoulder injuries in collegiate modern dance students, *Athl Ther Today* 14(4):43–46, 2009.
33. Shybut TB, Rose DJ, Strongwater AM: Second metatarsal physeal arrest in an adolescent flamenco dancer: A case report, *Foot Ankle Int* 29(8):859–862, 2008.
34. Cromie S, Greenwood JG, McCullagh JF: Does Irish-dance training influence lower-limb asymmetry? *Laterality* 12(6):500–506, 2007.
35. Bejjani FJ: Occupational biomechanics of athletes and dancers: A comparative approach, *Clin Podiatr Med Surg* 4(3):671–711, 1987.
36. Bejjani FJ, Halpern N, Pio A, et al: Musculoskeletal demands on flamenco dancers: A clinical and biomechanical study, *Foot Ankle* 8(5):254–263, 1988.
37. Kauther MD, Wedemeyer C, Kauther KM, et al: Breakdancer's "Headspin Hole": First description of a common overuse syndrome, *Sportverletz Sportschaden* 23(1):52–53, 2009.
38. Kauther MD, Wedemeyer C, Wegner A, et al: Breakdance injuries and overuse syndromes in amateurs and professionals, *Am J Sports Med* 37(4):797–802, 2009.
39. Winkler AR, Barnes JC, Ogden JA: Break dance hip: Chronic avulsion of the anterior superior iliac spine, *Pediatr Radiol* 17(6):501–502, 1987.
40. Cho CH, Song KS, Min BW, et al: Scaphoid nonunion in breakdancers: A report of 3 cases, *Orthopedics* 32(7):526, 2009.
41. Cho CH, Song KS, Min BW, et al: Musculoskeletal injuries in break-dancers, *Injury* 40(11):1207–1211, 2009.
42. McCauley A, Lamb KL: An assessment of the prevalence and correlates of injuries in Irish dancers [Abstract], *J Sports Sci* 22(3):251, 2004.
43. Henderson J, MacIntyre D: A descriptive survey of injury patterns in Canadian Premier Highland dancers, *Physiother Can* 58(1):61–73, 2006.
44. Pedersen ME, Wilmerding MV: Injury profiles of student and professional flamenco dancers, *J Dance Med Sci* 2(3):108–114, 1998.
45. Walls RJ, Brennan SA, Hodnett P,, et al.: Overuse ankle injuries in professional Irish dancers, *Foot Ankle Surg* 16(1):45–49, 2010.
46. Washington EL: Musculoskeletal injuries in theatrical dancers: Site, frequency, and severity, *Am J Sports Med* 6(2):75–98, 1978.
47. Leavesley RGE, Borthwick AM: Foot and lower-limb injury in ballet: Dancers' perspectives, *Br J Podiatry* 6(3):73–79, 2003.

48. Air M: Health care seeking behavior and perceptions of the medical profession among pre- and post-retirement age Dutch dancers, *J Dance Med Sci* 13(2):42–50, 2009.

49. Lai RYJ, Krasnow D, Thomas M: Communication between medical practitioners and dancers, *J Dance Med Sci* 12(2):47–53, 2008.

50. Tajet-Foxell B, Rose FD: Pain and pain tolerance in professional ballet dancers, *Br J Sports Med* 29(1):31–34, 1995.

51. Ramel E, Moritz U: Self-reported musculoskeletal pain and discomfort in professional ballet dancers in Sweden, *Scand J Rehabil Med* 26(1):11–16, 1994.

52. Anderson R, Hanrahan SJ: Dancing in pain: Pain appraisal and coping in dancers, *J Dance Med Sci* 12(1):9–16, 2008.

53. Rip B, Fortin S, Vallerand RJ: The relationship between passion and injury in dance students, *J Dance Med Sci* 10(1–2):14–20, 2006.

54. Macchi R, Crossman J: After the fall: Reflections on injured classical ballet dancers, *J Sport Behav* 19(3):221–234, 1996.

55. Adam MU, Brassington GS, Matheson GO: Psychological factors associated with performance-limiting injuries in professional ballet dancers, *J Dance Med Sci* 8(2):43–46, 2004.

56. Requa RK, Garrick JG: Do professional dancers have medical insurance? Company-provided medical insurance for professional dancers, *J Dance Med Sci* 9(3–4):81–83, 2005.

57. Weiss DS, Shah S, Burchette RJ: A profile of the demographics and training characteristics of professional modern dancers, *J Dance Med Sci* 12(2):41–46, 2008.

58. Ambegaonkar JP, Caswell SV: Dance program administrators' perceptions of athletic training services, *Athl Ther Today* 14(3):17–19, 2009.

59. Bronner S, Ojofeitimi S, Spriggs J: Occupational musculoskeletal disorders in dancers, *Phys Ther Rev* 8:57–68, 2003.

60. Askling C, Lund H, Saartok T, et al: Self-reported hamstring injuries in student-dancers, *Scand J Med Sci Sports* 12:230–235, 2002.

61. Kerr G, Krasnow D, Mainswaring L: The nature of dance injuries, *Med Prob Performing Artists* 7:25–29, 1992.

62. Bowling A: Injuries to dancers: Prevalence, treatment and perception of causes, *BMJ* 298:731–734, 1989.

63. Laws H: *Fit to dance 2*, London, 2005, Dance UK.

64. Sohl P, Bowling A: Injuries to dancers: Prevalence, treatment and prevention, *Sports Med* 9(5):17–22, 1990.

65. Rovere GD, Webb LX, Gristina AG, et al: Musculoskeletal injuries in theatrical dance students, *Am J Sports Med* 11(4):195–198, 1983.

66. Olsson I: A 2-year study of 77 dancers: Almost 90 per cent needed help because of injury, *Lakartidningen* 95(15):1689, 1998.

67. Arendt YD, Kerschbaumer F: Injury and overuse pattern in professional ballet dancers, *Z Orthop Ihre Grenzgeb* 141(3):349–356, 2003.

68. Ambegaonkar JP: Dance medicine: At the university level, *Dance Res J* 37(2):113–119, 2005.

69. Schon LC, Weinfeld SB: Lower extremity musculoskeletal problems in dancers, *Curr Opin Rheumatol* 8(2):130–142, 1996.

70. Negus V, Hopper D, Briffa NK: Associations between turnout and lower extremity injuries in classical ballet dancers, *J Orthop Sports Phys Ther* 35(5):307–318, 2005.

71. Hincapié CA, Morton EJ, Cassidy JD: Musculoskeletal injuries and pain in dancers: A systematic review, *Arch Phys Med Rehabil* 89:1819–1829, 2008.

72. Baker J, Scott D, Watkins K, et al: Self-reported and reported injury patterns in contemporary dance students, *Med Probl Perform Art* 25(1):10–15, 2010.

73. Van Mechelen W, Hlobil H, Kemper HC: Incidence, severity, aetiology and prevention of sports injuries: A review of concepts, *Sports Med* 14(2):82–99, 1996.

74. Ekstrand J, Karlsson J: The risk for injury in football. There is a need for a consensus about definition of the injury and the design of studies, *Scand J Med Sci Sports* 13(3):147–149, 2003.

75. Brooks JHM, Fuller CW: The influence of methodological issues on the results and conclusions from epidemiological studies of sports injuries: Illustrative examples, *Sports Med* 36(6):459–472, 2006.

76. Hodgson L, Gissane C, Gabbett TJ, et al: For debate: Consensus injury definitions in team sports should focus on encompassing all injuries, *Clin J Sport Med* 17(3):188–191, 2007.

77. Garrick JG: The frequency of injury, mechanism of injury, and epidemiology of ankle sprains, *Am J Sports Med* 5(6):241–242, 1977.

78. Bronner S, Ojofeitimi S, Mayers L: Comprehensive surveillance of dance injuries: A proposal for uniform reporting guidelines for professional companies, *J Dance Med Sci* 10(3–4):69–80, 2006.

79. Hamilton WG: Foot and ankle injuries in dancers, *Clin Sports Med* 7(1):143–173, 1988.

80. McLean SG, Samorezov JE: Fatigue-induced ACL injury risk stems from a degradation in central control, *Med Sci Sports Exerc* 41(8):1661–1672, 2009.

81. McLean SG, Fellin RE, Suedekum N, et al: Impact of fatigue on gender-based high-risk landing strategies, *Med Sci Sports Exerc* 39(3):502–514, 2007.

82. Chappell JD, Herman DC, Knight BS, et al: Effect of fatigue on knee kinetics and kinematics in stop-jump tasks, *Am J Sports Med* 33(7):1022–1029, 2005.

83. Gefen A: Biomechanical analysis of fatigue-related foot injury mechanisms in athletes and recruits during intensive marching, *Med Biol Eng Comput* 40(3):302–310, 2002.

84. Angioi M, Metsios GS, Koutedakis Y, et al: Physical fitness and severity of injuries in contemporary dance, *Med Prob Performing Artists* 24:26–29, 2009.

85. Twitchett E, Brodrick A, Nevill AM, et al: Does physical fitness affect injury occurrence and time loss due to injury in elite vocational ballet students? *J Dance Med Sci* 14(1):26–31, 2010.

86. Gamboa JM, Roberts LA, Maring J, et al: Injury patterns in elite preprofessional ballet dancers and the utility of screening programs to identify risk characteristics, *J Orthop Sports Phys Ther* 38(3):126–136, 2008.

87. Koutedakis Y, Khaloula M, Pacy PJ, et al: Thigh peak torques and lower-body injuries in dancers, *J Dance Med Sci* 1(1):12–15, 1997.

88. Grant G: *Technical manual and dictionary of classical ballet*, ed 3, New York, 1982, Dover Publications.

89. Barringer J, Schlesinger S: *The pointe book: Shoes, training and technique*, ed 2, Hightstown, NJ, 2004, Princeton Book Company.

90. Lee C: *Ballet in Western culture: A history of its origins and evolution*, New York, 2002, Routledge.

91. Gaynor Minden Inc: *10 Ergonomic Secrets*, 2009. Available at http://gaynorminden.com/tensecrets.php. Accessed August 5, 2009.

92. Bloch International: *thermoMorphtechnology*, 2009. Available at http://www.bloch-tmt.com/. Accessed August 5, 2009.

93. Novella TM: Pointe shoes: Fitting and selection criteria, *J Dance Med Sci* 4(2):73–77, 2000.

94. Teitz CC, Harrington RM, Wiley H: Pressures on the foot in pointe shoes, *Foot Ankle* 5(5):216–221, 1985.

95. Kadel N, Boenisch M, Teitz CC, et al: Stability of Lisfranc joints in ballet pointe position, *Foot Ankle Int* 26(5):394–400, 2005.

96. Solan MC, Moorman CT III, Miyamoto RG, et al: Ligamentous restraints of the second tarsometatarsal joint: a biomechanical evaluation, *Foot Ankle Int* 22(8):637–641, 2001.

97. Johnson A, Hill K, Ward J, et al: Anatomy of the Lisfranc ligament, *Foot Ankle Spec* 1(1):19–23, 2008.

98. American Academy of Orthopaedic Surgeons: *Joint motion: Method of measuring and recording*, Chicago, 1965, American Academy of Orthopaedic Surgeons.

99. Gerhardt JJ: *Documentation of joint motion*, ed 4, Portland, 1994, ISOMED.

100. Reese NB, Bandy WD: *Joint range of motion and muscle length testing*, ed 2, St Louis, 2010, Saunders Elsevier.

101. Hamilton WG, Hamilton LH, Marshall P, et al: A profile of the musculoskeletal characteristics of elite professional ballet dancers, *Am J Sports Med* 20(3):267–273, 1992.

102. Luke AC, Kinney SA, D'Hemecourt PA, et al: Determinants of injuries in young dancers, *Med Prob Performing Artists* 17(3):105–112, 2002.

103. Novella TM: Simple techniques for quantifying choreographically essential foot and ankle extents of motion, *J Dance Med Sci* 8(4):118–122, 2004.

104. Steinberg N, Hershkovitz I, Peleg S, et al: Range of joint movement in female dancers and nondancers aged 8 to 16 years, *Am J Sports Med* 34(5):814–823, 2006.

105. Wiesler ER, Hunter DM, Martin DF, et al: Ankle flexibility and injury patterns in dancers, *Am J Sports Med* 24(6):754–757, 1996.

106. Sammarco GJ, Burstein AH, Frankel VH: Biomechanics of the ankle: A kinematic study, *Orthop Clin North Am* 4(1):75–96, 1973.

107. Lundberg A, Goldie I, Kalin B, et al: Kinematics of the ankle/foot complex: Plantarflexion and dorsiflexion, *Foot Ankle* 9(4):194–200, 1989.

108. Bonnin JG: *Injuries to the ankle* (facsimile of the 1950 edition), Darien, CT, 1970, Hafner Publishing Co.

109. Kitaoka HB, Patzer GL: Clinical results of the Mayo total ankle arthroplasty, *J Bone Joint Surg Am* 78(11):1658–1664, 1996.

110. Kitaoka HB, Alexander IJ, Adelaar RS, et al: Clinical rating systems for the ankle-hindfoot, midfoot, hallux, and lesser toes, *Foot Ankle Int* 15(7):349–353, 1994.

111. Lundberg A: Kinematics of the ankle and foot: In vivo roentgen stereophotogrammetry, *Acta Orthop Scand* 60(Suppl 233):1–24, 1989.

112. Russell JA, Shave RM: Tri-color superimposition x-rays for evaluation of extreme ankle and foot motion in ballet dancers, *American Orthopaedic Society for Sports Medicine Annual Conference*, Keystone, Colorado, 2009.

113. Anderson KJ, LeCocq JF: Operative treatment of injury to the fibular collateral ligament of the ankle, *J Bone Joint Surg Am* 36(4):825–832, 1954.

114. Ferran NA, Maffulli N: Epidemiology of sprains of the lateral ankle ligament complex, *Foot Ankle Clin North Am* 11(3): 659–662, 2006.

115. Foetisch CA, Ferkel RD: Deltoid ligament injuries: Anatomy, diagnosis, and treatment, *Sports Med Arthrosc* 8:326–335, 2000.

116. Russell JA, McEwan IM, Koutedakis Y, et al: Clinical anatomy and biomechanics of the ankle in dance, *J Dance Med Sci* 12(3):75–82, 2008.

117. Nigg BM, Skarvan G, Frank CB, et al: Elongation and forces of ankle ligaments in a physiological range of motion, *Foot Ankle* 11(1):30–40, 1990.

118. Siegler S, Block J, Schneck CD: The mechanical characteristics of the collateral ligaments of the human ankle joint, *Foot Ankle* 8(5):234–242, 1988.

119. Renstrom P, Wertz M, Incavo S, et al: Strain in the lateral ligaments of the ankle, *Foot Ankle* 9(2):59–63, 1988.

120. Bahr R, Pena F, Shine J, et al: Ligament force and joint motion in the intact ankle: A cadaveric study, *Knee Surg Sports Traumatol Arthrosc* 6:115–121, 1998.

121. Colville MR, Marder RA, Boyle JJ, et al: Strain measurement in lateral ankle ligaments, *Am J Sports Med* 18(2):196–200, 1990.

122. Hamilton WG: Sprained ankles in ballet dancers, *Foot Ankle* 3(2):99–102, 1982.

123. Macintyre J, Joy EA: Foot and ankle injuries in dance, *Clin Sports Med* 19(2):351–368, 2000.

124. Shah S, Luftman J, Vigil DV: Stress injury of the talar dome and body in a ballerina: A case report, *J Dance Med Sci* 9(3):91–95, 2005.

125. O'Loughlin PF, Hodgkins CW, Kennedy JG: Ankle sprains and instability in dancers, *Clin Sports Med* 27(2):247–262, 2008.

126. Clippinger K: *Dance anatomy and kinesiology*, Champaign, IL, 2007, Human Kinetics.

127. Oztekin HH, Boya H, Nalcakan M, et al: Second-toe length and forefoot disorders in ballet and folk dancers, *J Am Podiatr Med Assoc* 97(5):385–388, 2007.

128. Tuckman AS, Werner FW, Bayley JC: Analysis of the forefoot on pointe in the ballet dancer, *Foot Ankle* 12(3):144–148, 1991.

129. Kravitz SR, Huber S, Murgia CJ, et al: Biomechanical study of bunion deformity and stress produced in classical ballet, *J Am Podiatr Med Assoc* 75(7):338–345, 1985.

130. Sammarco GJ, Cooper PS: Flexor hallucis longus tendon injury in dancers and nondancers, *Foot Ankle Int* 19(6):356–362, 1998.

131. Meck C, Hess RA, Helldobler R, et al: Pre-pointe evaluation components used by dance schools, *J Dance Med Sci* 8(2):37–42, 2004.

132. Howse AJG: *Dance technique and injury prevention*, ed 3, London, 2000, A & C Black.

133. Weiss DS, Rist RA, Grossman G: When can I start pointe work? Guidelines for initiating pointe training, *J Dance Med Sci* 13(3):90–92, 2009.

134. Shah S: Determining a young dancer's readiness for dancing on pointe, *Curr Sports Med Rep* 8(6):295–299, 2009.

135. Welsh TM, Rodriguez M, Beare LW, et al: Assessing turnout in university dancers, *J Dance Med Sci* 12(4):136–141, 2008.

136. Hardaker WT Jr., Erickson L: The pathogenesis of dance injury. In Shell CG, editor: *The dancer as athlete*, Champaign, IL, 1986, Human Kinetics Publishers.

137. Clippinger-Robertson K: A unique challenge: Biomechanical considerations in turnout, *JOPERD* 58(5):37–40, 1987.

138. Hamilton WG: Physical prerequisites for ballet dancers, *J Musculoskel Med* 3:61–66, 1986.

139. Thomasen E: *Diseases and injuries of ballet dancers*, Århus, Denmark, 1982, Universitetsforlaget I Århus.

140. Sammarco GJ: The dancer's hip, *Clin Sports Med* 2(3):485–498, 1983.

141. Hamilton D, Aronsen P, Løken JH, et al: Dance training intensity at 11-14 years is associated with femoral torsion in classical ballet dancers, *Br J Sports Med* 40(4):299–303, 2006.

142. Magee DJ: *Orthopedic physical assessment*, ed 5, Philadelphia, 2008, Saunders Elsevier.

143. Bauman PA, Singson R, Hamilton WG: Femoral neck anteversion in ballerinas, *Clin Orthop* 302:57–63, 1994.

144. Grossman G, Waninger KN, Voloshin A, et al: Reliability and validity of goniometric turnout measurements compared with MRI and retro-reflective markers, *J Dance Med Sci* 12(4): 142–152, 2008.

145. Grossman G: Measuring dancer's active and passive turnout, *J Dance Med Sci* 7(2):49–55, 2003.

146. Kadel NJ: Foot and ankle injuries in dance, *Phys Med Rehabil Clin N Am* 17 (4):813–826, 2006.

147. Micheli L: Back injuries in dancers, *Clin Sports Med* 2(3): 473–484, 1983.

148. Coplan JA: Ballet dancer's turnout and its relationship to self-reported injury, *J Orthop Sports Phys Ther* 32(11):579–584, 2002.

149. Hamilton WG: Stenosing tenosynovitis of the flexor hallucis longus tendon and posterior impingement upon the os trigonum in ballet dancers, *Foot Ankle* 3(2):74–80, 1982.

150. Kadel NJ, Micheli LJ, Solomon R: Os trigonum impingement syndrome in dancers, *J Dance Med Sci* 4(3):99–102, 2000.

151. Kleiger B: Anterior tibiotalar impingement syndromes in dancers, *Foot Ankle* 3(2):69–73, 1982.

152. Kleiger B: The posterior tibiotalar impingement syndrome in dancers, *Bull Hosp Jt Dis Orthop Inst* 47(2):203–210, 1987.

153. Peace KAL, Hillier JC, Hulme A, et al: MRI features of posterior ankle impingement syndrome in ballet dancers: A review of 25 cases, *Clin Radiol* 59:1025–1033, 2004.

154. O'Kane JW, Kadel N: Anterior impingement syndrome in dancers, *Curr Rev Musculoskel Med* 1(1):12–16, 2008.

155. Stoller SM, Hekmat F, Kleiger B: A comparative study of the frequency of anterior impingement exostoses of the ankle in dancers and nondancers, *Foot Ankle* 4(4):201–203, 1984.

156. Tsuruta T, Shiokawa Y, Kato A, et al: Radiological study of the accessory skeletal elements in the foot and ankle, *Nippon Seikeigeka Gakkai Zasshi* 55(4):357–370, 1981.

157. Lawson JP: Symptomatic radiographic variants in extremities, *Radiology* 157:625–631, 1985.

158. Kleinberg S: Supernumerary bones of the foot, *Ann Surg* 65(4):499–509, 1917.

159. Shands AR, Jr.: The accessory bones of the foot: An x-ray study of the feet of 1,054 patients, *South Med Surg* 93:326–336, 1931.

160. Geist ES: Supernumerary bones of the foot—A röntgen study of the feet of one hundred normal individuals, *J Bone Joint Surg Am* s2-12(3):403–414, 1915.

161. O'Rahilly R: A survey of carpal and tarsal anomalies, *J Bone Joint Surg Am* 35(3):626–642, 1953.

162. Gottlieb A: Post-traumatic os trigonum, *J Int Coll Surg* 26(1):80–82, 1956.

163. Stieda L: Ueber secundäre fusswerzelknochen, *Archiv für Anatomie, Physiologie und Wissenschaftliche Medizin* 36:108–111, 1869.

164. Hedrick MR, McBryde AM: Posterior ankle impingement, *Foot Ankle* 15(1):2–8, 1994.

165. Howse AJG: Posterior block of the ankle joint in dancers, *Foot Ankle* 3(2):81–84, 1982.

166. Brodsky AE, Khalil MA: Talar compression syndrome, *Am J Sports Med* 14(6):472–476, 1986.

167. Bureau NJ, Cardinal E, Hobden R, et al: Posterior ankle impingement syndrome: MR imaging findings in seven patients, *Radiology* 215:497–503, 2000.

168. Jourdel F, Tourne Y, Saragaglia D: Posterior ankle impingement syndrome: A retrospective study in 21 cases treated surgically, *Rev Chir Orthop Reparatrice Appar Mot* 91(3):239–247, 2005.

169. Golanó P, Vega J, Pérez-Carro L, et al: Ankle anatomy for the arthroscopist. Part II: Role of the ankle ligaments in soft tissue impingement, *Foot Ankle Clin N Am* 11:275–296, 2006.

170. Hamilton WG, Geppert MJ, Thompson FM: Pain in the posterior aspect of the ankle in dancers: Differential diagnosis and operative treatment, *J Bone Joint Surg Am* 78(10):1491–1500, 1996.

171. Lohrer H: Flexor hallucis longus tendon rupture as an impingement lesion induced by os trigonum instability, *Sportverletz Sportschaden* 20(1):31–35, 2006.

172. Karasick D, Schweitzer ME: The os trigonum syndrome: Imaging features, *Am J Roentgenol* 166:125–129, 1996.

173. Tey M, Monllau J, Centenera J, et al: Benefits of arthroscopic tuberculoplasty in posterior ankle impingement syndrome, *Knee Surg Sports Traumatol Arthrosc* 15(10):1235–1239, 2007.

174. Van Dijk CN: A 2-portal endoscopic approach for diagnosis and treatment of posterior ankle pathology, *Arthroscopy* 16(8):871–876, 2000.

175. Hillier JC, Peace K, Hulme A, et al: MRI features of foot and ankle injuries in ballet dancers, *Br J Radiol* 77:532–537, 2004.

176. Paterson RS, Brown JN, Roberts SNJ: The posteromedial impingement lesion of the ankle: A series of six cases, *Am J Sports Med* 29(5):550–557, 2001.

177. Fiorella D, Helms CA, Nunley JAI: The MR imaging features of the posterior intermalleolar ligament in patients with posterior impingement syndrome of the ankle, *Skeletal Radiol* 28:573–576, 1999.

178. Rosenberg ZS, Cheung YY, Beltran J, et al: Posterior intermalleolar ligament of the ankle: Normal anatomy and MR imaging features, *Am J Roentgenol* 165:387–390, 1995.

179. Koulouris G, Connell D, Schneider T, et al: Posterior tibiotalar ligament injury resulting in posteromedial impingement, *Foot Ankle Int* 24(8):575–583, 2003.

180. Hamilton WG: Posterior ankle pain in dancers, *Clin Sports Med* 27(2):263–277, 2008.

181. Ihle CL, Cochran RM: Fracture of the fused os trigonum, *Am J Sports Med* 10(1):47–50, 1982.

182. Labs K, Leutloff D, Perka C: Posterior ankle impingement syndrome in dancers: A short-term follow-up after operative treatment, *Foot Ankle Surg* 8:33–39, 2002.

183. Macquirriain J: Posterior ankle impingement syndrome, *J Am Acad Orthop Surg* 13(6):365–371, 2005.

184. Hamilton WG, Patel MM, Sibel RA: Impingement syndromes of the foot and ankle. In Porter DA, Schon LC, editors: *Baxter's the foot and ankle in sport*, ed 2, Philadelphia, 2008, Mosby.

185. Abramowitz Y, Wollstein R, Barzilay Y, et al: Outcome of resection of a symptomatic os trigonum, *J Bone Joint Surg Am* 85(6):1051–1057, 2003.

186. Kadel NJ: Excision of os trigonum, *Oper Tech Orthop* 14(1):1–5, 2004.

187. O'Donoghue DH: Impingement exostoses of the talus and tibia, *J Bone Joint Surg Am* 39(4):835–852, 1957.

188. Berberian WS, Hecht PJ, Wapner KL, et al: Morphology of tibiotalar osteophytes in anterior ankle impingement, *Foot Ankle Int* 22(4):313–317, 2001.

189. Tol JL, Verheyan CPPM, van Dijk CN: Arthroscopic treatment of anterior impingement in the ankle: A prospective study with a five- to eight-year follow-up, *J Bone Joint Surg Br* 83(1):9–13, 2001.

190. Tol JL, van Dijk CN: Etiology of the anterior ankle impingement syndrome: A descriptive anatomical study, *Foot Ankle Int* 25(6):382–386, 2004.

191. Tol JL, Verhagen RAW, Krips R, et al: The anterior ankle impingement syndrome: Diagnostic value of oblique radiographs, *Foot Ankle Int* 25(2):63–68, 2004.

192. Tol JL, van Dijk CN: Anterior ankle impingement, *Foot Ankle Clin N Am* 11:297–310, 2006.

193. Van Dijk CN: Anterior and posterior ankle impingement, *Foot Ankle Clin N Am* 11:663–683, 2006.

194. Nihal A, Rose DJ, Trepman E: Arthroscopic treatment of anterior ankle impingement syndrome in dancers, *Foot Ankle Int* 26(11):908–912, 2005.

195. Liebler WA: Injuries of the foot in dancers. In Bateman JE, editor: *Foot Science*, Philadelphia, 1976, WB Saunders.

196. Schneider HJ, King AY, Bronson JL, et al: Stress injuries and developmental change of lower extremities in ballet dancers, *Radiology* 113:627–632, 1974.

197. Umans HR: Ankle impingement syndromes, *Semin Musculoskel Radiol* 6(2):133–139, 2002.

198. Umans HR, Cerezal L: Anterior ankle impingement syndromes, *Semin Musculoskel Radiol* 12(2):146–153, 2008.

199. Van Dijk CN, Tol JL, Verheyen CCPM: A prospective study of prognostic factors concerning the outcome of arthroscopic surgery for anterior ankle impingement, *Am J Sports Med* 25(6):737–745, 1997.

200. Sanders TG, Rathur SK: Impingement syndromes of the ankle, *Magn Reson Imaging Clin North Am* 16(1):29–38, 2008.

201. Akseki D, Pinar H, Bozkurt M, et al: The distal fascicle of the anterior inferior tibiofibular ligament as a cause of anterolateral ankle impingement: Results of arthroscopic resection, *Acta Orthop Scand* 70(5):478–482, 1999.

202. Akseki D, Pinar H, Yaldiz K, et al: The anterior inferior tibiofibular ligament and talar impingement: a cadaveric study, *Knee Surg Sports Traumatol Arthrosc* 10:321–326, 2002.

203. Haller J, Bernt R, Seeger T, et al: MR-imaging of anterior tibiotalar impingement syndrome: Agreement, sensitivity and specificity of MR-imaging and indirect MR-arthrography, *Eur J Radiol* 58:450–460, 2006.

204. Van den Bekerom MPJ, Raven EEJ: The distal fascicle of the anterior inferior tibiofibular ligament as a cause of tibiotalar impingement syndrome: A current concepts review, *Knee Surg Sports Traumatol Arthrosc* 15:465–471, 2007.

205. Wolin I, Glassman F, Sideman S, et al: Internal derangement of the talofibular component of the ankle, *Surg Gynecol Obstet* 91(2):193–200, 1950.

206. Ferkel RD, Karzel RP, Del Pizzo W, et al: Arthroscopic treatment of anterolateral impingement of the ankle, *Am J Sports Med* 19(5):440–446, 1991.

207. Cerezal L, Abascal F, Canga A, et al: MR imaging of ankle impingement syndromes, *Am J Roentgenol* 181:551–559, 2003.

208. Kim S-H, Ha K-I: Arthroscopic treatment for impingement of the the anterolateral soft tissues of the ankle, *J Bone Joint Surg Br* 82(7):1019–1021, 2000.

209. Liu SH, Raskin A, Osti L, et al: Arthroscopic treatment of anterolateral ankle impingement, *Arthroscopy* 10(2):215–218, 1994.

210. Meislin RJ, Rose DJ, Parisien S, et al: Arthroscopic treatment of synovial impingement of the ankle, *Am J Sports Med* 21(2):186–189, 1993.

211. Jordan LK, III, Helms CA, Cooperman AE, et al: Magnetic resonance imaging findings in anterolateral impingement of the ankle, *Skeletal Radiol* 29:34–39, 2000.

212. Liu SH, Nuccion SL, Finerman G: Diagnosis of anterolateral ankle impingement: Comparison between magnetic resonance imaging and clinical examination, *Am J Sports Med* 25(3):389–393, 1997.

213. Rubin DA, Tishkoff NW, Britton CA, et al: Anterolateral soft-tissue impingement in the ankle: diagnosis using MR imaging, *Am J Roentgenol* 169:829–835, 1997.

214. Fong DT-P, Hong Y, Chan L-K, et al: A systematic review on ankle injury and ankle sprain in sports, *Sports Med* 37(1):73–94, 2007.

215. Hootman JM, Dick R, Agel J: Epidemiology of collegiate injuries for 15 sports: Summary and recommendations for injury prevention initiatives, *J Athl Train* 42(2):311–319, 2007.

216. Yeung MS, Chan KM, So CH, et al: An epidemiological survey on ankle sprain, *Br J Sports Med* 28(2):112–116, 1994.

217. Sharma P, Maffulli N: Tendon injury and tendinopathy: Healing and repair, *J Bone Joint Surg Am* 87(1):187–202, 2005.

218. Kaeding C, Best TM: Tendinosis: Pathophysiology and nonoperative treatment, *Sports Health* 1(4):284–292, 2009.

219. Kjær M, Langberg H, Heinemeier K, et al: From mechanical loading to collagen synthesis, structural changes and function in human tendon, *Scand J Med Sci Sports* 19(4):500–510, 2009.

220. Hodgkins CW, Kennedy JG, O'Loughlin PF: Tendon injuries in dance, *Clin Sports Med* 27(2):279–288, 2008.

221. Arndt AN, Komi PV, Brüggemann G-P, et al: Individual muscle contributions to the in vivo achilles tendon force, *Clin Biomech* 13:532–541, 1998.

222. Clement DB, Taunton JE, Smart GW: Achilles tendinitis and peritendinitis: Etiology and treatment, *Am J Sports Med* 12(3):179–184, 1984.

223. Miller BF, Hansen M, Olesen JL, et al: Tendon collagen synthesis at rest and after exercise in women, *J Appl Physiol* 102(2):541–546, 2007.

224. Hansen M, Koskinen SO, Petersen SG, et al: Ethinyl oestradiol administration in women suppresses synthesis of collagen in tendon in response to exercise, *J Physiol (Lond)* 586(12):3005–3016, 2008.

225. Hansen M, Miller BF, Holm L, et al: Effect of administration of oral contraceptives in vivo on collagen synthesis in tendon and muscle connective tissue in young women, *J Appl Physiol* 106(4):1435–1443, 2009.

226. Miller BF, Hansen M, Olesen JL, et al: No effect of menstrual cycle on myofibrillar and connective tissue protein synthesis in contracting skeletal muscle, *Am J Physiol Endocrinol Metab* 290(1):E163–168, 2006.

227. Hamilton WG: Tendonitis about the ankle joint in classical ballet dancers, *Am J Sports Med* 5(2):84–88, 1977.

228. Shybut G, Miller C: "Trigger toe" in a ballet dancer, *Med Prob Performing Artists* 20(2):99–102, 2005.

229. Kolettis GJ, Micheli LJ, Klein JD: Release of the flexor hallucis longus tendon in ballet dancers, *J Bone Joint Surg Am* 78(9):1386–1390, 1996.

230. Tamburrini O, Porpiglia H, Barresi D, et al: The role of magnetic resonance imaging in the diagnosis of the os trigonum syndrome, *Radiol Med (Torino)* 98(6):462–467, 1999.

231. Wredmark T, Carlstedt CA, Bauer H, et al: Os trigonum syndrome: A clinical entity in ballet dancers, *Foot Ankle* 11(6):404–406, 1991.

232. Goulart M, O'Malley MJ, Hodgkins CW, et al: Foot and ankle fractures in dancers, *Clin Sports Med* 27(2):295–304, 2008.

233. O'Malley MJ, Hamilton WG, Munyak J: Fractures of the distal shaft of the fifth metatarsal: Dancer's fracture, *Am J Sports Med* 24(2):240–243, 1996.

234. Evans A: "Dancer's fracture" —A clinical perspective, *Australas J Podiatr Med* 32(1):13–19, 1998.

235. Nunley JA: Fractures of the base of the fifth metatarsal: The Jones fracture, *Orthop Clin N Am* 32(1):171–180, 2001.

236. Jones R: Fracture of the base of the fifth metatarsal bone by indirect violence, *Ann Surg* 35(6):697–700.692, 1902.

237. Kadel NJ, Teitz CC, Kronmal RA: Stress fractures in ballet dancers, *Am J Sports Med* 20(4):445–449, 1992.

238. Warden SJ, Burr DB, Brukner PD: Repetitive stress pathology: Bone, In Magee DJ, Zachazewski JE, Quillen WS, editors: *Pathology and intervention in musculoskeletal rehabilitation*, St Louis, 2009, Saunders.

239. Micheli LJ, Sohn RS, Solomon R: Stress fractures of the second metatarsal involving Lisfranc's joint in ballet dancers: A new overuse injury of the foot, *J Bone Joint Surg Am* 67(9):1372–1375, 1985.

240. O'Malley MJ, Hamilton WG, Munyak J, et al: Stress fractures at the base of the second metatarsal in ballet dancers, *Foot Ankle Int* 17(2):89–94, 1996.

241. Muscolo L, Migues A, Slullitel G, et al: Stress fracture nonunion at the base of the second metatarsal in a ballet dancer, *Am J Sports Med* 32(6):1535–1537, 2004.

242. Albisetti W, Perugia D, De Bartolomeo O, et al: Stress fractures of the base of the metatarsal bones in young trainee ballet dancers, *Int Orthop* 34(1):51–55, 2010.

243. Lundon K, Melcher L, Bray K: Stress fractures in ballet: A twenty-five year review, *J Dance Med Sci* 3(3):101–107, 1999.

244. Nussbaum AR, Treves ST, Micheli LJ: Bone stress lesions in ballet dancers: Scintigraphic assessment, *Am J Roentgenol* 150(4):851–855, 1988.

245. Molnar M: Stress fracture of the second metatarsal: A case report, *J Dance Med Sci* 1(1):22–24, 1997.

246. Martinez SF, Murphy GA: Tibial stress fracture in a male ballet dancer: A case report, *Am J Sports Med* 33(1):124–130, 2005.

247. Ambegaonkar JP, Shultz SJ, Schulz MR: Anterior cruciate ligament injury in collegiate female dancers, *Athl Ther Today* 14(4):13–16, 2009.

248. Agel J, Arendt EA, Bershadsky B: Anterior cruciate ligament injury in National Collegiate Athletic Association basketball and soccer: A 13-year review, *Am J Sports Med* 33(4):524–531, 2005.

249. Gwinn DE, Wilckens JH, McDevitt ER, et al: The relative incidence of anterior cruciate ligament injury in men and women at the United States Naval Academy, *Am J Sports Med* 28(1):98–102, 2000.

250. Arendt EA, Agel J, Dick R: Anterior cruciate ligament injury patterns among collegiate men and women, *J Athl Train* 34(2):86–92, 1999.

251. Chappell JD, Creighton RA, Giuliani C, et al: Kinematics and electromyography of landing preparation in vertical stop-jump: Risks for noncontact anterior cruciate ligament injury, *Am J Sports Med* 35(2):235–241, 2007.

252. Orishimo KF, Kremenic IJ, Pappas E, et al: Comparison of landing biomechanics between male and female professional dancers, *Am J Sports Med* 37(11):2187–2193, 2009.

253. Winston P, Awan R, Cassidy JD, et al: Clinical examination and ultrasound of self-reported snapping hip syndrome in elite ballet dancers, *Am J Sports Med* 35(1):118–126, 2007.

254. Wahl CJ, Warren RF, Adler RS, et al: Internal coxa saltans (snapping hip) as a result of overtraining, *Am J Sports Med* 32(5):1302–1309, 2004.

255. Déslandes M, Guillin R, Cardinal É, et al: The snapping iliopsoas tendon: New mechanisms using dynamic sonography, *Am J Roentgenol* 190(3):576–581, 2008.

256. Jacobs M, Young R: Snapping hip phenomenon among dancers, *Am Correct Ther J* 32(3):92–98, 1978.

257. Blankenbaker DG, Tuite MJ: Iliopsoas musculotendinous unit, *Semin Musculoskel Radiol* 12(1):13–27, 2008.

258. Allen WC, Cope R: Coxa saltans: The snapping hip revisited, *J Am Acad Orthop Surg* 3(5):303–308, 1995.

259. Reid DC, Burnham RS, Saboe LA, et al: Lower extremity flexibility patterns in classical ballet dancers and their correlation to lateral hip and knee injuries, *Am J Sports Med* 15(4):347–352, 1987.

260. Da Silva AH, Bonorino KC: BMI and flexibility in ballerinas of contemporary dance and classical ballet, *Fitness Perf J* 7(1):48–51, 2008.

261. Beighton P, Horan F: Orthopaedic aspects of the Ehlers-Danlos syndrome, *J Bone Joint Surg Br* 51(3):444–453, 1969.

262. Klemp P, Stevens JE, Isaacs S: A hypermobility study in ballet dancers, *J Rheumatol* 11(5):692–696, 1984.

263. McCormack M, Briggs J, Hakim A, et al: Joint laxity and the benign joint hypermobility syndrome in student and professional ballet dancers, *J Rheumatol* 31(1):173–178, 2003.

264. Foss KDB, Ford KR, Myer GD, et al: Generalized joint laxity associated with increased medial foot loading in female athletes, *J Athl Train* 44(4):356–362, 2009.

265. Grahame R: Joint hypermobility and genetic collagen disorders: Are they related? *Arch Dis Child* 80(2):188–191, 1999.

266. Mishra MB, Ryan P, Atkinson P, et al: Extra-articular features of benign joint hypermobility syndrome, *Rheumatology (Oxford)* 35(9):861–866, 1996.

267. Klemp P, Chalton D: Articular mobility in ballet dancers: A follow-up study after four years, *Am J Sports Med* 17(1):72–75, 1989.

268. Briggs J, McCormack M, Hakim AJ, et al: Injury and joint hypermobility syndrome in ballet dancers—A 5-year follow-up, *Rheumatology (Oxford)* 48(12):1613–1614, 2009.

269. Andersson S, Nilsson B, Hessel T, et al: Degenerative joint disease in ballet dancers, *Clin Orthop* 238:233–236, 1989.

270. Brodelius Å: Osteoarthrosis of the talar joints in footballers and ballet dancers, *Acta Orthop Scand* 30:309–314, 1961.

271. Teitz CC, Kocoyne RF: Premature osteoarthrosis in professional dancers, *Clin J Sport Med* 8(4):255–259, 1998.

272. Van Dijk CN, Lim LSL, Poortman A, et al: Degenerative joint disease in female ballet dancers, *Am J Sports Med* 23(3):295–300, 1995.

273. Ambré T, Nilsson BE: Degenerative changes in the first metatarso-phalangeal joint of ballet dancers, *Acta Orthop Scand* 49:317–319, 1978.

274. Makhani JS: Lacerations of the lateral ligaments of the ankle, *J Int Coll Surg* 38(5):454–466, 1962.

275. Sarrafian SK: *Anatomy of the foot and ankle: Descriptive, topographic, functional,* ed 2, Philadelphia, 1993, JB Lippincott Company.

276. Stiehl JB: Biomechanics of the ankle joint. In Stiehl JB, editor, *Inman's joints of the ankle,* ed 2, Baltimore, 1991, Williams and Wilkins.

277. Logan BM, Singh D, Hutchings RT: *McMinn's color atlas of foot and ankle anatomy,* ed 3, Philadelphia, 2004, Mosby.

278. Christman RA: The normal foot and ankle. In Christman RA, editor: *Foot and ankle radiology,* St Louis, 2003, Churchill Livingstone.

279. Garrick JG: Early identification of musculoskeletal complaints and injuries among female ballet students, *J Dance Med Sci* 3(2):80–83, 1999.

280. Thomas H, Tarr J: Dancers' perceptions of pain and injury: Positive and negative effects, *J Dance Med Sci* 13(2):51–59, 2009.

281. Bennell KL, Khan KM, Matthews B, et al: Hip and ankle range of motion and hip muscle strength in young novice female ballet dancers and controls, *Br J Sports Med* 33:340–346, 1999.

282. Bennell KL, Khan KM, Matthews BL, et al: Changes in hip and ankle range of motion and hip muscle strength in 8-11 year old novice female ballet dancers and controls: A 12 month follow up study, *Br J Sports Med* 35:54–59, 2001.

283. Khan K, Roberts P, Nattrass C, et al: Hip and ankle range of motion in elite classical ballet dancers and controls, *Clin J Sport Med* 7(3):174–179, 1997.

284. Lin C-F, Su F-C, Wu H-W: Ankle biomechanics of ballet dancers in relevé en pointé dance, *Res Sports Med* 13:23–35, 2005.

285. Novella TM: An easy way to quantify plantarflexion in the ankle, *J Back Musculoskel Rehabil* 5:191–199, 1995.

The Athlete with Disability

Duane G. Messner

Introduction

Twenty to thirty years ago, on any given afternoon, a local charity organization would host a track meet for the "handicapped" at which an indiscriminate number of events would be offered. Participants would often compete in their street clothes and everyday wheelchairs, prostheses, or braces. Many competitors had never practiced or even attempted some of the events before the day of competition. However, everyone would have a day of fun and excitement.

Today, for the accomplished athlete with a disability, athletics is a world of aerodynamic wheelchairs and high-tech equipment costing thousands of dollars; scientific performance analysis; and year-round training for regional, national, and international competitions. The grassroots infrastructure of disabled athletics is still firmly in place, with charity groups, public schools, and local disabled sports organizations (DSOs) hosting improved, structured weekend competitions for novice- and intermediate-level competitors. In addition, the potential vertical growth of competition has flourished within disabled athletics for gifted and serious competitors.

During the past 30 years, disabled athletics has matured into a finely structured group of organizations dedicated to providing athletes of all disabilities with an equitable playing field for competition, while allowing individual athletes the opportunity to rise through the ranks of competition, depending on their athletic ability. Thanks to the relentless efforts of a persistent few, disabled competitors

Note: This chapter includes content from previous contributions by Kathleen A. Curtis, PhD, PT, and Robert S. Gailey Jr., MSEd, PT, as it appeared in the predecessor of this book—Zachazewski JE, Magee DJ, Quillen WS, editors: *Athletic injuries and rehabilitation*, Philadelphia, 1996, WB Saunders.

are beginning to enjoy the satisfaction of training, competing, and receiving the recognition so richly deserved yet frequently bestowed only on able-bodied athletes. Only recently have a few disabled athletes found themselves featured in the sports section of newspapers, magazines, and television. Unfortunately, the majority of the media still regards these talented athletes as "human interest" stories. This chapter provides a comprehensive overview of the complexities and challenges of disabled athletics, focusing on the enlightenment of rehabilitation providers as possible advocates in a variety of capacities. Most importantly, knowledgeable rehabilitation professionals can identify future disabled athletes and educate other professionals about the world of disabled athletics and the benefits for those who choose to get involved.

Organizational Structure of Disabled Athletic Events

The organizational structure of disabled athletic events appears complex to newcomers to disabled athletics. In most instances, the basic structure follows the same format used for able-bodied amateur athletics, with one exception. Because most DSOs arose to meet the needs of athletes with similar disabilities, disabled athletics has historically been governed by "disability-specific" organizations as opposed to "sport-specific" organizations as in able-bodied sports. For example, each of the eight DSOs offers track and field to its athletes; therefore, eight governing bodies exist for rules, competitions, and medal criteria (Table 28-1).[1] In contrast, in able-bodied sports in the United States, all track and field is governed by the national governing body (NGB), Track and Field USA.

Currently, many philosophic and structural changes are occurring at all levels of disabled athletics. Some sports are moving toward becoming entirely sport-specific with regard to organizational structure, whereas other more complex

Table 28-1

Competitive Sports and Recreation Activities Offered by US Disabled Sports Organizations

Sport	AAAD	DAAA	DSUSA	WSUSA	USABA	USCPAA	USLASA	SOI
Alpine skiing	X		X		X			X
Archery			X	X		X		
Basketball	X	X	X					X
Bocce						X	X	
Bowling	X					X		X
Canoeing			X					X
Cross country	X					X		X
Cycling	X		X		X	X		X
Diving	X							X
Equestrian						X		X
Figure skating								X
Floor hockey								X
Goal ball					X			
Gymnastics					X			X
Handball	X							
Ice hockey	X							
Judo					X			
Nordic skiing	X		X		X			X
Poly hockey								X
Powerlifting		X	X	X	X	X	X	X
Racquetball			X					
Road racing	X		X	X				X
Roller skating								X
Shooting	X	X	X	X		X	X	
Slalom				X		X	X	X
Soccer	X					X		X
Softball	X	X						X
Speed skating	X				X			X
Swimming	X	X	X	X	X	X	X	X
Table tennis	X	X	X	X		X	X	X
Team handball						X	X	X
Tennis	X		X	X				X
Track and field	X	X	X	X	X	X	X	X
Volleyball	X		X					X
Weight lifting			X	X				
Wrestling	X				X			

From Curtis KA, Gailey RS Jr: The athlete with a disability. Adapted from Paciorek MJ, Jones JA: Sports and recreation for the disabled: A resource manual, Indianapolis, 1989, Benchmark Press.

AAAD, American Athletic Association of the Deaf; *DAAA*, Dwarf Athletic Association of America; *DSUSA*, Disabled Sports USA (amputees); *SOI*, Special Olympics International (developmentally disabled); *USABA*, United States Association of Blind Athletes; *USCPAA*, United States Cerebral Palsy Athletic Association; *USLASA*, United States Les Autres Sports Association (other disabilities); *WSUSA*, Wheelchair Sports USA.

sports are weighing the advantages and disadvantages of such a change. The evolution of disabled sports has been rapid and appears to be gaining momentum. The organizational structure presented in this text will change to some degree in the future, as will some of the organizations' names, but the basic format will probably remain the same.

The International Olympic Committee (IOC) presides over all international Olympic-sanctioned sporting events and governing bodies. The parallel organization for the disabled is the International Paralympic Committee (IPC). The IPC's primary responsibility is to sanction disabled sporting events and act as a coordinating committee among the host city of the Paralympic Games and the six international DSOs (IDSOs), which are the Comite International des Sports des Soudes, Cerebral Palsy International Sports and Recreational Association, International Blind Sport Association, International Stoke-Mandeville Wheelchair

Sports Federation, International Sports Organization for the Disabled, and International Sport Federation for Persons with Mental Handicaps. Representation to the IDSOs is granted to DSOs from all countries that meet the criteria for membership. The IDSOs process information from participating countries and communicate directly to the IPC or the hosting Paralympic Games city. Policy and international rules for competition are governed by the IDSOs (Figure 28-1). The IOC works with member countries, which are represented by their individual national organizing committees (NOCs) and international sports federations. The United States Olympic Committee (USOC) is the NOC for the United States and is the coordinating body for amateur sports, with the primary purpose of preparing Olympic and Pan American Games teams. The five membership categories within the USOC are group A, Olympic/Pan American sports organizations, which includes the 42 NGBs for each sport; group B, community-based multisport organizations, armed forces, and education-based multisport organizations; group C, affiliated sport organizations; group D, state Olympic organizations; and group E, organizations of sport for the disabled (Figure 28-2).

The Committee on Sports for the Disabled currently recognizes six DSOs: American Athletic Association for the Deaf, Dwarf Athletic Association of America, United States Cerebral Palsy Athletic Association, United States Association for Blind Athletes, Wheelchair Sports USA (WSUSA), and Disabled Sports USA. The United States Les Autres Sports Association is currently not recognized by the USOC, but the organization contributes significantly to the disabled sports movement. Each of the US DSOs has representation to its respective international DSO as a voting member.

Classification of Athletes with Disabilities

Classification systems have existed almost as long as sports for persons with disabilities. The systems are intended to provide a means to ensure equitable competition, in which ability and skills, not degree of physical disability, are the variables among competitors. Accordingly, athletes of similar levels of disability are grouped together in a "class" designated for competition. Individuals in the same class compete against each other in individual sports, such as track and field or swimming. In team sports, athletes in various classes are allowed to compete as a team only in prescribed combinations, which serve to ensure that the most severely disabled players will not be excluded from the sport.

Classification Systems

Classification systems in disabled sports provide equitable competition when ability and skills are the variables for competition.

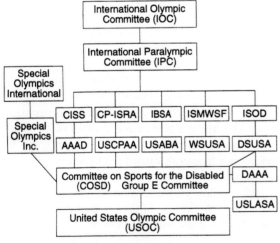

Figure 28-1
Organizational Chart for the International Sports Organizations. *AAAD,* American Athletic Association for the Deaf; *CISS,* Comité International des Sports des Soudes; *CP-ISRA,* Cerebral Palsy International Sports and Recreational Association; *DAAA,* Dwarf Athletic Association of America; *DSUSA,* Disabled Sports USA; *IBSA,* International Blind Sport Association; *IOC,* International Olympic Committee; *IPC,* International Paralympic Committee; *ISMWSF,* International Stoke-Mandeville Wheelchair Sports Federation; *ISOD,* International Sports Organization for the Disabled; *USABA,* United States Association for Blind Athletes; *USCPAA,* United States Cerebral Palsy Athletic Association; *USLASA,* United States Les Autres Sports Association; *WSUSA,* Wheelchair Sports USA. (From Curtis KA, Gailey RS Jr: The athlete with a disability. Adapted from Paciorek MJ, Jones JA: *Sports and recreation for the disabled: A resource manual,* Indianapolis, 1989, Benchmark Press.)

Traditionally, athlete classification was primarily a medical decision, based on the results of a physical examination of such criteria as neurological function, degree of visual deficit, or length of residual limbs. There were inherent problems in both the intent and the implementation of such systems. These systems classified athletes within a disability group for all sports in which they competed, regardless of the relative advantage of having certain functions for a particular sport. For example, a sport such as wheelchair racing requires considerably less trunk rotation for performance than a sport such as wheelchair basketball. In addition, the divisions between classes were arbitrary and did not reflect parallel increments in performance across all sports. Furthermore, it became apparent that as DSOs such as WSUSA tried to mix athletes with different disabilities in a classification system designed for spinal cord–injured athletes, the system clearly favored certain athletes. Weiss and Curtis[2] studied the distribution of disabilities across finalists in each class of competition at a national WSUSA multisport championship. They found that a disproportionate number of finalists were athletes with postpolio paralysis and athletes with amputations compared with the number of athletes with paraplegia and spina bifida in the organization. Athletes with cerebral palsy were also under-represented in the finalist groups.

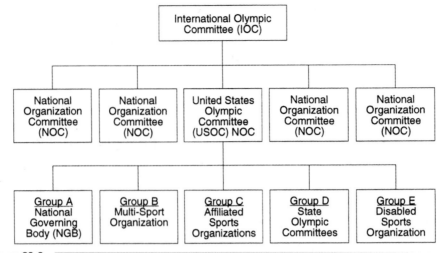

Figure 28-2
Organizational chart for the National Organization Committees. The United States Olympic Committee coordinates the five organizations identified and reports to the International Olympic Committee.

For some of these reasons, athletes within a DSO were prevented from competing against athletes from other DSOs, as each DSO developed separate meets for its national championships. At the world championship events, at which multiple DSOs represented various countries, amputees competing in wheelchairs had a different competition from paraplegics in wheelchairs for each distance of a track meet. In the 1988 Seoul Paralympics, this division by classification and by disability group resulted in more than 40 different 100-meter races being run. This was confusing and nonproductive for meet organizers, athletes, and spectators.

Dissatisfaction with classification systems has been the norm, rather than the exception, throughout the history of sports for the disabled. In the mid-1980s, Horst Strohkendl developed the first classification system that was based on observation of an athlete's function during actual wheelchair basketball competition rather than the athlete's neurological level.[3] Other sports have followed, in an effort to consolidate athletes by classification in their sports rather than by their disabilities. Sport-specific functional classification systems have now been developed for track and field, swimming, table tennis, and shooting.[4] For example, between the 1988 and 1992 Paralympics, a 10-class function classification system for swimming was implemented. This system combines cerebral palsy, amputee, and wheelchair athletes who would have competed in 25 classes in the 1992 Paralympic Games. The 10-class system is intended to reduce the time and organizational effort required to hold the competition. Despite the benefits of simplifying an athletic event, Richter and colleagues[5] argue that this system lacks reliability and validity by integrating disability groups and applying arbitrary criteria that disadvantage certain disability groups. Classification systems are currently in flux and are expected to evolve further as a result of the experiences in sport-specific functional classification. Performance and degree of disability do not always show a

direct relationship. In 2009, the International Paralympic Committee issued a position statement mandating the development of evidence-based classification systems related to health and functioning as advocated by the International Classification of Functioning, Disability and Health (ICF), and the use of selective sport classification.[6] To describe each classification system currently used goes beyond the scope of this chapter. Table 28-2 summarizes the various systems used in some competitive sports.

Rehabilitation professionals and physicians have traditionally been involved as classifiers in most DSOs, because traditional classification involved physical examination and disability assessment. These traditional observations still play a part in some functional classification systems, but more important now is the observation of athletic performance in the sport. Thus the role of the classifier in the era of functional classification is to observe performance in sports competition. Classification is frequently carried out by a team of classifiers, including medical personnel, sports technical experts, athletes, and coaches. Physical therapists are particularly well suited for this role because of their strengths in the observation of normal and abnormal movement.

Clinical Point

An ability of the classifier to observe movement carefully during functional performance is critical to the classification process.

Technical Assessment

Traditionally, a coach is responsible for the training of an athlete, and the medical team plays a supportive role, responding to injuries or implementing injury prevention programs.

Table 28-2

Classification Systems for Athletes with Disabilities

Organization	Sport	Classification System
DAAA, DSUSA, WSUSA, USABA, USABA, USCPAA, USLASA	Alpine skiing	10 classifications, based on type of ski equipment used
DSUSA, WSUSA, USLASA	Basketball (wheelchair)	3-class US system based on neurological function; 4-class international system based on functional trunk movement in wheelchair; combined classification points of players on court limited by rules
DSUSA	Cycling	3-class system, based on limb involvement
DAAA, DSUSA, WSUSA, USABA, USLASA	Powerlifting	Competition by weight classes
DAAA, DSUSA, WSUSA, USLASA	Swimming	10-class integrated system, with different classification for breast-stroke, backstroke, and freestyle
DSUSA, USLASA	Table tennis (standing)	5-class system for standing athletes
DSUSA, WSUSA, USLASA	Table tennis (wheelchair)	5 seated classes based on upper extremity and trunk function
DSUSA	Track and field (amputees, standing)*	9-class system based on upper- vs. lower-extremity involvement and level of amputation
DSUSA, WSUSA, USLASA	Track and field (wheelchair)	4 classes for track events; 7 seated classes for field events; 1 standing class for field events
DSUSA, USLASA	Volleyball (sitting)	All players must sit
DSUSA	Volleyball (standing)	8-class system; uses combined classification points of players on court
AAAD	All sports for AAAD	Must have hearing loss greater than 55 db in best ear
DAAA	All sports for DAAA	Eligibility based on height less than 5'0"
USABA	All sports for USABA†	3-class system, based on visual field and acuity
USCPAA	All sports for USCPAA‡	8-class system, based on level of function of extremities and ambulatory status
USLASA	All sports for USLASA§	6-class system, based on extremity and trunk function in sitting and standing competition
SOI	All	Participants compete in classes by age, gender, and ability level

AAAD, American Athletic Association of the Deaf; *DAAA,* Dwarf Athletic Association of America; *DSUSA,* Disabled Sports USA (amputees); *SOI,* Special Olympics International (developmentally disabled); *USABA,* United States Association of Blind Athletes; *USCPAA,* United States Cerebral Palsy Athletic Association; *USLASA,* United States Les Autres Sports Association (other disabilities); *WSUSA,* Wheelchair Sports USA.
*Bilateral above-knee amputees can compete in a wheelchair or standing.
†In cycling, athletes ride tandem.
‡In international swimming competition, an integrated system is used.
§Most athletes compete under specific functional classifications for wheelchair or ambulatory athletes.

Disabled athletes present a unique situation in which a growing number of therapists and other medical professionals have become involved in the training process. One reason for their involvement is that the coaching process of a disabled athlete must include some knowledge in the following areas: sport performance (the actual biomechanics of the event), pathology, kinesiology, pathokinesiology, adaptive physiology, prosthetics or orthotics, and motivational psychology. The criteria for coaching the disabled athlete go well beyond those required to coach an able-bodied athlete, in terms of assessing physical and technical methods for performance enhancement.

Areas to Consider When Performing Movement Analysis for Disabled Athletes

- Physiological laws related to the neuromuscular and musculoskeletal systems
- Mechanical laws based on Newton's Laws of Motion
- Physical environmental and external conditions
- Movements before and after the desired skill
- Mechanical efficiency of adaptive equipment
- Identify performance enhancement methods

Two approaches to the analysis of biomechanical events may be employed to study human movement. The first is the quantitative approach, which applies numerical values to describe all movements. This method is the most explicit, but it is complex, expensive, time consuming, and, for the average athlete, unnecessary. In contrast, the qualitative approach describes movement in non-numerical terms using observation, qualitative data, and applied physical principles as the foundation for interpretations made by the observer. Qualitative analysis is more easily employed than quantitative analysis. Qualitative analysis can be performed simply by general observation, memory of a performance, or use of videotape. Obviously, videotaped recordings provide a more accurate account of the movement being analyzed and can be reviewed to verify the impressions of the observer.[7]

The disability of the athlete adds another factor to the equation when attempting to enhance athletic performance and prevent injury. Each athlete presents with some form of biomechanical restriction: either a physical limitation, such as increased tone, weakened muscles, loss of range of motion, or vision loss, or the need for an additional mechanical device such as a wheelchair or prosthesis. A systematic assessment of each component of the athlete's sport must be made, as with able-bodied athletes, yet the therapist or coach must now take into consideration how each component of the skill being learned can be mastered by either physical or mechanical compensation. This is the challenge put before all those who work with disabled athletes, and that is what makes this work so exciting and gratifying.

Regardless of the approach—quantitative, qualitative, or a combination of the two—movement analysis must be performed in a systematic manner. The following is provided to give some insight into the performance enhancement process and the role that the medical professional can play.

Define the Movement or Skill to Be Analyzed

Before any analysis of movement can begin, the specific movement or skill to be analyzed must be defined. The more specifically the movement is defined, the greater the chance of success. For example, if a track sprinter is being analyzed, the first question that would have to be asked is what part of the sprint requires analysis? The start, mid-distance, or finish? Once the phase of the sprint has been determined, a host of sprinter components would have to be identified and assessed for that phase (Figure 28-3).

Identify the Biomechanical Principles That Govern the Desired Movement or Skill

Once the component parts of the sprint have been identified, the mechanical effects throughout the kinetic chain of the sprinter's body must be examined to determine the effect one body segment has on another. The mechanical effects can be the result of either internal or external influence. This

process can be either complex or general. In many cases, an educated coach can visually observe the majority of biomechanical constraints that may hinder an athlete's performance. Often an in-depth quantitative analysis only confirms what the coach has observed. The following is a brief outline suggesting the major topic areas that should be considered when performing a movement analysis:

The Physiological Laws That Relate to the Neuromuscular and Musculoskeletal Systems

The athlete's body size and weight, strength, range of motion, muscular tone, limb length, sensation, balance, coordination, agility, vision, hearing, endurance, and other physiological considerations that may be inherent to the type of disability or to the athlete's current physical condition must be analyzed. For example, athletes with quadriplegia or paraplegia are able to maximize their performance using different wheelchair strokes and trunk position as a result of the level of disability and the motor function available. Likewise, many swimmers with various disabilities find the backstroke to be faster for them than the crawl stroke and therefore choose the backstroke when competing in freestyle events.

The Mechanical Laws Based on Newton's Laws of Motion

The effects of physical laws such as gravity, friction, inertia, and momentum should be examined, especially as they relate to any physical compensation by an athlete. Likewise, mechanical advantages and disadvantages with regard to adaptive devices should be explored to determine the best modification for a particular athlete participating in a specific sport. Disabled athletics has been the catalyst for numerous technical advances as a result of modifications developed by athletes.

The Physical Environment and External Conditions

The playing surface (e.g., concrete, grass, wood, or synthetic surface) can have a tremendous effect on an athlete's performance. For example, a wheelchair racer may vary tire pressure with different track surfaces such as asphalt or a synthetic material. Every athlete must make important decisions based on environmental and external conditions. Another example would be a blind sprinter having the option of a sighted guide or a caller who provides auditory instruction to keep the athlete on line. In a noisy stadium, a caller may not be possible or too confusing, and a sighted guide would be mandatory.

The Movements Immediately Preceding or Following the Desired Skill

As with any movement skill, all the components of that skill build on each other and have a direct cause and effect. For example, all throwing performances depend on the windup, acceleration, release, and deceleration or follow-through phases. No one phase acts independently of the others.

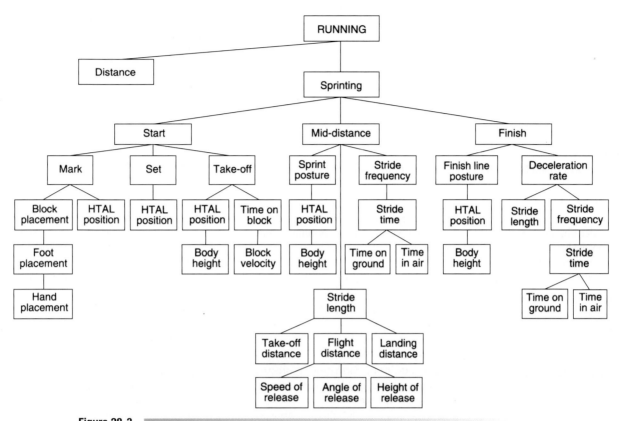

Figure 28-3

A model of the components of sprinting, divided into three phases: start, mid-distance, and finish. *HTAL*, Head, trunk, arm, and leg. (From Curtis KA, Gailey RS Jr: The athlete with a disability. Courtesy of Advanced Rehabilitation Therapy, Inc., Miami, FL.)

Therefore, if a cerebral palsy athlete has increased tone in the throwing arm (or anywhere throughout the body), one if not all of the throwing phases may be affected to some degree. As a result, alternative solutions that promote motion away from the limitations may enhance a throwing performance. Throwing the implement backward over the shoulder or sideways over the head may help increase the arc of motion during the acceleration or deceleration phase.

The Mechanical Efficiency of Adaptive Equipment

Once all the aspects of movement analysis have been completed, the evaluation team must ask how an adaptive device can provide a mechanical advantage to overcome a given limitation. Historically, the majority of innovative adaptive devices for disabled athletics have arisen through the efforts of disabled athletes themselves. One of the most significant advances in recent years has benefited lower-extremity amputees. Prosthetic designs have been developed to maximize athletic performance rather than just to facilitate walking. Contemporary socket designs take muscular efficiency into account, prosthetic knees meet the superior cadence demands placed on them, and newer foot materials and configurations optimize athletic performance. The same can be said about wheelchairs, orthotic devices, and other adaptive innovations that have been

introduced in recent years. Despite these achievements, there is still considerable room for improvement in this area.

Identify Performance-Enhancement Methods

Finally, after each of the component skills has been identified and the athlete's current level of performance has been evaluated, a program designed to improve the performance must be outlined. For a disabled athlete, training, equipment, and motivation are paramount when designing a strategy to prepare for competition. Performance enhancement in itself is a major topic of discussion. The following is a brief overview of some considerations for planning a training program for a disabled athlete:

Training Methods

Today there are as many different training programs for athletes as there are successful athletes who would like to share their secret to success. Many of these training methods are sound and well worth taking under advisement. Coaches and medical professionals must consider the nature of the athlete's disability and what, if any, limitations must be placed on the athlete to prevent injury or unnecessary medical complications. Although few disabled athletes have activity restrictions, there are many athletes who will benefit from preventive measures when participating in sports or training as outlined in Table 28-3.

Once any precautions are identified, the disabled athlete must begin a physical training program comparable to that of any able-bodied athlete. Similar training principles apply when selecting a strengthening, endurance, agility, speed, or any other type of program. Often a brief biomechanical analysis must be performed when creating a training program. If the athlete cannot use a traditional weight-training apparatus because of physical limitations, such as an inability to use the hands to grip, alternative methods, such as securing the

Table 28-3
Injuries and Disability-Specific Medical Conditions of Athletes with Disabilities

Problem	Prevention	Treatment
Chronic overuse syndromes (shoulder impingement, tendonitis, bursitis, carpal tunnel syndrome)	Taping, splinting, protective padding, proper wheelchair positioning, good technique	Rest; apply injury-specific principles of care; selective strengthening, muscle balancing, flexibility; analysis of technique
Overexertion (muscle strains)	Warm-up and stretching; proper conditioning and equipment	Rest; gradual progression of exercise program
Falls, physical contact (sprains, contusions)	Equipment safety; appropriate padding for sport; appropriate sport-specific spotting; qualified assistance/guides for athletes	Apply injury-specific principles of care; check for signs of fracture in athletes without movement or sensation
Blisters	Encourage callus formation; protective taping, gloves, padding, cushioning; adequate clothing	Apply injury-specific principles of care; be aware of areas that lack sensation; make prosthetic adjustments
Abrasions/lacerations	Check equipment for sharp or abrasive surfaces; wear protective clothing; use cushions or towels in all transfers; use mats on hard surfaces; camber wheelchair wheels	Apply injury-specific principles of care; be aware of areas that lack sensation
Decubitus ulcers and burns	Adequate cushioning; proper weight shifting; dry clothing; special precautions for areas without sensation; skin inspection; good nutrition and hygiene	Bed rest if necessary to remove all pressure from a weight-bearing surface; open wound care as necessary; check equipment
Hyperthermia	Minimize exposure to direct sun; provide shade; wear adequate clothing for insulation and maintain hydration; spray externally with water; avoid hot and humid conditions	Remove from ambient conditions; cool immediately; seek medical assistance
Hypothermia	Minimize exposure; wear adequate clothing, keeping head covered; maintain hydration; avoid exposure to cold and wet conditions	Cover and seek medical assistance
Autonomic dysreflexia	Encourage regular bowel and bladder habits in competitive situations	Lift to sitting position; search for source of stimulus, usually full bladder or bowel; attempt to relieve condition; this is a medical emergency
Orthostatic hypotension	Wear elastic stockings or corset supports; avoid heat	Recline in wheelchair or on ground/bed; encourage deep breathing
Seizures	Avoid stress, dehydration, extremes of temperatures, and fatigue	Protect head and keep airway open by jaw thrust; avoid putting objects in the mouth
Unexplained fever (often urinary tract infections)	Drink fluids; practice good hygiene for self-catheterization	Seek medical treatment
Allergies (bee sting, drug)	Notify medical personnel at competition site of potential problem; be prepared	Seek medical treatment
Eye injuries	Protective eyewear, goggles, safety glasses	Apply injury-specific principles of care

hand to the handle, may have to be employed. If environmental conditions such as poor weather prohibit a wheelchair athlete from performing the necessary road work for cardiovascular endurance, a roller trainer may be used. In short, the problem-solving process must continue with training as it does with competition, placing as few limitations on the athlete as possible.

Considerations for Planning a Training Program for Disabled Athletes

- Training method
- Equipment enhancement

Equipment Enhancement

As previously discussed, sport- and disability-specific adaptive equipment can enhance an athlete's performance in a number of ways. The selection and development of adaptive equipment for an individual athlete should be a collective decision, including the athlete, coach, therapist, orthotist, prosthetist, or equipment manufacturer.

Motivation

The motivation of a disabled athlete is no different from the motivation of an able-bodied athlete. As with all athletes, the intrinsic desires that compel an individual to succeed may vary, but the positive methods of motivation available to coaches remain the same. A discussion of the various motivational techniques that may be employed is beyond the scope of this chapter. Supportive personnel must develop a working relationship, and each must learn how to maintain the quest to strive for mutual goals and continued success. It is important to keep in mind that success is not always defined by winning.

Psychosocial Considerations

Sports involvement has been reported to have positive effects on the physical conditioning and self-image of adults with disabilities.[8] In fact, elite wheelchair athletes have psychological profiles that are similar to those of elite able-bodied athletes.[9] An athlete with a disability is likely to present similar challenges to medical professionals as an able-bodied athlete, with a few exceptions.

Depending on the age at the onset of the disability and the time since its onset, an athlete with a disability may still be actively engaged in the various stages of the coping process, such as denial, anger, or depression. Frustrations encountered in athletic competition or following an athletic injury may compound already existing feelings of loss or anger. An individual's ability to cope with outside stresses may vary widely, depending on the nature of the disability and the person's internal resources and social support

system. However, there is considerable evidence in the literature to support the premise that sports involvement among adults with disabilities promotes improved self-concepts and psychological well-being.[10]

Clinical Point

It is very important to assess the individual athlete's goals and pre-injury performance level and design realistic programs accordingly whether he or she is an able bodied or disabled athlete.

In addition, it is important to remember that disabled individuals may have different experiences with the health care system than their able-bodied counterparts. Their access to the health care system has traditionally been through rehabilitation medicine rather than sports medicine. The goals of the health professionals who treat these patients may vary from merely returning these individuals to an everyday level of performance to returning them to an elite athletic level.

Clinical Point

Injured disabled athletes should be seen as athletes with injuries who also happen to have permanent disabilities rather than disabled persons with injuries.

Some athletes with disabilities self-treat serious injuries rather than seeking medical assistance.[11,12] This may result in reinjury and the progression to chronic disability. Their training programs may also lack sufficient attention to flexibility and conditioning.[13] The sports rehabilitation team's ability to intervene and prevent chronic soft tissue changes, which increase further risk of injury, is of critical importance.

The active socialization and actual physical activity involved with sports participation may provide benefits for an individual with a disability. Active individuals with disabilities have been reported to have fewer problems with body image, a higher degree of physical function, and fewer medical complications than members of the inactive disabled population.[8,14,15]

It is also important to look at the skills developed through athletic participation. Athletics is an acceptable way to reintegrate with the community. Through athletic participation, there is a de-emphasis on the disability and a focus on goal-oriented objectives and resources. Athletic participation encourages the development of networking skills and interpersonal relationships that may be useful in work settings as well. An individual who participates in athletics becomes less dependent on society and makes more contributions to society. Athletes are motivated to raise funds for equipment and travel and are responsible for themselves during travel. This discipline often carries over to educational and employment endeavors.[16]

Like their able-bodied counterparts, some individuals with disabilities who participate in sports have substance abuse problems with alcohol or drugs. Many athletes with spinal cord injuries were initially injured in an alcohol- or drug-related incident.[17] Sports medicine professionals who work with athletes with disabilities need to be aware of the signs and symptoms of substance abuse and know the appropriate referrals to make.

Another segment of the population of athletes with disabilities has various cognitive and sensory disorders. Athletes who have sustained brain injuries sometimes exhibit behavior that is difficult to understand. Any athlete who becomes combative, abusive, or a danger to himself or herself or to other athletes should be removed to an area where he or she can refocus and calm down, away from any overstimulation that might add to the problem. Athletes who are unable to communicate verbally may use sign language or communication boards. Although not all athletes with disabilities are able to understand instructions, health professionals should not address a companion or coach instead of the athlete.

Common Injuries and Disability-Specific Medical Problems of Athletes with Disabilities

Preventive practices for disabled athletes are becoming a growing concern among coaches and medical staff alike. Coaches and athletes must be educated in proper warmup techniques, including stretching, elevating core body temperature, and sport-specific drills. Moreover, all athletes should be required to wear or use the recommended safety gear for every sport. Coaches and event organizers should also be obligated to provide certified or skilled spotters, sighted guides, or assistive personnel to ensure every athlete's safety during competition.

The health professional providing care to athletes with disabilities needs to be aware of common injuries and conditions that are inherent to certain disability groups. Table 28-3 provides information concerning prevention and treatment of common injuries and medical problems of athletes with disabilities. Table 28-4 presents the type and frequency of commonly reported injuries sustained by wheelchair athletes.

Table 28-4
Common Injuries of Wheelchair Athletes

	128 Adult Athletes, All Sports[11] (% of 291 Reported Injuries)	90 Adult Athletes, All Sports[18] (% of 346 Reported Injuries)	69 Pediatric Track Athletes[29] (% of Athletes Reporting)	19 Elite Adult Athletes[12] (% of 50 Reported Injuries)
Soft tissue injuries	33	32	34	52
Blisters	18	25	77	6
Lacerations/abrasions	17	27	38	24
Decubitus/pressure areas	7	3	14	Not reported
Arthritis/joint inflammation	5	1.5	Not reported	Not reported
Fractures	5	2	6	6
Head weakness/ numbness	5	Not reported	Not reported	Not reported
Bruises/contusions	Not reported	8	41	10
Temperature regulation disorders	3	Not reported	49	Not reported
Head injury/ concussion	2	2	Not reported	Not reported
Dental injury	1	1	Not reported	Not reported
Dislocation	Not reported	< 1	Not reported	Not reported
Eye injury	Not reported	< 1	Not reported	Not reported
Wheel burns	Included with lacerations	Not reported	71	Not reported
Other illness	Not reported	Not reported	Not reported	2

Injuries to Athletes Who Compete in Wheelchairs

Athletes with disabilities experience athletic injuries related to the specific risks and demands of their sport. Track, road racing, and wheelchair basketball are among the highest-risk sports for athletes who compete in wheelchairs.[11,18] Athletes who train more hours per week and for a longer period generally report more injuries than those who have a short-duration and less-intense training history.[11]

The most common injuries to athletes competing in wheelchairs are soft tissue injuries of the shoulder, elbow, and wrist; abrasions and contusions of the arms and hands; and blisters of the hands.[11,12] In addition, the spinal cord–injured population may experience some unique problems, including skin ulceration, temperature regulation disorders, and delayed recognition of injuries in areas that lack sensation.

Soft Tissue Injuries of Upper Extremities

Both novice and veteran wheelchair athletes experience chronic soft tissue problems of the upper extremities. Wheelchair basketball players often practice and play in excess of 15 to 20 hours per week during the basketball season. Elite road racers frequently have training schedules that entail total distances in excess of 100 miles per week. Propelling a wheelchair such distances requires specific repetitive upper extremity motion and therefore stresses the shoulder, elbow, and wrist joints. Rotator cuff injuries, bicipital tendinitis, shoulder impingement syndromes, lateral epicondylitis (tennis elbow), radial extensor muscle tendinitis, and carpal tunnel syndrome are common problems in wheelchair users.[11,19-23] The excessive forces imposed by weightbearing and continuous shoulder use are implicated in the development of chronic shoulder problems. Bayley and colleagues[24] reported shoulder intra-articular pressures to be 2.5 times greater than arterial pressure during wheelchair transfers. Impingement positioning is also frequent in this population, which must frequently engage in overhead activity, even to carry out daily activities.[25] Surgical decompression via acromioplasty has been reported to be effective in relieving chronic shoulder pain.[26,27] In addition to chronic soft tissue problems, osteonecrosis of the shoulder has been reported in wheelchair users.[28]

Poor flexibility may be a predisposing factor to the development of chronic shoulder problems. Wheelchair pushing stresses development of the chest, anterior shoulder, triceps, and biceps muscles. Specific stretching must be done before and after activity to emphasize flexibility in shoulder flexion, extension, horizontal abduction, and external rotation and to achieve full length of the triceps and biceps muscles, because they are two-joint muscles.

Strength training should emphasize achieving balance at the shoulder, specifically strengthening of the posterior shoulder, including the posterior deltoid, latissimus dorsi, external rotators, rhomboids, and middle and lower trapezius muscles. Many chronic soft tissue injuries can be prevented and managed by achieving such balance.

Athletes with chronic soft tissue problems of the shoulders or elbows may benefit from preventive use of ice after training. Preventive taping may also be useful with hand, wrist, and elbow problems. The well-known principles of rest, ice, compression, and elevation (RICE) apply to injuries sustained by athletes who compete in wheelchairs. The use of anti-inflammatory medications is also of value in assisting athletes with acute or chronic soft tissue problems. Stretching and strengthening are essential to prevent reinjury.

Abrasions and Contusions

When athletes use equipment such as wheelchairs, they are also at risk for accidental injury from incidental contact with the wheelchair parts.[11,29] For example, athletes frequently report friction burns of the inner arms from accidental contact with the large tires during the downstroke in pushing a racing wheelchair. Beginning athletes who are not using equipment that is specific for sports may attempt to train in wheelchairs with wheelchair brakes that are placed dangerously close to the wheelchair push rim. Traumatic injuries of the thumb can easily result from a slip forward during high-intensity pushing.

Simple preventive measures include protecting the upper arm from accidental contact with wheelchair tires, wearing gloves, and wearing a bicycle-type helmet to prevent head injury in the event of collision. Many athletes find it useful to protect the upper arm with the elasticized top of an athletic sock (Figure 28-4). All wheelchair parts or sharp surfaces that could accidentally result in a contact injury should be removed or covered with protective foam.

Blisters

Blisters are a frequent problem for most wheelchair athletes. Because the hands are used continuously for propulsion, athletes may experience frequent problems with blisters of the fingers and thumb from contact with the wheelchair push rim. Thick calluses may develop on the palm of the

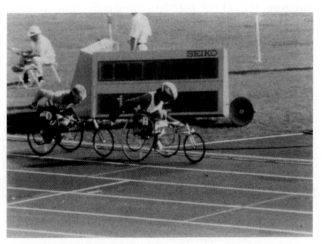

Figure 28-4
Wheelchair racers wear protection on the upper arms and use gloves.

hand; they can crack and result in painful fissures, open to infection.

Hands should be cleaned frequently and calluses filed with a pumice stone. Open cracks or fissures, blisters, and other abrasions should be managed with antibiotic creams and covered with bandages or dressings, as appropriate. Wheelchair athletes often develop symptoms of carpal tunnel syndrome from the repetitive trauma of wheelchair propulsion, causing compression in the carpal tunnel area.[11,30] Gloves are recommended for training and competition, but recent evidence questions their efficacy in preventing carpal tunnel syndrome.[30] Any athlete with symptoms of hand tingling or numbness should be referred for evaluation for carpal tunnel syndrome.

Leather batting gloves or handball gloves are most easily adapted and reinforced for wheelchair pushing, with layers of tape applied to the areas of highest pressure. Custom-designed leather mitts with reinforced neoprene use hook-and-loop fasteners to keep the hand in a closed position, creating a fist, and are widely used in road racing. This innovative glove design incorporates high-friction materials and maximizes the force generated during contact with the push rim. Because of the enhanced power available to the athlete, stroke dynamics have changed, and wrist and elbow injuries may decrease in frequency.

Lack of Protective Sensation

Spinal cord injury, multiple sclerosis, and other neurological disorders interfere with the normal protection that pressure, temperature, and pain sensation provide. Pressure points, especially under sitting areas, may lead to skin breakdown, ulceration, and infection. Insensitive skin must be inspected frequently.

Any time there is persistent redness of the skin, that area should have all pressure from sitting, clothes, or equipment relieved until the redness resolves and normal skin color returns. Otherwise, these areas may go on to ulcerate and may progress to serious infections. Athletes with open pressure sores should not participate in competition. Training should cease, and the athlete should avoid sitting or any position that may place him or her at risk for additional pressure damage, until the area is completely healed.

Athletes with chronic pressure sore problems may need customized seating systems that alleviate areas of pressure. Wheelchair cushions can be modified to accommodate an athlete's individual needs. If an athlete has chronic problems caused by positioning in the sports wheelchair, he or she should be referred to a physical or occupational therapist for evaluation and recommendations for possible adaptations.

Fractures account for less than 5% of all injuries sustained by wheelchair athletes.[11] However, osteoporosis is frequently associated with lower-extremity paralysis. As a result, athletes may be susceptible to lower-extremity fractures from relatively minor injuries. These fractures may go unnoticed because of the lack of sensation that would normally accompany a bony fracture. Therefore, following any injury, one must be aware of signs and symptoms such as abnormal body position, bruising, edema, or grinding sensations with movement. The athlete should be evaluated by x-ray examination to rule out a fracture, as movement of bony fragments may interfere with healing and cause further damage to muscles and blood vessels.

By using such simple preventive techniques, athletes who compete in wheelchairs can have safe and productive competitive careers.

Injuries of Athletes Who Compete Standing

Athletes with disabilities who compete while standing represent a variety of physical disabilities and sports interests. They often compete with disabilities such as upper and lower extremity amputations, visual deficits, and cerebral palsy. These athletes do not appear to be at greater risk for the common musculoskeletal problems associated with sports participation in the general population.[13] Although musculoskeletal problems may be no more frequent for athletes with disabilities, disability-related problems are seen among athletes who wear prostheses for running and athletes who sustain falls and other accidental injuries secondary to their disabilities or the use of assistive devices.

Abrasions and Blisters to Bony Prominences Within Prosthetic Socket

Many lower-extremity amputees run wearing prostheses. Common problems are skin breakdown, bruising, abrasion, blistering, skin rashes, and swelling on the residual limb, within the prosthetic socket, after or during exercise. These problems can sometimes be prevented by proper adjustment of prosthetic fit and alignment and prompt management of developing skin lesions.

Common sites for these problems in below-knee amputees are the fibula head, distal anterior end of the tibia, distal end of the fibula, medial and lateral femoral condyles, over the patella, and over scar tissue and poorly healed skin. Above-knee amputees may experience similar problems over the pubic or ischial rami, over the ischial tuberosities, at the distal lateral femur, over the greater trochanter, or over sites of scar tissue or poor healing.

Depending on the nature of the injury or trauma sustained, it may be appropriate to use a number of different management strategies. For bruising and blisters, the athlete can relieve friction by wearing additional (dry) stump socks or foam pads, or by applying abrasion protection products (e.g., Second Skin, Bioclusive, DuoDerm, Tegaderm, Ampu-Balm) over soft tissue areas that commonly break down as a result of continual friction. Unfortunately, in most cases the application of foam or leather padding may cause total-contact suction sockets to lose suction, and pistoning may result.

Ideally, the pads are used prophylactically prior to the event. However, often they are applied after a blister has formed to permit continued participation. Use of these protective pads must be monitored regularly, especially during long-distance events, because once the inner silicone gel dries out, the outer covering material can become a source of irritation.

It may be appropriate to use rest, ice, and compression and to decrease additional trauma to the limb through supported ambulation with crutches or a cane.

Compression Injuries

The absorption of ground reaction forces generated during support-limb impact in able-bodied athletes is accomplished by the mechanics of the foot-ankle complex, rotation of long bones, flexion of all lower-extremity joints, and insulation of muscle. Amputee runners lack many, if not all, of these shock-absorbing mechanisms and thus are prone to many "impact" or "compression" injuries. All these injuries are the result of the ground forces being transmitted to the socket via the prosthetic pylon. Above- and below-knee amputees often experience bruising over the bony prominences listed previously. In addition, above-knee amputees with ischial containment socket designs often complain of excessive pressure from the medial wall.

Recurrent skin problems, bruising, or recurrent tendinitis should lead to suspicion of prosthetic malalignment or a misfitting socket. The prosthetist, coach, and athlete should be able to work together to evaluate the athlete's needs and adjust or redesign an appropriate prosthesis. Modification of the patella tendon bar for below-knee amputees or modification of the height of the anterior or medial socket wall for above-knee amputees may provide some relief from compressive forces.

Falls

Accidental falls are likely to occur in runners with disabilities, as a result of uneven ground surfaces and environmental conditions. Falling is the most common cause of hand abrasions. Ambulatory athletes with disabilities may use special equipment such as prostheses, crutches, and canes, which are subject to fatigue and sudden breakdown, especially in the face of the uncommon stress associated with athletics. Blind runners present an obvious problem in that they lack the visual acuity to detect environmental hazards in their path. Sighted guides are critical to their optimal and safe performance.

Some athletes with disabilities wear bicycle helmets when running to provide an extra measure of safety, if they have problems with footing or balance. Athletes who use assistive devices such as crutches or canes should check for cracks or fissures in metal shafts or rubber tips prior to use.

All athletes with disabilities should take the same precautions recommended to athletes in the general population to help prevent accidents. Wearing reflective clothing at night,

running defensively when there are cars or bicycles present, carrying identification that includes pertinent medical information, and dressing appropriately for a workout will help improve safety margins.

It is strongly recommended that athletes with disabilities train with other athletes or groups who can provide companionship, support, and an extra measure of safety. Volunteers who run with blind athletes especially must be able to concentrate on obstacles and sudden environmental changes, as well as individual athletic needs and performance.

Low Back Pain

Some athletes with disabilities also experience chronic low back pain. Athletes with tightness of the hip flexor muscles often compensate with increased mobility in the lumbar spine. Amputees often overuse the lumbar spine as a compensatory mechanism. Because of the forces transmitted through a rigid, unforgiving prosthesis, amputees, especially above-knee amputees, must compensate for the lack of lower-extremity joint flexion with excessive lumbar spine lateral flexion and extension (Figure 28-5). Greater lateral lumbar flexion is observed during early support, and increased lumbar extension is observed during late support

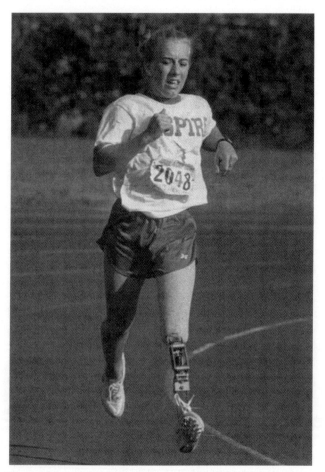

Figure 28-5
Above-knee amputee sprinter.

as the maximal hip extension is being achieved. As a result of daily ambulation and running, an imbalance in back musculature, as well as a functional scoliosis, may be observed in many amputees.

Muscle balancing, stretching, and traditional prophylactic low back pain measures may be employed to assist an athlete experiencing low back pain as the result of excessive lumbar movement or hip flexor tightness.

Bursitis

Rarely, amputees complain of bursa pain from socket irritation. On these occasions, below-knee amputees most frequently experience prepatellar, infrapatellar, or pretibial bursa pain. Above-knee amputees complain of ischial and trochanteric bursitis. Bursitis, when it occurs in amputees, is often the result of poor prosthetic fit. Necessary prosthetic modifications should be made.

Knee Injuries

Athletes with cerebral palsy often show genu valgum and mechanical instability at the knee. In addition, quadriceps muscles may be spastic and tight. Even though knee instability and muscle imbalance may be present, it is not clear that these predispose such athletes to a higher risk of injury.

Below-knee and Syme amputees may be considered vulnerable to many more knee injuries than actually occur because of the rigid lever constituted by the prosthesis. Most socket designs bring the medial and lateral wall well above the knee joint line, reducing the chance of collateral ligament injury. In most cases, the residual limb pulls away from the socket rather than being fixed within the socket.

Jumping events such as the long jump put amputees at the greatest risk of knee injury. Occasionally, hyperextension injuries occur as a result of the body's forward momentum over a fixed prosthesis and residual limb.

Injuries to the Sound Limb

In amputee athletes, the sound limb often sustains injuries as a result of the stresses endured by compensating for the prosthetic limb. Frequently, chronic hamstring problems arise as a result of the altered hip flexion of both lower extremities.

The sound limb foot also must adapt to the additional weightbearing that is often associated with amputees who hop on and use the sound limb more than the prosthetic limb. Some individuals develop plantar fasciitis, stretched plantar ligaments, or foot imbalances such as pronation because of the additional abnormal forces.

Treatment of injuries to runners with disabilities should follow the same principles and guidelines that apply to able-bodied and sighted runners. RICE, sport orthotics, athletic taping, and sports rehabilitation are all effective techniques for treating the musculoskeletal problems of runners with disabilities.

Injuries to the Upper Extremities in Crutch Users

Some lower-extremity amputees prefer to compete without a prosthesis, using crutches to assist in their mobility. As with all crutch users, care must be taken to avoid hand and wrist injuries such as carpal tunnel problems at the wrist and neurovascular compression at the axilla. Athletes who use crutches should be encouraged to use and frequently replace rubber padding on hand grips and under axillae.

Energy Requirements for Amputee Runners

The metabolic cost of ambulation has been well documented as being 15% to 30% higher for transtibial amputees while walking at a pace 10% to 40% slower than nonamputees[31-38] and 40% to 65% higher for transfemoral amputees who ambulate at a pace 15% to 50% slower than nonamputees.[38-41] The discrepancy in metabolic cost of ambulation is directly related to age, cause of amputation, length of residual limb, and prosthetic design.[38,42,43] To date, no studies have been published examining the metabolic cost of amputee running, but it appears that a considerable physiological demand is placed on amputee runners for several reasons. In addition to the reasons previously stated, alteration of the normal kinematics of the running gait, such as a transfemoral amputee's inability to flex the prosthetic knee during stance or the lack of normal foot-ankle motions, increases the physiological demands.[44-48] There are also kinetic and musculoskeletal disadvantages, such as the fact that an amputee's knee musculature absorbs only 1.4 times as much energy as it generates, compared with 3.6 times as much for a nonamputee jogger.[44,46] Increased demands are placed on the sound limb as well; for example, the sound limb is responsible for approximately 90% of the total energy generated during running.[44] The loss of the amputated limb also decreases the total body surface area available for physiological thermoregulation for cooling the body.

> **For Amputee Athletes**
>
> - Metabolic costs are greater
> - Physiological demands are greater
> - Greater stress is placed on the sound limb (both biomechanically and physiologically)

Collectively, all these influences can increase the physiological demands placed on an amputee runner and result in greater fatigue, potential hyperthermia, and injuries related to musculoskeletal imbalances. Hyperthermia is rarely a problem in running events, because 1500 meters is the longest distance permitted in international amputee track competition. However, there are a few amputee marathon runners and a great number of cyclists who could be at risk for developing hyperthermia.

Rehabilitation of Sports Injuries

The rehabilitative management of disabled athletes is similar to that of any other athlete. The rehabilitation must be a comprehensive program designed to return the disabled athlete to his or her sport with the greatest degree of function and in the shortest time possible. Just as an able-bodied athlete's program must be progressive and functional, so must a disabled athlete's rehabilitation program. Therefore, a general rehabilitation program should include warm-up, strengthening, flexibility, coordination, proprioception, balance, speed, agility, and muscular and cardiovascular endurance and conclude with a cool-down period. Some exercises may have to be adapted to meet the needs of the individual athlete.

One such adaptation is for cardiorespiratory endurance training. Athletes with sympathetic nervous system involvement, such as individuals with neurological lesions above T4, have diminished heart rate and blood pressure responses to exercise. This diminished sympathetic response limits the use of heart rate and blood pressure as effective indicators of exercise intensity. Age-adjusted formulas for calculating target heart rates cannot be used easily with this population. Therefore, exercise prescriptions for these athletes may include parameters of speed, duration, frequency, or mechanical resistance rather than using a target heart rate to vary intensity.

Clinical Caution

For disabled athletes with neurological lesions above T4, diminished sympathetic response limits heart rate and blood pressure use as effective indications of exercise intensity.

It is also important to note that an athlete with a disability is often unable to rest an injury completely because of the demands for continued daily function. For example, a wheelchair athlete who sustains a shoulder injury is unable to rest because demands of everyday mobility require the use of the shoulder joint. An amputee who injures the sound limb will have increased difficulty with ambulation if the prosthetic limb becomes the dominant limb. To regain the ability to perform everyday tasks, the temptation to increase the use of the injured extremity prematurely may increase recovery time and the risk of injury. Alternatives to daily activities, rehabilitation, and training methods designed to reduce the risk of insult to the injured limb should be explored by the physical therapist and athlete.

Education and Injury Prevention

Educating athletes as to the most effective means of prevention is an important task for both coaching and sports medicine staff. Common-sense coaching and sports medicine techniques; familiarization with the disability by the athlete, coach, and volunteers; planned workouts; and consideration of safety can help prevent injuries, minimize risks, and ensure success.

Disability-Specific Medical Problems

In addition to injuries, pre-existing medical conditions, the requirements of sport participation, and environmental conditions expose athletes with disabilities to the risk of specific medical problems.

Temperature Regulation Disorders

Exposure to heat and cold often provides unique challenges to an athlete with a disability.[49] The athlete may be intolerant to conditions that would not particularly trouble an able-bodied athlete, because of sensory impairments, sympathetic nervous system dysfunction, and inadequate body mechanisms for cooling or warming. In addition, specific medications (tranquilizers, diuretics, sedative-hypnotics, alcohol, sympathomimetics, anticholinergics, and thyroid replacement drugs) predispose an athlete to problems with temperature regulation.

Clinical Point

Thermal injuries and temperature regulation are common problems in all athletes with disabilities.

Equipment and surfaces such as asphalt or metal may heat up in the sun and cause burns to a person without sensation. Similarly, individuals with paralyzed limbs often have impaired circulation, with a tendency to develop swelling of their feet, because their muscles do not assist in venous return. There is also a relatively lower blood flow to the skin and deep tissues. This makes the limb more susceptible to sunburn or frostbite, and even lesser degrees of heat or cold may cause serious deep tissue damage.

In addition, in spinal cord injury and in multiple sclerosis, there are problems with regulation of core body temperature caused by a loss of normal blood flow regulation via the central nervous system. Athletes with quadriplegia often report heat and cold intolerance.[11] This is compounded by an inability to sweat below the level of a spinal cord injury. Many medications used for pain, depression, allergy, bladder dysfunction, high blood pressure, and other problems also interfere with normal sweating.

Hypothermia

Tolerance to cold is affected by an athlete's level of physical fitness, percentage of body fat, wind, and water immersion. There are adverse effects on athletic performance if the body's core temperature drops. Early symptoms of hypothermia include weakness, fatigue, clumsy movements, slurring speech, and a decreased shivering response. Later symptoms are collapse and unconsciousness. Hypothermia is potentially serious, or even fatal, because it may result in cardiac arrhythmias and dysfunction of other body systems.[50] The risk of hypothermia is greatly increased by exercising in extremely cold weather, especially if there is a high windchill factor or the athlete does not pay attention to skin and clothes wetness.

An athlete who has had a spinal cord injury (usually competing in a wheelchair or sit-ski) may not have sensation below the level of the neurological lesion to feel cold extremities. In addition, normal mechanisms of piloerection (goose bumps), shivering, and circulatory shunting for warming may not take place. This is especially a problem when it is both cold and wet. Even temperatures at approximately 50°F (10°C) may be a problem for an athlete with a spinal cord injury above the midthoracic level.[49]

The following general principles apply to prevent hypothermia in an athlete with a disability. Protective clothing should be worn whenever possible, and the clothing should keep the athlete comfortable during the activity. Multiple layers of clothes should be used to take advantage of air trapped between the layers. The innermost layer should carry moisture away from the body, as cooling occurs more rapidly if the skin surface is wet. Polypropylene and cotton are recommended materials. In addition, the head should be covered to prevent heat loss, because as much as 25% of heat loss can occur from the head especially if it is uncovered. Wearing hats and helmets when training or competing in cold weather is essential to maintain body temperature.

Athletes should be encouraged to drink adequate fluids. Thirst is an unreliable indicator of the state of hydration, and athletes may become as quickly dehydrated in cold, dry climates as in hot climates. Water is lost with hard breathing and perspiration under cold conditions as well as hot conditions.

Those athletes who are predisposed to cold intolerance should take special precautions during training and competition. Athletes with a past history of cold injury (e.g., frostbite) may suffer further trauma. Older athletes may have poorer circulation to the extremities and may be subject to greater intolerance to cold. In addition, an athlete who has a communication or cognitive disorder may not be able to communicate symptoms of cold intolerance readily. Special attention must be given to making sure that these athletes are well supervised to recognize potential problems.

Special attention should be given to awareness of environmental conditions (e.g., windchill factor, wet conditions), wearing appropriate clothing and head covering, hydration, and training intensity and duration. After training or competition, the athlete should go to a warm, dry environment and remove cold or wet garments and dress in warm, dry garments so that there is no postexercise lowering of the body temperature. Superficial frostbite can be treated by placing the affected area under a warmer body part or by blowing warm air onto the body part.[50] The most effective treatment for an athlete with hypothermia is medically supervised rewarming by using thermal blankets, intravenous fluid replacement, and warm baths. Hypothermia can be a life-threatening condition, requiring prompt medical attention.[51] The principles of treating a hypothermic athlete with a disability are essentially the same as for treating athletes without disabilities, with added awareness of the possibility of pre-existing sensory and autonomic nervous system dysfunction.

Hyperthermia

Intolerance to heat is exacerbated by the environmental temperature and humidity. Mild symptoms of heat illness are characterized by muscle cramps after exercising in the heat. More severe heat illness results in heat exhaustion, and the athlete may complain of headache, nausea, vomiting, lightheadedness, weakness, cramps, and general malaise. Most severe is heatstroke, in which the athlete's body temperature may rise dangerously high. The athlete's performance will deteriorate, and he or she may become confused and disoriented and may faint. He or she may not sweat normally and may experience personality changes. This athlete is at risk for multiple organ damage, which can be prevented with quick treatment.

Athletes with disabilities should exercise extreme caution when high temperatures are accompanied by high humidity. High humidity prevents cooling of the body by normal sweating. High ambient temperatures do not allow for heat dissipation from the body to the environment. In warm climates, under these conditions, athletes and coaches should plan training and competitions in the early morning or evening hours to prevent exposure to peak heat conditions.

Clothing should be worn to provide shade and hold moisture for heat loss. Light clothing, in light colors, with "breathable" fibers are the best attire for exercise in very hot conditions. Disabled athletes should be encouraged to wear shirts and clothing designed to act as a sunscreen, instead of removing them in hot conditions, because of the added protection. Clothing can provide protection from the sun's rays as well as assist with cooling by holding moisture close to the skin.

Sunscreens should be used whenever athletes will be exposed to the sun. An athlete with a spinal cord injury may have a particularly increased risk of sunburn in areas without sensation because of circulatory changes. Although sunscreens are helpful in protecting against sunburn, water-resistant sunscreens can also make the athlete more susceptible to heat intolerance by impeding perspiration. Thus, care should be taken to cover only those areas exposed to the sun, especially in athletes who may not perspire normally.

Athletes with disabilities sometimes lack physiological mechanisms for cooling. Athletes with spinal cord injuries (especially quadriplegia) and others with neurological dysfunction above the level of the first thoracic segment (T1) are particularly susceptible to heat intolerance. These athletes do not sweat below the level of the neurological lesion and therefore cannot lower their body temperature by this form of heat exchange.

Close monitoring and preventive measures, such as spraying the surface of the face, neck, upper trunk, and arms with water from a spray bottle, should be routine. Although there is no evidence that spraying with water lowers the core temperature of normal athletes, the experience of spinal cord–injured athletes seems to support that this is a useful practice. Even more important, however, is staying out of the sun and wearing protective clothing.

Special attention should be paid during field event competition, which may involve hours of waiting in hot, sunny conditions. Athletes should be encouraged to rest in shaded, cooler, well-ventilated areas prior to and following competition.

Athletes who have medical conditions that predispose them to heat intolerance should be closely monitored. Older athletes and young children may also experience more severe problems. In addition, athletes with heart disease, diabetes, high blood pressure, and sweat gland dysfunction may have a higher incidence of heat illness. Of course, any athlete who has an acute problem such as an infection, nausea, vomiting, fever, diarrhea, fatigue, or preexisting dehydration may be particularly intolerant to the heat. These individuals should refrain from training and competition until the acute condition improves. Close monitoring of clothing, fluid intake, and body temperature is essential to the safe participation of high-risk athletes in extreme environmental conditions.

Any athlete showing signs of heat intolerance should be removed to a shaded, cool, well-ventilated area and treated for heat illness. Any athlete displaying headache, lightheadedness, or general malaise in the heat should discontinue exercise and be taken to a shaded, well-ventilated area. Medical attention is essential to cool the athlete as quickly as possible. Fluid replacement and cooling at the neck, groin, and armpits are often adequate to reverse symptoms, although more extensive treatment may be indicated.

Athletes who have communication or cognitive disorders may not communicate symptoms of heat intolerance readily. Special attention must be given to making sure that these athletes are well supervised to recognize potential problems. Fluid replacement should be offered frequently by coaches or staff to all cognitively impaired athletes to prevent heat illness.

Hydration

Thirst is an unreliable indicator of the state of hydration. Athletes should be encouraged to drink water continually, regardless of thirst, and to avoid salt tablets and undiluted electrolyte solutions. Athletes should drink at least 1 liter (approximately a quart) of water 1 to 2 hours before competition or training and half a liter (16 oz or 500 cc) of water 15 to 30 minutes before the event. Fluid replacement should continue at a rate of at least 400 to 500 cc (13 to 16 oz) every 15 to 30 minutes during training or competition. Following practice or competition, the athlete should continue with 1 to 2 liters (0.3 to 0.5 gallons) of fluid.[51]

Cool (45°–55°F or 7.2°–12.8°C) water is the best form of fluid replacement for events lasting less than 1 hour, as they tend to be more rapidly absorbed than warm water.[51] Glucose and electrolyte solutions and carbohydrate polymer solutions may be beneficial in events lasting more than 1 hour, as they delay the onset of fatigue. Solutions should be of a concentration of less than 10%; a concentration of 6% to 8% is ideal. If an athlete drinks electrolyte solutions or sweetened drinks, he or she should be sure that the drink is well diluted or should drink an equal amount of water. Alcoholic beverages and caffeine-containing beverages should be avoided because they cause further dehydration.

Certain athletes with developmental disabilities may not be able to reliably monitor their own fluid intake. Coaches should be especially cognizant of the fluid needs of this population of cognitively impaired athletes. It may be helpful to monitor the athlete's weight daily in hot conditions and increase fluid replacement accordingly. Any change in weight greater than 2% daily may indicate dehydration and should be treated accordingly.

Some athletes with disabilities restrict water intake because of bladder incontinence. Coaches need to ensure that athletes have access to adequate bathroom facilities rather than risk heatstroke caused by poor fluid intake in hot weather.

Bladder Dysfunction

Athletes with neurological disorders such as spinal cord injury or multiple sclerosis often have a neurogenic bladder. Because the bladder does not always empty properly or completely, bladder infections, bladder stones, and bladder obstruction are common to wheelchair athletes with neurogenic bladder.

Those who have indwelling catheters to drain the bladder and, to a lesser degree, those who use catheters to drain the bladder on an intermittent schedule usually have frequent, if not constant, bacteria in their urine. When bacteria invade the bladder wall, the infection can spread into the kidneys and blood stream, causing severe illness and death. Therefore, any infection needs prompt treatment with antibiotics. Athletes should refrain from competition and training for at least 8 hours after the initiation of antibiotic treatment and should be without a fever for at least 24 hours before resuming participation.

To prevent recurrent bladder infection, athletes should ensure adequate fluid intake to flush the bladder regularly. They must also have access to clean areas to allow good technique to avoid contamination during the handling and use of catheters and connecting tubing and bags.

If catheter tubing becomes blocked, the athlete may develop a bladder obstruction and be unable to urinate. Bladder obstruction can obstruct blood flow back to the heart by pressure on the inferior vena cava, or cause abnormally high blood pressure by stimulation of reflex activity. If bladder obstruction precipitates autonomic dysreflexia, blood pressure can rise dangerously high and even cause a cerebral hemorrhage. Also, rapid relief of an obstruction may cause a precipitous drop in blood pressure and result in shock damage to the heart or kidneys. Exercise may exacerbate these problems.

Hypotension

Wheelchair athletes with multiple sclerosis and spinal cord injury may experience hypotension with rapid position changes, caused by the inability of the sympathetic nervous system to accommodate for a rapidly shifting blood volume. Infections from pressure sores may also cause pressure drop. Pain, antispasticity, antiseizure, and bladder and bowel medications may all affect blood pressure regulation. This may cause problems in endurance activities and even lead to lightheadedness or fainting.

If an athlete in a wheelchair experiences lightheadedness caused by hypotension, the individual should be helped into a recumbent position or the wheelchair should be tipped back. These maneuvers will help increase venous return. Gentle pressure on the abdomen with deep breathing may also be helpful. If problems with lightheadedness continue, the athlete should be referred to a physician for evaluation of the problem.

Hypertension

Autonomic dysreflexia is a serious problem of spinal cord–injured athletes whose lesions are above the midthoracic level. This reflexive process, causing massive sympathetic outflow, often begins from an obstruction of bowel or bladder.

Clinical Caution

Any spinal cord–injured athlete with sudden hypertension or pounding headache should be suspected of having autonomic dysreflexia.

Autonomic dysreflexia is a medical emergency. The individual should assume or remain in a sitting position if possible to minimize blood pressure changes. The bladder should be emptied and the bowel evacuated; the condition should then be re-evaluated. Immediate medical intervention should follow if the hypertension has not resolved.

Recent studies have revealed that many elite wheelchair athletes with quadriplegia routinely self-induce autonomic dysreflexia to increase sympathetic outflow and improve performance during competition.[52,53] With autonomic dysreflexia, the athlete experiences uncontrollably high hypertension, which may lead to cerebral hemorrhage and death. "Boosting" via clamping a catheter or inducing a painful stimulus is a dangerous and foolhardy practice and should be discouraged among all athletes.

Blood Flow

Some muscle and joint diseases have associated problems with spasm of the arteries of the hands and feet that may be induced by cold. Edema or swelling in paralyzed limbs may be increased by generalized increased blood flow with exercise or prolonged sitting with straps around the legs or trunk. If blood flow is obstructed, there may be problems with venous return and development of thrombophlebitis. Persistent swelling in a leg that does not get better with elevation may indicate thrombophlebitis, although symptoms usually occur without warning. Fragments of the thrombus may break off, resulting in pulmonary embolus, often a life-threatening complication.

Edema should resolve with elevation of the extremities. Redness or heat in the area can signify a serious problem. Edema of the lower extremities should be treated by removing obstructive straps and reclining and elevating the limbs above the heart. Individuals with persistent edema with signs of inflammation should be properly evaluated for infectious processes or thrombophlebitis and treated appropriately.

Dysphagia

Athletes with cerebral palsy sometimes present with dysphagia or difficulty swallowing. An athlete with dysphagia may drool saliva from the mouth, which can cause a great deal of fluid loss. In addition, an athlete who has difficulty swallowing may choke on water or soft drinks.

Because an athlete with dysphagia is at risk for losing fluids by drooling, coaches and supportive personnel should ensure that the athlete has access to fluids that are easy to swallow and that straws are available. Generally, athletes with dysphagia are able to swallow frequent small amounts of thicker liquids, such as juices, more easily than water. Because dehydration may be a problem, avoiding exposure to the sun is also important.

Dysarthria

Dysarthria, or difficulty controlling the oral and vocal musculature to speak, may be seen in the cerebral palsy and brain-injured populations. Although many athletes have both dysphagia and dysarthria, the two conditions are not always present together. An athlete with dysarthria may not be able to express his or her needs quickly or in a way that is easy to understand. Health professionals should be careful not to assume, however, that expressive problems also mean that the athlete does not understand. They should take the time to communicate simply and directly. It may help to speak clearly and slowly, using simple, direct instructions.

Aphasia

Brain-injured athletes and a small percentage of cerebral palsy athletes may present with aphasia. This is a problem either in receiving and processing the verbal information presented (usually fluent aphasia) or in formulating a verbal message to be expressed (usually nonfluent aphasia).

It may be helpful to use writing or gestures to communicate if there is a language problem. Those with significant communication problems may need to communicate through a coach. Always use direct communication with the athlete first, before communicating through another person. Athletes with pre-existing medical problems should carry written instructions or wear Medic-Alert bracelets at all times in the event that a coach or team member is not present and an emergency arises.

Behavioral Problems

With the overstimulation of athletic competition, some brain-injured athletes may become agitated, excited, or occasionally hostile or abusive. Specific intervention techniques to remove the athlete from the situation and redirect his or her attention may help reduce distress. It may be helpful to isolate the athlete from the stimulus in a medical tent or other quiet area. Attempting to reason, argue, or debate may only make the situation worse and provoke a more agitated response. It is usually helpful to redirect the athlete's attention.

Seizure Disorders

Some cerebral palsy athletes have a history of seizure disorders. Seizures do not often occur during sports competition because the state of metabolic acidosis that frequently accompanies hypoxia stabilizes neuronal membranes. The most likely time for a seizure to occur is during travel and other times of stress, dehydration, and extremes of temperature. Seizure activity should be suspected following a syncopal episode in which there is no other explanation.

Routine safety measures apply during seizure activity to protect the head and airway. Following the seizure or in the postictal period, it is important to do a neurological examination to look for deficits, signs of head injury, contusions, or neck pain. The athlete may be confused and should be encouraged to rest. Hospitalization is required only if the seizure activity is new or different from that experienced previously. A coach or other responsible party should, however, check the athlete's responsiveness every 2 hours for the first 24 hours.

A medication history and schedule should be reviewed, as athletes often forget to take seizure medications such as phenytoin (Dilantin), carbamazepine (Tegretol), or phenobarbital in the excitement of travel and competition. Fatigue and dehydration may also precipitate the onset of seizure activity and may need to be addressed.

Considerations for Travel with Disabled Athletes

There are numerous areas in which sports medicine applies to athletes and teams that are traveling for competition. A medical staff member with a group of athletes with disabilities has many significant roles in the pretrip planning, as well as providing services during the competition.

Pretrip Health Screening and Emergency Contact Information

Athletes should complete forms that include current name and address, physician's name and address, emergency contacts, insurance coverage, past medical history, a list of current medications, and current medical problems. Some organizations and teams require that athletes have a physical examination within 3 to 6 months of departure. It is also important to have a mechanism to ensure that other medical problems have not developed in the interim between sending in the medical information and the departure date. Infections, pressure sores, traumatic injuries, seizures, or hospitalizations that have occurred in this interim period require attention by the medical staff to determine the current stability of the athlete's condition and his or her fitness for travel and competition.

Education on Doping for International Competitions

Athletes with disabilities are subject to the same antidoping regulations as able-bodied athletes, regardless of their medical problems. Athletes need to be educated about banned over-the-counter and prescription medications. In the United States, if an athlete is taking a medication that is banned, the athlete needs to call the USOC Drug Hotline (1-800-233-0393) in Colorado Springs, Colorado to discuss alternatives. The athlete then needs to consult with the athlete's physician to determine which nonbanned medications could be substituted. Athletes with disabilities must be especially careful, because even traces of prescription medications such as sympathomimetics, antihypertensives, diuretics, corticosteroids, or pain medications routinely prescribed in the management of their chronic medical conditions may result in a positive drug test. It is critical that alternative non-banned medications be prescribed well in advance of the competition, as some banned medications can be detected in the urine as long as several months after the last dose was taken. It is also important to remember that all over-the-counter medications and prescription medications that the medical team brings should meet the USOC or SMSCC guidelines as well.

Pretrip Information and Planning

Athletes who are traveling must bring sufficient medications and supplies, such as catheters and gloves, for their care for the duration of the trip. This needs to be emphasized in writing to all athletes, as medications, services, and supplies are often difficult to find in other countries. State Department and Centers for Disease Control advisories for pretrip immunizations should be followed. Athletes and staff must receive this information several months prior to departure, in many cases, to achieve desired immunity.

Jet Lag Education

Athletes traveling through several time zones often experience problems with eating and sleep cycles because of the abrupt time change. These changes can affect performance dramatically. To minimize changes, athletes are encouraged to change watches to the destination time zone immediately on departure. They are encouraged to sleep and wake at a time appropriate for the destination. Meals should also be adjusted accordingly. Athletes are encouraged to stay well hydrated and to use natural light, rather than stimulants such as caffeine, to assist in staying awake during the day in the new time zone. Sleep cycles should remain at 6 to 8 hours, and athletes should avoid the temptation to take long naps during midday. Alcohol should be avoided during the trip because of its depressant and diuretic effects.

Attention to Hydration and Nutrition Outside North America

Athletes may not tolerate all food and water in other countries, and water and food may not meet standards of sanitation. Unlabeled water sources, in particular, may not be safe for consumption. It is important to provide a clean water source for the athletes' hydration needs, which may mean that the team must immediately purchase cases of bottled water to be kept in the housing area and brought to the competition site. Athletes should be aware of when it is essential to drink bottled water and to be cautious about food choices. Food from street vendors in any country should be avoided. Ice made from contaminated water is often overlooked and may cause serious gastrointestinal problems when added to bottled water.

Athlete nutrition may suffer from changes in diet. With decreased protein intake, immune system function may be compromised.[54] It is a good idea to advise athletes to bring a supply of high-protein food sources from home for emergencies and for supplementation of the local diet. Choices such as nuts, trail mix, peanut butter, cans of tuna fish, and small packages of cereal may provide protein to supplement the diet at the competition site.

Equipment for Travel

Medical staff who are traveling with groups of athletes with disabilities should bring a well-stocked trainer's bag, including first-aid supplies and emergency equipment (Box 28-1). It is helpful to have electrical stimulation and ultrasound units that are battery operated, can be recharged, or run on local current. Because voltages (and wall plugs) often vary, staff should be prepared with a variety of adapters and converters. It is often easier to use a battery-operated unit and bring a supply of batteries.

Foreign Facilities

It is important to remember that the facilities for treating athletes or acquiring ice in other countries may be quite different from those at home. A treatment room may not be available, and a medical staff person must sometimes improvise by providing treatment on the team bus, in the athlete's room, or on a bench at a sport venue. Ice is frequently not as available as it is in North America.

The medical staff must be aware of the mechanism for managing a serious injury or problem. Emergency services and contacts should be established, and the local hospital identified. Local organizers should provide emergency systems access at competition sites and a mechanism for doing so at the housing site as well. In cases of severe injury or illness, the US or Canadian consulate may be able to assist with information on local resources to provide appropriate care to injured or ill athletes.

Injury Management Principles
Serious Injuries

Serious injuries or illnesses may require hospitalization. It is important to remember that medical personnel are not usually licensed to practice in other countries. Plans for transport of injured or ill athletes should be established early. An athlete who is seriously ill in a foreign country is often hospitalized in an environment where he or she may not speak the same language and the standards for treatment

Scissors: 7-inch tape scissors, small suture scissors
Tape cutter
Fingernail cutter
Penlight
Tongue forceps
Tweezers
1-inch adhesive tape (2-3)
1½-inch adhesive tape (6-8)
½-inch adhesive tape (2)
2-inch elastic tape (2-3)
1-inch dermal tape (1-2)
Elastic wraps 2-inch, 4-inch, 6-inch (2 each)
Contact lens solution
Eye wash
Taping base (Tuf Skin spray)
Tape underwrap (4-6)
Gauze pads (4 × 4, 3 × 3, large) (4–6 each)
Telfa pads (nonadherent, various sizes) (2–3 each)
Finger splints
Petroleum jelly
Antiseptic soap
Aspirin, acetaminophen, ibuprofen
Antacid (liquid or tablets)
Bandages (various sizes)
Steri-strips (butterfly bandages are second choice)
Cotton-tipped applicators
Padding: cotton; sponge (miscellaneous) ¼ and ½ inch; only felt (miscellaneous) ¼ and ½ inch
Fungicide ointment
Alcohol and/or Betadine swabs
Antibacterial cream
Plastic bags for ice or instant cold packs
Moleskin
Second Skin Blister Pak
Peroxide, 6 oz
Ampu Balm
Sterile catheters
Sterile and nonsterile rubber gloves
Mirror (small)
Thermometer (oral)
Sunscreen lotion (seasonal/location)
Small spray bottle
Triangular bandage or sling
Pocket cardiopulmonary resuscitation mask or shield
Portable, battery-operated ultrasound and electrical stimulation units

may differ markedly. It is usually beneficial to evacuate a seriously injured athlete as soon as it is medically advisable.

Minor Injuries

Even minor injuries and illnesses that occur at the competition site may affect athlete participation in competition. It is inadvisable for an athlete with a fever to compete under

any circumstances. Injuries that may become worse with continued physical activity should be identified. Athletes and coaching staff should be educated about the serious sequelae of continued activity. Medical staff members should enforce precautions and activity restrictions as needed and look to the team administrative leaders for support of those recommendations.

Organization of Disabled Athletic Events

The logistics of hosting and organizing an event for disabled athletes is an enormous task. The process of organizing an event is not a topic specific to this chapter, but clinicians are frequently asked to assume many roles when they become involved with event organizing committees. Most commonly, they are asked to provide medical coverage or, if certified as a classifier, to classify athletes or assume the role of a technical consultant. Boxes 28-2, 28-3, and 28-4 list the specific needs of organizing, medical, and classification committees, respectively.

Conclusion

The past 30 years have shown significant advancements in sport for disabled athletes. The scope of this progress can be attributed to many organizations.

Newer methods of teaching adaptive sports have spread through activities ranging from alpine skiing to shooting, cycling, horseback riding, and fishing. In the United States, the inclusion of persons with disabilities in this variety of activities can be attributed to organizations such as Professional Ski Instructors of America, US Tennis, US Sailing,

Sponsorship
Medical
Classification
Technical, event, and officiating
Manpower
Accommodations
Meals and refreshments
Transportation
Registration and packets
Command post (on-site information center)
Awards
Computer operations
Correspondence
Entertainment
Equipment
Outfitters
Athlete assistance
Public relations and marketing

US Water Skiing, US Kayaking and Canoeing, USA Volleyball, USA Track and Field, and Professional Association of Diving Instructors among others. These organizations have educated their coaching staffs in the adaptations necessary for successful participation and competition in their respective sports. Concurrent with the expanded knowledge and adaptation of coaching techniques for persons with disabilities has been the development and refinement of adaptive sports equipment using the latest technology in materials and engineering. Complementing advances in technology were the adoption of rules changes by governing organizations that opened up competition and reconciled the changes in competition fostered by technological innovation.

Who would have conceived 30 years ago that a paraplegic might race down a ski slope at 60 miles per hour (97 km/hr) or that an above-knee amputee could complete a 360° aerial on a snowboard? Could the authors and readers of this original chapter published circa 1995 have envisioned an individual pushing a lightweight sport wheelchair through a grueling 26-mile marathon in less than 1 hour and 30 minutes, faster than their able-bodied counterparts?

With all of these developments in coaching techniques, rules modifications, and equipment technologies, extraordinary performances by those with a disability have become ubiquitous within our society.

Sports medicine team members involved with disabled athletes have the ability to serve in many roles. The traditional role of providing emergency and rehabilitative medical care is only a fraction of the contribution that may be offered. Classifying, coaching, consulting with coaches, officiating, organizing, and administering are some of the many functions that medical personnel have the professional training and expertise to perform to enhance the overall performance of disabled athletes. Another integral responsibility that must be assumed by medical professionals is the education and recruitment of athletes through hospitals, rehabilitation centers, and other medical facilities where potential disabled athletes can be educated as to the availability of various sports organizations and quality training programs.

References

1. Paciorek MJ, Jones JA: *Sports and recreation for the disabled: A resource manual*, Indianapolis, 1989, Benchmark Press.
2. Weiss M, Curtis KA: Controversies in medical classification of wheelchair athletes. In Sherrill C, editor: *Sports and disabled athletes*, Champaign, IL, 1986, Human Kinetics.
3. Strohkendl H: The new classification system for wheelchair basketball. In Sherrill C, editor: *Sports and disabled athletes*, Champaign, IL, 1986, Human Kinetics.
4. Curtis KA: Sport-specific functional classification for wheelchair athletes, *Sports 'n' Spokes* 17:45–48, 1991.
5. Richter KJ, Adams-Mushett C, Ferrara MS, McCann BC: Integrated swimming classification: A faulted system, *APAQ* 9: 5–13, 1992.
6. Tweedy SM, Vanlandewijck YC: International Paralympic Committee position stand—background and scientific principles of classification in paralympic sport, *Br J Sports Med* 2009, in press.
7. Hay JG: *The biomechanics of sports techniques*, Englewood Cliffs, NJ, 1985, Prentice-Hall.
8. Goldberg G, Shephard RJ: Personality profiles of disabled individuals in relation to physical activity patterns, *J Sports Med* 22:477–484, 1982.
9. Horvat M, French R, Henschen K: A comparison of the psychological characteristics of male and female able-bodied and wheelchair athletes, *Paraplegia* 24:115–122, 1986.
10. Sherrill C, Silliman L, Gench B, Hinson M: Self-actualisation of elite wheelchair athletes, *Paraplegia* 28:252–260, 1990.
11. Curtis KA, Dillon DA: Survey of wheelchair athletic injuries: Common patterns and prevention, *Paraplegia* 23:170–175, 1985.
12. Ferrara MS, Davis RW: Injuries to elite wheelchair athletes, *Paraplegia* 28:335–341, 1990.
13. Ferrara MS, Buckley WE, McCann BC, et al: The injury experience of the competitive athlete with a disability: Prevention implications, *Med Sci Sports Exerc* 24:184–188, 1992.

14. Curtis KA, McClanahan S, Hall KM, et al: Health, vocational, and functional status in spinal cord injured athletes and nonathletes, *Arch Phys Med Rehabil* 67:862–865, 1986.

15. Stotts KM: Health maintenance: Paraplegic athletes and nonathletes, *Arch Phys Med Rehabil* 67:109–114, 1986.

16. Shephard RJ: Benefits of sport and physical activity for the disabled: Implications for the individual and for society, *Scand J Rehabil Med* 23:51–59, 1991.

17. Sweeney FF, Foote JE: Treatment of drug and alcohol abuse in spinal cord injured veterans, *Int J Addict* 17:897–904, 1982.

18. McCormack DAR, Reid DC, Steadward RD, Syrotuik DG: Injury profiles in wheelchair athletes: Results of a retrospective survey, *Clin J Sport Med* 1:35–40, 1991.

19. Aljure J, Eltorai I, Bradley WE, et al: Carpal tunnel syndrome in paraplegic patients, *Paraplegia* 23:182–186, 1985.

20. Gellman H, Sie I, Waters RL: Late complications of the weight-bearing upper extremity in the paraplegic patient, *Clin Orthop Rel Res* 233:132–135, 1988.

21. Burnham R, Newell E, Steadward R: Sports medicine for the physically disabled: The Canadian team experience at the 1988 Seoul Paralympic Games, *Clin J Sport Med* 1:193–196, 1991.

22. Sie I, Waters RL, Adkins RH, Gellman H: Upper extremity pain in the post rehabilitation spinal cord injured patient, *Arch Phys Med Rehabil* 73:44–48, 1992.

23. Burnham RS, Steadward RD: Upper extremity peripheral nerve entrapments among wheelchair athletes: Prevalence, location and risk factors, *Arch Phys Med Rehabil* 75:519–524, 1994.

24. Bayley JC, Cochran TP, Sledge CB: The weightbearing shoulder-impingement syndrome in paraplegics, *J Bone Joint Surg Am* 69:676–678, 1987.

25. Burnham RS, May L, Nelson E, Steadward R: Shoulder pain in wheelchair athletes—The role of muscle imbalance, *Am J Sports Med* 21:238–242, 1993.

26. Robinson MD, Hussey RW, Ha CY: Surgical decompression of impingement syndrome in the weight-bearing shoulder, *Arch Phys Med Rehabil* 74:324–332, 1993.

27. Neer CS: Anterior acromioplasty for the chronic impingement syndrome in the shoulder, *J Bone Joint Surg Am* 54:41–50, 1972.

28. Barber DB, Gall NG: Osteonecrosis: An overuse injury of the shoulder in paraplegia: Case report, *Paraplegia* 29:423–426, 1991.

29. Wilson PE, Washington RL: Pediatric wheelchair athletics: Sports injuries and prevention, *Paraplegia* 31:330–337, 1993.

30. Burnham RS, Chan M, Hazlett C, et al: Acute median nerve dysfunction from wheelchair propulsion: The development of a model and study of the effect of hand protection, *Arch Phys Med Rehabil* 75:513–518, 1994.

31. Ganguli S, Datta SR, Chatterjee BB: Metabolic cost of walking at different speeds with patellar tendon bearing prosthesis, *J Appl Physiol* 36:440–443, 1974.

32. Gonzalez EG, Corcoran PJ, Reyes RL: Energy expenditure in below-knee amputees: Correlation with stump length, *Arch Phys Med Rehabil* 55:111–119, 1974.

33. Molen NH: Energy/speed relation of below-knee amputees walking on motor-driven treadmill, *Int Z Angew Physiol* 31:173–185, 1973.

34. Pagliarulo MA, Waters R, Hislop HJ: Energy cost of walking of below-knee amputees having no vascular disease, *Phys Ther* 59:538–542, 1979.

35. Torburn L, Perry J, Ayyappa E, Shanfield SL: Below-knee amputee gait with dynamic elastic response prosthetic feet: A pilot study, *J Rehabil Res Dev* 27:369–384, 1990.

36. Waters RL, Perry J, Antonelli EE, et al: Energy cost of walking of amputees: The influence of level of amputation, *J Bone Joint Surg Am* 58:42–46, 1976.

37. Waters RL, Yakura JS: The energy expenditure of normal and pathological gait, *Crit Rev Phys Med* 1:183, 1989.

38. Fisher SV, Gullickson G: Energy cost of ambulation in health and disability: A literature review, *Arch Phys Med Rehabil* 59:121–132, 1978.

39. Huang CT, Jackson JR, Moore NB, et al: Amputation: Energy cost of ambulation, *Arch Phys Med Rehabil* 60:18–24, 1979.

40. James U: Oxygen uptake and heart rate during prosthetic walking in healthy male unilateral above-knee amputees, *Scand J Rehabil Med* 5:71–80, 1973.

41. Traugh GH, Corcoran PJ, Rudolpho LR: Energy expenditure of ambulation in patients with above-knee amputations, *Arch Phys Med Rehabil* 56:67–71, 1975.

42. Flandry E, Beskin J, Chambers R, et al: The effects of the CAT-CAM above-knee prosthesis on functional rehabilitation, *Clin Orthop* 239:249–262, 1989.

43. Gailey RS, Lawrence D, Burditt C, et al: The CAT-CAM socket and quadrilateral socket: A comparison of energy cost during ambulation, *Prosthet Orthot Int* 17:95–100, 1993.

44. DiAngelo DJ, Winter DA, Dhanjoo N, Newcombe WR: Performance assessment of the Terry Fox jogging prosthesis for above-knee amputees, *J Biomech* 22:543–558, 1989.

45. Enoka RM, Miller DI, Burgess EM: Below-knee amputee running gait, *Am J Phys Med* 61:68–84, 1982.

46. Winter DA, Sienko SE: Biomechanics of below-knee amputee gait, *J Biomech* 21:361–367, 1988.

47. Smith AW: A biomechanical analysis of amputee athlete gait, *Int J Sports Biomech* 6:262–282, 1990.

48. Czerniecki JM, Gitter A, Munro C: Joint moment and muscle power output characteristics of below knee amputees during running: The influence of energy storing prosthetic feet, *J Biomech* 24:63–75, 1991.

49. Corcoran PJ: Sports medicine and the physiology of wheelchair marathon racing, *Orthop Clin North Am* 11:697–716, 1980.

50. Arnheim DD: *Modern principles of athletic training*, ed 6, St Louis, 1985, Times Mirror/Mosby College Publishing.

51. Roy S, Irvin R: *Sports medicine: Prevention, evaluation, management and rehabilitation*, Englewood Cliffs, NJ, 1983, Prentice-Hall.

52. Burnham R: *Boosting self-induced autonomic dysreflexia in wheelchair athletes*, Paper presented at Vista '93 Conference, Jasper, Alberta, Canada, May 19, 1993.

53. Raymond S: *Using dysreflexia to enhance athletic performance: An athlete's opinion*, Paper presented at Vista '93 Conference, Jasper, Alberta, Canada, May 19, 1993.

54. Good RA, Lorenz BA: Nutrition, immunity, aging, and cancer, *Nutr Rev* 46:62–67, 1988.

SELECTED REHABILITATION NEEDS OF THE MASTERS ATHLETE

James W. Matheson and Robert C. Manske

Introduction

Sports medicine is often described as the treatment and care of competitive athletes. Yet any clinician currently practicing sports medicine will tell you that this is only a part of the definition. If asked, he or she will state that sports medicine is a philosophy. This philosophy is defined by the patient's will to get back to the specific desired physical activity. The attitude of the clinician factors into this definition as well. The role of the sports medicine clinician is to engage, educate, and facilitate the patient's ability to reach his or her goal. Whether the patient is a star high school basketball player competing for a full college scholarship or a 75-year-old grandmother who wants to cross-country ski with her grandchildren, both are highly motivated individuals who want to return to their sports. Both need the expertise of a sports medicine clinician.

The world's population is aging. The median age of the global population is increasing because of a decline in fertility and a 20-year increase in the average lifespan during the second half of the twentieth century.[1] These factors, combined with elevated fertility in many countries during the two decades after World War II (i.e., the "Baby Boom" generation), will result in increased numbers of persons aged 65 years or older between 2010 and 2030.[2] Worldwide, the average lifespan is expected to extend another 10 years by 2050.[1]

In the United States, the proportion of the population aged 65 years or older is projected to increase from 12.4% in 2000 to 19.6% by 2030.[3] By the numbers, the population aged older than 65 years is expected to increase from approximately 35 million in 2000 to an estimated 71 million in 2030. The number of persons aged 80 years or older is expected to increase from 9.3 million in 2000 to 19.5 million in 2030. Internationally, the worldwide population aged 65 years and older is projected to increase by approximately 550 million to 973 million,[3] increasing from 6.9% to 12% worldwide (Table 29-1).[2]

As a result of the population aging and increased lifespan, more and more people are retiring in their mid to late 60s with plans to engage in physical activity such as golf, tennis, hiking, swimming, weightlifting, and other forms of both aerobic and anaerobic exercises. Recently, the US federal government has issued its first-ever Physical Activity Guidelines for Americans.[4] They describe the types and amounts of physical activity that offer substantial health benefits to Americans of all ages. The driving force behind these guidelines is the overwhelming body of research and opinion that moderate exercise and daily physical activity is a valuable intervention in preventing and controlling disease and chronic illness.[4-9] There is also a large consensus in medical opinion that moderate exercise in the senior population may markedly reduce the age-related declines in musculoskeletal function.

Clinical Point

Moderate exercise in the senior population may reduce age-related decline in musculoskeletal function.

The new Physical Activity Guidelines recommend what is considered the "minimum" activity requirements for general fitness. It is unknown if the growing older population

Table 29-1

United States and World Estimated Population

Location and Age	Dates	
	2000	2030
% Age > 65	12.4	19.6
US # Age > 65 (millions)	35	71
US #Age > 80 (millions)	9.3	19.5
Int % Age > 65	6.9	12.0
Int # Age > 65 (millions)	550	973

Data from Kinsella K, Velkoff V: An aging world, US Census Bureau, Editor, Washington, DC, 2001, US Government Printing Office; and US Census Bureau: International database. Table 094. Midyear population, by age and sex. Available from: http://www.census.gov/ population/www/projections/natdet-D1A.html.

%, Percentage; *#*, number; *Int*, international; *US*, United States.

will follow the new guidelines. Currently, the activity level of many older Americans falls short of the guideline recommendations. However, there exists a subgroup of the aging population that exceeds these new activity requirements. These active individuals represent the upper end of the functional spectrum among older adults. These are the masters athletes.

Masters athletes are competitors who exceed a minimum age specific to each sport and who participate in competitive events designed for master athletes.[10] Some of these events include the Senior Sports Classics, the World Veterans Games, and the events sponsored by the National Senior Games Association (NSGA) in the United States. The competitive events for the 2009 National Senior Games included 18 different sports: archery, badminton, basketball, bowling, cycling, golf, horseshoe, race walk, racquetball, road race, shuffleboard, softball, swimming, table tennis, tennis, track and field, triathlon, and volleyball. The NSGA holds local and state games for seniors across the nation to encourage seniors to become active and get involved. These local and state games are estimated to have 350,000 senior athlete participants annually.[11] To participate in the Senior Games, an athlete must be at least 50 years old.[11] The minimum age of a masters athlete varies according to the extent to which youth is required for success. For example, in swimming, the minimum masters athlete age is 25 and in rowing it is 27.[10] In track and field, masters athletes are considered those older than 35 years; in race walking they must exceed 40. Selected outdoor track world records for male and female master athletes in the 100 m are shown in Table 29-2.

Masters athletes who have pursued lifelong sports activities do not want to alter activity levels or recreational plans following a recent diagnosis of osteoarthritis (OA) or a surgical procedure. These "veteran" athletes do not want or need clinicians to tell them that they can no longer be as active as they have been in the past. They want clinicians who treat them no differently than athletes several decades younger. This is the challenge to the sports medicine practitioner. Returning masters athletes to their activities is challenging and involves a specific understanding of the physiological changes that occur within the aging musculoskeletal system. This chapter begins by discussing the physiological effects that are altered in the aging athlete. The selected topics of OA and overuse tendinopathy will be discussed. Common treatment interventions and the research evidence supporting these interventions is emphasized. Last but certainly not least, considerations for those returning to athletics following total joint replacement is addressed.

Table 29-2

World Masters Outdoor Track and Field World Records at 100 Meters

Age Group	Marks	Athlete Name	Country	Age	Meet Date
Men 45	10.72	Willie Gault	USA	45	6/24/2006
Women 45	11.34	Merlene Ottey	SLO	47	8/12/2008
Men 55	11.44	William Collins	USA	57	4/25/2008
Women 55	13.30	Philippa Raschker	USA	55	8/10/2002
Men 65	12.37	Stephen Robbins	USA	65	8/2/2008
Women 65	14.10	Nadine O'Connor	USA	65	6/30/2007
Men 75	13.54	Bruno Kimmel	GER	75	7/10/2009
Women 75	15.91	Paula Schneiderhan	GER	75	9/6/1997
Men 85	16.16	Suda Giichi	JPN	85	8/23/1998
Women 85	19.83	Nora Wedemo	SWE	86	8/21/1999
Men 95	21.44	Friederich E. Mahlo	GER	95	9/7/2007
Women 90	23.18	Nora Wedemo	SWE	90	8/9/2003
Men 100	30.86	Philip Rabinowitz	RSA	100	7/10/2004

Data from http://www.usatf.org/statistics/records/masters_outdoorTF_world.asp, accessed on 04/04/2010.

GER, Germany; *JPN,* Japan; *RSA,* Russia; *SLO,* Slovenia; *SWE,* Sweden; *USA,* United States.

In April, 2010, a team physician consensus statement was published in *Medicine and Science in Sports and Exercise* entitled "Selected Issues for the Masters Athlete and the Team Physician: A Consensus Statement" that provides a guide to the care and treatment of these athletes for selected conditions.[12]

Physiological Effects of Aging on the Masters Athlete

Progressive loss of muscle strength and endurance resulting in a loss of athletic performance and function has traditionally been accepted as a consequence of aging. However, several studies have shown that a significant portion of these losses in function may be musculoskeletal adaptations to physical inactivity.[13-19] These studies have shown that high-intensity training in the frail elderly can lead to a significant increase in their ability to resume activities of daily living (ADLs). Masters athletes continue to challenge this concept of age-related decline and may serve as a model from whom a better understanding may be gained of the inevitable senescent changes that occur.

Changes in Body Composition in the Masters Athlete

Body composition comprises body fat and fat free mass, which includes skin, bone, internal organs, and muscle mass.[20] In our relatively sedentary society, it is typical to gain approximately 1 pound (0.5 kg) a year between the ages of 25 and 65 years. This increase in girth is attributable to fat mass and generally occurs in the peritoneum, which puts older adults at greater risk for diabetes and heart disease. Occurring concomitantly with the expansion of the waistline, a reduction in lean mass begins in middle age, primarily of skeletal muscle and bone. Even in men and women who are rigorously active throughout the course of a lifetime (e.g., masters athletes), there is a change in body composition reflecting the expected increase in fat mass and the related loss of lean mass.[15] A cross-sectional comparison of sedentary women indicates that percentage body fat is higher in 50- to 60-year-old women (42.1%) compared with women in their twenties (27.1%) and seventies (36.7%). The absolute quantity of body fat of masters athletes is similar to that of young, active women and lower than that of sedentary 50- to 60-year-old women. Cross-sectional data indicate that the percentage of body fat for masters athletes is relatively constant at approximately 28% between the ages of 35 and 75.[21] In masters athletes, the percentage of body fat varies by sport. Those participating in long-distance track events have a lower percentage body fat (23.5%) than those participating in short-distance track events (28.8%).[21] For the same age span, masters athletes have a lower rate of decline (7.5%) in lean muscle mass than the general population (25%-30%).[21-23] Thus, maintenance of a high level of physical activity throughout the lifespan allows masters athletes to have a slower increase in body fat and preserve lean mass to a greater extent than the general population.

Changes in Muscle Structure and Function in the Masters Athlete

The primary function of skeletal muscle is for movement and generation of force. This function occurs at both the macroscopic and microscopic level. Muscle fibers are classified as type I, type IIa, and type IIb fibers. Type I fibers, also known as "slow-twitch" fibers, are more resistant to fatigue than types IIa or IIb, also known as "fast-twitch" fibers. In comparison with slow-twitch fibers, fast-twitch fibers fatigue faster and are mainly anaerobic. It is generally accepted that slow-twitch fibers are mainly used for endurance, whereas fast-twitch fibers are used for speed and power. In regard to hypertrophy (muscle growth), fast-twitch fibers grow faster and larger than slow-twitch fibers.

Sarcopenia is of profound importance for the maintenance of posture, locomotion, and the ability to perform ADLs.[24] Arm, leg, and back strength decline at an overall rate of 8% per decade, starting in the third decade of life. It is important to note that the rate of decline is not linear, but is slightly slower early in the decline and accelerates late in life. Healthy men and women in their seventh and eighth decades of life demonstrate average reductions of 20% to 40% in maximal isometric strength.[24,25] From a functional perspective, the age-associated reduction of quadriceps muscle strength is such that the average 80-year-old is at or near the minimum level of strength required to rise from a chair.[26,27]

Clinical Point

Sarcopenia is the progressive decline of muscle mass, force generation, and quality associated with aging.

This age-associated decline in muscular force generation also negatively affects the performance capacity of the masters athlete. The loss in muscle mass and subsequent loss of muscle force is the consequence of an actual decline in the number of muscle fibers present and the atrophy of many of the remaining fibers, particularly among the fast-twitch or type II fibers. This preferential decline in type II fiber area also affects the ability to recruit muscles quickly, which makes athletic activities requiring explosive power (e.g., sprinting, jumping) more difficult. Despite these senescent changes in muscle tissue, masters athletes continue to perform at a level much higher than their sedentary counterparts.

Clinical Point

Aging combined with inactivity leads to loss of muscle mass and muscle force. It is the result of a decrease in number of muscle fibers and atrophy of remaining fibers especially fast-twitch (type II) muscle fibers.

In a study of elite weightlifters, aged 18 to 82 years, researchers examined changes in muscle structure. Results are shown in Figure 29-1.[28] It is apparent that after age 50, there is a consistent loss of muscle fiber size. Of note is the oldest lifter, who had fiber areas that were comparable to those of five physical therapy students who were biopsied as controls. These data suggest that a large portion of fiber atrophy that occurs with aging may be due to inactivity. However, the data also illustrate that despite rigorous training, the masters athlete cannot maintain fiber hypertrophy with advancing age.[28]

During the past 20 years, scientists have investigated the underlying mechanisms for the reduction in strength with age.[24,25,28-30] At present, it appears that there is no single cellular or molecular mechanism that can explain the total reduction in strength. It is conceivable that age-related weakness may be caused partly by a decreased central drive, and thus a decline in ability to voluntarily activate a muscle. The threshold of excitability of the corticospinal tract increases progressively with age and is significantly higher in the older adult. Although this increased threshold of activation influences performance, masters athletes continue to push their musculoskeletal systems to the limit and to provide evidence of the true physiological limitations of muscle force and structure in the active older adult (see Table 29-2).

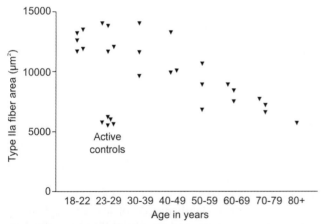

Figure 29-1

Muscle fiber area in master lifters. Muscle biopsies from the vastus lateralis muscle of 22 master athletes aged 18 to 82 years and 5 physical therapy students who exercise recreationally. Only type IIa fiber areas are presented as this fiber type represented approximately 75% of the total in the lifters. (From Brown M: Effects of aging-growth changes and lifespan concerns (40+). In Magee DJ, Zachazewski JE, Quillen WS, editors: Scientific foundations and Principles of Practice in Musculoskeletal Rehabilitation, p 307, St. Louis, 2007, Saunders.)

Changes in Tendon Structure in the Masters Athlete

With aging, there are mechanical and structural changes in tendon tissue, including increased collagen cross-linking, decreased content of glycosaminoglycans and water, and increased stiffness.[31] Strocchi and colleagues[32] reported that changes in the Achilles tendon included a decrease in the collagen fibril diameter, an increase in fibril density, a decrease in the number of tenocytes, and a loss of the waviness (crimp) noted in a young tendon not under tensile load. Birch and colleagues[33] reported that the ultimate stress values (mega Pascal) of Achilles tendon decreased with age. However, other researchers have reported that although tendons from healthy older adults show these changes, there is no evidence of degenerative changes in tendons as seen in tendinosis.[34,35] It is possible, however, that the mechanical and structural changes in tendons with age may predispose the tendon to tendinopathy or tendon rupture.

Age-Related Changes in Tendon

- Increased collagen crosslinking
- Decreased glucosaminoglycans
- Decreased water
- Increased stiffness
- Decreased fiber diameter
- Increased fibril density
- Decreased tenocytes
- Loss of crimp

Cardiorespiratory Fitness in the Masters Athlete

As with skeletal muscle and body composition, senescent changes occur in the cardiopulmonary system. Decreases in maximal oxygen consumption, exercise economy, and the exercise intensity at which a high fraction of the maximal oxygen consumption can be sustained (lactate threshold) are considered factors that result in a decline in performance of the masters athlete.[36-40] A detailed discussion of these factors is beyond the scope of this chapter; however, because maximal oxygen consumption appears to be the most influential factor in cardiorespiratory fitness in the masters athlete, it is briefly discussed. Maximum oxygen uptake (VO_2 max) is the gold-standard measure of cardiorespiratory fitness. VO_2 max represents the upper limit of "aerobic" power or performance. Maximal oxygen consumption is generally considered to be a primary determinant of endurance exercise performance among young, endurance-trained athletes.[38,41] VO_2 max declines approximately 10% per decade after age 25 to 30 years in healthy, sedentary men and women.[39,42-44] Unlike the other physiological variables previously discussed, endurance exercise–trained men and women demonstrate greater "absolute" (1 mL/kg per 1 min) rates of decline in VO_2 max with age than healthy sedentary adults.[40,42,44,45] It is suspected that this is a result of these athletes having greater baseline levels of VO_2 max as young adults and a proportionally greater loss of exercise with aging compared with sedentary adults.[44,45] Based on current scientific research, a progressive reduction in VO_2 max appears to be the primary physiological mechanism associated with declines in endurance performance in the masters athlete.

Age-Related Structural Changes in the Cardiovascular System

Heart
- Myocardium
  - Increased wall thickness
  - Accumulation of lipofuscin
  - Increased elastin, fat, and collagen
- Endocardium
  - Thickened areas composed of elastic, collagen, and muscle fibers
  - Fragmentation and disorganization of elastic, collagen, and muscle fibers
- Conduction system
  - Atrophy and fibrosis of left bundle branches
  - Decreased number of sinoatrial node pacemaker cells
- Valves
  - Thickening and calcification

Vasculature
- Increased size (primarily of proximal vessels)
- Increased wall thickness (primarily of distal vessels)
- Increased connective tissue and lipids in subendothelial layer
- Atrophy of elastic fibers in medial layer
- Disorganization and degeneration of elastin and collagen

From Irwin S: *Cardiopulmonary physical therapy: A guide to practice*, ed 4, St Louis, 2004, Mosby.

Clinical Point

Maximum oxygen uptake decreases approximately 10% per decade after 25 to 30 years of age in sedentary adults.

Flexibility

As was true with muscle tissue, the connective tissue elements that make up tendon, capsule, muscle, fascia, and aponeurosis also undergo senescent changes. The quantity of change of the collagen, elastin, and other elements influence the response of these tissues to the physical stresses of athletic activity. A result of these age-related tissue changes is a decrease in the passive viscoelastic properties or "flexibility" of the connective tissue elements.

Connective tissue tends to increase with age in proportion to muscle mass, to become less hydrated, and to change its relative composition of collagen and elastin, all of which contribute to its increased density and rigidity. Aging results in a decrease in the amount of insoluble collagen and total collagen. Both of these have been correlated with decreases in the tensile strength of tendons and increases in the stiffness of tendons.[46] The result of this change is an increase in passive mechanical resistive torque in response to stretching of the connective tissues in and around an involved joint complex, a condition that contributes to joint stiffness resulting in range of motion (ROM) loss. Clinically, *flexibility* is defined as the ROM around a joint. Research suggests that flexibility decreases with age (approximately 20% to 30% between 30 to 70 years of age).[46] This may make it harder for the masters athlete to adequately move easily into ranges required for his or her desired sports activity.

Clinical Point

Flexibility decreases approximately 20% to 30% between 30 and 70 years of age.

In summary, the sports medicine professional needs to have a basic understanding of the senescent changes that occur in the injured masters athlete. The challenge to the clinician is to determine how these changes may influence clinical decision making. A general understanding of the age-related physiological changes that occur in the masters athlete is necessary for the design and implementation of effective therapeutic interventions in this special population.

Osteoarthritis and the Masters Athlete

OA affects more than 20 million individuals in the United States. This figure is expected to double during the next two decades. Based on radiographic criteria, OA occurs in 30% of affected individuals aged 45 to 65 years and in more than 80% by their eighth decade of life, although many individuals are asymptomatic.[47] The likelihood of developing OA increases with age and the disease is equally common among men and women aged 45 to 55 years. After age 55 years, the disease becomes more common in women. OA is a disease process that causes progressive hyaline articular cartilage loss and may cause underlying bone to develop outgrowths (osteophytes) and bony sclerosis.[48-50]

OA is categorized as either *primary* or *secondary*. Primary OA has an unknown cause and is thought to lead to joint destruction caused by an articular cartilage defect, whereas secondary OA is thought to occur as a result of previous trauma, hemarthrosis, infection, osteonecrosis, or some other condition.[51] The pathological process of OA generally results in the following characteristics: (1) erosion of hyaline articular cartilage covering long bones; (2) sclerosis, or thickening, of bone under articular cartilage in an attempt at a reparative process, (3) formation of bone spurs or osteophytes (Figure 29-2).[28,52]

Knee Osteoarthritis

OA of the knee is known to cause more symptoms and disability than OA affecting any other joint in the body.[53,54] Approximately 80% of those with knee OA will develop a varus deformity caused by medial joint compartment narrowing, with the remaining patients demonstrating a valgus knee angulation (~5% to 10%) or no angulation (~5% to 10%).[55] Many masters athletes have secondary knee OA because of ligamentous, cartilage or bone injuries received when participating in sports at a younger age. Several studies have shown a substantial increased risk of knee OA in individuals with a history of anterior cruciate ligament rupture, meniscal tears, and fractures.[56-61] Given the increased participation in

varsity sports by today's boys and girls, it is commonplace for several athletes each year to have a significant ligament injury requiring surgery. Although many of these athletes are able to return to their sports, few clinicians take into consideration the future risk of OA in these athletes.

Imaging of Knee Osteoarthritis

The primary means of evaluation of OA is plain-film radiography. However, a strong correlation between radiographic severity and loss of function has not been shown. According to Moskowitz,[62] arthritis is demonstrated in 90% of the population by the age of 40 when viewing weightbearing joints such as knees, hips, and ankles. What complicates this picture is that many of these individuals may show evidence of OA on a radiograph, but have absolutely minimal or no symptoms. Often there is a poor correlation between pain and actual structural damage.[63] Some of this disparity may be due to the fact that radiographs do not image synovitis or bone marrow edema.[64] Bedson and Croft[65] reported several other reasons for this disparity between radiograph evidence and function, including (1) insufficient radiographic views to estimate the association between degeneration and pain, (2) the wide variation in definitions of *pain* that may result in discrepancy between the score and the amount of evidence of OA, and (3) the nature of the study population. Therefore, the prevalence of OA, when

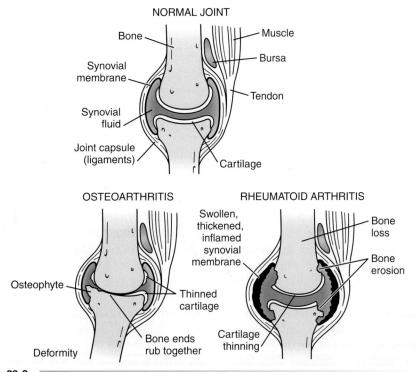

Figure 29-2

Typical osteoarthritic changes that may occur with advancing age. Severe erosion of articular cartilage results in bone on bone, altered biomechanics at the joint, an increase in joint friction or resistance to movement, and frequently pain and swelling. (From Brown M: Effects of aging-growth changes and lifespan concerns (40+). In Magee DJ, Zachazewski JE, Quillen WS, editors: Scientific Foundations and Principles of Practice in Musculoskeletal Rehabilitation, p 307, St. Louis, 2007, Saunders.)

assessed by radiographs, may be much higher than those actually experiencing pain and disability.[66] Knee-specific OA has been shown to be present more often when both patellofemoral and tibiofemoral joints are affected, creating more pain.[67]

One of the major diagnostic criteria for arthritis is the symptom of joint pain. Articular cartilage itself is not innervated, so where is the pain coming from? The general consensus is that the pain is a result of inflammation of the synovium, medullary hypertension, microfractures of the underlying subchondral bone, stretching of periosteal nerve endings caused by sclerosis, osteophyte formation, or excessive stretching of ligaments and spasm of muscles surrounding the affected joint.[68] Symptoms of OA include pain and stiffness in and around the joint, osteophyte formation, cartilage degeneration, joint malalignment, weightbearing difficulty, muscle spasm, weakness, and ROM loss.

Radiographic Evidence of Osteoarthritis[68]

- Decreased joint space (cartilage degeneration)
- Sclerosis of subchondral bone
- Osteophyte formation at joint margins
- Subchondral cyst formation
- Genu varum or valgum joint deformity

Rehabilitation Exercises for Knee Osteoarthritis

Rehabilitation for those with lower-extremity OA should include all facets of training including flexibility, mobility, muscle strengthening, endurance training, and cardiovascular training. Consideration of each of these training aspects is critical when designing a rehabilitation plan of care for the aging athlete.

The goals of any specific rehabilitation program should depend on the individual athlete's specific needs. For the aging athlete, this includes ROM, strengthening, and endurance training. Lower-extremity strength training allows the muscular system to work to attenuate impact loads, provide needed joint stability, and support independent function.[69] The American College of Sports Medicine has determined several specific muscle groups that should be emphasized with a strengthening program for older adults to maintain independence in ADLs. These muscle groups include the hip extensors, knee extensors, ankle plantar flexors, and ankle dorsiflexors.[9] Exercises for these muscle groups should be done at functional speeds and using functional patterns specific to the athlete's needs.[70-72]

There appears to be significant consensus with respect to the efficacy of exercise in the case of knee OA.[73-78] Because ROM of affected joints may be limited due to pain, muscle spasm, or soft tissue contractures, motion and flexibility

exercises are a crucial part of any program for those with OA. Although joints should never be passively forced through a range, gentle ROM, joint mobilizations, and stretching exercises should be performed with each exercise session.[79-81]

Both loss of knee flexion and extension can be affected in knee OA, although knee flexion is usually limited to a greater degree. The restoration of full extension is critical for the establishment of a normal gait pattern and an adequate of flexion is needed for sport-specific activities. Although the masters athlete with knee OA may only complain about knee pain and loss of motion, the clinician needs to consider loss of mobility of the entire trunk and lower extremity. Examining mobility of the lumbar spine, hip, ankle, and foot is an important part of the physical examination of a masters athlete with knee pain. Limitations in the lumbopelvic or lower-extremity kinetic chain may need to be addressed.[80,81]

Mobilization techniques specific to the knee include dorsal and anterior glides of the tibia on the femur; medial and lateral rotation of the tibia on the femur; and superior, inferior, and lateral patellofemoral glides. For masters athletes with restricted motion at the knee or hip, combining a home exercise program with skilled manual therapy appears to work best. Deyle and colleagues[79,82] determined that providing a home program in addition to manual therapy was more effective in increasing overall function, decreasing pain and stiffness, and requiring less medication use at a 1-year follow-up. In this study, clinicians were encouraged to evaluate and treat any ROM limitations in the lumbar spine, hip, ankle or foot if it was believed that this would improve knee function.[79,82] A more recent study has shown that the pain-pressure threshold was significantly increased following anterior and posterior glide tibiofemoral joint mobilizations as compared with manual contact or no contact.[83] For more information on this topic, see Chapter 27, "Physical Rehabilitation After Total Knee Arthroplasty," in *Pathology and Interventions in Musculoskeletal Rehabilitation*, Volume 3 of this series.

Unloading Braces and Insoles for Knee Osteoarthritis

The majority of knee OA affects the medial compartment of the knee, which bears greater than 60% of the load during weightbearing.[84-86] As the medial joint compartment becomes more arthritic, a loss of medial joint space is observed on radiographs and eventually visually, with the patient exhibiting a varus or bowlegged knee deformity. To offset or "unload" the medial compartment, especially during physical activity, two biomechanical interventions have been suggested.

A specialized "counterforce" knee brace may be custom fit to the patient. Typically, the athlete is measured and then the brace is made with an intrinsic valgus correction of 2° to 3°. Often, via a small hex wrench or key, the athlete can increase the valgus force by several additional degrees. This allows some individual customization of the brace during different physical activities. Biomechanical analysis has shown that wearing a valgus unloading brace can alter pain, joint position sense, strength, and function in the older athlete.[87-90] The hypothesis surrounding the brace effectiveness has been the fact that if a brace can place the knee with medial joint space narrowing in neutral or a slight valgus alignment, normal biomechanical loading may be restored. In addition, recent evidence appears to illustrate that pain relief may also be a result from diminished muscle co-contractions rather than from so-called medial compartment unloading.[91] Using a knee unloading brace is not always feasible in the older athlete with knee OA. Custom unloading braces are very expensive and often are not fully covered by insurance. Other comorbidities, body size, and body shape may also prohibit the success of an unloading brace. In addition, prolonged brace wear can cause skin breakdown and leg pain. Empirically, it appears the unloading brace works best for the athlete who can wear the brace for his or her desired athletic activity, but does not necessarily need it for ADLs.

As an adjunct or as an alternative, the clinician may consider the use of a laterally wedged insole for the masters athlete with medial compartment knee OA. For this to be effective, the athlete cannot have significant ankle instability. Too much ankle laxity will result in any changes made at the rearfoot not being transmitted up the kinetic chain. Are lateral insoles effective? Using insoles to statically alter the knee in a more upright position by placing the calcaneus in a position of valgus, Sasaki[84,85] and Yasuda reduced the mechanical load on the medial joint surface. These two studies and others illustrate that a laterally wedged insole may be effective in reducing pain and improving function in individuals with medial compartment OA.[92-97] This insole research has yielded some interesting findings. At present, it appears that a laterally wedged, full-length orthotic is more effective than a heel wedge alone,[92-94] that the wedged insole should not be used with heeled footwear,[98] and that having the patient self-select wedge size based on numeric pain ratings before and after wedge use is best.[97] An additional benefit of using a wedged insole is that it is significantly less expensive than a custom unloading brace. Further research is needed to identify which individuals would benefit from an unloading brace and a wedged insole.

Viscosupplementation Therapy in Knee Osteoarthritis

Many palliative treatments in the form of viscosupplementation have become available to help reduce symptoms associated with articular cartilage degradation. These come in the form of intra-articular injections with hyaluronic acid. Hyaluronic acid is a normal component of synovial fluid, which bathes the articular surfaces of the normal knee. In an arthritic knee, this molecule is depleted by a factor of 2 or 3 because of dehydration and dilution.[99] Recommended injection schedules depend on preparations used. For Hylan G-F 20, an injection weekly for 3 weeks is recommended, whereas for sodium hyaluronan, the recommended dosage is an injection weekly for 3 to 5 weeks.[99] Most of the clinical studies on the use of injectable hyaluronic acid are inconsistent. Early studies demonstrated relief of symptoms and benefit from this form of treatment,[100-103] although others did not.[104,105] Problems abound with these early studies including heterogenicity of patient populations, different formulations of injected preparations, and different treatment regimens.[99]

Despite these problems in research methodology, several meta-analyses indicate that viscosupplementation has a therapeutic effect on pain, function, and patient global assessment.[106-108] A limitation of these multiple studies is that, to date, the effect of a placebo response on study participants has not been fully analyzed and that adverse effects of the injections have been reported.[109]

One of the problems with use of injectable viscosupplementation is the accurate placement of intra-articular needle. Jackson and colleagues,[110] using fluoroscopic confirmation of needle position, found that accurate placement was very difficult. When using an anterolateral approach, only 71% of injections were performed in the correct position. Injection site pain and discomfort is another common complication seen with injectable hyaluronate. Although hyaluronate injections are used frequently when treating symptoms of OA, the potentially high placebo effect with the use of hyaluronate injections warrants further study before the true efficacy of this intervention can be determined.

Hip Osteoarthritis

The most common predisposing factor for hip OA is age.[111-113] Hip arthritis is common and occurs in up to 4% to 6% of the population.[114] Risk factors for hip OA include systemic issues such as ethnicity, age, gender, hormonal status, genetics, bone density, and nutrition. Local biomechanical risk factors include joint injury, obesity, occupation, sports participation, physical activity, altered joint biomechanics, and muscle weakness.[115] Hip OA is more common in laborers than those with sedentary jobs. This probably is accounted for by stress caused by heavy lifting and carrying in those occupations.[114,116-118] Previous hip injury is also associated with hip OA.[110,118] Cooper and colleagues[119] reported that the odds ratio for hip OA when having a previous hip injury as 4.3 (95%, confidence interval 2.2-8.4). In addition, patients with OA of one hip are at increased risk of developing OA in the opposite hip.[120] A masters athlete's previous occupation may determine his or her risk of hip OA. Numerous studies in Europe and the United States have found a higher prevalence of hip OA in men whose occupation involves repetitive lifting of heavy loads.[121-124] Suspected occupational risk factors for hip OA have been suggested, including regular heavy lifting, operating machinery, and walking on uneven ground.[124-131]

One of the problems in diagnosing hip OA is that symptoms can be vague and not localized solely to the hip region. As other areas afflicted with OA, the severity of OA in the hip may not exactly correlate with the degree of damage seen radiographically. Pain and symptoms associated with hip OA tend to be of much greater degree than radiographic evidence seems to justify, whereas symptoms may also be moderate in the presence of severe radiographic changes.

In hip OA, the entire joint structure and function is affected with joint capsular changes (shortening and lengthening) along with subsequent articular cartilage degeneration.[132] Later in the disease process, osteophytes or bone spurs may develop from excessive tensile force on the hip joint capsule or from abnormal pressure on the articular cartilage.[132,133] Other changes also develop, including sclerosis of the subchondral bone from increased focal pressure, and in some cases, cyst formation.[134] Muscle weakness often develops around the hip joint with OA,[135] specifically the abductor muscles in the hip.[136] The hip abductor weakness progressively weakens in the later stages of hip OA, which may create a Trendelenburg gait pattern.[137]

Recently, several studies have found an association between acetabular labral tears and the early onset of hip OA.[138-140] This is important to understand as the aging athlete may have had previous injuries or lower-level symptoms of hip discomfort that may have gone on for years without formal treatment.

Rehabilitation of Hip Osteoarthritis

Rehabilitation for hip OA includes therapeutic exercise and manual therapy. Manual therapy techniques may be beneficial for those with restricted hip capsular mobility. Hoeksma and colleagues[141] performed a clinical trial assessing the effectiveness of manual therapy compared with exercise therapy in those with hip OA. Successful outcomes were found in 81% of those receiving manual therapy compared with only 50% in the exercise group. Positive effects related to improvements of pain, hip function, and ROM lasted up to 29 weeks.

Evidence shows that those with hip OA have limitation in strength of the hip musculature and limitations in ROM as compared with those with no hip problems.[137,142] One of the earliest signs of hip OA is restriction of hip ROM. Altman and colleagues have described hip flexion of 115° or less and medial rotation less than 15° to be prevalent in patients with hip OA.[112] Birrell and colleagues have noted that an increased number of restricted planes of ROM increases the specificity of ruling in hip OA as the actual diagnosis.[143] Therefore, the mainstay of conservative treatment must include increasing limited motion and strength. Limitations in rotation can be restored by use of joint mobilization and passive stretching of the hip musculature. If these limitations

are simply from disuse and are from muscle-tendon unit shortening, passive stretching should suffice. This is likely not the case in the masters athlete. If, however, these limitations are from hip capsular attenuation, joint mobilizations may be more beneficial. Joint mobilization techniques may be required in all planes, but most commonly will involve increasing hip flexion and hip medial rotation in those with hip OA.

Although evidence for the use of manual therapy for hip OA is limited, there are several studies that do support its use. Hoeksma and colleagues demonstrated the superiority of manual therapy plus exercise over exercise in isolation for hip OA.[141] Furthermore, a case series from MacDonald and coauthors described outcomes of individual patients treated with manual physical therapy and exercise for hip OA.[144] This case series reported reductions in pain and an increase in hip ROM in subjects with hip OA.

Proximal stability of the hip is required for almost all weightbearing activities. Studies indicate that patients with hip OA have decreased strength compared with nonarthritic control subjects.[137,145] Initial exercises can begin in the hook lying position because of the effects of gravity and pain that could occur with full weightbearing. Once exercises are tolerated in hook lying, advancement to progressive resistive exercises via machine weights or isotonic exercises may commence.

Does Running Increase the Risk of Hip or Knee Osteoarthritis in the Masters Athlete?

Many have questioned if running can increase the risk of hip and knee OA. Multiple studies have attempted to answer this question. Some studies have reported that running, especially in excess, does increase the risk of OA.[146,147] Other investigations have shown no influence of distance running on OA.[148-150] In several studies, moderate distance running has been reported to perhaps have a protective effect in preventing the development of hip OA.[151,152] At present, the preponderance of data seems to indicate that long-distance running in moderation does not appear to increase the risk of hip or knee OA in healthy individuals and that running may even have a protective effect on the risk of OA. Previous trauma to the hip or knee, whether the result of injury or overuse, excessive running above the individual's physical threshold, and intrinsic anatomical instability in the joints may accelerate the onset of OA. The clinician should weigh the risks of running against the cardiovascular and musculoskeletal benefits of running.

Surgical Treatment for Hip Osteoarthritis

Surgical treatment for hip OA includes but is not limited to arthroscopic or open procedures. Arthroscopic surgery is less invasive and is indicated for pathological conditions of the hip such as symptomatic tears of the labrum, ligamentum teres injuries, snapping hip syndrome, and removal of loose bodies. Open procedures commonly performed include a variety of total hip arthroplasty (THA) treatments. With advances in surgical techniques and high-performance prosthetic components, many aging athletes are able to return to an acceptable level of sports both recreational and competitive following THA. For more information on this topic see Chapter 26, "Physical Rehabilitation After Total Hip Arthroplasty," in *Pathology and Intervention in Musculoskeletal Rehabilitation*, Volume 3 in this series.

Glenohumeral Osteoarthritis

In addition to weightbearing joints, OA affects the shoulder in an estimated 20% of the elder population.[153] This rate is well below that of other locations in the body, but its effects appear to be just as debilitating and are a common cause of depression, anxiety, activity limitations, and job performance decrements.[154] Treating glenohumeral arthritis in the masters athlete requires providing adequate pain relief and restoration of ROM and function. Full-thickness articular cartilage defects in the shoulder have limited capacity to heal.[155] Multiple causes of articular cartilage abnormalities in the glenohumeral joint occur and include avascular necrosis, chondrolysis, idiopathic focal defects, OA, osteochondritis dissecans, postsurgical cartilage abnormalities (iatrogenic injuries and post-traumatic defects).[155-157] Numerous risk factors abound for shoulder OA and include age, genetics, sex, weight, joint infection, history of shoulder dislocation, previous injury, overhead sports, or heavy labor.[158] Similar to the knee, OA of the shoulder can occur as either a primary or secondary process. Although primary OA of the shoulder occurs as a gradual onset of pain, athletes may remember an inciting event or injury that created symptoms. Secondary OA occurs as the result of some trauma or damage to the glenohumeral joint. Degeneration of the glenohumeral joint is a difficult condition for the masters athlete. This is especially true of athletes who participate in overhead sports such as baseball, tennis, swimming, or volleyball. However, competitors in cycling, football, basketball, and soccer may also find themselves with severe post-traumatic, postreconstruction, or primary cartilage loss in their shoulders. Unfortunately, this may lead to impeded performance in these elder athletes.

Shoulder OA presents as a gradual onset of pain, crepitus with decreased motion in those older than 50 years of age who may have a history of previous shoulder surgery.[159] Classic signs and symptoms include pain, weakness, and limited shoulder lateral rotation secondary to anterior soft tissue contracture.[160] Rotator cuff integrity may be difficult to determine in the presence of pain, and this can make an exact diagnosis difficult. Diagnostic imaging reveals joint space narrowing, humeral osteophytes, and posterior subluxation of the humeral head.[161,162]

Secondary OA from trauma in the shoulder is often due to history of dislocation or subluxation. During a subluxation or dislocation, excessive forces may be imparted to the cartilage of the humeral head and glenoid fossa. Depending on the mechanism of injury, the result may be either a classical Hill-Sachs lesion or, if dislocated posteriorly, a reverse Hill-Sachs lesion. These injuries can cause articular cartilage to disrupt from bone or cause an osteochondral compression defect. Recent evidence concludes that arthritic changes after a dislocation are due to the age of the patient, the time of insult, and the span of time between insult and treatment after injury.[163,164] Primary OA of the shoulder is generally due to more chronic causes such as rotator cuff disease. Up to 76% of patients with cartilage lesions of the shoulder have associated rotator cuff degeneration or tears, whereas only 19% of subjects without cartilage problems experience rotator cuff degeneration or tears.[157] This is probably caused by progressive wear and the fact that the rotator cuff tendons have areas of reduced blood supply, making them more vulnerable to degeneration with increased age.[165] As with treatment of knee and hip OA, there are several medical treatment options, including rehabilitation, supplementation, medicine, and surgery. At present, there is no way in which the natural progression of OA can be altered.

Rehabilitation Interventions for Shoulder Osteoarthritis

Rehabilitation depends on whether the OA is treated conservatively or following surgical procedures. Conservative treatment of shoulder OA begins with activity modification and pain control, followed by progressive ROM and strengthening exercises. Pain reduction can be attempted through the use of numerous modalities. Limited evidence exists regarding the best modality for glenohumeral OA. Moist heat and electrical stimulation may help alleviate symptoms, but is generally not long lasting. Use of these modalities may allow soft tissue relaxation, allowing more ease with obtaining or regaining valuable shoulder ROM. Although ROM of the shoulder is important, clinicians must remember that the patient's arthritic glenohumeral joint surfaces may not be congruent. Aggressive attempts at increasing ROM may exacerbate an already irritated condition. Therefore, working within a pain-free motion may be more beneficial.[166] Because shoulder joint stiffness is a poor prognostic indicator for surgical outcomes, its avoidance should be adequately addressed in conservative rehabilitation.[160]

Strengthening within the nonpainful range of shoulder motion is beneficial as some physiological overflow may occur. Particular emphasis on the rotator cuff muscles and scapular stabilizers is important because these muscles provide a strong foundation on which upper-extremity movement can occur. Because some of these patients may have chronic rotator cuff arthropathy, strength gains may be minimal or slow at best. Conservative treatments should be exhausted before attempts at surgery are considered. For more information on this topic, see Chapter 25, "Shoulder Arthroplasty," in *Pathology and Intervention in Musculoskeletal Rehabilitation*, Volume 3 in this series.

Surgical Treatments for Glenohumeral Osteoarthritis

Surgical intervention of glenohumeral OA includes arthroscopic debridement, capsular release, glenoidplasty, corrective osteotomies, and interposition arthroplasty. In younger, active patients aged 55 to 60 with moderate pain and associated motion restrictions, arthroscopic debridement with a capsular release may provide significant improvement. The debridement component of surgery will clean out the joint, removing loose bodies, cartilage flaps, or fraying. The capsular release can restore joint mobility and unload the articular joint surfaces of the humeral head. Older patients with more severe joint destruction may require a shoulder arthroplasty because of pain and loss of function that was not corrected by conservative means. If both the glenoid and the humeral head have seen destruction, a total joint arthroplasty is performed, and when only the humeral head has been damaged, a hemiarthroplasty is the treatment of choice.

Osteochondral allograft and autograft procedures have been used predominantly in the knee and hip for years. Recent surgical advances have allowed use of osteochondral allografting and autografting, which may prove to be a beneficial form of surgical treatment for glenohumeral OA.[167-169]

Although OA is known to be a painful joint condition that limits an athlete's function, conservative treatment methods and selected surgical alternatives can be used judiciously in an effort to help active older adults to maintain a healthy lifestyle. Although at times expectations for activities and specific sports participation may need to be adjusted, most can still participate in active sports recreationally and at times even competitively.

Tendinopathy in the Masters Athlete

Primary disorders of tendons are common and constitute a high proportion of referrals of the sports medicine clinician. Certain tendons are particularly vulnerable to degenerative pathological conditions; these include the Achilles,[170] patella,[171] proximal or high hamstring,[172] gluteus medius,[173] rotator cuff,[174] and common wrist flexor and extensor tendons.[175] It is important to note that both high hamstring and gluteus medius tendinopathy are often misdiagnosed as piriformis syndrome or trochanteric bursitis respectively.[172,173] The sports medicine–trained clinician should be aware of this as misdiagnosis can prevent the masters athlete from receiving the appropriate treatment in a timely manner.

Tendon pain is a common condition in the masters athlete and can cause lasting disability. Significant advances have been made in understanding the pathophysiological characteristics of these conditions. Histopathological evidence, together with advances in imaging techniques, has made clinicians more appreciative of the degenerative nature of these conditions. Traditionally, treatments have placed a heavy emphasis on anti-inflammatory strategies, which are often inappropriate. Recently, however, significant advances in the practical management of tendon disorders have been made. In particular, the advent of "eccentric loading" training programs has revolutionized the treatment of Achilles and patellar tendinopathy in some athletes.

Tendonitis versus Tendinosis and Tendinopathy

It is common practice among health care professionals to use the term *tendinitis* indiscriminately to describe all pathological conditions of the tendon. However, the suffix *-itis* is a Greek element used to denote inflammation. Multiple histopathological studies have indicated that the pathological process in most painful tendons is degenerative rather than inflammatory.[176-179] Accordingly, use of the term *tendinitis* appears to be inappropriate in most cases when describing the pathological condition underlying tendon pain. Several experts have suggested that the term *tendinitis* be abandoned in favor of the term *tendinosis,* which describes a degenerative tendon condition.[178-180] This distinction regarding pathological conditions of the tendon was first described by Puddu and colleagues[181] with regard to classifying Achilles tendon pain. Fredberg[179] challenged the concept of tendon pain as primarily a degenerative condition, suggesting that a lack of inflammatory cells may not mean the lack of an inflammatory process. To definitively distinguish between *-itis* and *-osis,* the diseased tissue must be biopsied and subjected to histopathological testing. Given that such histological studies are not common clinical practice, it is most appropriate for the sports medicine clinician to describe tendon pain as *tendinopathy.*

Tendon Pain

A significant challenge in providing intervention to patients with tendinopathy or fasciopathy is in understanding the potential sources of pain. In the traditional histopathological model, tendon pain was considered an inflammatory problem, hence the term *tendinitis.* However, as previously discussed, there is a lack of inflammatory cells in chronically painful tendons; this observation applies not only to the Achilles tendon, but to other problematic tendons including the patellar, rotator cuff, and wrist extensor tendons.[180] There is some evidence that there may be a neurochemical aspect of tendinopathy pain. Alfredson and Lorentzon[177] found higher concentrations of glutamate in painful tendons, including Achilles tendon, extensor carpi radialis brevis tendon, and patellar tendon, and reported the presence of glutamate receptor sites in nerve endings associated with painful tendons. Using immunohistochemical analyses of painful Achilles tendons, Schubert and colleagues[182] found sprouting of substance P–positive nerve fibers, which may explain the transmission of the tendon pain.

Historically, the mechanical model of tendon pain has implicated that pain is a consequence of repetitive loading of the tendon, resulting in collagen disruption.[183] In the past decade, several imaging studies have seriously questioned this model. First, studies on patellar tendons[184-187] and Achilles tendons[170] have shown that the tendon can be partially disrupted without pain, or painful without disruption.[188,189] Other research on pathological conditions of the tendon at the shoulder and ankle has found the location of a pathological tendon condition is not in the region subjected to the highest tensile forces, but rather in a region of relative stress shielding where tensile forces are lower.[190,191] These findings are inconsistent with a model that describes excessive tensile forces as a primary stimulus for pathological conditions of the tendon. To explore new avenues of examination and intervention for tendinopathy, clinicians must recognize that research findings are contrary to a traditional view of pathological conditions of the tendon as inflammatory conditions caused by repetitive tensile stress on the tendon. If we continue to allow such a traditional view to persist, attempts to relieve tensile stress or reduce inflammation will continue to result in frustration for clinicians and patients alike.

Treatment of Tendinopathy in the Masters Athlete

Management of tendinopathy should address both intrinsic and extrinsic factors identified in the physical examination. Correction of training errors, cross-training, and active rest are common recommendations made in the early stages of rehabilitation. A multitude of treatment interventions exist for treating tendinopathy, although more research is necessary to determine their efficacy and effectiveness.

Manual Therapy for Tendinopathy

There are several manual therapies popular in the treatment of tendon disorders, the two most common being friction massage and augmented soft tissue mobilization (ASTM). Made popular by Cyriax, deep transverse friction massage (DTFM) is a part of many clinical tendinopathy programs. A Cochrane review in 2002[192] examined the available evidence for DTFM. There were only two randomized controlled trials of sufficient quality to be included: one on the treatment of lateral epicondylalgia and the other on the iliotibial band syndrome. Neither of these two trials demonstrated a lasting benefit versus the control group for either pain or functional status.[192] Therefore, at present, no conclusions can be drawn concerning the use or nonuse of DTFM for the treatment of tendinopathy. A second popular technique is that of ASTM.[193,194] This is an intervention that involves the use of ergonomically designed instruments that theoretically assist clinicians in treatment of areas exhibiting excessive soft tissue fibrosis.[195,196] Following each ASTM treatment, the patient completes a stretching and strengthening program. Both DTFM and ASTM are thought to stimulate blood supply in the vicinity of the tendinopathy and this is thought to promote healing of the affected tendon. However, studies in this area are lacking and currently no high-quality evidence exists for or against the use of these two manual therapy interventions for treatment of tendinopathy.

Eccentric Training for Tendinopathy

One of the most exciting outcomes of tendinopathy research has been the positive findings of eccentric exercise as a treatment for chronic tendinopathy. Eccentric loading exercises involve active lengthening of the muscle tendon unit. Eccentric training as a treatment for chronic tendinopathy is not a new concept.[197,198] The original Achilles tendinopathy eccentric exercise protocol published by Stanish and colleagues[198] in 1986 has been expanded and improved. In the protocol by Alfredson and colleagues,[199] the patient groups were required to perform three sets of 15 repetitions of eccentric heel lowering at a slow speed with the knee straight and bent, twice per day for 12 weeks. The control group was required to perform concentric exercises (active shortening of the muscle tendon unit). As opposed to performing pain-free eccentric heel lowering per the original Stanish protocol,[198] in the Alfredson protocol, resistance was increased to the point at which performance of the exercise became painful but not disabling. The subjects were instructed to increase the resistance used once the exercise became pain-free. High levels of patient satisfaction were seen in the eccentric loading groups (82%) and all 12 participants returned to their sports activities. In subsequent long-term follow-up (mean 3.8 years) Alfredson and co-workers have confirmed both the initial good results and a statistically significant reduction of tendon thickening and resolved neovasculation.[200,201] One problem with the Alfredson protocol was that it was less successful for patients with insertional Achilles tendinopathy.[202] Initially, it was thought that this was because of differences in pathological conditions; however, this appears to be untrue.[203] Jonsson and colleagues have reported that modifying the Alfredson protocol by performing the eccentric Achilles exercises on the floor instead of off a step improves success in those with insertional Achilles tendinopathy.[204] These researchers hypothesize that the avoidance of excessive passive dorsiflexion in weightbearing prevents soft tissue impingement between tendon, bursa, and bone at the calcaneal tendon. In addition, investigators have determined that the need to avoid sports activity during eccentric training for Achilles tendinopathy is not necessary. Silbernagel and colleagues investigated whether any difference in outcomes could be found between those subjects who rested and those who continued their sports activity.[205] The exercise training group was allowed, with the use of a pain-monitoring model, to continue Achilles tendon–loading activity, such as running and jumping, whereas the active rest group had to stop such activities during the first 6 weeks. No negative effects could be demonstrated from continuing Achilles tendon–loading activity, with the use of a pain-monitoring model, during treatment.[205] This is important as it allows the clinician, with some confidence, to permit loading activity during rehabilitation. This may allow better adherence to the rehabilitation program by the athlete if he or she does not feel that the health professional is taking away the desired activity. The eccentric training program described by Silbernagel and colleagues is shown in Box 29-1.[205]

The success of eccentric training for Achilles tendinopathy has fostered efforts to determine whether eccentric training will work for other tendinopathies. Two small studies on the use of eccentric exercises on a decline board for treatment of patella tendinopathy have shown positive results.[206,207] A pilot study has also been performed showing some positive results using eccentric exercises in patients with supraspinatus tendinopathy.[208] Despite these promising results, questions remain.[209] Why eccentric training appears to work is uncertain. The eccentric programs also seem to be of more benefit for active individuals.[200] These programs require highly motivated people (e.g., the masters athlete) who are also willing to perform multiple repetitions, twice daily, 7 days a week for 12 weeks, and this will not suit all patients. Although results appear promising, future research is still needed to support the use of eccentric exercise in the management of tendinopathy.

Injection Therapy for Tendinopathy

A systematic review of corticosteroid injection for lateral epicondylalgia found a total of 12 trials suitable for analysis. The review authors concluded that corticosteroid injection was effective in the short term (2 to 6 weeks) but that in the long term, there was no difference in outcome when compared with those not receiving injections.[210,211] There are several case reports of tendon rupture following corticosteroid injection,[212-215] particularly involving the Achilles tendon.[214,215] Because of the concerns surrounding tendon integrity following steroid injection, the mounting evidence shows that the use of intratendinous injections is contraindicated. In contrast, evidence surrounding peritendinous

---

Box 29-1 Silbernagel's Achilles Tendinopathy Protocol

Phase 1: Weeks 1 to 2

Patient Status: Pain and difficulty with all activities, difficulty performing 10 one-legged toe raises

Goal: Start to exercise, gain understanding of the injury and of the pain-monitoring model

Treatment Program: Perform exercises daily
- Pain monitoring model information and advice on exercise activity
- Circulation exercises (moving foot up and down)
- Two-legged toe raises standing on the floor (three sets × 10-15 repetitions per set)
- One-legged toe raises standing on the floor (3 × 10)
- Sitting toe raises (3 × 10)
- Eccentric toe raises standing on the floor (3 × 10)

Phase 2: Weeks 2 to 5

Patient Status: Pain with exercise, morning stiffness, pain when performing toe raises

Goal: Start strengthening

Treatment Program: Perform exercises daily
- Two-legged toe raises standing on edge of stair (3 × 15)
- One-legged toe raises standing on edge of stair (3 × 15)
- Sitting toe raises (3 × 15)
- Eccentric toe raises standing on edge of stair (3 × 15)
- Quick-rebounding toe raises (3 × 20)

Phase 3: Weeks 3 to 12 (longer if needed)

Patient Status: Handled the phase 2 exercise program, no pain distally in tendon insertion, possibly decreased or increased morning stiffness

Goal: Heavier strength training, increase or start running or jumping activity

Treatment Program: Perform exercises daily and with heavier load two to three times per week
- One-legged toe raises standing on edge of stair with added weight (3 × 15)
- Sitting toe raises (3 × 15)
- Eccentric toe raises standing on edge of stair with added weight (3 × 15)
- Quick-rebounding toe raises (3 × 20)
- Plyometric training

Phase 4: Week 12 to 6 Months (longer if needed)

Patient Status: Minimal symptoms, morning stiffness not every day, can participate in sports without difficulty

Goal: Maintenance exercise, no symptoms

Treatment Program: Perform exercises two to three times per week
- One-legged toe raises standing on edge of stair with added weight (3 × 15)
- Eccentric toe raises standing on edge of stair with added weight (3 × 15)
- Quick-rebounding toe raises (3 × 20)
- One-legged toe raises standing on edge of stair with added weight (3 × 15)
- Eccentric toe raises standing on edge of stair with added weight (3 × 15)
- Quick-rebounding toe raises (3 × 20)

From Silbernagel KG, Thomeé R, Eriksson BI, Karlsson J: Continued sports activity, using a pain-monitoring model, during rehabilitation in patients with Achilles tendinopathy: A randomized controlled study, *Am J Sports Med* 35(6):897-906, 2007.

steroid injections is lacking, and at present no recommendations for or against their use can be made.

In contrast to corticosteroid injections, four other injection therapies are currently being used in the treatment of tendinopathy. These are prolotherapy,[216-218] sclerosing polidocanol,[219-222] autologous whole-blood and platelet-rich plasma (PRP) injections.[223-227] Prolotherapy (proliferative injection therapy) involves injecting an inactive irritant solution into the tendon for the purpose of strengthening weakened connective tissue and alleviating musculoskeletal pain. Although several injection agents have been used, hyperosmolar dextrose and morrhuate sodium are the most common.[216-218] Polidocanol is a vascular sclerosant. In treating tendinopathy, it is used to sclerose areas of high intratendinous blood flow. These areas of high blood flow, or neovascularity, are thought to be associated with the underlying mechanism of lateral epicondylalgia and other overuse tendinopathies.[219-222] Autologous whole blood and the blood product PRP have been used as injectants for tendinopathy with the aim of promoting (via cellular mediators) healing in areas of tendon degeneration. PRP is prepared from autologous whole blood, which is centrifuged to concentrate platelets in plasma. It is thought that the platelet-derived growth factors in the PRP may improve soft tissue healing within the damaged tendon.[223-227] Unlike steroid injections, these injections theoretically try to address the new model of tendinopathy as being a pathological entity without inflammation. Despite initial positive results in pilot studies, these new injection therapies need further analysis. Rigorous controlled studies of sufficient sample size with validated patient reported outcome and radiological measures are needed to determine long-term effectiveness and safety, and whether these techniques can play a definitive role in the management of tendinopathy.[227]

Topical Glyceryl Trinitrate for Tendinopathy

One group of researchers has recently completed several randomized controlled trials examining the effect of topical glyceryl trinitrate in the treatment of Achilles, wrist extensor, and supraspinatus tendinopathies.[228-231] These researchers have shown long-term benefits of topical glyceryl trinitrate use 3 years after the cessation of therapy.[229] The reasons for these positive findings are uncertain, although current speculation is that the topical gel may cause local vasodilatation that may lead to an increased local blood supply. To be validated clinically, these positive results need to be repeated by other research groups. It is also important to realize that in each of these studies, the use of the topical gel or patch was not done in isolation but rather in addition to eccentric strengthening and stretching.

The practicing sports medicine clinician needs to be aware of the current research investigating manual therapy, eccentric exercise, and injection therapy for the treatment of tendinopathy. Likely a staged, multimodality program is best. However, the most effective tendinopathy treatment algorithm to return the masters athlete to sport remains elusive.

Sports Activity in the Masters Athlete Following Total Joint Arthroplasty

For many masters athletes, joint pain and dysfunction can pose an insurmountable obstacle in their pursuit to continue sports activities. In severe pathological conditions of the joint, total joint arthroplasty offers a viable option to reduce pain and improve function. Although basic functional tasks are often attainable after surgery, restrictions on sporting activity after the procedures remain unclear.

Historically, the medical community has viewed postarthroplasty physical activity with caution. Several studies have implicated heavy or moderate activity to be a cause of surgical revision in joint arthroplasty. Chandler and colleagues[232] reported that 62% of subjects who participated in moderate or heavy activities after a THA displayed increased incidence of prosthetic loosening. Others have found that patients who participated in high-impact activities had the highest rates of revision surgery.[233]

Despite evidence of potential complications, patients with total joint arthroplasty are more commonly pursuing sports activity following surgery. Bradbury and colleagues[234] noted 65% of total knee arthroplasty (TKA) patients returned to sports activities after surgery, although many chose lower-impact and less physically demanding activities. Examples in popular sports culture reveal successful rehabilitation of high-profile sports figures overcoming total joint arthroplasty and returning to competition at the professional level. Professional golfer Jack Nicklaus received a THA in 1999 and returned to the Senior Pro Tour within 4 months. He continued to compete until 2005. Bo Jackson was at the height of his professional baseball and football career when he had a THA in the early 1990s. Jackson returned to play for 2 years of professional baseball before eventually retiring. These athletes have challenged the physical limits after joint arthroplasty and brought notoriety to sports activity following total joint arthroplasty.

Although exceptions do exist, candidates for total joint arthroplasty are generally middle-aged to elderly.[235] Patients in this age group are more susceptible to serious health conditions such as cardiovascular disease, diabetes, and osteoporosis. Physical activity is an important factor in reducing the risk of such diseases. For many adults, participation in various sports and athletic activities offer a vehicle to a healthy lifestyle. Ries and colleagues[236,237] reported improved cardiovascular function in patients who had undergone knee or hip arthroplasty compared with their presurgical status.

Total Hip Arthroplasty

Age and activity level are important aspects to consider when discussing THA. Younger, active individuals may place high demands on the implants and may place themselves at risk for implant failure and subsequent revision. It appears that activity level is the most variable patient-related factor and may explain why some implants last longer.[238] Joint load must be considered when discussing postarthroplasty activity levels with patients. If patients resume activities that place high loads on the joint, wear and tear may increase exponentially.[239,240] Because cardiovascular fitness is an important preventative measure, it is important to determine at what level masters athletes can return to activities that promote this. Speed walking appears to be a good alternative to running, while still providing for cardiovascular fitness. Compressive loads at the hip joint are 4 to 4.5 times the athlete's body weight when power walking.[239] Jogging or running will increase hip joint compressive forces to greater than 5 times the athlete's body weight. Unfortunately, there are many activities without documented evidence on joint forces and loads. Kuster[239] suggests the following guidelines: during daily activities, loads of 3 to 4 times the athlete's body weight may apply; while in sporting activities, loads of 5 to 10 times the athlete's body weight may occur. Other considerations include weight training, which will increase loads, and endurance activities in which load depends on speed.

Clinical Points

Activity level, and type and amount of joint loading are better parameters than age when determining implant longevity following total joint arthroplasty.

Patients who have been active and athletically skilled prior to THA will have the greatest chance for returning to a high level of skilled activity postoperatively. Individuals with increased athletic ability typically display less joint forces than those who are less skilled. Attempting to learn a new athletic skill is unlikely to be successful and may put the patient at risk for injury after surgery.

What specific recommendations exist for returning to exercise and sports activities following total joint arthroplasty? Most literature reviews are based on personal opinion rather than prospective studies. In general, low-impact activities are tolerated well by patients given that forces and wear will be lower relative to high-impact exercise and sport. As impact and torsional loading increase during high-impact sports and exercise, relative risk associated with activity increases as well.[239,241] Surgeons and residents at the Mayo Clinic[242] surveyed themselves and reviewed the literature regarding return to athletics following THA. They determined that orthopedic surgeons should suggest the following low-impact sports to their patients who are interested in returning to sports: sailing, swimming, scuba diving, cycling, golf, and bowling. They advise against high-impact activities such as running, water skiing, football, baseball, basketball, hockey, handball, karate, soccer, and racquetball. In 1999, Healy and colleagues[243] conducted a survey of 54 members of The Hip Society to determine their recommendations for athletics and sport participation following hip arthroplasty surgery. The survey was completed by Society members and they were asked to rate 42 different sports as either recommended or allowed, allowed with experience, no opinion, and not recommended. See Table 29-3 for a list of these activities and recommendations.[243]

Table 29-3
Activities Following Total Hip Arthroplasty—1999 Hip Society Survey

Recommended/Allowed	Allowed with Experience	Not Recommended	No Conclusions Made
Ballroom dancing	Bowling	Baseball/softball	Fencing
Bicycling (stationary)	Bicycling (road)	Basketball	Ice skating
Croquet	Canoeing	Football	Jazz dancing
Doubles tennis	Cross-country skiing	Gymnastics	Square dancing
Golf	Hiking	Handball	
Horseshoes	Horseback riding	High-impact aerobics	
Shooting	Low-impact aerobics	Hockey	
Shuffleboard		Jogging	
Swimming		Lacrosse	
Walking		Racquetball	
		Rock climbing	
		Singles tennis	
		Soccer	
		Squash	
		Volleyball	

Modified from Healy WL, Iorio R, Lemos MJ: Athletic activity after joint replacement, *Am J Sports Med* 29(3):382, 2001.

Golf has been widely studied and the majority of surgeons permit or do not discourage patients to return to golf after THA, but it is recommended that patients use a cart while playing. Mallon and colleagues[244-247] determined that surgeons allow patients to return to golf 19.5 weeks after surgery. Golfers surveyed stated that their driving distance decreased 3.3 yards and their handicap increased by 1.1 strokes after THA. These golfers played an average of 3.7 times per week and were followed for 3 or more years. At an average follow-up time of 61 months, hybrid and uncemented total hip arthroplasties were associated with less loosening as determined by radiograph when compared with cemented total hip arthroplasties. No differences in pain during or after golf were noted.[244-247]

Mont and colleagues[235] evaluated tennis following THA. For 58 tennis players who had 75 THA surgeries, only 14% of the patients stated that their physician approved of their return to tennis. Of these patients, 21% specifically had the surgery to return to tennis and they did so after approximately 7 months. These individuals played three times per week and maintained their presurgical national tennis ranking. Revision was necessary for 4% of these patients at a mean of 8 years after their initial hip arthroplasty.

Healy and colleagues[243] suggest that patient education is crucial when addressing treatment options and expectations regarding return to activity and sport. Emphasizing the importance of previous activity and athletic skill, preoperative rehabilitation, proper choice of components and procedure, adherence to precautions, and surgeon skill and experience on THA outcomes are essential. Setting realistic expectations for return to sport and emphasizing the risks and benefits of specific activities is also important. For the active patient, Healy and his colleagues[243] recommend a cementless acetabular component, a hemispheric titanium porous-coated implant inserted with an under-ream press-fit technique and supplemental screw fixation, with a minimum polyethylene thickness of 6 mm. Femoral components for active patients may be cemented or cementless. For cemented techniques they recommend cobalt-chrome implants with the proper femoral offset for restoration of abductor biomechanics. Second-generation cementing techniques with vacuum mixing are also used. For cementless techniques, a cobalt-chrome tapered wedge stem with porous coating is inserted with the appropriate offset. A 28-mm ball is used to balance wear and stability factors.[243]

Patient Education Following Total Joint Arthroplasty is Essential and Should Include:

- Treatment options
- Treatment expectations regarding return to activity and sport
- Pre- and postoperative rehabilitation
- Adherence to precautions
- Risks and benefits of specific activities
- Maintenance of cardiovascular fitness

Regarding physical activity, patients should be motivated to maintain appropriate cardiovascular fitness levels. Cardiovascular exercise is beneficial for the THA patient for many other reasons including general health, prevention of cardiac problems, and for improvement of bone quality and implant fixation. Low-impact aerobic exercise suggestions that allow for increased heart rate are the most appropriate. Aerobics are completed 3 to 4 days per week for 30- to 40-minute sessions. Whether the patient wants to return to recreational or competitive sports is ultimately up to him or her, although prudent guidance from the surgeon and rehabilitation clinician physical therapist is essential. For these individuals, skiing, tennis, and hiking can be suggested, along with consideration of their previous athletic participation. Recommendations that help reduce joint forces are essential to reducing hip joint loading. These include using ski poles when hiking; skiing on flat, groomed runs; and cross-country skiing techniques. Many of these masters athletes will push the durability and longevity of arthroplasty implants by engaging in high-demand sports and activities that repetitively cycle the implant with and without excessive loads. Health care professionals must learn from these situations as well as engage in further research to assist in determining what activities are appropriate and possible for the aging athlete following THA.

Total Knee Arthroplasty

As with masters athletes with a THA, considerations to the prosthetic wear and joint-loading forces during sports activity following TKA is important. Normal and fast walking speeds have joint loads estimated at 2.8 and 4.3 times body weight, respectively. Power walking results in tibiofemoral compressive joint forces of 4 to 4.5 times the athlete's bodyweight.[240] An estimated load during slow jogging is 7.5 to 8 times the athlete's body weight for male patients and 8.5 to 9 times the athlete's body weight for women. Knee joint moments increase with increasing speed, resulting in knee joint loads of 10 or more times the athlete's body weight with jogging.[240] Cycling has demonstrated increasing compressive forces with increasing workload. Saddle height can also influence joint load; the higher the saddle, the lower the compressive force. Cycling demonstrates a tibiofemoral joint load of 1.2 times the athlete's bodyweight.[240] Hiking is another activity patients may want to participate in after TKA. Downhill walking places large loads on the knee joint. Fast downhill walking has demonstrated loads up to 8 times the athlete's body weight. The use of ski poles is recommended to reduce these joint loading forces by as much as 20%. Unfortunately, there are many activities without documented evidence on joint forces and loads. Kuster and Stachowiak[240] report that during daily activities, loads of 3 to 4 times the athlete's body weight may apply, whereas in sporting activities, loads of 5 to 10 times the athlete's body weight may occur. Other considerations include weight training, which will increase loads, and endurance activities, in which load depends on speed.

Clinical Point

Use of ski poles or walking sticks can reduce lower limb joint loading forces by up to 20%.

Recommendations for Return to Sport after Total Knee Arthroplasty

Bradbury and colleagues[234] evaluated participation in sports after TKA. They demonstrated that 65% of their patients who participated in regular exercise before TKA returned to sports after the procedure. The majority of these patients returned to low-impact sports (91%), although some (20%) returned to higher-impact activities such as tennis. Of 42 patients who underwent simultaneous bilateral TKA, 20 participated in sports prior to surgery. Of those 20 patients, 15 (75%) returned to sports following completion of their rehabilitation program. Healy and colleagues[243] surveyed members of The Knee Society regarding recommendations for athletics and sports participation following TKA. Table 29-4 illustrates the results of this survey.

Mallon and Callaghan[246] investigated members of The Knee Society and active golfers who had a TKA. Of the surveyed surgeons, 92% did not discourage patients from playing golf after knee arthroplasty, nor did they note increased complications in those patients returning to golf.

More than half of these surgeons also suggested that patients use a golf cart after knee arthroplasty. The golfers evaluated played an average of almost four rounds of golf a week. At a 3-year follow-up, the golfers noted that their handicap increased an average of 4.6 strokes and their driving distance decreased an average of 12 yards. The majority of these golfers did use golf carts and 84% did not have pain when playing golf, but did complain of mild ache after playing. Right-handed golfers with left TKA experienced more discomfort associated with playing golf than those following a right TKA. This was likely due to the rotational stresses required on the left knee during a right-handed golf swing.

Diduch and colleagues[248] evaluated outcomes of TKA in young, active patients. The mean age of patients was 51 years and 24% regularly participated in strenuous activities such as tennis, skiing, bicycling, farm, or construction work. All but two of the 88 patients experienced increased activity levels postoperatively. The average survivorship of the prosthesis for this group was 94% at 18-year follow-up. Despite the active lifestyles of these patients, loosening was not a problem. Healy and colleagues[243] recommend an anteromedial arthrotomy with a cemented and minimally constrained PCL-sacrificing or PCL-substituting condylar knee implant for active patients requiring a TKA. They use intramedullary femoral instrumentation and extramedullary tibial instrumentation to achieve the correct tibiofemoral alignment of 5° to 7.0°. The femoral component should be made of cobalt-chrome with a rounded condylar geometry and conforming patellofemoral joint. The tibial implant is modular and made of titanium with a high-molecular-weight polyethylene insert at least six to eight mm thick. It is recommended that patients avoid recreational and

Table 29-4

Activities Following Total Knee Arthroplasty—1999 Knee Society Survey

Recommended/Allowed	Allowed with Experience	Not Recommended	No Conclusions Made
Bowling	Bicycling (road)	Baseball/softball	Downhill skiing
Bicycling (stationary)	Canoeing	Basketball	Fencing
Croquet	Cross-country skiing	Football	Inline skating
Dancing (ballroom, square, jazz)	Doubles tennis	Gymnastics	Weight lifting (free weights)
Golf	Hiking	Handball	
Horseback riding	Ice skating	High-impact aerobics	
Horseshoes	Rowing	Hockey	
Low-impact aerobics	Speed walking	Jogging	
Shooting	Weight lifting (machines)	Lacrosse	
Shuffleboard		Racquetball	
Swimming		Rock climbing	
Walking		Singles tennis	
		Soccer	
		Squash	
		Volleyball	

Modified from Healy WL, Iorio R, Lemos MJ: Athletic activity after joint replacement, *Am J Sports Med* 29(3):384, 2001.

athletic activity until their quadriceps and hamstrings are sufficiently rehabilitated in physical therapy.[243] Masters athletes are counseled to maintain cardiovascular fitness with activities such as swimming and cycling. If a masters athlete wishes to participate in more aggressive activities, the patient should be assisted in making reasonable choices.

Total Shoulder Arthroplasty

Although hip and knee total joint arthroplasty remain common procedures in orthopedics, total shoulder arthroplasty (TSA) is less prevalent. The total number of hip and knee joint arthroplasties performed annually is nearly 20 times that of TSA.[249] Trends in pain relief and patient satisfaction tend to mirror those found in joint arthroplasty of the hip and knee. Subjectively, 92% of patients describe their shoulder as "much better" or "better" following TSA.[250]

Recommendation for Return to Sport after Total Shoulder Arthroplasty

To assess the appropriateness of athletic activity, one must consider the sport being pursued following TSA. A survey of the American Society of Shoulder and Elbow Surgeons reported by Healy and colleagues[243] revealed recommendations of appropriate sports activity following TSA. These results are illustrated in Table 29-5. None of the recommended sports were classified as contact sports and were relatively low-impact with respect to the upper extremity. Most activities also involved primarily a uniplanar movement of the shoulder. Bowling, horseshoes, and cross-country skiing are all sports that require primarily sagittal plane movement of the shoulder. In addition, the stress to the dynamic stabilizers during the deceleration phase of these activities is partially negated by gravitational forces.

Mitchell and colleagues[251] examined the mechanics of the shoulder during the golf swing for amateur senior golfers and established normative data characterizing shoulder motion. Key components of the golf swing required 119° horizontal adduction, 94° of vertical elevation during the backswing, and 59° lateral rotation during the follow-through for the nondominant arm. The dominant shoulder required 48° of lateral rotation during the backswing and 103° elevation with 108° horizontal adduction during the follow-through. The expectation of a patient wishing to return to golf would require that he or she be able to achieve these ranges of motion against gravity and hold these positions against resistance. Table 29-6 compares the normal ROM after TSA to the normal ROM needed for a golf swing in an older amateur golfer. These expectations may be less attainable in patients having a TSA because of rotator cuff deficiency and more realistic in patients with isolated OA.[252]

Jensen and Rockwood[253] studied 24 golfers following TSA. Of the 24 golfers, 23 were able to return to golf. The average return to golf took 4.5 months. No radiographic evidence of component loosening was noted compared with nongolfers at follow-up evaluations ranging between 2 to 10 years postoperatively. Handicap scores of these patients were reported to improve on average by five strokes. Members of the American Society of Shoulder and Elbow Surgeons were surveyed regarding the risks involved with playing golf after a TSA. Of those surveyed, 91% recommended patients return to golf and believed there was no increased risk of postoperative complications by playing golf.[243]

In regard to tennis, the survey demonstrated an interesting contradiction. Doubles tennis was recommended, but no conclusion was made about singles tennis.[243] Ground strokes would appear to be appropriate if adequate strength

Table 29-5
Activities Following Total Shoulder Arthroplasty—1999 American Shoulder and Elbow Society Survey

Recommended/Allowed	Allowed with Experience	Not Recommended	No Conclusions Made
Bicycling (road or stationary)	Downhill skiing	Football	Baseball/softball
Bowling	Golf	Gymnastics	Fencing
Canoeing	Ice skating	Hockey	Handball
Croquet	Shooting	Rock climbing	High-impact aerobics
Cross country skiing			Horseback riding
Dancing (ballroom, square, jazz)			Lacrosse
Doubles tennis			Racquetball
Horseshoes			Roller or inline skating
Jogging			Rowing
Low-impact aerobics			Soccer
Shuffleboard			Singles tennis
Speed walking			Volleyball
Swimming			Weight training

Modified from Healy WL, Iorio R, Lemos MJ: Athletic activity after joint replacement, *Am J Sports Med* 29(3):386, 2001.

Table 29-6

Comparison of Shoulder Range of Motion During the Golf Swing with Range of Motion Following Total Shoulder Arthroplasty

Shoulder ROM	Horizontal Adduction	Elevation	Lateral Rotation
Dominant shoulder ROM during the golf swing	108°	103°	48°
Non-dominant shoulder ROM during the golf swing	119°	94°	59°
Shoulder ROM following total shoulder arthroplasty	Not available	90°	47°

Data from Mitchell K, Banks S, Morgan D, Sugaya H: Shoulder motions during the golf swing in male amateur golfers, *J Orthop Sports Phys Ther* 33(4):196-203, 2003; and Wilcox RB, Arslanian LE, Millett P: Rehabilitation following total shoulder arthroplasty, *J Orthop Sports Phys Ther* 35(12):821-836, 2005.
ROM, Range of motion.

and dynamic control was demonstrated in the affected shoulder below shoulder height. Traditional serving mechanics may have to be altered secondary to predictable elevation and rotational motion loss following TSA. This may require even more involvement of the muscles of the legs and torso to generate power needed to perform an effective tennis stroke. As a result, a complete evaluation of the patient's trunk and lower extremities with regard to strength, mobility, and proprioception is critical in making an appropriate recommendation for the return to sport. Overhead sports pose interesting challenges. It is well known that athletes involved in throwing and racquet sports tend to have differences in rotational ROM, specifically with significant increases in lateral rotation of the dominant side.[254,255] Optimal lateral rotation as reported in the literature following TSA averages only 60°.[252] This is far below averages seen in overhead athletes. In addition, limitations in rotator cuff strength may further hinder the ability to attain sport-specific positions and stabilize the shoulder in such positions. Follow-through and deceleration phases of overhead throwing require significant force from the rotator cuff. Inadequate eccentric strength of these muscles increases the risk of injury and the inherent stability of the shoulder.[255]

Because of the factors listed previously, it seems unlikely that many patients having TSA of their throwing arm would be physically able to perform such tasks. The sports medicine team should consider that loss of functional lateral rotation ROM may manifest itself in other biomechanical compensations. Trunk rotation may become excessive to counteract the lack of shoulder rotation. In this instance,

strength and mobility of the lumbar and thoracic spine may become an important factor in making an appropriate recommendation on postoperative throwing. Other muscles of the legs and arms may compensate for shoulder weakness. The patient may also alter throwing mechanics with a pushing motion similar to throwing a shot put. This requires less rotation of the shoulder and uses more of the triceps and pectoralis major musculature to propel the ball. For those masters athletes wishing to pursue throwing sports, it is recommended that they have pain free anti-gravity control of the arm in elevated and laterally rotated position and that they demonstrate dynamic control of not only the shoulder, but of the trunk and lower body as well.

Total Ankle Arthroplasty

In the past, athletic activity following total ankle arthroplasty (TAA) has been strongly discouraged.[256] In 1994, Kitaoka and colleagues[257] reported an overall prosthetic survivorship of 65% at 10 years postoperatively, but only a 42% prosthetic survivorship in a subgroup of patients younger than 57 years old. Prosthetic loosening caused by the shearing forces during athletic activity is of most concern regardless of cement or uncemented fixation.[258] Pivoting and cutting maneuvers risk dislocation and malleoli fractures caused by the lack of ligamentous integrity and dynamic strength that is often compromised with ankle surgery. Normal postoperative ROM of combined dorsiflexion and plantar flexion is often significantly less than what is considered normal. The limited ROM would likely hinder and dramatically change the mechanics of the entire lower limb, including the foot, ankle, knee, and hips. Ankle stability, functional ROM, strength, and balance require careful assessment before returning to any sport activity. Low-impact activities with primarily movement in the sagittal plane logically put the patient at lower risk for complications.

The emergence of newer surgical techniques is promising. Wood and Deakin[259] reported a revision rate at 5 years to be approximately 7% in a sample of 200 ankles. Anderson and colleagues[260] retrospectively followed patients with TAA using the Scandinavian total ankle replacement prosthesis between the years 1993 and 1999, and reported 30% of the patients required a revision for their TAA, but noted the patients who underwent surgery later had much greater success. Valderrabano and colleagues[261] examined 147 patients (28 to 86 years of age) 2 to 4 years following TAA. Patient satisfaction, ROM, American Orthopaedic Foot and Ankle Society hindfoot score, radiological assessment, rate, level, and type of sports activity were recorded and compared with the patient's preoperative results. At follow-up, excellent and good outcomes were reported in 83% of cases and 69% of patients were pain free. The mean ROM preoperatively was 21° and after TAA, it was 35°. Before surgery, 36% of the patients were active in sports; after surgery, this percentage rose significantly to 56%. Overall, sports-active patients with a TAA showed better functional results than did inactive ones.[261]

Timing of Return to Sport After Total Joint Arthroplasty

Determining when a total joint arthroplasty patient is ready to return to sport is essential. Whether it is directly determined by the treating clinician or physician or self-initiation, a conservative approach is prudent. Functional and acceptable ROM that allows for athletic or exercise movements is necessary, as is well-balanced muscle strength across the joints involved. Ensuring that the older athlete has good balance in bilateral and unilateral stance is very important for those returning to sports. If balance and postural stability are compromised, risk of injury during sport may increase. Sport-specific rehabilitation exercises should be added to the plan of care when the athlete has passed specific examination- and performance-based criteria. Eventually, it is necessary to put the masters athlete through more rigorous testing to ensure he or she is ready to return to sport.

As the world of sports medicine has evolved, so has the context in which athletes are defined. Athletes span the entire life cycle, and the traditional age-related boundaries by which athletes are confined have expanded. Athletic careers and recreation in sports may not be terminated by a joint arthroplasty procedure. Although there appears to be some inherent risk to performing sports following arthroplasty, low-impact and noncontact sports are usually appropriate and generally are encouraged by physicians. Newer surgical techniques and prosthetic materials have shown greater durability and have decreased postoperative complications. Overall survivorship of arthroplasty procedures demonstrates satisfactory results between 15 to 20 years in the literature. In many procedures, press fit or uncemented fixation is recommended for younger, active patients. Press fit or uncemented fixation provides less initial fixation, but allows bone ingrowth for a strong, long-term fixation and preserves greater bone integrity in cases in which a future revision is needed.

As medical science advances to provide individuals with greater longevity, expectations of function and recreation will continue to grow as well. Patients who undergo total joint arthroplasty are not necessarily limited to a sedentary lifestyle. The methods and technology in the areas of joint arthroplasty will continue to evolve, and so will the possibilities to return to physical activity and athletics.

Conclusion

The population of masters athletes will continue to increase as the world's population ages. Better health care and technology is allowing the continuation of athletic activity in individuals well into their golden years. Because of the physiological changes associated with aging, the masters athlete requires a knowledgeable health professional who can balance patient safety with return to sport. These masters athletes require greater counseling, closer follow-up, and scrutiny of the physiological demands and musculoskeletal stresses of their desired sport. Ultimately, clinicians and masters athletes must find a balance between a return to participation, safety, and a lifelong enjoyment of their sport.

References

1. United Nations: *Report of the second world assembly on aging,* Madrid, Spain, 2002.
2. Kinsella K, Velkoff V: *An aging world,* US Census Bureau, Editor, Washington, DC, 2001, US Governement Printing Office.
3. US Census Bureau: International database. Table 094. Midyear population, by age and sex. Available from: http://www.census.gov/population/www/projections/natdet-D1A.html.
4. Physical Activity Guidelines Advisory Committee: Physical Activity Guidelines Advisory Committee Report, Washington, DC, 2008, US Department of Health and Human Services.
5. Warburton DE, Katzmarzyk PT, Rhodes RE, Shephard RJ: Evidence-informed physical activity guidelines for Canadian adults, *Can J Public Health* 98(Suppl 2): S16–68, 2007.
6. Kushi LH, Byers T, Doyle C, et al: American Cancer Society Guidelines on Nutrition and physical activity for cancer prevention: reducing the risk of cancer with healthy food choices and physical activity, *CA Cancer J Clin* 56(5):254–281; quiz 313–314, 2006.
7. Williams PT: Vigorous exercise, fitness and incident hypertension, high cholesterol, and diabetes, *Med Sci Sports Exerc* 40(6): 998–1006, 2008.
8. Lee IM, Skerrett PJ: Physical activity and all-cause mortality: What is the dose-response relation? *Med Sci Sports Exerc* 33 (6 Suppl):S459–471; discussion S93–94, 2001.
9. Mazzeo RS, Cavanagh P, Evans WJ, et al: American College of Sports Medicine Position Stand. Exercise and physical activity for older adults. *Med Sci Sports Exerc* 30(6):992–1008, 1998.
10. Spiduso WW, Francis KL, MacRae PG: *Physical dimensions of aging,* ed 2, Champaign, IL, 2005, Human Kinetics.
11. National Senior Games Association, 2009 01/06/2009 [cited 2009 January 7]; Welcome page NSGA. Available from: http://www.nsga.com/DesktopDefault.aspx.
12. Team Physician Consensus Statement: Selected issues for the master athlete and the team physician: A consensus statement. *Med Sci Sports Exerc* 42(4):820–833, 2010.
13. Chin APMJ, van Uffelen JG, Riphagen I, van Mechelen W: The functional effects of physical exercise training in frail older people: A systematic review, *Sports Med* 38(9):781–793, 2008.
14. Daniels R, van Rossum E, de Witte L, et al: Interventions to prevent disability in frail community-dwelling elderly: A systematic review, *BMC Health Serv Res* 8(1):278, 2008.
15. Evans WJ: Effects of exercise on body composition and functional capacity of the elderly, *J Gerontol A Biol Sci Med Sci* 50 Spec No:147–150, 1995.
16. Fiatarone MA, Marks EC, Ryan ND, et al: High-intensity strength training in nonagenarians. Effects on skeletal muscle, *JAMA* 263(22):3029–3034, 1990.
17. Fielding RA: The role of progressive resistance training and nutrition in the preservation of lean body mass in the elderly, *J Am Coll Nutr* 14(6):587–594, 1995.

18. Hess JA, Woollacott M: Effect of high-intensity strength-training on functional measures of balance ability in balance-impaired older adults, *J Manip Physiol Ther* 28(8):582–590, 2005.

19. Seynnes O, Fiatarone Singh MA, Hue O, et al: Physiological and functional responses to low-moderate versus high-intensity progressive resistance training in frail elders, *J Gerontol A Biol Sci Med Sci* 59(5):503–509, 2004.

20. Going S, Williams D, Lohman T: Aging and body composition: Biological changes and methodological issues, *Exerc Sport Sci Rev* 23:411–458, 1995.

21. Kavanagh T, Shephard RJ: Can regular sports participation slow the aging process? Data on masters athletes, *Phys Sports Med* 18:94–104, 1990.

22. Grimby G: Physical activity and effects of muscle training in the elderly, *Ann Clin Res* 20(1–2):62–66, 1988.

23. Grimby G: Muscle performance and structure in the elderly as studied cross-sectionally and longitudinally, *J Gerontol A Biol Sci Med Sci* 50 Spec No:17–22, 1995.

24. Thompson LV: Skeletal muscle adaptations with age, inactivity, and therapeutic exercise, *J Orthop Sports Phys Ther* 32(2):44–57, 2002.

25. Thompson LV: Effects of age and training on skeletal muscle physiology and performance, *Phys Ther* 74(1):71–81, 1994.

26. Chandler JM, Duncan PW, Kochersberger G, Studenski S: Is lower extremity strength gain associated with improvement in physical performance and disability in frail, community-dwelling elders? *Arch Phys Med Rehabil* 79(1):24–30, 1998.

27. Weiner DK, Long T, Hughes MA, et al: When older adults face the chair-rise challenge. A study of chair height availability and height-modified chair-rise performance in the elderly, *J Am Geriatr Soc* 41(1):6–10, 1993.

28. Brown M: Effects of aging—growth changes and lifespan concerns. In Magee DJ, Zachazewski JE, Quillen WS, editors: *Scientific foundations and principles of practice in musculoskeletal rehabilitation*, Philadelphia, 2007, Saunders.

29. Brown M, Sinacore DR, Host HH: The relationship of strength to function in the older adult, *J Gerontol A Biol Sci Med Sci* 50 Spec No:55–59, 1995.

30. Thompson LV: Age-related muscle dysfunction, *Exp Gerontol* 44(1–2):106–111, 2009.

31. Tuite DJ, Renstrom PA, O'Brien M: The aging tendon, *Scand J Med Sci Sports* 7(2):72–77, 1997.

32. Strocchi R, De Pasquale V, Guizzardi S, et al: Human Achilles tendon: Morphological and morphometric variations as a function of age, *Foot Ankle* 12(2):100–104, 1991.

33. Birch HL, Smith TJ, Tasker T, Goodship AE: Age related changes to mechanical and matrix properties in human Achilles tendon, *Transactions of the 47th Annual Meeting of the Orthopaedic Research Society*, San Francisco, CA, 2001.

34. Maffulli N, Barrass V, Ewen SW: Light microscopic histology of achilles tendon ruptures, A comparison with unruptured tendons, *Am J Sports Med* 28(6):857–863, 2000.

35. Maffulli N, Ewen SW, Waterston SW, et al: Tenocytes from ruptured and tendinopathic achilles tendons produce greater quantities of type III collagen than tenocytes from normal achilles tendons. An in vitro model of human tendon healing, *Am J Sports Med* 28(4):499–505, 2000.

36. Heath GW, Hagberg JM, Ehsani AA, et al: A physiological comparison of young and older endurance athletes, *J Appl Physiol* 51(3):634–640, 1981.

37. Hagberg JM, Coyle EF: Physiological determinants of endurance performance as studied in competitive racewalkers, *Med Sci Sports Exerc* 15(4):287–289, 1983.

38. Joyner MJ: Physiological limiting factors and distance running: Influence of gender and age on record performances, *Exerc Sport Sci Rev* 21:103–133, 1993.

39. Tanaka H, Seals DR: Invited review: Dynamic exercise performance in masters athletes: Insight into the effects of primary human aging on physiological functional capacity, *J Appl Physiol* 95(5):2152–2162, 2003.

40. Tanaka H, Seals DR: Endurance exercise performance in Masters athletes: Age-associated changes and underlying physiological mechanisms, *J Physiol* 586(1):55–63, 2008.

41. Coyle EF: Integration of the physiological factors determining endurance performance ability, *Exerc Sport Sci Rev* 23:25–63, 1995.

42. Fitzgerald MD, Tanaka H, Tran ZV, Seals DR: Age-related declines in maximal aerobic capacity in regularly exercising vs. sedentary women: a meta-analysis, *J Appl Physiol* 83(1):160–165, 1997.

43. Tanaka H, Desouza CA, Jones PP, et al: Greater rate of decline in maximal aerobic capacity with age in physically active vs. sedentary healthy women, *J Appl Physiol* 83(6):1947–1953, 1997.

44. Pimentel AE, Gentile CL, Tanaka H, et al: Greater rate of decline in maximal aerobic capacity with age in endurance-trained than in sedentary men, *J Appl Physiol* 94(6):2406–2413, 2003.

45. Eskurza I, Donato AJ, Moreau KL, et al: Changes in maximal aerobic capacity with age in endurance-trained women: 7-yr follow-up, *J Appl Physiol* 92(6):2303–2308, 2002.

46. Zachazewski JE: Range of motion and flexibility. In Magee DJ, Zachazewski JE, Quillen WS, editors: *Scientific foundations and principles of practice in musculoskeletal rehabilitation*, Philadelphia, 2007, Saunders.

47. Altman RD, Lozada CJ: Clinical features of osteoarthritis. In Hochberg MC, Weinblatt ME, Silman AJ, et al, editors: *Practical rheumatology*, St Louis, 2004, Mosby.

48. Felson DT, Chaisson CE, Hill CL, et al: The association of bone marrow lesions with pain in knee osteoarthritis, *Ann Intern Med* 134(7):541–549, 2001.

49. Felson DT, Gale DR, Elon Gale M, et al: Osteophytes and progression of knee osteoarthritis, *Rheumatology* (Oxford) 44(1):100–104, 2005.

50. Felson DT, Lawrence RC, Dieppe PA, et al: Osteoarthritis: New insights. Part 1: The disease and its risk factors, *Ann Intern Med* 133(8):635–646, 2000.

51. Boissonnault WG, Goodman CC: Bone, joint and soft tissue disorders. In Goodman CC, Boissonnault WG, editors: *Pathology: Implications for the physical therapist*, Philadelphia, 2000, Saunders.

52. Hoare K, Donahoe KM: Alteration of musculoskeletal function. In McCance KL, Huether SE, editors: *Pathophysiology: The biologic basis for disease in adults and children*, St Louis, 1990, Mosby.

53. Felson DT, Zhang Y, Hannan MT, et al: The incidence and natural history of knee osteoarthritis in the elderly. The Framingham Osteoarthritis Study, *Arthritis Rheum* 38(10):1500–1505, 1995.

54. Felson DT, Naimark A, Anderson J, et al: The prevalence of knee osteoarthritis in the elderly. The Framingham Osteoarthritis Study, *Arthritis Rheum* 30(8):914–918, 1987.

55. Cameron H, Brotzman SB: The arthritic lower extremity. In Brotzman SB, Wilk KE, editors: *Clinical orthopedic rehabilitation*, Philadelphia, 2003, Mosby.

56. Neyret P, Donell ST, DeJour D, DeJour H: Partial meniscectomy and anterior cruciate ligament rupture in soccer players. A study with a minimum 20-year followup, *Am J Sports Med* 21(3):455–460, 1993.

57. Neyret P, Donell ST, Dejour H: Results of partial meniscectomy related to the state of the anterior cruciate ligament. Review at 20 to 35 years, *J Bone Joint Surg Br* 75(1):36–40, 1993.

58. Honkonen SE: Degenerative arthritis after tibial plateau fractures, *J Orthop Trauma* 9(4):273–277, 1995.

59. Lundberg M, Thuomas KA, Messner K: Evaluation of knee-joint cartilage and menisci ten years after isolated and combined ruptures of the medial collateral ligament. Investigation by weight-bearing radiography, MR imaging and analysis of proteoglycan fragments in the joint fluid, *Acta Radiol* 38(1):151–157, 1997.

60. Roos H, Laurén M, Adalberth T, et al: Knee osteoarthritis after meniscectomy: Prevalence of radiographic changes after twenty-one years, compared with matched controls, *Arthritis Rheum* 41(4):687–693, 1998.

61. Gillquist J, Messner K: Anterior cruciate ligament reconstruction and the long-term incidence of gonarthrosis, *Sports Med* 27(3): 143–156, 1999.

62. Moskowitz RW: Clinical and laboratory findings in osteoarthritis. In Koopman WJ, editor: *Arthritis and allied conditions: A textbook of rheumatology*, Baltimore, 1997, Williams and Wilkins.

63. Hannan MT, Felson DT, Pincus T: Analysis of the discordance between radiographic changes and knee pain in osteoarthritis of the knee, *J Rheumatol* 27(6):1513–1517, 2000.

64. Flores RH, Hochberg MC: Definitions and classifications of osteoarthritis. In Brandt KD, Doherty M, Lohmander LS, editors: *Osteoarthritis,* Oxford, UK, 2003, Oxford University Press.

65. Bedson J, Croft PR: The discordance between clinical and radiographic knee osteoarthritis: A systematic search and summary of the literature, *BMC Musculoskelet Disord* 9:116, 2008.

66. Fisher NM: Osteoarthritis, rheumatoid arthritis, and fibromyalgia. In Myers JN, Herbert WG, Humphrey R, editors: *Clinical exercise physiology. Musculoskeletal, neuromuscular, neoplastic, immunologic, and hematologic conditions,* Philadelphia, 2002, Lippincott Williams and Wilkins.

67. Szebenyi B, Hollander AP, Dieppe P, et al: Associations between pain, function, and radiographic features in osteoarthritis of the knee, *Arthritis Rheum* 54(1):230–235, 2006.

68. Brandt KD: Nonsurgical management of osteoarthritis, with an emphasis on nonpharmacologic measures, *Arch Fam Med* 4(12):1057–1064, 1995.

69. Felson DT, Lawrence RC, Hochberg MC, et al: Osteoarthritis: New insights. Part 2: Treatment approaches, *Ann Intern Med* 133(9):726–737, 2000.

70. Hurley MV, Scott DL: Improvements in quadriceps sensorimotor function and disability of patients with knee osteoarthritis following a clinically practicable exercise regime, *Br J Rheumatol* 37(11):1181–1187, 1998.

71. Fisher NM, Pendergast DR, Gresham GE, Calkins E: Muscle rehabilitation: Its effect on muscular and functional performance of patients with knee osteoarthritis, *Arch Phys Med Rehabil* 72(6):367–374, 1991.

72. O'Reilly SC, Muir KR, Doherty M: Effectiveness of home exercise on pain and disability from osteoarthritis of the knee: A randomised controlled trial, *Ann Rheum Dis* 58(1):15–19, 1999.

73. Bennell KL, Hinman RS, Metcalf BR, et al: Efficacy of physiotherapy management of knee joint osteoarthritis: A randomised, double blind, placebo controlled trial, *Ann Rheum Dis* 64(6): 906–912, 2005.

74. Fransen M, McConnell S, Bell M: Exercise for osteoarthritis of the hip or knee, *Cochrane Database Syst Rev* (3):CD004286, 2003.

75. Devos-Comby L, Cronan T, Roesch SC: Do exercise and self-management interventions benefit patients with osteoarthritis of the knee? A metaanalytic review, *J Rheumatol* 33(4):744–756, 2006.

76. Roddy E, Zhang W, Doherty M, et al: Evidence-based recommendations for the role of exercise in the management of osteoarthritis of the hip or knee—The MOVE consensus, *Rheumatology* (Oxford) 44(1):67–73, 2005.

77. Van Baar ME, Dekker J, Oostendorp R, et al: The effectiveness of exercise therapy in patients with osteoarthritis of the hip or knee: A randomized clinical trial, *J Rheumatol* 25(12): 2432–2439, 1998.

78. Iwamoto J, Takeda T, Sato Y: Effect of muscle strengthening exercises on the muscle strength in patients with osteoarthritis of the knee, *Knee* 14(3):224–230, 2007.

79. Deyle GD, Henderson NE, Matekel RL, et al: Effectiveness of manual physical therapy and exercise in osteoarthritis of the knee. A randomized, controlled trial, *Ann Intern Med* 132(3): 173–181, 2000.

80. Currier LL, Froehlich PJ, Carow SD, et al: Development of a clinical prediction rule to identify patients with knee pain and clinical evidence of knee osteoarthritis who demonstrate a favorable short-term response to hip mobilization, *Phys Ther* 87(9):1106–1119, 2007.

81. Cliborne AV, Wainner RS, Rhon DI, et al: Clinical hip tests and a functional squat test in patients with knee osteoarthritis: Reliability, prevalence of positive test findings, and short-term response to hip mobilization, *J Orthop Sports Phys Ther* 34(11):676–685, 2004.

82. Deyle GD, Allison SC, Matekel RL, et al: Physical therapy treatment effectiveness for osteoarthritis of the knee: A randomized comparison of supervised clinical exercise and manual therapy procedures versus a home exercise program, *Phys Ther* 85(12):1301–1317, 2005.

83. Moss P, Sluka K, Wright A: The initial effects of knee joint mobilization on osteoarthritic hyperalgesia, *Man Ther* 12(2):109–118, 2007.

84. Sasaki T, Yasuda K: Clinical evaluation of the treatment of osteoarthritic knees using a newly designed wedged insole, *Clin Orthop Relat Res* (221):181–187, 1987.

85. Yasuda K, Sasaki T: The mechanics of treatment of the osteoarthritic knee with a wedged insole, *Clin Orthop Relat Res* (215):162–172, 1987.

86. Andriacchi TP: Dynamics of knee malalignment, *Orthop Clin North Am* 25(3):395–403, 1994.

87. Finger S, Paulos LE: Clinical and biomechanical evaluation of the unloading brace, *J Knee Surg* 15(3):155–158; discussion 159, 2002.

88. Lindenfeld TN, Hewett TE, Andriacchi TP: Joint loading with valgus bracing in patients with varus gonarthrosis, *Clin Orthop Relat Res* (344):290–297, 1997.

89. Pollo FE, Otis JC, Backus SI, et al: Reduction of medial compartment loads with valgus bracing of the osteoarthritic knee, *Am J Sports Med* 30(3):414–421, 2002.

90. Self BP, Greenwald RM, Pflaster DS: A biomechanical analysis of a medial unloading brace for osteoarthritis in the knee, *Arthritis Care Res* 13(4):191–197, 2000.

91. Ramsey DK, Briem K, Axe MJ, Snyder-Mackler L: A mechanical theory for the effectiveness of bracing for medial compartment osteoarthritis of the knee, *J Bone Joint Surg Am* 89(11): 2398–2407, 2007.

92. Nakajima K, Kakihana W, Nakagawa T, et al: Addition of an arch support improves the biomechanical effect of a laterally wedged insole, *Gait Posture* 29(2):208–213, 2009.

93. Kuroyanagi Y, Nagura T, Matsumoto H, et al: The lateral wedged insole with subtalar strapping significantly reduces dynamic knee load in the medial compartment gait analysis on patients with medial knee osteoarthritis, *Osteoarthritis Cartilage* 15(8):932–936, 2007.

94. Kerrigan DC, Lelas JL, Goggins J, et al: Effectiveness of a lateral-wedge insole on knee varus torque in patients with knee osteoarthritis, *Arch Phys Med Rehabil* 83(7):889–893, 2002.

95. Crenshaw SJ, Pollo FE, Calton EF: Effects of lateral-wedged insoles on kinetics at the knee, *Clin Orthop Relat Res* (375): 185–192, 2000.

96. Ogata K, Yasunaga M, Nomiyama H: The effect of wedged insoles on the thrust of osteoarthritic knees, *Int Orthop* 21(5):308–312, 1997.

97. Butler RJ, Marchesi S, Royer T, Davis IS: The effect of a subject-specific amount of lateral wedge on knee mechanics in patients with medial knee osteoarthritis, *J Orthop Res* 25(9):1121–1127, 2007.

98. Toda Y, Tsukimura N: Influence of concomitant heeled footwear when wearing a lateral wedged insole for medial compartment osteoarthritis of the knee, *Osteoarthritis Cartilage* 16(2): 244–253, 2008.

99. Brockmeier SF, Shaffer BS: Viscosupplementation therapy for osteoarthritis, *Sports Med Arthrosc* 14(3):155–162, 2006.

100. Dixon AS, Jacoby RK, Berry H, Hamilton EB: Clinical trial of intra-articular injection of sodium hyaluronate in patients with osteoarthritis of the knee, *Curr Med Res Opin* 11(4):205–213, 1988.

101. Puhl W, Bernau A, Greiling H, et al: Intra-articular sodium hyaluronate in osteoarthritis of the knee: A multicenter, double-blind study, *Osteoarthritis Cartilage* 1(4):233–241, 1993.

102. Dougados M, Nguyen M, Listrat V, Amor B: High molecular weight sodium hyaluronate (hyalectin) in osteoarthritis of the knee: A 1 year placebo-controlled trial, *Osteoarthritis Cartilage* 1(2):97–103, 1993.

103. Lohmander LS, Dalén N, Englund G, et al: Intra-articular hyaluronan injections in the treatment of osteoarthritis of the knee: A randomised, double blind, placebo controlled multicentre trial. Hyaluronan Multicentre Trial Group, *Ann Rheum Dis* 55(7): 424–431, 1996.

104. Henderson EB, Smith EC, Pegley F, Blake DR: Intra-articular injections of 750 kD hyaluronan in the treatment of osteoarthritis: A randomised single centre double-blind placebo-controlled trial of 91 patients demonstrating lack of efficacy, *Ann Rheum Dis* 53(8):529–534, 1994.

105. Dahlberg L, Lohmander LS, Ryd L: Intraarticular injections of hyaluronan in patients with cartilage abnormalities and knee pain. A one-year double-blind, placebo-controlled study, *Arthritis Rheum* 37(4):521–528, 1994.

106. Lo GH, LaValley M, McAlindon T, Felson DT: Intra-articular hyaluronic acid in treatment of knee osteoarthritis: A meta-analysis, *JAMA* 290(23):3115–3121, 2003.

107. Wang CT, Lin J, Chang CJ, et al: Therapeutic effects of hyaluronic acid on osteoarthritis of the knee. A meta-analysis of randomized controlled trials, *J Bone Joint Surg Am* 86(3): 538–545, 2004.

108. Bellamy N, Campbell J, Robinson V, et al: Viscosupplementation for the treatment of osteoarthritis of the knee, *Cochrane Database Syst Rev* (2):CD005321, 2005.

109. Arrich J, Piribauer F, Mad P, et al: Intra-articular hyaluronic acid for the treatment of osteoarthritis of the knee: Systematic review and meta-analysis, *CMAJ* 172(8):1039–1043, 2005.

110. Jackson DW, Evans NA, Thomas BM: Accuracy of needle placement into the intra-articular space of the knee, *J Bone Joint Surg Am* 84(9):1522–1527, 2002.

111. Tepper S, Hochberg MC: Factors associated with hip osteoarthritis: Data from the First National Health and Nutrition Examination Survey (NHANES-I), *Am J Epidemiol* 37(10):1081–1088, 1993.

112. Altman R, Alarcón G, Appelrouth D, et al: The American College of Rheumatology criteria for the classification and reporting of osteoarthritis of the hip, *Arthritis Rheum* 34(5): 505–514, 1991.

113. Quintana JM, Arostegui I, Escobar A, et al: Prevalence of knee and hip osteoarthritis and the appropriateness of joint replacement in an older population, *Arch Intern Med* 168(14): 1576–1584, 2008.

114. Felson DT, Zhang Y: An update on the epidemiology of knee and hip osteoarthritis with a view to prevention, *Arthritis Rheum* 41(8):1343–1355, 1998.

115. Garstang SV, Stitik TP: Osteoarthritis: Epidemiology, risk factors, and pathophysiology, *Am J Phys Med Rehabil* 85 (11 Suppl):S2–11; quiz S12–4, 2006.

116. Lievense A, Bierma-Zeinstra S, Verhagen A, et al: Influence of work on the development of osteoarthritis of the hip: A systematic review, *J Rheumatol* 28(11):2520–2528, 2001.

117. McAlindon TE, Wilson PW, Aliabadi P, et al: Level of physical activity and the risk of radiographic and symptomatic knee osteoarthritis in the elderly: The Framingham study, *Am J Med* 106(2):151–157, 1999.

118. Coggon D, Croft P, Kellingray S, et al: Occupational physical activities and osteoarthritis of the knee, *Arthritis Rheum* 43(7):1443–1449, 2000.

119. Cooper C, Inskip H, Croft P, et al: Individual risk factors for hip osteoarthritis: Obesity, hip injury, and physical activity, *Am J Epidemiol* 147(6):516–522, 1998.

120. Vossinakis IC, Georgiades G, Kafidas D, Hartofilakidis G: Unilateral hip osteoarthritis: Can we predict the outcome of the other hip? *Skeletal Radiol* 37(10):911–916, 2008.

121. Vingård E, Hogstedt C, Alfredsson L, et al: Coxarthrosis and physical work load, *Scand J Work Environ Health* 17(2): 104–109, 1991.

122. Vingård E, Alfredsson L, Malchau H: Osteoarthrosis of the hip in women and its relation to physical load at work and in the home, *Ann Rheum Dis* 56(5):293–298, 1997.

123. Vingård E, Alfredsson L, Goldi I, Hogstedt C: Occupation and osteoarthrosis of the hip and knee: A register-based cohort study, *Int J Epidemiol* 20(4):1025–1031, 1991.

124. Maetzel A, Mäkelä M, Hawker G, Bombardier C: Osteoarthritis of the hip and knee and mechanical occupational exposure—A systematic overview of the evidence, *J Rheumatol* 24(8): 1599–1607, 1997.

125. Croft P, Coggon D, Cruddas M, Cooper C: Osteoarthritis of the hip: An occupational disease in farmers, *BMJ* 304(6837): 1269–1272, 1992.

126. Walker-Bone K, Palmer KT: Musculoskeletal disorders in farmers and farm workers, *Occup Med* (Lond) 52(8):441–450, 2002.

127. Holmberg S, Stiernström EL, Thelin A, Svärdsudd K: Musculoskeletal symptoms among farmers and non-farmers: A population-based study, *Int J Occup Environ Health* 8(4):339–345, 2002.

128. Thelin A: Hip joint arthrosis: An occupational disorder among farmers, *Am J Ind Med* 18(3):339–343, 1990.

129. Thelin A, Holmberg S: Hip osteoarthritis in a rural male population: A prospective population-based register study, *Am J Ind Med* 50(8):604–607, 2007.

130. Thelin A, Jansson B, Jacobsson B, Ström H: Coxarthrosis and farm work: A case-referent study, *Am J Ind Med* 32(5):497–501, 1997.

131. Thelin A, Vingard E, Holmberg S: Osteoarthritis of the hip joint and farm work, *Am J Ind Med* 45(2):202–209, 2004.

132. Lloyd-Roberts GC: The role of capsular changes in osteoarthritis of the hip joint, *J Bone Joint Surg Br* 35(4):627–642, 1953.

133. Altman RD, Hochberg M, Murphy WA Jr, et al: Atlas of individual radiographic features in osteoarthritis, *Osteoarthritis Cartilage* 3 Suppl A:3–70, 1995.

134. Karachalios T, Karantanas AH, Malizos K: Hip osteoarthritis: What the radiologist wants to know, *Eur J Radiol* 63(1):36–48, 2007.

135. Steultjens MP, Dekker J, van Baar ME, et al: Muscle strength, pain and disability in patients with osteoarthritis, *Clin Rehabil* 15(3):331–341, 2001.
136. Rasch A, Byström AH, Dalen N, Berg HE: Reduced muscle radiological density, cross-sectional area, and strength of major hip and knee muscles in 22 patients with hip osteoarthritis, *Acta Orthop* 78(4):505–510, 2007.
137. Arokoski MH, Arokoski JP, Haara M, et al: Hip muscle strength and muscle cross sectional area in men with and without hip osteoarthritis, *J Rheumatol* 29(10):2185–2195, 2002.
138. Ganz R, Parvizi J, Beck M, et al: Femoroacetabular impingement: A cause for osteoarthritis of the hip, *Clin Orthop Relat Res* (417):112–120, 2003.
139. McCarthy JC, Noble PC, Schuck MR, et al: The Otto E Aufranc Award: The role of labral lesions to development of early degenerative hip disease, *Clin Orthop Relat Res* (393):25–37, 2001.
140. McCarthy JC, Noble PC, Schuck MR, et al: The watershed labral lesion: Its relationship to early arthritis of the hip, *J Arthroplasty* 16(8 Suppl 1):81–87, 2001.
141. Hoeksma HL, Dekker J, Ronday HK, et al: Comparison of manual therapy and exercise therapy in osteoarthritis of the hip: A randomized clinical trial, *Arthritis Rheum* 51(5):722–729, 2004.
142. Arokoski MH, Haara M, Helminen HJ, Arokoski JP: Physical function in men with and without hip osteoarthritis, *Arch Phys Med Rehabil* 85(4):574–581, 2004.
143. Birrell F, Croft P, Cooper C, et al: Predicting radiographic hip osteoarthritis from range of movement, *Rheumatology* (Oxford) 40(5):506–512, 2001.
144. MacDonald CW, Whitman JM, Cleland JA, et al: Clinical outcomes following manual physical therapy and exercise for hip osteoarthritis: A case series, *J Orthop Sports Phys Ther* 36(8):588–599, 2006.
145. Rasch A, Dalen N, Berg HE: Test methods to detect hip and knee muscle weakness and gait disturbance in patients with hip osteoarthritis, *Arch Phys Med Rehabil* 86(12):2371–2376, 2005.
146. Marti B, Knobloch M, Tschopp A, et al: Is excessive running predictive of degenerative hip disease? Controlled study of former elite athletes, *BMJ* 299(6691):91–93, 1989.
147. Vingård E, Alfredsson L, Goldie I, Hogstedt C: Sports and osteoarthrosis of the hip. An epidemiologic study, *Am J Sports Med* 21(2):195–200, 1993.
148. Panush RS, Schmidt C, Caldwell JR, et al: Is running associated with degenerative joint disease? *JAMA* 255(9):1152–1154, 1986.
149. Konradsen L, Hansen EM, Sondergaard L: Long distance running and osteoarthrosis, *Am J Sports Med* 18(4):379–381, 1990.
150. Lane NE, Oehlert JW, Block DA, Fries LF: The relationship of running to osteoarthritis of the knee and hip and bone mineral density of the lumbar spine: A 9 year longitudinal study, *J Rheumatol* 25(2):334–341, 1998.
151. Kettunen JA, Kujala UM, Kaprio J, Sarna S: Health of master track and field athletes: A 16-year follow-up study, *Clin J Sport Med* 16(2):142–148, 2006.
152. Kettunen JA, Kujala UM, Kaprio J, et al: Lower-limb function among former elite male athletes, *Am J Sports Med* 29(1):2–8, 2001.
153. Matsen FA, Rockwood CA, Wirth MA, et al: Gleno-humeral arthritis and its management. In Rockwood CA, Matsen FA, Wirth MA, Lippitt SB, editors: *The shoulder,* Philadelphia, 2004, WB Saunders.
154. Memel D, Francis K: The Disability Discrimination Act: an opportunity more than a threat, *Br J Gen Pract* 50(461):950–951, 2000.
155. Siebold R, Lichtenberg S, Habermeyer P: Combination of microfracture and periostal-flap for the treatment of focal full thickness articular cartilage lesions of the shoulder: A prospective study, *Knee Surg Sports Traumatol Arthrosc* 11(3):183–189, 2003.
156. McCarty LP, Cole BJ: Nonarthroplasty treatment of glenohumeral cartilage lesions, *Arthroscopy* 21(9):1131–1142, 2005.
157. Ruckstuhl H, de Bruin ED, Stussi E, Vanwanseele B: Post-traumatic glenohumeral cartilage lesions: A systematic review, *BMC Musculoskelet Disord* 9:107, 2008.
158. Millett PJ, Gobezie R, Boykin RE: Shoulder osteoarthritis: Diagnosis and management, *Am Fam Physician* 78(5):605–611, 2008.
159. Iannotti JP, Kwon YW: Management of persistent shoulder pain: A treatment algorithm, *Am J Orthop* 34(12 Suppl):16–23, 2005.
160. WIlliams MD, Edwards RB: Glenohumeral arthritis in the athlete: Evaluation and algorithm for management, *Op Tech Sports Med* 16:2–8, 2008.
161. Neer CS: Replacement arthroplasty for glenohumeral osteoarthritis, *J Bone Joint Surg Am* 56(1):1–13, 1974.
162. Walch G, Ascani C, Boulahia A, et al: Static posterior subluxation of the humeral head: An unrecognized entity responsible for glenohumeral osteoarthritis in the young adult, *J Shoulder Elbow Surg* 11(4):309–314, 2002.
163. Buscayret F, Edwards TB, Szabo I, et al: Glenohumeral arthrosis in anterior instability before and after surgical treatment: Incidence and contributing factors, *Am J Sports Med* 32(5):1165–1172, 2004.
164. Hovelius L, BG Augustini, H. Fredin, et al: Primary anterior dislocation of the shoulder in young patients. A ten-year prospective study, *J Bone Joint Surg Am* 78(11):1677–1684, 1996.
165. Neer CS, Craig EV, Fukuda H: Cuff-tear arthropathy, *J Bone Joint Surg Am* 65(9):1232–1244, 1983.
166. Burbank KM, Stevenson JH, Czarnecki GR, Dorfman J: Chronic shoulder pain: Part II. Treatment, *Am Fam Physician* 77(4):493–497, 2008.
167. Nowinski RJ, Schiffern SC, Burkhead WZ: Biological resurfacing of the glenoid: Longer term results and newer innovations, *Semin Arthroplasty* 16:274–280, 2005.
168. Ball CM, Galatz LM, Yamaguchi K: Meniscal allograft interposition arthroplasty for the arthritic shoulder: Description of a new surgical technique, *Tech Shoulder Elbow Surg* 2:247–254, 2001.
169. Brislin KJ, Savoie FH, Field LD: Surgical treatment fo glenohumeral arthritis in the young patient, *Tech Shoulder Elbow Surg* 5:165–169, 2004.
170. Maffulli N, Kenward MG, Testa V, et al: Clinical diagnosis of Achilles tendinopathy with tendinosis, *Clin J Sport Med* 13(1):11–15, 2003.
171. Crossley KM, Thancanamootoo K, Metcalf BR, et al: Clinical features of patellar tendinopathy and their implications for rehabilitation, *J Orthop Res* 25(9):1164–1175, 2007.
172. Fredericson M, Moore W, Guillet M, Beaulieu C: High hamstring tendinopathy in runners: Meeting the challenges of diagnosis, treatment, and rehabilitation, *Phys Sports Med* 33(5).32–43, 2005.
173. Lequesne M, Mathieu P, Vuillemin-Bodaghi V, et al: Gluteal tendinopathy in refractory greater trochanter pain syndrome: Diagnostic value of two clinical tests, *Arthritis Rheum* 59(2):241–246, 2008.
174. Lewis JS: Rotator cuff tendinopathy, *Br J Sports Med* 43(4):236–241, 2009.
175. Bisset L, Paungmali A, Vicenzino B, Beller E: A systematic review and meta-analysis of clinical trials on physical interventions for lateral epicondylalgia, *Br J Sports Med* 39(7):411–422; discussion 422, 2005.

176. Maffulli N, Wong J, Almekinders LC: Types and epidemiology of tendinopathy, *Clin Sports Med* 22(4):675–692, 2003.

177. Alfredson H, Lorentzon R: Intratendinous glutamate levels and eccentric training in chronic Achilles tendinosis: A prospective study using microdialysis technique, *Knee Surg Sports Traumatol Arthrosc* 11(3):196–199, 2003.

178. Khan KM, Cook JL, Kannus P, et al: Time to abandon the "tendinitis" myth, *BMJ* 324(7338):626–627, 2002.

179. Fredberg U: Tendinopathy—Tendinitis or tendinosis? The question is still open, *Scand J Med Sci Sports* 14(4):270–272, 2004.

180. Maffulli N, Khan KM, Puddu G: Overuse tendon conditions: Time to change a confusing terminology, *Arthroscopy* 14(8):840–843, 1998.

181. Puddu G, Ippolito E, Postacchini F: A classification of Achilles tendon disease, *Am J Sports Med* 4(4):145–150, 1976.

182. Schubert TE, Weidler C, Lerch K, et al: Achilles tendinosis is associated with sprouting of substance P positive nerve fibres, *Ann Rheum Dis* 64(7):1083–1086, 2005.

183. Rees JD, Wilson AM, Wolman RL: Current concepts in the management of tendon disorders, *Rheumatology* (Oxford) 45(5):508–521, 2006.

184. Cook JL, Khan K M, Zoltan Z S, et al: Prospective imaging study of asymptomatic patellar tendinopathy in elite junior basketball players, *J Ultrasound Med* 19(7):473–479, 2000.

185. Cook JL, Kiss ZS, Khan KM: Patellar tendinitis: The significance of magnetic resonance imaging findings, *Am J Sports Med* 27(6):831, 1999.

186. Major NM, Helms CA: MR imaging of the knee: Findings in asymptomatic collegiate basketball players, *AJR Am J Roentgenol* 179(3):641–644, 2002.

187. Cook JL, Khan KM, Harcourt PR, et al: Patellar tendon ultrasonography in asymptomatic active athletes reveals hypoechoic regions: A study of 320 tendons. Victorian Institute of Sport Tendon Study Group, *Clin J Sport Med* 8(2):73–77, 1998.

188. Cook JL, Khan KM, Kiss ZS, et al: Reproducibility and clinical utility of tendon palpation to detect patellar tendinopathy in young basketball players. Victorian Institute of Sport tendon study group, *Br J Sports Med* 35(1):65–69, 2001.

189. Shalaby M, Almekinders LC: Patellar tendinitis: The significance of magnetic resonance imaging findings, *Am J Sports Med* 27(3):345–349, 1999.

190. Almekinders LC, Weinhold PS, Maffulli N: Compression etiology in tendinopathy, *Clin Sports Med* 22(4):703–710, 2003.

191. Bey MJ, Ramsey ML, Soslowsky LJ: Intratendinous strain fields of the supraspinatus tendon: Effect of a surgically created articular-surface rotator cuff tear, *J Shoulder Elbow Surg* 11(6):562–569, 2002.

192. Brosseau L, Casimiro L, Milne S, et al: Deep transverse friction massage for treating tendinitis, *Cochrane Database Syst Rev* (4):CD003528, 2002.

193. Melham TJ, Sevier TL, Malnofski MJ, et al: Chronic ankle pain and fibrosis successfully treated with a new noninvasive augmented soft tissue mobilization technique (ASTM): A case report, *Med Sci Sports Exerc* 30(6):801–804, 1998.

194. Sevier TL, Wilson JK: Treating lateral epicondylitis, *Sports Med* 28(5):375–380, 1999.

195. Davidson CJ, Ganion LR, Gehlsen GM, et al: Rat tendon morphologic and functional changes resulting from soft tissue mobilization, *Med Sci Sports Exerc* 29(3):313–319, 1997.

196. Gehlsen GM, Ganion LR, Helfst R: Fibroblast responses to variation in soft tissue mobilization pressure, *Med Sci Sports Exerc* 31(4):531–535, 1999.

197. Nirschl RP: The etiology and treatment of tennis elbow, *J Sports Med* 2(6):308–323, 1974.

198. Stanish WD, Rubinovich RM, Curwin S: Eccentric exercise in chronic tendinitis, *Clin Orthop Relat Res* (208):65–68, 1986.

199. Alfredson H, Pietila T, Jonsson P, et al: Heavy-load eccentric calf muscle training for the treatment of chronic Achilles tendinosis, *Am J Sports Med* 26(3):360–366, 1998.

200. Alfredson H, Cook J: A treatment algorithm for managing Achilles tendinopathy: New treatment options, *Br J Sports Med* 41(4):211–216, 2007.

201. Ohberg L, Lorentzon R, Alfredson H: Eccentric training in patients with chronic Achilles tendinosis: Normalised tendon structure and decreased thickness at follow up, *Br J Sports Med* 38(1):8–11, 2004.

202. Fahlström M, Jonsson P, Lorentzon R, Alfredson H: Chronic Achilles tendon pain treated with eccentric calf-muscle training, *Knee Surg Sports Traumatol Arthrosc* 11(5):327–333, 2003.

203. Maffulli N, Testa V, Capasso G: Similar histopathological picture in males with Achilles and patellar tendinopathy, *Med Sci Sports Exerc* 36(9):1470–1475, 2004.

204. Jonsson P, Alfredson H, Sunding K, et al: New regimen for eccentric calf-muscle training in patients with chronic insertional Achilles tendinopathy: Results of a pilot study, *Br J Sports Med* 42(9):746–749, 2008.

205. Silbernagel KG, Thomeé R, Eriksson BI, Karlsson J: Continued sports activity, using a pain-monitoring model, during rehabilitation in patients with Achilles tendinopathy: A randomized controlled study, *Am J Sports Med* 35(6):897–906, 2007.

206. Purdam CR, Jonsson P, Alfredson H, et al: A pilot study of the eccentric decline squat in the management of painful chronic patellar tendinopathy, *Br J Sports Med* 38(4):395–397, 2004.

207. Young MA, Cook JL, Purdam CR, et al: Eccentric decline squat protocol offers superior results at 12 months compared with traditional eccentric protocol for patellar tendinopathy in volleyball players, *Br J Sports Med* 39(2):102–105, 2005.

208. Jonsson P, Wahlström P, Öhberg L, Alfredson H: Eccentric training in chronic painful impingement syndrome of the shoulder: Results of a pilot study, *Knee Surg Sports Traumatol Arthrosc* 14(1):76–81, 2006.

209. Cook J, Purdam CR: Is tendon pathology a continuum? A pathology model to explain the clinical presentation of load-induced tendinopathy, *Br J Sports Med* 43(6):409–416, 2009.

210. Assendelft W, Green S, Buchbinder R, et al: Tennis elbow, *Clin Evid* (11):1633–1644, 2004.

211. Assendelft WJ, Hay EM, Adshead R, Bouter LM: Corticosteroid injections for lateral epicondylitis: A systematic overview, *Br J Gen Pract* 46(405):209–216, 1996.

212. Clark SC, Jones MW, Choudhury RR, Smith E: Bilateral patellar tendon rupture secondary to repeated local steroid injections, *J Accid Emerg Med* 12(4):300–301, 1995.

213. Lambert MI, St Clair Gibson A, Noakes TD: Rupture of the triceps tendon associated with steroid injections, *Am J Sports Med* 23(6):778, 1995.

214. Jones JG: Achilles tendon rupture following steroid injection, *J Bone Joint Surg Am* 67(1):170, 1985.

215. Kleinman M, Gross AE: Achilles tendon rupture following steroid injection. Report of three cases, *J Bone Joint Surg Am* 65(9):1345–1347, 1983.

216. Scarpone M, Rabago DP, Zgierska A, et al: The efficacy of prolotherapy for lateral epicondylosis: A pilot study, *Clin J Sport Med* 18(3):248–254, 2008.

217. Fullerton BD: High-resolution ultrasound and magnetic resonance imaging to document tissue repair after prolotherapy: A report of 3 cases, *Arch Phys Med Rehabil* 89(2):377–385, 2008.

218. Rabago D, Best TM, Beamsley M, Patterson J: A systematic review of prolotherapy for chronic musculoskeletal pain, *Clin J Sport Med* 15(5):376–380, 2005.

219. Willberg L, Sunding K, Ohberg L, et al: Sclerosing injections to treat midportion Achilles tendinosis: A randomised controlled study evaluating two different concentrations of Polidocanol, *Knee Surg Sports Traumatol Arthrosc* 16(9):859–864, 2008.

220. Alfredson H, Ohberg L, Zeisig E, Lorentzon R: Treatment of midportion Achilles tendinosis: Similar clinical results with US and CD-guided surgery outside the tendon and sclerosing polidocanol injections, *Knee Surg Sports Traumatol Arthrosc* 15(12):1504–1509, 2007.

221. Zeisig E, Ohberg L, Alfredson H: Sclerosing polidocanol injections in chronic painful tennis elbow-promising results in a pilot study, *Knee Surg Sports Traumatol Arthrosc* 14(11):1218–1224, 2006.

222. Hoksrud A, Ohberg L, Alfredson H, et al: Ultrasound-guided sclerosis of neovessels in painful chronic patellar tendinopathy: A randomized controlled trial, *Am J Sports Med* 34(11):1738–1746, 2006.

223. Moon YL, Jo SH, Song CH, et al: Autologous bone marrow plasma injection after arthroscopic debridement for elbow tendinosis, *Ann Acad Med* Singapore 37(7):559–563, 2008.

224. James SL, Ali K, Pocock C, et al: Ultrasound guided dry needling and autologous blood injection for patellar tendinosis, *Br J Sports Med* 41(8):518–521; discussion 22, 2007.

225. Suresh SP, Ali KE, Jones H, Connell DA: Medial epicondylitis: is ultrasound guided autologous blood injection an effective treatment? *Br J Sports Med* 40(11):935–939; discussion 9, 2006.

226. Mishra A, Pavelko T: Treatment of chronic elbow tendinosis with buffered platelet-rich plasma, *Am J Sports Med* 34(11):1774–1778, 2006.

227. Rabago D, Best TM, Zgierska A, et al: A systematic review of four injection therapies for lateral epicondylosis: Prolotherapy, polidocanol, whole blood and platelet rich plasma, *Br J Sports Med* 43(7):471–481, 2009.

228. Paoloni JA, Murrell GA, Burch R, et al: Randomised, double blind, placebo controlled, multicentre dose-ranging clinical trial of a new topical glyceryl trinitrate patch for chronic lateral epicondylosis, *Br J Sports Med* 43(4):299–302, 2009.

229. Paoloni JA, Murrell GA: Three-year followup study of topical glyceryl trinitrate treatment of chronic noninsertional Achilles tendinopathy, *Foot Ankle Int* 28(10):1064–1068, 2007.

230. Paoloni JA, Appleyard RC, Nelson J, Murrell GA: Topical glyceryl trinitrate application in the treatment of chronic supraspinatus tendinopathy: A randomized, double-blinded, placebo-controlled clinical trial, *Am J Sports Med* 33(6):806–813, 2005.

231. Paoloni JA, Appleyard RC, Nelson J, Murrell GAC: Topical glyceryl trinitrate treatment of chronic noninsertional achilles tendinopathy. A randomized, double-blind, placebo-controlled trial, *J Bone Joint Surg Am* 86(5):916–922, 2004.

232. Chandler HP, Reineck FT, Wixson RL, McCarthy JC: Total hip replacement in patients younger than thirty years old. A five-year follow-up study, *J Bone Joint Surg Am* 63(9):1426–1434, 1981.

233. Kilgus DJ, Dorey FJ, Finerman GAM, Amstutz HC: Patient activity, sports participation, and impact loading on the durability of cemented total hip replacements, *Clin Orthop Relat Res* (269):25–31, 1991.

234. Bradbury N, Borton D, Spoo G, Cross MJ: Participation in sports after total knee replacement, *Am J Sports Med* 26(4):530–535, 1998.

235. Mont MA, LaPorte DM, Mullick T, et al: Tennis after total hip arthroplasty, *Am J Sports Med* 27(1):60–64, 1999.

236. Ries MD, Philbin EF, Groff GD, et al: Effect of total hip arthroplasty on cardiovascular fitness, *J Arthroplasty* 12(1):84–90, 1997.

237. Ries MD, Philbin EF, Groff GD, et al: Improvement in cardiovascular fitness after total knee arthroplasty, *J Bone Joint Surg Am* 78(11):1696–1701, 1996.

238. Schmalzried TP, Callaghan JJ: Wear in total hip and knee replacements, *J Bone Joint Surg Am* 81(1):115–136, 1999.

239. Kuster MS: Exercise recommendations after total joint replacement: A review of the current literature and proposal of scientifically based guidelines, *Sports Med* 32(7):433–445, 2002.

240. Kuster MS, Stachowiak GW: Factors affecting polyethylene wear in total knee arthroplasty, *Orthopedics* 25(2 Suppl):S235–S242, 2002.

241. Clifford PE, Mallon WJ: Sports after total joint replacement, *Clin Sports Med* 24(1):175–186, 2005.

242. McGrory BJ, Stuart MJ, Sim FH: Participation in sports after hip and knee arthroplasty: Review of literature and survey of surgeon preferences, *Mayo Clin Proc* 70(4):342–348, 1995.

243. Healy WL, Iorio R, Lemos MJ: Athletic activity after joint replacement, *Am J Sports Med* 29(3):377–388, 2001.

244. Mallon WJ, Liebelt RA, Mason JB: Total joint replacement and golf, *Clin Sports Med* 15(1):179–190, 1996.

245. Mallon WJ, Callaghan JJ: Total joint replacement in active golfers, *J South Orthop Assoc* 3(4):295–298, 1994.

246. Mallon WJ, Callaghan JJ: Total knee arthroplasty in active golfers, *J Arthroplasty* 8(3):299–306, 1993.

247. Mallon WJ, Callaghan JJ: Total hip arthroplasty in active golfers, *J Arthroplasty* 7 Suppl:339–346, 1992.

248. Diduch DR, Insall JN, Scott WN, et al: Total knee replacement in young, active patients. Long-term follow-up and functional outcome, *J Bone Joint Surg Am* 79(4):575–582, 1997.

249. Fortin PR, Clarke AE, Joseph L, et al: Outcomes of total hip and knee replacement: Preoperative functional status predicts outcomes at six months after surgery, *Arthritis Rheum* 42(8):1722–1728, 1999.

250. Nicholls MA, Selby JB, Hartford JM: Athletic activity after total joint replacement, *Orthopedics* 25(11):1283–1287, 2002.

251. Mitchell K, Banks S, Morgan D, Sugaya H: Shoulder motions during the golf swing in male amateur golfers, *J Orthop Sports Phys Ther* 33(4):196–203, 2003.

252. Wilcox RB, Arslanian LE, Millett P: Rehabilitation following total shoulder arthroplasty, *J Orthop Sports Phys Ther* 35(12):821–836, 2005.

253. Jensen KL, Rockwood CA: Shoulder arthroplasty in recreational golfers, *J Shoulder Elbow Surg* 7(4):362–367, 1998.

254. Schmidt-Wiethoff R, Rapp W, Mauch F, et al: Shoulder rotation characteristics in professional tennis players, *Int J Sports Med* 25(2):154–158, 2004.

255. Meister K: Injuries to the shoulder in the throwing athlete. Part one: Biomechanics/pathophysiology/classification of injury, *Am J Sports Med* 28(2):265–275, 2000.

256. McGuire MR, Kyle RF, Gustilo RB, Premer RF: Comparative analysis of ankle arthroplasty versus ankle arthrodesis, *Clin Orthop Relat Res* (226):174–181, 1988.

257. Kitaoka HB, Patzer GL, Ilstrup DM, Wallrichs SL: Survivorship analysis of the Mayo total ankle arthroplasty, *J Bone Joint Surg Am* 76(7):974–979, 1994.

258. Kofoed H, Sorensen TS: Ankle arthroplasty for rheumatoid arthritis and osteoarthritis: Prospective long-term study of cemented replacements, *J Bone Joint Surg Br* 80(2):328–332, 1998.

259. Wood PL, Deakin S: Total ankle replacement. The results in 200 ankles, *J Bone Joint Surg Br* 85(3):334–341, 2003.

260. Anderson T, Montgomery F, Carlsson A: Uncemented STAR total ankle prostheses. Three to eight-year follow-up of fifty-one consecutive ankles, *J Bone Joint Surg Am* 85(7):1321–1329, 2003.

261. Valderrabano V, Pagenstert G, Horisberger M, et al: Sports and recreation activity of ankle arthritis patients before and after total ankle replacement, *Am J Sports Med* 34(6):993–999, 2006.

APPLIED SPORTS INJURY EPIDEMIOLOGY

Mitchell J. Rauh, Caroline A. Macera, and Stephen W. Marshall

Introduction

The number of people who participate in sport is very large. In the United States, more than 400,000 collegiate athletes participated in sports (174,534 women and 233,830 men) during the 2006-2007 collegiate years.[1] At the high school level, sport participation has continued to grow during the past two decades with more than 7.3 million athletes (3,021,807 girls, 4,321,103 boys) participating in the 2006-2007 interscholastic sport seasons.[2] For women, participation in the United States has increased significantly since the passage of Title IX in 1972. Since then, a 190% increase has been observed for collegiate women athletes as compared with a 23% increase for male collegiate athletes. The change has been even more dramatic at the high school level, with a 928% increase in participation for girl athletes compared with only an 18% increase for their male counterparts.

Although involvement in competitive organized sports bestows many health benefits and rewards such as medals and scholarships, it also carries the risk of injury. The increase in the number of participants in sports poses special problems for medical professionals and sports injury researchers who monitor, treat, and recommend preventive measures to minimize injuries. Negative consequences of sports-related musculoskeletal injuries among athletes may result in reduced playing time or possible loss of an entire season of sports participation. In the long-term, injuries may lead to chronic musculoskeletal problems and osteoarthritis,[3-6] limiting the ability to experience pain-free mobility or participate in fitness-enhancing activities later in life.[7]

Athletes and those who work with them, including sports medicine professionals, coaches, and school- or sport-governing bodies, should be aware of the following general epidemiological determinants of sports injury incidence: Is the risk of injury greater in some sports than others? What

body parts or type of injuries are most common in a sport? In what sports are severe or season-ending injuries likely to occur? Do some physical, environmental, or sport-related factors increase the likelihood of injury? Can certain injuries be prevented? If so, how? Finally, of the preventive measures available, how many are effective? The goals of sports injury epidemiology are to provide information to these questions.

General Epidemiological Determinants of Sport Injury Incidence

- Is the risk of injury greater in certain sports?
- What parts of the body are more likely to be injured?
- What types of injuries are more likely to occur?
- What sports are more inherently dangerous?
- In what sports do more severe injuries occur more often?
- What factors increase the likelihood of injury?
- Can injuries be prevented?
- Are preventive measures effective?

Sports Injury Epidemiology

The epidemiologist in sports medicine is concerned with quantifying injury occurrence (how much) with respect to who is affected by injury, where and when injuries occur, and their outcome for the purpose of explaining why and how injuries occur and identifying strategies to control and prevent them.[8] Equally important, sports injury epidemiology should inform the development of interventions and provide a means of testing their effectiveness.

Definition of Sports Injury Epidemiology

Sports injury epidemiology is the study of the distribution and determinants of sports injuries for the purpose of identifying and implementing measures to prevent their development.[8]

Purpose and Organization of this Chapter

The purpose of this chapter is to provide clinicians and researchers with a basic introduction to fundamentals of epidemiological methods as applied to sports injury. The first section of the chapter provides an applied approach to principles and methods in sports injury epidemiology. The second section provides a summary of the injury prevention process, including recent descriptive sports injury rate patterns for selected interscholastic and collegiate sports, an overview of risk factors in selected high school sports, and a brief discussion of injury prevention studies. It is hoped that this chapter will provide the reader with essential tools to better understand, and perhaps conduct, research in this field.

Study Designs

The science of epidemiology is devoted to the study of health conditions in human populations. To understand these processes, most of which occur outside the laboratory setting, a series of study designs and related statistics have been developed. Sports injuries are an excellent example of the type of diseases or conditions that epidemiologists study. To understand and interpret data on sports injuries, a basic understanding of study design and related terms is necessary. There are two basic types of study designs: descriptive and analytical. *Descriptive studies* (i.e., case-series and cross-sectional) are used primarily for understanding the scope of the problem and identifying trends, whereas *analytical studies* (i.e., case-control, case-crossover, and prospective cohort) are used for assessing risk and identifying risk factors. The research question to be answered should drive the choice of study design. This section outlines the major study designs, the potential use of each design, and the questions that can be answered with each design. More detailed information can be found in a basic epidemiology or biostatistics text, such as *Modern Epidemiology*.[9]

Table 30-1 shows the general types of study designs that are used in the epidemiology of sports injuries. Some of these studies only count injuries and do not make inferences as to cause, whereas others use different approaches to estimate risk, rates, or risk factors. The gold standard of study designs is the randomized control trial (RCT), but not all injuries are amenable to that level of study. Often, initial evidence to make a case for a more comprehensive study is often obtained by conducting series of studies that build a body of knowledge around a general area of inquiry. The types of study designs are discussed in the following sections.

Case Series

Often the most direct way to obtain information on sports-related injuries is to get lists of people who have been injured. These lists can come from such places as clinics, medical sites, and schools. From these lists, it is also possible to collect additional information on the injury event, its severity, the tasks surrounding the event, use of protective gear if any, and other elements to further describe the injured population. However, without uninjured people for comparison, there is no way to identify risk factors for injury. Case series are useful for getting an idea of the scope of the problem. For example, if there are no tibial stress

Table 30-1

Types of Study Designs

Study Design	Uses	Population
Case series	To assess the scope of a problem	Injured persons
Cross-sectional	To determine the prevalence of a problem in a defined population	All persons or a sample of persons in a defined area (school, county, state)
Case-control	To evaluate risk factors among injured and noninjured persons	Injured persons and representative controls (uninjured persons)
Case-crossover	To evaluate proximal risk factors, usually acute, among injured persons	Injured persons
Prospective (cohort)	To assess incidence of an injury To evaluate cause and effect	Uninjured cohort with assessment of exposure
Randomized control trial	Gold standard of study designs To assess incidence of injury, risk factors, and causality To assess prevention strategies	Uninjured cohort with assessment of exposure and random assignment to treatment groups

fractures during a year of clinic visits, then it is not feasible to design a study to look at risk factors for tibial stress fractures in this population. However, if there were 2 tibial stress fractures in 1 year and 24 tibial stress fractures in the next year, without denominator data one has no way of knowing whether this is even an important increase. If one can estimate a denominator and determine that this represents an increase in tibial stress fractures, one still cannot look for risk factors because one does not have an uninjured group for comparison. In summary, case series can often help the clinician or researcher generate ideas for sports injury studies that need to be done and can help plan for care, but they are very limited in terms of their ability to track trends or identify risk factors for prevention.

Cross-Sectional

Studies that are conducted on a random sample of a target population provide valuable information on the prevalence of (or percentage of the target population currently experiencing) certain diseases, conditions, or risk factors. A cross-sectional study on concussions, for example, can be conducted on a target population of high school athletes.[10] If information is requested of all high school athletes (both injured and uninjured), then there is a denominator to use to calculate the number of concussions that have occurred. In time, the rates of concussions can be calculated from multiple cross-sectional studies to observe trends. This can be useful information to determine if there are unusual increases in concussions, but cross-sectional studies have limited ability to identify risk factors for concussion injuries because all of the information on injuries and behaviors or equipment use is collected at the same time. Therefore, there is no way to know which came first—the risk factor (not wearing protective gear) or the injury (which generated a need to wear protective gear). Other study designs are used to assess risk factors.

Case-Control

One example of a study design that can be used to assess risk factors is the case-control study. In this design, cases (for example, injured athletes) are selected, and then comparable controls (uninjured athletes) are selected so that the two groups can be compared on possible risk factors. For example, one may be interested in studying female high school athletes who incurred or did not incur an anterior cruciate ligament (ACL) injury during a basketball or soccer game.[11] For each person with an ACL injury (a case), another soccer or basketball player without an ACL injury would be selected as a "control." Then potential risk factors could be explored. For example, did hamstrings or quadriceps muscle strength vary among cases and controls? There are many advantages of the case-control design. These studies

are usually relatively cheap to conduct because there is no waiting time for an injury to occur. The downside of this efficiency is that the researchers have to find a way to document retrospectively the potential risk factors, such as playing time. It is also not possible to obtain rates of injury or to assess severity of injury with this type of study design. The particular outcome (in this case, degree of ACL injury) must be clearly identified prior to conducting the study and this may prove to be a limitation if the researchers decide they want to study a slightly different outcome (such as any knee ligament injury) while the study is in progress. This design is only useful for studying risk factors that are not affected by injury, such as genomics, or anatomical characteristics. If the injury changes the risk factor, this design cannot be used.[12] If the investigator is relying on self-reported data, then recall bias is another problem with case-control studies. Recall bias occurs if cases remember their risk factor data with greater clarity than controls.

The most fundamental point concerning case-control studies is that controls serve as a sample from the population in which the cases occurred. The control and the case groups should come from the same core "source population." They should *not* be two random groups of patients who have no logical relationship to one another. This simple rule is often ignored. The first step in designing a case-control study is to identify the source population from which the cases arose. This could be all basketball or soccer players in a geographical area, for example. Then work out how to draw a sample from this population—for example, from team members or lists of league members. These are the controls. If the investigator cannot identify the core source population of the cases, perhaps another type of study design should be considered.

Clinical Point

For case control studies, the case group and control group must come from the same core "source population."

Case-Crossover

In certain situations, it is possible for a case to serve as its own control, thus eliminating potential biases (such as recall) inherent in traditional case-control studies. With this type of study, it is possible to assess whether the injury was preceded by something that happened immediately prior to the injury. The injured person would be assessed for deviations from usual activity in a period at some point prior to the injury. Because each person serves as his or her own control, the problems of finding an appropriate control group are not present. For certain acute injuries, this is a very strong design that maximizes efficiency. It is well-suited for studying transient factors that have an immediate or near-immediate effect on injury, for example, fatigue or hormonal factors.

Prospective Cohort

One of the strongest study designs for assessing risk factors is the prospective cohort study. In this design, a healthy group of athletes is followed for a period of time (usually a season or until an injury occurs). Baseline information can include potential risk factors and, at follow-up, comparisons can be made to see if the injury risk is similar among athletes with different initial exposures. For example, to study the effect of a particular type of helmet on the occurrence of concussions among college athletes, a prospective cohort study could follow two groups of athletes during the season: those who wore the special helmet and those who wore the traditional helmet. Then the rate of new concussions in each helmet group could be compared, thus making some conclusions about the efficacy of the new helmet in preventing or reducing concussion injuries. The key characteristic of this type of study is that the risk factor (in this case helmet use) is identified prior to the injury (in this case concussion).[13] Although this type of study is very powerful in its ability to identify potential risk factors, evaluate the performance of interventions, and identify the incidence (new cases) of an injury, it is also very costly because it requires a large sample size and a period of follow-up time before an injury occurs. For a relatively rare injury (such as concussion), thousands of athletes need to be followed to have a sufficient sample size to attain statistical power. Thus, for injuries with a low rate of incidence, a case-control study might be more feasible.

Clinical Point

The key feature and strength of the prospective cohort study, as compared with other observational epidemiological designs, is that the risk factor is identified prior to the injury.

Randomized Control Trial

An RCT is a special case of the prospective study that randomly assigns healthy subjects to a "treatment" or "control" group. For example, to assess the benefits of wearing a special protective helmet among college football players, randomly selected athletes would wear these special helmets while other athletes would wear traditional head gear. If all other factors were the same (e.g., playing time, other equipment), then one would expect the rate of concussions to be lower among the athletes with the special helmets compared with athletes with the standard head gear. In practice, it is often easier to randomize at the level of the team or school, rather than to randomize individuals. This is called *cluster-randomization,* and it does decrease the statistical power of the study, further increasing the need for large numbers of athletes to be studied.

An RCT study designed by Gilchrist and colleagues[14] to prevent ACL injury in women collegiate soccer players illustrates the power of this study design. In this study, National Collegiate Athletic Association (NCAA) division I women's soccer teams were randomly assigned to a treatment or control group. The treatment group participated in a program that included stretching and strengthening activities three times a week during the season while the control group did their usual activities. This study was able to document a reduction in ACL injuries occurring during practice and games throughout the 2002 season. In spite of the strength of these types of studies, which are considered the gold standard of study designs, they are often difficult to carry out in practice. First of all, the random assignment is difficult to achieve. For studies assessing types of equipment, for example, it is difficult to randomly assign special equipment to an individual because players on the same team have different equipment (and it may be difficult to ensure that everyone wears the assigned equipment). As mentioned previously, if randomization is done on a team or school level, then a much larger sample size is needed because the unit of measurement becomes the team or school rather than the subject. This leads to a more complex statistical analysis plan. Finally, if the intervention is a knee brace or a training program, it is often difficult or impossible to blind subjects and study staff as to which athletes are in the treatment group and which are in the control group. Thus, double-blind RCTs are rare in sports medicine.

In summary, there are several types of study designs, each with specific advantages and disadvantages (Table 30-2). The time factor may be an important consideration in conducting a specific study and in understanding one that has been conducted (Figure 30-1). For example, case series studies are collected in the present and use records that are available for other purposes, which makes data collection very time efficient. However, without a control group only limited inferences can be drawn. A cross-sectional study includes those with and without injury, but because all data are collected in the present, it is possible to look for associations within the sample but not to identify risk factors. Case-control and case-crossover studies provide a comparison group, but the temporal sequence of the risk factor and the outcome (injury) may be harder to identify. The prospective cohort and the randomized clinical trial study designs are the most powerful studies from which to draw inferences about cause and effect (risk factors), but these are also the most difficult to conduct and can be quite expensive and take a long time to complete.

Table 30-2

Advantages and Disadvantages of Various Study Designs

Study Design	Advantages	Disadvantages
Case series	Easy to conduct Can use existing records Gives scope of the problem Generates hypotheses for further study	No control group, so no comparisons can be made Cannot give incidence data Cannot give risk factor data
Cross-sectional	Inexpensive (data collected at one time) Many sampling techniques available Can evaluate many exposures or outcomes Can provide prevalence data Can identify injury trends using repeated cross-sectional studies	Selective survival and recall Cannot establish cause and effect Cannot calculate risk or incidence Not appropriate for rare injuries Cannot study natural history of injuries
Case control	Well suited for rare injuries Relatively quick and inexpensive Existing records may be used to document past exposure No risk to subjects because data are obtained after injury has occurred Allows study of multiple potential causes of injury	Relies on recall or existing records for past exposures Validation of exposure often impossible Appropriate control group difficult to obtain Can estimate risk but cannot determine rates of injuries
Case crossover	Same advantages as for case-control studies Substantially reduces biases in control groups Particularly appropriate for acute injuries	Same disadvantages as for case-control studies May not be an appropriate design depending on the injury
Prospective cohort	Provides information on exposure prior to injury Provides rates of progression and natural history of injury Can study multiple effects of exposure Can assess causality Can provide incidence rates Can identify risk factors	Relatively expensive to conduct May require long follow-up or large number of subjects Less practical for rare injuries
Randomized control trial	Same advantages of prospective cohort design Gold standard of study designs Can monitor the effectiveness of different prevention protocols	Same disadvantages as prospective cohort design Ethical issues with random assignment Compliance may be a problem

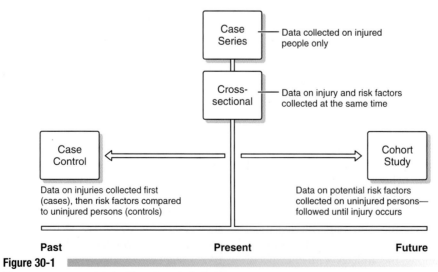

Figure 30-1

Time sequence associated with various study designs.

Incidence and Prevalence

Definition

Incidence and prevalence are fundamental concepts in sports injury epidemiology. However, these concepts are frequently misunderstood, even to the point at which the terms *prevalence* and *incidence* are sometimes used interchangeably. The definitions are very simple, and are summarized in the following text.

Main Measures of Sports Injury Frequency

- *Incidence:* Number of new injury occurrences in a population at risk in the time period
- *Prevalence:* Total number of injury occurrences in a population at risk at a given time

---

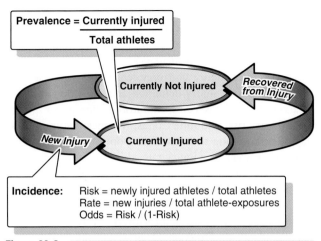

Figure 30-2

Relationship between prevalence and incidence.

Prevalence is the proportion of currently injured athletes in a sports population. For example, in a high school, the prevalence of injury is the proportion of athletes who are currently injured on any given day. For a specific sports team, prevalence is the proportion of players unable to play or practice because of injury on a particular day (this information is often presented in a "coach's report"). Note that *prevalence* is defined at a specific moment in time—it provides a "snapshot" of the *current status* of the athletes: who is injured and who is not.

Incidence measures the occurrence of *new injuries* in the population. Incidence tells how quickly the noninjured become injured, for example, the pace at which new injuries occur. Incidence, unlike prevalence, has an implicit dimension of time. To measure incidence, one must define a subset of the population that is not currently injured (i.e., those that are not prevalent injuries), and then prospectively monitor this subgroup to determine how many of them become injured during a defined time. *Incidence* is defined by the length of time for which subjects are monitored, the number of people being monitored, and the number of new cases.

Figure 30-2 provides a simple model that illustrates the relationship between incidence and prevalence. In this diagram, a group of athletes—for example, all NCAA athletes at a college—has been divided into two groups: those currently free of injury *(top circle)* and those who are currently injured *(bottom circle)*. The total number of NCAA athletes at the college is the sum of the two circles (all noninjured and all injured athletes).

In Figure 30-2, prevalence is defined by the size of the lower circle relative to the size of both circles combined. That is, it is the number currently injured *(bottom circle)* divided by the total number of athletes (size of both circles

together). Note that prevalence is sometimes referred as the *prevalence rate;* however, prevalence is actually a proportion. It ranges from zero (no one injured) to one (everyone injured). The prevalence can never be less than zero or greater than one. *Incidence* is defined by the pace at which athletes move from a noninjured state to an injured state. This is the "flow" from the noninjured group *(top circle)* to the injured group *(bottom circle)*, as indicated by the *descending left hand arrow.* As athletes heal, they leave the injured group *(bottom circle)* and return to the noninjured group *(top circle)*. This assumes that the injuries are recoverable (i.e., nonfatal). Three measures of incidence are of interest:

1. Injury rate (incidence rate or incidence density)—the number of new cases per unit of athlete-time at risk
2. Injury risk (incidence proportion or cumulative incidence)—the proportion of athletes who are injured at least once during a defined interval of time (such as a season)
3. Injury odds—risk divided by 1 minus risk

Each of these measures is discussed in more detail later in this section. For the moment, it is sufficient to note that the numerator for injury risk and injury odds is injured athletes, whereas the numerator for injury rate is injuries. Thus, athletes who have more than one injury during the monitoring period contribute multiple events to the calculation of injury rate, but only once to the calculation of injury risk and odds. Unfortunately, the field has historically been very confused about these three incidence measures, and some researchers incorrectly refer to *risks* as *rates.*[15]

Note that prevalence can be high even when incidence is low, and vice versa. This is because prevalence is a function of both incidence and healing time. Thus, if the average healing time is long, even very low incidence can lead to high prevalence. Likewise, if the average healing time is short, prevalence may be low even if incidence is high.

Prevalence, itself, cannot directly tell one anything about how frequently new cases occur in the population. However, if one knows the average healing time, then one can deduce something about incidence.

To define incidence and prevalence, one needs a clear and unambiguous injury definition and some denominator data on the athletes being monitored. For injury prevalence, injury risk, and injury odds, this means some simple way of determining the size of the population at risk (such as a team roster). For injury rate, this means some mechanism for tracking the number of team sessions (e.g., games and practices) for the athletes being monitored.

Earlier, the importance of having a study design that is appropriate for the research question that a study is addressing was stressed. However, even if the study design is correct, additional problems can occur. Two particularly important areas in sports injury epidemiology are the study's *injury definition,* and the collection of *denominator data* on exposure to athletic participation. Methodological errors in either of these areas can result in serious flaws in a study. The next two subsections discuss these important areas in more detail.

Injury Definition

Injury definition refers to the criteria used to include an injury in the study. An injury definition should be clear and unambiguous. A wide range of injury definitions have been used in the literature. Most injury definitions involve some minimal criteria for time lost from participation in the sport. For example, a researcher might decide to include only those injuries that caused the athlete to miss at least a week of participation. Injury definitions also often involve some minimal criteria for clinical attention, such as requiring a physician's assessment. Some studies use different criteria for different injuries. The North Carolina High School Athletic Injury Study, for example, defined an *injury* as "a result of participation in a high school sport that either limited the student's full participation in the sport the day following the injury or required medical attention by a health care professional (i.e., athletic trainer, physician, nurse, emergency medical technician, emergency room personnel, or dentist)."[16] In addition, all fractures, concussions, and eye injuries were included because the researchers considered those injuries to be serious.

The fact that there is no standard, universal definition of *injury* makes it exceedingly difficult to compare different studies. As an example, Table 30-3 lists a sequence of rugby injury studies from the 1980s and 1990s.[17-26] As can be seen, the definition of *injury* used in these studies varied widely, and included criteria such as (1) prevented play for any period, (2) required any health care, (3) prevented play for any period *or* required any health care, (4) prevented play 7 days or more, and (5) prevented play 7 days or more *and* required health care.

Given the huge variations in the definitions of *injury* used, it is not surprising that the injury rates reported by these studies also vary widely. Note that the variation in injury rates is due to more than just the variations in injury definitions. It is also due to differences in the methods used to collect the injury data, and to underlying differences in the real incidence of injury in the different populations under study.

There is no obvious solution to the problem of injury definitions that vary between studies. Definitions that involve access to health care are plagued by the problem that different populations have widely differing levels of access to health care. Most NCAA Division I teams, for example, have ready access to clinical services through the provision of certified athletic trainers (ATCs), whereas many high schools and recreational club athletes have very limited access to on-site services. Definitions that involve time lost from the sport are even more problematic. A sprained ankle that is a debilitating injury for a track athlete might only be a mild inconvenience in crew (rowing). Furthermore, chronic injuries such as low back pain or bone stress reactions may cause considerable distress for the athlete without resulting in any time lost from the sport. There are profound differences in physiological and psychological make-up between athletes—some athletes might be able to play with an injury that would be debilitating to another athlete. There are wide variations in clinician management of some injuries. For example, two concussions that have identical severity and presentation might be managed very differently by different clinicians. One might become a lost-time injury and the other might not.

> **Clinical Point**
>
> An explicit and clear injury definition should be reported in every study.

In summary, the best possible recommendation is simply that every study should have an explicit and clear injury definition and that the injury definition should be reported in all publications from the study data. If the goals of the study are broad-based injury surveillance, it is highly preferable to provide a qualified primary data collector, such as an ATC, at the data site, if one does not already exist. It is also preferable to capture all injuries that require evaluation, not just those that result in lost time.

Denominator Data

In general, regardless of how good the injury data is, it is meaningless unless some denominator data is also collected. At a minimum, the denominator should at least quantify the number of athletes in the population under study. However,

Table 30-3

Studies of Injury in Rugby Showing Effect of Variations in Study Methodology

Study	Year	Country	Population	Definition of Injury	Data Collection Method	No. of Injuries	Rate per 100 Player-Years
Nathan et al.[17]	1983	South Africa	High school boys	Prevented play > 7 days	Interview players who missed games	79	16.99
Sugerman[18]	1983	Australia	High school boys	Prevented play or school	Teacher and coach report	258	114.67
Roux et al.[19]	1987	South Africa	High school boys	Prevented play > 7 days and all concussion	Teacher and coach report; some personal visits	495	10.31
Davidson[20]	1987	Australia	High school boys	Required medical care	School physician or nurse in central location	1444	10.56
Clark et al.[21]	1990	South Africa	Adult men	Prevented play > 7 days or medical care	Self-administered form; contact at club	114	95.00
Dalley et al.[22]	1992	New Zealand	Mixed age and gender	Required medical care	Club and team contacts	921	8.37
Hughes and Fricker[23]	1994	Australia	Adult men	Prevented play or required medical care	Team trainer	133	110.83
Garraway and Macleod[24]	1995	Scotland	Adult men	Prevented play	Club contact; volunteer observers	358	29.44
Lee and Garraway[25]	1996	Scotland	High school boys	Prevented play	School contact	210	12.32
Bird et al.[26]	1998	New Zealand	Mixed age and gender	Prevented play or required medical care	Weekly telephone follow-up of all players	569	159.83

detailed denominator data collection can become exceedingly time-consuming. Fortunately, denominator data can often be approximated (or estimated) from pre-existing sources of information, such as team rosters and practice schedules.

An important point about the denominator is that injury risk and injury odds only require simple head counts of the number of athletes under observation and the definition of the length of the monitoring (or follow-up period). Injury rate, on the other hand, requires a much more detailed accounting of the number of games and practices in which the athletes participate. Despite this considerable obstacle, most researchers prefer injury rate to injury risk because injury rate has the ability to account for differences between athletes in their denominator, and allows the researcher to identify risk factors and compare sports in a manner that is scientifically more rigorous.

The most common type of denominator used in injury rate studies is "athlete-exposures." Athlete-exposures is computed by summing up the total number of athletes who participated in every game and every practice during the monitoring or follow-up period. Although it is not immediately obvious, athlete-exposures is a type of measurement that epidemiologists refer to as "person-time." Thus, although athlete-exposures is typically presented as counts, it is in fact conceptually measured in units of time. Some researchers go the extra step of multiplying the count of athlete-exposures by the average number of minutes per exposure; however, this is an approximation of the true athlete-time. Only in a very few settings—for example, in professional basketball[27]—can participation truly be tracked at the individual level in terms of minutes and seconds. Thus, athlete-exposures has become the "industry standard," despite the fact that important methodological details of its estimation remain underdeveloped (see discussion later in this chapter).

Clinical Point

Athlete-exposures is the preferred denominator to help increase comparisons of injury rates across sport studies. Comparisons of risks across sports often use athletes (rather than athlete-exposures) in the denominator. Although use of risks is rare in the literature, they are important and their use should be encouraged.

To date, most studies have attempted to do the best possible job of collecting denominators with the limited resources available. However, collecting denominator data is a thankless task and the sports injury epidemiology field is distinguished by a lack of creativity or originality to the issue of denominator data collection. Much denominator data is probably not as accurate as the researchers would have liked. In general, there is a desperate need for methodological research to streamline the collection of denominator data without sacrificing data quality.

Injury Risk and Injury Odds

Injury risk is the number of injured athletes divided by the total number of athletes. The unit of analysis is the athlete. Athletes who have multiple injuries are counted only once in the numerator of injury risk. *Risk* is the same as *probability*, and therefore risk must always be a positive number and can never exceed 1.

Table 30-4 presents two example calculations of injury risk, injury odds, and injury rate. The data (originally presented by Knowles and colleagues[15]) are taken from two real high school teams enrolled in the North Carolina High School Athletic Injury Study: a football team and a volleyball team. On the football team, 22 of the 36 athletes were injured; therefore, the injury risk for this season was 22 of 36, or 61%. Thus, the average risk of injury on this team in this season was 61%. Put another way, the probability of being injured in this season playing football at this school was 0.61 or just over 6 out of 10.

It is very important that the period for which the athletes are followed is specified, because a 10-season risk is obviously going to be much larger than a 1-season risk. The way to report injury risk is to always state the monitoring period, for example, "the risk of injury in a season of football is 61%." One should never state "the injury risk was 61%" without also specifying the period.

Table 30-4

Comparing the Three Measures of Injury Incidence (Risk, Odds, and Rate)

	Football (One Season for One High School Team)	Volleyball (One Season for One High School Team)	Football Team vs. Volleyball Team	Comment
Athletes	36	17		
Injuries	44	5		
Injured athletes	22 (Two injuries per injured athlete)	5 (one injury per injured athlete)		
Athlete-exposures	3,860 (107 exposures per athlete)	741 (44 exposures per athlete)		
Injury risk	$\frac{22}{36} = 61.1\%$ The average risk of being injured in a football season is 61%.	$\frac{5}{17} = 29.4\%$ The average risk of being injured in a volleyball season is 29%.	Risk ratio = 2.1 Footballers have twice the risk of injury, per season, relative to volleyballers.	Useful for parents, athletes, administrators
Injury odds	$\frac{0.611}{1-0.611} = 1.57 : 1$ The average odds of being injured in a football season is 1.6 to 1 (approximately 3:2).	$\frac{0.294}{1-0.294} = 0.42 : 1$ The average odds of being injured in a volleyball season is approximately 0.4 to 1 (approximately 1:2).	Odds ratio = 3.7 Footballers have nearly four times greater odds of injury, per season, relative to volleyballers.	Tracks close to the risk ratio if risk is 10% or less; otherwise useless
Injury rate	$\frac{44}{3860} = 11.3$ per 1,000 athlete-exposures The average rate of injury on the football team is 11.3 per 1000 athlete-exposures.	$\frac{5}{741} = 6.8$ per 1000 athlete-exposures The average rate of injury on the volleyball team is 6.8 per 1000 athlete-exposures.	Rate ratio = 1.7 Footballers have nearly twice the rate of injury, per game or practice, relative to volleyballers.	Useful for scientists

To compute a 95% confidence interval (CI) for injury risk in this study, take 0.611 and add and subtract 1.96 × 0.08125. Then multiply by 100 to get 45% and 77%. Where do these numbers come from? The 1.96 is a standard multiplier used to compute 95% CIs and it is taken from the bell-shaped normal curve. The 0.08125 is called the standard error of injury risk and is computed as:

$$\sqrt{\frac{0.611 \times (1-0.611)}{36}}$$

in which 36 is the number of athletes on the team (the denominator of injury risk). The scientific interpretation of this interval is that if the study was repeated 100 times, and 100 estimated injury risks were computed, 95% of them would contain the true (unobservable) injury risk. When communicating with nonscientists, it is sufficient to point out that the estimate of 61% is subject to statistical error and state that there is a 95% probability—on average—that the CI (45% to 77%) contains the true injury risk.

Note that the numerator and denominator of injury risk are counts of athletes—the count of injured athletes divided by the count of total athletes. Historically, some researchers have divided the count of *injuries* by the total athletes. This calculation is not a risk, odds, or rate. It has no meaning as a *personal* measure of injury incidence. However, it is useful from the standpoint of allocation of clinical resources. For this reason, the term *clinical incidence* has been suggested for this measure.[15]

Injury odds is simply injury risk divided by 1 minus risk. The odds of injury for the football season in Table 30-4 was 0.61 ÷ (1 − 0.61) or 1.57 to 1. The usefulness of injury odds is simply that it can be a useful surrogate for injury risk in some situations in which risk cannot be estimated directly (such as case-control studies). Other than that, odds has no direct use.

Note that the term *risk* is used very loosely in science. For example, if a surveillance study found that football had twice the injury rate of volleyball, people might say "the risk is twice as high in football." However, the fact that the *rate* is twice as high in football does not mean that the *risk* is twice as football.

Injury Rate

Injury rate is the number of injuries divided by the total number of athlete-exposures. The unit of analysis is the injuries. Athletes who have multiple injuries are counted multiple times—once for each injury—in the numerator of injury rate. A rate must always be a positive number and it has no upper bound, that is, it can exceed 1.

Note that one divides *injured athletes* by total athletes to get **injury risk,** and one divides *injuries* by athlete-exposures to get **injury rate.** One should not divide injuries by athletes if one's goal is to measure the personal incidence of injury.

In Table 30-4, note that there are 44 injuries on the football team, and 3860 athlete-exposures during the follow-up period. Therefore, the injury rate per 1000 athlete-exposures is:

$$\frac{44}{3860} \times 1000 = 11.3$$

The choice of multiplier - 1000 - is arbitrary. Its purpose is simply to make the result more readable. To compute a 95% CI for the injury rate, one simply divides 44 by 3860 to get 0.0113, and then adds and subtracts 1.96 × 0.001718 to get 0.0079 and 0.0147, and multiply both numbers by 1000. The resulting 95% CI is 7.9 to 14.7. As with injury risk, the interpretation of this interval is that if the study was repeated 100 times, and 100 injury rates were computed, 95% of them would contain the true (unobservable) injury rate. More informally, there is a 95% probability—on average—that this interval contains the true injury rate.

Note that there were 12 athletes having a single injury, four athletes having two injuries, and six athletes having three injuries, and one unfortunate athlete having six injuries. All of these injuries are used in calculation of the injury rate, and this is an important advantage of injury rate over injury risk: it uses all the injury data, whereas multiple injuries on the same athlete are not reflected in injury risk. Injury risk uses only the 22 "first injuries"—the first injury for each athlete during the follow-up period.

Note that a single event, such as a collision on the field of play, can give rise to more than one injury. For example, if two soccer players collide in midair when trying to head the ball, one could be concussed and the other might suffer a fractured clavicle. Should the one event, or the two injuries, be used in the numerator of the injury rate? It depends on the purposes of the study, but, in general, both should be used, because injury rate should be the rate of incident injuries, not the rate of events that give rise to injuries. Technically, these multiple events are not statistically independent; however, this is a minor issue and typically can be safely ignored as most injury events do not give rise to multiple injuries.

Another issue is whether only "new" injuries should be used in the calculation of injury rate and injury risk, or whether the "reinjuries" to a body part (i.e., the athlete had previously sustained an injury) should be included. As with the other aspects of injury definition, limiting the range of injuries that are to be included is fraught with peril, and there are no standard clinical criteria for defining a reinjury to the same body part. Thus, the injury rate (or risk) measure should typically include all injuries, both "new" and "reinjuries." However, if there are multiple injuries to the same body part during the course of the follow-up period, the conditional risk methods discussed in the following section should be used.

Conditional Risk for Multiple Injuries

Injury rate contains an implicit assumption that the rate of injury is similar for all athletes on a team. However, some athletes will experience no injuries and others will experience multiple injuries. As mentioned previously, in the example of the football team given in Table 30-4, one football player sustained six injuries in a season, while 14 of his teammates sustained no injuries at all. Why is this? Factors such as human behavior and playing style may contribute, as may the position played, the fitness of the individual, and any anatomical or physiological weakness. The method of *conditional risk* can be used to explore these influences. This method simply consists of repeating the injury risk calculation but conditioning on the presence of a prior injury. Thus, the injury risk referred to previously ($22 \div 36 = 61.1\%$) is actually the injury risk for the first injury. An injury risk for a second injury can be computed as follows: the risk of second injury, given a first injury, is $10 \div 22 = 45.5\%$ (note that the denominator for this risk is the numerator of the injury risk for the first injury). Rauh and colleagues explored the patterns and causes of multiple injuries in detailed analyses, and concluded that nearly one quarter of high school female athletes had multiple injuries.[28] They called more attention to the problem of multiple injuries as it indicates that (1) some sport positions have a higher risk for multiple injuries, (2) some players are at greater risk for injury time (athlete-exposure) because of player skill or smaller team size, (3) some sports increase the risk of injury for all body regions, (4) the contact or noncontact nature of the sport influences injuries, or (5) inadequate rehabilitation (that is, sending the athlete back to practice or game before the injury is appropriately healed) influences injuries. However, a large sample size is needed for this type of analyses.

Clinical Point

Some athletes may be at greater risk for incurring multiple injuries. Some factors that may increase their risk include:
- Sport positions that may have a higher injury risk
- Players who may be at greater risk because of their skill level or having to play on a small team size
- Sports that increase risk of injury to all body regions
- Contact/noncontact nature of some sports
- Return to activity before rehabilitation of their injury has been appropriately completed

---

Measuring the Effect of a Risk Factor

Incidence and prevalence are important, but ultimately, one wants to be able to identify risk factors and measure the effect of interventions. Ratio measures are often used to

accomplish this. Table 30-4 includes some example calculations for the risk ratio, odds ratio, and rate ratio, for the hypothetical scenario that one might want to compare the injury incidence in football to the injury incidence in volleyball. To do this, one simply divides the risk (or odds or rate) in football by the risk (or odds or rate) in volleyball. In this example, volleyball is the "reference" category.

Main Measures of Effect of a Factor on Injury Incidence

- Risk ratio
- Rate ratio
- Odds ratio

The odds ratio is widely used in the sports medicine literature, largely because logistic regression has become a popular tool for analysis of binary data. Odds approximates risk if risk is less than 10%, and thus odds ratios will be very similar to risk ratios in this range. However, if risk is more than 10%, odds ratios will not track closely to risk ratios, and they should be used with caution. Note how the odds ratio in the example is 3.7—very different from the risk ratio of 2.1—because the risk is much more than 10% (29.4% in volleyball, 61.1% in football). Also note that the risk ratio (2.1) and the rate ratio (1.7) are reasonably close. They diverge only because there are more athletes with multiple injuries in football (10) than in volleyball (0) and because there are more exposures per athlete in football (107) than in volleyball (44).

The risk ratio is good metric for parents and athletes who are seeking an answer to questions such as, "How much greater is my risk of injury if I play one sport compared with another sport this season?" The fact that the risk ratio does not account for multiple injuries or differing number of exposures per athlete is a strength of the risk ratio, because these factors are beyond the control of the athlete. The rate ratio, on the other hand, is a scientifically more precise means to compare sports, because it accounts for those two factors.

Statistical Methods

Table 30-5 lists some common statistical methods. The choice of statistical method is mainly driven by the goals of the study and the study design. The analysis should always address the basic research questions and be appropriate to the design of the study. A statistician or biostatistician should be consulted if there is any doubt about these factors. Assuming they are addressed, the type of data often becomes an important factor, and so Table 30-5 tabulates various methods by the type of data—continuous or categorical.

Table 30-5

Statistical Analyses Overview

Dependent Variable (Outcome Measure)	Independent Variable (Predictors or Risk Factors)	Recommended Statistical Analysis	
		Nonparametric	Regression
Continuous (e.g., BMI, age, VO_2 max)	Continuous (e.g., BMI, age, VO_2 max)	Correlation coefficient	Linear regression
	Categorical (e.g., sex, injury history, menstrual dysfunction status)	Student t-test	ANOVA
Categorical* (e.g., sex, injury history, menstrual dysfunction status)	Continuous (e.g., BMI, age, VO_2 max)	Trend test	Logistic or binomial regression
	Categorical (e.g., sex, injury history, menstrual dysfunction status)	Chi-square test	Logistic or binomial regression
Injury rate* (continuous count)	Continuous and categorical	Chi-square test	Poisson/negative binomial regression
Time-to-injury (continuous survival time)	Continuous or categorical	Log-rank test	Proportional hazards (Cox) model

*Two types of continuous data that require special methods
ANOVA, Analysis of variance; *BMI,* body mass index; *VO_2 max,* maximum oxygen consumption.

Continuous data are measurements such as body height or miles run per week, whereas categorical data are binary, nominal, or ordinal measures, such as sex, race, or sprain status (e.g., first degree, second degree, third degree).

Multivariate Regression

Multivariate regression is an important tool in sports injury epidemiology, because it allows the researcher to account for nonrandomized covariates that potentially might confound an analysis. The solutions ("beta coefficients") produced by a regression model have useful interpretations: linear regression produces means, binomial regression produces risk ratios, logistic regression produces odds ratios, and Poisson regression produces rate ratios. A variant of Poisson regression named *negative binomial regression* is often used for injury rates. Finally, the popular Cox model (proportional hazards regression) is used if the outcome measure is a time-to-event variable (such as number of days to injury).

In all cases, these measures can be adjusted for the confounding effect of other factors simply by including the relevant factors, including covariates, in the model. Caution is required, however. Regression models are not a panacea, and will give misleading results if variables are entered into the model without thought. It is good advice to develop a written analysis plan and make sure that the regression models (and all statistics) directly address the aims of the study in a logical and coherent fashion. In particular, the thoughtless inclusion of interaction terms in a regression model can often produce highly misleading and confusing results.

P Values and Confidence Intervals

There is widespread use of p values in the biomedical sciences, and p values and hypotheses can provide a useful means for quantifying study findings, especially in randomized studies. However, researchers have become overly dependent on the p value and hypothesis test when interpreting the results of their studies. This is dangerous, because p values can be very misleading in some situations.[29-32] Researchers in any area of sports injury medicine should not depend solely on p values when interpreting their data. They should also consider and report meaningful measures of effect (e.g., means, or rate ratios) that provide a context for the p values. A statistically significant finding may have little or no clinical meaning, and there is no way to know this if only the p value is reported.

In addition, the authors recommend reporting CIs for all major findings in any study. A profound limitation of the p value is that it combines two pieces of information—the precision of the study, and the magnitude of the treatment effect—that really should be kept separate. The CI allows the precision of the study to be quantified as separate piece of information, to be considered alongside the magnitude of effect.

P values can be particularly misleading when reported as a simple inequality (e.g., $p > 0.05$), rather than as a numerical value (e.g., $p = 0.06$). It is important that sports injury researchers are able to distinguish a p value of 0.06 from a p value of 0.99, because these two results represent very different sets of findings and would probably have different implications. The truth is that $p = 0.06$ has much more in common with $p = 0.04$ than it does with $p = 0.99$. Perhaps, with the addition of a few more subjects, or a slightly different random sample, the $p = 0.06$ result would become $p = 0.04$, purely because of slight improvements in study precision (statistical power). However, the blind adherence to rules of hypothesis testing would mislead one to conclude that the $p = 0.06$ result and the $p = 0.99$ result convey the same information, whereas the $p = 0.04$ finding is somehow vastly different from the $p = 0.06$ result - clearly, a ludicrous situation. Sadly, many investigators downplay, or even disregard, potentially useful findings simply because the result failed to attain the somewhat arbitrary cut-off criteria ($p = 0.05$) used for statistical significance.

Clinical Point

The reporting of confidence intervals is encouraged as a supplement or even replacement for p values. Confidence intervals allow the investigator to consider the precision and the magnitude of effect as two separate items, whereas the p value collapses these items into a single summary measure.

General Injury Surveillance Systems

Sports injury surveillance or reporting systems exist to serve a variety of functions. The data collected may be used to estimate the total burden of morbidity or mortality, or to identify risk factors and high-risk groups in sport populations.[33] This information can also be used as a basis for safety decision making and for the allocation of health care and other resources. Finally, the data may serve as an outcome measure for research on injury prediction and form the basis for assessing the effectiveness of interventions aimed at injury prevention.[33]

During the past three decades, a wide variety of injury surveillance systems have been developed to assess sport-related injury. Table 30-6 summarizes selected surveillance systems by design type, years of existence, data collected and source of data.[16,34-46] The systems vary in the method used in the reporting of athletic injuries. Some systems are based on the reporting of a specific injury type, whereas others are sport-specific. Some systems are aimed at specific athletic populations, whereas other systems survey the general population. An important issue in distinguishing between these systems is to determine the design used for collecting the data.[33] The design is what places limitations on how data may be interpreted and how it may be used. In general, two design types are used: case-series and cohort.[33] Each design type has its strengths and limitations.

Case-Series Design

The case-series design approach is the least complex. The advantages of this approach are that data on a variety of injury or diseases can be easily collected in many settings, cost

is low, and frequency data can be generated.[33] This approach can be useful when there is a low occurrence of injury but the injury type is severe or catastrophic as in head and spinal cord injuries. However, there are several distinct disadvantages to the case-series approach.[33] First, it is usually impossible to determine the completeness of reporting (i.e., if all or only some injuries are reported). This may lead to inaccurate conclusions. Second, the setting in which the data is collected can introduce a bias in the injury profile. These systems tend to identify acute and more severe sport-related injuries, which limits the generalizability of the data. For example, reporting on snowboarding injuries, the number of injuries occurring in the general population would be underestimated but the severity of injury may be overestimated. Third, and probably the main disadvantage of the case-series approach is that these systems do not collect data on noninjured athletes or participants or exposure. Thus, because the population at risk and exposure information is not collected, risk and causal associations cannot be determined.

Cohort Design

In contrast to the case-series design, sports injury surveillance systems collect data on a group of uninjured athletes (a cohort) at the beginning of the study and follow them forward in time. Thus, the main advantage of the cohort design is that it offers the ability to examine characteristics between injured and noninjured athletes.[33] Accordingly, the researcher can estimate both injury rates and injury risk (injury rate ratio).[33] Thus, cohort systems can determine casual associations from the data. In sports injury, as previously mentioned in the section on denominator data, the most commonly used measure of participation is the *athletic exposure (AE)*, in which one AE is one athlete participating in a practice or game. The disadvantages of these systems are the time and costs associated with collecting the exposure information.

Cohort Personal-Estimation versus Cohort Team-Estimation

There are two types of cohort design systems based on their method of how exposure data (denominator) is collected. In the cohort design with personal-measurement system, the total amount of AE is based on the sum of all *individual* athlete participations (i.e., an athlete is credited with an AE only if he or she actually participates in a practice or game). Thus, athletes are not credited with an AE if they missed or did not participate in a practice because of injury or noninjury reasons. This method is more time consuming but allows the ability to record varying amounts of participation (exposure) for each athlete, providing a more precise injury rate or risk estimate. In contrast, the systems that use the cohort design with team estimation estimate individual exposure rather than measuring it directly. The exposure for a given situation is calculated as the number of players multiplied by

Table 30-6
Sports Surveillance Systems

Surveillance System	Years of Existence	Data Collected	Source of Data
Case-Series Design			
National Electronic Surveillance System [34]	1972-present	All injuries	Hospital emergency department injury records
National Football Head & Neck Injury Registry[35]	1975-present	Football head and neck injuries	Survey, direct contact with athlete, parent, or school official at colleges and high schools
National Center for Catastrophic Sports Injury Research[36]	1982-present	Any severe injury incurred during high school– or college-sponsored sport events	Coaches, athletic trainers, athletic directors, executive officers of state and national athletic organizations, a national newspaper clipping service, and professional associates of the researchers
Children's Hospital Injury, Research and Prevention Program[37]	1989-present	All injuries in persons younger than 20 years of age	Hospital records
Cohort Team-Estimation			
National Athletic Injury Reporting System[38]	1974-1983	Sport-related injuries, participation data (AEs)	Injury report form completed by medical personnel and athletic trainers from professional teams, colleges, and high schools
Canadian Athletic Injury/ Illness Reporting System[39]	1979-1986	Sport-related injuries, participation data (AEs)	Injury report form completed by medical personnel or athletic trainers from professional teams, colleges, and high schools (teacher and coach)
NCAA Injury Surveillance System[40]	1982-present	Sport-related injuries, participation data (AEs)	Injury report form completed by athletic trainers from US colleges
Sports Injury Monitoring System[41]	?-present	Sport-related injuries and participation data (AEs)	Injury report form completed by medical personnel and athletic trainers from professional teams and colleges
National High School Athletic Injury Registry[42]	1985-?	Sport-related injuries and participation data (AEs)	Injury report form completed by athletic trainers from US high schools
Big Ten Conference[43]	1986-present	Sport-related injuries and participation data (AEs)	Injury report form completed by medical personnel and athletic trainers from Big Ten Conference colleges
University of North Carolina High School Athletic Injury Registry[16]	1996-2000	Sport-related injuries and participation data (AEs)	Injury report form completed by athletic trainers from 100 North Carolina (US) high schools
High School Sports-Related Injury Surveillance Study[44]	2005-present	Sport-related injuries and participation data (AEs)	Injuries reported by athletic trainers from 100 US high schools (nationally representative) weekly via Internet-based surveillance system
Cohort Personal-Estimation			
Athletic Health Care System[45]	1978-1995	Sport-related injuries and participation data (AEs)	Injury report form completed by athletic trainers or coaches from Washington state (US) high schools
Canadian Intercollegiate Sport Injury Registry[46]	1993-present	Sport-related injuries and participation data (AEs)	Injury and medical report forms and weekly exposure sheet completed by athletic trainers from Canadian Collegiate sports

AE, Athletic exposure; *NCAA,* National Collegiate Athletic Association.

the number of games or practices. The main advantage of this approach is the data collection is significantly minimized (e.g., need to count only the number of team players and total number of practices and games from the team roster for the entire season or any specified amount of time). In addition, injury risk can be computed for the team. However, there are some disadvantages with the team-estimation method. First, it assumes that all team members are "exposed" on each and every practice and game throughout the season. Thus, athletes who (1) start the season late, (2) do not complete the entire season because of injury or noninjury reasons, or, (3) miss several or many practices or games because of absences or injury are still credited with the same amount of exposures. Similarly, in many sports, although most players participate in each practice, many non–first team members may not participate in games. However, in this team-estimation system, those who did not play or participate in the game are still awarded a game exposure. In summary, injury rates calculated from the cohort team-estimation system may underestimate the true injury rate or injury risk as compared with the cohort personal-estimation method. For example (Table 30-7), in a study of 423 high school cross-country runners, Rauh and colleagues[47] reported an injury rate of 17 injuries per 1000 AEs using the cohort personal-estimation method whereby only practices and competitions in which runners actually participated (absences and time loss from injury days not counted in exposure estimation) were counted. If the study had used the cohort team-estimation method, the injury rate would have been observed as 13.7 injuries per 1000 AEs. Thus, using the cohort team-estimation method, there would have been an excess of 4510 total AEs (practices: 3683, competitions: 827) because of counting exposures for practices or competitions in which all runners did not participate. This would have caused an underestimation of almost four injuries per 1000 AEs. This difference could be important when comparing rates with other studies or when making important decisions regarding program planning for health care allocation.

It is unlikely that one universal system will fit all the needs of injury reporting in all populations and settings. Thus, a general sports injury surveillance system can be useful for answering questions about the incidence and severity of the sports injury problem in various subsets of a population.[48] Such a general sports injury surveillance system requires easy-to-use, uniform, and unambiguous definitions of the variables. If the purpose of the surveillance system is to identify causal factors or to assess the effectiveness of preventative measures, then the sports injury surveillance system should be tailored to the specific research situation.[48] Some important components of sports injury systems as recommended by Finch[49] are presented in Box 30-1.

Clinical Point

Sports injury data are important for a number of reasons. It is important that definitions of injury and collection of meaningful exposure data be determined and agreed on before injury surveillance activities are undertaken. In addition, the system should also collect information in a form that is of relevance across a broad range of potential users of the data: sports participants themselves, sport medicine physicians, other sports medicine professionals and researchers, coaches, trainers, and sports administrators.[49]

Box 30-1 Recommended Components of a Sports Injury Surveillance System[49]

- The sports activity the injured person was engaging in at the time of the injury (e.g., football, running)
- The location where the injury was incurred (e.g., football field, basketball course, running surface)
- The particular activity initiating the injury (e.g., pitching, tackling)
- What went wrong? (e.g., collided with another player)
- The level of supervision of the initiating activity (e.g., recreation vs. competition, organized sporting event)
- The nature of the injury (e.g., sprain, fracture, concussion)
- The body regions injured (e.g., head, shoulder, knee)
- The severity of the injury (e.g., number of participation days lost, emergency department visit)
- The characteristics of the injured person (e.g., age, gender, race, etc.)
- The places of the presentation and referral for treatment (hospital emergency room, physical therapist, athletic trainer)
- Sports participation data (e.g., number of exposures, hours, or minutes spent in an activity, competition vs. training)
- The use of sports injury countermeasures (e.g., modified rules, protective equipment, clothing, appropriate training)

Table 30-7

Example of Cohort Personal-Estimation versus Cohort Team-Estimation in High School Cross-Country Runners

Design Type	Injuries	Athletic Exposures	Rate
Cohort Personal-Estimation			
Practices	272	15447	17.6
Competitions	44	3161	13.9
Total	316	18608	17.0
Cohort Team-Estimation			
Practices	272	19130	14.2
Competitions	44	3,988	11.0
Total	316	23118	13.7

Data from Rauh MJ, Koepsell TD, Rivara FP et al: Epidemiology of musculoskeletal injuries among high school cross-country runners, *Am J Epidemiol* 163(2):151-159, 2006.

Injury Prevention

The reduction of sport injuries would have a major effect on quality of life through the maintenance and promotion of physical activity. There is epidemiological evidence that physical fitness level is a significant predictor of all-cause mortality, morbidity, and disease-specific morbidity (e.g., cardiovascular disease, diabetes, cancer).[50-52] There is recent evidence that sports injuries, particularly knee injuries, result in an increased risk of osteoarthritis.[53] Thus, there is a significant public health effect associated with sports injuries and future development of osteoarthritis and other diseases associated with decreased levels of physical activity.

> **Clinical Point**
>
> Minimizing the occurrence of injury would help maintain the benefits of sport participation at all ages, including good health, greater self-esteem, relaxation, competition, socialization, teamwork, fitness, and greater motor skill development.

A four-step approach has been proposed by van Mechelen and colleagues[54,55] to study injury prevention (Figure 30-3). First, surveillance (as discussed in the previous section) must be used to measure the extent or magnitude of injury in a given sport population. Second, the causes of injury or risk factors must be identified. The third step is to introduce prevention measures that are likely to reduce future risk and severity of sports injuries. Such measures should be based on information on the causal factors and injury mechanisms as identified in the second step. Finally, the effect of the measures must be evaluated by repeating the first step, which can be achieved by RCTs, other intervention studies, or by time-trend analysis of injury patterns.

Step 1: Basic Descriptive Sports Injury Epidemiology

There are two inter-related types of epidemiological research: descriptive and analytical. Quantifying injury occurrence (i.e., how much) with respect to who is affected, where and when injuries occur, and what is the injury outcome is referred to as *descriptive epidemiology*. Explaining why and how injuries occur and identifying strategies to control and prevent them is referred to *analytical epidemiology.*[8,56]

For the purposes of this chapter, the authors have limited their summary of descriptive epidemiology to sport injuries occurring in selected collegiate and high school sports. The search included published studies of collegiate and high school sport injuries in the United States that reported incidence risk (i.e., number of injured athletes per total number of injured athletes, and number of total injuries per total number of injured athletes) and incidence rate (i.e., total number of injuries per 1000 AEs) for males and females. Because of the large sample sizes, their prospective longitudinal nature, and the systematic manner in which the data was collected, the literature search for collegiate athletes was limited to findings of the NCAA Injury Surveillance Summary (1988-1989 to 2003-2004). The authors limited the literature search of high school studies to prospective studies during the relatively similar time frame (1987-2007). The epidemiological literature of sports injuries should be evaluated in light of the restrictive nature of the overview.

Sports with Highest Injury Incidence

High School. A summary of studies reporting overall (i.e., practice and games combined) incidence for girls' and boys' high school sports is shown in Table 30-8 and Table 30-9, respectively. Girls' incidence (i.e., number of injured athletes per athletes, injury rate per 100 athlete seasons, and injury rate per 1000 AEs) are presented for basketball,[41,44,57-62] cross-country running,[47,59,63,64] field hockey,[41,62] gymnastics,[59,62] lacrosse,[65] soccer,[41,44,58,59,62,66] softball,[41,44,58,59,62] swimming,[59,62] tennis,[59,62] track and field,[58,59,62,67] and volleyball.[41,44,58,59,62] Studies reporting incidence (i.e., number of injured athletes per athletes, and injury rate per 100 athlete seasons, injury rate per 1000 AEs) for boys' high school sports include baseball,[41,44,58,59,62,68] basketball,[41,44,57-59,61,62] cross-country running,[47,59,63,64] football,[41,44,58,59,62,69-72] gymnastics,[59,62] lacrosse,[65] soccer,[41,44,58,59,62,66] swimming,[59,62] tennis,[59,62] track and field,[58,59,62,67] volleyball,[59] and wrestling.[41,44,58,59,62,73]

Using Tables 30-8 and 30-9, the highest rates of injury per 1000 AEs are found for girls' high school sports in cross-country running (range: 4.3 to 19.6), soccer (range: 2.34 to 5.3), basketball (range: 1.28 to 4.4), and field hockey (3.7).

Text continued on p. 752

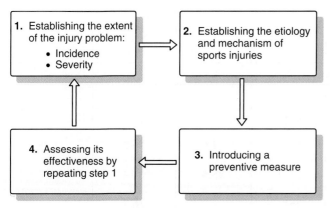

Figure 30-3
Four-step sequence of injury prevention research model proposed by van Mechelen and colleagues.[54,55] (From van Mechelen W, Hlobil H, Kemper HCG: Incidence, severity, aetiology and prevention of sports injuries: A review of concepts, *Sports Med* 14(2):84, 1992.)

Table 30-8

A Comparison of Injury Rates in Prospective Studies of Girls' Selected High School Sports

Study	Data Collection	Duration	Number of Participants	Number of Injuries	Number of Injured Athletes/N	Injury Rate/ 100 Athlete Seasons	Injury Rate/ 1000 Athletic Exposures
Basketball							
Borowski et al. (2008)[57]	DM	2 years	DNP	745	—	—	2.08
Comstock et al. (2006)[44]	DM	1 year	DNP	—	—	—	2.01
Knowles et al. (2006)[58]	IRF	3 seasons	714	151	15.0	21.1	1.28
Powell et al. (1999)[41]	AT	3 years	6083	1748	23.0	28.7	4.4
Beachy et al. (1997)[59]	AT	8 years	587	144	—	24.5	—
Gomez et al.(1986)[60] and Messina et al. (1999)[61]	DM	1 year	890	436	49.0	—	3.6
McLain and Reynolds (1989)[62]	DM	1 year	45	14	31.0	31.0	—
Cross-Country Running							
Plisky et al. (2007)[63]	AT/IRF	1 season	46	11	21.7	23.9	4.3
Rauh et al. (2006)[47]	IRF	1 season	186	157	41.9	84.4	19.6
Rauh et al. (2000)[64]	IRF	15 seasons	1202	776	34.0	64.6	16.7
Beachy et al. (1997)[59]	AT	8 years	787	164	—	20.8	—
Field Hockey							
Powell et al. (1999)[41]	AT	3 years	2805	510	15.8	18.2	3.7
McLain and Reynolds (1989)[62]	DM	1 year	46	3	6.5	6.5	
Gymnastics							
Beachy et al. (1997)[59]	AT	8 years	177	23	—	13.0	—
McLain and Reynolds (1989)[62]	DM	1 year	24	11	45.8	45.8	—
Lacrosse							
Hinton et al. (2005)[65]	AT	3 seasons	2658	371	—	14.0	2.54
Soccer							
Yard et al. (2008)[66]	AT	2 years	744	—	—	—	2.34
Comstock et al. (2006)[44]	DM	1 year	DNP	DNP	—	—	2.36
Knowles et al. (2006)[58]	IRF	3 seasons	748	121	14.6	16.2	2.35
Powell and Barber-Foss (1999)[41]	AT	3 years	6642	1771	25.6	31.4	5.3
Beachy et al. (1997)[59]	AT	8 years	683	251	—	36.7	—
McLain and Reynolds (1989)[62]	DM	1 year	72	12	16.7	16.7	—

Table 30-8

A Comparison of Injury Rates in Prospective Studies of Girls' Selected High School Sports—cont'd

Study	Data Collection	Duration	Number of Participants	Number of Injuries	Number of Injured Athletes/N	Injury Rate/ 100 Athlete Seasons	Injury Rate/ 1000 Athletic Exposures
Softball							
Comstock et al. (2006)[44]	DM	1 year	—	—	—	—	1.13
Knowles et al. (2006)[58]	IRF	3 seasons	829	125	8.6	15.1	0.96
Powell and Barber-Foss (1999)[41]	AT	3 years	5435	910	14.4	16.7	3.5
Beachy et al. (1997)[59]	AT	8 years	448	84	—	18.8	—
McLain and Reynolds (1989)[62]	DM	1 year	54	7	13.0	13.0	—
Swimming							
Beachy et al. (1997)[59]	AT	8 years	402	21	—	5.2	—
McLain and Reynolds (1989)[62]	DM	1 year	41	0	0.0	0.0	—
Tennis							
Beachy et al. (1997)[59]	AT	8 years	297	40	—	13.5	—
McLain and Reynolds (1989)[62]	DM	1 year	30	1	3.3	3.3	—
Track and Field							
Knowles et al. (2006)[58]	IRF	3 seasons	1266	90	6.0	7.1	1.18
Beachy et al. (1997)[59]	AT	8 years	1531	425	—	27.8	—
McLain and Reynolds (1989)[62]	AT	1 season	65	12	18.5	18.5	—
Watson and DiMartino (1987)[67]	I/Q	1 season	78	11	14.1	14.1	—
Volleyball							
Comstock et al. (2006)[44]	DM	1 year	DNP	DNP	—	—	1.64
Knowles et al. (2006)[58]	IRF	3 seasons	1100	154	7.6	14.0	1.31
Powell and Barber-Foss (1999)[41]	AT	3 years	4222	601	14.9	14.2	1.7
Beachy et al. (1997)[59]	AT	8 years	525	86	—	16.4	—
McLain and Reynolds (1989)[62]	DM	1 year	64	11	17.2	17.2	—

AT, Athletic trainer reports; *DM,* direct monitoring; *DNP,* data not provided; *I,* interview; *IRF,* injury report form; *Q,* questionnaire.

Table 30-9

A Comparison of Injury Rates in Prospective Studies of Selected Boys' High School Sports

Study	Data Collection	Duration	Number of Participants	Number of Injuries	Number of Injured Athletes/N	Injury Rate/100 Athlete Seasons	Injury Rate/1000 Athletic Exposures
			Baseball				
Collins and Comstock (2008)[68]	DM	2 years	DNP	431	—	—	1.26
Comstock et al. (2006)[44]	DM	1 year	DNP	DNP	—	—	1.19
Knowles et al. (2006)[58]	IRF	3 seasons	1084	140	12.9	12.9	0.95
Powell and Barber-Foss (1999)[41]	AT	3 years	6502	861	11.8	13.2	2.8
Beachy et al. (1997)[59]	AT	8 years	571	132	—	23.1	—
McLain and Reynolds (1989)[62]	DM	1 year	68	10	15.0	15.0	—
			Basketball				
Borowski et al. (2008)[57]	DM	2 years	—	773	—	—	1.83
Comstock et al. (2006)[44]	DM	1 year	DNP	DNP	—	—	1.89
Knowles et al. (2006)[58]	IRF	3 seasons	1266	186	14.7	14.7	2.32
Messina et al. (1999)[61]	DM	1 season	973	543	—	—	3.2
Powell and Barber-Foss (1999)[41]	AT	3 years	6831	1933	22.5	28.3	4.8
Beachy et al. (1997)[59]	AT	8 years	541	185	—	34.2	—
McLain and Reynolds (1989)[62]	DM	1 year	57	21	36.8	36.8	—
			Cross-Country Running				
Plisky et al. (2007)[63]	AT/IRF	1 year	59	6	10.2	10.2	1.7
Rauh et al. (2006)[47]	IRF	1 season	235	159	35.7	67.7	15.0
Rauh et al. (2000)[64]	DM	15 seasons	2031	846	26.0	41.7	10.9
Beachy et al. (1997)[59]	AT	8 years	501	108	—	21.6	—
			Football				
Comstock et al. (2006)[44]	DM	1 year	DNP	DNP	—	—	4.36
Knowles et al. (2006)[58]	IRF	3 seasons	3323	1064	32.0	32.0	3.54
Rameriz et al. (2006)[69]	DM	2 seasons	5118	1700	25.5	33.2	—
Turbeville et al. (2003)[70]	AT/Coach	2 years	717	132	14.1	18.4	3.20
Powell and Barber-Foss (1999)[41]	AT	3 years	21122	10557	34.6	50.0	8.1
Beachy et al. (1997)[59]	AT	8 years	1278	984	—	77.0	—
DeLee and Farney (1992)[71]	AT	1 season	4399	2228	—	50.6	—
Prager et al. (1989)[72]	AT	4 seasons	598	251	—	42.0	—
McLain and Reynolds (1989)[62]	DM	1 year	179	109	60.9	60.9	—
			Gymnastics				
Beachy et al. (1997)[59]	AT	8 years	177	23	—	13.0	—
McLain and Reynolds (1989)[62]	DM	1 year	20	8	40.0	40.0	—

Table 30-9

A Comparison of Injury Rates in Prospective Studies of Selected Boys' High School Sports—cont'd

Study	Data Collection	Duration	Number of Participants	Number of Injuries	Number of Injured Athletes/N	Injury Rate/100 Athlete Seasons	Injury Rate/1000 Athletic Exposures
			Lacrosse				
Hinton et al. (2005)[65]	AT	3 seasons	3870	615	—	15.9	2.89
			Soccer				
Yard et al. (2008)[66]	DM	2 years	780	—	—	—	2.44
Comstock et al. (2006)[44]	DM	1 year	DNP	DNP	—	—	2.43
Knowles et al. (2006)[58]	IRF	3 seasons	1304	252	19.3	19.3	2.81
Powell and Barber-Foss (1999)[41]	AT	3 years	7539	1765	20.2	23.4	4.6
Beachy et al. (1997)[59]	AT	8 years	757	312	—	41.2	—
McLain and Reynolds (1989)[62]	DM	1 year	99	13	13.1	13.1	—
			Swimming				
Beachy et al. (1997)[59]	AT	8 years	294	15	—	5.1	—
McLain and Reynolds (1989)[62]	DM	1 year	40	0	0.0	0.0	—
			Tennis				
Beachy et al. (1997)[59]	AT	8 years	291	21	—	7.2	—
McLain and Reynolds (1989)[62]	DM	1 year	32	0	0.0	0.0	—
			Track and Field				
Knowles et al. (2006)[58]	IRF	3 seasons	1003	74	7.4	7.4	1.06
Beachy et al. (1997)[59]	AT	8 years	1205	342	—	28.4	—
McLain and Reynolds (1989)[62]	AT	1 season	70	7	10.0	10.0	—
Watson and DiMartino (1987)[67]	I/Q	1 season	156	30	19.2	19.2	—
			Volleyball				
Beachy et al. (1997)[59]	AT	8 years	500	78	—	15.6	—
			Wrestling				
Comstock et al. (2006)[44]	DM	1 year	DNP	DNP	—	—	2.50
Knowles et al. (2006)[58]	IRF	3 seasons	1515	168	11.1	11.1	1.49
Pasque and Hewett (2000)[73]	I/Q	1 season	418	219	15.1	52.4	6.0
Powell and Barber-Foss (1999)[41]	AT	3 years	8117	2910	26.7	35.9	5.6
Beachy et al. (1997)[59]	AT	8 years	594	391	—	65.8	—
McLain and Reynolds (1989)[62]	DM	1 year	65	26	40.0	40.0	—

AT, Athletic trainer reports; *DM*, direct monitoring; *DNP*, data not provided; *I*, interview; *IRF*, injury report form; *Q*, questionnaire.

For boys' high school sports, the highest injury rates per 1000 AEs are reported in cross-country running (range: 1.7 to 15.0), football (range: 3.2 to 8.1), and wrestling (range: 1.49 to 7.6). It should be noted that although injury rates per 1000 AEs were not reported for gymnastics, swimming, tennis, and men's volleyball, the reported injury rates per 100 athletes in these sports were low.

Caution should be used when making comparisons of incidence rates across studies because of study differences and methodological limitations, including varying sample sizes, differing definitions of *injury* and methods of data collection, and variable data collection periods. Thus, in light of these methodological differences, it may be more appropriate to compare injury rates across sports within a multiple-sport study that has used the same study injury definition and data collection methods (i.e., designated data collectors for injuries and participation [athletic] exposures) consistently across all sports. Only three multisport studies reported injury rates per 1000 AEs during the past two decades.[41,44,58] In all three studies, football had the highest overall injury rate for boys and soccer had the highest incidence rate of injury for girls' sports (Figure 30-4). In general, softball and baseball had the lowest incidence injury rates for girls' and boys' sports, respectively. However, not all high school sports were included in these studies, especially girls' and boys' cross-country running that have reported high injury rates per 1000 AEs.[47,64]

Clinical Point

Clinicians and researchers should carefully consider the following methodological issues when making comparisons of injury incidence across studies:

- Different injury definitions
- Type of denominator use
- Varying sample sizes
- Different methods of data collection
- Variable data collection periods

Collegiate. At the collegiate level, women's soccer had the highest incidence rate injury followed by men's wrestling and soccer between 1988 to 2004 (Figure 30-5).[40] Men's baseball and women's softball had the lowest incidence of injury, which is similar to the high school level.

Gender Differences

High School. A comparison of high school studies providing incidence rates per 1000 AEs for both girls and boys in same sports is provided in Table 30-10. Significantly higher incidence rates were reported for girls than boys in softball,[41] basketball,[57] cross-country running,[47,64] and soccer.[41] None of the studies reported injury rates that were significantly higher for boys as compared with girls in same sports.

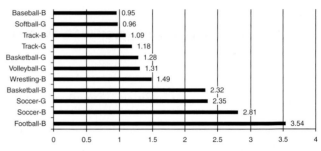

Injury Rates per 1000 AEs: Knowles et al., *Am J Epidem* 2006 (58)

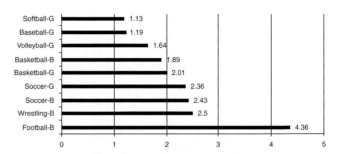

Injury Rates per 1000 AEs: Comstock et al., *MMWR* 2006 (44)

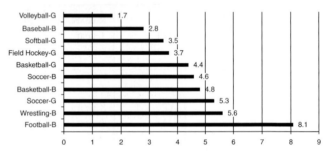

Injury Rates per 1000 AEs: Powell & Barber-Foss, *J Athl Train* 1999 (41)

Figure 30-4

A comparison of injury rates in prospective studies of selected high school sports. Girls *(G)*, Boys *(B)*.

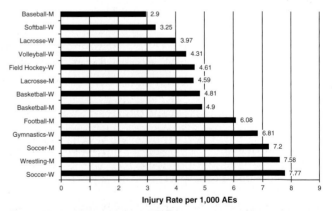

Injury Rate per 1,000 AEs

Figure 30-5

A comparison of injury rates in selected National Collegiate Athletic Association (NCAA) collegiate sports: 16-year longitudinal study of NCAA collegiate men's and women's sports.[40] Women *(W)*, men *(M)*.

Table 30-10

A Comparison of Injury Rates in Prospective Studies of Similar Girls' and Boys' High School Sports

Study	Injury Rate		Girls/Boys Rate Ratio	95% CI
	Girls	Boys		
Softball and Baseball				
Comstock et al. (2006)[44]	1.13	1.19	0.95	(0.77-1.17)
Knowles et al. (2006)[58]	0.96	0.95	1.01	DNP
Powell and Barber-Foss (1999)[41]	3.5	2.8	1.27	(1.16-1.40)*
Basketball				
Borowski et al. (2008)[57]	2.08	1.83	1.14	(1.03-1.26)*
Comstock et al. (2006)[44]	2.01	1.89	1.06	(0.92-1.23)
Knowles et al. (2006)[58]	1.28	2.32	0.55	DNP
Gomez et al. (1986)[60] and Messina et al. (1999)[61]	3.6	3.2	1.13	(0.99-1.28)
Powell and Barber-Foss (1999)[41]	4.4	4.8	1.02	(0.96-1.09)
Cross-Country Running				
Plisky et al. (2007)[63]	4.3	1.7	2.50	(0.85-8.23)
Rauh et al. (2006)[47]	19.6	15.0	1.30	(1.04-1.64)*
Rauh et al. (2000)[64]	16.7	10.9	1.52	(1.38-1.68)*
Lacrosse				
Hinton et al. (2005)[65]	2.54	2.89	0.88	(0.77-1.00)
Soccer				
Yard et al. (2008)[66]	2.34	2.44	1.03	(0.93-1.14)
Comstock et al. (2006)[44]	2.36	2.43	0.97	(0.84-1.13)
Knowles et al. (2006)[58]	2.35	2.81	0.84	DNP
Powell and Barber-Foss (1999)[41]	5.3	4.6	1.15	(1.08-1.23)*
Track and Field				
Knowles et al. (2006)[58]	1.18	1.06	1.11	DNP

CI, Confidence interval; *DNP,* data not provided (denominator) to determine confidence intervals.
*$p \leq 0.05$.

Collegiate. At the collegiate level, although incidence rates of injury were significantly higher among women than men in soccer (rate ratio [RR] = 1.08, 95% CI: 1.05-1.11) and softball (RR = 1.12, 95% CI: 1.08-1.16), men had a significantly higher incidence injury rate in lacrosse than women (RR = 1.15, 95% CI: 1.11-1.21) (Figure 30-6).[40] The incidence of injury was similar for women's and men's basketball.

Exposure (Practice versus Competition or Games) Setting

High School. Most studies on participation setting have reported on percent of injury in practice and competitions or games. Studies reporting competition and practice injury rates per 1000 AEs for girls' and boys' high school sports are presented in Table 30-11. The incidence rates were consistently higher in competition and games than practice for girls' basketball,[41,44,57,60,61] field hockey,[41] soccer,[41,44,66] and softball.[41,44] For boys, the rate of injury was consistently greater in competition and games than practices for baseball,[41,44,68] basketball,[41,44,57,61] football,[41,44,70] lacrosse,[65] and wrestling.[41,44,73] In several girls' and boys' cross-country running studies,[47,64] and in girls' lacrosse[65] and volleyball[41] the incidence of injury was higher in practices than in competition/games.

Collegiate. As shown in Table 30-12, the incidence rates of injury were higher in games than in practices for all women's and men's collegiate sports.[74-86] The risk of incurring an injury

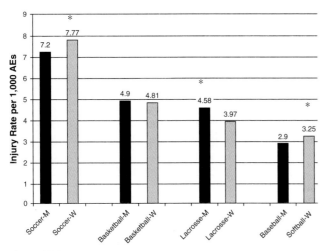

Figure 30-6

A comparison of injury rates among similar men's and women's selected National Collegiate Athletic Association (NCAA) collegiate sports: 16-year longitudinal study of NCAA collegiate men's and women's sports.[40] Women *(W)*, men *(M)*, *$P \leq 0.0001$.

during a game rather than in a practice was greatest (i.e., three to four times greater) for men's baseball,[75] lacrosse,[82] and wrestling,[86] and men's and women's soccer.[83,84]

Body Location

Determining which anatomical sites are most commonly injured is vital as it informs sports medicine personnel which body sites will likely need more attention during preparticipation musculoskeletal screening and preventative strategies.

High School. A percent comparison of injuries by body location reported in girls' and boys' high school sports are presented in Table 30-13 and Table 30-14.[41,47,57,61,64-71,73,87-89] With the exception of boys' baseball and wrestling, these tables indicate that the lower-extremity body region incurred the greatest percentage of injuries. In general, the ankle and knee are the most commonly injured lower-extremity sites, except in cross-country and track and field in which injuries primarily occur at the lower leg and knee. Upper extremity injuries are most common in girls' softball and boys' baseball and wrestling. In general, the shoulder was the most common upper-extremity injury area in these three sports, followed by the elbow, forearm, and wrist injuries, although the actual percent of injury for these areas are difficult to determine as they were frequently combined together when reported. Boys' lacrosse and wrestling had the highest frequency of injuries involving the head-face and neck-spine. For girls' sports, a high percentage of head and spine injuries were also reported in field hockey[41] and softball.[87]

Collegiate. Table 30-15 and Table 30-16 present percent comparisons of injuries by body location calculated from women's and men's collegiate sports between 1988 and 2004. Similar to the interscholastic level, the lower-body region had the highest percent of injury for all women's

and men's collegiate sports with the exception of men's baseball. The ankle was the most common lower-extremity injury for basketball,[76,77] gymnastics,[80] lacrosse,[81,82] men's soccer,[84] and volleyball,[85] whereas the knee was more common for field hockey,[78] football,[79] softball,[74] and women's soccer.[83] Women's softball[74] and baseball[75] had the highest percent of upper-extremity injury, with the shoulder most commonly affected. The percent of head and spine injuries are highest in wrestling,[86] field hockey,[78] and women's lacrosse,[81] with the head and face being the most commonly injured sites. Gymnastics,[80] volleyball,[85] and wrestling[86] have the highest percent of injuries in the trunk region, with the lower back being the most commonly injured body site.

Severity of Injury

Injury severity can consist of a broad spectrum of injuries from abrasions to fractures to injuries that result in permanent functional disability or even death. Injury severity can be expressed by one or more of the following: injury type, time loss, clinical outcome (e.g., reinjury, catastrophic injury), and economic cost. Assessment in each of the following areas is important in identifying the extent of the problem.

Four Methods to Assess Injury Severity
• Injury type
• Time loss
• Clinical outcome
• Economic cost

Injury Type

Identification of common injury types is important, because, like body location, it alerts sports medicine personnel to injuries that may need special attention (e.g., ACL injuries), and it directs researchers in identifying and testing related risk factors and preventive measures.[90] Most studies report injury types in general terms, such as *sprain* or *fracture*, without providing specifics (e.g., grade of sprain, fracture type), especially at the high school level.

High School. The most commonly reported injuries across most high school sports are sprain, strains, and contusions; followed by lacerations, fractures, and inflammation, depending on sport and gender.[41,57,61,65,66,68-70,73] A slightly different trend was found in track and field, in which muscle strains and inflammations were reported as more common.[67] Although concussions are generally the least common severe injury reported, a higher occurrence of concussions than fractures have been reported in soccer[66] and girls' lacrosse.[65] Although the proportion of concussion injuries were similar between boys' and girls' soccer players,[66] male lacrosse players were three times more likely to incur a concussion injury than female lacrosse players (incidence rate ratio = 2.99 [1.65-5.79]).[65]

Table 30-11

A Comparison of Injury Rates in Competition and Practice Settings in Selected High School Sports (per 1000 AEs)

Study	Girls			Boys		
	Competition	Practice	C/P Ratio	Competition	Practice	C/P Ratio
Baseball						
Collins and Comstock (2008)[68]	—	—	—	1.89	0.85	2.22
Comstock et al. (2006)[44]	—	—	—	1.78	0.79	2.3
Powell and Barber-Foss (1999)[41]	—	—	—	5.6	1.8	3.1
Basketball						
Borowski et al. (2008)[57]	3.66	1.43	2.55	2.93	1.38	2.12
Comstock et al. (2006)[44]	3.60	1.37	2.6	2.98	1.46	2.0
Gomez et al. (1996)[60] and Messina et al. (1999)[61]	16.0	2.0	8.0	16.9	1.8	9.4
Powell and Barber-Foss (1999)[41]	7.9	3.2	2.5	7.1	3.4	2.1
Cross-Country Running						
Rauh et al. (2006)[47]	12.5	21.1	0.59	15.0	15.0	1.0
Rauh et al. (2000)[64]	11.9	11.2	1.07	5.6	8.0	0.7
Field Hockey						
Powell and Barber-Foss (1999)[41]	4.9	3.2	1.5	—	—	—
Football						
Comstock et al. (2006)[44]	—	—	—	12.09	2.54	4.78
Turbeville et al. (2003)[70]	—	—	—	13.12	1.31	10.01
Powell and Barber-Foss (1999)[41]	—	—	—	26.4	5.3	5.0
Lacrosse						
Hinton et al. (2005)[65]	1.48	2.28	0.65	4.44	1.40	3.17
Soccer						
Yard et al. (2008)[66]	5.34	1.21	4.40	4.26	1.51	3.83
Comstock et al. (2006)[44]	5.21	1.10	4.7	4.22	1.58	2.7
Powell and Barber-Foss (1999)[41]	11.4	3.1	3.7	10.2	2.5	4.1
Softball						
Comstock et al. (2006)[44]	1.77	0.87	2.0	—	—	—
Powell and Barber-Foss (1999)[41]	5.9	2.7	2.2	—	—	—
Volleyball						
Comstock et al. (2006)[44]	1.92	1.48	1.3	—	—	—
Powell and Barber-Foss (1999)[41]	1.2	2.8	0.4	—	—	—
Wrestling						
Comstock et al. (2006)[44]	—	—	—	3.93	2.04	1.9
Pasque and Hewett (2000)[73]	—	—	—	9.0	5.0	1.8
Powell and Barber-Foss (1999)[41]	—	—	—	8.2	4.8	1.7

AE, Athletic exposure; *C/P Ratio*, competition to practice ratio.

Table 30-12

A Comparison of Injury Rates in Game and Practice Settings in Selected Collegiate Sports (per 1000 AEs)*

Study	Women			Men		
	Game	Practice	G/P Ratio	Game	Practice	G/P Ratio
Softball						
Marshall et al.[74]	4.3	2.7	1.59	—	—	—
Baseball						
Dick et al.[75]	—	—	—	5.78	1.85	2.96
Basketball						
Agel et al.,[76] Dick et al.[77]	7.68	3.99	1.92	9.9	4.3	2.30
Field Hockey						
Dick et al.[78]	7.87	3.70	2.13	—	—	—
Football						
Dick et al.[79]	—	—	—	9.62	3.80	2.53
Gymnastics						
Marshall et al.[80]	15.19	6.07	2.50	—	—	—
Lacrosse						
Dick et al.,[81] Dick et al.[82]	7.15	3.30	2.17	12.58	3.24	3.88
Soccer						
Dick et al.,[83] Agel et al.[84]	16.4	5.20	3.15	18.75	4.34	4.32
Volleyball						
Agel et al.[85]	4.58	4.10	1.12	—	—	—
Wrestling						
Agel et al.[86]	—	—	—	26.4	5.7	4.63

AE, Athletic exposure; *G/P ratio,* game/practice ratio.
*16-year longitudinal study of the National Collegiate Athletic Association Collegiate Men's and Women's Sports.

Collegiate. Although there is some small variation by sport, gender, and exposure type (i.e., practice or game), the most frequently reported injuries at the collegiate level are sprains, strains, and contusions.[91] Ligamentous injuries to the ankle were the most common injury occurrence (14.9% of all injuries, 0.83 per 1000 AEs), regardless of sport or exposure type. More than 27,000 ankle ligament sprains were reported in 16 sports during 16 academic years, yielding an average of approximately 1700 per year. Although spring football (1.34 per 1000 AEs) had the highest rates of ankle ligament sprains, these injuries accounted for approximately one quarter of all injuries in men's (1.30 per 1000 AEs) and women's basketball (1.15 per 1000 AEs) and women's volleyball (1.01 per 1000 AEs). During this same period, approximately 5000 ACL injuries (0.15 per 1000 AEs) were reported for average of 313 per year. Football had the highest number of reported ACL knee injuries (fall 2159 [0.18 per 1000 AEs], spring 379 [0.33 per 1000 AEs], 53% of all reported ACLs). Three of the four sports with the highest rates of ACL injuries were women's sports: gymnastics,

Table 30-13

A Percent Comparison of Injuries by Body Location Among Selected Girls' High School Sports

Study	Basketball			Cross-Country		Field Hockey	Lacrosse	Soccer		Softball		Track and Field	Volleyball	
	Borowski et al.[57]	Messina et al.[61]	Powell and Barber-Foss[41]	Rauh et al.[64]	Rauh et al.[47]	Powell and Barber-Foss[41]	Hinton et al.[65]	Powell and Barber-Foss[41]	Yard et al.[66]	Powell and Barber-Foss[41]	Rechel et al.[87]	Watson and DiMartino[67]	Powell and Barber-Foss[41]	Rechel et al.[87]
Number of injuries	745		1748	776	157	510	370	1771	DNP	910	DNP	11	628	DNP
Head/Face/Neck/Spine	*14.2*	*7.5*	*11.0*	*0.0*	*0.0*	*16.6*	*14.9*	*9.7*	*14.6*	*11.2*	*19.5*	*0.0*	*4.5*	*3.9*
Head	14.2[a]	7.5	11.0[a]			16.6[a]	14.1	9.7[a]	14.6	11.2[a]			4.5[a]	
Neck/spine							1.6							
Upper Extremity	*12.0*	*13.1*	*12.7*	*0.0*	*0.0*	*15.8*	*15.2*	*6.4*	*6.1*	*39.2*	*36.1*	*0.0*	*20.8*	*18.8*
Shoulder	2.5[b]	2.8	2.4[b]			3.1[b]	4.1	1.9[b]	1.3	16.3[b]			9.4[b]	
Upper arm														
Elbow							1.6[h]		4.2[k]					
Forearm	9.5[c]	2.3[f]	10.3[c]			12.7[c]		4.5[c]		22.9[c]			11.4[c]	
Wrist		8.0					9.5[i]							
Hand/fingers														
Trunk	*4.0*	*7.1*	*6.4*	*2.8*	*5.9*	*4.9*	*4.0*	*4.5*	*4.8[j]*	*5.5*	*1.7*	*18.1*	*11.4*	*12.5*
Chest		0.9		0.0	0.0		0.0					0.0		
Abdomen				0.0	0.0		0.0					0.0		
Back		6.2		2.8	5.9		4.0					18.1		
Lower extremity	*67.7*	*69.8*	*68.9*	*96.2*	*94.1*	*58.8*	*64.2*	*78.7*	*74.5*	*43.6*	*42.7*	*81.9*	*62.5*	*64.8*
Hip/groin	8.7[d]	9.4[g]	16.8[d]	7.8	13.6	21.8[d]	4.1	25.8[d]	1.6	18.0[d]		0.0	9.6[d]	
Upper leg/thigh				4.8	5.9		4.1		11.7			18.2		
Knee	18.2	19.7	15.7	19.5	17.8	13.7	21.4	19.4	21.8	10.8		9.1	11.1	
Lower leg	4.9	4.4		38.3	45.0		6.5		7.8			27.3		
Ankle	35.9[e]	31.0	36.4[e]	15.8	7.7	23.3[e]	25.1	33.5[e]	24.7	14.8[e]		27.3	41.8[e]	
Foot		5.3		10.0	4.1		3.0		6.9			0.0		
Other	*2.2*	*2.5*	*1.1*	*1.0*	*0.0*	*3.3*	*1.9*	*0.7*	*0.8*	*0.5*	*0.0*	*0.0*	*0.4*	*0.0*

DNP, data not provided.

a Includes head, neck and spine injuries.
b Includes shoulder and arm injuries.
c Includes forearm, wrist, and hand injuries.
d Includes hip, thigh, and leg injuries.
e Includes ankle and foot injuries.
f Includes arm and wrist injuries.
g Includes hip and thigh injuries.
h Includes upper arm, elbow, and forearm injuries.
i Includes wrist and hand injuries.
j Includes torso, spine, and neck.
k Includes upper arm, elbow, forearm, wrist, and hand injuries.

Table 30-14

A Percent Comparison of Injuries by Body Location Among Selected Boys' High School Sports

Study	Baseball		Basketball			Cross-Country			
	Collins and Comstock[68]	Powell and Barber-Foss[41]	Borowski et al.[57]	Messina et al.[61]	Powell and Barber-Foss[41]	Rauh et al.[64]	Rauh et al.[47]	DeLee and Farney[71]	Powell and Barber-Foss[41]
Number of injuries	431	861	773	543	1933	846	159	2228	10557
Head/Face/ Neck/Spine	*16.5*	*10.8*	*12.8*	*13.6*	*13.3*	*0.0*	*0.0*	*10.0*	*15.5*
Head/face	15.8	10.8[a]	12.8[a]	13.6	13.3[a]			9.0	15.5[a]
Neck/spine	0.7							1.0	
Upper extremity	*39.9*	*44.3*	*12.2*	*16.8*	*13.8*	*0.0*	*0.0*	*23.0*	*26.2*
Shoulder	15.5	19.7[b]	2.8[b]	6.1	2.4[b]			11.0	12.0[b]
Upper arm	1.2								
Elbow	7.2							4.0	
Forearm	2.1	24.6[c]	9.4[c]	3.4[f]	11.4[c]				14.2[c]
Wrist	3.7								
Hand	10.2			8.8				8.0	
Trunk	*5.8*	*7.2*	*7.1*	*6.1*	*7.7*	*3.4*	*2.4*	*9.0*	*8.6*
Chest	1.6			0.4		0.0	0.0	0.0	
Abdomen	0.5					0.0	0.0	0.0	
Back	3.7			5.7		3.4	2.4	9.0	
Lower extremity	*35.7*	*37.5*	*65.4*	*60.4*	*64.8*	*94.2*	*97.6*	*55.0*	*47.7*
Hip/groin	1.8	14.5[d]	8.2[d]	10.5[g]	14.4[d]	5.5	9.8	7.0	16.7[d]
Upper leg/ Thigh	7.6					8.5	4.3		
Knee	8.6	10.5	10.6	9.7	11.1	24.3	25.8	20.0	15.1
Lower leg	3.0		3.4	4.4		29.2	31.3	8.0	
Ankle	14.2	12.5[e]	43.2[e]	31.9	39.3[e]	18.4	19.0	18.0	15.9[e]
Foot	0.5			3.9		8.3	7.4	2.0	
Other	*2.1*	*0.1*	*2.4*	*3.9*	*0.4*	*2.4*	*0.0*	*2.0*	*2.0*

[a]Includes head, neck, and spine injuries.
[b]Includes shoulder and arm injuries.
[c]Includes forearm, wrist, and hand injuries.
[d]Includes hip, thigh, and leg injuries.
[e]Includes ankle and foot injuries.
[f]Includes arm and wrist injuries.
[g]Includes hip and thigh injuries.
[h]Includes upper arm, elbow, forearm, and wrist injuries.
[i]Includes torso, spine, and neck injuries.
[j]Includes lower leg, ankle, and foot injuries.
[k]Includes upper arm, elbow, and forearm injuries.
[l]Includes upper leg and lower leg injuries.
[m]Includes wrist and hand injuries.
[n]Includes upper arm, elbow, forearm, wrist, and hand injuries.

Football			Lacrosse	Soccer		Track and Field	Wrestling		
Rameriz et al.[69]	Shankar et al.[88]	Turbeville et al.[70]	Hinton et al.[65]	Powell and Barber-Foss[41]	Yard et al.[66]	Watson and Dimartino[67]	Pasque and Hewett[73]	Powell and Barber-Foss[41]	Yard et al.[89]
1724	1881	132	615	1765	1524	30	219	2910	387
18.6	11.5	14.4	18.6	8.7	13.1	0.0	19.0	16.5	16.2
13.6	11.5[a]	8.3	15.8	8.7[a]	13.1		8.0	16.5[a]	9.4
5.0		6.1	2.8				11.0		6.8
23.2	29.1	18.9	22.1	8.2	7.3	6.6	42.0	32.6	39.2
	12.4	9.1[k]	8.5	2.4[b]	2.2	3.3	24.0	18.4[b]	18.6
	7.4[h]	2.3[k]	2.9[k]		5.1[n]	0.0			1.8
						3.3	7.0		10.1
				5.8[c]		0.0		14.2[c]	0.0
		3.0	10.7[m]			0.0	11.0[m]		1.7
	9.3	4.5				0.0			7.0
13.0	11.6[i]	4.6	7.6	6.5	5.2[i]	13.3	8.0	11.9	12.0
1.4		7.8	0.0			0.0			
6.6		0.0	0.0			0.0			
5.0		3.8	7.6			13.3			
45.1	46.9	62.1	49.9	76.6	73.0	80.1	31.0	27.2	32.3
	9.3[g]	3.0	2.6	28.0[d]	5.1	16.6		5.4[d]	4.5[g]
		27.3[l]	7.7		14.6	3.4	3.0[l]		
	15.2	19.7	15.5	15.1	15.4	23.3	17.0	14.8	15.4
			5.2		7.6	16.7			2.9
	22.4[j]	9.8	16.1	33.5[e]	22.0	16.7	11.0[e]	7.0[e]	8.4
		2.3	2.8		8.3	3.4			1.1
0.1	1.1	0.0	2.0	0.2	1.4	0.0	0.0	11.7	0.4

Table 30-15

A Percent Comparison of Injuries by Body Location Among Selected Women's Collegiate Sports

Study	Basketball	Field Hockey	Gymnastics	Lacrosse	Soccer	Softball	Volleyball
	Agel et al.[76]	Dick et al.[78]	Marshall et al.[80]	Dick et al.[81]	Dick et al.[83]	Marshall et al.[74]	Agel et al.[85]
Number of injuries*	9792	3145	2621	3242	10714	5153	6692
Head/Face/Neck/Spine	*11.4*	*15.6*	*7.0*	*15.8*	*9.1*	*12.0*	*4.8*
Head/face	10.7	14.9	3.2	15.3	8.5	10.9	3.6
Neck/spine	0.7	0.7	3.8	0.5	0.6	1.1	1.2
Upper extremity	*12.5*	*13.3*	*17.4*	*7.2*	*5.5*	*34.2*	*20.4*
Shoulder	3.9	2.3	6.3	2.8	2.1	13.3	10.9
Upper arm	0.1	0.2	0.4	0.2	0.1	1.3	0.3
Elbow	1.0	0.5	3.9	0.5	0.4	4.0	1.7
Forearm	0.3	0.7	0.9	0.2	0.2	2.0	0.3
Wrist	1.2	0.8	2.7	0.7	0.7	2.5	1.8
Hand/fingers	6.0	8.8	3.2	2.8	2.0	11.1	5.4
Trunk	*5.6*	*5.7*	*13.8*	*4.7*	*5.3*	*6.5*	*10.9*
Chest	0.7	0.7	0.8	0.5	0.9	1.0	0.5
Abdomen	0.1	0.1	0.5	0.1	0.2	0.3	1.8
Back	4.8	4.9	12.5	4.1	3.2	5.2	8.6
Lower extremity	*70.7*	*63.7*	*61.8*	*72.0*	*80.1*	*47.0*	*63.4*
Hip/groin	4.0	7.4	3.5	5.8	7.0	3.4	4.5
Upper leg/thigh	5.5	15.6	4.5	13.0	18.0	9.0	7.1
Knee	21.1	15.9	17.7	16.6	20.1	14.5	15.0
Lower leg	4.7	6.0	5.2	9.8	7.5	4.7	3.4
Ankle	26.9	12.4	18.8	20.1	20.0	12.0	26.3
Foot	8.5	6.4	12.1	6.7	7.5	3.4	7.1
Other	*0.1*	*1.7*	*0.1*	*0.3*	*0.9*	*0.3*	*0.5*

*Number of injuries that specified a body part.

soccer, and basketball (0.33, 0.28, 0.23 per 1000 AEs, respectively). Although ACL injuries accounted for only 3% of all injuries, 88% of these injuries resulted in 10 or more days of time loss. The rate of ACL injury increased 1.3% on average during the 16-year period.

Overall, 9150 concussions, or a rate of 0.94 concussions per 1000 AEs, were reported among the 16 collegiate sports between 1988 and 2004.[91] The rate of concussion increased significantly by 7% on average during this period. The rate of concussion ranged from 0.07 (men's baseball) to 0.91 (women's ice hockey) per 1000 AEs. Football had the largest number of reported concussions (n = 5016) with higher rates in spring (0.54 per 1000 AEs) than in fall (0.37 per 1000 AEs) football. Higher rates of concussion were reported among women than men for basketball, hockey, soccer, and softball.

Clinical Point

Sprains, strains, and contusion are the most commonly reported type of injury at high school and collegiate levels.

Time Loss

An often used and useful measure of injury severity in the sports injury literature is the duration of restriction from athletic performance. Although the length of time lost because of sports injury likely provides the most precise indication of the consequences of injury to an athlete,[55] it is recognized that subjective factors such as personal motivation, peer influence, or coaching staff reluctance may determine if and when athletes return to play.[90] In addition, as shown in Table 30-17, there is presently no consensus on what amount of time loss constitutes the degree of severity of an injury. In general, *time loss* has been defined as any injury that restricts the athlete from completing a practice or competitive event or prevents the athlete from returning to a subsequent practice or competitive event with an unrestricted participation status.[47,92] At the high school level, although time-loss severity classifications of mild (< 8 days), moderate (8 to 21 days), or major (≥ 22) have been advocated to standardize injury severity,[41] others have used different classifications (1 to 4 days, 5 to 14 days, 15 or more days, respectively[47,64] or 1 to 6 days, 7 to 21 days, 22 or more days, respectively[44,66]). Beachy and colleagues[59] also included a fourth category of no time lost. The lack of

Table 30-16

A Percent Comparison of Injuries by Body Location Among Selected Men's Collegiate Sports

Study	Baseball	Basketball	Football	Lacrosse	Soccer	Wrestling
	Dick et al.[75]	Dick et al.[77]	Dick et al.[79]	Dick et al.[82]	Agel et al.[84]	Agel et al.[86]
Number of injuries*	8089	11659	82716	4696	12583	9448
Head/Face/Neck/Spine	*8.3*	*12.7*	*10.9*	*8.8*	*9.3*	*17.6*
Head/face	7.7	12.0	7.1	7.1	8.6	12.9
Neck/spine	0.6	0.7	3.8	1.7	0.7	4.7
Upper extremity	*46.8*	*12.5*	*21.7*	*21.3*	*6.2*	*23.3*
Shoulder	20.7	3.7	13.3	12.3	2.9	14.1
Upper arm	1.5	0.1	0.4	0.5	0.1	0.4
Elbow	10.3	1.1	1.5	1.1	0.5	4.1
Forearm	1.9	0.2	0.4	0.8	0.3	0.5
Wrist	3.2	2.0	1.1	1.5	0.6	0.7
Hand/fingers	9.2	5.4	5.0	5.1	1.8	3.5
Trunk	*6.4*	*6.7*	*5.8*	*6.5*	*4.4*	*8.9*
Chest	1.1	0.6	1.6	2.0	1.1	4.6
Abdomen	0.5	0.2	0.3	0.4	0.4	0.2
Back	4.8	5.9	3.9	4.1	2.9	4.1
Lower extremity	*38.2*	*67.8*	*59.4*	*63.1*	*79.1*	*37.0*
Hip/groin	3.6	6.2	5.6	6.9	8.0	1.6
Upper leg/thigh	11.1	6.3	11.0	15.7	17.8	1.8
Knee	7.5	14.3	19.9	15.0	16.0	22.4
Lower leg	3.9	3.2	3.3	5.0	7.4	1.0
Ankle	9.3	29.1	15.0	16.0	20.5	8.2
Foot	2.8	8.7	4.6	4.5	9.4	2.0
Other	*0.3*	*0.3*	*2.2†*	*0.3*	*1.0*	*13.2*

*Number of injuries that specified a body part.
†92.4% of others were general body-related injuries.

consensus in reporting severity of injury has been apparent at the collegiate level. Although Powell and Dompier[93] used the classification of less than 8 days, 8 to 21 days, and 22 or more days to describe mild, moderate, and major time-lost injuries, an NCAA compendium of 16 sports used less than 10 days or 10 or more days to denote severity of injury.[40] Thus, these differences in definitions make the comparability within and across competitive levels difficult.

Clinical Point

Because there is no standard definition of what constitutes the degree of severity of an injury, in terms of amount of time loss, making comparisons within and across sport studies can be difficult.

High School. Of the few studies that have reported time lost from injury, most indicated that the majority of injuries in girls' and boys' high school sports are minor in nature (see Table 30-17).[41,44,47,57,64,66,68] One study compared time loss relative to AE or gender. Rechel and

colleagues[87] reported that a significantly greater proportion of competition injuries (19.2%) resulted in more than 3 weeks of time loss than injuries that occurred in practice (15%) (proportion ratio [PR] = 1.28, 95% CI: 1.08-1.52). Competition injuries were more likely to result in 3 or more weeks of time loss or the end of the athletes' season than practice injuries in baseball (23.9% vs. 6.9%; PR = 3.47, 95% CI: 1.48-8.11) and girls' volleyball (21.3% vs. 7.4%; PR = 2.88; 95% CI: 1.01-8.24). Finally, in two separate studies of cross-country runners, Rauh and colleagues,[47,64] reported that girls had significantly higher rates of injuries resulting in 15 or more days of time lost (RR = 1.5, 95% CI: 1-2.2; RR = 3.2, 95% CI: 1.4-8, respectively) or out-for-season (RR = 1.8, 95% CI: 1.2-2.6; RR = 3.3, 95% CI: 1-14.5, respectively) than boys.

Collegiate. As shown in Table 30-18, most injuries that occurred in practices or games resulted in nine or fewer participation days lost for both women's and men's sports.[74-81,83-86] The distribution of injuries resulting in 10 or more days of time loss was slightly higher during games for most sports with the exception of spring football[79] and men's lacrosse.[82]

Table 30-17

Percent Comparison of Severity Rates in Selected High School Sports

Study	Girls			Boys		
	Minor	Moderate	Major	Minor	Moderate	Major
Baseball						
Collins and Comstock (2008)[68]*	—	—	—	50.3	31.0	6.7
Comstock et al. (2006)[44]†	—	—	—	50.0	35.0	15.0
Powell and Barber-Foss (1999)[41]‡	—	—	—	69.0	18.5	12.5
Basketball						
Borowski et al. (2008)[57]*	G: 49.6	28.3	7.4	56.4	28.9	6.4
	P: 45.7	33.4	10.5	54.4	29.4	8.0
Comstock et al. (2006)[44]†	46.0	30.0	19.0	52.0	28.0	15.0
Powell and Barber-Foss (1999)[41]‡	72.1	15.4	12.4	75.5	14.5	9.9
Cross-Country Running						
Rauh et al. (2006)[47]§	71.0	16.2	12.8	67.9	20.0	12.1
Rauh et al. (2000)[64]§	62.9	20.0	17.1	63.8	28.2	8.0
Field Hockey						
Powell and Barber-Foss (1999)[41]‡	79.6	13.3	7.1	—	—	—
Football						
Comstock et al. (2006)[44]†	—	—	—	48.0	28.0	19.0
Powell and Barber-Foss (1999)[41]‡	—	—	—	72.5	16.3	11.2
Soccer						
Yard et al. (2008)[66]†	53.9	29.2	16.9	57.9	28.9	13.2
Comstock et al. (2006)[44]*	48.0	32.0	15.0	55.0	27.0	14.0
Powell and Barber-Foss (1999)[41]‡	72.5	15.4	12.1	74.6	15.0	10.4
Softball						
Comstock et al. (2006)[44]†	55.0	28.0	14.0	—	—	—
Powell and Barber-Foss (1999)[41]‡	77.1	15.1	7.8	—	—	—
Volleyball						
Comstock et al. (2006)[44]†	58.0	25.0	12.0	—	—	—
Powell and Barber-Foss (1999)[41]‡	75.0	17.1	7.8	—	—	—
Wrestling						
Comstock et al. (2006)[44]*	—	—	—	45.0	27.0	24.0
Powell and Barber-Foss (1999)[41]‡	—	—	—	67.4	17.8	14.8

G, Games; P, practices.

*Borowski et al.[57] and Collins and Comstock[68]: Minor < 1 week, Moderate 1-3 weeks, Major > 3 weeks.

†Comstock et al.[44]: Estimated from figure (categories do not add up to 100% because of nonreporting of injuries); Yard et al.[66]: Minor 1-6, Moderate 7-21, Major 22+ days.

‡Powell and Barber-Foss[41]: Minor < 8 days, Moderate 8-21 days, Major 22+ days.

§Rauh et al.[47,64]: Minor 1-4 days, Moderate 5-14 days, Major 15+ days.

Table 30-18

Percent Comparison of Game and Practice Injuries Resulting in 10 or Days Lost in Selected Collegiate Sports

Study	Women (≥ 10 days lost)		Men (≥ 10 days lost)	
	Games	Practices	Games	Practices
Softball				
Marshall et al.[74]	24.8	22.0	—	—
Baseball				
Dick et al.[75]	—	—	25.2	25.0
Basketball				
Agel et al.,[76] Dick et al.[77]	25.3	23.6	18.0	18.0
Field Hockey				
Dick et al.[78]	15.0	13.0	—	—
Football				
Dick et al.[79]	—	—	27.0	Fall: 24.9 Spring: 33.5
Gymnastics				
Marshall et al.[80]	34.0	32.0	—	—
Lacrosse				
Dick et al.,[81] Dick et al.[82]	21.9	23.9	21.0	21.0
Soccer				
Dick et al.,[83] Agel et al.[84]	21.8	16.5	18.7	14.6
Volleyball				
Agel et al.[85]	23.0	19.0	—	—
Wrestling				
Agel et al.[86]	—	—	34.0	28.0

Longitudinal, 16-year study of National Collegiate Athletic Association Collegiate Men's and Women's Sports.

Reinjury

At all levels of sport, players may return to full participation before their injury has completely recovered.[94] The unresolved residual symptoms from the previous injury may predispose the athlete to reinjury at the same or a different site.[64,95,96] Some recent studies indicate that previous injury may be a significant factor for an injury in high school sports.[47,69,97]

High School. Few studies have reported the incidence of reinjury to the same body part in high school sports, with percent estimates in a variety of sports ranging from 8.4% to 49.0%.[41,47,64,97] Incidence rates have ranged from 1.2 per 100 person-session hours in football[69] to 37.6 per 1000 AEs in cross-country.[64] Although the risk of reinjury in a study of five girls' team sports ranged from 0.9 to 1.1,[28] the risk of reinjury in girls' cross-country was four times greater.[64] Body parts with the highest risk of reinjury were the shoulder (softball, volleyball), knee (field hockey, softball, volleyball), and lower leg (basketball, volleyball). Soccer players were 1.3 times more likely to reinjure their ankle ($p = 0.02$). The likelihood of rotator cuff strain reinjuries was two to three times higher for softball and soccer players, respectively, and volleyball players were almost three times more likely to reinjure their ACLs. The reoccurrence of hamstring strains and shin splints were significant for field hockey and volleyball players, respectively, in contrast with injuries found in girls' cross-country (RR = 4.3).[64] In cross-country, the shin and knee have the highest rates of reinjury.[47,64]

Collegiate. To date, collegiate studies have not reported rates for reinjury on a comprehensive scale.

Catastrophic Injury

Catastrophic injuries are rare but severely debilitating events. The most comprehensive review of catastrophic injuries comes from the National Center for Catastrophic Sports Injury Research (NCCSI).[36] Data on catastrophic injury among high school and collegiate sports have been monitored by the NCCSI since 1982. According to the NCCSI, catastrophic injuries are considered direct (i.e., injuries that result directly from participation in the skills of the sport) and indirect (i.e., injuries that were caused by systemic failure as a result of exertion while participating in a sport activity or by a complication that was secondary to a nonfatal injury). Catastrophic injuries are also divided into three classifications: fatal, nonfatal (i.e., permanent, severe functional disability), and serious (i.e., no permanent functional disability but severe injury—e.g., cervical vertebral fracture with no paralysis).

High School. According to the NCCSI's twenty-fifth annual report, during the 25-year period from the fall of 1982 through the spring of 2007, a total of 1303 catastrophic injuries were associated with high school sports.[36] This indicates that approximately one out of every 100,000 (0.89 per 100,000) high school athlete suffers some type of catastrophic injury. Of these, 864 were direct (0.59 per 100,000) and 439 indirect (0.30 per 100,000) injuries. Of these, 580 (0.39 per 100,000) were fatal, 370 (0.25 per 1000 participants) were nonfatal and 353 (0.24 per 100,000) were considered serious. The rate of any catastrophic injury was almost five times greater for boys' sports (1.22 per 100,000; n = 1173 injuries) than in girls' sports (0.25 per 100,000; n = 130 injuries). Football had the greatest number of catastrophic injuries for all high school sports. However, when assessing the risk by incidence rates (i.e., number of injuries per total number of athlete at risk), for both boys' and girls' sports, the rates are highest for gymnastics and ice hockey for direct injuries, and water polo for indirect injuries.

Collegiate. During the 25-year period from the fall of 1982 through the spring of 2007, a total of 306 catastrophic injuries were reported in college sports.[36] This indicates that almost 4 of every 100,000 (3.81 per 100,000) college athletes suffered a catastrophic injury. Of these, 204 were direct (2.54 per 100,000) and 102 indirect (1.27 per 100,000) injuries. Of these, 100 (1.51 per 100,000) were fatal, 65 (0.81 per 1000 participants) were nonfatal, and 120 (1.49 per 100,000) were considered serious. The rate of any catastrophic injury was similar between men's sports (74.1 per 100,000; n = 182 injuries) and women' sports (77.9 per 100,000; n = 124 injuries). Football also

had the greatest number of catastrophic injuries for all collegiate sports. When assessing the risk by incidence rates, gymnastics and ice hockey had the highest rates for direct injuries for both men's and women's sports. However, for indirect injuries, the highest rates were found for rowing and basketball in men's sports, and gymnastics in women's sports.

Step 2: Identification of Risk Factors

A critical step in injury sequence is to establish the causes. This includes obtaining information on why a particular athlete may be at risk in a given situation (i.e., risk factors) and how the injuries happen (i.e., injury mechanisms). Furthermore, a comprehensive understanding of injury causation needs to address the multifactorial nature of sports injuries. Meeuwisse[98] developed a model to account for all factors involved. As shown in Figure 30-7, although an injury may appear to have been caused by a single inciting event, it may result from a complex interaction between athlete-related internal (intrinsic) and external (extrinsic) environmental risk factors.[98-101] Intrinsic risk factors (e.g., age, gender, body composition, previous injury, or psychosocial factors) may influence the risk of sustaining injuries, predisposing the athlete to injury. Once the athlete is predisposed to injury, extrinsic factors (e.g., sports equipment, rules, weather, or

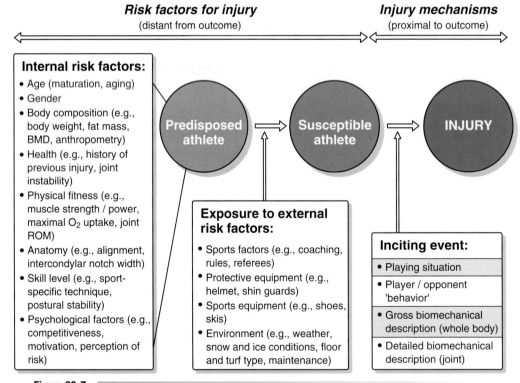

Figure 30-7

A comprehensive injury causation model developed by Bahr and Krosshaug[99] based on the epidemiological model of Meeuwisse[98] and the biomechanical model of McIntosh.[100] (From Bahr R, Krosshaug T: Understanding the injury mechanisms—A key component to prevent injuries in sport, *Br J Sports Med* 39(6):327, 2005.)

field conditions) may make the athlete more susceptible to injury. Although the presence of both intrinsic and extrinsic factors make the athlete more vulnerable to injury, the presence of these factors may not be sufficient to cause injury. The cumulative number and interaction of these factors "set up" the athlete for injury in a given situation, and an inciting event (e.g., playing situation, player behavior, biomechanical description) is the final link in the chain that causes the injury occurrence.[98,99]

> ### Clinical Point
>
> Although an injury may appear to have been caused by a single inciting event, it typically has resulted from a complex interaction between athlete-related internal (intrinsic) and external (extrinsic) environmental risk factors.

Risk factors can also be divided into modifiable and nonmodifiable factors.[99,101] Modifiable risk factors are those that can be altered by injury prevention strategies to reduce injury rates.[102-104] Nonmodifiable risk factors cannot be altered, but still may affect the relationship between modifiable risk factors and injury. Although nonmodifiable risk factors such as age, gender, and previous injury may be worthy of consideration in studies of sport injury prediction and prevention, it is important to study factors that are potentially modifiable, such as physical training, flexibility, balance and proprioception, or psychological and social factors.[101,104] For the purposes of this chapter, risk factors that have been subjected to statistical tests for association or predictive value in prospective or retrospective studies of high school sports are summarized in Table 30-19.

Nonmodifiable Intrinsic Factors

Gender. In studies of high school athletes, in sports played by both sexes, there is evidence that girls may be at greater risk of injury, including softball vs. baseball,[105] basketball,[61,105] cross-country running,[47,64,106] lacrosse,[65] and soccer.[66,97] The reasons for girls being at greater risk of injury may be related to lower skill level, training differences, or some physiological or neuromuscular factor.

Previous Injury. Although an important aspect of injury prevention is to minimize the risk of the athlete's initial (first) injury, an equal goal is to minimize the occurrence of a previous (subsequent) injury to the same (reinjury) body location or additional injuries to new body locations.[28,41,47,58,64,95] Several high school studies have shown prior history of injury to be a risk factor for future injury.[28,47,58,64,70,107] The risk of subsequent injury has been reported significantly greater than the risk of the initial (first) occurrence in multiple studies of cross-country runners.[28,47,64] As mentioned previously, the effect of reinjury to the same body part or injury type is evident (see the

"Reinjury" section in the discussion of "Severity of Injury" earlier in this chapter), particularly for some injury types such as concussion or ankle sprain in which a history of concussion or ankle injury is a significant predictor of future concussion or ankle sprain in high school football players.[108,109] These findings suggest an underestimation of the severity of the primary injury, inadequate rehabilitation, or premature return to sports activity.[28,64,96] Subsequent injuries at a different site might be indicative of kinetic chain dysfunction.[95] Previous injuries can lead to fibrosis, with adhesions and limited joint motion and function. Long-standing joint injuries resulting in chronic instability, or even a slight effusion, can result in reflex inhibition of the muscles and secondary alteration of body biomechanics. Restricted motion (hypomobility) will increase stresses on other areas, and joint instability may result in muscle atrophy and increased compensatory stresses on other areas.[95]

Age, Grade Level, and Experience Level. The relationship between age, grade, or experience levels appears to be sport-specific. Two football studies indicated that the older or more experienced players were more likely to incur an injury.[69,70] In a study of 418 wrestlers, Pasque and Hewett[73] found that older, experienced athletes sustained more injuries. These studies suggested that older or more experienced athletes are at increased risk because of increased playing time, increased aggressiveness, or increased likelihood of attempting a high-risk skill. In contrast, Emery and colleagues[110] reported a significantly higher injury rate among younger (younger than 14) soccer players than older (younger than 18) players. They reported that this finding may be due to physiological differences or under-reporting of injuries, particularly minor injuries, among older players. The greatest risk was found among the elite playing divisions in the younger-than-14 and younger-than-16 age groups. They reported that the increased risk was likely due to increased intensity of play in higher divisions. Finally, in several studies of cross-country runners,[47,63] age, grade, level, or running experience were not associated with increased risk of injury.

Nonmodifiable Extrinsic Factors

Sport Type. As discussed in the section on overall incidence, sport-specific rates for high school sports indicate that the highest rates of injury per 1000 AEs are found for girls' high school sports in cross-country running,[47,63,64] soccer,[41,44,58,66] basketball,[41,44,60,61] and field hockey.[41] For boys' high school sports, the highest injury rates per 1000 AEs are in football,[41,44,58,70] cross-country running,[47,63,64] and wrestling.[41,44,58,73] The high incidence rate of injury in both girls' and boys' cross-country running is likely related to the repetitive nature of motor pattern activity in combination with the varying sport surfaces for training and competing. The relatively high incidence injury rates for football, wrestling, soccer, basketball, and field hockey are likely because these sports involve direct player contact and a large amount of pivoting, jumping, and quick-burst and sprinting activities.

Table 30-19

Risk Factor Studies for Selected High School Sports

Study	Duration	Number of Participants	Significant Intrinsic Risk Factors	Significant Extrinsic Risk Factors
Baseball/Softball				
Powell and Barber-Foss (2000)[105]	3 seasons	635 (F: 311, M: 324)	Gender (girls)	Position (pitching)
Basketball				
Plisky et al. (2006)[111]	1 season	235 (F: 105, M: 130)	Poor dynamic balance for lower-extremity injury	
McGuine et al. (2000)[109]	2 seasons	301 (F: 91, M: 210)	Poor balance (higher postural sway) for ankle sprains	Setting (increased risk of injury during competition) for boys and girls
Messina et al. (1999)[61]	1 season	1863 (F: 890, M: 973)	Gender (girls) for any knee or ACL injury	
Powell and Barber-Foss (2000)[105]	3 seasons	801 (F: 395, M: 406)	Gender (girls) for overall knee injury and ACL injury	
Cross-Country Running				
Rauh et al. (2007)[112]	1 season	393 (F: 171, M: 222)	Q-angle $\geq 20°$ associated with any injury for girls, knee and ≥ 8 days-lost injuries Q-angle $\geq 15°$ with any injury (males) Q-angle right-left $\geq 4°$ difference with any injury, shin injury, and ankle foot injury (males)	
Plisky et al. (2007)[63]	1 season	105 (F: 46, M: 59)	High BMI and gender (females) with MTSS injury	
Rauh et al. (2006)[47]	1 season	421 (F: 186, M: 235)	Gender (female) Q-angle $\geq 20°$ Previous summer running injury (females) Any prior running injury (males)	Setting (increased risk of injury in practice vs. competition) Girls only
Bennett et al. (2001)[106]	1 season	125 (F: 68, M: 57)	Greater navicular drop and gender (females) predicted MTSS	
Rauh et al. (2000)[64]	15 seasons	3233 (F: 1202, M: 2031)	Gender (female)	Setting (increased risk of injury in practice vs. competition)
Football				
Garlock et al. (2009)[120]	4 seasons	283 football players, 256 soccer players (125 females, 131 males)		Playing surface (grass)
Ramirez et al. (2006)[69]	2 seasons	5118 males	Increased years of experience Increased grade level (12th)	Setting (increased risk of injury in competition versus practice) Position (offensive/defensive backfield) Playing surface (artificial turf) Weather (foggy, rain, clear night)
Tyler et al. (2006)[107]	3 seasons	152 males	For ankle sprains: Previous injury Overweight	Previous injury and ankle tape

Table 30-19

Risk Factor Studies for Selected High School Sports—cont'd

Study	Duration	Number of Participants	Significant Intrinsic Risk Factors	Significant Extrinsic Risk Factors
Meyers and Barnhill (2004)[119]	5 seasons	NA		No difference in injury rates between FieldTurf and grass surface Weather (hot days on FieldTurf)
Schulz et al. (2004)[108]	3 seasons	15,802 athletes (total # football not provided)		History of concussion
Turbeville et al. (2003)[70]	1 season	1092 males	History of injury	Setting (males more likely to be at increased risk of injury in competition than females) Position (lineman) Increased playing experience
Gunnoe et al. (2001)[116]	2 seasons	331 males	Total and negative life changes	
Gomez et al. (1998)[114]	1 season	215 males	High % body fat and high BMI with lower-extremity injury	
Lacrosse				
Hinton et al. (2005)[65]	5 seasons	6528 (F: 2658, M: 3870)	Gender (boys)	Setting (increased risk of injury for boys in competition than girls) Setting (increased risk of injury for girls in practice than boys)
Webster et al. (1999)[121]	2 seasons	1386 females		Protective eyewear reduced forehead and periorbital injuries
Soccer				
Yard et al. (2008)[66]	2 seasons	1524 (F: 744, M: 780)	Gender (girls) increased risk of knee ligament sprains during games Player-to-player contact during competition Noncontact mechanisms during practices	Setting (increased risk of injury in competition vs. practice) Setting (increased risk of knee ligament sprain during practice—girls only)
Emery et al. (2005)[110]	1 season (Canada)	317 (F: 164, M: 153)	Gender (girls) for knee ligament sprain Previous injury Competition (elite) Age (younger) with minor injury	Setting (increased risk of injury in competition vs. practice)
Wrestling				
Pasque and Hewett (2000)[73]	1 season	418 males	Increased wrestling experience Age (older) Decreased ligament laxity with shoulder injury	Setting (increased risk of injury in competition vs. practice)
Combined Sports				
Knowles et al. (2006)[58]	3 seasons	15,038 (F: 5801, M: 9237)	Gender (males) History of injury	Increased playing experience
Hewett et al. (2005)[113]	1 season	205 females	Increased dynamic valgus Increased knee abduction movement	

ACL, Anterior cruciate ligament; *BMI*, body mass index; *F*, female; *M*, male; *MTSS*, medial tibial stress syndrome; *NA*, not applicable.

Sport Position. Few studies have compared risk of injury by sport position. In a study of 1092 football players, Turbeville et al.[70] reported that lineman were almost two times more likely to incur an injury than nonlineman. In contrast, among 5100 football players, Ramirez and colleagues[69] found that offensive backfield (i.e., quarterback, running back, full back, wide receiver) and defensive backfield (i.e., cornerback, defensive back, linebacker, safety) players had a 20% higher risk of injury when compared with linemen. They reported that the level of physical activity in a specified position coupled with player's physique was an important marker for risk. Offensive linemen, who are often larger in size, station their bodies to block or tackle, whereas backfielders move with greater speed. The transmission of energy forces from larger lineman to backfielders, or halfbacks being tackled rather than blocking, may increase the risk of injury to backfielders. Finally, when looking at the same position by gender, Powell and Barber-Foss[105] reported that pitchers in boys' baseball were injured more often in practices and games than girls' softball pitchers ($p = 0.001$). Hence, future research should address biomechanical and training activities that might explain the increased risk difference. Further, as few studies have examined the risk of injury by position in team sports, or by event type (e.g., swimming, track and field, tennis), more studies are warranted in this area.

Clinical Point

In terms of injury prevention, a higher priority should be placed on studying factors that are potentially modifiable (alterable) rather than nonmodifiable (unalterable) factors.

Potentially-Modifiable Intrinsic Factors

Neuromuscular. Several recent studies suggest that dynamic balance may increase the risk of injury. Plisky and colleagues[111] found that a decreased normalized right composite reach distance and greater anterior right and left reach distance difference on the Star Excursion Balance Test predicted lower-extremity injury in girl and boy basketball players, respectively. These findings are consistent with those reported by McGuine and colleagues,[109] who reported that basketball players with poor balance were more susceptible to ankle injury.

Anatomical and Biomechanical. Two lower-extremity anatomical measures have been found to be associated with running injuries. In a prospective study of 421 cross-country runners, Rauh and colleagues[112] reported that a large Q-angle ($\geq 20°$ for girls and $\geq 15°$ for boys), was associated with a twofold increased risk of injury. Runners with a large Q-angle were almost six times more likely to incur a knee injury.[112] Bennett and colleagues[106] reported

that a large navicular drop predicted injury among cross-country runners, especially among girl runners. However, Plisky and colleagues[63] found no relationship between cross-country runners with a greater navicular drop (≥ 10 mm).

Two biomechanical measures of neuromuscular control have predicted ACL risk in a prospective study of female soccer, basketball, and volleyball players. Hewett and colleagues[113] found that female athletes with increased dynamic valgus and high abduction loads at the knee were at increased risk of an ACL injury.

Body Composition. In some sports, such as football, athletes try to increase their size or weight to become more effective players. However, the evidence suggests that increased weight and size may increase the likelihood of injury. Gomez and colleagues[114] reported that a high body fat and increased body mass index (BMI) were associated with lower-extremity injury among football players. Similarly, two other football studies reported that being overweight, as indicated by BMI, increased the risk for ankle sprains.[107,115]

In sports such as cross-country and gymnastics, a large BMI has been thought to increase the risk of injury.[47,102] A study of 105 cross-country runners by Plisky and colleagues[63] provides some support. They found that runners with a higher BMI (20.2-21.6) were five times more likely to incur a medial tibial stress syndrome (MTSS) injury than runners with a lower BMI (18.8-20.1). However, a study of 421 cross-country runners found no association between high BMI ($\geq$ seventy-fifth percentile) and running injury.[47]

Psychosocial. Limited evidence exists on the role of psychosocial variables and risk of injury. Using a modified version of the Life Events Survey for Collegiate Athletes, Gunnoe and colleagues[116] found that football players with higher levels of preseason total and negative lifestyle changes were more likely to incur an injury during the season.

Potentially-Modifiable Extrinsic Factors

Exposure and Setting. Evidence from cohort studies during the past two decades suggest that for most girls' and boys' high school sports the risk of injury is higher during competition or games than in practice for baseball and softball,[41,44,68] basketball,[44,57,61] field hockey,[41] football,[41,44,69,70] soccer,[41,44,66,97] and wrestling.[41,44,73] However, in cross-country running[47] and girls' volleyball,[41] the incidence of injury has been reported higher in practices than in competitions or games. In lacrosse, the rates vary by gender, with the risk of injury being higher in games for boys and during practices for girls.[65] In the latter study, the authors suggested that the finding was likely because boys are allowed more purposeful contact than girls during competitions and games, which increases their risk of injury, particularly to the neck, shoulder, arm, and trunk.

The proportion of injuries is greater in practice than competition or games in most high school and collegiate sports.

This finding is likely due to the greater amount of time spent in practice compared with competition.[41,87] On a practical basis, this relationship indicates the need for a strong program of early recognition and treatment of practice-related injuries to potentially minimize game-related injuries.[41] However, the findings from competition levels indicate the rates of injury are actually greater during competition than practices in most sports. The higher rates of injury during competition or games may be due to increased play intensity,[110] increased legal and illegal contact,[117,118] and increased exposure to high-risk activities (e.g., tackling in football).[87] The increased rate of game injuries suggests a need to incorporate drills of potentially high-risk situations into practice under controlled conditions in an effort to decrease competition- or game-related injuries.[87]

Environment. Few studies have assessed the effect of environmental conditions on risk of injury among high school athletes. Regarding playing surface, the findings appear equivocal. Meyers and Barnhill[119] compared the injury rates on FieldTurf and natural grass during games among high school football players during a 5-year period and found no significant difference. Conversely, during a 2-year period, Garlock and colleagues[120] found that the injury risk was 1.3 and 1.94 times greater for football and girls' soccer players, respectively, on natural grass than FieldTurf ($p < 0.0001$). In a study of 5118 football players, Ramirez and colleagues[69] found that playing on an artificial turf surface increased the risk of injury 1.6-fold (95% CI: 1.3-1.9) as compared with natural grass. They also reported that playing on a wet or muddy surface was also significantly associated with risk of injury (RR: 1.2, 95% CI: 1–1.5). Finally, in a study of 421 cross-country runners, Rauh and colleagues[47] reported that running on a concrete surface or irregular terrain significantly increased the risk of injury 12% for each mile run.

Two studies have found associations between weather conditions and injury among football players. Ramirez and colleagues[69] reported that playing in foggy, rainy, or clear night conditions increased the risk of injury when compared with playing on sunny days. Meyers and Barnhill[119] reported a significantly higher incidence of injury (62.8%) during hot days on FieldTurf when compared with natural grass (50.9%).

Equipment. Protective equipment devices are often worn by high school athletes in many sports. Current evidence from three studies reported equivocal findings on the risk of injury. Webster and colleagues[121] assessed the rate of head and facial injuries in 1386 female lacrosse players and reported that the risk of certain head and facial injuries were lower in players that wore protective eyewear, especially during games. Partly, as a result of this evidence, female lacrosse players must now wear eye protection during games.[65] Tyler and colleagues[107] observed an increased risk of injury in football players who used ankle braces or tape compared with players who did not. Further, the increased

risk of injury was found among athletes who had incurred a previous ankle sprain. Yang and colleagues[122] reported that high school athletes who used protective equipment were less likely to incur a lower-extremity injury. However, the protective effect was largely attributed to protective knee pad use. Athletes who used braces and who did not have a history of knee or ankle injury were more likely to incur an ankle or knee injury.

Coaching Experience and Education. It has been speculated that coaches with more educational training or experience are more likely to implement training methods or teach techniques to minimize the number of injuries among their athletes. Only a few studies have examined this relationship at the high school level. Schulz and colleagues[123] found a lower risk of injury among competitive cheerleaders whose coaches had a college degree and more years of coaching experience compared with cheerleaders whose coaches had only a high school diploma and few years of experience. Conversely, in a similar study of athletes in multiple sports, Schulz and colleagues[108] reported no difference in risk of concussion injury among athletes who coaches had a master's degree than athletes whose coaches did not have a master's degree.

Step 3: Injury Prevention Programs—What Works and Does Not Work

A summary table (Table 30-20) provides a snapshot of the level of evidence for a variety of interventions.[124] Some of the interventions in the "proven" column are sometimes based on only one positive study, or are still contentious (as in the case of ACL injury prevention programs). Nevertheless, this table provides a sense that there is a large number of "proven" interventions. However, there has been little translational research to date on how best to implement more widespread use of these interventions.

The authors stress that just because an intervention is proven in one study, it does not mean that research on that topic should be halted. In fact, it should encourage a whole new phase of research, dealing with how to encourage athletes to adopt the intervention, in addition to studies that replicate the original trial or extend the intervention to a new population. An example of this occurred with a series of studies of safety bases in softball and baseball.[125-127] These studies demonstrated the effectiveness of safety bases in recreational youth, recreational adult, and elite softball. It is clear from these studies that use of safety bases should be encouraged at all levels of the game. It is curious, however, that the line of research addressing safety bases phased out in the 1990s. One would expect that these studies would have generated follow-up research on how best to get safety bases adopted by as many users as possible (i.e., behavioral change research).

Table 30-20

Examples of Injury Prevention Intervention in Common Activities

Activity	Proven	Promising/Potential	Not Evaluated, Insufficient or Conflicting Evidence
Baseball/softball	Breakaway bases Reduced-impact balls Face guards/Protective eyewear	Batting helmets Pitch count	Chest protectors
Basketball	Protective eyewear Mouthguards	Ankle disk training Semirigid ankle stabilizers (especially with history of ankle instability)	Preventive knee braces
Bicycling	Helmet use (Educational campaigns, laws, and subsidies all increase use)	Bike paths/lanes Retractable handlebars	Lighting on bike trails
Football	Helmets and other equipment Ankle braces rather than taping Minimizing cleat length Rule changes (no spearing, etc.) Playing field maintenance Preseason conditioning Cross training reduces overuse Coach training/experience	Limiting practices with contact	Preventive knee braces Body pads
General	Fitness/conditioning	Return to play guidelines Attention to training parameters	Pre-exercise stretching Coaching factors related to injury prevention
Ice hockey	Helmet with full face shield down Rules: fair play, no checking from behind, no high sticking Increased ice size	Enforcement of rules Discouraging fighting	Body pads
Inline skating/skateboarding Playgrounds	Wrist guards Knee/elbow pads Shock-absorbing surfacing Height standards Maintenance standards	Helmets	
Running/jogging Skiing/snowboarding	Altered training regimen Training to avoid risk situations Binding adjustment Wristguards in snowboarding	Shock absorbing insoles Helmets	Reflective clothing
Soccer	Anchored, padded goal posts Shin guards Movement training: (Proprioceptive, neuromuscular & plyometric training) Strength training		Head gear "Fair Head" rule

From Gilchrist J, Saluja G, Marshall SW: Interventions to prevent sports and recreation-related injury. In Doll LS, Bonzo SE, Mercy JA, Sleet DA: *Handbook of injury and violence prevention*, New York, 2007, Springer.

Conclusion

The epidemiology of sports injuries is an important area of research for all ages and expertise levels, for both recreational and competitive sports. It is clear from this review that there is limited information on injury rates, injury location, injury type, and injury severity, particularly at the high school level. Presently, it is difficult to compare injury incidence estimates among published high school studies for two main reasons: (1) investigators have used different methods for collecting injury data, different injury definitions, different ways of defining and collecting data on time at risk (i.e., exposure), and different ways of estimating incidence; and (2) investigators do not report their methods in sufficient detail. Clearly, a standard operational definition of *injury* needs to be determined to make any meaningful comparisons across studies. At a minimum, the authors suggest the use of a denominator that specifies actual daily practice and competitive events participated in without restriction of injury. This would provide an injury rate (per 1000 AEs) that would account for varying lengths of season and allow for better comparisons of injury risk by gender, athletic event, injury setting, body location, injury type, and other sports. The authors also recommend that there is a need to establish large-scale high school injury surveillance systems that use the same standardized definitions and data collection methods for injuries and AE data similar to that collected by the NCAA. Data collected in this manner would help to improve its consistency and trustworthiness to assess trends, identification and examination of risk factors, and assessment of preventive measures. Large-scale systems should be comprehensive to include sports such as cross-country, field hockey, lacrosse, swimming and diving, tennis, and track and field, for which there is a scarcity of descriptive studies.

Although the authors only reviewed risk factors at the high school level, it is clear that there are few prospective cohort and case-control studies that have adequately examined potential risk factors for injury at this level. The review indicates that the evidence provides the most support for gender (i.e., girls—particularly knee injuries), previous injury, and game settings as risk factors. There is also some support for poor dynamic balance, anatomical alignment, coaching inexperience, older age and greater playing experience, playing surface, and weather conditions. Future research should examine multiple potential risk factors within a single study and assess how their interactions affect the risk of injury.

The authors' review indicated that injury prevention efforts are promising in many competitive and recreational sports. There are an increasing number of injury prevention studies that indicate that the use of a protective helmet and other equipment, rule changes, and preseason conditioning significantly reduce the risk of injury. Recent studies of the effect of neuromuscular training and reduction of ACL injuries among high school and collegiate athletes highlight these efforts.

Although this chapter has illustrated that significant efforts have been made in the past several decades to better understand trends and risk factors for injury, as well as what might work to minimize injury, the authors would like to point out that it only has captured the "tip of the iceberg" on what still needs to be done in sports injury epidemiology. For example, more athletes, in the past few decades, have begun to specialize and train year round in a particular sport, but it is not known if change in training has increased their risk of acute and overuse injuries. Another understudied question is whether the combination of preseason screening examinations to identify potential risk factors and enforcement of policies not to allow injured athletes to return to play until fully rehabilitated would result in a reduction in future injuries. Finally, since Title IX, the number of females participating in competitive sports has steadily increased in the past few decades, and is likely to continue as more opportunities for scholarship or monetary awards and media exposure (at the professional level) are provided. As shown in this chapter, higher rates of injury have been found among women than men competing in the same sport. Future research is needed to learn what factors might explain this discrepancy. Because there is increasing evidence that the onset of osteoarthritis may occur at an earlier age due to a sport-related injury,[5,6] and that fear of injury may lead to inactivity as an adult,[128] finding answers to these and other important questions will be pressing issues for current and future sports injury epidemiologists.

References

1. National Collegiate Athletic Association: *1981-82-2006-07 NCAA sports sponsorship and participation rates report*, accessed November 27, 2008, from http://www.ncaapublications.com/p-4124-participation-rates-1981-82-2006-07-ncaa-sports-sponsorship-and-participation-rates-report.aspx.
2. *National Federation of State High School Association 2006-2007 Survey*. High school sports participation increases again; girls exceed three million for first time. Press release: 09/05/07, accessed November 13, 2007, from http://www.nfhs.org/participation.
3. Lohmander LS, Englund PM, Dahl LL, Roos EM: The long-term consequence of anterior cruciate ligament and meniscus injuries: Osteoarthritis, *Am J Sports Med* 35(10):1756–1769, 2007.
4. Roos EM: Joint injury causes knee osteoarthritis in young adults, *Curr Opin Rheumatol* 17(2):195–200, 2005.
5. Lohmander LS, Ostenberg A, Englund M, Roos H: High prevalence of knee osteoarthritis, pain, and functional limitations in female soccer players twelve years after anterior cruciate ligament injury, *Arthritis Rheum* 50(10):3145–3152, 2004.
6. Von Porat A, Roos EM, Roos H: High prevalence of osteoarthritis 14 years after an anterior cruciate ligament tear in male soccer players: A study of radiographic and patient-relevant outcomes, *Ann Rheum Dis* 63(3):269–273, 2004.

7. Garrick JG, Requa RK: Sports and fitness activities: The negative consequence, *J Am Acad Orthop Surg* 11(6):439–443, 2003.

8. Caine CG, Caine DJ, Lindner KJ: The epidemiologic approach to sports injuries. In Caine DJ, Caine CG, Lindner KJ, editors: *Epidemiology of sports injuries,* Champaign, 1996, Human Kinetics.

9. Rothman KJ, Sander G, Lash TL: *Modern epidemiology,* ed 3, Philadelphia, 2008, Lippincott Williams & Wilkins.

10. Gessel, LM, Fields SK, Collins CL, et al: Concussions among United States high school and collegiate athletes, *J Athl Train* 42(4):495–503, 2007.

11. Myer GD, Ford KR, Barber-Foss KD, et al: The relationship of hamstring and quadriceps strength to anterior cruciate ligament injury in female athletes, *Clin J Sports Med* 19(1):3–8, 2009.

12. Schootman M, Powell JW, Torner JC: Study designs and potential biases in sports injury research: The case-control study, *Sports Med* 18(1):22–37, 1994.

13. Collins M, Lovell MR, Iverson GL, et al: Examining concussion rates and return to play in high school football players wearing newer helmet technology: A three-year prospective cohort study, *Neurosurgery* 58(2):275–286, 2006.

14. Gilchrist J, Mandelbaum BR, Melancon H, et al: A randomized controlled trial to prevent noncontact anterior cruciate ligament injury in female collegiate soccer players, *Am J Sports Med* 36(8):1476–1483, 2008.

15. Knowles SB, Marshall SW, Guskiewicz KM: Estimating rates and risks in sports injury research, *J Athl Train* 41(2):201–215, 2006.

16. Weaver NL, Mueller FO, Kalsbeek WD, Bowling JM: The North Carolina high school athletic injury study: Design and methodology, *Med Sci Sports Exerc* 31(1):176–182, 1999.

17. Nathan M, Goedeke R, Noakes TD: The incidence and nature of rugby injuries experienced at one school during the 1983 rugby season, *S Afr Med J* 64(4):132–137, 1983.

18. Sugerman S: Injuries in an Australian schools Rugby Union season, *Aust J Sports Med Exerc Sci* 15:5–14, 1983.

19. Roux CE, Goedeke R, Visser GR, et al: The epidemiology of schoolboy rugby injuries, *S Afr Med J* 71(5):307–313, 1987.

20. Davidson RM: Schoolboy rugby injuries, 1969-1986, *Med J Aust* 147(3):119–120, 1987.

21. Clark DR, Roux C, Noakes TD: A prospective study of the incidence and nature of injuries to adult rugby players, *S Afr Med J* 77(11):559–562, 1990.

22. Dalley DR, Laing DR, Rowberry JM, Caird MJ: Rugby injuries: An epidemiological survey, Christchurch 1980, *N Z J Sports Med* 10:5–17, 1982.

23. Hughes DC, Fricker PA: A prospective survey of injuries to first-grade rugby union players, *Clin J Sports Med* 4(4):249–256, 1994.

24. Garraway M, Macleod D: Epidemiology of rugby football injuries, *Lancet* 345(8963):1485–1487, 1995.

25. Lee AJ, Garraway WM: Epidemiological comparison of injuries in school and senior rugby, *Br J Sports Med* 30(3):213–217, 1996.

26. Bird YN, Waller AE, Marshall SW, et al: The New Zealand Rugby Injury and Performance Project V. Descriptive epidemiology of a season of rugby injury, *Br J Sports Med* 32(4):319–325, 1998.

27. Lombardo S, Sethi PM, Starkey C: Intercondylar notch stenosis is not a risk factor for anterior cruciate ligament tears in professional male basketball players: An 11-year prospective study, *Am J Sports Med* 33(1):29–34, 2005.

28. Rauh MJ, Macera CA, Ji M, Wiksten DL: Subsequent injury patterns in girls' high school sports, *J Athl Train* 42(4):486–494, 2007.

29. Poole C: Low p-values or narrow confidence intervals: Which are more durable? *Epidemiology* 12(3):291–294, 2001.

30. Marshall SW: Testing with confidence: The use (and misuse) of confidence intervals in biomedical research, *J Sci Med Sport* 7(2):135–137, 2004.

31. Wolfe R, Cumming G: Communicating the uncertainty in research findings: Confidence intervals, *J Sci Med Sport* 7(2):138–143, 2004.

32. Cordova ML: Giving clinicians more to work with: Let's incorporate confidence intervals into our data, *J Athl Train* 42(4):445, 2007.

33. Meeuwisse WH, Love EJ: Athletic injury reporting: Development of universal systems, *Sports Med* 24(3):184–204, 1997.

34. Duvall DP: *The National Electronic Injury Surveillance System: A description of its role in the U.S. Consumer Product Safety Commission,* Division of Hazard and Injury Data Systems, U.S. Consumer Product Safety Commission, 1990.

35. Torg JS, Vegso JJ, O'Neill MJ, Sennett B: The epidemiologic, pathologic, biomechanical, and cinematographic analysis of football-induced cervical spine trauma, *Am J Sports Med* 18(1):50–57, 1990.

36. *National Center for Catastrophic Sport Injury Research (NCCSI): 25th Annual Report,* NCCSI, 2008. Accessed Jan 25, 2009, at http://www.unc.edu/depts/nccsi/AllSport.htm.

37. Mackenzie SG, Pless IB: CHIRPP: Canada's principal injury surveillance program. Canadian Hospitals Injury Reporting and Prevention Program, *Inj Prev* 5(3):208–213, 1999.

38. Levy IM: Formation and sense of the NAIRS athletic injury surveillance system, *Am J Sports Med* 16 (Suppl 1):S132–S133, 1988.

39. Pelletier R: *Canadian Athletic Injury/Illness Reporting System: CAIRS 1 recorder's handbook,* Ottawa, 1992, University of Ottawa.

40. Dick R, Agel J, Marshall SW: National Collegiate Association Injury Surveillance System Commentaries: Introduction and methods, *J Athl Train* 42(2):173–182, 2007.

41. Powell JW, Barber-Foss KD: Injury patterns in selected high school sports: A review of the 1995-1997 seasons, *J Athl Train* 34(3):277–284, 1999.

42. Powell JW: National High School Injury Registry, *Am J Sports Med* 16 (Suppl):S134–S166, 1988.

43. Big Ten Sports Injury Reporting System, *Am J Sports Med* 16 (Suppl):S166–S200, 1988.

44. Comstock RD, Knox C, Yard E, Gilchrist J: Sports-related injuries among high school athletes—United States, 2005–06 school year, *MMWR* 55(38):1037–1040, 2006.

45. Rice SG: Development of an injury surveillance system: Results from a longitudinal study of high school athletes. In Ashare AB, editor: *Safety in ice hockey,* vol 3, West Conshocken, 2000, American Society for Testing and Materials.

46. Meeuwisse WH, Love EJ: Development, implementation, and validation of the Canadian Intercollegiate Sport Injury Registry, *Clin J Sport Med* 8(3):164–177, 1998.

47. Rauh MJ, Koepsell TD, Rivara FP, et al: Epidemiology of musculoskeletal injuries among high school cross-country runners, *Am J Epidemiol* 163(2):151–159, 2006.

48. Van Mechelen W: Sports injury surveillance systems. One size fits all? *Sports Med* 24(3):164–168, 1997.

49. Finch CF: An overview of some definitional issues for sports injury surveillance, *Sports Med* 24(3):157–163, 1997.

50. Blair SN, Kohl HW, Barlow CE, et al: Changes in physical fitness and all-cause mortality: A prospective study of healthy and unhealthy men, *JAMA* 273(14):1093–1098, 1995.

51. Jebb S, Moore M: Contribution of a sedentary lifestyle and inactivity to the etiology of overweight and obesity: Current evidence and research issues, *Med Sci Sports Exerc* 31(11 Suppl):S154–S541, 1999.

52. Paffenbarger RS, Kampert JB, Lee IM, et al: Changes in physical fitness and other lifestyle patterns influence longevity, *Med Sci Sports Exerc* 26(7):857–865, 1994.

53. Koh J, Dietz J: Osteoarthritis in other joints (hip, elbow, foot, ankle, toes, wrist) after sports injuries, *Clin Sports Med* 24(1):57–70, 2005.

54. Van Mechelen W, Hlobil H, Kemper HCG: How can sports injuries be prevented? *Nationaal Instituut voor Sport GezondheidsZorg publicatie*, nr 25E, Papendal, 1987.

55. Van Mechelen W, Hlobil H, Kemper HCG: Incidence, severity, aetiology and prevention of sports injuries: A review of concepts, *Sports Med* 14(2):82–99, 1992.

56. Robertson LS: *Injury epidemiology*, New York, 1992, Oxford University Press, Inc.

57. Borowski LA, Yard EE, Fields SK, Comstock RD: The epidemiology of US high school basketball injuries, 2005–2007, *Am J Sports Med* 36(12):2328–1235, 2008.

58. Knowles SB, Marshall SW, Bowling JM, et al: A prospective study of injury incidence among North Carolina high school athletes, *Am J Epidemiol* 164(12):1209–1221, 2006.

59. Beachy G, Akau CK, Martinson M, Olderr TF: High school sports injuries. A longitudinal study at Punahou School: 1988 to 1996, *Am J Sports Med* 25(5):675–681, 1997.

60. Gomez E, DeLee JC, Farney WC: Incidence of injury in Texas girls' high school basketball, *Am J Sports Med* 24(3):686–687, 1986.

61. Messina DF, Farney WC, DeLee JC: The incidence of injury in Texas high school basketball. A prospective study among male and female athletes, *Am J Sports Med* 27(3):294–299, 1999.

62. McLain LG, Reynolds S: Sports injuries in high school, *Pediatrics* 84(3):446–450, 1989.

63. Plisky MS, Rauh MJ, Heiderscheit B, et al: An epidemiological investigation of medial tibial stress syndrome among high school cross country runners, *J Orthop Sports Phys Ther* 37(2):40–47, 2007.

64. Rauh MJ, Margherita AJ, Koepsell TD, et al: High school cross country running injuries: A longitudinal study, *Clin J Sports Med* 10(2):110–116, 2000.

65. Hinton RY, Lincoln AE, Almquist JL, et al: Epidemiology of lacrosse injuries in high school-aged girls and boys: A 3-year prospective study, *Am J Sports Med* 33(9):1305–1314, 2005.

66. Yard EE, Schroeder MJ, Fields SK, et al: The epidemiology of United States high school soccer injuries, 2005.2007, *Am J Sports Med* 36(10):1930–1937, 2008.

67. Watson MD, DiMartino PP: Incidence of injuries in high school track and field athletes and its relation to performance ability, *Am J Sports Med* 15(3):251–254, 1987.

68. Collins CL, Comstock RD: Epidemiological features of high school baseball injuries in the United States, 2005–2007. *Pediatrics* 121(6):1181–1187, 2008.

69. Ramirez M, Schaffer KD, Shen H, et al: Injuries to high school football athletes in California, *Am J Sports Med* 34(7):1147–1158, 2006.

70. Turbeville SD, Cowan LD, Owen WL, et al: Risk factors for injury in high school football players, *Am J Sports Med* 31(6):974–980, 2003.

71. DeLee JC, Farney WC: Incidence of injury in Texas high school football, *Am J Sports Med* 20(5):575–580, 1992.

72. Prager BI, Fitton WL, Cahill BR, Olson GH: High school football injuries: A prospective study and pitfalls of data collection, *Am J Sports Med* 17(5):681–685, 1989.

73. Pasque CB, Hewett TE: A prospective study of high school wrestling injuries, *Am J Sports Med* 28(4):509–515, 2000.

74. Marshall SW, Hamstra-Wright KL, Dick R, et al: Descriptive epidemiology of collegiate women's softball injuries: National Collegiate Athletic Association Injury Surveillance System, 1988-1989 through 2003-2004, *J Athl Train* 42(2):286–294, 2007.

75. Dick R, Sauers EL, Agel J, et al: Descriptive epidemiology of collegiate men's baseball injuries: National Collegiate Athletic Association Injury Surveillance System, 1988–1989 through 2003-2004. *J Athl Train* 42(2):183–193, 2007.

76. Agel J, Olsen DE, Dick R, et al: Descriptive epidemiology of collegiate women's basketball injuries: National Collegiate Athletic Association Injury Surveillance System, 1988-1989 through 2003-2004, *J Athl Train* 42(2):202–210, 2007.

77. Dick R, Hertel J, Agel J, et al: Descriptive epidemiology of collegiate men's basketball injuries: National Collegiate Athletic Association Injury Surveillance System, 1988-1989 through 2003-2004, *J Athl Train* 42(2):194–201, 2007.

78. Dick R, Hootman JM, Agel J, et al: Descriptive epidemiology of collegiate women's field hockey injuries: National Collegiate Athletic Association Injury Surveillance System, 1988–1989 through 2003–2004, *J Athl Train* 42(2):211–220, 2007.

79. Dick R, Ferrara MS, Agel J, et al: Descriptive epidemiology of collegiate men's football injuries: National Collegiate Athletic Association Injury Surveillance System, 1988–1989 through 2003–2004, *J Athl Train* 42(2):221–233. 2007.

80. Marshall SW. Covassin T. Dick R, et al: Descriptive epidemiology of collegiate women's gymnastics injuries: National Collegiate Athletic Association Injury Surveillance System, 1988–1989 through 2003–2004, *J Athl Train* 42(2):234–240, 2007.

81. Dick R, Lincoln AE, Agel J, et al: Descriptive epidemiology of collegiate women's lacrosse injuries: National Collegiate Athletic Association Injury Surveillance System, 1988–1989 through 2003–2004, *J Athl Train* 42(2):262–269, 2007.

82. Dick R, Romani WA, Agel J, et al: Descriptive epidemiology of collegiate men's lacrosse injuries: National Collegiate Athletic Association Injury Surveillance System, 1988–1989 through 2003–2004, *J Athl Train* 42(2):255–261, 2007.

83. Dick R, Putukian M, Agel J, et al: Descriptive epidemiology of collegiate women's soccer injuries: National Collegiate Athletic Association Injury Surveillance System, 1988–1989 through 2003–2004, *J Athl Train* 42(2):278–285, 2007.

84. Agel J, Evans TA, Dick R, et al: Descriptive epidemiology of collegiate men's soccer injuries: National Collegiate Athletic Association Injury Surveillance System, 1988–1989 through 2003–2004, *J Athl Train* 42(2):262–277, 2007.

85. Agel J, Palmeri-Smith RM, Dick R, et al: Descriptive epidemiology of collegiate women's volleyball injuries: National Collegiate Athletic Association Injury Surveillance System, 1988–1989 through 2003–2004, *J Athl Train* 42(2):295–302, 2007.

86. Agel J, Ransone J, Dick R, et al: Descriptive epidemiology of collegiate men's wrestling injuries: National Collegiate Athletic Association Injury Surveillance System, 1988–1989 through 2003–2004, *J Athl Train* 42(2):303–310, 2007.

87. Rechel JA, Yard EE, Comstock RD: An epidemiologic comparison of high school sports injuries sustained in practice and competition, *J Ath Train* 43(2):197–204, 2008.

88. Shankar P, Fields SK, Collins CL, et al: Epidemiology of high school and collegiate football injuries in the United States, 2005–2006, *Am J Sports Med* 35(8):1295–1303, 2008.

89. Yard EE, Collins C, Dick RW, Comstock RD: An epidemiologic comparison of high school and college wrestling injuries, *Am J Sports Med* 36(1):57–64, 2008.

90. Caine D, Caine C, Maffuli N: Incidence and distribution of pediatric of sport-related injuries, *Clin J Sport Med* 16(6):500–513, 2006.

91. Hootman JM, Dick R, Agel J: Epidemiology of collegiate injuries for 15 sports: Summary and recommendations for injury prevention initiatives, *J Athl Train* 42(2):311–319, 2007.

92. Rice SG, Schlotfeldt JD, Foley WE: The Athletic Health Care and Training Program. A comprehensive approach to the prevention and management of athletic injuries in high schools, *West J Sports Med* 142(3):352–357, 1985.

93. Powell JW, Dompier TP: Analysis of injury rates and treatment patterns for time-loss and non-time loss injuries among collegiate student athletes, *J Athl Train* 39(1):56–70, 2004.

94. Fuller CW, Bahr R, Dick R, Meeuwisse WH: A framework for recording recurrences, reinjuries, and exacerbations in injury surveillance, *Clin J Sports Med* 17(3):197–200, 2007.

95. Renstrom PA: Mechanism, diagnosis, and treatment of running injuries, *Instr Course Lect* 42:225–234, 1993.

96. Lysens R, Steverlynck A, van der Awuweele Y, et al: The predicatability of sports injuries, *Sports Med* 1(1):6–10, 1984.

97. Emery CA, Meeuwisse WH: Survey of sport participation and sport injury in Calgary and area high schools, *Clin J Sports Med* 16 (1):20–26, 2006.

98. Meeuwisse WH: Assessing causation in sport injury: A multifactorial model, *Clin J Sport Med* 4(3):166–169, 1994.

99. Bahr R, Krosshaug T: Understanding the injury mechanisms—A key component to prevent injuries in sport, *Br J Sports Med* 39(6):224–229, 2005.

100. McIntosh AS: Risk compensation, motivation, injuries, and biomechanics in competitive sport, *Br J Sports Med* 39(1):2–3, 2005.

101. Bahr R, Holme I: Risk factors for sports injuries—A methodological approach, *Br J Sports Med* 37(5):384–392, 2003.

102. Caine D, Maffulli N, Caine C: Epidemiology of injury in child and adolescent sports: Injury rates, risk factors and prevention, *Clin Sports Med* 27(1):19–50, 2008.

103. Meeuwisse WH: Predictability of sports injuries: What is the epidemiological evidence? *Sports Med* 12(1):8–15, 1991.

104. Emery CA: Injury prevention and future research. In Maffuli N, Caine DJ, editors: *Epidemiology of pediatric sports injuries*, Medicine and Sport Science, Basil, 2005, Karger.

105. Powell JW, Barber-Foss KD: Sex related injury patterns among selected high school sports, *Am J Sports Med* 28(3):385–391, 2000.

106. Bennett J, Reinking M, Pluemer B, et al: Factors contributing to the development of medial tibial stress syndrome in high school runners, *J Orthop Sports Phys Ther* 31(9):504–510, 2001.

107. Tyler TF, McHugh MP, Mirabella MR, et al: Risk factors for non-contact ankle sprains in high school football players: The role of previous ankle sprains and body mass index, *Am J Sports Med* 34(3):471–475, 2006.

108. Schulz MR, Marshall SW, Mueller FO, et al. Incidence and risk factors for concussion in high school athletes, North Carolina, 1996–1999, *Am J Epidemiol* 160(10):937–944, 2004.

109. McGuine TA, Greene JJ, Best T, Leverson G: Balance as a predictor of ankle injuries in high school basketball players, *Clin J Sports Med* 10(4):239–244, 2000.

110. Emery CA, Meeuwisse WH, Hartmann SE: Evaluation of risk factors for injury in adolescent soccer: Implementation and validation of an injury surveillance system, *Am J Sports Med* 33(12):684–687, 2005.

111. Plisky PJ, Rauh MJ, Kaminski TW, Underwood FB: Star Excursion Balance Test as a predictor of lower extremity injury in boys and girls high school basketball players, *J Orthop Sports Phys Ther* 36(12):911–919, 2006.

112. Rauh MJ, Koepsell TD, Rivara FP, et al: Quadriceps angle and risk of injury among high school cross country runners, *J Orthop Sports Phys Ther* 37(12):725–733, 2007.

113. Hewett TE, Myer GD, Ford KR, et al: Biomechanical measures of neuromuscular control and valgus loading of the knee predict anterior cruciate ligament injury risk in female athletes: A prospective study, *Am J Sports Med* 33(4):492–501, 2005.

114. Gomez JE, Ross SK, Calmbach WL, et al: Body fatness and increased injury rates in high school football linemen, *Clin J Sport Med* 8(2):115–120, 1998.

115. McHugh MP, Tyler TF, Tetro DT, et al: Risk factors for non-contact ankle sprains in high school athletes: The role of hip strength and balance ability, *Am J Sports Med* 34(3):464–470, 2006.

116. Gunnoe AJ, Horodyski M, Tennant LK, Murphey M: The effects of life events on incidence of injury in high school football players, *J Athl Train* 36(2):150–155, 2001.

117. Stuart MJ: Gridiron football injuries, *Med Sport Sci* 49:62–85, 2005.

118. Guskiewicz KM, Weaver NL, Padua DA, Garrett WE Jr: Epidemiology of concussion in collegiate and high school football players, *Am J Sports Med* 28(5):643–650, 2000.

119. Meyers MC, Barnhill BS: Incidence, causes, and severity of high school football injuries on FieldTurf versus natural grass: A 5-year prospective study, *Am J Sports Med* 32(7):1626–1638, 2004.

120. Garlock PG, Rauh MJ, Hummel-Berry K, Bateman MJ: Injury rates on FieldTurf and natural grass for high school football and soccer, *Med Sci Sports Exerc* 41(5):S587, 2009.

121. Webster DA, Bayliss GV, Sparado JA: Head and face injuries in scholastic women's lacrosse with and without eyewear, *Med Sci Sports Exerc* 31(7):938–941, 1999.

122. Yang J, Marshall SW, Bowling JM, et al: Use of discretionary protective equipment and rate of lower extremity injury in high school athletes, *Am J Epidemiol* 161(6):511–519, 2005.

123. Schulz MR, Marshall SW, Yang J, et al: A prospective cohort study of injury incidence and risk factors in North Carolina high school competitive cheerleaders, *Am J Sports Med* 32(2): 396–405, 2004.

124. Gilchrist J, Saluja G, Marshall SW: Interventions to prevent sports and recreation-related injury. In Doll LS, Bonzo SE, Mercy JA, Sleet DA, editors: *Handbook of injury and violence prevention*, New York, 2007, Springer.

125. Janda DH, Bir C, Kedroske B: A comparison of standard vs. breakaway bases: An analysis of a preventative intervention for softball and baseball foot and ankle injuries, *Foot Ankle Int* 22(10):810–816, 2001.

126. Janda DH, Wojtys EM, Hankin FM, Benedict ME: Softball sliding injuries. A prospective study comparing standard and modified bases, *JAMA* 259(12):1848–1850, 1988.

127. Sendre, RA, Keating TM, Hornak, JE, Newitt PA: Use of the Hollywood Impact Base and standard stationary base to reduce sliding and base-running injuries in baseball and softball, *Am J Sports Med* 22(4):450–453, 1994.

128. Schneider S, Seither B, Tönges S, Schmitt H: Sports injuries: Population based representative data on incidence, diagnosis, sequela, and high risk groups, *Br J Sports* 40(4):334–339, 2006.

Index

Page numbers followed by *f* refer to illustrations; page numbers followed by *t* refer to tables; page numbers followed by *b* refer to boxes.

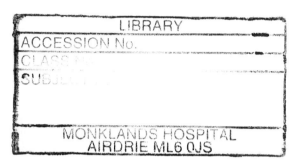